Little, Brown's Personalized Five-Week
Countdown *Key* to NCLEX Success

A timetable to use in preparing for the NCLEX-RN
How to prepare step-by-step:

Introduction to Timetable

Reviewing is easy when you follow this step-by-step countdown to the exam date you selected.

Whether your hectic schedule makes the NCLEX-RN test date come up sooner than you realized, or you've been putting off preparing for the exam, or you're just eager to begin the review process, this timetable is designed for *you!*

You can do focused, effective self-study in only 5 weeks. Just think—the day before your chosen exam date, you will rest assured, knowing that you have methodically covered everything you need to pass the test!

Begin your plan:

1. *Decide when you will take the exam.* Choose a date that will allow 5–6 weeks before you're scheduled to take the licensure exam. This will give your school time to submit the required verification and documentation of your eligibility to take the exam to your state Board of Registered Nursing (BRN). At the same time, the state BRN will process your application, and you will use the time to study.

2. Take the *Pre Test* in this book.

3. *Evaluate* your strengths and weaknesses based on your Pre Test scores. The problem areas you should focus on are those in which you scored below 75% correct.

4. *Prioritize your review time* by starting with your most problematic *client need* area (Safe, Effective Care Environment; Physiologic Integrity; Psychosocial Integrity; or Health Promotion and Maintenance).

5. *Count back 5 weeks* on your calendar from the exam date and block off *what* subject areas you will review *when* and for *how long*. Model your own study plan after the following timetable:

Total Days	Total Weeks	Subject Areas	Units
10	2	Nursing Care of the Acutely Ill and the Chronically Ill Adult	2
		Common Diagnostic Procedures, Treatments, and Nursing Care	5
		Review of Pharmacology	4
		Review of Nutrition	3
5	1	Nursing Care of Children and Families	8
5	1	Nursing Care of the Childbearing Family	7
3–5	1	Nursing Care of Behavioral and Emotional Problems Throughout the Life Span	6
		Ethical and Legal Aspects in Nursing	9
1–2	—	Practice Test	10
		Final Test	11
		Computer Test (on disk)	

Unit 2					
Units 3,4,5					
Unit 8					
Unit 7					
Units 6,9	Units 10,11, Disk			EXAM	

See reverse side for a guide to creating your own review plan based on your *Pre Test* results.

This material taken from Sally L. Lagerquist, ed. *Little, Brown's NCLEX-RN Examination Review*. Boston: Little, Brown, 1996.

Little Brown's
Countdown Key to Review for the NCLEX-RN

Below is a sample review plan that you should use, based on your **Pre Test** results, as a model for your own review plan. In this sample, the student's most problematic area is *Nursing Care of the Acutely Ill and the Chronically Ill Adult*, followed by *Nursing Care of Children and Families*. (The student scored less than 75% correct in both subject areas on the **Pre Test**.) The student's strengths are in the *Nursing Care of the Childbearing Family* and *Nursing Care of Behavioral and Emotional Problems Throughout the Life Span* subject areas. (The student scored 75% or more correct in these subject areas on the **Pre Test**.) **Remember, this is a** *model* **of how to plan your own study.**

5 weeks before the exam

- ☑ Carefully and thoroughly READ and highlight *Unit 2. Nursing Care of the Acutely Ill and the Chronically Ill Adult*. Pay special attention to lab values, diagnostic procedures, *italic print*, **bold print**, charts, figures, nursing care plan/implementation sections for each condition, and content on positions and tubes.

4 weeks before the exam

- ☑ Carefully and thoroughly READ and highlight *Unit 3. Review of Nutrition, Unit 4. Review of Pharmacology,* and *Unit 5. Common Diagnostic Procedures, Treatments, and Nursing Care*. Pay special attention to nursing care plan/implementation sections.

- ☑ Take the *exam questions* at the end of Units 2–5.

Note: If your score is still **less** than 75% correct—like it was on the **Pre Test**—determine what your problem areas are according to **concepts** (e.g., mobility), **body systems** (e.g., musculoskeletal), and **conditions** (e.g., fractures).

- ☑ Go back to the content outline and re-read the sections on your problem areas in Units 2, 3, 4, and 5.

3 weeks before the exam

- ☑ Carefully and thoroughly READ and highlight *Unit 8. Nursing Care of Children and Families*. Pay special attention to charts, figures, and nursing care plan/implementation sections.

- ☑ Take the *exam questions* at the end of Unit 8.

Note: If your score is still **less** than 75% correct—like it was on the **Pre Test**—evaluate which age groups and conditions were the problem areas.

- ☑ Go back and re-read these identified problem areas.

2 weeks before the exam

- ☑ As a quick review, READ *Unit 7. Nursing Care of the Childbearing Family*. Primarily focus on charts; figures; diagnostic procedures; and physiologic and emotional adaptations related to pregnancy, labor, birth, postpartum, newborn, and health teaching.

- ☑ Take the *exam questions* at the end of Unit 7.

Note: If your score is still **greater** than 75% correct—like it was on the **Pre Test**—identify any areas that you want or need to *refresh* your knowledge in.

- ☑ Re-read any areas in Unit 7 that you want a "quick refresher" in.

1 week before the exam

- ☑ Quickly READ *Unit 6. Nursing Care of Behavioral and Emotional Problems Throughout the Life Span* and *Unit 9. Ethical and Legal Aspects in Nursing*. In Unit 6, focus mainly on therapeutic and nontherapeutic communication, psychopharmacology, and nursing care plan/implementation sections.

- ☑ Take the *exam questions* at the end of Units 6 and 9.

Note: If your score is still **greater** than 75% correct, identify any particular content areas that you want a quick review in.

- ☑ Re-read any topics in Units 6 and 9 that you want to brush up on.

- ☑ Now take the integrated *Practice Test* if you scored **less** than 75% correct in **any** of the end-of-the-unit tests.

Note: Score your answers. If your total score on this integrated practice test was **less** than 75% correct, identify which steps of the *nursing process* and categories of *human functions* were your problem areas. In the Answers/Rationale, the first two codes listed with each question identify the areas of nursing process and human function tested by the question.

- ☑ Refer to *Appendix C. Index: Questions Related to Nursing Process* and retake the *questions* in **all** the units (across the board and in all subject areas) that cover the steps of the nursing process that were your weakest areas.

- ☑ Refer to *Appendix I. Index: Questions Related to Categories of Human Functions* and retake the *questions* in **all** the units (across the board and in all subject areas) that cover the categories of human functions that were your weakest areas.

- ☑ NOW TAKE THE FINAL TEST

Note: Score yourself. You can stop studying and celebrate if you get 75% or more correct. (If you score is significantly lower than 65% correct, you may need more time to continue this step-by-step review process. You may consider audio, video, or live reviews to supplement your study.)

 Complete your review by taking the **Computer Test** that comes free with this book.

Reward yourself for a job well done. You have done it all!

Little, Brown's
NCLEX-RN
Examination Review

Little, Brown's
NCLEX-RN
Examination Review

Edited by
Sally L. Lagerquist, RN, MS

Written by
Irene M. Bobak, RN, PhD, FAAN

Professor Emerita, Women's Health and Maternity Nursing, San Francisco State University, San Francisco

Geraldine C. Colombraro, RN, MA, PhD candidate

Assistant Dean, Center for Continuing Education in Nursing and Health Care, Lienhard School of Nursing, Pace University, Pleasantville, NY

Sally L. Lagerquist, RN, MS

Former Instructor of Undergraduate, Graduate, and Continuing Education in Nursing, University of California, San Francisco, School of Nursing; President, Review for Nurses, Inc., and RN Tapes Company, San Francisco

Robyn M. Nelson, RN, DNSc

Professor of Nursing, California State University, Sacramento, CA

Janice Horman Stecchi, RN, EdD

Dean, College of Health Professions, University of Massachusetts Lowell, Lowell, MA

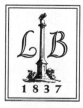

Little, Brown and Company
Boston   New York   Toronto   London

A modified version of this text was previously published as *Addison-Wesley's Nursing Examination Review* by Addison-Wesley Nursing, A Division of The Benjamin/Cummings Publishing Company, Inc. Copyright © 1991.

Library of Congress Cataloging-in-Publication Data

Little, Brown's NCLEX-RN examination review / edited by Sally L.
Lagerquist ; authors, Irene M. Bobak . . . [et al.].
    p.   cm.
    Includes index.
    ISBN 0-316-51279-6
    1. Nursing—Examinations, questions, etc.   I. Lagerquist, Sally
L.   II. Bobak, Irene M.
    [DNLM: 1. Nursing—examination questions.   WY 18.2 L778 1996]
RT55.L57   1996
610.73′076—dc20
DNLM/DLC
for Library of Congress   95-49688
                                               CIP

Printed in the United States of America
MV-NY

Editorial: Evan R. Schnittman, Suzanne Jeans
Production Editor: Katharine S. Mascaro
Copyeditors: Mary Babcock, Ann Calandro
Indexer: Alexandra Nickerson
Production Supervisor: Cate Rickard
Designer: Virginia Pierce
Cover Designer: Martucci Studio

To Tom, my Aquarian husband:
Without your gifts of loving patience and humor, the power of your belief in what I was doing, and the energy of your optimism, I wouldn't have had 28 years of "chicken soup" that warmed my heart. Here's to when life will be full of Saturdays for us!

To our daughter, Elana:
Your sensitivity, creativity, and gentle self have been a source of our pride and joy in all that you are, in all that you have done. As you go forward with your own dreams, we'll be there for you with love, care, and support.

To our son, Kalen:
In celebration of your graduation from the University of California, San Diego, we take time to honor our Svensk pojke. As you go from "yesterday" straight into "tomorrow," I want you to know how grateful I have been all these years for your enthusiasm for learning, and especially for your giving, caring, family-oriented ways.

To my co-authors and friends, Irene, Gerrie, Robyn, and Jan:
A heart full of thanks for years of being there for me in solid friendship, ever-caring, and sharing your expertise as we pioneered and trailblazed together in many overwhelming projects. Without the four of you, I wouldn't have ventured onto the "roads less travelled."

To all nurses and soon-to-be colleagues:
May you use all the power that you have to be all that you can, to make a difference in other people's lives. We offer you this book as a tool to your success in passing the NCLEX-RN.

Sally L. Lagerquist

To the memory of my parents, Susan and Joseph Bobak, who provided a good beginning.

To my family and friends, who encourage me and cheer me on.

To my colleagues, who supply the professional inspiration.

To my students, who motivate me.

Irene M. Bobak

To my husband, Bruce, who has always been there for me whenever I needed him; you have given me Magik all my life!

To my children, Jon and Jacki, with thanks for sharing your childhood with me; I look forward to sharing whatever the future will bring to all of us!

To my newest daughter, Tori, welcome to our family!

And finally, to all of the nursing students and new graduates who will use this book, I hope that your chosen profession of nursing will give you all the joy, pride, and personal satisfaction that I have been blessed with!

Geraldine C. Colombraro

Completion of a project such as this book is never done in isolation (although sometimes it might be easier, how lonely it would be). I was never alone because I had the presence of my husband, Dean; calls from my daughters, Kelly and Tina; food from my mother-in-law, Ruth; and encouragement from my parents, Gordon and Patty. May the road to professional nursing practice be a bit easier as a result of this book.

Robyn M. Nelson

To the memory of my mother, Esther Horman, R.N., my nurse role model. Special thanks to my husband, Dave; sons, Dave, Bill, and Joe; and my dad, Joe Horman, for all their help and support.

Janice Horman Stecchi

To my aunt, Mary Estok, who cared enough.

Marianne K. Zalar

Contents

Preface

With a conceptual framework based on client needs, covered by *categories of human functions,* and emphasizing *nursing process, Little, Brown's NCLEX-RN Examination Review* differs significantly from other nursing review books.

Proven Results

This book has evolved from more than **25 years of experience** in presenting nursing exam review courses throughout the United States. These courses emphasize a comprehensive review of *commonalities* in client care throughout the life span and in a variety of clinical settings. The content, the framework, the sequence of topics, the test-taking guidelines, and the practice exam questions and answers in this book have been tested during the past 25 years with *actual examination candidates* who have passed the RN licensure exam with highly successful results. **This gives the material an authenticity and relevance that is difficult to attain in any other way.**

Conceptual Framework

The conceptual framework of this book concentrates on nursing concerns for *client needs* and the essential requirements for safe, effective, competent nursing care. The text emphasizes *practical application* of clinically relevant data. Each unit is organized in terms of the eight categories of human functions (which are subtopics of the four *client needs*): (1) Protective; (2) Sensory-Perceptual; (3) Comfort, Rest, Activity, and Mobility; (4) Nutrition; (5) Growth and Development; (6) Fluid-Gas Transport; (7) Psychosocial-Cultural, and (8) Elimination functions. (See Appendix G for definitions of these key terms, and Appendices H and I for an index to these key categories in the **text** and **test questions.**) Separate units emphasize the content areas of *nutrition; pharmacology; common diagnostic procedures, treatments, and nursing care;* and *ethical and legal aspects in nursing.*

Special Features

There are many special features in this book that make it stand out from all other nursing review books. The most unique features to help you prepare for exams are a section on **memory aids** (Appendix L), and lists of **common abbreviations and clinical signs** (Appendices J and K) that provide quick and interesting ways to review. In the Orientation section of Unit 1, you'll also find **testing tips and relaxation exercises,** along with more memorizing ideas. Other features include:

- A practice **computer test** for self-assessment and familiarization with the NCLEX-RN computer testing format.
- Many **easy-to-use and easy-to-find** tables summarize information for *quick* review and emphasize nursing responsibilities in a *visual* way.
- Boxed lab data, **diagnostic tests** indicated by a ⚗, **drug information** indicated by a ⬤, and **nursing care and treatments** indicated by a ▶ in the margin for quick reference. Also, **nursing diagnoses, positions, diets,** and **nursing procedures** are *italicized* for visual reinforcement.
- Easy-to-find **content divisions** are marked with black page tabs at the outer margin of each page.
- Unique **indexes to content and test questions** related to specific **categories of human functions** (Appendices H and I) and **client needs** (Appendices E and F), as well as an index to **test questions** at the end of each unit that cover specific steps of the **nursing process** (Appendix C). These indexes are based on the official **NCLEX-RN Test Plan** and especially useful in facilitating review for **repeat exam-takers.**
- Emphasis on **all five steps of the nursing process,** especially *health teaching* and specific *outcome criteria for evaluation* of the effectiveness of nursing care.

- Current NANDA-approved *nursing diagnoses* as a structure for presenting nursing interventions.
- A thorough **question-and-answer review** at the end of *each unit,* in a nursing process format reflecting diverse cultural influences.
- Boxes preceding main headings throughout the units for students to "check off" once they have mastered the topic.

Little, Brown's NCLEX-RN Examination Review incorporates the latest knowledge and current trends in nursing practice, and parallels the latest NCLEX-RN Test Plan. All content has been submitted to outstanding educators and nursing practitioners for their review and critique. We would like to express our appreciation to this editorial review panel for their contributions, which make this book the best to use for *complete* nursing review.

In Unit 1, **Orientation and Pre Test,** you will find suggestions on how to use this book and how to plan your study, information about the NCLEX-RN, *test-taking tips and strategies,* help with memorization, and relaxation exercises. At the end of this unit is the **Pre Test,** to use as self-assessment before reading the nursing content units that follow.

Unit 2, **Nursing Care of the Acutely Ill and the Chronically Ill Adult,** presents content under appropriate categories of human functions. *Risk factors* have been identified for all conditions, *goals of nursing* are clearly stated, and a brief description of *pathophysiology* has been incorporated with each condition. *Tables* on fluid and electrolyte imbalances, acid-base disorders, assessment differences with valvular defects, hazards of immobility, complications of diabetes, and malignant disorders supplement the *condensed* and *consolidated content.* The up-to-date content also includes acquired immune deficiency syndrome, Lyme disease, compartment syndrome, Crohn's disease, ulcers, external fixation devices for fractures, and lithotripsy. Assessment of the *older adult* includes material on the normal changes of aging. The *many tables, charts,* and *diagrams* include cardiac dysrhythmias, comparison of causes of chest pain, burn care, the Glasgow Coma scale, breast and testicular self-exams, chest drainage, comparison of hepatitis types, postoperative complications, enteric and universal precautions, respiratory isolation, care of the adult patient with medical and surgical emergencies, pain assessment, preventing TPN complications, and TPN dressing changes. *Nursing interventions* are grouped according to the goal of care and identify appropriate treatments and drug therapies. More detailed discussions follow in two special units on *pharmacology* (Unit 4) and *treatments* (Unit 5).

Unit 3, **Review of Nutrition,** contains unique information regarding ethnic food patterns, nutritional needs of the elderly, religious and ethnic food preferences, and cultural disease treatments involving food. Special and therapeutic diets are featured.

Unit 4, **Review of Pharmacology,** contains drug classifications and drug treatments with emphasis on **nursing implications.** Pediatric medication adminis-

tration, obstetric analgesia, and psychotropic and mind-altering substances are included.

Unit 5, **Common Diagnostic Procedures, Treatments, and Nursing Care,** includes content on commonly used tubes, intravenous therapy, fluid and electrolyte therapy, oxygen therapy, positioning, and colostomy care, as well as many other diagnostic procedures commonly tested on NCLEX-RN.

Unit 6, **Nursing Care of Behavioral and Emotional Problems Throughout the Life Span,** presents psychiatric disorders that have been organized under DSM-IV guidelines. We have included *thorough* coverage of suicide precautions, midlife crises, mental health of the elderly, substance abuse, panic disorders, posttraumatic disorder, amnestic disorders, personality disorders, sleep and eating disturbances, and affective disorders. Content includes a detailed section on psychiatric emergencies and therapeutic communication techniques.

Unit 7, **Nursing Care of the Childbearing Family,** is streamlined and up-to-date; it contains the most exam-relevant content for both pregnancy and care of the neonate. The unit includes *detailed* information regarding many important diagnostic tests, such as chorionic villi sampling and biophysical profile testing, to identify the woman and fetus at risk. We include the latest information on emergency care in labor and birth, perinatal acquired immune deficiency syndrome, sexually transmitted diseases, and preterm labor. We provide information regarding new drug therapies during the perinatal period recommended for the at-risk infant. *Client teaching* and *nursing interventions* are delineated for each of these areas of practice. The question and answer sections also address these advances in technology and care.

Unit 8, **Nursing Care of Children and Families,** includes much up-to-date information concerning cardiac, respiratory, orthopedic systems, and communicable diseases, that has been synthesized into table format for *easier reading, recall, and application* to client care. Diagrams show genetic transmission of sickle cell anemia and hemophilia, tracheoesophageal fistulas, and the dislocated hip in an infant. Coverage is provided for Reye's syndrome; Kawasaki disease; and salicylate, Tylenol, and lead poisoning. Content includes normal development concerns and parental counseling, as well as appreciation of cultural diversity in assessment and nursing interventions.

Unit 9, **Ethical and Legal Aspects in Nursing** contains a special section on bioethics and client rights.

Appendices in this book include indexes to content and test questions related to specific *client needs* (Appendices E and F) and *categories of human functions* (Appendices H and I), and to test questions related to specific steps of the *nursing process* (Appendix C). These indexes, which are not found in any other book, provide immediate, easy reference to topics from the NCLEX-RN Test Plan exam that are covered in this book. Other appendices cover lab values, common abbreviations, common clinical signs, and fun-to-use memory aids.

Four Unique Self-Evaluation Tools

This book contains four special, *integrated* tests to help you assess your knowledge before taking the NCLEX-RN. The **Pre Test** at the end of Unit 1 is intended for students to take after reading the Orientation section, but *before* reading the rest of this book. It is a pre-assessment tool to let you find your areas of strength and weakness before beginning focused study. The **Practice Test** is intended to be taken *after* reviewing the material in this book to evaluate your progress. The **Final Test,** the third exam tool, will assess your readiness to take NCLEX-RN and identify any last-minute knowledge gaps.

Use the practice **Computer Test** anytime in your preparation when you need extra practice or want to become familiar with the NCLEX-RN testing format.

In addition to these four tests, there are **review questions and answers following each unit.** Their purpose is to help students *review each content area separately* before taking the integrated tests. All questions at the *end of units* and in the integrated tests have been field-tested for several years with students—a diverse group of candidates who have successfully passed the exam—from all over the United States. These questions have also been reviewed by an editorial panel for appropriateness. The Answers/Rationale sections in each unit contain detailed explanations about why a particular answer is best and *why* the other options are incorrect. We expect that these special integrated tests, end-of-unit review questions, and corresponding answer sections will prove to be invaluable review tools for each and every student.

In the answers for each of the end-of-unit review question sections, and for the **Pre Test, Practice Test, Final Test,** and **Computer Test,** you will find a three-part code to help you understand exactly what is being tested by each question. The code refers to the step of the *nursing process,* the *category of human function,* and the *client need* that applies to that question. See the code legend on the first page of each Answers/Rationale section. The **Computer Test** will track these codes for you, to identify your problem areas. Use these codes as a guide for review when you find you did not select the best answer. **The codes are unique to this book;** they are an added study tool to help you assess your strengths and pinpoint problem areas as you prepare for the NCLEX-RN.

S.L.L.
I.M.B.
G.C.C.
R.M.N.
J.H.S.
M.K.Z.

Acknowledgments

To Evan Schnittman, our Little, Brown editor:

Without your visionary, exuberant ways, this book wouldn't have become a joyful reality.

You saw, you believed, you made it happen! Your energy and delightful quick wit added to all else that made you the best editor.

To Bonnie Bergstrom, our very own editor:

You have been the pivotal point that kept it all together for us in seeing this book all the way through. Months of eye-strain, tons of "post-its," countless refills of graphite in your editing pencil are but a few inklings of what you put into this book. We are so very appreciative of your commitment to excellence and incredible eye for editing details. Thank you for always making adjustments to meet the needs and varying styles of your five authors.

To Suzanne Jeans (Senior Editorial Assistant) and Katie Mascaro (Production Editor):

Thank you for your upbeat, encouraging voices over the phone, always accommodating, very supportive of us, and willing to go that extra way to make this project "do-able."

Contributing Authors

Irene M. Bobak, RN, PhD, FAAN
Professor Emerita, Women's Health and Maternity Nursing, San Francisco State
  University, San Francisco

Geraldine C. Colombraro, RN, MA, PhD candidate
Assistant Dean, Center for Continuing Education in Nursing and Health Care,
  Lienhard School of Nursing, Pace University, Pleasantville, NY

Sally L. Lagerquist, RN, MS
Former Instructor of Undergraduate, Graduate, and Continuing Education in
  Nursing, University of California, San Francisco, School of Nursing; President,
  Review for Nurses, Inc., and RN Tapes Company, San Francisco

Robyn M. Nelson, RN, DNSc
Professor of Nursing, California State University, Sacramento, CA

Janice Horman Stecchi, RN, EdD
Dean, College of Health Professions, University of Massachusetts Lowell, Lowell, MA

Marianne K. Zalar, RN, EdD
Clinical Specialist in Nursing Research, Department of Nursing, Palo Alto Veterans
  Administration Medical Center, Palo Alto, CA

Little, Brown's
NCLEX-RN
Examination Review

Unit 1

Orientation and Pre Test

Orientation

❏ How To Use This Review Book as a Study Guide

Although nursing students may know that they are academically prepared to take the computer adaptive National Council Licensure Examination (NCLEX-RN), many find that reviewing nursing content for the licensure examination itself presents special concerns about *what* and *how* to study.

Some typical concerns about *what to study* are reflected in the following questions:

- Since there will be up to 265 questions on the exam, and every candidate gets a different exam, how does one select what is the most important content for review? How does one narrow the focus of study and distinguish the relevant from the irrelevant material?
- What areas should be emphasized?
- How detailed should the review be?
- How does one know what areas to review first?
- Should basic sciences, such as anatomy, physiology, microbiology, and nutrition, be included in the study?

Concerns relating to *how to study* include:

- How does one make the best of limited review time to go over content that may be in lecture and clinical notes compiled during 2 to 4 years of schooling?
- Is it best to review from all the major textbooks used in nursing school?
- Should material be memorized, or should one study from broad principles and concepts?

We have written this nursing review book with the *general* intent of assisting nurses in identifying what

they need to study in a format designed to use their study time effectively, productively, and efficiently while preparing for the examination.

The contributing authors have selected content and developed a style of presentation that has been tested by thousands of nursing students attending review courses coordinated by the editor in various cities throughout the United States. *Little, Brown's NCLEX-RN Review* is the result of this study.

This review book can be used in a variety of ways: (a) as a *starting point* for review of essential content specifically aimed at NCLEX or Canadian exam preparation, (b) as an *end point* of studying for the examinations, (c) as an *anxiety-reduction tool,* (d) as a general guide and *refresher* for nurses not presently in practice, and (e) as a guide for graduates of *foreign* nursing schools.

As a Starting Point

This text can be used in early review when a longer study period is needed to *fill in gaps* of knowledge. One cannot remember something if one does not know or understand it. A lengthy review before the exam allows students time to rework and organize notes accumulated during 2 to 4 years of basic nursing education. In addition, an early review allows time for *self-evaluation.* We have provided questions and answers to help students identify areas requiring further study and to help them *integrate* unfamiliar material with what they already know.

As an End Point

This text can also be used for a *quick review* (a) to *promote retention and recall* and (b) to aid in determining *nursing actions* appropriate to specific health situations. During the time immediately preceding the examination, the main objective might be to *strengthen previous learning* by refreshing the memory. Or a brief overview may serve to *draw together* the isolated points under key concepts and principles in a way that shows their relationships and relative importance.

As an Anxiety-Reduction Tool

In some students, anxiety related to taking examinations in general may reach such levels that it causes students to be unproductive in study and to function at a lower level during the actual examination. Sections of this text are directed toward this problem and provide simple, *practical approaches to the reduction of general anxiety.* For anxiety specifically related to unknown aspects of the licensure examination itself, the section on the *structure, format, and mechanics of the RN examination* might bring relief through its focus on basic examination information.

For anxiety related to lack of confidence or skill in test-taking "know-how," the special section on *test-taking techniques* may be helpful.

As a General Study Guide and as a Refresher for Nurses Not Presently in Practice

Many nursing students will find this review book useful throughout their education as a general study guide as they prepare patient care plans and study for midterm and final exams. It will help them put information into perspective as they learn it. And nurses who have not been in practice for several years will find it a useful reference tool and review device.

As a Guide for Graduates of Foreign Nursing Schools

Nurses who are foreign educated can use this book to serve their special needs.

1. To check their experiences, skills, and knowledge for *equivalency* to those of nursing candidates from U.S. programs, in terms of their ability to deliver effective and safe health care as determined by U.S. standards of practice.
2. To identify cultural differences in perception of patient needs and nursing responses and actions.
3. To obtain state board of nursing addresses, to find out requirements and procedures to apply to take the RN licensure exam in their state.
4. To learn about the structure and format of the exam.
5. To learn how to prepare for the exam.
6. To practice taking tests made up of multiple choice questions.
7. To assess the level of language difficulty in reading the exam.

If you are a foreign-educated nurse and wish to compare your preparation with that of U.S.-educated nurses, you will find that the practice questions with detailed answers that are included at the end of each major content unit can serve as an effective self-assessment guide. If you find that you need further in-depth

study after taking the practice test and reviewing the essential content presented in outline format throughout the book, you may wish to seek assistance from review courses or self-paced review on audiocassette tapes. In addition, Unit 4 may help you review drugs used in the U.S. that may be called by other names outside the U.S.

Cultural differences may be one cause of incorrect answers stemming from your different perception of patients' needs or nursing action. In addition, Unit 9 contains the code of ethics and standards of nursing practice and legal aspects that pertain to nursing *in the U.S.* We suggest that the foreign-educated nurse become familiar with these sections to determine what is *emphasized* in this country. Appendix D addresses important client needs.

To assist the nurse in making contact with Boards of Registered Nursing, the inside front cover contains a directory of addresses to write for information about each state's specific requirements for application to take the RN licensing exam.

This Orientation unit is designed to help the foreign-educated nurse know what to expect during the exam, what the exam structure and format will be like, what content will be covered, and how it will be scored. It will also help him or her learn how to study for the test, how to take a multiple choice test, and how to reduce test-taking anxiety.

If you are not familiar with or proficient in taking exams with multiple choice questions, the approximately 1000 sample test questions in this book will provide you with sufficient practice for taking such a test.

If you are concerned about your ability to read and comprehend English as it might be used in the exam, first check yourself by looking at the exam questions in this book. The terms used here are those used in the health care field and are considered to be those a nurse needs to know and use. If the vocabulary is different from yours or is difficult, consult local colleges for courses in *English as a second language (ESL courses).*

Where To Begin

In using this review book to prepare for the licensure examination, the nurse must:

1. Be prepared mentally.
    a. Know the purpose of the examination.
    b. Know the purpose of reviewing.
    c. Anticipate what is to come.
    d. Decide on a good study method—set a study goal before beginning a particular subject area (number of pages, for example); plan the length of the review period by the amount of material to be covered, not by the clock.
2. Plan the work to be done.
    a. Select one subject at a time for review, and establish and follow a sequence for review of each subject.
       (1) Answer the practice questions following the outline of the selected subject area. (Set a time limit, as pacing is important.)

(2) Compare your answers with those provided following the questions as a means of evaluating areas of competence.

b. Identify those subjects that will require additional concentrated study in this review book as well as in basic textbooks.

c. Study the review text outlines, noting headings, subheadings, and *italics* and **boldface** type for emphasis of relative importance.

d. Study the content presented in chart format to facilitate memorization, understanding, and application.

e. Repeat the self-evaluation process by taking the test again.

f. Look up the answers for the correct response to the multiple choice questions. Do not memorize the answers. Read the rationale explaining *why* it was the correct response. (These explanations serve to correct as well as reinforce. Understanding the underlying principles also serves as an aid in applying the same principles to questions that may be based on similar rationale, but phrased differently on the actual examination.)

g. If necessary, refer to basic textbooks to relearn any unclear aspects of anatomy, physiology, nutrition, or basic nursing procedures. Look up unfamiliar terminology in a medical dictionary.

While Reviewing

1. Scan the outline for main ideas and topics.
   a. Do not try to remember verbatim what is on each page.
   b. Paraphrase or explain this material to another person.
2. Refer to basic textbooks for details and illustrations as necessary to recall specific information related to basic sciences.
3. Integrate reading with experience.
   a. Think of examples that illustrate the key concepts and principles.
   b. Make meaningful associations.
   c. Look for implications for nursing actions as concepts are reviewed.
4. Take notes on the review outline—use stars and arrows, underscore, highlight with highlighter pens, and write comments in margins, such as "most important" and "memorize," to reinforce the relative importance of points of information.

After Reviewing

1. Repeat the self-evaluation process as often as necessary to gain mastery of content essential to safe nursing practice.
2. Continue to refer to major textbooks to fill in gaps where greater detail or in-depth comprehension is required.
3. Look for patterns in your selection of responses to the multiple choice practice questions—identify sources of difficulty in choosing the most appropriate answers.

❏ Key Points To Recall for Better Study

1. *Schedule*—study time should be scheduled so that review begins close to the time at which it will be used. Retention is much better following a well-spaced review. It may be helpful to group material into small learning segments. Study goals should be set before beginning each period of study (number of pages, for example).
2. *Organize*—many students have better retention of material after they have reorganized and re-learned it.
3. *Rephrase and explain*—try to rephrase material in your own words or explain it to another person. Reinforce learning through repetition and usage.
4. *Decide on order of importance*—organize study time in terms of importance and familiarity.
5. *Use mechanical memory aids*—mnemonic (memory) devices simplify recall. For example, in "On Old Olympus's Towering Top a Finn and German Viewed Some Hops," the first letter of each word identifies the first letter of a cranial nerve. (See Appendix L.)
6. *Association*—associate new material with related concepts and principles from past experience.
7. *Original learning*—if an unfamiliar topic is presented, do more than review. Seek out sources of additional information.
8. *Make notes*—look for key words, phrases, and sentences in the outlined review material, and mark them for later reference.
9. *Definitions*—look up unfamiliar terms in a dictionary or the glossary of a basic text, or in Appendix J.
10. *Additional study*—refer to other textbook references for more detailed information.
11. *Distractors*—keep a pad of paper on hand to jot down extraneous thoughts; get them out of the mind and onto the paper.

❏ Memorization: Purpose and Strategies

You'll need to memorize some items before you can rapidly assess or apply that knowledge to a particular situation; for example, you need to be able to recall the standard and lethal doses of a drug before deciding to administer it. Items you should memorize include, but are not limited to:

1. Names of common drugs.
2. Lethal and therapeutic doses.
3. Lab norms and values.
4. Growth and development norms.
5. Foods high or low in iron, protein, sodium, potassium, or carbohydrates.
6. Conversion formulas.
7. Anatomic names.
8. List of cranial nerves and their innervations.

To facilitate memorizing these and other essentials, here are some strategies.

1. Before you work on training your mind to remember, you must *want* to remember the material.
2. You cannot memorize something that you do not understand; therefore, *know* your material.
3. Visualize what you want to memorize; picture it; draw a picture.
4. Use the familiar to provide vivid mental pictures, to peg the unfamiliar.
   a. When needing to remember a *sequence,* use your body to turn material into a picture. Draw a person, then list the first item to be memorized on top of the head, the next item on the forehead, and so on for nose, mouth, neck, chest, abdomen, thighs, knees, and feet.
   b. Use what you already know to tie in with what you want to remember; make it memorable.
   c. Use as pegs the unexpected, the exaggerated. Weird imagery is easiest to recall.
5. Use the blank-paper technique:
   a. Place a large blank sheet on the wall.
   b. After you have studied, draw on the blank paper what you remember.
   c. When you have drawn all that you can recall, check with the book and study what you did correctly and incorrectly.
   d. Take another sheet and do it again. Purpose: to reinforce what you already know and work with what you want to remember.
6. Make up and use mnemonic devices to help you remember the important elements (see Appendix L).
7. Repetitively explain to another person the material you want to memorize.
8. Saturate your environment with the material you want to memorize.
   a. Purpose: to overcome the mind's tendency to ignore.
   b. Tape facts, formulas, concepts on walls.
9. Above all, feel confident in your ability to memorize!

❑ The Mechanics of the National Council Licensure Examination for Registered Nurses–Computer Adaptive Test (NCLEX-RN)

As of April 1994, the licensure examination for registered nurses is administered year-round by computer, in an adaptive format: NCLEX-RN. Frequently, candidates for the exam have many questions about the structure and format of the test itself and the rules and regulations concerning the examination procedure.

As an aid to reducing apprehension and time spent on speculation, this section is intended to provide information that candidates need, in outline form; the last segment offers a "question-and-answer" format for specific questions frequently asked by nursing students.

This information was verified as correct at the time that it was compiled from information provided by the National Council of State Boards of Nursing, Inc., and other parties involved in the testing. If you have further questions, contact the board of nursing in your state (see listing on inside front cover).

I. What NCLEX is
   A. National Council Licensure Examination, developed and administered by the National Council of State Boards of Nursing, Inc., with services provided by Educational Testing Service (ETS) and Sylvan Learning Systems.
   B. Tests for minimum nursing competence according to a national standard.
   C. Pass/fail result; must pass to be issued license from state board of registered nursing.
   D. National exam. Application procedure and licensing requirements are determined by each state board and may differ from state to state.

II. CAT: How it works
   A. Stands for "computer adaptive testing."
   B. "Adaptive" because the computer estimates the candidate's ability after each question; the next question is chosen based on the candidate's estimated ability so far. The test is therefore "adapted" to each candidate; everyone takes a different, "customized" test.
   C. Estimated ability is recalculated after each question until it is precise enough to determine whether the candidate is above or below minimum competence level, in all areas of the test plan. The test will stop as soon as this is determined.
   D. Example: The first question is of a fairly easy level. The candidate answers correctly, so the computer estimates that the candidate's ability level is above the level of this question and selects a harder question; or if the candidate answers incorrectly, it selects an easier question, to pinpoint where the candidate's ability level lies, in each area of the test plan.

III. Some specifics
   A. Format
      1. Multiple choice questions, each with four options.
      2. One question at a time appears on screen, with question stem on the left and options on the right, or with background information on the left and question stem with options on the right (Figure 1.1).
      3. Each question stands alone (no "scenarios" with several spin-off questions); no question will relate to information given in previous questions.
   B. Answering
      1. As candidate chooses the answer to each question, he or she will be asked to confirm that answer, *or* can change that answer before confirming.

2. Must answer every question (no penalty for guessing; will simply count as a correct or incorrect answer and adjust difficulty of next question accordingly).
3. Cannot go back to previous questions either to review or change answers (because *subsequent* questions are administered based on *previous* answers).

C. Number of questions
1. 75–265, including about 15 "tryout" questions which are not scored (these are questions being field tested for use on future exams).
2. Depends on number needed to determine whether candidate is definitely above or definitely below minimum competence level.
3. Taking only the minimum can mean **either pass or fail;** it indicates that it took fewer questions to determine whether this candidate is above or below minimum competence, but does not indicate which!

D. Timing
1. No time limit for each question.
2. Maximum time for test is 5 hours.
3. A 10-minute break is mandatory after 2 hours; an optional 10-minute break may be taken after another 1½ hours.

E. The test will stop when any *one* of the following occurs:
1. A "pass" or "fail" determination can be made.
2. The maximum number of questions has been taken (265).
3. The test has lasted for 5 hours.

F. The computer
1. Computer experience will not be necessary.
2. Only two keys will be used, one to move down the list of options and another to select and confirm answer choice; all other keys will be "turned off."
3. Candidate receives a brief orientation with sample questions before beginning the exam.

■ **FIGURE 1.1 Computer screen.**

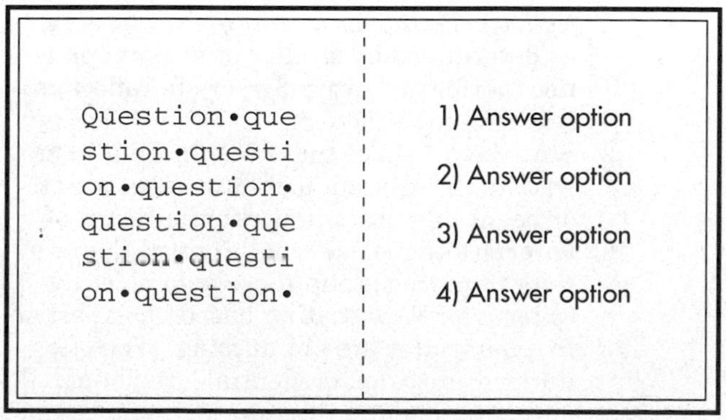

Question•question•question•question•question•question•question•question•question•question•	1) Answer option
	2) Answer option
	3) Answer option
	4) Answer option

IV. Administration
A. Application and scheduling
1. Involves three parties: the state board of nursing, Educational Testing Service (ETS), and Sylvan Learning Systems.
2. Candidate applies to the board of nursing in the state in which licensing is desired; must meet requirements of that state board. (Some state boards may require an administrative fee.)
3. Candidate must also register with ETS to take the exam, and pay a test fee. (**NOTE:** These procedures differ in some states, including Florida, Illinois, Massachusetts, and New York; candidates should follow instructions from state board.)
4. After state board determines eligibility and fees are received, ETS mails candidate an *Authorization To Test* (ATT) and information on available Sylvan Technology Centers, which serve as testing sites (at least one per state; some states have many more).
5. Candidate contacts Sylvan Technology Center (or other designated test site) to set up testing appointment (6 d/wk, 15 h/d, in 5-h time slots). Sunday appointments *may* be available in peak testing periods. Candidates may test at any test center in any state (they do not have to take the test in the same state to which they have applied for licensure).
6. After testing, results are communicated to state board to which the candidate applied, which mails results to candidate (time frame will differ by state). Candidates who do not pass will receive diagnostic profiles, indicating performance in each area of the test plan relative to the passing standard, and information about retesting.

B. Test environment: Sylvan Technology Center test sites
1. Up to 15 workstations, each with computer terminal, desk lamp, work surface, and scratch paper.
2. Designed for security, monitored by a proctor as well as by videotape.
3. Candidate must present *Authorization To Test* and two signed pieces of identification, one with picture; candidate must sign in and be thumbprinted and photographed.
4. Lockers or other secured storage provided; personal items restricted in testing room.

V. Test plan, development
A. Test plan*
1. *Client needs* and the *nursing process* are the bases, or "dimensions," for the test plan. See Tables 1.1 and 1.2.
2. Health needs of clients: About half of the test plan emphasizes meeting the clients'

*Source: National Council of the State Boards of Nursing.

physical needs in actual or potentially life-threatening, chronic, or recurring *physiologic* conditions and the needs of clients who are at risk for complications or untoward effects of treatment. Subcategories include (1) physiologic adaptation, (2) reduction of risk potential, and (3) provision of basic care.

The second highest category in emphasis, *safe, effective care environment,* focuses on (1) coordinated care, (2) environmental safety, and (3) safe and effective treatment and procedures.

The next category in terms of emphasis is *health promotion and maintenance,* covering (1) growth and development throughout the life span, (2) self-care and integrity of support systems, and (3) prevention and early treatment of disease.

Finally, 8–16% of the test plan concerns *psychosocial coping and adaptation* in stress- and crisis-related situations throughout the life cycle.

3. Nursing process (nursing behaviors): The exam places approximately equal emphasis on each step of the nursing process, as applied to client situations from all stages in the life cycle and to common health problems in all the major health areas and based on current morbidity studies.

4. Levels of cognitive ability: Most items are at the *application* and *analysis* level (application of principles, ideas, theories; and analysis of data to set priorities and see relationships), but include knowledge and comprehension.

5. Categories of nursing knowledge and other concepts that are commonly tested:

■ **TABLE 1.1**   **Exam Weight Given to Each Category of Health Needs of Clients Based on Job Analysis Study 1992–93**

Client Health Needs Tested	Percentage of Test
Safe, effective care environment	15–21
Physiologic integrity	46–54
Psychosocial integrity	8–16
Health promotion and maintenance	17–23

■ **TABLE 1.2**   **Exam Weight Given to Steps of Nursing Process (Nursing Behaviors)**

Nursing Behavior Tested	Percentage of Test
Assessment	17–23
Analysis	17–23
Planning	17–23
Implementation	17–23
Evaluation/outcome criteria	17–23

a. Nursing fundamentals (see Unit 5).
b. Nutrition and diet therapy (see Unit 3).
c. Pharmacology (see Unit 4).
d. Communicable diseases (see Unit 8).
e. Psychosocial aspects (see Unit 6).
f. Natural and behavioral sciences (integrated into all units).
g. Normal growth and development (see Units 6 and 8).
h. Basic human needs (see Unit 6).
i. Individual coping mechanisms (see Unit 6).
j. Actual or potential health problems (see Units 2, 7, and 8).
k. Effect of age, sex, culture, ethnicity, and religion on health needs (sociocultural components) are integrated into all units; for special emphasis on dietary implications, see Unit 3.
l. Ways by which nursing can assist individuals to maintain health and cope with health problems (see *nursing care plan / implementation* sections in *each* unit).
m. Legal and ethical aspects of nursing, accountability (see Unit 9).
n. Life cycle (consult the Contents to see how the conceptual framework for this book is organized by life cycle).
o. Patient environment (there is continual reference throughout this book related to protection from harm against airborne irritants, cold, and heat; identification of environmental discomforts such as noise, odors, dust, and poor ventilation; elimination of potential *safety hazards;* maintenance of environmental order; and *cleanliness*).

B. Development
1. The Examination Committee of the National Council prepares the test plan, which is approved by the delegates representing the state boards of nursing. It is designed to reflect the knowledge and skills needed for *minimum competence by a newly licensed nurse to be a safe and effective practitioner in entry-level nursing,* as determined by studies of nursing practice (performed every 3 years to reflect current nursing practice).

2. State boards take turns nominating item writers (faculty, clinical nurse specialists, or beginning practitioners); the Board of Directors of the National Council then selects from this group those who meet the criteria for item writing based on expertise in a particular area of nursing, type of nursing program, credentials, regional balance, etc. The item writers write questions based on common clinical situations and

according to the test plan. Then the questions are researched and reviewed by a panel of experts (nominated by the state boards), by those state boards that choose to review, and by the National Council's Examination Committee.

3. Finally, the questions are field tested to eliminate questions that may be ambiguous, irrelevant, or not equally applicable to all regions of the U.S. (Each candidate taking NCLEX will take 15 of these "tryout" questions, mixed in with the regular questions; they will *not* count toward that candidate's performance.) The data gained through field testing are also used to analyze and determine the difficulty level of a question.

C. Passing standard: The passing standard is *criterion referenced;* this means that there is no fixed percentage of candidates that pass or fail. Passing depends solely on performance in relation to the level of minimum competence. The passing standard is reviewed every 3 years.

VI. Frequently asked questions and answers about NCLEX-RN

A. Test questions, test plan

1. *How many questions will there be?* You will take anywhere from 75 to 265 multiple choice questions. (See III. Some specifics, p. 4.)

2. *Where do the questions come from?* The state boards of nursing nominate item writers, who must meet various criteria. (See V.B. Development, p. 6.)

3. *Will there be questions involving conditions with which I may not have had experience in my nursing program?* Most of the questions are about patients with conditions familiar to you and are representative of common health problems on a national basis. Some questions may relate to nursing problems with which you may not have had prior experience; their purpose is to test your ability to *apply* knowledge of specific principles from the physical, biologic, and social sciences to *new* situations.

4. *Can a question have more than one answer?* No. Only *one* of the four options is the *best* answer. You will not be able to choose more than one option as your answer.

5. *Will I get partial credit for selecting the next-to-the-best answer?* No. Your answer will be treated only as correct or incorrect.

6. *If everyone takes a different test, how can it be fair?* Each candidate is tested according to the *same test plan,* and the *same passing standard.* It may simply require more items to reach a stable pass/fail determination for one candidate, while another may

require fewer questions to demonstrate competence level.

7. *Do diploma, associate, and baccalaureate graduates all take the same test? What about graduates from schools outside the U.S.?* All candidates are held to the *same test plan and passing standard,* and take the "same test." (Of course, due to the nature of CAT, each will receive an "individualized" test, without regard to degree, or to state or country of education.)

8. *Does the exam differ by state?* The exam is a national exam; all candidates are held to the *same test plan and passing standard,* and take questions from the same pool. (Again, through CAT, each candidate receives an "individualized" test, but without regard to state.)

9. *How is the exam different from the old "paper-and-pencil" test?* The purpose, test plan, and nursing knowledge and skills tested *did not change* significantly with the advent of CAT (there were minor adjustments to the test plan in October 1995, unrelated to the change to computer testing). The *main differences* lie in the efficiency of the computerized testing (maximum of 5 hours and 265 questions, compared to the old 2-day test with up to 372 questions) and the adaptive nature, which precludes skipping questions and changing answers.

B. Taking the test/after the test

1. *Can I skip questions?* No. You must answer each question in order to move on to the next. You also will not be able to return to previous questions to try them again or change the answer (because *subsequent* questions are administered based on *previous* answers).

2. *What if I just don't know the answer?* Use the tips in Twenty Strategies in Answering Questions, p. 10, to make your best guess. You will need to answer the question in order to move on to the next question.

3. *When will I know my results? Will the computer tell me?* You will not learn your pass/fail status at the testing center; the results will be communicated directly to your state board of nursing, who will mail the results to you. The time frame may differ from state to state, but most candidates should receive their results within 2 to 4 weeks after taking the exam. **NOTE:** Taking only the minimum number of questions, or taking the maximum, is not an indication of whether you have passed or failed. It merely indicates that a lesser, or greater, number of items was required to reach a determination.

4. *What percentage must I answer correctly to pass?* Because of the nature of CAT, a per-

centage rate is *not* used to determine passing or failure. The test determines whether you are above or below standard competence by determining not the *number* of questions you answer correctly, but rather the *difficulty level* you can consistently answer correctly. The process of administering harder or easier questions, as described in II. CAT: How it works, p. 4, continues until you reach the level where you answer approximately 50% of the questions correctly. **NOTE:** When practicing with questions of mixed difficulty, such as those in this book, you may wish to use 75% correct as a "benchmark" goal for yourself.

5. *If I do not pass, can I retest only those areas of the test plan in which I tested poorly?* No. The whole exam is on a pass/fail basis.

6. *Can I repeat the exam before I get my results?* No.

7. *How many times can the exam be repeated, and when?* The National Council allows you to repeat the exam a maximum of four times per year, but not more than once in any 90-day period; however, each state board may set its own, more restrictive time limits and retake requirements.

8. *Who grants the nursing license?* The license is granted by the state board of nursing to which you applied and for which you took the exam.

9. *I will be repeating the exam; how do I know what to study?* A good place to start is Appendices C, F, and I. On your diagnostic profile from NCLEX, find the area(s) of client needs and nursing process in which your performance was lowest; then use the appendices in this book to find specific page numbers and question numbers to begin focused study in what you need, in preparation for repeating the exam.

C. Testing facilities

1. *Can I bring any materials into the examination room?* There are severe restrictions on personal items allowed in the examination room; you will be provided with a locker or other secure place for your belongings. Do *not* take any study materials (books, notes, calculators, etc.) or cameras into the examination building.

2. *How many people will take the test at the same time?* Up to 15 people may be at computer workstations in your testing room; however, they may not all be taking the NCLEX, as Sylvan Learning Systems also offers other services.

3. *When and where will I take the test?* After you receive your authorization (ATT), you need to contact a Sylvan Technology Center facility to set up your own testing ap-

pointment (6 d/wk, 15 h/d, in 5-h time slots). There is at least one facility per state, although most states have many more.

4. *What accommodations are available for candidates with disabilities?* All test centers are accessible to candidates with disabilities. Other accommodations will be made only with the prior authorization of the board of nursing; contact your state board *prior* to submitting your application.

❏ How To Prepare for and Score Higher on Exams

The Psychology of Test Taking

Many nursing students know the nursing material on which they are being tested, and can demonstrate their nursing skills in practice, but do not know how to prepare themselves for taking and passing examinations.

It is not just a matter of taking exams but of *knowing how* to take them, taking steps to ensure you can function at full capacity, and utilizing the allotted time in the most productive way. You must learn to use strategy and judgment in answering questions, and to make educated guesses when you are not sure of the right answer.

This section offers practical suggestions to help ensure you are "at your best" on exam day, and discusses practical strategies for eliminating wrong answers and for increasing your chances of selecting the best ones.

Prepare Physically and Mentally

1. *On the morning of an exam, avoid excessive oral intake of products that act as diuretics for you.* If you know that coffee or cigarettes, for example, increase urgency and frequency, it is best to limit their intake. Undue physiologic discomforts can distract your focus from the exam at hand.

2. *Increase your oral intake of foods high in glucose and protein.* These foods reportedly have been helpful to some examinees for keeping up their blood-sugar level. This may enhance your concentration and problem-solving ability at the times when you most need to function at a high level. On the other hand, avoid carbohydrates such as doughnuts, which slow down thinking.

3. *Prior to examination days, avoid eating exotic or highly seasoned foods to which your system may not be accustomed.* Avoid possible gastrointestinal distress when you least need it!

4. *Use hard candy or something similar* during a test, if it is allowed in the exam room, to help relieve the discomfort of a dry mouth related to a state of anxiety.

5. *Wear comfortable clothes that you have worn before.* The day of an exam is not a good time to wear new clothes or footwear that may prove to be constricting, binding, or uncomfortable, especially at the waistline and shoulder seams.

6. Anxiety states can bring about rapid increases and decreases in body temperature. *Wear clothing that can be shed or added on.* For example, you might bring a sweater that can be put on when you feel chilled or removed when your body temperature fluctuates again.

7. *Women need to be prepared for late, irregular, or unanticipated early onset of menses* on exam day, a time of stress.

8. Exam jitters can elicit anxiety-like reactions, both physiologic and emotional. Since anxiety tends to be contagious, *try to limit your contacts with those who are also experiencing exam-related anxiety or who elicit those feelings in you.*

9. *The night before an exam is a good time to engage in a pleasurable activity* as a means of anxiety reduction. You need stamina and endurance for sitting, thinking, and reacting. Give yourself a chance for restful, not energy- or emotion-draining, activities in the days before an exam.

10. *Try a relaxation process* if anxiety reaches an uncomfortable level that cannot be channeled into the service of learning (see How To Reduce Anxiety, pp. 11–12).

11. When you arrive home after an exam, *jot down content areas that were unfamiliar to you.* This may serve as a key focus for review.

Tips for NCLEX-RN

1. Get an early start on the day you take the examination, to avoid raising your anxiety level before the actual exam starts. Allow yourself time for delays in traffic and in public transportation or for finding a parking place. Even allow for a dead battery, flooded engine, flat tire, or bus breakdown. If you are unfamiliar with the area in which the test center is located, find it the day before.

2. Remember that *you do not need to get all the answers right to pass.* The exam is designed to test for *minimum* competence; demonstrating a higher level will not earn a special designation on your license, or any other bonus. Moreover, due to the adaptive nature of the test, you will probably reach a level where you are answering only 50% of the questions correctly; this is *normal* for this test and *should not* in itself be taken as an indication of poor performance (you may be answering 50% of the *very difficult* questions correctly)!

3. Since you cannot skip questions and go back to them, or go back to change answers, it is important that you simply *do the best you can* on a particular question, using the Twenty Strategies in Answering Questions, p. 10, and *move on.* The adaptive test will give you another chance to show your competence, should you get that question wrong.

4. Remember that although you cannot change answers you have already "confirmed," you *may change your answer during the selection process.* As you make your answer selection, you will *choose* an answer (by pressing the enter key once) and then *confirm* it (by pressing the key a second time); you will be able to change your mind *before confirming* your answer choice.

5. Although the exam uses different levels of difficulty to estimate your competence level, *do not try to figure out the difficulty level* of each question; likewise, do not try to keep track of the number of questions you are answering. You will only distract yourself and raise your anxiety. Again, simply answer each question to the best of your ability and move on.

6. When taking practice questions, it is a good idea to *aim for an average of 1 minute per question,* so that you will be at a speed to finish the exam even if you *do* need to take the maximum number of questions. For the actual exam, however, the 5-hour time limit is not a problem for most candidates, so go ahead and *take the time to work through a difficult problem,* and make use of the scratch paper provided (but *don't* dwell on a question you "just can't get!").

Tips for Other (Pencil-and-Paper) Tests and Exams

1. *Answer the easy questions first.* Too often students focus on 1 question for 10 minutes, for example, instead of going on to answer 20 additional questions during this time. The main goal in this type of exam is to answer correctly as many questions as possible.

2. *Your first hunch is usually a good one.* Pay attention to your intuition, which may indicate which answer "feels" best.

3. *Be wise about the timing.* Divide your time. For example, if you have 90 questions and 1½ hours for the test, aim for an average of 1 question per minute. Keep working! Do not lose time looking back at your answers.

4. *If you cannot decide between two multiple choice answers, make a note of the numbers of the two choices.* This will narrow down your focus when you come back to this question. Leave the question; do not spend much time on those in doubt. When you have completed the test, go back and spend more time on those with which you had trouble.

5. *Exercise care and caution when using electronically scored answer sheets or booklets.* It is essential that you use only the type of pencil or ink specified in the instructions. If erasing is possible, be sure to erase completely; a mere trace might throw out the answer.

6. When using a separate answer sheet or booklet, be especially careful to *mark your answer in the space for the correct question number.* It might be helpful to say to yourself as you answer each question, "Choice No. 4 to question No. 3," to make sure that the right answer goes with each question number.

7. *Stay the entire time allotted.* If you complete the test early, check your answers. On a second look, after you have completed the test, you may find something that you are *now sure* you marked in er-

ror the first time. If you were undecided between two possible answers on any questions, use leftover time to reconsider those answers. (Also, look for and erase stray marks, if using electronically scored answer sheets.)

Twenty Strategies in Answering Questions

If you can intelligently eliminate false answers, you can reduce a four-answer question to a two-answer one and thereby make your chances as good as those in the true-false type of question; that is, odds will favor your guessing half of the answers correctly.

We think that the following pointers will assist you to narrow down your choices intelligently.

1. *Always, all, never, none.* Answers that include global words such as these should be viewed with caution because they imply that there are no exceptions. There are very few instances in which a correct answer is that absolute. Any suggested answer, such as in the following:

   Nurses should exercise caution in interviewing alcoholics because:
   1. Alcoholics *always* exaggerate.
   2. Alcoholics are *never* consistent.

   should be looked at with care because any exception will make that a false response. A more reasonable answer to the preceding might be "Alcoholics may not be reliable historians."

2. *Broadest, most comprehensive answers.* Choose the answer that includes all the others, which is referred to here as the "umbrella effect." For example, in answering the question:

   A main nursing function in group therapy is to:
   1. Help patients give and receive feedback in the group.
   2. Encourage patients to bring up their concerns.
   3. Facilitate group interaction among the members.
   4. Remind patients to address their comments to the group.

   Number 3 is the best choice because all the other choices fall under it.

3. Test how *reasonable* the answer is by posing a specific situation to yourself. For example, the question might read, "The best approach when interviewing children who have irrational fears is to: (1) Help them analyze why they feel this way." Ask yourself if it is reasonable to use Freudian analysis with 2-year-old children.

4. *Focus on the patient.* Usually the reason for doing something with a patient is *not* to preserve the good reputation of the doctor, hospital, or nurse or to enforce rules. Wrong choices would focus on enlisting the patient's cooperation for the purpose of fulfilling orders or because it is the rule. On seeing a patient out of bed against orders, instead of just saying, "It's against doctor's orders for you to get up," you might better respond by focusing on how the patient is reacting to the restriction on his mobility, by saying, for example, "I can see that you want to get up and that it is upsetting to you to be in bed now. Let me help you get back to bed safely and see what I can do for you."

5. *Eliminate any answer that takes for granted that anyone is unworthy or ignorant.* For example, in the question, "The patient should not be told the full extent of her condition because . . . ," a poor response would be, "she would not understand."

6. *Look for the answer that may be different from the others.* For example, if all choices but one are stated in milligrams and that one reads, "1 g," that choice may be a distractor. In that case, you can narrow your selection to the other choices.

7. Read the question carefully to see if a *negative* modifier is used. If the question asks, "Which of the following is least helpful," be sure to gear your thinking accordingly. Emphasize a key word like *least* as you read the questions.

8. *Do not look for a pattern* in the correct answers. If you have already selected answer option number 3 for several questions in a row, do not be reluctant to choose option 3 again, if you think that it is the correct response.

9. *Look for the choices that you know are either correct or incorrect.* You can save time and narrow your selection by using this strategy.

10. In eliminating potentially wrong answers, remember to look for examples of what has been included in the *nontherapeutic response* list in Unit 6, Nursing Care of Behavioral and Emotional Problems Throughout the Life Span.

11. Wrong choices tend to be either *very brief* or *very long and involved.*

12. Better choices to select are those responses that (a) focus on *feelings* (unless safety is at stake!): "How did that make you feel?" (b) *reflect* the patient's comments: "You say that made you angry," (c) communicate *acceptance* of the patient by the nurse rather than criticism or a value judgment, (d) *acknowledge* the patient: "I see that you are wincing," and (e) stay in the *here-and-now*: "What will help now?" Examples of better choices can be found in the *therapeutic responses* list in Unit 6, Nursing Care of Behavioral and Emotional Problems Throughout the Life Span.

13. Look for the *average, acceptable, safe, common, "garden variety"* responses, not the "exception to the rule," esoteric, or controversial responses.

14. Eliminate the response that may be the best for a *physician* to make. Look for an *RN role-appropriate* response; for example, *psychiatrists* analyze the *past,* and *nurses* in general focus on *present* feelings and situations.

15. *Look for similarities and groupings* in responses and the one-of-a-kind key idea in multiple choice responses. For example:

At which activity would it be important to protect the patient who is on phenothiazines from the side effects of this drug?
1. Sunday church services.
2. A twilight concert.
3. A midday movie in the theater.
4. A luncheon picnic on the hospital grounds.

Choices 1, 2, and 3 all involve indoor activities. Choice 4 involves outdoor exposure during the height of the sun's rays. Clients need to be protected against photosensitivity and burns when on phenothiazines.

16. Be sure to note whether the question asks for what is the *first* or *initial* response to be made or action to be taken by the nurse. The choices listed may all be correct, but in this situation selecting the response with the *highest priority* is important.

17. When you do not know the specific facts called for in a question, use your *skills of reasoning;* for example, when an answer involves amounts or time (mainly numbers) and you do not know the answer and cannot find any basis for reasoning (all else being equal), avoid the extreme responses (the highest or lowest numerical values).

18. *Give special attention to questions in which each word counts.* The purpose of this type of question may be not only to test your knowledge but also to see if you can read accurately and find the main point. In such questions, each answer may be a profusion of words, but there may be one or two words that make the critical difference.

19. All else being equal, select the response that you best *understand.* Long-winded statements are likely to be included as distractors and may be a lot of words signifying little or nothing, such as "criteria involved in implementing conceptual referents for standardizing protocol."

20. *Apply skim-reading techniques.* Read the question quickly. Pick out *key* words (write them down, if that is helpful to you). Translate, into *your own* words, the gist of what is asked in the question. You might close your eyes at this point and see if the answer "pops" into mind. *Then,* skim the answer choices, looking for the response that corresponds to what first came into your mind. Key ideas or themes to look for in responses have been covered in this section—look for a "feeling" response, acceptance, acknowledgment of the patient, and reflection, for example.

❏ How To Reduce Anxiety

Most people have untapped inner resources for achieving relaxation and tension-release in stressful situations (such as during an examination) when they need to function at their highest potential. The goal of this discussion is to help you experience a self-guided approach to reducing your anxiety level to one that is compatible with learning and high performance.

In anxiety-producing settings whenever you feel overwhelmed or blocked, a fantasy experience can be of help in mastering the rising anxiety by promoting a feeling of calm, detached awareness, and a sense of deeper personal coping resources. Through the fantasy you can gain access to a zone of *tranquility* in the center of your being. Guided imagery often carries with it feelings of serenity, warmth, and comfort.

Fantasy experiences are, of course, highly individual. Techniques that help one person experience serenity may frustrate another. Try out the self-guided experiences suggested here, make up your own, and select ones that are best for you. There are endless possibilities for fantasy journeys. The best approach is to work with whatever fantasy occurs to you at the moment. The ideas for a journey presented here are meant to be a springboard for variations of your own.

A fantasy will be more effective if you take as comfortable a physical position as possible, with eyes closed and attention focused on the inner experience. Get in touch with physical sensations, your pattern and rate of breathing, your heartbeat, and pressure points of your body as it comes in contact with the chair and floor.

When you take a fantasy journey by yourself, it is important for you to read over the instructions several times so that you will be able to recall the overall structure of the fantasy. *Then,* close your eyes and take your trip without concern for following the instructions in detail.

Progressive Relaxation

Relaxation approaches are used in a variety of anxiety states whenever stress interferes with the ability to function.

Progressive relaxation training was originated in 1929 by Dr. Edmund Jacobson. It is a technique for attaining self-control over skeletal muscles in order to induce low-level tonus in the major muscle groups. The approach involves learning systematically and sequentially to tense and relax various muscle groups throughout the body.

The *objectives* of this approach are to soothe nerves, combat hypertonus in muscles, and substitute relaxing activities for stressful ones in order to feel comfortable in and more alert to the internal and external environments.

The *theory* behind this method takes as its basis the idea that muscular relaxation and anxiety states produce directly opposite physiologic effects and thus cannot coexist. In other words, it is not possible to be tense in any body part that is completely relaxed.

The *physiologic changes* during relaxation include decreased oxygen consumption, decreased carbon dioxide elimination, and decreased respiratory rate.

The basic factors vital to eliciting a relaxation response include:

1. *Quiet setting*—eliminate unnecessary internal and external stimuli.

2. *Passive, "let-it-happen" attitude*—empty your mind of thoughts and distractions.
3. *Comfortable position*—sit or recline in one position for 20 minutes or so.
4. *Constant stimulus on which to focus*—a repetitive sound, constant gaze on an object or image, or attention to one's own breathing pattern.

Relaxation training is a procedure that can be defined, specified, and memorized until you can go through the exercises mechanically. If you regularly practice relaxation, you will be able to cope more effectively with difficult situations by reaping the physiologic and psychological benefits of a balanced and relaxed state.

Instructions

■ Sit comfortably in a chair. Shut your eyes and chase your thoughts for a minute; go where your thoughts go.
■ Then, let the words go. Become aware of how you *feel,* here and now, not how you would like to feel.
■ Shift your awareness to your feet. Do not move them. Become aware of what they are doing.
■ Spend 20 to 30 seconds focusing progressively on different parts of your body. Relax each part in turn:

Relax each of your toes; the tops of your feet; the arch of each foot; the insteps, balls, and heels; and your ankles, calves, knees, thighs, and buttocks. Become aware of how your body is contacting the chair in which you are sitting. Let go of your abdominal and chest muscles; relax your back. Release the tension in your shoulders, arms, elbows, forearms, wrists, hands, and each finger in turn; relax the muscles in your throat, lips, and cheeks. Wrinkle your nose; relax your eyelids and eyebrows (first one and then the other); relax the muscles in your forehead and top and back of your head. Relax your whole body.

Concentrate on your breathing: become aware of how you breathe. Allow yourself to inhale and exhale in your usual way. Become aware of the depth of your breathing. Are you expanding the lungs all the way? Or is your breathing shallow? Increase your depth of breathing. Now focus on the rate at which you are breathing. See if you can slow the rate down. When you breathe in, can you feel an inflow of energy that fills your entire body?

■ Now concentrate on the sounds in the room.
■ Focus on how you feel right now.
■ Slowly open your eyes.

Suggestions for Additional Experiential Vignettes

■ Imagine yourself leaving the room. In your mind's eye go through the city and over the fields. Come to a meadow covered with fresh, new grass and flowers. Look out on the meadow and focus on what you see, hear, smell, and feel. Walk through the meadow. See the length and greenness of the grass; see the brilliance and feel the warmth of the sunlight.
■ For a more expansive feeling, visualize a mountain in the distance. Fantasize going to the country and slowly ascending a mountain. Walk through a forest. Climb to the top until at last you reach a height where you can see forever. Experience your awareness.
■ Focus on a memory of a beautiful place you have been to, enjoyed, and would like to enjoy again. Be there; experience it.
■ Imagine that you are floating on your back down a river. It may help at first to breathe deeply and feel yourself sinking. Visualize that you are coming out on a gentle river that is slowly winding its way through a beautiful forest. The sun is out and the rays feel warm on your skin. You pass trees and meadows of beautiful flowers. Smell the grass and flowers. Hear the birds. Look up in the blue sky; see the lazy tufts of clouds floating by. Leave the river and walk across the meadow. Enjoy the grass around your ankles. Come to a large tree . . .

Fill in the rest of the trip—what do you see now? Where do you want to go from here?

Sally L. Lagerquist

Pre Test

❑ Introduction

The **Pre Test** is an *initial assessment* tool intended to help you to assess your strengths and weaknesses in your ability to apply the material you have learned in specific clinical areas to any nursing situation. By taking the **Pre Test,** you can focus your subsequent review of content, based on your own analysis of your results.

We suggest that you take the **Pre Test** before you read any of the content units in this book. After taking the **Pre Test,** you should:

1. Score your answers.
2. Take another look at the questions where your answer was wrong.
3. Identify the clinical areas where you need further review, i.e., Childhood and Adolescence, Behavioral and Emotional, etc.

4. Read those specific content units in detail.
5. Then test yourself again on the **Practice Test**.

❑ Questions

1. The nurse can quickly assess volume depletion in a patient with ulcerative colitis by:
   1. Measuring the quantity and specific gravity of the patient's urine output.
   2. Taking the patient's blood pressure first supine, then sitting, noting any changes.
   3. Comparing the patient's present weight with weight on a previous admission.
   4. Administering the oral water test.
2. Physical assessment of a patient admitted for a bronchoscopy revealed a thin, muscular man with rhonchi and wheezes in the left lung and some wheezes in the right lower lobe. Rhonchi and wheezes are due to:
   1. Total obstruction of small bronchioles.
   2. Partial obstruction of bronchi and bronchioles.
   3. Fluid in the alveoli.
   4. Inflammation of the pleura.
3. Which of the following best describes the metabolic functions of the liver?
   1. Detoxification of endogenous and exogenous substances.
   2. Fluid volume control and acid-base balance.
   3. Erythrocyte and leukocyte breakdown.
   4. Concentration and storage of bile.
4. In response to a patient's questions regarding the cause of glomerulonephritis, the nurse explains that acute glomerulonephritis is the result of:
   1. Acute infection of the kidney by gram-negative bacteria.
   2. An immune response of the glomerular membrane to protein of the beta-hemolytic streptococcus.
   3. Destruction of the glomerular membrane by gram-positive streptococci.
   4. Ischemia of glomerular capillary and vasa recta.
5. A patient who is scheduled for repair of bilateral inguinal hernias has a history of obesity, smoker's cough, and heavy lifting following a previous inguinal hernia repair. The *most* likely cause for the herniation is:
   1. Intestinal obstruction.
   2. Failure of resected muscles in previous operations to heal properly.
   3. Chronic cough and vigorous exercise.
   4. Obesity.
6. The nurse knows that the function of the gallbladder is to:
   1. Synthesize and manufacture bile.
   2. Collect, concentrate, and store bile.
   3. Collect and dilute bile.
   4. Regulate bile flow into the duodenum.
7. The most accurate description the nurse could give a colleague about a thyroid scan is that it:
   1. Assists in differentiating between primary and secondary hypothyroidism.
   2. Demonstrates increased uptake of radioactive iodine in areas of possible malignancy.
   3. Demonstrates decreased uptake of radioactive iodine in areas of possible malignancy.
   4. Measures the effect of TSH on thyroid function.
8. A stat cesarean birth is ordered for a woman in labor; her husband is with her. The *primary* priority of the nurse at this time would be to:

   1. Obtain an operation permit.
   2. Attempt to alleviate the couple's anxiety.
   3. Monitor maternal and fetal signs closely.
   4. Provide emotional and physiologic support.
9. The nurse knows that a decreased hematocrit occurs in chronic renal failure because:
   1. Secretion of erythropoietin factor by the diseased kidney is decreased.
   2. Chronic hypertension tends to suppress bone marrow centers.
   3. Metabolic alkalosis tends to increase red blood cell fragility.
   4. Excretion of red blood cells in the urine is increased.
10. A routine preoperative assessment for the patient having vein ligation and stripping would include the following laboratory studies:
    1. VDRL, NA, K, Cl.
    2. Prothrombin time, ALT[SGOT], VDRL.
    3. UA, CBC, prothrombin time.
    4. WBC, VDRL, serum glucose.
11. The nurse finds a marijuana joint under an adolescent patient's pillow. After being confronted, the patient promises not to smoke marijuana again if the nurse will not report the incident. The nurse fears that the patient is being manipulative. The *most* therapeutic nursing intervention when working with manipulative patients is to:
    1. Make decisions for them.
    2. Reinforce use of alternative behaviors.
    3. Set rigid limits.
    4. Confront them in front of others.
12. A multiparous woman is admitted to the birth unit for induction of labor. The nurse performing Leopold's maneuvers notes that uterine tonicity is normal and the presenting part (the sacrum) is high, not engaged. The nurse expects that medical management will probably consist of:
    1. Delaying induction until the presenting part is at 0 station.
    2. Piper forceps–assisted vaginal birth.
    3. Spontaneous, vaginal birth.
    4. Cesarean birth.
13. The nurse knows that acetonuria develops in diabetes due to:
    1. Excessive oxidation of fatty acids for energy, which increases ketones in glomerular filtrate.
    2. Osmotic diuresis, accompanying elevation in serum-glucose levels, which decreases exchange of electrolytes in renal tubules.
    3. Failure of sodium-hydrogen ion exchange mechanism in the renal tubules to secrete excess hydrogen ions.
    4. Increased volatile H^+ ions and decreased nonvolatile H^+ ions in the glomerular filtrate.
14. A woman experienced an incomplete spontaneous abortion. After evacuation of the uterus, an oxytocic agent is ordered to prevent hemorrhage. An ergot product (e.g., ergonovine) is ordered. The nurse knows that ergot products are contraindicated:
    1. Until the uterus is emptied.
    2. When the woman is normotensive.
    3. If her religion proscribes the use of blood products.
    4. If she is a candidate for receiving $Rh_o(D)$ immune globulin.
15. A diabetic woman gives birth to an 8-pound 11-ounce boy at 38 weeks. On her first postpartum day, she is eating a full diet and her insulin has been cut to one-third of the dosage during pregnancy. The night nurse

is making rounds and wants to assess the sleeping woman for signs indicating her response to the lowered insulin dosage. Which indicates this woman is hyperglycemic?

1. A flash of light in her face does not elicit a squint or turn of the head.
2. She seems restless, her face is flushed, her pulse is rapid, and her respirations are deep.
3. She is perspiring profusely.
4. She awakens with a headache.

16. The nurse expects hyperkalemia on assessment to occur in chronic renal dysfunction because:
    1. As metabolic acidosis increases, the kidneys selectively secrete more H^+ than K^+ in exchange for Na^+.
    2. As edema forms, sodium diffuses into the interstitial space and is balanced by increased serum potassium.
    3. Respiratory compensation for metabolic acidosis tends to increase K^+ reabsorption by the kidneys.
    4. The nausea and vomiting that occur with metabolic acidosis tend to increase serum potassium to compensate for chloride losses.

17. A patient has second-degree burns of the left leg and thigh. The nurse plans to help prevent contractures in the burned leg by:
    1. Maintaining abduction of the left leg, extension of the left knee, and flexion of the left ankle.
    2. Maintaining adduction of the left leg and extension of the left knee and ankle.
    3. Maintaining abduction of the left leg and flexion of the left knee and ankle.
    4. Maintaining adduction of the left leg, flexion of the left knee, and extension of the left ankle.

18. A truss is a pad of firm material that is placed over a hernial opening and held in place with a belt. When should the nurse apply a hernia truss on a patient?
    1. After the patient gets out of bed but before engaging in strenuous activity.
    2. After the hernia has been reduced, with the patient lying down with feet elevated.
    3. At any time, whether or not the hernia has been reduced, to prevent further extrusion of the bowel.
    4. Not at all, for physicians no longer recommend the use of a truss, because athletic supporters are sufficient in preventing further herniation.

19. To correctly administer a Mantoux test, the nurse would inject 5 TU (tuberculin units) of PPD (purified protein derivative) of tuberculin:
    1. Intradermally.
    2. Subcutaneously.
    3. Intramuscularly.
    4. Subdermally.

20. If bile flow into the duodenum is obstructed, absorption of fat-soluble vitamins is reduced. Which of the following complications would the nurse therefore observe?
    1. Peripheral neuritis.
    2. Scurvy.
    3. Increased bleeding tendencies.
    4. Macrocytic anemia.

21. The preoperative nursing care plan for a patient having cataract surgery includes:
    1. Keeping the patient flat in bed.
    2. Applying eye patches to both eyes.
    3. Orienting the patient to the environment and nursing personnel.
    4. Teaching the patient eye-drop instillation.

22. Following a thyroid scan with ^{131}I for a thyroid nodule, the nurse should plan for:
    1. No special radiation precautions.
    2. Full radiation precautions to be instituted, including segregating the patient in a private room.
    3. Radiation precautions that are limited to urine and feces.
    4. Full radiation precautions to be instituted for 8 hours (the half-life of ^{131}I).

23. To prevent displacement of radium implants in the cervix, the nurse should position the patient:
    1. With the foot of the bed elevated.
    2. Flat in bed.
    3. With the head elevated 45 degrees (semi-Fowler's).
    4. On the side only.

24. A woman in labor is moved into the Cesarean room. Her husband enters the room and appears anxious. The nurse should ask him:
    1. "How are you feeling?"
    2. "Are you feeling up to this?"
    3. "Would you rather wait outside?"
    4. "Can I get you anything?"

25. The parents of an infant who has a unilateral cleft lip and palate are anxious to have surgery performed to repair the deformities. The most appropriate response to the couple's request for surgery would be to:
    1. Reinforce what the physicians have told the parents.
    2. Inform the parents that the lip may be repaired when their baby is 2–3 months old and the palate repaired at 18 months.
    3. Refer the couple to the surgeon.
    4. Tell the couple that surgery may be performed when their baby weighs at least 10 pounds.

26. A total thyroidectomy is ordered following discovery of a cold nodule. In this case of *hyperthyroidism* versus malignancy, the nurse anticipates that the patient will have:
    1. A complete thyroidectomy also.
    2. A partial thyroidectomy (approximately one-half of the thyroid is removed).
    3. A partial thyroidectomy (approximately five-sixths of the thyroid is removed).
    4. Administration of thyroid medication.

27. Besides jaundice of the sclera and skin, what other clinical parameters might indicate biliary obstruction in the patient?
    1. Increased systolic and diastolic pressures.
    2. Frequent eructation between meals.
    3. Darkened urine and clay-colored stools.
    4. Longitudinal ridging of the fingernails.

28. A patient who has a long-term history of smoking and a smoker's cough is scheduled for bilateral herniorrhaphy. Which preoperative nursing action will be a priority?
    1. Explanation of the surgical procedure.
    2. Respiratory hygiene measures and instructions in deep breathing.
    3. Discussion of postoperative nursing care measures.
    4. Assurance that pain medication will be available whenever needed.

29. A patient has been NPO for the last 12 hours in preparation for an IVP (intravenous pyelogram), and has been complaining of thirst. The specific gravity of his urine has been averaging 1.008. The nurse's explanation for these signs and symptoms is:
    1. The hypothalamus is stimulating increased secretion of ADH.
    2. Extracellular fluid has become hypo-osmolar.

3. The kidneys are no longer able to concentrate urine, making the extracellular fluid hyperosmolar.

4. Most patients complain of thirst after fluid restriction.

30. Which contributes to the development of ascites in cirrhosis of the liver?
    1. Portal hypertension, venous dilatation, and stasis.
    2. Increased hepatic synthesis of albumin.
    3. Decreased serum levels of aldosterone and ADH.
    4. Increased blood volume causing increased blood hydrostatic pressure in the capillary bed.

31. The nurse explains to a patient that a bronchoscopy is:
    1. An X-ray procedure that allows for multiple views of the lungs.
    2. A procedure utilizing a lighted mirror lens to observe the walls of the trachea, mainstem bronchus, and major bronchial tubes.
    3. A diagnostic test during which a radiopaque substance is inserted into the tracheobronchial tree for clear visualization.
    4. A needle puncture of the lung mass, identified on an X-ray with aspiration of cells for microscopic examination.

32. With severe diarrhea, electrolytes as well as fluids are lost. The nurse would conclude that the patient is experiencing hypokalemia if which of the following were observed?
    1. Spasms, high T waves on ECG, irregular pulse.
    2. Kussmaul breathing, thirst, furrowed tongue.
    3. Apathy, weakness, GI disturbance.
    4. Pitting edema, confusion, bounding pulse.

33. A woman anticipating a stat cesarean birth expresses some concern over feeling the incision and experiencing pain. The most appropriate response would be:
    1. "You will feel nothing at all."
    2. "You may feel some pressure in the area during surgery."
    3. "You may feel slight pain when the incision is made."
    4. "If you feel any pain, it is only your imagination."

34. After discharge following ileostomy surgery, a patient calls the nurse at the hospital to report the sudden onset of abdominal cramps, vomiting, and watery discharge from the ileostomy. What should the nurse advise?
    1. Call the physician if symptoms persist for 24 hours.
    2. Take 30 mL of m.o.m. (milk of magnesia).
    3. NPO until vomiting stops.
    4. Call the physician immediately.

35. To safely transport a patient who has chest tube drainage to the X-ray department to assess the degree of lung reexpansion, the nurse would:
    1. Remove the chest tubes, immediately covering the incision site with a sterile petrolatum gauze to prevent air from entering the chest.
    2. Disconnect the drainage bottles from the chest tubes, covering the catheter tip with a sterile dressing to prevent contamination.
    3. Send the patient to X ray with the chest tube clamped but still attached to the drainage system to prevent air from entering the chest wall if the bottles are accidentally broken.
    4. Send the patient to X ray with the chest tube attached to the drainage system, taking precautions to prevent interruption in the system.

36. Which statement would the nurse make to differentiate ketoacidosis from insulin shock?

1. Deep and rapid respirations are characteristic of ketoacidosis, whereas slow, shallow respirations are characteristic of insulin shock.
2. Acetone breath characterizes ketoacidosis, whereas the breath of the patient in insulin shock is frequently fetid.
3. Warm, dry, flushed skin and loss of turgor characterize the patient with ketoacidosis, whereas the skin of the patient with insulin shock is usually pale, cool, and diaphoretic.
4. Apprehension, irritability, and combative behavior occur with ketoacidosis, whereas the patient in insulin shock is more likely to be confused, lethargic, or comatose.

37. The nurse explains to the patient and family that because of excessive bleeding, an emergency hysterectomy will need to be performed:
    1. Upon completion of the necessary surgical preparation.
    2. Immediately.
    3. Within 24 hours.
    4. At the start of the next surgical day.

38. The nurse can anticipate a marked improvement in the patient's prognosis if a hepatic coma lasts no longer than:
    1. 24 hours.
    2. 36 hours.
    3. 48 hours.
    4. 72 hours.

39. The effectiveness of peritoneal dialysis will be measured by:
    1. Serum potassium less than 3.5 mEq/L and serum sodium greater than 148 mEq/L.
    2. Unchanged quantity and specific gravity of urine.
    3. BUN less than 20 mg/dL, serum creatinine less than 1.2 mg/dL.
    4. Moderately soft abdomen and dullness on percussion.

40. After explaining peritoneal dialysis procedures to a patient and the family and obtaining a signed operative permit, the nurse's next action is to:
    1. Have the patient empty the bladder.
    2. Position the patient in a comfortable supine position.
    3. Weigh the patient and record vital signs.
    4. Cleanse and drape the abdomen.

41. Of the following activities of daily living, which should the nurse recommend that a patient who has had a bilateral hernia repair avoid after discharge?
    1. Driving to and from work.
    2. Walking 3 miles a day.
    3. Washing and polishing the car.
    4. Carrying out the garbage cans.

42. A patient has had a spinal anesthetic. In the recovery room, it will be important that the nurse immediately position this patient:
    1. On the side to prevent obstruction of airway by tongue.
    2. Flat on the back.
    3. On the back, with knees flexed 15 degrees.
    4. Flat on the stomach, with head turned to side.

43. After positioning a patient who has had spinal anesthesia, the recovery room nurse initially should make which observation?
    1. Status of reflexes.
    2. Vital signs.
    3. Patient's level of consciousness.
    4. Integrity of airway.

44. While instructing a postoperative cholecystectomy patient about diet, the nurse would inform the patient that:
    1. The diet will not include fatty food for at least 1 year.
    2. After approximately 3 months polyunsaturated fats can be added to the diet.
    3. There are no specific dietary restrictions in the postoperative period, but the patient will be more comfortable if large, fatty meals are avoided.
    4. The diet will be limited to 20 g of fat per day.

45. While assisting a patient who has had a thyroidectomy to dangle at the bedside on the first postoperative evening, the most appropriate nursing action would be to:
    1. Support the patient under the axilla while bringing the feet over the bedside.
    2. Bring the patient's feet to the side of the bed and support the back of the neck while assisting the patient to assume a sitting position.
    3. Allow the patient to assume the sitting position at the patient's own pace, unassisted unless necessary.
    4. Bring the patient's feet to the side of the bed, then pull the patient forward.

46. New parents of a baby with a cleft lip and palate are experiencing a reactive depression in response to the birth of their infant, who is in the high-risk newborn nursery. The primary difference between a reactive depression and an endogenous depression is that in a reactive depression:
    1. There is substantial weight loss, usually over 10 pounds.
    2. The individual does not respond to environmental stimuli.
    3. The individual generally feels worse as the day progresses.
    4. The precipitating event is usually difficult to identify.

47. An Apgar score of 4 at 1 and 5 minutes indicates that the neonate's condition is:
    1. Excellent.
    2. Good.
    3. Fair.
    4. Poor.

48. A toddler who fractured the right femur in a car accident is placed in Bryant's traction and admitted to the hospital. During the first night in the hospital, the toddler lies still in the crib, sucks a thumb, and occasionally sobs quietly in a monotone voice. The nurse should interpret these behaviors to mean that the toddler:
    1. Wants his or her mother.
    2. Might prefer to sleep in a bed.
    3. Probably does not sleep through the night at home.
    4. May be experiencing painful muscle spasms due to the fracture.

49. Most accidental pregnancies in couples using "natural" family planning methods have been related to unprotected intercourse *prior* to ovulation. Which of the following factors explains why pregnancy may be achieved by unprotected intercourse during the preovulatory period?
    1. Spermatozoal viability.
    2. Ovum viability.
    3. Tubal motility.
    4. Secretory endometrium.

50. Parents of an infant with deformities may use which of the following defense mechanisms in attempting to cope with their anxiety?
    1. Fixation.
    2. Displacement.
    3. Conversion.
    4. Sublimation.

51. The parents of an infant born with a cleft lip and palate express concern about caring for their infant. They are especially worried about paying excessive hospital bills because insurance has set limits. The most appropriate nursing action would be to:
    1. Refer the couple to a social worker.
    2. Validate the couple's perceived needs.
    3. Discuss alternatives with the couple.
    4. Implement health teaching regarding the physical care of the infant.

52. The nurse suggests that premenopausal breast self-examinations are best carried out:
    1. During the middle of the menstrual cycle.
    2. On the first day of each month.
    3. One week after the onset of menses.
    4. The week before the onset of menses.

53. In preparing a patient for an IV cholangiogram, it is important for the nurse to ascertain:
    1. If the patient has ever had the procedure before.
    2. If the patient has any known allergies, particularly to fish or other iodine-containing substances.
    3. If the patient's epigastric discomfort occurs only with fatty-food ingestion.
    4. If there is a family history of gallstones.

54. The nurse suspects abdominal wound dehiscence, and lifts the edges of the patient's dressings. The nurse notes that the wound edges are entirely separated. What is the *next* nursing action?
    1. Tell the patient to remain quiet and not to cough.
    2. Offer the patient a warm drink to promote relaxation.
    3. Position the patient in a chair with the feet elevated.
    4. Apply a scultetus bandage.

55. Which of the following signs and symptoms are *least* likely to occur during peritoneal dialysis if fluid drainage is inadequate?
    1. A negative balance between the amount drained and the amount instilled.
    2. Confusion, lethargy, and coma.
    3. Moist crackles and rhonchi.
    4. Flattened neck veins in a supine position.

56. Which nursing action is designed to reduce ammonia intoxication in a patient with bleeding esophageal varices who is jaundiced, edematous, and in a hepatic coma?
    1. Active and passive range-of-motion exercises to prevent venous stasis.
    2. Tap-water enemas to remove blood that may still be in the gut from the bleeding esophageal varices.
    3. Administration of insulin and glucagon to reduce serum-potassium levels.
    4. Holding all antibiotic medications so that the action of the intestinal bacteria on protein is enhanced.

57. In analyzing the BBT record of a woman who has a normal 30-day cycle, on which of the following days would the nurse expect to find evidence of ovulation?
    1. Day 5 or 6.
    2. Day 13 or 14.
    3. Day 16 or 17.
    4. Day 28 or 29.

58. The nurse explains to a patient's family that the surgical treatment *most* often implemented for excessive vaginal bleeding due to uterine fibroids is:
    1. Panabdominal hysterectomy.
    2. Vaginal hysterectomy.

3. Dilatation and curettage.
4. Abdominal hysterectomy.

59. Following surgery, a diabetic patient complains of nausea and appears lethargic and flushed. BP 108/78, P 100, R 24 and deep. The first nursing action should be:
1. Call the attending physician.
2. Check the patient's blood glucose.
3. Administer an antiemetic.
4. Decrease the patient's IV infusion rate.

60. Passive arm exercises are instituted on a patient's left arm 4 hours after lobectomy surgery. The nurse assists with these exercises to prevent which dysfunction?
1. Hyperflexion of the wrist.
2. Ankylosis of the shoulder.
3. Flexion of the elbow.
4. Spasticity of the intercostal muscles.

61. The nurse initiates ileostomy teaching with a patient during the early postoperative period. The primary objective of this procedure is:
1. To facilitate maintenance of intake and output records.
2. To control unpleasant odors.
3. To prevent excoriation of the skin around the stoma.
4. To reduce the risk of postoperative wound infection.

62. When teaching families about cleft lip and palate, the nurse would need to be aware that:
1. Cleft lip occurs most frequently in girls.
2. Cleft palate occurs most frequently in boys.
3. Cleft lip and palate almost always occur simultaneously.
4. Cleft lip and palate are both influenced by hereditary factors.

63. A pregnant woman was instructed to report signs and symptoms of preterm labor. The nurse knows that the woman failed to follow instructions about evaluating her signs and symptoms when she telephoned *before* she:
1. Waited to see if uterine contractions were occurring every 10 minutes.
2. Assessed that her contractions continued after she emptied her bladder.
3. Drank a glass of water for hydration.
4. Rested in bed on her side for 1 hour.

64. The Trendelenburg test is frequently used to evaluate the competence of venous valves. Prior to administering the test, the nurse tells the patient that this test will consist of:
1. Walking back and forth so the nurse can observe venous changes during walking.
2. Injecting a contrast medium into the veins and taking multiple X rays the dye flows in the veins.
3. Stripping a superficial vein, occluding flow, and then releasing the vein and observing the direction of filling.
4. Elevating the involved leg to empty the veins, applying a tourniquet to the upper thigh while the patient is standing, and then removing the tourniquet to observe the filling of the superficial veins.

65. A woman anticipating a stat cesarean birth for a fetus in transverse lie questions the nurse about the type of incision the physician will use in her operation. The nurse should realize that this woman's *primary* concern involves the possibility of:
1. Infection.
2. Bleeding.
3. Scarring.
4. Rupture.

66. A patient asks the nurse whether marijuana is addictive. The most appropriate response by the nurse would be:
1. "It is addictive."
2. "It causes a psychological dependence."
3. "It is not addictive."
4. "It is physiologically addictive."

67. Following the insertion of a catheter into the abdominal cavity, warmed dialyzing solution is allowed to run rapidly (10–20 minutes) into the abdominal cavity. The nurse warmed the solution to body temperature to prevent abdominal pain and to:
1. Expand the molecules and increase the osmotic gradient.
2. Increase dilation of the peritoneal vessels, thereby increasing urea clearance.
3. Decrease the likelihood of peritonitis due to constriction of peritoneal vessels.
4. Expedite the movement of the dialyzing solute into the abdomen.

68. Preoperative teaching measures unique to the patient having a thyroidectomy should encompass:
1. Active flexion exercise of the neck, special coughing instructions, voice rest, and antithyroid medications postoperatively.
2. Active flexion and extension neck exercises, deep breathing and coughing, and thyroid replacement when necessary.
3. Instruction on supporting the back of the neck when repositioning and/or ambulating, and avoiding hyperextension and flexion of the neck when coughing.
4. Instruction on supporting the back of the neck when ambulating and/or repositioning and active flexion exercises of the neck.

69. The nurse will plan to read the reaction to an intradermal tuberculin test in:
1. 6–12 hours.
2. 12–24 hours.
3. 24–48 hours.
4. 48–72 hours.

70. Which are precautionary nursing measures to be used when caring for a patient being treated with internal radioisotopes?
1. Maintain strict patient isolation, and limit professional contact with patient.
2. Limit exposure, and maximize distance between patient, professional, and family.
3. Position the patient in a prone position, and restrict turning to mealtimes only.
4. Maintain the legs in a flexed position to decrease the likelihood of dislodgement.

71. The nurse explains to a patient who is diagnosed with cirrhosis that the anemia is the result of:
1. Increased RBC fragility due to folic acid deficiencies from inadequate dietary intake.
2. Decreased efficiency of Kupffer cells in the liver.
3. Increased blood-ammonia levels.
4. Decreased amino acid breakdown and synthesis.

72. A postoperative diabetic patient's vital signs are: BP 108/78, pulse 100, respirations 24 and deep. IV intake has been 2100 mL and urine output 2000 mL. The nurse recognizes that the patient is experiencing:
1. Increased ADH release in response to physiologic stress of surgery.
2. Decreased ECF (extracellular fluid) volume due to osmotic diuresis.
3. A hypo-osmolar fluid imbalance.
4. Circulatory overload.

73. Following bronchoscopy, what is the nurse's most important observation?
    1. Blood pressure, pulse, and temperature.
    2. Color and consistency of sputum.
    3. Function of the tenth cranial nerve.
    4. Presence of urticaria.

74. The nurse knows that emergency procedures increase the surgical risk to the patient because:
    1. The surgery is performed immediately.
    2. There is little time for psychological/physical preparation.
    3. There is decreased physiologic stress.
    4. The anesthesia of choice is different for emergency surgery.

75. Care of the patient on peritoneal dialysis must allow a dwell time, or equilibration period, of the dialyzing fluid, which is normally:
    1. 10–15 minutes.
    2. 20–30 minutes.
    3. 50–60 minutes.
    4. More than 1 hour.

76. The Billings method (or cervical mucus method) of natural family planning incorporates patient examination of cervical mucus. Which of the following characteristics should the nurse teach are typical of the cervical mucus during the "fertile" period of the menstrual cycle?
    1. Thick, cloudy.
    2. Thin, clear, good spinnbarkeit.
    3. Yellow, sticky.
    4. Absence of ferning.

77. An elderly patient asks about the type of anesthesia used for cataract surgery. The nurse replies that this surgery is generally performed using a:
    1. Local.
    2. General.
    3. Intravenous.
    4. Rectal.

78. A patient has frequent stools, with poor oral intake of both fluids and solids. While administering the ordered parenteral hyperalimentation, it is important to remember that hyperalimentation solutions are:
    1. Hypotonic solutions used primarily for hydration when hemoconcentration is present.
    2. Hypertonic solutions used primarily to increase osmotic pressure of blood plasma.
    3. Alkalyzing solutions used to treat metabolic acidosis, thus reducing cellular swelling.
    4. Hyperosmolar solutions used primarily to reverse negative nitrogen balance.

79. A newborn's Apgar score at 1 and 5 minutes is 4. The nurse assisting with the care of this newborn should realize the *primary* goal is to:
    1. Establish an airway.
    2. Maintain an adequate temperature.
    3. Reassure the parents.
    4. Monitor the infant's vital signs.

80. The nurse concludes from a patient's assessment and history of muscle fatigue and ankle swelling that vein-stripping is indicated, because of:
    1. Advancing varicosities and cosmetic reasons.
    2. Stasis ulceration and thrombophlebitis.
    3. Lymphedema and Raynaud's disease.
    4. Advancing varicosities only.

81. Besides omission of food and fluids by mouth, other nursing considerations in the preparation of a patient for IVP would include:
    1. Ingestion of contrast medium the morning of the procedure.

2. Administration of cathartics or enemas to improve visualization of contrast medium in renal structures.
    3. A low-protein and low-salt diet the evening before to increase hyperosmolarity of ECF.
    4. Institution of an intravenous line to maintain fluid and electrolyte balance.

82. The nurse explains to a postoperative diabetic patient that regular or crystalline insulin is utilized as an adjunct to NPH therapy because:
    1. There is increased tissue metabolism with surgery.
    2. Insulin production is decreased even further with the stress of surgery.
    3. Physiologic and psychological stress increases serum-glucose levels via sympathetic nervous system stimulation.
    4. An increased insulin load is necessary to prevent hyperkalemia.

83. Three days after successful resuscitation from cardiac arrest after myocardial infarction, the patient states to the nurse, "I'm all washed up. I don't think I'll ever be the same man again." The nurse's best response to this statement would be:
    1. "Most patients who have been as ill as you feel that way."
    2. "How do you feel you have changed from before your illness?"
    3. "Getting depressed won't help you get better."
    4. "Tell me more."

84. The nurse recognizes dyspnea as:
    1. Increased awareness of respiratory effort.
    2. Decreased alveolar ventilation.
    3. Increased rate and depth of respiration.
    4. Decreased oxygen saturation of venous blood.

85. A teenage patient in a substance abuse facility feels very isolated from his peer group because he has been placed in an adult unit. In planning care for this patient, which would be most effective?
    1. Assisting the patient to develop a working relationship with a 51-year-old patient.
    2. Encouraging friends to visit frequently.
    3. Asking the adolescent what he enjoys doing.
    4. Establishing a one-to-one relationship with the patient.

86. A patient asks what type of anesthesia is usually used during vein-stripping. The nurse tells the patient to expect:
    1. Local.
    2. Topical.
    3. Regional.
    4. General.

87. A patient with a history of many years of smoking and a smoker's cough is scheduled for bilateral herniorrhaphy. Which type of surgical anesthesia may be most appropriate for this situation?
    1. General.
    2. Intravenous.
    3. Spinal.
    4. Local infiltration.

88. Pulmonary function testing on a patient with a long history of smoking revealed a vital capacity within normal limits but a reduced forced expiratory volume (FEV_1). The nurse explains to the family that this means that the patient:
    1. Has difficulty moving air in and out of the lungs.
    2. May have some airway obstruction.
    3. Has weakened expiratory muscles of respirations.
    4. May have some areas of atelectasis in the lungs.

89. A patient has a long leg cast due to a fractured right tibia and fibula. Which of the following is an appropriate exercise for this patient to engage in to prevent complications of immobility?
    1. Quadriceps setting.
    2. Extension of the right knee.
    3. Passive range of motion of the hip.
    4. Flexion of the right knee.

90. The nurse concludes that a Mantoux test result is positive if the following is present:
    1. An induration of 10 mm or more.
    2. An induration of 10 cm or more.
    3. An induration of 5–9 mm.
    4. A hivelike vesicle.

91. In providing emotional support for a couple whose infant is unhealthy or has an abnormality, the nurse should realize that at first they will probably:
    1. Wish to talk with other couples who have experienced the same circumstances.
    2. Wish to be left alone, unless they seek out someone to talk to.
    3. Need reassurance and emotional support.
    4. Avoid discussing the situation at this time.

92. In assessing the acid-base status of a patient diagnosed with glomerulonephritis, the nurse would be alert to the following signs of metabolic acidosis:
    1. Hyperreflexia, paresthesias, and tetany.
    2. Giddiness, irregular respiratory pattern, and moist, cool skin.
    3. Muscle weakness, and numbness and tingling in the extremities.
    4. Lethargy, disorientation, and increased rate and depth of respirations.

93. On the second day after a lobectomy, the fluid in the suction bottle's glass tube ceases to fluctuate. The nurse knows that this most likely indicates:
    1. The chest tube is plugged by fibrin or a clot.
    2. There is an air leak in the system.
    3. Pulmonary edema has occurred due to increased blood volume in remaining lung tissue.
    4. The patient's position needs to change to facilitate drainage.

94. What side effects would a patient demonstrate if he or she received hyperalimentation solution at too rapid an infusion rate?
    1. Cellular dehydration and potassium depletion.
    2. Circulatory overload and hypoglycemia.
    3. Hypoglycemia and hypovolemia.
    4. Potassium excess and congestive heart failure.

95. Which nursing action is *least* likely to assist parents to adjust to the psychological trauma of the birth of a deformed child?
    1. Encouraging verbalization of anxiety, fears, and concerns.
    2. Explaining all treatments and prognosis.
    3. Interacting normally with the infant.
    4. Expressing sympathy.

96. Nursing measures that should decrease the incidence of hemorrhage after thyroidectomy are:
    1. Frequent checking of dressing, semi-Fowler's position, and ice packs to neck.
    2. Frequent checking of dressing, supine position, and ice packs to neck.
    3. Frequent checking of dressing, coughing every 2 hours, and moist packs to neck.
    4. Frequent checking of dressings and maintenance of neck flexion.

97. The nurse must assess past medical history and use of medications for any surgical candidate. Which drugs can negatively interfere with anesthesia or contribute to postoperative complications?
    1. Anticoagulants and antihypertensives.
    2. Anticoagulants and insulin.
    3. Digoxin and thiazide diuretics.
    4. Vitamins and mineral replacements.

98. Anticipatory guidance planned for a diabetic woman who has just given birth includes health teaching regarding self-care health maintenance actions in the postpartum period. She wants to breastfeed her baby. Which should be emphasized as part of her postpartum instructions?
    1. Breastfeeding is contraindicated because it stimulates gluconeogenesis.
    2. Her caloric needs will decrease during the postpartum period, so she must be alert for signs of hyperglycemia.
    3. She should breastfeed the baby before feeding herself so that she can relax; stress inhibits the flow of breast milk.
    4. She must prevent hypoglycemia because it can inhibit the let-down reflex and decrease her milk supply.

99. To assess accurately a patient's functional and vocational rehabilitation potential with myasthenia gravis, the nurse must *first* ascertain:
    1. The degree of physical and emotional stress in the patient's present occupation.
    2. The activities of daily living that cause the greatest degree of muscle weakness and fatigue.
    3. The patient's understanding of and attitude toward myasthenia gravis, as well as the ability to cope with activity restrictions.
    4. Whether or not the patient's current occupation allows opportunities to sit down and rest when necessary.

100. The nurse tells a patient that NPH insulin reaches its peak action:
    1. 4 hours after injection.
    2. 6–12 hours after injection.
    3. 12–14 hours after injection.
    4. 15–18 hours after injection.

101. A patient has multiple fractures of both legs; treatment includes bedrest with skeletal traction. The nursing intervention that would be *most* effective in prevention of footdrop would be use of:
    1. A bed cradle.
    2. A footboard.
    3. Passive range of motion every shift.
    4. A trochanter roll.

102. While providing care for a newborn with a cleft lip and palate, the nurse must also be aware of the parents' feelings. Both appear stunned. However, they are still in touch with reality and are asking appropriate questions focused on the newborn's condition. The couple is functioning at what level of anxiety at this time?
    1. Mild.
    2. Moderate.
    3. Severe.
    4. Panic.

103. Which nursing action is inappropriate in the preparation of a patient for *oral* cholecystography?
    1. Administering a fat-free diet the evening before the test.
    2. Administering Telepaque (iopanoic acid) tablets in 5-minute intervals 1 hour after supper.

3. Administering at least 6 oz of water with each Tele-paque (iopanoic acid) tablet.

4. Allowing the patient, after ingesting the tablets, to drink water until midnight, then NPO.

104. A preoperative *nursing priority* for a patient having a tracheostomy is:
1. Establishing postoperative communication.
2. Drawing blood for serum-electrolyte and blood gas determinations.
3. Inserting a Foley catheter and attaching it to dependent drainage.
4. Doing a surgical prep of the neck and upper chest wall.

105. The nurse explains to a patient that the purpose of intermittent positive-pressure breathing (IPPB) with normal saline is to maintain patent airways and to mobilize secretions. To accomplish this, IPPB exerts:
1. Positive pressures on inspiration.
2. Negative pressures on inspiration.
3. Positive pressures on expiration.
4. Negative pressures on expiration.

106. A 3-month-old infant brought unconscious to the ER by the parents was pronounced dead. The mother becomes hysterical, crying uncontrollably. The father asks the nurse to "do something." The most appropriate nursing action would be:
1. Providing the patients with privacy.
2. Obtaining an order for a tranquilizer.
3. Sitting quietly with the couple.
4. Asking the mother to calm down.

107. A pregnant woman tells the nurse that she has a family history of cystic fibrosis and wonders if her unborn child is at risk for this disorder. The nurse's response is based on knowledge that most inborn errors of metabolism are:
1. Autosomal-dominant inherited disorders.
2. Autosomal-recessive inherited disorders.
3. X-linked recessive inheritance disorders.
4. Multifactorial inheritance disorders.

108. The drainage period during peritoneal dialysis generally takes 20 minutes, though this may vary from patient to patient. If fluid is not draining properly, the nurse can facilitate return by:
1. Turning the patient to a prone position.
2. Manipulating the indwelling catheter.
3. Elevating the head of the bed, thereby increasing intraabdominal pressures.
4. Elevating the foot of the bed, thereby increasing abdominal pressures and gravity flow.

109. The nurse needs to know that the essential purpose of the water-sealed drainage system for a postop patient following a lower left lobectomy is to:
1. Prevent early precipitous reinflation of the lung.
2. Drain off excess fluid and air, thereby promoting reestablishment of negative intrapleural pressures.
3. Drain off excess fluid and air, thereby promoting reestablishment of positive intrapleural pressures.
4. Decrease atelectasis in unaffected lung tissue and to monitor blood loss.

110. In providing nursing care for the infant who is postop for cleft lip repair, the nurse should:
1. Place the infant in a prone position to facilitate drainage.
2. Avoid moving the infant too much in order to keep from dislodging the Logan bar.
3. Cleanse the suture area frequently to prevent scarring.

4. Encourage the infant to cry to promote adequate lung aeration.

111. Muscular twitching and hyperirritability of the nervous system indicate tetany (hypocalcemia). The nurse can assess for this complication by:
1. Checking the urine calcium.
2. Palpating the calf muscle, with the ankle hyperflexed.
3. Tapping the facial nerve just proximal to the ear.
4. Checking for ankle clonus.

112. Which problem should the nurse expect following uterine isotope insertion?
1. Bladder atony.
2. Constipation.
3. Foul-smelling vaginal discharge.
4. Loss of sexual libido.

113. Preoperative nursing measures for a patient having a cholecystectomy due to cholelithiasis and cholecystitis include:
1. Observing for bruising or easy bleeding due to potential prothrombin deficiency.
2. Informing the patient of the purpose of the postoperative Jackson-Pratt drain.
3. Providing relief for abdominal discomfort by placing a heating pad on the upper abdomen.
4. Providing a low-carbohydrate diet to stimulate release of glycogen stores in the liver.

114. The following is the best single nursing measure of fluid volume status in a patient with chronic renal dysfunction:
1. Skin turgor.
2. Vital signs.
3. Daily weights.
4. Intake and output.

115. The nurse discusses available methods for family planning with the patient. Which method acts by preventing implantation of the zygote if fertilization occurs?
1. Tubal ligation.
2. Intrauterine device.
3. Oral contraceptives.
4. Diaphragm and spermicidal jelly.

116. Which recreational activity for a hospitalized adolescent would be most appropriate for the nurse to support?
1. A television to watch in the two-bed hospital room.
2. Schoolwork that can be brought to the hospital.
3. A board game such as checkers or backgammon.
4. Various novels the adolescent wants to read.

117. Women who tend to delay seeking medical advice after discovering a lump in the breast are displaying what common defense mechanism?
1. Suppression.
2. Denial.
3. Repression.
4. Intellectualization.

118. When can the nurse expect a patient who is receiving NPH insulin to *most* likely have a hypoglycemic reaction?
1. Before lunch (10–11 A.M.).
2. Early afternoon (1–3 P.M.).
3. Late afternoon (4–7 P.M.).
4. After supper (8–10 P.M.).

119. The physician has left orders to deflate a patient's Sengstaken-Blakemore tube, used to stop esophageal bleeding, for 5 minutes every 12 hours to prevent esophageal erosion. Two hours following the second reinflation, the patient suddenly becomes severely dyspneic and dusky. The nurse should:

1. Call a code blue (cardiac arrest).
2. Deflate the balloons.
3. Decrease the traction on the tube where it enters the nose.
4. Irrigate the tube with ice-cold saline to facilitate movement of the balloons into the stomach.

120. The nurse explains that the surgical preparation for a patient scheduled for bilateral herniorrhaphy would include cleansing and shaving:
1. The entire abdomen from just below the nipple line to the mid-thigh.
2. The entire abdomen from the axilla to the pubis.
3. From the waistline of the abdomen to below both knees.
4. Lower abdomen, the pubic area, perineum, and inner sides of thighs and buttocks.

121. Postoperative coughing and deep breathing may become a nursing problem following cholecystectomy because:
1. Patients having abdominal surgery are prone to pulmonary complications.
2. Patients with biliary surgery tend to breathe shallowly to prevent pain and discomfort.
3. Many people tend to be thoracic breathers rather than diaphragmatic breathers.
4. Patients with upper-abdominal surgery usually have a nasogastric tube in place, which inhibits deep breathing.

122. A newborn is admitted to the high-risk neonatal nursery. The father requests permission to see the mother and baby immediately. The most appropriate nursing response would be to:
1. Take him to see the mother.
2. Inform him that they both need their rest.
3. Refer him to the mother's physician.
4. Allow him to go see the infant.

123. Which statement is correct regarding nursing care of a patient receiving hyperalimentation?
1. The patient's urine should be tested for glucose acetone every 8–12 hours.
2. The hyperalimentation subclavian line may be utilized for CVP readings and/or blood withdrawal.
3. Occlusive dressings at the catheter insertion site are changed every 48 hours using the clean technique.
4. Records of intake and output and daily weights should be kept.

124. During the procedure to remove the opacified lens, an iridectomy will also be performed. The nurse tells the patient that this procedure is done:
1. To prevent secondary glaucoma from developing in the postoperative period.
2. To increase pupillary dilatation postoperatively.
3. To facilitate circulation and postoperative healing.
4. To prevent corneal scarring during the procedure.

125. In a closed chest drainage system (Pleur-evac), the nurse knows that:
1. The first chamber establishes the suction pressure and the second chamber collects the drainage.
2. The first chamber establishes the suction pressure and the second is attached to motor suction.
3. The first chamber collects the drainage and the third chamber provides easy access for removing drainage specimens.
4. The first chamber collects the drainage and the second contains the water seal.

126. Women selecting oral contraceptives as their chosen method of family planning should be instructed to notify the clinic if they develop symptoms of potential problems. Which symptom requires prompt evaluation?
1. Mild to moderate nausea during the first few days on the medication.
2. Chloasma.
3. Leg cramps and/or headaches.
4. Breast tenderness and weight gain.

127. In anticipation of emergency complications after thyroidectomy, which nursing measure is essential in the postoperative period?
1. Having calcium gluconate available for possible tetany.
2. Having a thoracentesis tray available to reduce edema.
3. Having a tracheostomy tray available for possible airway obstruction.
4. Having pressure dressings available for possible hemorrhage.

128. A patient's skin test and sputum smear and culture are positive. The chest X ray demonstrated four small lesions and one of moderate density. Diagnosis: tuberculosis. Respiratory isolation is initiated by the nurse. This means:
1. Both patient and attending nurse must wear masks at all times.
2. Full isolation; that is, caps and gowns are required during the period of contagion.
3. Nurse and visitors must wear masks until chemotherapy is begun. Patient is instructed in cough and tissue techniques.
4. Gloves are worn when handling the patient's tissues, excretions, and linen.

129. The physician recommends an inpatient, short-term drug treatment program for an 11-year-old with a substance abuse problem. The adolescent's father becomes very hostile and states, "My child is no addict and isn't going to be put away in any crazy house." To assess the father's reaction to the physician's recommendation, the nurse should realize that the father is:
1. Expressing anger about the accurate diagnosis.
2. Denying that his child is a drug abuser.
3. Projecting the blame elsewhere.
4. Looking for another, better solution.

130. The laboratory data of a preoperative patient recorded an Hgb of 8.5. What is the nurse's *first* responsibility?
1. To attach the lab report to the chart.
2. To hang a unit of blood.
3. To notify the physician immediately.
4. To chart the report in the nurses' notes.

131. The nurse explains to a patient that methyldopa acts to decrease hypertension by:
1. Dilating peripheral blood vessels and increasing renal flow.
2. Depleting norepinephrine at postganglionic synapses.
3. Inhibiting formation of dopamine, a precursor of norepinephrine.
4. Depressing reticular activating system activity.

132. The mother of a newborn on an apnea monitor tells the nurse that her baby looks so frail and sick. The best response for the nurse to make is:
1. "Your baby does have a life-threatening illness."
2. "Have you seen many newborns?"
3. "Try not to think of your baby like that. Think positive!"
4. "I know how you must feel. It can be very scary to see your baby looking like this."

133. A patient refuses to cough after surgery "because it hurts." The nurse's action would be to:
    1. Administer an analgesic and wait a few minutes.
    2. Assist the patient to sit up on the side of the bed and splint the incision with a pillow during coughing.
    3. Allow the patient to rest this time, but inform the patient that coughing will be expected the next time.
    4. Increase fluid intake so as to loosen secretions and ease expectoration.

134. The postoperative nursing care plan following vein-stripping would include which of the following?
    1. Administration of anticoagulants to prevent clotting.
    2. Elastic stockings/bandages from toe to groin.
    3. Sitting in a chair.
    4. Bedrest for 48 hours after surgery.

135. On her third postpartum day, a diabetic woman prepares to return home with her new infant. Which of the following is the priority information to be discussed with this woman before she leaves the hospital?
    1. The statistical probability of her infant developing diabetes.
    2. The type of medical and obstetric problems that may occur in subsequent pregnancies.
    3. Coping strategies with her new baby and her disease in the immediate postpartum period.
    4. Follow-up medical visits for both the infant and herself in the next 6 weeks.

136. The patient returns to the surgical unit following a bilateral hernia repair. The nurse observes that his scrotum is quite swollen. The *first* nursing action is to:
    1. Notify the surgeon stat.
    2. Elevate the scrotum on a rolled towel and apply ice bags.
    3. Administer prn pain medication.
    4. Encourage vigorous deep breathing and coughing.

137. A patient with chest tubes returns to the unit. The first nursing measure concerning the closed chest drainage system is:
    1. Milking the tubing to prevent accumulation of fibrin and clots.
    2. Raising the bottle to bed height to accurately assess the meniscus level.
    3. Attaching the chest tubes to the bed linen to ensure that airflow and drainage are unhindered by kinks.
    4. Marking the time and the amount of drainage in the collection bottle.

138. Which is a complication of thyroidectomy?
    1. Hypercalcemia.
    2. Respiratory obstruction.
    3. Elevated serum T_4.
    4. Paralytic ileus.

139. The nurse implements which precaution when caring for a neonate born to a woman who is HIV positive?
    1. The nurse should wear gloves until all blood and amniotic fluid have been removed.
    2. The woman should be encouraged to breastfeed.
    3. The HIV-positive father should have limited contact with the child.
    4. The parents should be encouraged to place the infant for adoption since the outlook for the mother is poor.

140. After the birth of an abnormal or unhealthy infant, the nurse should expect the parents' initial reactions to include:
    1. Depression.
    2. Apathy.
    3. Withdrawal.
    4. Anger.

141. A postoperative cholecystectomy patient has a T-tube connected to gravity drainage. The nurse knows that the purpose of the T-tube is to:
    1. Maintain patency of the common bile duct.
    2. Reduce the occurrence of postoperative hemorrhage.
    3. Prevent infection.
    4. Reduce bile flow into the duodenum.

142. A patient being admitted for modified radical mastectomy was restless and had the following vital signs: BP, 186/110 mm Hg; pulse, 90 bpm; respirations, 22; and temperature, 98.4°F. A half-hour later the nurse retakes the patient's vital signs: BP, 132/86 mm Hg; pulse, 80 bpm; and respirations, 16. The patient's initial elevated BP indicated:
    1. She may be an individual who is highly sensitive to sympathetic nervous system stimulation.
    2. She is emotionally labile and will need to be assessed closely in the postoperative period.
    3. She is psychologically unprepared for surgery and a psych consult is in order.
    4. She is denying the possible loss of her breast.

143. A patient diagnosed with cirrhosis has been placed on a moderate-protein, high-carbohydrate, high-calorie, low-salt diet. Which statement would the nurse select as the best rationale for this diet?
    1. Since the liver may not be able to detoxify proteins, carbohydrates are substituted to meet metabolic and nutritional needs.
    2. Proteins are given in sufficient amount to facilitate tissue repair. High-carbohydrate diet prevents further weight loss and spares proteins from energy metabolism. Sodium restriction facilitates management of fluid imbalances.
    3. High-protein foods are harder to digest and also have a high sodium content. Carbohydrates are more palatable and will more quickly correct the patient's weight loss.
    4. High-carbohydrate diets, particularly if they contain adequate fiber, are more likely to decrease dyspepsia and diarrhea. Sodium is always restricted when the patient is edematous.

144. Neomycin is administered by the nurse prior to ileostomy surgery:
    1. To decrease the incidence of postoperative atelectasis due to decreased depth of respirations.
    2. To increase the effectiveness of the body's immunologic response following surgical trauma.
    3. To reduce the incidence of wound infections by decreasing the number of intestinal organisms.
    4. To prevent postoperative bladder atony due to catheterization.

145. A patient has been diagnosed with cirrhosis and placed on a diet. One nursing measure that might increase the patient's acceptance of the diet is to:
    1. Sit with the patient until he or she has eaten everything.
    2. Give a family member the responsibility of seeing that the patient eats.
    3. Feed the patient yourself.
    4. Offer frequent, small feedings instead of three large ones.

146. The most important postoperative activity a thoracic surgical patient performs is:
    1. Arm exercises to prevent shoulder ankylosis.

2. Deep breathing and coughing up of sputum to prevent airway obstruction.

3. Leg exercises to prevent thrombophlebitis due to prolonged bedrest.

4. Deep breathing only to prevent undue suture stress while maintaining ventilation.

147. A patient becomes extremely lethargic following administration of meperidine HCl 100 mg IM for pain. What is the most appropriate nursing action?

1. Give only 50 mg of meperidine next time pain medication is required.

2. Administer an oral preparation of meperidine instead of the intramuscular preparation.

3. Consult with physician about decreasing the amount of pain medication ordered.

4. Endeavor to prolong the time between medication dosages by employing alternative pain relief strategies.

148. Postoperatively, a cataract patient should be positioned:

1. In a semi-Fowler's position.

2. In a prone position only.

3. On the back or on the unoperated side.

4. On the operative side.

149. To evaluate a woman's understanding of the use of a diaphragm for family planning, the nurse asks her to explain, in her own words, how she will use the appliance. Which response indicates a need for further health teaching?

1. "I really need to use the diaphragm and jelly most during the middle of my menstrual cycle."

2. "The diaphragm must be left in place for at least 6 hours after intercourse."

3. "I may need a different size diaphragm if I gain or lose more than 20 pounds."

4. "I should check the diaphragm carefully for holes everytime I use it."

150. In observing the drainage from the T-tube during a cholecystectomy patient's early postoperative period, the nurse would notify the physician if:

1. The drainage contained blood during the first 2–4 hours after surgery.

2. The drainage was less than 500 mL on the first postoperative day.

3. The drainage turned greenish brown in color.

4. The drainage was more than 500 mL on the fourth postoperative day.

151. When a toddler's mother comes to visit, the toddler clings to the nurse, who is washing her, and refuses to look at her mother. How should the nurse explain this behavior to the mother?

1. The toddler is upset because her mother left her at the hospital.

2. The toddler is spoiled and needs firm, consistent limits set for her.

3. The toddler has adjusted to the nurse and is doing fine.

4. The toddler may be trying to make her mother jealous of the nurse.

152. A couple asks to see their baby, who is in a high-risk newborn nursery. The most appropriate nursing action would encompass:

1. Assessing and analyzing the couple's level of readiness.

2. Arranging for the couple to see and hold their baby immediately.

3. Teaching the couple what to expect.

4. Preparing the couple for what to expect while making the arrangements for visitation.

153. Paracentesis is a minor surgical procedure done at the bedside; its purpose is to remove ascitic fluid. After explaining the procedure to the patient, the *next* nursing action would be to:

1. Position the patient in a chair or in high Fowler's position.

2. Instruct the patient to void.

3. Take vital signs.

4. Drape the abdomen with sterile towels.

154. Following ileostomy, the nurse would expect the drainage appliance to be applied to the stoma:

1. 24 hours later, when edema has subsided.

2. In the operating room.

3. After the ileostomy begins to function.

4. When the patient is able to begin self-care procedures.

155. The best explanation the nurse could give for the signs and symptoms (edema, joint pain, oliguria, muscle cramps, and lethargy) a patient with a history of renal disease has on admission would be:

1. Renal ischemia due to increase in circulating toxins and chronic hypertension.

2. A decrease in the number of functioning nephrons, which further decreases glomerular filtration.

3. Increased water and salt loss due to flushing effect in the diseased kidney tubules.

4. Water and salt retention due to insufficient renal blood flow.

156. One potential complication of an abdominal hysterectomy is abdominal distention. Postoperative nursing measures designed to *avoid* abdominal distention are:

1. Auscultation of the abdomen for bowel sounds.

2. Abdominal massage and bedrest.

3. Insertion of nasogastric and rectal tubes and ambulation, as ordered.

4. Progression of postoperative diet.

157. The most appropriate plan for immediate follow-up care for a family whose baby has died would include:

1. Referring the family to a psychotherapist.

2. Arranging for the social worker to visit the family.

3. Asking the family to identify their needs.

4. Assessing the family's need for follow-up care.

158. Ten hours after bilateral hernia surgery, a male patient has not been able to void, despite repeated efforts, including standing to void. He states he feels like he could void but just can't seem to get his stream started. The nurse should:

1. Try getting him up in a standing position once again.

2. Insert a Foley catheter stat.

3. Run water while he attempts to use the urinal.

4. Consult with his physician to obtain either a medication or catheterization order.

159. Since ascitic fluids are rich in serum proteins, the nurse would observe for which of the following complications following a paracentesis?

1. Disequilibrium.

2. Hypotension.

3. Hypoalbuminuria.

4. Paralytic ileus.

160. A patient receiving internal radiation therapy for treatment of adenocarcinoma complains of nausea and a general feeling of weakness. The patient's stools are loose. The nurse might suspect:

1. Extension of the cancer to the abdominal contents.

2. Radiation syndrome.

3. Electrolyte imbalances.
4. Depression.

161. Signs and/or symptoms of postthyroidectomy respiratory obstruction vary with the degree of severity. Early warnings observed by the nurse might include:
    1. Hoarseness and weakness of the voice.
    2. Stridor and cyanosis.
    3. Vague feeling of choking, difficulty swallowing, and fullness of the throat.
    4. Pale nailbeds, disorientation, and combative behavior.

162. Objective data seen with hypoglycemic reactions include:
    1. Irritability, confusion, and lethargy.
    2. Increased temperature and flushing of skin.
    3. Muscle tremors and hyperreflexia.
    4. Decreased blood pressure and fatigue.

163. Which of the following activities of daily living must a patient be instructed to avoid to prevent complications upon returning home following cataract removal?
    1. Self-feeding.
    2. Self-dressing.
    3. Adjusting shoelaces.
    4. Ambulating.

164. A woman who had rheumatic fever at age 8 is admitted in labor 4 days before her EDB. If implemented during labor and birth, which of the following would *increase* the stress on her heart?
    1. Helping her maintain a semirecumbent position.
    2. Monitoring her pulse more frequently than her other vital signs.
    3. Preparing her for regional anesthesia (epidural).
    4. After complete dilatation, coaching her to bear down only once per contraction.

165. Which instruction would be *inappropriate psychological* instruction for a thoracic surgery patient regarding the surgery and postoperative care?
    1. Explain that he or she will be surrounded, for example, by chest tubes, oxygen equipment, and IV infusions, and that these are routine.
    2. Tell the patient that he or she will have periods of rest but will be awakened approximately every 2 hours for turning, coughing, and deep breathing.
    3. Assure the patient that he or she will receive medication that will assist in relieving the discomfort.
    4. Assure the patient that anesthesia will not have any untoward effects on respiratory status.

166. Nursing measures to eliminate the cause of joint pain from chronic renal failure would include:
    1. Using Amphogel (aluminum hydroxide) to lower the elevated blood phosphate that occurs with renal failure.
    2. Preparing for dialysis to decrease serum-creatinine levels.
    3. Increasing the patient's activity level.
    4. Implementing a low-purine diet to decrease uric-acid level.

167. The physician orders a magnesium sulfate infusion for a woman with preeclampsia. Which assessment is most important when administering this drug?
    1. Monitoring the serum-magnesium level every 8 hours.
    2. Evaluating the apical heart rate every 4 hours.
    3. Counting the respiratory rate every hour.
    4. Auscultating bowel sounds before meals.

168. A patient is treated with isoniazid (INH) 300 mg PO, and rifampin (RMP). Which of the following vitamins would the nurse expect this patient to receive to prevent the peripheral neuritis that may occur with INH therapy?
    1. Ascorbic acid (vitamin C).
    2. Pyridoxine (vitamin B_6).
    3. Vitamin E.
    4. Vitamin B_{12}.

169. The nurse explains to a patient that urinary retention may be a problem after spinal anesthesia because:
    1. Conduction of autonomic nervous system impulses as well as central nervous system impulses is inhibited.
    2. Sensation and motor responses are decreased.
    3. Patients tend to secrete less ADH with spinal anesthesia than they do with general anesthesia.
    4. Vasomotor depression, which occurs with spinal anesthesia, reduces the glomerular filtration rate.

170. During discharge teaching with a post–abdominal hysterectomy patient, the nurse should include the following instruction:
    1. Avoid sitting for long periods of time.
    2. Evacuate bowels daily.
    3. Restrict sexual activity for 6 months after hysterectomy.
    4. Avoid all household chores for 2 months.

171. The labor room nurse decides to intervene when the fetal heart rate (FHR) pattern indicates:
    1. A baseline range of 110–160 bpm.
    2. Absence of variability.
    3. Early decelerations.
    4. Mild variable decelerations.

172. The nurse would explain to a patient that elevation of the foot of the bed after vein-stripping surgery is done to:
    1. Decrease pain.
    2. Aid venous return.
    3. Increase blood supply to feet.
    4. Make the patient more comfortable.

173. Which goals would be described as the highest nursing priority to a patient recovering from ileostomy surgery?
    1. Relief of pain to promote rest and relaxation.
    2. Assisting the patient with self-care activities.
    3. Maintenance of fluid, electrolyte, and nutritional balances.
    4. Skin care and control of odors.

174. A woman's initial reaction to seeing her infant in the high-risk neonatal nursery is to cry and tremble slightly. The most appropriate nursing intervention would be to:
    1. Remove her from the area immediately.
    2. Monitor her for vital signs.
    3. Allow her to cry.
    4. Ask her what she is feeling.

175. On the fourth postoperative day, the surgeon orders a cholecystectomy patient's T-tube clamped for 1 hour prior to the first solid meal. The nurse explains to this patient that the purpose of clamping the T-tube is to:
    1. Inhibit excessive bile drainage during meals.
    2. Allow bile to flow into the duodenum and aid digestion.
    3. Relieve abdominal distention and promote normal peristalsis.
    4. Assess the patency of the common bile duct.

176. What ECG changes would you anticipate a chronic renal failure patient to demonstrate on assessment, given a potassium level of 6.5 mEq/L?
    1. Peaked T waves.
    2. Flattened T waves.

3. ST-segment depression.
4. ST-segment elevation.

177. In reviewing an infant's admission history, the nurse should know that intussusception most typically presents with which two signs or symptoms?
1. Currant-jelly stools and paroxysmal abdominal pain.
2. Olive-shaped mass in the right upper quadrant and projectile vomiting.
3. Obstinate constipation and increasing abdominal girth.
4. Excessive amounts of mucus and abdominal distention.

178. The nurse can anticipate that the amount of ascitic fluid removed during a paracentesis will generally be:
1. 500 mL.
2. 1000 mL.
3. 2000 mL.
4. 3000 mL.

179. The husband of a woman having a radical modified mastectomy has arrived early to be with his wife before surgery. After his wife leaves for the operating room, the nurse would *initially*:
1. Tell him to go on to work and come back in the early evening, when his wife is likely to be more responsive.
2. Explain that, following surgery, his wife will be taken to the recovery room, but the surgeon will contact him when the procedure is over.
3. Get him a cup of coffee and tell him to make himself comfortable, as it will be some time before his wife returns to her room.
4. Encourage him to express his feelings and concerns so as to plan for postoperative family teaching.

180. One week after surgery, a patient was fitted with cataract glasses. Which of the following nursing statements would best prepare this patient for adjusting to these glasses?
1. "The cataract lenses magnify objects so that they will seem closer to you than they really are."
2. "While your central vision may be somewhat distorted, you will be able to see well peripherally."
3. "These lenses will enable you to see as well as you did before the cataract formed."
4. "The lenses on these glasses are quite narrow, and therefore you may have some double vision."

181. Upon returning from the recovery room, a postthyroidectomy patient begins to complain of a choking sensation. The immediate nursing action should be to:
1. Elevate the head to high Fowler's.
2. Suggest the patient suck on some ice chips.
3. Assess the wound and dressing for increased swelling, and loosen dressing if necessary.
4. Call the physician.

182. The blood gases of a patient with chronic renal failure reveal: pH, 7.36; PO_2, 90; PCO_2, 34; serum bicarbonate, 20 mEq/L. The nurse's interpretation would be:
1. Metabolic acidosis.
2. Compensated metabolic acidosis.
3. Respiratory alkalosis with metabolic compensation.
4. Metabolic acidosis with minimal respiratory compensation.

183. Four days after admission for cirrhosis of the liver, a patient began to bleed from an esophageal varix. The earliest indications of bleeding noted by the nurse would include:
1. Tachycardia, restlessness, and pallor.
2. Tachycardia, lethargy, and flushing.

3. Sudden drop in blood pressure of 10 mm Hg or more.
4. Increasing combativeness and widening pulse pressure.

184. Initially, a new mother is reluctant to touch or hold her son, who is in a high-risk newborn nursery. She says, "I don't know what to do. He's so small, so helpless. He looks so awful." Crying, she turns into her husband's arms. Which nursing diagnosis is the *least* accurate interpretation of her behavior?
1. Altered parenting.
2. Ineffective family coping: compromised.
3. Impaired verbal communication.
4. *High risk for* altered family processes.

185. Objective assessment data indicating circulatory overload in a chronic renal failure patient would include:
1. Neck vein distention, apprehension, soft eyeballs.
2. Periorbital edema, distended neck veins, moist crackles.
3. Increased blood pressure, flattened neck veins, shock.
4. Decreased pulse pressure, cool, dry skin, decreased skin turgor.

186. On the fifth postoperative day, a patient who has had abdominal surgery complains of a "giving" sensation around the wound when walking about. After assisting the patient back in bed, the nurse notes that the dressing covering the incision is saturated with clear, pink drainage. The nurse should suspect:
1. Late hemorrhage.
2. Dehiscence.
3. Infection.
4. Evisceration.

187. The nurse working with a SIDS (sudden infant death syndrome) family should:
1. Be knowledgeable about various theories of psychotherapy.
2. Have extensive experience working with dying patients.
3. Be able to identify personal feelings about death.
4. Be able to suppress personal feelings about death.

188. The nurse knows that a Sengstaken-Blakemore tube is primarily used to:
1. Prevent bleeding by applying pressure to the esophageal varices.
2. Prevent accumulation of blood in the GI tract, which could precipitate hepatic coma.
3. Stop bleeding by applying pressure to the cardiac portion of the stomach and against the esophageal varices.
4. Reduce transfusion requirements.

189. Which postoperative instruction for an abdominal hysterectomy patient includes *inaccurate* information?
1. Monitor vaginal drainage and report any color changes.
2. Expect that vaginal discharge will diminish and cease gradually.
3. Plan on contraception, considering her ovaries are still intact.
4. Expect that menses will no longer occur.

190. While the T-tube is clamped, the nurse should observe a patient after a cholecystectomy for signs of:
1. Abdominal discomfort or pain.
2. Eructation.
3. Jaundice.
4. Increased respiratory rate.

191. Although chemotherapy renders a TB patient noninfectious within days to a few weeks, barring side effects, the patient is instructed by the nurse to continue INH therapy for:
    1. 6 months.
    2. 1 year.
    3. 2 years.
    4. The rest of the patient's life.

192. Prior to lobectomy surgery for squamous cell carcinoma of the left lower lobe, pulmonary function tests are done and blood is drawn for blood gas analysis to establish baseline data on a patient admitted with fever, tachypnea, productive cough, rhonchi and wheezes, and a smoking history that covered 30 years. Given the respiratory symptomatology, which outcome would the nurse expect to find?
    1. Increased vital capacity and respiratory acidosis.
    2. Decreased vital capacity and respiratory alkalosis.
    3. Increased total lung capacity and metabolic acidosis.
    4. Decreased FEV_1 and respiratory acidosis.

193. When teaching the parents about the care of their baby with a cleft lip and palate, the nurse should inform them that:
    1. It is important to use a nipple with large holes to make sucking easier.
    2. The infant will have difficulty feeding because the baby cannot create a vacuum in the mouth.
    3. The infant should be given small amounts of formula while being maintained in a supine position to facilitate feeding.
    4. It is important to isolate the infant from others to prevent possible infection.

194. After presenting a brief class on various methods of family planning to students in a health course, the nurse administers a post test. If teaching has been effective, which statement should the students select as true?
    1. To be effective, rhythm requires avoiding intercourse during the last week of the menstrual cycle.
    2. Couples using coitus interruptus may become pregnant accidentally due to escape of preejaculatory fluid containing spermatozoa.
    3. Spermicidal jellies are highly effective whether used alone or with a diaphragm.
    4. The intrauterine device is the most effective method of contraception.

195. The nurse would recognize signs of hypovolemia, which include:
    1. Dry mucous membranes and soft eyeballs.
    2. Decreased hematocrit and hemoglobin.
    3. Decreased pulse rate and widened pulse pressure.
    4. Dyspnea and crackles.

196. Newborn assessment revealed a scaphoid-shaped abdomen. The nurse knows that this finding suggests a:
    1. Diaphragmatic hernia.
    2. Normal newborn abdomen.
    3. Imperforate anus.
    4. Gastroschisis or omphalocele.

197. During a predischarge teaching session, the nurse tells a patient who has had vein ligation surgery that elastic stockings are best applied:
    1. Before rising in the morning, to prevent pooling of blood in the lower extremities.
    2. After showering and application of skin care to the legs, to prevent undue dermal irritation.
    3. After 15 minutes of vigorous leg exercises designed to increase blood flow.

    4. Only when the patient plans to be standing for an extended period of time because undue constriction of the veins can cause a recurrence of varicosities.

198. Which assessment finding provides data to validate an 8-week gestation?
    1. Fundal height.
    2. Auscultation of fetal heart tones.
    3. Positive radioimmunoassay (RIA) test.
    4. Leopold maneuvers.

199. On the third postoperative day, a postmastectomy patient voiced concern about her husband's reaction to her surgery. Which approach by the nurse is most likely to minimize this patient's concern?
    1. Emphasizing the lifesaving aspects of her surgery.
    2. Explaining that depression and anxiety are common behaviors following radical surgery.
    3. Interviewing the husband to ascertain his real reaction to his wife's surgery.
    4. Encouraging her to identify the strengths in her relationship with her husband.

200. The nurse must be alert to the development of spontaneous bleeding (ecchymoses) in cirrhosis due to:
    1. Rupture of esophageal varices.
    2. Decreased synthesis of blood-clotting factors by the liver.
    3. Failure of the gut to absorb water-soluble vitamins needed to promote coagulation.
    4. Decreased venous pressures and slow blood flow.

❏ Answers/Rationale

1. **(2)** Postural blood pressure readings are an excellent mode for assessing volume depletion. If the systolic blood pressure decreases more than 10 mm Hg and there is a concurrent increase in the pulse rate, a volume depletion problem is indicated. Urine output and specific gravity **(No. 1)** are better measures of the adequacy of fluid volume replacement than of fluid volume depletion. Comparing the prior and present weight of the patient **(No. 3)** will give the nurse an estimate of the slow catabolism of body stores that occurs with ulcerative colitis. There is no oral water test **(No. 4)**. **AS,8,PhI**

2. **(2)** Rhonchi and wheezes occur when there is partial obstruction of the bronchi or bronchioles. These sounds are due to the increased vibration of air molecules as they pass over these obstructions. **No. 1** is incorrect because total obstruction would produce *no* sounds. **No. 3** is incorrect because the sounds produced by fluid in the alveoli are the finer, less harsh sounds generally referred to as crackles. **No. 4** is incorrect because inflammation of the pleura creates a grating sound referred to as a friction rub. **AN,6,PhI**

3. **(1)** Liver functions are many and varied, including detoxification of chemicals (estrogen, adrenocorticoids, aldosterone, drugs, poisons, and heavy metals); synthesis of plasma proteins (albumin, fibrinogen, globulin) and several clotting factors (prothrombin, factor VII); stor-

---

Key to codes following rationales Nursing process: **AS**, Assessment; **AN**, Analysis; **PL**, Plan; **IMP**, Implementation; **EV**, Evaluation. Category of human function: **1**, Protective; **2**, Sensory-perceptual; **3**, Comfort, Rest, Activity, and Mobility; **4**, Nutrition; **5**, Growth and Development; **6**, Fluid-Gas Transport; **7**, Psycho-Social-Cultural; **8**, Elimination. Client need: **SECE**; Safe, Effective Care Environment; **PhI**, Physiologic Integrity; **PsI**, Psychosocial Integrity; **HPM**, Health Promotion/Maintenance. See appendices for full explanation.

age of glycogen, iron, and vitamins (A, D, E, K, and B_{12}); gluconeogenesis (glucose from amino acids and fats); and deamination of amino acids. Fluid volume control and acid-base balance are functions of the *kidney* (**No. 2**). Most erythrocyte and leukocyte breakdown occurs in the *spleen* (**No. 3**). The *gallbladder* concentrates and stores bile (**No. 4**), and the liver is involved with synthesis and secretion of bile. **AN,4,PhI**

4. (2) Acute glomerulonephritis is an autoimmune response to an antigen produced by beta-hemolytic streptococci. Antibodies produced to fight the antigen also react against the glomerular tissue. This causes proliferation and swelling of endothelial cells in the glomerular capillary wall and results in passage of blood cells and protein into the glomerular filtrate. Acute glomerular nephritis is not the result of direct infection (**Nos. 1 and 3**) or of hypoxia (**No. 4**). **IMP,8,PhI**

5. (3) Coughing, vigorous exercise, and straining or lifting increase intraabdominal pressures, which tend to extrude the intestines through weakened areas of the abdominal wall. This patient's history includes all of the above. Other causes of hernia include combinations of **Nos. 1, 2, and 4**; *alone* they are less likely causes. **AN,8,PhI**

6. (2) The functions of the gallbladder are to collect, concentrate, and store bile, which is produced by the *liver, not* by the gallbladder (**No. 1**). Bile reaches the gallbladder via the hepatic duct, which later joins the cystic duct emanating from the gallbladder to form the common bile duct. The common bile duct joins the pancreatic duct, which opens into the duodenum. Bile is not diluted (**No. 3**). No. 4 is incorrect because contraction of the gallbladder and therefore flow of bile are stimulated by the hormone cholecystokinin, which is secreted by the duodenal mucosa when food enters the duodenum. **AN,4,PhI**

7. (3) A thyroid scan utilizes the uptake of ^{131}I by the thyroid gland to determine the size, shape, and function of the gland. Also identified are areas of increased uptake (hot areas), indicating increased metabolic function, as in hyperthyroidism, not malignancy (**No. 2**), and areas of decreased or no uptake (cold areas), which are associated with malignancy. **Nos. 1 and 4** both describe the TSH stimulation test. **IMP,3,PhI**

8. (4) This is the most appropriate response because it attempts to provide total intervention for all parties involved. **No. 1** is essentially the physician's role. It would be almost impossible to alleviate the couple's anxiety at this time (**No. 2**). The most appropriate intervention is to assist the couple to cope with their anxiety as effectively as possible. **No. 3** is essential, but it neglects the psychological needs of the woman and her family. **PL,7,PsI**

9. (1) The kidneys secrete the erythropoietin factor, which stimulates the bone marrow to produce red blood cells. In chronic kidney disease, secretion of this factor decreases as greater portions of the kidney are destroyed by the disease process. Hypertension does not suppress bone marrow centers (**No. 2**), because local blood flow regulators tend to compensate over the long run by supplying tissue with adequate blood flow for metabolic purposes. Unlike metabolic acidosis, metabolic alkalosis does not increase RBC fragility (**No. 3**). Frank bleeding into the urine is uncommon in chronic renal disease (**No. 4**). **AN,8,PhI**

10. (3) For patients having elective surgery, *routine* preoperative laboratory studies generally include a complete blood count, urinalysis, and prothrombin time. Some

institutions also require a VDRL. The urinalysis provides information about specific gravity (indicating the ability of the kidney to concentrate and dilute urine); the presence of albumin or pus, indicating renal infection; and the presence of sugar and acetone. The CBC detects the presence of anemia, infection, allergy, and leukemia. Prothrombin time (increased) may indicate a need for preoperative vitamin K therapy. Electrolytes (**No. 1**), enzymes such as ALT[SGOT] (**No. 2**), and serum glucose (**No. 4**) are ordered *only if* the patient's history or physical condition warrants a more complete workup. **AS,6,PhI**

11. (2) Many times, manipulative patients are not aware of any other mechanisms for fulfilling their needs. Teaching them to identify manipulative behaviors may help them to avoid being manipulative and to eventually adopt more appropriate means for meeting their needs. The patients should be *involved* in the decision-making process (**No. 1**). Limits must be *realistically* established (**No. 3**). Public confrontation (**No. 4**) may only exacerbate the power struggle. **PL,7,PsI**

12. (4) For this woman, a cesarean birth may be expected. With the fetus in breech presentation, there is a risk of prolapsed cord if membranes rupture in early labor (the presenting part is not engaged as yet). Induction (**No. 1**) may not be considered since the presenting part is the sacrum and it is high. Vaginal birth (**No. 2**) may not be considered; however, if breech birth is vaginal, Piper forceps are used to assist in the birth of the after-coming head. Spontaneous vaginal birth (**No. 3**) may not be possible for this woman. **PL,6,SECE**

13. (1) When excessive quantities of fatty acids are oxidized, blood buffer systems may become exhausted. Ketoacidosis develops and acetone bodies are excreted in the urine. In an emergency room situation, diabetic acidosis can be recognized not only by the increased rate and depth of respirations (Kussmaul's respirations) but also by the odor of acetone on the breath. Neither osmotic diuresis (**No. 2**) nor failure in the sodium-hydrogen ion exchange (**No. 3**) causes acetonuria. In the latter case, failure to excrete excess hydrogen ions would decrease urinary acids. Volatile hydrogen ions (CO_2) are excreted by the lungs; a decrease in nonvolatile hydrogen ions in the glomerular filtrate (**No. 4**) would move the pH of the urine toward the alkaline side. **AN,6,PhI**

14. (1) Ergot products such as ergonovine, which contract the uterus and cervix, are contraindicated until the uterus is emptied to avoid retention of placental fragments or tissue. Retained fragments predispose to uterine relaxation and puerperal infection. No. 2 is incorrect because ergot products are not given to women if they are *hypertensive* because of the vasoconstrictive properties of these products. Ergot products are *not* blood products (**No. 3**). No. 4 is incorrect because ergot products are *not contraindicated* if she is also a candidate for $Rh_o(D)$ immune globulin (i.e., she is Rh negative, Coombs negative, and pregnancy had progressed past 10 weeks since the last menstrual cycle). **EV,5,HPM**

15. (2) The woman who seems restless, with flushed face, rapid pulse, and rapid deep respirations, is exhibiting signs of hyperglycemia. No. 1 is incorrect because failure to react to a flash of light in the face is associated with an insulin reaction (hypoglycemia). No. 3 is wrong because diaphoresis during sleep is associated with insulin reactions. No. 4 is wrong because headaches are associated with insulin reactions. **AN,4,HPM**

16. **(1)** Hyperkalemia tends to develop in renal dysfunction for two reasons: In the kidneys, more hydrogen ions than potassium ions are selectively secreted in exchange for sodium ions, and decreasing glomerular filtration and urine output tends to decrease the excretion of all electrolytes and waste products of metabolism. Potassium does not move out of the cell to balance sodium shifts in edema **(No. 2)**, nor does respiratory alkalosis affect potassium reabsorption in the kidneys **(No. 3)**. Nausea and vomiting **(No. 4)** cause hypokalemia. **AN,8,PhI**

17. **(1)** To prevent contractures, the affected limb is kept straight (knee extension) and slightly abducted (to prevent pressure in hip joint), and the foot is supported (ankle flexion) to prevent footdrop. **Nos. 2, 3, and 4** are incorrect because all or part of each response could produce a contracture. **PL,3,HPM**

18. **(2)** A truss should be applied *before* the patient gets out of bed or after the hernia has been reduced, by having the patient lie down with the feet elevated in bed or in the bath. If the hernia cannot be reduced, the truss should not be applied **(Nos. 1 and 3)**. Although the truss is not a cure for a hernia and its use is not as common as it once was, it is far more effective in keeping a hernia reduced than is an athletic supporter **(No. 4)**. **AN,3,SECE**

19. **(1)** The PPD for the Mantoux test is injected intradermally on the polar aspect of the forearm. If the test is correctly administered, a pale elevation similar to a mosquito bite should be apparent. **Nos. 2, 3, and 4** are not used for this test. **IMP,1,SECE**

20. **(3)** Fat-soluble vitamins, particularly vitamin K, are poorly absorbed in the absence of bile. Decreased absorption of vitamin K results in decreased levels of circulating prothrombin, thus reducing normal clotting levels. Peripheral neuritis **(No. 1)** occurs with vitamin B_6 deficiencies, and scurvy **(No. 2)** occurs with deficiency in vitamin C; these are *water-soluble* vitamins. Macrocytic anemia **(No. 4)** is consistent with a vitamin B_{12} deficiency, which may be due to lack of intrinsic factor in the stomach. **AN,4,SECE**

21. **(3)** Even though the patient will have only one eye patched after surgery, familiarization with the physical environment and with nursing personnel will decrease the occurrence of disorientation (this is especially important with elderly patients). It is not necessary to keep the patient flat in bed before or after surgery **(No. 1)**. Patches **(No. 2)** are not generally applied to both eyes. Eye-drop instillations **(No. 4)** are part of the *postoperative* or predischarge teaching plan. **PL,2,PhI**

22. **(1)** Following an injection of the small dose of ^{131}I used in a thyroid scan, no radiation precautions are necessary. Full radiation precautions **(No. 2)** are utilized for radium implants. **No. 3** may be employed when ^{131}I therapy is utilized to control and reduce hypersecretion by the thyroid (*hyperthyroidism*). **No. 4** is not an example of normal radiation therapy policy. **PL,3,SECE**

23. **(2)** Patients with radioactive implants should be positioned flat in bed to prevent dislodgement of the vaginal packing. The patient may roll to the side for meals, but the upper body should not be raised more than 20 degrees. **Nos. 1, 3, and 4** are incorrect because these positions are more likely to change the position of the cobalt seeds. **IMP,1,SECE**

24. **(1)** This is an open-ended question that allows the husband to identify what his needs are at this time. **No. 2** is too threatening. **No. 3** assumes he cannot tolerate the situation, which is unfair. **No. 4** is unrealistic because the nurse has many responsibilities at this time. In addition, the husband would have to leave the room anyway to drink or take anything. **IMP,7,PsI**

25. **(1)** This is the most appropriate response congruent with the nurse's role. **No. 2** is the physician's role. The nurse should accurately reinforce the information the physician gives the couple. In addition, the information is incomplete, in that the initial repair of the palate may begin as early as 6 months or as late as 2 years, depending on the condition of the infant. **No. 3** avoids answering the couple's question and may stimulate an increase in anxiety. **No. 4** is the physician's role. **IMP,7,PsI**

26. **(3)** Surgical treatment of hyperthyroidism involves a subtotal thyroidectomy in which approximately five-sixths of the thyroid tissue is removed. While this procedure does not cure hyperthyroidism, it reduces the amount of circulating thyroid hormone by reducing the amount of functioning tissue. **No. 1**, complete or total thyroidectomy, is *rarely* done for hyperthyroidism today but *is* indicated for thyroid malignancy. **No. 2**, removal of half of the thyroid, would leave enough functioning hyperactive tissue to prevent diminution of symptoms in the patient. **No. 4** is incorrect because the patient with hyperthyroidism needs no additional thyroid hormone; he or she receives antithyroid medications such as propylthiouracil (PRU) or methimazole (Tapazole) to reduce both circulating and stored thyroid hormone. **AN,3,SECE**

27. **(3)** Obstruction of the bile duct will cause elevated serum and urine bilirubin (dark urine) as well as a decreased amount of urobilinogen in the feces (clay-colored stools). Bilirubin is an end product of hemoglobin breakdown. Normally it is conjugated in the liver and secreted, in the bile, into the intestines, where it is converted into urobilinogen and excreted in the stools. **No. 1** is incorrect because biliary obstruction itself does not directly affect blood pressure. However, if the obstruction is acute and accompanied by pain, changes in blood pressure in response to increased sympathetic tone can be expected. **No. 2** is incorrect because between-meal eructation is a symptom of ulcer disease. Eructation in gallbladder disease occurs after eating, particularly if large amounts of fat have been ingested. **No. 4** is also incorrect; longitudinal ridging of the fingernails is a sign seen frequently in anemia. **AS,4,PhI**

28. **(2)** This patient's smoking history and history of chronic cough necessitate directing preoperative nursing measures toward clearing the respiratory tract of excess secretions that might lead to postoperative complications. Besides oral hygiene, the following may be instituted or ordered before surgery: postural drainage, incentive spirometers, IPPB, and mucolytic agent. Since postoperative coughing is contraindicated with hernia repairs, removal of secretions is a priority, as is instruction in deep-breathing techniques. **Nos. 1, 3, and 4**, though *not top priority,* are correct and should also be included in the preoperative teaching plan. **AN,6,SECE**

29. **(3)** This patient's urine specific gravity indicates that the kidneys have lost their ability to concentrate urine. Therefore the patient has a greater water loss than would normally be expected. ADH secretion **(No. 1)** would produce an elevated specific gravity. **No. 2** is incorrect because water loss without concomitant electrolyte loss causes the extracellular fluids to become hyperosmolar (that is, the patient is dehydrated). **No. 4** is incorrect because hyperosmolarity of ECF causes the

thirst receptors in the hypothalamus to shrink (which stimulates the thirst mechanism). **IMP,6,PhI**

30. **(1)** The portal system becomes obstructed, causing a rise in portal venous pressure and portal hypertension, venous dilatation, and stasis. In cirrhosis, there is *decreased* hepatic synthesis of albumin, not increased **(No. 2)**, and *increased* levels of aldosterone, not decreased **(No. 3)**. Blood volumes are *decreased,* not increased **(No. 4)**, while total body fluid is increased due to the physiologic effects of hypoproteinemia (decreased serum proteins). These factors, plus increasing obstruction of the portal vein, cause fluids, electrolytes, and serum proteins to move out of the vascular compartment and into the intestines. The abdomen provides a large potential space for the accumulation of these fluids. **AN,4,PhI**

31. **(2)** Bronchoscopy provides direct visualization of the airways by utilizing a long, slender, hollow instrument through which a light is reflected. Bronchoscopy can be utilized for diagnostic purposes, for removal of foreign objects, for removal of mucous plugs, or for obtaining a biopsy or bronchial washings for cytology. **No. 1** is an example of a fluoroscopic exam. **No. 3** characterizes a bronchogram, and **No. 4**, a lung biopsy. **IMP,6,SECE**

32. **(3)** Potassium deficit leads to decreased muscular function, causing muscle weakness, decreased intestinal motility, and a variety of GI symptoms (vomiting, abdominal distention, flatulence). There is also decreased neuromuscular irritability, which contributes to apathy, lethargy, and mental confusion. **No. 1** is partially correct (spasms or tetany and irregular pulse), but high T waves occur in *hyperkalemia;* low flat waves occur in hypokalemia. **No. 2** is incorrect because the symptoms indicated would likely be seen in metabolic acidosis and dehydration. Hyperkalemia would be expected. Pitting edema and bounding pulse **(No. 4)** are seen in fluid overload, which would be consistent with hyperkalemia and renal impairment. Confusion does occur in hypokalemia. **AS,6,PhI**

33. **(2)** The effect of the anesthesia will be closely checked prior to making the incision, and the level of anesthesia will be monitored throughout the procedure. Many times the woman will complain of tightness or pressure in the area where the physician is working **(No. 1)**. No significant pain should be felt as long as the anesthesia is closely monitored and maintained **(No. 3)**. **No. 4** is inappropriate because it makes her feel that she should not complain about pain even if she actually does feel it. **IMP,7,PsI**

34. **(4)** Abdominal cramps, vomiting, and watery or no discharge are signs of intestinal obstruction, a complication that requires immediate medical intervention. **Nos. 1, 2, and 3** are incorrect, not only because they can delay appropriate medical intervention but also because they increase the risk of severe fluid and electrolyte imbalance. Although obstruction of an ileostomy is a rare problem, a very small stoma or one that is contracted may need to be dilated regularly so that the little finger can be inserted easily. **IMP,4,PhI**

35. **(4)** Normal functioning of chest tubes is maintained, and the drainage system is transported below the level of the chest. Chest tubes are not removed **(No. 1)** to facilitate transportation of the patient; they are removed only after the physician is satisfied with the degree of reexpansion. Removing the chest tubes from the suction drainage system **(No. 2)** will result in an equalization of intrapleural pressures with atmospheric pressures, thus also increasing the risk of pneumothorax.

Current practice precludes the clamping of the chest tubes **(No. 3)**. It is believed that clamping increases the risk of a tension pneumothorax because air may enter the intrapleural space during inspiration but cannot escape during expiration. **IMP,6,SECE**

36. **(3)** Hypoglycemic or insulin reactions are the result of decreased circulatory serum glucose to the brain. This stimulates epinephrine release. Early symptoms include cold, clammy skin, nervousness, tremors, numbness of the hands or around the lips, and cardiac palpitations. Later symptoms may mimic alcoholic intoxication, such as staggering gait, slurring of words, combative behavior, or uncontrolled weeping. As hypoglycemia deepens, the patient may develop convulsions and coma. **No. 1** is incorrect, in that respirations in insulin shock, though shallow, are increased. **No. 2** is incorrect because the breath of the patient in insulin shock is noncontributory, not fetid. Fetid breath may occur with liver failure or poor dental hygiene. Behavioral responses in **No. 4** are switched; that is, confusion and lethargy are common with ketoacidosis, and cold, clammy skin is consistent with insulin shock. **AN,4,PhI**

37. **(1)** Emergency surgery must be performed to save the life of the patient, save the function of an organ or limb, remove a damaged organ or limb, or stop hemorrhage. Few emergency situations are so urgent as to require immediate response **(No. 2)**, eliminating the necessary laboratory data to evaluate the patient's physiologic response to the situation. Surgical preparation would be completed within 24 hours **(No. 3)**, but this is not the *best* answer. True emergency situations cannot be postponed to the following surgical day **(No. 4)**. **IMP,1,SECE**

38. **(1)** Prognosis is generally poor if hepatic coma lasts longer than 24 hours. Other measures that have been utilized to decrease serum ammonia and allow for regeneration of hepatocytes include hemodialysis, exchange blood transfusions, and administration of lactalose, which, when degraded in the large bowel, decreases the pH of the feces, thus preventing formation of ammonia and promoting its excretion. **Nos. 2, 3, and 4** all exceed the 24-hour threshold. **AN,2,PhI**

39. **(3)** A BUN of less than 20 mg/dL and serum creatinine less than 1.2 mg/dL would be optimal outcome measures for this patient (that is, within normal range). Nos. 1, 2, and 4 are incorrect because a serum K^+ of less than 3.5 mEq/L would be indicative of hypokalemia and a serum Na^+ above 148 mEq/L indicates hypernatremia **(No. 1)**; quantity of urine output *should increase* to over 500 mL/24 hours **(No. 2)**; and the abdomen should be soft and tympanic to percussion, so dullness to percussion in the abdomen is consistent with *fluid excess* **(No. 4)**. **EV,8,SECE**

40. **(3)** Before the dialysis procedure is started, baseline information needs to be collected so that the therapy can be accurately evaluated. Baseline information will include vital signs, body temperature, weight, ECG, and electrolyte levels. If the patient does not have a Foley catheter (often by this time he or she does because of the need to assess hourly outputs), then the patient is asked to void. Following voiding, the patient is positioned in a supine or low Fowler's position and the abdomen is prepared and draped. **Nos. 1, 2, and 4** are actions subsequent to No. 3. **IMP,8,PhI**

41. **(4)** All straining and lifting should be avoided for at least 3 weeks to prevent undue stress on the sutures. Other less strenuous activities, such as **Nos. 1, 2, and**

3, are appropriate, though good body mechanics should be reviewed with the patient. **PL,3,PhI**

42. **(2)** To avoid the complication of a painful spinal headache that can last for several days, the patient is kept flat in a supine position for approximately 4–12 hours postoperatively. Headaches are believed due to the seepage of cerebral spinal fluid from the puncture site. By keeping the patient flat, cerebral spinal fluid pressures are equalized, which avoids trauma to the neurons. **No. 1** is the position for patients having general anesthesia. **No. 3** is incorrect because knees are flexed. **No. 4** is the position for patients with head traumas. **IMP,1,SECE**

43. **(2)** Patients who have had spinal anesthesia have varying degrees of hypotension due to the vasodepressor effect of the anesthetic agent on the autonomic nervous system. Reflexes **(No. 1)** will be depressed in the lower extremities because of the anesthetic and should be checked *after* circulatory status. However, sensory impulses remain blocked longer than motor activity, so safety measures should be instituted to prevent injury from bedding, poor positioning, or sources of heat. Since the patient is awake with a spinal anesthetic, level of consciousness **(No. 3)** and airway integrity **(No. 4)** are lower priorities than circulatory status. **AS,1,PhI**

44. **(3)** There are no specific dietary restrictions following cholecystectomy. Patients are advised, however, to avoid foods high in fats. Most patients tend to avoid these foods anyway because they are more comfortable if they do so. Generally, after about 3 months, patients may begin to experiment with certain foods to ascertain their tolerance to them. **No. 1** is incorrect because some fat is allowed in the diet at all times. **No. 2** is incorrect because fats are not limited to those classified as polyunsaturates. **No. 4** is incorrect because fats are allowed in the postcholecystectomy diet, to tolerance. **IMP,4,PhI**

45. **(2)** The patient who has had thyroid surgery should be assisted in supporting the head and neck whenever the position is changed during the first 3 postoperative days. Supporting the head is particularly important during early ambulation procedures, when sudden movement may result in hyperextension of the neck. **Nos. 1, 3, and 4** are incorrect because none of these responses takes into account the need to prevent hyperextension of the neck. **IMP,3,SECE**

46. **(3)** This is characteristic of a reactive depression. The individuals experiencing an endogenous depression usually feel worse in the morning but better as the day progresses. There is usually a weight loss of less than 10 pounds **(No. 1)**. The individuals usually respond to environmental stimuli **(No. 2)**. The precipitating event is usually an identifiable stressor, such as the birth of an unhealthy baby **(No. 4)**. **AN,7,PsI**

47. **(3)** An Apgar score of 4–6 indicates the infant is in fair condition. "Excellent" **(No. 1)** is not a category in the Apgar score. "Good" **(No. 2)** is a score of 7–10. "Poor" **(No. 4)** is a score of 0–3. **EV,5,HPM**

48. **(1)** Toddlers will most likely experience separation anxiety when separated from parents. In the "despair" phase, the child appears to be mourning the apparent loss of the parent, as evidenced by nonverbal behavior cues such as monotone crying, regressive behavior (thumb sucking), and sleep disturbances. If this child were experiencing muscle spasms due to her fracture **(No. 4)**, she would most likely scream out in severe pain intermittently. The other explanations for her behavior **(Nos. 2 and 3)** do not take her developmental level into account. **AN,5,HPM**

49. **(1)** Sperm deposited during intercourse may remain viable for about 3 days. If ovulation occurs during this period, conception may result. **No. 2** is incorrect because the ovum is present only *after* ovulation. **No. 3** is wrong because tubal motility is important in the union of ovum and sperm (and transport of the zygote) *after ovulation*. **No. 4** is wrong because the uterine endometrium becomes secretory postovulation. **EV,5,HPM**

50. **(2)** Both parents will probably attempt to place the blame for their infant's deformities on someone or something else, such as "inadequate prenatal care," "bad counseling," or "God's wish." **No. 1** involves a state in which personality development is arrested in one or more aspects at a level short of maturity. **No. 3** involves unconsciously translating psychic problems into physical symptoms. **No. 4** involves channeling a destructive or instinctual impulse that is socially unacceptable into a socially acceptable behavior, such as coping with anger by participating in sports that require the release of a lot of energy. **AN,7,PsI**

51. **(2)** It is important to assess and validate the parents' perceived needs in order to plan care effectively. The parents may need a social worker as well as a public health nurse, speech pathologist, audiologist, etc. Therefore it is essential to make an accurate and continual assessment of the family's needs **(No. 1)**. Alternatives **(No. 3)** may be more appropriately identified after performing a total assessment. Health teaching **(No. 4)** is necessary, but it must be based on an assessment and validation of the family's needs as well as of their level of readiness. **PL,7,PsI**

52. **(3)** Breast self-examinations are best done the week following onset of menses. The breasts are then the softest, and any lumps not associated with hormonal changes are more evident. **No. 1** is incorrect because breast changes due to hormonal changes, such as fullness or tenderness, may occur at this time, obscuring possible pathology. **No. 2** is a good idea (that is, having a regular time or pattern for examination), but does not take into account the normal breast-tissue changes during the menstrual cycle. **No. 4** is incorrect for the same reason as No. 1. **IMP,1,SECE**

53. **(2)** The contrast medium utilized in IV cholangiograms, like that used in intravenous pyelograms, contains iodine. It is important to ascertain before the test whether the patient is aware of any allergy to iodine. Saltwater fish generally leave a high iodine content, so it is helpful to ascertain if the patient has an allergy to fish, and if so, to what kind. **No. 1** is helpful in planning patient teaching. **Nos. 3 and 4** are less specific responses that provide interesting, though not essential, data. **AS,1,SECE**

54. **(1)** The patient should remain quiet in a low Fowler's or horizontal position. He or she should be cautioned not to cough so as not to extrude any intestines by increasing intraabdominal pressures. The physician should be notified next. Remain with the patient, reassuring him or her, monitoring vital signs, and having others bring equipment such as an IV setup, nasogastric tube, and suction equipment. The surgeon should also be notified that the patient will be returning to the operating room. The patient should be kept NPO **(No. 2)** in the above position **(No. 3)** and the dressing left in place to prevent evisceration **(No. 4)**. **IMP,1,SECE**

55. **(4)** Flattened neck veins in a supine position are characteristic of hypovolemia. Inadequate drainage would

result in fluid retention and hypervolemia. Indications of fluid retention include inadequate fluid drainage (greater intake than output), increased blood pressure, and signs of congestive heart failure, for example, *distended* neck veins, increased dependent edema, crackles, and decreased mentation (**Nos. 1, 2, and 3**). **EV,8,PhI**

56. **(2)** Ammonia is formed in the intestines by the action of intestinal bacteria on proteins. Tap-water enemas may be given to remove protein-rich blood that has resulted from bleeding esophageal varices. Since ammonia is formed during muscle contraction, active range-of-motion exercises are contraindicated (**No. 1**). To prevent skin breakdown in a patient who is jaundiced and edematous, passive exercises, turning, and frequent skin care are indicated. In an effort to reduce serum-ammonia levels, potassium levels need to be increased, not reduced (**No. 3**), because potassium is necessary for cerebral metabolism of ammonia. Antibiotics that are poorly absorbed by the intestines, such as neomycin, are given, rather than withheld (**No. 4**), to decrease the intestinal flora that manufacture ammonia. **IMP,4,PhI**

57. **(3)** Ovulation occurs most commonly 14 days *prior* to the next menstrual period. In a 30-day cycle, this would be day 16 or 17. Answers **1 and 2** are incorrect because they describe a time prior to normal ovulation; **No. 4** is wrong because ovulation occurs prior to the last week of the menstrual cycle. **AS,5,HPM**

58. **(4)** An abdominal hysterectomy is generally the treatment of choice for uterine fibroids with excessive vaginal bleeding. If the ovaries are not pathologic, there is no reason for surgical removal. **No. 1**, panabdominal hysterectomy, involves the removal of the uterus, fallopian tubes, and ovaries and is usually performed for extensive endometriosis or carcinoma. A vaginal hysterectomy (**No. 2**) is the treatment of choice for a prolapsed uterus, and a D&C (**No. 3**) is primarily a diagnostic tool, not a measure to control excessive uterine bleeding. **IMP,5,SECE**

59. **(2)** Before notifying the physician (**No. 1**), it is necessary to collect the data, blood sugar and urine sugar and acetone, on which the physician will base the insulin order. The physician should also be notified of the patient's vital signs and intake and output. Generally, urinary output is depressed for about 36 hours after surgery due to increased circulating levels of ADH. Given that the patient has also had insensible water loss (respirations and perspiration), the assessment data strongly indicate dehydration or hypovolemia. An antiemetic (**No. 3**) may be administered if nausea persists *after* blood sugar and fluid balance are rectified. The physician may order an increase in the amount and rate of intravenous fluids (contrary to **No. 4**). **AN,4,PhI**

60. **(2)** Arm exercises are initiated to prevent ankylosis of the shoulder. Most patients tend to splint incisional discomfort by limiting movement on the affected side. This protective mechanism may lead to "frozen shoulder," or ankylosis. Therefore, it is important to initiate movement early to maintain muscle tone and joint integrity. **No. 1** is an example of wristdrop due to poor positioning of wrist joints. **No. 3** is usually a normal finding, although it may occur with improper positioning with upper motor neuron lesions. Intercostal muscle spasticity (**No. 4**) is rare and is not due to positioning. **IMP,1,SECE**

61. **(3)** The primary objective of stoma care is to prevent skin irritation and excoriation. The stoma and surrounding skin should be washed with mild soap and water, rinsed thoroughly, and patted dry. The ostomy appliance should be fitted close to the stoma to further prevent skin irritation. Although fecal material is measured as output (**No. 1**), this procedure is secondary to control of skin damage. A tight-fitting seal on the drainage bag and a well-ventilated room will decrease odor problems (**No. 2**). Likewise, a tight-fitting appliance will prevent contamination of the abdominal incision (**No. 4**). **PL,8,SECE**

62. **(4)** The exact cause of the failure of the embryonic structures of the face to form a union is unclear. However, there is a significant familial pattern, and a hereditary factor is involved. Cleft palate is seen more frequently in girls, whereas cleft lip is seen more frequently in boys (**Nos. 1 and 2**). Although cleft lip and palate sometimes do occur together (**No. 3**), in many cases they occur independently. **AN,5,HPM**

63. **(3)** The woman should have waited to telephone until she had assessed her signs and symptoms *after* drinking three to four 8-oz glasses of water for hydration. She is correct to call when her contractions are every 10 minutes (**No. 1**), to call after she emptied her bladder (**No. 2**), and to call after she rested in bed for 1 hour (**No. 4**). **EV,5,HPM**

64. **(4)** The Trendelenburg test evaluates the competency of the superficial veins. The patient is asked to elevate the involved leg to empty the veins. A tourniquet is then applied lightly to occlude the superficial veins. The patient is then asked to stand, the tourniquet is removed, and the direction and degree of vein-filling are observed. **No. 1** is also a test of venous competence: Ordinarily, distended veins decrease markedly during walking because muscular contractions facilitate venous flow in deeper veins. **No. 2** describes a phlebography, and **No. 3** is a test generally used on the jugular vein when pump failure is suspected. **IMP,6,SECE**

65. **(3)** Usually with a transverse lie the classic or longitudinal incision is used, and the woman is concerned about her body image. **Nos. 1, 2, and 4** may be concerns, but they are not usually primary in the woman's mind. **AN,7,HPM**

66. **(2)** There is a physical tolerance, but the dependence is purely psychological. **Nos. 1 and 3** are imprecise; and **No. 4** is incorrect because this drug is not physiologically addictive. **IMP,7,PsI**

67. **(2)** The dialysate is warmed to body temperature before administration to minimize discomfort and optimize clearance of waste products. Warming the fluid tends to dilate the peritoneal vessels, increasing the amount of urea that passes through the membrane. It has little effect on the osmotic gradient (**No. 1**), does not prevent peritonitis, which is secondary to infection (**No. 3**), and does not speed infusion time (**No. 4**), although it does make it more comfortable. **PL,8,SECE**

68. **(3)** To prevent undue stress on the suture line and underlying surgical repair, the patient is taught to support the back of the neck when repositioning and to avoid both hyperextension and flexion of the neck. **No. 1** is incorrect because active flexion of the neck is avoided and because after a total thyroidectomy the patient will receive thyroid medications to prevent hypothyroidism and to maintain a euthyroid state. **No. 2** is also incorrect due to the focus on active flexion and extension neck exercises, which would put undue stress on the suture line. **No. 4** is partially correct;

however, again, active flexion exercises are contraindicated. **IMP,3,SECE**

69. **(4)** The Mantoux test is read in 48–72 hours. Color is observed, and the injection site is palpated for induration. Reading the test in less than 48 hours may lead to inaccurate interpretation **(Nos. 1, 2, and 3)**. **EV,1,SECE**

70. **(2)** It is not necessary to isolate a patient with radioactive implants **(No. 1)**, but to prevent undue exposure to radiation contacts, contact time should be brief and distance between the patient and others maximized. Specific instructions as to the amount of time permitted with the patient and the safe distance should be posted. **Nos. 3 and 4** are incorrect because the best position for the patient is supine. **IMP,1,SECE**

71. **(1)** Anemia occurs in cirrhosis due to (a) erythrocyte destruction in the engorged spleen, (b) gastrointestinal blood losses, and (c) folic acid deficiencies from inadequate dietary intake. Kupffer cells **(No. 2)** line the venous sinusoids in the liver and are primarily macrophagic. **Nos. 3 and 4** are incorrect because decreased amino acid breakdown and synthesis result in increasing serum-ammonia levels, which may further inhibit dietary intake. **AN,6,SECE**

72. **(2)** The patient's vital signs and urine output reflect a decrease in extracellular volume secondary to osmotic diuresis. Increased ADH release *decreases* urinary output **(No. 1)**. A hypo-osmolar fluid imbalance is one in which there is more water than solute in the extracellular fluid compartment **(No. 3)**. Like circulatory overload **(No. 4)**, symptoms of a hypo-osmolar imbalance include widened pulse pressure, increased blood pressure, distended neck veins, and respiratory crackles. **AN,6,PhI**

73. **(2)** After bronchoscopy the patient generally produces a large amount of sputum that must be observed carefully for signs of hemorrhage, particularly if a biopsy specimen has been taken during the procedure. Although the sputum is generally blood streaked, any pronounced bleeding should be reported immediately. Patency of the airway is the *first priority*. **Nos. 1 and 3** are also observations made after a bronchoscopy. Vital signs are observed until stable, and food and fluids are withheld until the gag reflex returns. **No. 4**, urticaria, does not occur following bronchoscopy, though it may after a bronchogram if the patient reacts to the iodine-based dye. **AS,6,PhI**

74. **(2)** Few surgeries warrant immediate treatment **(No. 1)**; however, the urgency of the situation does decrease preparation time. Consequently, the patient's physiologic stress will increase, not decrease **(No. 3)**, placing greater demands on metabolic functions and increasing the risk of complications. Emergency surgery does not compromise the use of general anesthesia **(No. 4)**. It is imperative to ascertain before an emergency surgery the time, type, and amount of the last oral intake, as gastric lavage or suctioning may be necessary to prevent aspiration during the surgery. Generally patients are NPO 12 hours before surgery. **AN,1,SECE**

75. **(2)** Generally, the dwell time of the dialysate is 20–30 minutes, occasionally longer. The dwell time as well as the instillation and outflow times are prescribed by the physician according to the patient's needs. Ten to 15 minutes **(No. 1)** is too short a time to allow for diffusion of waste products. Equilibrium between dialysate and body fluids occurs in 15–30 minutes. Longer times **(Nos. 3 and 4)** are not necessary. **IMP,1,SECE**

76. **(2)** Under high estrogen levels, during the period surrounding ovulation, the cervical mucus becomes thin, clear, and elastic (spinnbarkeit), facilitating sperm passage. **No. 1** is incorrect because cervical mucus becomes thicker and opaque under progesterone stimulation after ovulation. **No. 3** is wrong because cervical mucus is essentially colorless, and postovulation, under progesterone stimulation, it becomes thick and sticky. **No. 4** is wrong because ferning is absent during the postovulatory period. **IMP,5,HPM**

77. **(1)** Local anesthesia is used in cataract surgery, not only because this surgery is a short procedure but also because most patients are elderly, with one chronic disease or more, which may be exacerbated by general anesthesia **(No. 2)**. Intravenous anesthesia **(No. 3)** with thiopental sodium (Pentothal) is most frequently used when unconsciousness is desirable for short procedures or when an anesthetic induction is desired for general anesthesia. Rectal anesthesia **(No. 4)**, though rarely used today, has been employed to induce short-term anesthesia in children. **IMP,2,SECE**

78. **(4)** Parenteral hyperalimentation solutions are hyperosmolar solutions containing amino acids, 10–25% glucose, multivitamins, and electrolytes. These solutions are administered through large veins such as the subclavian to avoid the inflammation or thrombosis that these hyperosmolar solutions tend to cause in peripheral veins. These solutions are given to patients with disturbances of *ingestion,* digestion, or absorption that are combined with excessive catabolism. Hypotonic solutions **(No. 1)** have osmolality less than blood plasma osmotic pressures and cause fluids to enter the cells. They are used for fluid replacement when some sodium is also necessary. **No. 2** is partially correct, in that hyperalimentation solutions are hypertonic; that is, they have an osmolarity greater than that of the plasma. However, the goal of hyperalimentation is not to reduce cellular swelling but to *reverse negative nitrogen balance.* Hypertonic solutions utilized to reduce cellular swelling are indicated in water intoxication and/or severe sodium depletion. Rapid infusion of hyperalimentation solution, however, will cause cellular dehydration. **No. 3** is incorrect because it is *not* a hyperosmolar fluid. **IMP,6,SECE**

79. **(1)** Ensuring adequate oxygenation of the infant's system is the number one priority to sustain life. **Nos. 2, 3, and 4** are all appropriate *secondary* goals. **PL,6,PhI**

80. **(1)** Vein-stripping is done not only for advancing varicosities but also for cosmetic reasons. Vein-stripping is *not* done for thrombophlebitis **(No. 2)**, though it is done for stasis ulcerations following successful healing of the ulcer. **No. 3** is incorrect because lymphedema is due to blockage of lymph channels and Raynaud's disease is a syndrome that affects the *arterial* vasculature. **No. 4** is incomplete. **AN,6,PhI**

81. **(2)** The evening before an intravenous pyelogram (IVP), the patient is administered oral cathartics or enemas to clean the bowel of fecal material and flatus, thereby improving visualization of the kidneys and ureters. The radiopaque dye used in this procedure is injected by a physician in the radiology department, not by the nurse prior to the procedure **(No. 1)**. **No. 3** is *not* part of IVP preparation. If the patient is having difficulty maintaining fluid volume balance, an intravenous infusion *may* be initiated to prevent dehydration, but it is not standard **(No. 4)**. **PL,8,SECE**

82. **(3)** Glycogenolysis and therefore serum-glucose levels are increased due to the stresses of surgery. To control

blood-glucose levels and prevent ketoacidosis, secondary to increased tissue metabolism (**No. 1**), regular insulin is given in doses adjusted according to the results of urine tests (rainbow or sliding scale). Regular insulin may be given alone until results of urine tests for glucosuria and ketonuria stabilize or as a supplement along with an intermediate-acting insulin such as NPH. **No. 2**, decreased insulin production, results from the extent of the patient's dysfunction, not the stress of surgery. Insulin does facilitate the movement of potassium across the cellular membrane, thus preventing hyperkalemia (**No. 4**), but this is not the *best* answer. **AN,4,PhI**

83. (2) Life-threatening illnesses, especially those with complications resulting in prolonged recuperative periods, provoke alterations in body image. To assist a patient experiencing altered body image, the nurse needs to ascertain how the patient viewed his or her body previously and how he or she views it now. Doing this may unleash a torrent of feeling from the patient, which may help the nurse discover ways to help the patient cope. **Nos. 1 and 3**, while acknowledging this patient's mood, tend to cut off further response from the patient. **No. 4** is too open-ended. **IMP,7,PsI**

84. (1) *Dyspnea* is a term that describes the patient's subjective awareness of increased respiratory effort. The increased work of breathing may indeed be *related* to alveolar hypoventilation (**No. 2**), which *results* in an increased rate and depth of respiration (**No. 3**). Oxygen saturation (**No. 4**) shows whether the *circulation* is normal or tissue demands have changed. **AN,6,PhI**

85. (3) This allows the patient some control over his care and makes the patient feel that the staff is interested in meeting his needs. **No. 1** is inappropriate unless they have a common interest. Frequent visits should initially be *dis*couraged (**No. 2**) to avoid the possibility of receiving drugs from the outside. **No. 4** may be appropriate; however, it is not as important as allowing the patient some control over his own care. **PL,7,PsI**

86. (4) Vein-stripping is a painful and tiresome procedure and, for the patient's comfort, is almost always done under general anesthesia. **No. 1** is incorrect because local anesthesia is limited to small areas such as with laceration repair. Topical anesthesia (**No. 2**) only decreases pain sensation in mucous membranes. And, since the incisions for vein-stripping are made in the groin as well as the ankle, regional anesthesia (**No. 3**) would be impractical. Vein-stripping could also be done using spinal anesthesia. **IMP,6,SECE**

87. (3) Since the patient has a history of chronic cough, and since hernias can be repaired with spinal anesthesia, this approach may have the least amount of risk for postoperative complications. General anesthesia (**No. 1**) has the greatest risk for respiratory complications after surgery. Intravenous (**No. 2**) and local infiltration (**No. 4**) would not supply the depth of anesthesia needed to complete the repair. **PL,1,SECE**

88. (2) Timed forced expiratory volume measures the functional ability of an individual to remove air from his or her lungs. Reduction in FEV_1 is usually due to airway obstruction from excess mucus. Vital capacity measures the individual's ability to move a volume of air in and out of the lungs (**No. 1**). Though inadequate innervation of the intercostals (**No. 3**) would also reduce the FEV_1, there is nothing in this case study to indicate that this patient has neuromuscular problems. Atelec-

tasis (**No. 4**) is determined by X ray, clinical symptomatology, and blood gases. **IMP,6,PhI**

89. (1) Quadriceps-setting exercise is an appropriate activity to prevent complications of immobility. Range-of-motion exercises for joints not enclosed in the cast are encouraged. The primary purpose of the cast is to immobilize those joints above and below the fracture site; therefore extension (**No. 2**) and flexion (**No. 4**) of the knees are inappropriate. **No. 3** is not correct because passive range of motion is *not as effective as active* range of motion in the prevention of complications of immobility. **PL,3,SECE**

90. (1) An induration of 10 mm or more (not cm, as in **No. 2**) is considered a positive reaction. The skin is generally reddened. Indurations of 5–9 mm (**No. 3**) are considered doubtful reactions. Individuals with doubtful reactions should be retested, unless they have had a known contact with persons with tuberculosis. Indurations of less than 5 mm are considered negative reactions. The reaction is not hivelike (**No. 4**). **EV,1,SECE**

91. (3) Initially this couple will be unable to make appropriate decisions regarding their own needs. They need tender support, empathy, and reassurance to assist them in coping with this stress. **No. 1** may be appropriate at a later time. **No. 2** is incorrect because this couple is probably incapable of seeking out someone to talk or to listen to. They need guidance. If left alone, they may isolate themselves, withdraw, and become depressed. Avoidance (**No. 4**) is nontherapeutic; the problems must be faced eventually. **EV,7,PsI**

92. (4) Lethargy, disorientation, and increased rate and depth of respirations are clinical manifestations of metabolic *acidosis*. As hydrogen ion concentration rises, the central nervous system is depressed, causing the patient to become increasingly lethargic and slower in his or her responses. Likewise, the lungs endeavor to compensate for a metabolic acidosis by increasing both the rate and depth of respirations. Serum bicarbonates provide an estimate of metabolic components of acid-base balance. The level of these ions is controlled by the kidney's ability to secrete hydrogen ions and actively reabsorb bicarbonate ions. Decreased levels of bicarbonate indicate metabolic acidosis, and increased levels of serum bicarbonate indicate metabolic alkalosis. **Nos. 1, 2, and 3** are symptoms of *alkalosis*. **AS,6,PhI**

93. (1) Fluid in the long tube of the suction bottle will cease to fluctuate when the tubing is plugged by fibrin or a clot and/or when negative intrapleural pressures have been reestablished and the lung has reexpanded. The likelihood of lung reexpansion on the second postoperative day is quite small. Therefore, it is necessary to check the tubing for fibrin, clots, or severe kinking. If the tubing is kinked, it needs to be repositioned. Milking of the tube may be ordered if fibrin or clots are suspected. **No. 2** is incorrect because an air leak is indicated by bubbling in the water-sealed suction bottle. Pulmonary edema (**No. 3**) would be reflected in dyspnea, orthopnea, crackles, and pink, frothy sputum. **No. 4** is not entirely incorrect since the patient's position may be such that the chest tubes are unnecessarily looped or kinked and repositioning the patient may facilitate flow; however, it is *not* the *best* answer. **EV,6,SECE**

94. (1) The primary effect of rapid infusion of hyperalimentation solutions is cellular dehydration due to osmosis of water from the cell in response to vascular hyperosmolarity. Occasionally circulatory overload (**No.**

2) does occur, but with hyperglycemia. When infusion rates are rapid, supplementary insulin should be administered to prevent the effects of hyperglycemia. Hypoglycemia (**No. 3**) may occur if the infusion rate is suddenly decreased because the body generally adapts to hyperosmolar solutions by increasing insulin release from the pancreas. However, *hypervolemia,* not hypovolemia, generally occurs. Potassium *depletion,* not excess (**No. 4**), also results. **EV,6,PhI**

95. (4) Expressing sympathy is *least* likely to assist the family to adjust, whereas empathy and understanding *are* effective in providing emotional support to families in crisis. **No. 1** is wrong because the family *may* need to openly communicate their anxiety, fears, and concerns about the baby in order to begin positive coping. **No. 2** is wrong because understanding the treatment being given and the potential for a successful surgical repair *may* aid them in coping with their fears. **No. 3** is wrong because staff attitudes in working with compromised infants *do* affect parental perceptions of the infant. **PL,7,PsI**

96. (1) Nursing measures designed to reduce the occurrence of postthyroidectomy hemorrhage include frequent checks of the dressings and bedclothes under the patient, semi-Fowler's position to prevent hyperextension of the neck, and ice packs to reduce hematoma formation and edema. **No. 2** is partially correct; however, the supine position would increase edema because it prevents gravity drainage of the wound site. **No. 3** is incorrect because coughing will increase stress on the sutures unless the head and neck are well supported, and moist packs tend to increase local blood flow, which in turn tends to increase edema formation in this patient. **No. 4** is incorrect because flexion-like hyperextension puts increased stress on the suture line. **IMP,3,SECE**

97. (1) Anticoagulants increase bleeding time and tendency to hemorrhage. Antihypertensives such as reserpine, hydralazine, and methyldopa potentiate the hypotensive effects of anesthetic agents, thereby creating problems with maintenance of blood pressure. Thiazide diuretics may induce potassium depletion and lead to respiratory depression during anesthesia. **Nos. 2, 3, and 4** are incorrect because neither insulin, digoxin, nor vitamins and minerals potentiate the central nervous system depression due to anesthesia. **EV,1,SECE**

98. (4) Hypoglycemia does inhibit the let-down reflex and interfere with successful breastfeeding. Further, maintaining a stable serum-glucose concentration is important to maternal health. **No. 1** is incorrect because breastfeeding exerts a positive effect on diabetes, reducing blood-sugar levels by transferring glucose from serum to the breast for conversion to lactose; energy is expended in milk production. **No. 2** is wrong because her caloric needs will *increase* with lactation; insulin dosage must be adjusted to maintain optimum serum-glucose levels. **No. 3** is wrong because hypoglycemia jeopardizes both successful breastfeeding and maternal status. **IMP,5,HPM**

99. (3) Before assessing and planning any rehabilitation program, the nurse must *first* assess the patient's and the family's understanding of and attitudes toward myasthenia, as well as their emotional response and coping abilities. *Before* ascertaining any further information about job stresses (**Nos. 1 and 4**) and/or life-style (**No. 2**), any unusual fears, misconceptions, or problems relating to the patient's condition need to be identified and dealt with. It may be necessary to utilize the skills of a psychiatric nurse specialist, health psychologist, or psychiatrist to evaluate the situation and assist in planning interventions. **AS,3,HPM**

100. (2) NPH is an intermediate-acting insulin with an onset time of 2 hours, peak action in 6–12 hours, and a duration of action of 24 hours. **No. 1** is the peak action time for regular insulin. **Nos. 3 and 4** are within the range for long-acting insulins. **IMP,4,PhI**

101. (2) Keeping the foot in the correct anatomic position is the *best* method of preventing footdrop, and a footboard is best when the patient is in traction. A bed cradle (**No. 1**) is effective in keeping pressure off the legs and feet. Passive range of motion (**No. 3**) is most effective in preventing contractures. A trochanter roll (**No. 4**) is most effective in preventing external rotation of the hip. **IMP,3,SECE**

102. (2) The couple is able to perceive events and communicate their concerns, although there is overt tension present. **No. 1** is usually indicated by restlessness and increased alertness. **No. 3** is indicated by an increase in physical symptoms (headaches, nausea, dizziness, etc.) and perceiving only details. **No. 4** is indicated by an inability to communicate or function. **AN,7,PsI**

103. (3) Iopanoic acid (Telepaque) tablets are administered 1 hour after eating a fat-free meal (**No. 1**), one at a time and in 5-minute intervals (**No. 2**), with a minimal amount of water (usually 8 oz) to swallow *all* the tablets. Water is allowed until bedtime (**No. 4**), but food is withheld to allow as much dye as possible to concentrate in the gallbladder. The next morning an initial X ray is taken, after which the patient is given a fatty meal, and several more pictures are taken to observe the functioning of the gallbladder. **PL,4,SECE**

104. (1) Since tracheostomy inhibits the patient from talking, it is essential to establish a mode of postoperative communication so that the patient can express needs. The mode chosen should be communicated to the rest of the staff so that the approach to the patient is consistent. Blood work (**No. 2**) may or may not be ordered before tracheostomy, though blood gas analysis is frequently ordered to establish baseline data in order to evaluate the effectiveness of the intervention. Inserting a Foley catheter (**No. 3**) is not a priority *unless* urinary output has decreased. A standard surgical prep (**No. 4**), cleansing and shaving the operative area, is not done before tracheostomy. However, the physician does cleanse the area with an antiseptic before performing the tracheostomy. **AN,7,PsI**

105. (1) IPPB facilitates the flow of air deep into the lungs by exerting pressures greater than atmospheric pressure (positive pressure) on inspiration. The patient needs to learn to take slow, controlled inspirations to prevent hyperventilation. **Nos. 2, 3, and 4** are incorrect because negative inspiratory pressures are consistent with CPAP or PEEP ventilatory systems, and pressures normally become more negative as the patient exhales. **AN,6,SECE**

106. (3) It is essential that the nurse be readily available to provide physiologic, sociologic, and psychological support when needed. The father has requested assistance; therefore, although privacy (**No. 1**) is important, remaining with the couple to provide support and guidance is paramount. **No. 2** may not be appropriate unless sitting with the couple does not decrease the mother's anxiety. **No. 4** will probably be ineffective. Furthermore, she may need to feel that it is OK to express her feelings, and the nurse should encourage her to be as open as possible. **PL,7,PsI**

107. **(2)** Usually inborn errors of metabolism are autosomal-recessive inherited disorders; that is, if a woman with the disorder has a child with a man who carries the recessive gene, there is a chance for her child to exhibit the disorder. **Nos. 1, 3, and 4** are incorrect, because this disorder is autosomal-*recessive* (individuals carrying the gene are not aware of it until two people with the gene have a child who exhibits the disorder), *not* a *sex*-linked disorder, and not a multifactorial inheritance disorder. **AN,5,PhI**

108. **(3)** The cumulative inflow and outflow records should show an outflow equal to or in excess of the amount instilled. The amount of excess outflow allowed is also determined by the physician; this rarely exceeds 200 mL per cycle. Occasionally, drainage is less than expected. Nursing measures to enhance outflow include turning the patient from side to side, elevating the head of the bed (increases intraabdominal pressures), and/or gently massaging the abdomen. If the problem continues, notify the physician before initiating another cycle; she or he may attempt to clear the catheter by rotation or by probing it for fibrin clots **(No. 2)**. **Nos. 1 and 4** will not improve flow. **IMP,3,SECE**

109. **(2)** The primary purpose of the water-sealed drainage system is to remove excess fluid and air from the pleural space, thereby speeding reinflation of the lung, reestablishing normal negative intrapleural pressure, and preventing the development of pneumothorax in the unaffected lung. Secondarily, water-sealed drainage enables the nurse to monitor blood loss. **Nos. 1 and 3** are incorrect because both effects are the opposite of those intended. **No. 4** is incorrect because atelectasis is caused by insufficient removal of secretions from the bronchial tree. **AN,6,SECE**

110. **(3)** The prevention of scarring is essential. All crusts should be cleaned away as gently as possible, and the area should be cleansed frequently to prevent infection. The infant should be placed on the back or side and minimally restrained to prevent him or her from turning onto the face. The side position is preferred in order to prevent the aspiration of mucus or the regurgitation of milk **(No. 1)**. The infant needs to be repositioned frequently to lessen the danger of hypostatic pneumonia **(No. 2)**. Crying should be minimized as much as possible to avoid unnecessary strain on the suture line **(No. 4)**. **PL,1,SECE**

111. **(3)** Tetany caused by hypocalcemia can be assessed for by briskly tapping the facial nerve, which is located near the middle of the masseter muscle just proximal to the ear lobe (Chvostek's sign). A positive reaction occurs when there is facial-muscle contraction, which includes a twitch of the upper lip on that side. Checking urine-calcium levels **(No. 1)** is not helpful in assessing for early signs of hypocalcemia because urine-calcium levels are dependent not only on parathormone excretion but also on oral intake. **No. 2** describes Homans' sign, which is used to determine the presence of deep-vein thrombosis. **No. 4** is a late sign of hypocalcemia. **AS,2,PhI**

112. **(3)** During treatment (total insertion time varies from 48–144 hours), vaginal discharge may become foul-smelling due to tissue destruction; however, perineal care is generally not allowed due to the danger of dislodging the needles. Frequently, patients find this quite distressing. A douche given under low pressure following removal of the applicator helps to reduce this side effect of therapy. Bladder atony **(No. 1)** is a rare complication; diarrhea, rather than constipation **(No. 2)**, is

more likely to occur. Sexual libido **(No. 4)** following this therapy seems more dependent on the relationship of the partners before therapy than on the therapy itself. **AS,8,SECE**

113. **(1)** Fat-soluble vitamins, particularly vitamin K, are poorly absorbed in the absence of bile. This leads to decreased levels of circulating prothrombin, thus reducing normal clotting and increasing the tendency to bleed. Patients will have a T-tube postoperatively, not a Jackson-Pratt drain **(No. 2)**. Heating pads **(No. 3)** are not used to relieve the abdominal discomfort of cholelithiasis and cholecystitis since they have little effect on reducing spasms of deeper organs. Instead, antispasmodics are used. A high-carbohydrate diet, rather than a low-carbohydrate one **(No. 4)**, would be given to build up glycogen stores in the liver. **AS,6,PhI**

114. **(3)** The single best measure for assessing fluid volume status is daily weights. Significant water loss must occur before there are changes in skin turgor **(No. 1)**. Similarly, blood pressure **(No. 2)** may not reflect changes in fluid volume status if the fluid is sequestered in the interstitial spaces (edema formation). Finally, intake and output measures are important **(No. 4)** but generally do not reflect insensible water losses (water lost per respiration and diaphoresis) and are not always as sensitive to decreases in urine output in chronic renal dysfunction as they are in more acute illnesses. **AS,6,PhI**

115. **(2)** Intrauterine devices (IUDs) are believed to prevent conception. The copper-bearing IUD damages sperm in transit to fallopian tubes. The progesterone-bearing IUD causes progestin-related effects on cervical mucus and endometrial maturation. **No. 1** is incorrect because tubal ligation prevents union of sperm and egg by closing the passage. **No. 3** is wrong because oral contraceptives prevent maturation of the graafian follicle and expulsion of the egg. **No. 4** is wrong because the diaphragm and spermicidal jelly serve as mechanical and chemical barriers to prevent viable sperm from gaining access to the egg. **AN,5,HPM**

116. **(4)** Provide activities the patient enjoys. **No. 1** does not promote intellectual stimulation and may disturb the roommate. Furthermore, the nurse has not validated whether the patient enjoys watching television. **No. 2** is not a recreational activity. The nurse does not yet know whether the patient enjoys board games **(No. 3)**, and they also require a suitable partner. **PL,5,HPM**

117. **(2)** Denial is a very strong defense mechanism used to allay the emotional effects of discovering a potential threat. Although denial has been found to be an effective mechanism for survival in some instances, such as during natural disasters, it may result in greater pathology in a woman with potential breast carcinoma. Suppression **(No. 1)** occurs when the individual recognizes the threat but consciously refuses to think about it. Repression **(No. 3)** is an unconscious mechanism that keeps the knowledge of the threat from coming to one's conscious awareness. Intellectualization **(No. 4)** occurs when the individual attempts to consciously allay anxiety by attributing symptoms to other possible causes, such as cystic breast disease. However, the patient who intellectualizes does not attempt to deny the possibility that a more serious pathology may be present. **AN,7,PsI**

118. **(3)** The patient receiving NPH insulin is most likely to experience a hypoglycemic reaction in the late afternoon. Several factors may be involved, such as increased physical activity or inadequate dietary intake.

Patients should be instructed to carry gumdrops or Life-savers as a source of quickly absorbed carbohydrates should symptoms occur. **Nos. 1, 2, and 4** are not as likely. **AN,4,SECE**

119. **(2)** Symptoms of severe respiratory distress indicate that the tube has dislodged and is obstructing the airway. Reestablishing an airway is the first priority: Deflate the balloons using a syringe. Following deflation, the doctor should be notified to assess the patient's condition and determine ongoing medical therapy. A code blue **(No. 1)** would be called only after establishing the airway. Traction on the Sengstaken-Blakemore tube should be increased or decreased **(No. 3)** only by the attending physician. Iced saline **(No. 4)** is no longer used for irrigation during active bleeding, and this problem is respiratory, not hemorrhagic. **IMP,6,SECE**

120. **(1)** The skin preparation area for hernia repair includes the entire abdomen from just below the nipple line to the mid-thigh. It includes all pubic hair visible when the legs are together, and should extend to the bedline on each side. **No. 2** is an example of an abdominal prep when the incision is above the umbilicus. **No. 3** is a lower-extremities prep for surgeries such as a femoral arterial graft. **No. 4** is a perineal prep used for vaginal or rectal surgeries. **IMP,1,SECE**

121. **(2)** Patients having upper-abdominal surgery tend to breathe shallowly after surgery in order to splint incisional discomfort. Consequently, these patients need both assistance and encouragement to breathe deeply and cough. Splinting of the incisional area by the nurse helps, as well as planning deep breathing and particularly coughing times to follow the administration of a pain reliever. **Nos. 1 and 3** are correct statements but not the best answers. Patients having abdominal surgery tend to guard against coughing as it increases intraabdominal pressures and incisional discomfort. Many people do tend to be thoracic breathers and need to be taught abdominal or diaphragmatic breathing in the preoperative period. **No. 4** is incorrect, because NG tubes do not inhibit deep breathing; rather, they tend to increase oral respirations, which causes drying of the oral mucous membranes. **AN,6,PhI**

122. **(1)** It is important for the couple to be able to rely on each other at this time. They need time to communicate and to begin to cope with their feelings. As long as the mother's vital signs are stable, it may be most therapeutic to allow the father into the recovery room. **No. 2** isolates the father from all significant others. **No. 3** evades the problem and does not alleviate any anxiety. **No. 4** is a physician's decision, and the infant is probably still being worked up and treated at this time. **IMP,7,PsI**

123. **(4)** Intake and output records, as well as daily weights, provide important measures of the effectiveness of the treatment and are good monitors of fluid balance. Urine testing **(No. 1)** is done to detect glycosuria every 4–6 hours. In the event glycosuria occurs, the physician should be notified. The physician may order insulin coverage or a decrease in the flow rate. Blood withdrawal and CVP readings **(No. 2)** are contraindicated because infusion rates must be kept constant to avoid the formation of clots in the catheter. If the catheter insertion site remains dry, dressings are changed every 48 hours utilizing strict aseptic technique, not just clean technique **(No. 3)**. Gloves and masks are used during the dressing change and while the IV tubing and filter are changed. **IMP,6,SECE**

124. **(1)** An iridectomy, or removal of a wedge from the iris, is performed with cataract removal to prevent the forward push of the aqueous humor from blocking the canal of Schlemm, which would produce a secondary glaucoma. Iridectomy does not affect pupillary dilatation **(No. 2)**, facilitate retinal circulation **(No. 3)**, or prevent corneal scarring **(No. 4)**. **IMP,2,SECE**

125. **(4)** In a closed chest drainage system (Pleur-evac), the first chamber collects the drainage from the patient's chest, the second chamber provides the water seal to reestablish negative pressure, and the third chamber is attached to the suction. **No. 1** is incorrect because the third chamber establishes the suction and the first chamber collects the drainage. **No. 2** is incorrect because it is the third chamber that is associated with the suction, not the first and second. **No. 3** is incorrect because the self-sealing diaphragm for drainage sampling is in the first chamber. **AN,1,SECE**

126. **(3)** Women should be instructed to contact the clinic doctor or nurse if they have leg cramps or headaches (signs of possible thrombophlebitis caused by the hypercoagulability that occurs under estrogen/progesterone stimulation). **No. 1** is incorrect because mild to moderate nonpathologic nausea may occur during the first few days on oral contraceptives as the body adjusts to the elevated hormone levels. **No. 2** is wrong because chloasma, the "mask of pregnancy," is merely hyperpigmentation related to the high hormone levels. **No. 4** is wrong because breast tenderness and weight gain are nonpathologic and are associated with an increased tendency to retain fluid in the interstitial spaces. **AN,1,HPM**

127. **(3)** Maintenance of an adequate airway is always the primary goal of nursing care. Respiratory obstruction is a very serious complication; therefore it is wise to have both an emergency tracheostomy set and suctioning apparatus available at the bedside of the patient who has had a thyroidectomy. **No. 1** is also correct, but it is not the best answer since the onset of this complication is more gradual. With adequate nursing observation, it can be handled before it becomes life-threatening. **No. 2** is incorrect because thoracentesis is utilized to remove excess fluid from the *pleural* space. The correct nursing strategy for postoperative bleeding **(No. 4)** is to notify the *physician immediately*. **PL,6,SECE**

128. **(3)** Proper handling of sputum is essential to allay droplet transference of bacilli in the air. Patients need to be taught to cover their nose and mouth with tissues when sneezing or coughing. Chemotherapy generally renders the patient noninfectious within days to a few weeks, usually before cultures for tubercle bacilli are negative. Until chemical isolation is established, many institutions require the patient to wear a mask when visitors are in the room or when the nurse is in attendance. Patients should be in a well-ventilated room, without air recirculation, to prevent air contamination. **Nos. 1, 2, and 4** are unnecessary precautions. **IMP,1,SECE**

129. **(2)** He is attempting to cope with his anxiety by denying reality. He may also be angry **(No. 1)**, but his behavior and verbalization indicate denial. It is through the use of denial that he is displacing the blame **(No. 3)**, so denial is the more appropriate answer. He is unable to think clearly enough to seek any type of intervention **(No. 4)**; he is reacting rather than problem solving. **AN,7,PsI**

130. **(3)** The initial response would be to notify the physician of the critical hemoglobin (oxygen-carrying pro-

tein) level. A hemoglobin of 10 is desirable for the patient, decreasing the deleterious risks of general anesthetic and hypovolemic shock. The lab slip is then attached to the chart (**No. 1**). Most likely a blood transfusion will be ordered before surgery (**No. 2**), but there is no order yet. The nurse's actions will be charted on the nurse's notes (**No. 4**), but charting is *not* the *first* priority. **AN,6,PhI**

131. (**3**) Methyldopa acts to decrease blood pressure by inhibiting the formation of dopamine, thus decreasing the amount of norepinephrine that is secreted in adrenergic synapses. Decreased adrenergic stimulation results in decreased vasoconstriction, which causes peripheral vascular resistance. **No. 1** is an example of the effects of hydralazine; **No. 2**, of guanethidine SO_4; and **No. 4**, of diazepam. **IMP,6,PhI**

132. (**2**) New parents, especially parents of infants with health problems, may need help focusing on what is normal and healthy in their infant. Discussing how their baby compares with other infants and focusing on the baby's strengths will help parents to focus on these important aspects of development. To tell this mother that her baby has a "life-threatening illness" (**No. 1**) could be very frightening and not at all helpful to her at this time. False reassurance (**No. 3**) and stating you "know how she feels" (**No. 4**) are also not therapeutic responses. **IMP,7,PsI**

133. (**2**) Sitting the patient up allows for deeper ventilation, and splinting of the incisional area reduces incisional discomfort. **No. 1** is also correct but not specific enough. Generally 20–30 minutes should elapse before instituting coughing techniques following administration of an analgesic, to allow for the full effects of the drug. **No. 3** is incorrect unless the patient is in a good deal of pain; if so, the patient should be medicated, then coughed. **No. 4** is incorrect because oral intake is withheld until bowel activity is reestablished. Secretions can be kept mobilized by frequent turning and deep breathing. **IMP,6,SECE**

134. (**2**) The legs of the patient undergoing vein-stripping are wrapped from foot to groin with elastic bandages. Anticoagulants (**No. 1**) are not routinely ordered following surgery, although analgesics will be ordered for pain. Sitting in a chair (**No. 3**) is contraindicated because the pressure this position exerts behind the knees and at the hips impedes venous return and increases dependent venous pressures. **No. 4** is incorrect because the patient is usually ambulated the day of vein-stripping surgery to enhance venous return by way of muscle contraction. **PL,1,SECE**

135. (**3**) The primary goal is to prepare the new mother with diabetes to care for her infant while effectively managing her disease. **No. 1** is incorrect because it will not ensure adequate home health maintenance of mother and infant. **No. 2** is incorrect because potential problems will vary, depending on many factors such as maternal age, and it does not address the primary health maintenance goal. **No. 4** is incorrect because, although follow-up care is an important aspect of discharge teaching, it is subsumed under the broader goal of discussing coping strategies for managing diabetes. **PL,1,HPM**

136. (**2**) Postoperative inflammation and edema underlie the frequent occurrence of scrotal swelling after indirect hernia repair. This complication is very painful, and any movement by the patient results in discomfort. Elevating the scrotum on rolled towels or providing support with a suspensory helps to reduce edema.

Ice bags facilitate pain relief. **No. 1** is inappropriate, as this is not an emergency side effect of surgery. Pain medication (**No. 3**) may also be administered, but vigorous coughing (**No. 4**) is contraindicated following herniorrhaphy. **IMP,3,SECE**

137. (**4**) The first nursing measure should be to mark the time and the amount of drainage in the collection bottle to ensure a baseline measurement for further observations. The milking of chest tubes (**No. 1**) is a matter of debate at this time. Although the process of stripping or milking does assist in the removal of fibrin and clots from the chest tubes, compression of the tubes also increases intrapleural pressures by preventing the movement of air and fluid. Whether the chest tubes are milked or not will depend on institutional or individual physician's policies. **No. 2** is incorrect because the drainage system is always kept in a dependent position to maintain gravity flow of air and fluids. The nurse's next measure is to secure the tubes to the bed linen (**No. 3**) to prevent kinking or unnecessary looping of the drainage tubes, which would hinder the flow of air and fluid. **IMP,6,SECE**

138. (**2**) Respiratory obstruction, hemorrhage, tetany, and laryngeal nerve injury are the major complications following thyroid surgery. *Hypocalcemia,* not hypercalcemia (**No. 1**), is a complication resulting from damage to the parathyroid glands during surgery. Serum T_4 will be *decreased* or absent, *not* elevated (**No. 3**), and the patient will need replacement therapy because no thyroid hormone is secreted once the total thyroid gland is removed. **No. 4** is not a good answer. Since the integrity of the gastrointestinal tract is not interrupted during thyroid surgery, paralytic ileus is a *rare* complication. **AN,3,PhI**

139. (**1**) Universal precautions specify that all health care providers should wear gloves until all blood and amniotic fluid have been removed. Since transmission of the virus may occur via breast milk, breastfeeding is discouraged (**No. 2**). **Nos. 3 and 4** are incorrect because the parents are encouraged to bond with the child and the nurse needs to support all positive parental feelings. **IMP,1,SECE**

140. (**4**) This couple is experiencing an actual loss and will probably exhibit many of the same symptoms as a person who has lost someone to death. **Nos. 1, 2, and 3** will most likely occur at some later time. **EV,7,PsI**

141. (**1**) The purpose of the T-tube is to maintain the patency of the bile duct after surgery. Localized edema in the surgery area tends to obstruct the outflow of bile, which is continuously being synthesized by the liver. The T-tube does not directly prevent postoperative hemorrhage (**No. 2**) or postoperative wound infection (**No. 3**). A secondary effect of this procedure is that bile flow is directed away from the duodenum (**No. 4**). **AN,4,PhI**

142. (**1**) Anxiety, like pain, glucose imbalance, or changes in blood pressure, stimulates discharge of the sympathetic nervous system. In some patients this increased adrenergic discharge results in moderate to severe increases in systolic and diastolic pressures that decrease to normal levels when emotional equilibrium is restored. The patient may be emotionally labile (**No. 2**), but at this time there are insufficient data to make this judgment. She is fearful, but that does not mean she is unprepared for this surgery (**No. 3**). Should her anxiety remain high, however, the attending physician should be notified. Though the patient may be attempting to employ denial (**No. 4**), her emotional response

(restlessness and increased blood pressure) indicates this defense mechanism is ineffective in allaying her present anxieties **(No. 4)**. **EV,7,PsI**

143. **(2)** The diet of a cirrhotic patient should provide ample protein for tissue repair, at least 0.5 g/lb. Some modification occurs *if* serum-ammonia levels are elevated **(No. 1)**. Sufficient carbohydrate intake is needed to sustain weight and prevent proteins from being utilized for energy, *not for the reason* stated in **No. 3**. **No. 4** is partially correct. Salt is restricted to assist in decreasing edema formation. However, the reason for high-carbohydrate foods is as discussed above. Fluids may also be restricted to 1000–1500 mL/d. Vitamin supplements, particularly fat-soluble vitamins (A, D, and K), are usually prescribed because of decreased bile production for their absorption and because of the inability of the liver to store them successfully. Initially, if the patient has a very poor appetite, liquid protein supplements such as Sustagen may be given. Frequent, small feedings may also increase intake. **PL,4,PhI**

144. **(3)** Neomycin is administered preoperatively because it is a poorly absorbed antibiotic and therefore is effective in reducing the number of intestinal organisms that may cause infection of the suture line. Neomycin is not effective in reducing postoperative atelectasis **(No. 1)**. Prevention of atelectasis is dependent on adequate pulmonary hygiene (deep breathing and coughing up of secretions) in the postoperative period. **No. 2** is correct, but it is not the *best* answer, because the ability of the body to ward off infection is a result of the decrease in intestinal organisms. **No. 4** is incorrect because bladder atony is generally due to decreased parasympathetic outflow and bladder tone secondary to anesthesia. **AN,8,PhI**

145. **(4)** Frequent, small meals do not visually overwhelm the patient and they require less energy for ingestion. Because patients with cirrhosis frequently have very poor appetites, the nurse may have to be very creative in approaches to ensure adequate nutritional intake. **Nos. 1, 2, and 3** take the responsibility away from the patient and increase his or her dependency. **IMP,4,PsI**

146. **(2)** Postoperatively, deep breathing and particularly coughing up of sputum are the most important activities engaged in by the patient after chest surgery. These activities reduce bronchotracheal secretions, prevent atelectasis, and promote adequate ventilation. Although **Nos. 1 and 3** are also important in preventing postoperative complication, airway integrity is always the *first* priority. **No. 4** is employed for patients having herniorrhaphies. **IMP,6,SECE**

147. **(3)** Although most patients are able to rest more comfortably and even sleep after administration of a narcotic, extreme or prolonged lethargy indicates that the medication dose may be too large. The physician should be consulted for both a change of dose and/or route of administration **(Nos. 1 and 2)**. Alternative modes of pain relief can and should be instituted if the patient's discomfort is not severe, but not as a delaying tactic **(No. 4)** when the issue is the appropriateness of a specific medication dose. **IMP,2,PhI**

148. **(3)** Postoperatively the cataract patient may be placed in a flat or low Fowler's position on the back or turned to the unoperated side. Turning the patient to the operated side **(No. 4)** or raising the head of the bed **(No. 1)** increases the stress on the sutures and may lead to hemorrhage. The patient may assume a prone position with the head turned to the unoperated side **(No. 2)**, though most patients find a side-lying position more comfortable. **PL,2,SECE**

149. **(1)** The woman must understand that, although the "fertile" period is approximately mid-cycle, hormonal variations do occur and can result in early or late ovulations. To be effective, the diaphragm should be inserted prior to every intercourse. **No. 2** is incorrect because the diaphragm must be left in place for a minimum of 6 hours after intercourse. Premature removal may permit passage of viable sperm. **No. 3** is incorrect because marked variations in weight may result in the need for a larger or smaller appliance. **No. 4** is wrong because pin holes in the diaphragm may permit viable sperm to pass the barrier. **EV,5,HPM**

150. **(4)** Normally drainage from the T-tube averages 300–500 mL during the first few days after surgery and then gradually decreases; the tube is generally removed in 7–10 days. By the fourth postoperative day, flow has usually begun to decrease. Excessive drainage at this time should be reported as it indicates possible reobstruction of the duct. **Nos. 1, 2, and 3** are normal postoperative findings. **AN,6,PhI**

151. **(1)** After a settling-in period, the toddler experiencing separation anxiety may enter the phase of "denial," covering up painful feelings toward parents and seeming to turn instead to others, such as the nurse. Although it may seem like the toddler is doing fine **(No. 3)**, she is actually denying feelings that are too painful to deal with just now. At her age, she is not trying to make her mother jealous **(No. 4)**; neither does she need discipline **(No. 2)**. **AN,5,HPM**

152. **(4)** It is essential that the couple be prepared for what they will see. However, it is equally as important for them to be able to see, touch, and hold their infant as soon as possible, to begin the attachment process. **No. 1** merely delays the couple's seeing their infant. The nurse continually assesses the parents' readiness while caring for the infant. Parents *do* need some preparation prior to seeing their infant **(No. 2)**. Teaching without immediate parent-child contact can increase the parents' anxiety **(No. 3)**. **PL,7,PsI**

153. **(2)** After explaining the procedure to the patient, the nurse should first instruct the patient to void. This prevents accidental nicking or perforation of the bladder during the procedure. The patient is positioned in a chair or in high Fowler's position in bed **(No. 1)**, after the vital signs have been taken to establish baseline information **(No. 3)** and the abdomen is prepared **(No. 4)**. **IMP,6,PhI**

154. **(2)** The stoma drainage bag is applied in the operating room. Drainage from the ileostomy contains secretions that are rich in digestive enzymes and highly irritating to the skin. Protection of the skin from the effects of these enzymes is begun at once. Skin exposed to these enzymes even for a short time becomes reddened, painful, and excoriated. **Nos. 1, 3, and 4** are incorrect because they would result in skin irritation. **IMP,8,SECE**

155. **(2)** Chronic renal failure symptomatology is due to a decrease in the number of functioning nephrons, with resultant decrease in glomerular filtration due to the extension of the disease process. **No. 1** is incorrect because the cause of the renal failure was likely related to intrarenal damage from acute glomerulonephritis. **Nos. 3 and 4** are incorrect because the patient has moved from the second stage of chronic kidney disease (renal insufficiency, characterized by water diuresis and mild azotemia) to renal failure, which is characterized by acidosis, marked electrolyte imbalances, fluid

retention, anemia, and increases in serum urea, uric acid, and creatinine. **AN,8,PhI**

156. **(3)** Manipulation of abdominal contents during surgery produces inhibition of peristalsis for 24–48 hours. Measures to avoid potential distention could include insertion of a nasogastric tube before surgery and continuous postsurgical suction until peristalsis returns; rectal tubes can be inserted to remove excess air in the lower colon; and early ambulation promotes return of gastrointestinal functioning. Auscultation of the abdomen for return of bowel sounds **(No. 1)** will be necessary in assessing the return and degree of peristalsis. Abdominal massage is *not* recommended **(No. 2)**. *When* bowel sounds return, oral intake **(No. 4)** may be started. **PL,1,SECE**

157. **(4)** Immediately following a death, the nurse must assess and validate the family's needs for follow-up care. It is important to look at their past ability to cope with stress, how effective these coping mechanisms were, and so forth. However, initially the family will be unable to communicate their feelings and perceptions due to their high level of anxiety. **No. 1** may be necessary if the family is unable to cope effectively with their anxiety. **No. 2** would depend on the individual family's needs. **No. 3** may be appropriate once the family is able to communicate their feelings and needs. **PL,7,PsI**

158. **(4)** If all the secondary measures have been tried and the patient's bladder is distended, the physician should be notified if he or she has not left a catheterization order. Occasionally, drugs such as neostigmine bromide (Prostigmin) are ordered to stimulate bladder contractions before resorting to catheterization. **No. 1** will only tire the patient more. Catheters should not be inserted without an order **(No. 2)**, nor should the patient be unduly fatigued by continuing to try other measures **(No. 3)** that most likely were unsuccessful prior to this point in time. The bladder should not be allowed to become overdistended. **IMP,8,SECE**

159. **(2)** Hypotension and shock can occur during or after paracentesis. Fluid from the vascular compartment shifts into the abdomen to replace fluids that are withdrawn. This complication can be minimized if withdrawal of ascitic fluid is limited to 1000 mL and/or if lost fluid is replaced by administration of salt-poor albumin. To assess for this complication, vital signs are taken every 15 minutes during the procedure and afterward until stable, then every hour for 4 hours. Disequilibrium **(No. 1)** occurs with rapid removal of wastes during renal dialysis. Hypoalbuminuria (no protein in urine) is a normal physical finding; therefore **No. 3** is incorrect. Paralytic ileus **(No. 4)** is rarely a complication of this procedure. **AN,6,PhI**

160. **(2)** Local radiation is generally used under four conditions: The tumor is relatively well defined, a larger dose of radiation can be delivered than by an external source, there is a critical need to reduce involvement of other tissue, and the site is accessible for introduction of seeds or implants. As a result of cobalt implantation, diarrhea may occur due to radiation-induced toxicosis of the mucous membranes of the large bowel. Diarrhea may be painful as well as profuse and bloody. **No. 1** is incorrect because the rationale for doing an implant is that the tumor is generally well defined. The effects of severe diarrhea may indeed be electrolyte imbalance **(No. 3)**, but this is not the cause in this situation. **No. 4** may indeed be occurring, but is not the basis for the patient's present symptoms. **AN,3,PhI**

161. **(3)** In early respiratory obstruction, the patient generally complains of a feeling of fullness or a choking sensation. Swallowing difficulties are fairly common due to tracheal irritation; however, difficulty in swallowing in conjunction with a choking sensation is indicative of airway obstruction. **No. 1**, hoarseness and weakness of the voice, is common and is secondary to edema of the larynx. **No. 2**, stridor and cyanosis, is a late sign of airway obstruction. **No. 4**, disorientation and combative behaviors, is indicative of severe anoxia. **AS,6,SECE**

162. **(3)** Hypoglycemic or insulin reactions are the result of decreased circulatory serum glucose to the brain. This stimulates epinephrine release. Early symptoms include cold, clammy skin, nervousness, tremors, numbness of the hands or around the lips, and cardiac palpitations. Later symptoms may mimic alcoholic intoxication, such as staggering gait, slurring of words, combative behavior, or uncontrolled weeping. As hypoglycemia deepens, the patient may develop convulsions and coma. **Nos. 1, 2, and 4** are symptoms of ketoacidosis, which acts to depress the central nervous system. **AS,4,PhI**

163. **(3)** Bending to adjust shoelaces would increase intraocular pressures and should therefore be *avoided* during the early postoperative period; the ambulating client should wear slip-on shoes or slippers to avoid bending or stooping. Other activities to avoid include coughing, brushing the teeth, shaving, and vomiting. Self-feeding **(No. 1)** *is* encouraged, to help reduce the patient's perception of helplessness, though food may need to be cut up for the patient to reduce exertion. Self-dressing **(No. 2)** and ambulation **(No. 4)** *are* permitted. **IMP,2,HPM**

164. **(4)** Bearing down is too strenuous for the pregnant cardiac patient. **No. 1** is incorrect because relaxation in a semirecumbent position reduces the workload on the heart. **No. 2** is wrong because frequent monitoring may help identify increased pulse rate as an early sign of cardiac decompensation. **No. 3** is wrong because regional anesthesia *reduces* pain and the physiologic response to pain, which may cause cardiac decompensation. It also pools blood in the lower extremities, thereby preventing the rapid increase in cardiac output that immediately follows birth. **AN,6,HPM**

165. **(4)** The rationale for turning, coughing, and deep breathing every 1–2 hours is to rid the lungs of the side effects of anesthesia. Inhalant anesthetics, like cigarette smoke, irritate the mucous membranes lining the bronchi, increasing mucous production. It is exceedingly important that the patient understand that these activities are important in mobilizing and removing these excess secretions. Failure to remove them may lead to atelectasis or hypostatic pneumonias. **Nos. 1, 2, and 3** are all appropriate interventions. **PL,6,SECE**

166. **(4)** Increased circulating levels of uric acid, an end product of purine metabolism, are responsible for the patient's goutlike joint discomfort. Thus the diet will exclude foods high in purines (e.g., high-protein foods, organ meats). Hyperphosphatemia does occur in the third stage of chronic kidney disease. Normally this would stimulate the parathyroid gland to increase parathormone, thus raising calcium levels and lowering phosphate **(No. 1)**. However, in chronic renal failure the kidney fails to produce a metabolite of vitamin D, which effectively reduces parathormone activity, lowering serum-calcium levels. Amphogel (an aluminum hydroxide preparation) is given to bind the phosphate excreted in the bowel **(No. 1)**. Dialysis is used to decrease the serum-creatinine level, which causes central

nervous system depression (**No. 2**). Joint pain is usually related to inflammation or trauma rather than decreased activity level. Increasing activity (**No. 3**) might aggravate the pain. **AN,4,PhI**

167. (**3**) Respiratory depression is a cardinal sign of magnesium toxicity. **No. 1** is incorrect because individual variations in respiratory depression are observed at the same serum-magnesium level. **No. 2** is incorrect because respiratory compromise normally precedes depressed cardiac function and is a late sign of magnesium toxicity. **No. 4** is incorrect because, although decreased peristalsis can occur with a magnesium infusion, it is not the most important assessment to make. **AS,1,PhI**

168. (**2**) Pyridoxine (vitamin B₆) 25–50 mg a day is ordered prophylactically to prevent symptoms of peripheral neuritis. Serious side effects of INH therapy are rare. **Nos. 1, 3, and 4** have no effect on peripheral neuritis. **IMP,4,PhI**

169. (**1**) Urinary retention following spinal anesthesia is due to blockage of autonomic nervous system fibers, which innervate the bladder and sensory perception. **No. 2**, though correct, is not as complete as No. 1. All patients secrete ADH postoperatively because of the surgical insult. However, ADH reduces the volume of urine (**No. 3**), as does lowered blood pressure (**No. 4**), but neither causes urinary retention. **AN,8,SECE**

170. (**1**) Sitting for long periods of time and wearing constrictive clothing tend to increase pelvic congestion. Daily bowel movements (**No. 2**) are not necessary as long as a normal pattern is achieved. It is important to reinforce the physician's instructions that sexual activity may be resumed within a specific period of time, usually 6–8 weeks. Six months (**No. 3**) is too long. Paced and gradual ambulation aids in increasing venous return and general strength. Complete avoidance of chores for 2 months (**No. 4**) is not necessary. Lifting of heavy objects, however, may injure the incision site and promote bleeding. **IMP,1,SECE**

171. (**2**) Absence of variability (a smooth baseline) is an ominous sign of potential fetal distress. It can result from fetal hypoxia and acidosis and certain drugs that depress the central nervous system. A baseline range of 110–160 bpm is within normal limits (**No. 1**). Early decelerations (from head compression) are of no clinical significance (**No. 3**). Mild variable decelerations are usually remedied by changing the woman's position (**No. 4**). **EV,6,SECE**

172. (**2**) Elevation of the foot of the bed enhances venous return and reduces edema by utilizing the force of gravity. Pain is decreased (**No. 1**) as the edema is reduced. **No. 3** is incorrect because raising the foot of the bed should not greatly affect arterial blood flow. Reducing edema is what makes the patient more comfortable (**No. 4**). **IMP,6,SECE**

173. (**3**) Postoperatively the potential for severe fluid and electrolyte imbalances exists for several reasons: (a) the ileostomy drainage contains large amounts of sodium and water, (b) postsurgical diuresis increases both water and potassium excretion, and (c) nasogastric suction further decreases fluid and electrolytes by preventing their normal reabsorption. **Nos. 1, 2, and 4** are also important measures in this patient's postoperative care; however, maintenance of fluid and electrolyte balance is most critical. **PL,8,SECE**

174. (**3**) Crying is an appropriate, expected, and natural response. **Nos. 1, 2, and 4** all invade the woman's need for privacy at this time. **IMP,7,PsI**

175. (**2**) The T-tube is clamped prior to eating to increase bile flow into the duodenum and assist in the digestion of fats. **No. 1** is incorrect because the act of eating normally stimulates bile secretion, and clamping of the T-tube will not inhibit its flow except to the dependent drainage bag. **No. 3** is incorrect because bile does not affect peristalsis, although inadequate bile flow can result in abdominal distention. **No. 4** is also correct, though it is not the best answer. If the patient is able to tolerate clamping of the T-tube, then bile is flowing normally into the duodenum and the duct is patent. **IMP,4,SECE**

176. (**1**) Increased serum potassium (hyperkalemia) causes the T waves to lose their normal, rounded configuration and become more pointy or peaked (the difference in shape between a mountain and a mound); therefore **No. 2** is incorrect. ST segments are not significantly affected by this electrolyte imbalance (**Nos. 3 and 4**). **AS,6,PhI**

177. (**1**) Severe, crampy, intermittent pain accompanies the progressive telescoping of the bowel wall found in intussusception; as this progresses, the stools become bloody and full of mucus ("currant jelly"). An olive-shaped mass in the right upper quadrant and projectile vomiting (**No. 2**) are found in pyloric stenosis. Obstinate constipation and increasing abdominal girth (**No. 3**) are found in Hirschsprung's disease. Excess mucus and abdominal distention (**No. 4**) are found in tracheoesophageal fistula. **AS,8,PhI**

178. (**2**) Hypotension and shock can occur during or after paracentesis. Fluid from the vascular compartment shifts into the abdomen to replace fluids that are withdrawn. This complication can be minimized if withdrawal of ascitic fluid is limited to 1000 mL and/or if lost fluid is replaced by administration of salt-poor albumin. To assess for this complication, vital signs are taken every 15 minutes during the procedure and afterward until stable, then every hour for 4 hours. **Nos. 1, 3, and 4** are incorrect amounts. **AN,6,PhI**

179. (**2**) After the patient has left for surgery, family members should be told the approximate time the patient will be in surgery and that from there the patient will go to the recovery room until awake and all vital signs are stable. Clarify that delays may occur and that the induction of, as well as the emergence from, anesthesia takes time. **Nos. 1 and 3** are incorrect because family members should be allowed to decide whether they will stay or go and come back later. If family members decide to wait, direct them to a waiting area where they can be comfortable. Assure them that you will direct the surgeon to them after the surgery is finished. **No. 4** is not an initial action. The nurse does answer any questions and/or concerns the family members may have, being as supportive as possible. **IMP,7,PsI**

180. (**1**) Patients should be informed that the cataract glasses will magnify objects; this not only causes distortions in the shape of an object but also may result in color distortions. The spatial changes that result from these lenses may cause the patient to underreach for an object or have difficulty walking and climbing stairs. Peripheral vision is decreased (**No. 2**), so the patient needs to be taught to turn the head and utilize the central vision provided by the lenses. **Nos. 3 and 4** are incorrect because the magnification created by these lenses (up to 35%) is not similar to the size perception before the cataract formed, nor do they cause double vision. **IMP,2,SECE**

181. (3) An immediate response to the choking sensation is assessment of the surgical site by examining under the dressing. If the area appears edematous, loosen the dressing and have someone remain with the patient. Elevating the head to a high Fowler's position (**No. 1**), though the preferred position for improving ventilation of the lung, will not reduce upper-airway obstruction. **No. 2** is inappropriate for this situation and may actually increase the patient's distress. Notify the physician (**No. 4**), who might order the sutures or clips to be removed, *after* assessing the surgical site. **IMP,6,SECE**

182. (2) This patient's blood gases indicate mild acidosis. pH is still within normal limits. **No. 1** is incorrect because the remaining functional nephrons and the lungs have been able to compensate for the increase in circulating hydrogen ions. If respiratory alkalosis (**No. 3**) were the underlying pathology, the pH would demonstrate alkalosis (pH above 7.40). **No. 4** is incorrect because the patient does have respiratory alkalosis, but it represents respiratory compensation rather than the primary pathologic mechanism. **AN,6,PhI**

183. (1) The earliest clinical signs of bleeding include restlessness, pallor, tachycardia, and cooling of the skin. These symptoms occur as the result of vasoconstriction (increased sympathetic stimulation) in order to maintain venous return and cardiac output. **No. 2** represents symptoms of ketoacidosis. When the vasoconstrictive mechanisms discussed above are no longer effective, the blood pressure begins to fall (**No. 3**). It is essential to identify bleeding early because liver cells are very susceptible to ischemia. **No. 4** may occur with increases in intracranial pressure. **AS,6,PhI**

184. (3) The mother *is* communicating her feelings of distress at seeing her physiologically compromised son. **No. 1** is wrong because interference with the bonding process may affect later parenting. **No. 2** is wrong because the mother is demonstrating her inability to cope with the situation at present. **No. 4** is wrong because the family system is unable to meet the neonate's emotional needs at present due to being overwhelmed by their own reactions to the baby. **AN,7,PsI**

185. (2) Symptoms of circulatory overload result from varying degrees of cardiac decompensation, with blood backing up into the pulmonary (moist crackles) and systemic circuits (neck vein distention, dependent edema, periorbital edema, and hepatomegaly). Symptoms of circulatory *failure* or hypovolemia include apprehension, soft eyeballs, flattened neck veins, shock, decreased pulse pressure, and poor skin turgor (**Nos. 1, 3, and 4**). **AS,6,PhI**

186. (2) Given the patient's complaint and evidence of pink drainage, the nurse should suspect dehiscence. Dehiscence is characterized by a gush of pink serous drainage and a parting of the wound edges. Dehiscence generally occurs in the fifth to seventh day following surgery, due to increased intraabdominal pressures from flatus, coughing, retching, or inadequate tissue support. Late hemorrhage (**No. 1**) would be accompanied by signs of shock such as decreased blood pressure, rapid pulse, and diaphoresis. Wound infection (**No. 3**) would be characterized by pain, redness, and fever. Evisceration (**No. 4**) occurs after dehiscence when loops of intestine escape through the opened incision. **AN,1,PhI**

187. (3) It is important for all health team members to be in touch with their feelings about death and dying in order to help the family work through *their* feelings. **Nos. 1 and 2** may help the nurse teach the family to express their feelings, but No. 3 is still primary. **No. 4** is inappropriate because suppression may lead to avoidance and to the ineffective resolution of feelings. **PL,7,PsI**

188. (3) The Sengstaken-Blakemore tube is a triple-lumen tube composed of a catheter that goes to the stomach for suctioning, a lumen that ends in a gastric balloon, and a lumen that ends in an esophageal balloon. The *primary* purpose of this tube is to stop bleeding by applying pressure to the cardiac portion of the stomach and against the esophageal varices. Thus, **No. 1** is only partially correct. The *secondary* purposes of the tube are (a) to prevent accumulation of blood in the gastrointestinal tract (**No. 2**), which could precipitate hepatic coma, and (b) to reduce blood transfusion requirements (**No. 4**). **PL,6,SECE**

189. (3) Once the uterus is removed, the woman is infertile and contraception is *not* necessary. **Nos. 1, 2, and 4** *should* be included in the teaching plan. Following a hysterectomy, the vaginal flow is usually brownish in nature and will gradually diminish and cease. If the flow continues and is obviously red in nature, the physician must be notified. These signs could indicate a bleeding vessel. Menses will be absent following removal of the uterus. **IMP,5,HPM**

190. (1) Following clamping of the T-tube, observe the patient for signs of abdominal distress, pain, nausea, chills, or fever. These symptoms may be due to a localized reaction to the bile, edema, or obstructed flow. Severe abdominal pain may indicate leakage of bile into the peritoneal cavity. Eructation (**No. 2**) or burping may occur after eating if bile flow was insufficient. Jaundice (**No. 3**) is a late symptom of biliary obstruction. An increased respiratory rate (**No. 4**) may occur if the patient has abdominal discomfort, pain, or nausea. **AS,3,PhI**

191. (3) Since tubercle bacilli multiply very slowly, and since antitubercular drugs are bacteriostatic, not bactericidal, the patient must continue therapy for at least 2 years to allow time for the body's defenses to contain the organisms. Six months (**No. 1**) would be insufficient treatment. Individuals who have been inspected for tuberculosis but who do not have evidence of active disease are treated prophylactically with INH for a 1-year period (**No. 2**). **No. 4** is an excessive length of time. **IMP,1,SECE**

192. (2) Space-occupying lesions and pneumonia tend to decrease vital capacity by reducing inspiratory capacity. In order to maintain arterial oxygen levels, the respiratory rate is increased, which results in excess CO_2 excretion by the lungs (respiratory alkalosis). It is important to remember that patients can be hypoxic ($\downarrow PO_2$) but not hypercapnic ($\uparrow CO_2$—respiratory acidosis) because of the facility with which carbon dioxide passes through the respiratory membrane. **No. 1** is incorrect because the patient's pathology tends to decrease, *not* increase, vital capacity. The total lung capacity (**No. 3**) is usually increased with the hyperinflation of obstructive airway disease. Even though the patient has an extensive smoking history, neither the health history nor the physical assessment findings indicate hyperinflation (chronic cough, barrel chest). **No. 4** is partially correct and partially incorrect. With extensive rhonchi and wheezes, the nurse would expect a slight to moderate decrease in the forced expiratory volume in 1 second (FEV_1); however, the respiratory rate and lack of other symptoms (lethargy, easy fatigue) tend to contradict the occurrence of respiratory acidosis. **EV,6,PhI**

193. **(2)** The nurse must meet the parents at their level of readiness while at the same time providing them with enough information to allow them to care adequately for the infant. Sucking needs to be *avoided* in an infant with a cleft palate because of the possibility of aspiration and because the infant will not be allowed to suck postoperatively **(No. 1)**. A special nipple or feeder is helpful, such as Lamb's nipple or Brecht feeder. The infant should be fed in an *upright* position to decrease the likelihood of aspiration **(No. 3)**. The infant needs to be isolated *only* from those individuals with *infectious* diseases such as colds or chickenpox **(No. 4)**. The infant should be treated as normally as possible to stimulate growth and development. **IMP,4,HPM**

194. **(2)** Withdrawal of the penis prior to orgasm is not reliable as a method of birth control because fluid containing semen, stored in the prostate or Cowper's glands, may release viable sperm around or into the vaginal canal before ejaculation. **No. 1** is incorrect because the rhythm method of birth control requires avoiding intercourse around the time of ovulation (approximately 14 days *prior* to next menses). **No. 3** is incorrect because spermicidal jellies are most effective when used in *conjunction* with the barrier diaphragm. **No. 4** is wrong because *oral* contraceptives provide the most effective modern method of contraception when used appropriately. **EV,5,HPM**

195. **(1)** Decreases in body fluids lead to dryness of mucous membranes and softness of eyeballs. Weight loss and decreased urinary output would also be present. **No. 2** is incorrect because hemoglobin and hematocrit are elevated due to hemoconcentration. **No. 3** is incorrect because the pulse *elevates* to increase blood flow to vital organs; and crackles and dyspnea **(No. 4)** would be present in fluid *overload.* **AS,6,PhI**

196. **(1)** A scaphoid-shaped abdomen suggests a diaphragmatic hernia. The newborn abdomen should have a symmetric, slightly rounded contour. Diaphragmatic hernia is the most urgent of the neonatal emergencies. The abdominal viscera are in the thoracic cavity. If extensive, the viscera in the thoracic cavity during embryonic life prevent the normal development of pulmonary tissue. **No. 2** is incorrect because a normal newborn abdomen should have a symmetric, slightly rounded contour. Imperforate anus does not manifest with a scaphoid-shaped abdomen **(No. 3)**. **No. 4** is incorrect because gastroschisis is an abdominal wall defect at the base of the umbilical stalk, and omphalocele is a congenital defect resulting from failure of the abdominal wall or muscles to close and leads to herniation of abdominal contents through the navel. **AN,5,HPM**

197. **(1)** Elastic stockings are applied before standing up in order to prevent stagnation of blood in the lower extremities. If the patient has been standing or exercising **(No. 3)**, he or she should sit in a chair, with legs elevated, for at least 15 minutes before applying the stockings. Elastic stockings should be removed *regularly,* both to inspect the skin and to provide skin care **(No. 2)**. The patient should be cautioned not to sit or stand in any one position for a prolonged period of time **(No. 4)**. Stockings should fit properly and be kept wrinkle free because when improperly used they can cause venous stasis, the condition they are designed to prevent. **IMP,3,SECE**

198. **(3)** Serum radioimmunoassay (RIA) is accurate within 7 days of conception. This test is specific for HCG, and accuracy is not compromised by confusion with LH levels. **No. 1** is incorrect because the pregnant uterus is not palpable at or above the pubic symphysis before 12-week gestation. **No. 2** is incorrect because fetal heart tones are not audible by present methods before 9–12 weeks (Doppler) or 20 weeks (fetoscope). **No. 4** is wrong because Leopold maneuvers are neither possible nor applicable until much later in pregnancy. **AS,5,HPM**

199. **(4)** Initial intervention when patients are reacting to the loss of a significant body part is to encourage verbalization of their fears and to assist them in identifying how they see the change in their body image as well as how it may affect their relationships. One of the most important factors in the mastectomy patient's response to surgery is the reaction of her husband or the person with whom she is intimately involved. **Nos. 1 and 2** tend to cut off communication in this instance. Many partners are very supportive; others are not. It is therefore also important to assist the partners to talk with each other, not just to the nurse, to acknowledge feelings and concerns **(No. 3)**. The patient needs the reassurance of the partner's love and support to work through her own emotional reaction and begin the work of recovery. **IMP,7,PsI**

200. **(2)** Ecchymoses occur in cirrhosis due to decreased synthesis of clotting factors as well as decreased vitamin K storage. Dilatation and slow blood flow in veins cause the formation of spider angiomas (particularly on the upper chest), palmar redness, and varicosities (esophageal and rectal are common). Esophageal hemorrhage **(No. 1)** results in the *vomiting* of bright red blood. Vitamin K is fat soluble, *not* water soluble **(No. 3)**. Venous pressures will increase, *not* decrease **(No. 4)**, due to mechanical obstruction in the liver, which results in increased capillary fragility. **AN,6,PhI**

Unit 2

Nursing Care of the Acutely Ill and the Chronically Ill Adult

❑ Assessment, Analysis, and Nursing Diagnosis of the Adult

Assessment is the process of gathering a comprehensive database about the patient's present, past, and potential health problems, as well as a description of the patient as a whole in his or her environment. It includes a comprehensive nursing history, a physical examination, and laboratory/X-ray data, and it concludes with the formulation of nursing diagnoses.

Subjective Data

Nursing History

The nursing history obtains data for planning and implementing nursing actions.

I. **General information:** reason for admission; duration of present illness; previous hospitalization; history of illnesses; diagnostic procedures prior to admission; allergies—type and severity of reactions; medications taken at home—over-the-counter and prescription.

II. **Information relative to growth and development:** age; menarche—age at onset; heavy menses; dysmenorrhea; vaginal discharge; date of last Pap smear; pregnancies; abortions; miscarriages.

III. **Information relative to psychosocial functions:** feelings (anger, denial, fear, anxiety, guilt, life-style changes); language barriers; family support; spiritual needs; history of trauma/rape.

IV. **Information relative to nutrition:** appetite—normal, changes; dietary habits; food preferences or intolerances; difficulty swallowing or chewing; dentures; use of caffeine/alcohol; weight changes; excessive thirst, hunger, sweating.

V. **Information relative to fluid and gas transport:** difficulty breathing; shortness of breath; history of cough/smoking; colds; sputum; swelling of extremities; chest pain; palpitations; varicosities; excessive bruising; blood transfusions; excessive bleeding.

VI. **Information relative to protective functions:** skin problems—rash, itch; current treatment; unusual hair loss.

VII. **Information relative to comfort, rest, activity, mobility:** usual activity (ADL); present ability and restrictions; rest and sleep pattern; weakness; joint or muscle stiffness, pain, or swelling; occupation; interests.

VIII. **Information relative to elimination:** bowel habits; changes—constipation, diarrhea; ostomy; emesis; nausea; voiding—retention, frequency, dysuria, incontinence.

IX. **Information relative to sensory/perceptual functions:** pain—verbal report; quality, location; precipitating factors; duration; limitations in vision (glasses), hearing, touch, smell; orientation to person, place, time; confusion; headaches; fainting; dizziness; convulsions.

Objective Data

◆ I. **Physical assessment**—requires knowledge of normal findings, organization, and keen senses, i.e., visual, auditory, touch, smell. For abnormal findings, refer to the *Assessment* section of each health problem discussed under the categories of human functioning.

A. *Components*

1. *Inspection*—uses observations to detect deviations from normal.
2. *Auscultation*—to perceive and interpret sounds arising from various organs, particularly heart, lungs, and bowel.
3. *Palpation*—used to assess for discomfort, temperature, pulsations, size, consistency, and texture.
4. *Percussion*—technique used to elicit vibrations produced by underlying organ structures; used less frequently in nursing practice.
   a. Flat—normal percussion note over muscle or bone.
   b. Dull—normal percussion note over organs such as liver.
   c. Resonance—normal percussion note over lungs.
   d. Tympany—normal percussion note over stomach or bowel.

B. *Sequence**

1. *General appearance*—well or poorly developed or nourished. Color (black, white, jaundiced, pale). In distress (acutely or chronically)?
2. *Vital signs*—blood pressure (which arm or both, orthostatic change). Pulse (regular or irregular, orthostatic change). Respirations (labored or unlabored, wheeze). Temperature (axillary, rectal, or oral). Weight. Height.
3. *Skin, hair, and nails*—pigmentation, scars, lesions, bruises, turgor. Describe or draw rashes.
   a. Skin color:
      Red—fever, allergic reaction, CO poisoning.
      White (pallor)—excessive blood loss, fright.
      Blue (cyanosis)—hypoxemia, peripheral vasoconstriction.
      Mottled—cardiovascular embarrassment.
   b. Skin temperature:
      Hot, dry—excessive body heat (heat stroke).
      Hot, wet—reaction to increased internal or external temperature.
      Cool, dry—exposure to cold.
      Cool, clammy—shock.
4. *Nodes*—any cervical, supraclavicular, axillary, epitrochlear, inguinal lymphadenopathy? If so, size of nodes (in cm), consistency (firm, rubbery, tender), mobile or fixed.
5. *Head*—scalp, skull (configuration), scars, tenderness, bruits.
6. *Eyes:*

   a. **External eye.** Conjunctivae, sclerae, lids, cornea, pupils (including reflexes), visual fields, extraocular motions.
   b. **Fundus.** Disk, blood vessels, pigmentation.
7. *Ears*—shape of pinnae, external canal, tympanic membrane, acuity, air conduction versus bone conduction (*Rinne test*), lateralization (*Weber's test*).
8. *Nose*—septum, mucosa, polyps.
9. *Mouth and throat*—lips, teeth, tongue (size, papillation), buccal mucosa, palate, tonsils, oropharynx.
10. *Neck*—suppleness. Trachea, larynx, thyroid, blood vessels (jugular veins, carotid arteries).
11. *Chest and lungs:*
    a. **Inspection.** Contour, symmetry, expansion.
    b. **Palpation.** Expansion, rib tenderness, tactile fremitus.
    c. **Percussion.** Diaphragmatic excursion, dullness.
    d. **Auscultation.** Crackles, rhonchi, rubs, wheezes, egophony, pectoriloquy.
       (1) Use diaphragm or bell. Normal sounds over alveoli—*vesicular.* Large airway or abnormal sounds—*bronchial or bronchovesicular.* Adventitious sounds—*crackles or wheezes.*
       (2) *Crackles*—discontinuous noises heard on auscultation; caused by popping open of air spaces; usually associated with increased fluid in the lungs; *formerly called rales and rhonchi.*
       (3) *Wheezes*—high-pitched, whistling sounds made by air flowing through narrowed airways.
12. *Heart:*
    a. **Inspection.** Point maximal impulse, chest contour.
    b. **Palpation.** Point maximal impulse, thrills, lifts, thrusts.
    c. **Auscultation.** Heart sounds, gallops, murmurs, rubs. Use diaphragm for high-pitched sounds of normal heart sounds (S_1 and S_2) and bell for abnormal sounds (S_3 and S_4).
13. *Breasts*—symmetry, retraction, lesions, nipples (inverted, everted), masses, tenderness, discharge.
14. *Abdomen:*
    a. **Inspection.** Scars (draw these), contour, masses, vein pattern.
    b. **Auscultation.** Bowel sounds, rubs, bruits. Use diaphragm. Auscultate after inspection and before palpation and percussion. Listen to each quadrant for at least 1 min. If bowel sounds

---

*From Judge R, Zuidema G, Fitzgerald F. *Clinical Diagnosis* (5th ed). Boston; Little, Brown, 1989. Pp 30–31.

are present, they will be heard in lower right quadrant (area of ileocecal valve).

    c. **Percussion**—organomegaly, hepatic dullness.

    d. **Palpation**—tenderness, masses, rigidity, liver, spleen, kidneys.

    e. **Hernia**—femoral, inguinal, ventral.

  15. *Genitalia:*

    a. **Male.** Penile lesions, scrotum, testes. Circumcised?

    b. **Female.** Labia, Bartholin's and Skene's glands, vagina, cervix. Bimanual of internal genitalia.

  16. *Rectum*—perianal lesions, sphincter tone, tenderness, masses, prostate, stool color, occult blood.

  17. *Extremities*—pulses (symmetry, bruits, perfusion). Joints (mobility, deformity). Cyanosis, edema. Varicosities. Muscle mass.

  18. *Back*—contour spine, tenderness. Sacral edema.

  19. *Neurologic:*

    a. **Mental status.** Alertness, memory, judgment, mood.

    b. **Cranial nerves** (I–XII).

    c. **Cerebellum.** Gait, finger–nose, heel–shin, tremors.

    d. **Motor.** Muscle mass, strength deep-tendon reflexes. Pathologic or primitive reflexes.

    e. **Sensory.** Touch, pain, vibration. Heat and cold as indicated.

II. General—provides information on the patient as a whole.

  A. *Race, sex, apparent age* in relation to stated age.

  B. *Nutritional status*—well hydrated and developed or obesity, cachexia—include weight.

  C. *Apparent health status*—general good health or mild, moderate, severe debilitation.

  D. *Posture and motor activity*—erect, symmetric, and balanced gait and muscle development or ataxic, circumducted, scissor, or spastic gait; slumped or bent-over posture; mild, moderate, or hyperactive motor responses.

  E. *Behavior*—alert; oriented to person, time, place; hears and comprehends instructions, or tense, anxious, angry; uses abusive language; slightly or largely unresponsive; delusions, hallucinations.

  F. *Odors*—noncontributory, or acetone, alcohol, fetid breath, incontinent of urine or feces.

◆**III. Health assessment of the older adult**

  A. *Skin:*

    1. Decrease in elasticity → wrinkles and lines, dryness.

    2. Loss of fullness → sagging.

    3. Wasting appearance due to generalized loss of adipose and muscle tissue.

    4. Decrease of adipose tissue on extremities, redistributed to hips and abdomen in middle age.

    5. Bony prominences become visible.

    6. Excessive pigmentation → age spots.

    7. Dry skin and deterioration of nerve fibers and sensory endings → pruritus.

    8. Pallor and blotchiness because of decreased blood flow.

    9. Overgrowth of epidermal tissue leads to lesions (some benign, some premalignant, some malignant).

  B. *Nails:*

    1. Dry, brittle.

    2. Increased susceptibility to fungal infections.

    3. Decreased growth rate.

    4. Toenails thick, difficult to cut.

  C. *Hair:*

    1. Loss of pigment → graying, white.

    2. Decreased density of hair follicles → thinning of hair.

    3. Baldness due to decreased blood flow to skin and decreased estrogen production.

      a. Hair distribution thin on scalp, axilla, pubic area, upper and lower extremities.

      b. Decreased facial hair in *men.*

    4. Increased facial (chin, upper lip) hair in *women* due to decreased estrogen production.

  D. *Eyes:*

    1. Loss of soluble protein with loss of lens transparency → development of *cataracts.*

    2. Decrease in pupil size limits amount of light entering the eye → elderly need more light to see.

    3. Decreased pupil reactivity → decrease in rate of light changes to which a person can readily adapt.

    4. Diminished night vision due to decreased accommodation to darkness and dim light.

    5. Shrunken appearance due to loss of orbital fat.

    6. Blink reflex—slowed.

    7. Eyelids—loose.

    8. Visual acuity—decreased.

    9. Peripheral vision—diminished.

    10. Visual fields—diminished.

    11. Lens accommodation—decreased; requires corrective lenses.

    12. *Presbyopia*—lens may lose ability to become convex enough to accommodate to nearby objects; starts at age 40 (*farsightedness*).

    13. Color—fades.

    14. Conjunctiva—thins, looks yellow.

    15. Increased intraocular pressure leads to glaucoma.

E. *Ears:*
1. Changes in cochlea—decrease in average pitch of sound.
2. Hearing loss—greater in left ear than right; greater in higher frequencies than in lower.
3. Tympanic membrane—atrophied, thickened, causing hearing loss.
4. Presbycusis—progressive loss of hearing in old age.

F. *Mouth:*
1. Dental caries.
2. Poor-fitting dentures.
3. Cancer of the mouth—increased risk.
4. Decrease in taste buds → inability to taste sweet/salty foods.
5. Olfactory bulb atrophies → decreased ability to smell.

G. *Cardiovascular:*
1. Blood pressure increased due to lack of elasticity of vessels → increased resistance to blood flow; decreased diameter of arteries.
2. Atherosclerotic plaques → thrombosis.
3. Valves become sclerotic, less pliable → reduced filling and emptying.
4. Diastolic murmurs heard at base of heart.
5. Loss of elasticity, decreased contractility → decreased cardiac output.
6. Pumping action of the heart is reduced due to changes in the coronary arteries → pooling of blood in systemic veins and shortness of breath.
7. Dysrhythmias due to disturbance of the autonomic nervous system.
8. Extremities—pedal pulses weaker due to arteriosclerotic changes; colder extremities, mottled color.

H. *Respiratory:*
1. Efficiency reduced with age.
2. Greater residual air in lungs after expiration.
3. Decreased vital capacity.
4. Decreased capacity to cough because of weaker expiratory muscles.
5. Decreased ciliary activity → stasis of secretions → susceptibility to infections.
6. Dyspnea on exertion (DOE) due to oxygen debt in the muscles.
7. Reduced chest wall compliance.

I. *Breasts:*
1. Atrophy.
2. Cancer risk—increased with age.

J. *Gastrointestinal:*
1. Pernicious anemia due to lack of intrinsic factor.
2. Gastric motility—decreased.
3. Esophageal peristalsis—decreased.
4. Hiatal hernia—increased incidence.
5. Digestive enzymes—gradual decrease of ptyalin (which converts starch), pepsin and trypsin (which digest protein), lipase (fat-splitting enzyme).

6. Absorption—decreased.
7. Constipation due to improper diet.

K. *Endocrine:*
1. Basal metabolism rate lowered → decreased temperature.
2. Cold intolerance.
3. *Females:* decreased ovarian function → increased gonadotropins.
4. Decreased renal sensitivity to ADH → unable to concentrate urine as effectively as younger persons.
5. Decreased clearance of blood glucose after meals → elevated postprandial blood glucose.
6. Risk of diabetes mellitus increased with age.

L. *Urinary:*
1. Renal function—impaired due to poor perfusion.
2. Filtration—impaired due to reduction in number of functioning nephrons.
3. Urgency and frequency: *men*—often due to prostatic hypertrophy; *women*—due to perineal muscle weakness.
4. Nocturia—both men and women.
5. Urinary tract infection—increased incidence.
6. Incontinence—especially with dementia.

M. *Musculoskeletal:*
1. Muscle mass—decreased.
2. Bony prominences—increased.
3. Demineralization of bone.
4. Shortening of trunk due to narrowing of intervertebral space.
5. Posture—normal; some kyphosis.
6. Range of motion—limited.
7. Osteoarthritis—related to extensive physical activities and joint use.
8. Gait—altered.
9. Osteoporosis related to menopause, immobilization, elevated levels of cortisone.
10. Calcium, phosphorus, and vitamin D decreased.

N. *Neurologic:*
1. Voluntary, automatic reflexes—slowed.
2. Sleep pattern—changes.
3. Mental acuity—changes.
4. Sensory interpretation and movement—changes.
5. Pain perception—diminished.
6. Dexterity and agility—lessened.
7. Reaction time—slowed.
8. Memory—past more vivid than recent memory.
9. Depression.
10. Alzheimer's disease.

O. *Sexuality:*
1. Women
   a. Estrogen production—decreased with menopause.
   b. Breasts atrophy.
   c. Vaginal secretions—reduced lubricants.

d. Sexuality—drive continues; sexual activity declines.
2. Men
  a. Testosterone production—decreased.
  b. Testes—decrease in size; decreased sperm count.
  c. Libido and sexual satisfaction—no changes.

IV. Routine laboratory studies—see Appendix A for normal ranges.
  A. *Hematology*
    1. Complete blood count—detects presence of anemia, infection, allergy, and leukemia.
    2. Prothrombin time—increase may indicate need for vitamin K therapy.
    3. Serology (VDRL)—determines presence of syphilis; false positives may indicate collagen dysfunctions.
  B. *Urinalysis*
    1. Specific gravity—measures ability of kidney to concentrate urine. Fixed specific gravity indicates renal tubular dysfunction.
    2. Albumin and pus—indicate renal infection.
    3. Sugar and acetone—presence indicates metabolic disorder.
  C. *Chest X ray*—detects tuberculosis or other pulmonary dysfunctions, as well as changes in size and/or configuration of heart.
  D. *Electrocardiogram (ECG)*—detects rhythm and conduction disturbances, presence of myocardial ischemia or necrosis, and ventricular hypertrophy.
  E. *Blood chemistries*—detect deviation in electrolyte balance, presence of tissue damage, and adequacy of glomerular filtration.

Assessment is followed by analysis of data and formulation of a nursing diagnosis. Possible nursing diagnoses for each category of human functioning are given in the following sections.

❏ Growth and Development*

Young Adulthood (20–30 Years of Age)

I. Stage of development—psychosocial stage: intimacy versus isolation.
II. Physical development
  A. At the *height* of bodily vigor.
  B. *Maximum* level of strength, muscular development, height, and cardiac and respiratory capacity; also, period of peak sexual capacity for males.

*Adapted from Saxton D, et al. *Addison–Wesley Manual of Nursing Practice*. Menlo Park, CA: Addison–Wesley, 1983.

III. Cognitive development
  A. Close to *peak* of intelligence, memory, and abstract thought.
  B. Maximum ability to solve problems and learn new skills.
IV. Socialization
  A. Has a vision of the future and imagines various possibilities for self.
  B. Defines and tests out what can be accomplished.
  C. Seeks out a mentor to emulate as a guiding, though transitional, figure; the mentor is usually a mixture of parent, teacher, and friend who serves as a role model to support and facilitate the developing vision of self.
  D. Grows from a beginning to a fuller understanding of own authority and autonomy.
  E. Transfers an interest into an occupation or profession; crucial work choice may be made after one has knowledge, judgment, and self-understanding, usually at the end of young adulthood; when the choice is deferred beyond these years, valuable time is lost.
  F. Experiments with and chooses a life-style.
  G. Forms mature peer relationships with the opposite sex.
  H. Overcomes guilt and anxiety about the opposite sex and learns to understand the masculine and feminine aspects of self as well as the adult concept of roles.
  I. Learns to take the opposite sex seriously and may choose someone for a long-term relationship.
  J. Accepts the responsibilities and pleasures of parenthood.

Adulthood (31–45 Years of Age)

I. Stage of development—psychosocial stage: generativity versus self-absorption.
II. Physical development
  A. Gradual decline in biologic functioning, although in the late 30s the individual is still near peak.
  B. Period of peak sexual capacity for females occurs during the mid-30s.
  C. Distinct sense of bodily decline occurs around 40 years of age.
  D. *Circulatory* system begins to slow somewhat after 40 years of age.
III. Cognitive development
  A. Takes longer to memorize.
  B. Still at peak in abstract thinking and problem solving.
  C. Generates new levels of awareness.
  D. Gives more meaning to complex tasks.
IV. Socialization
  A. Achieves a realistic self-identity.
  B. Perceptions are based on reality.
  C. Acts on decisions and assumes responsibility for actions.
  D. Accepts limitations while developing assets.

E. Delays immediate gratification in favor of future satisfaction.

F. Evaluates mistakes, determines reasons and causes, and learns new behavior.

G. Struggles to establish a place in society.
   1. Begins to settle down.
   2. Pursues long-range plans and goals.
   3. Has a stronger need to be responsible.
   4. Invests self as fully as possible in social structure, including work, family, and community.

H. Seeks advancement by improving and using skills, becoming more creative, and pursuing ambitions.

Middle Life (46–64 Years of Age)

I. **Stage of development**—psychosocial stage: continuation of generativity versus self-absorption.

II. **Physical development**
   A. Failing *eyesight,* especially for close vision, may be one of the first symptoms of aging.
   B. Hearing loss is very gradual, especially for low sounds; hearing for *high-pitched* sounds is impaired more readily.
   C. There is a gradual loss of *taste* buds in the 50s and gradual loss of sense of *smell* in the 60s, causing the individual to have a diminished sense of taste.
   D. *Muscle strength* declines because of decreased levels of estrogen and testosterone; it takes more time to accomplish the same physical task.
   E. *Lung* capacity is impaired, which adds to decreased endurance.
   F. The *skin* begins to wrinkle, and hair begins graying.
   G. *Postural changes* take place because of loss of calcium and reduced activity.

III. **Cognitive development**
   A. *Memory* begins to decline slowly around the age of 50 years.
   B. It takes longer to *learn* new tasks, and old tasks take longer to perform.
   C. *Practical judgment* is increased due to experiential background.
   D. May tend to withdraw from mental activity or overcompensate by trying the impossible.

IV. **Socialization**
   A. The middle years can be very rewarding if previous stages have been fulfilled.
   B. The years of responsibility for raising children are over.
   C. Husbands and wives usually find a closer bond.
   D. There is less financial strain for those with steady employment.
   E. Individuals are usually at the height of their careers; the majority of leaders in their field are in this age group.
   F. Self-realization is achieved.
      1. There is more inner direction.

2. There is no longer a need to please everyone.
3. Individual is less likely to compare self with others.
4. Individual approves of self without being dependent on standards of others.
5. There is less fear of failure in life because past failures have been met and dealt with.

Early Late Years (65–79 Years of Age)

I. **Stage of development**—psychosocial stage: ego integrity and acceptance versus despair and disgust.

II. **Physical development**
   A. Continues to decrease in vigor and capacity.
   B. Has more frequent aches and pains.
   C. Likely to have at least one major illness.

III. **Cognitive development**
   A. Mental acuity continues to slow down.
   B. Judgment and problem solving remain intact, but the processes may take longer.
   C. May have problems in remembering *names* and *dates.*

IV. **Socialization**
   A. Individual is faced with the reality of the experience of physical decline.
   B. Physical and mental changes intensify the feelings of aging and mortality.
   C. Increasing frequency of death and serious illness among friends, relatives, and associates reinforces further the concept of mortality.
   D. Constant reception of medical warnings to follow certain precautions or run serious risks adds to general feeling of decline.
   E. Individual is less interested in obtaining the rewards of society and is more interested in utilizing own inner resources.
   F. Individuals feel that they have earned the right to do what is important for self-satisfaction.
   G. Retirement allows time for expression of own creative energies.
   H. Overcomes the splitting of youth and age; gets along well with adolescents.
   I. Learns to deal with the reality that only old age remains.
   J. Provides moral support to grandchildren; more tolerant of grandchildren than was of own children.
   K. Tends to release major authority of family to children while holding self in the role of consultant.

Later Years (80 Years of Age and Older)

I. **Stage of development**—psychosocial stage: continuation of ego integrity and acceptance versus despair and disgust.

II. Physical development

A. Additional sensory problems occur, including diminished sensation to *touch and pain.*

B. Increase in loss of muscle tone occurs, including *sphincter* (urinary and anal) control.

C. Individual is insecure and unsure about orientation to *space* and sense of *balance,* which may result in falls and injury.

III. Cognitive development

A. Has better memory for the *past* than the present.

B. *Repetition* of memories occurs.

C. Individual may use *confabulation* to fill in memory gaps.

D. Forgetfulness may lead to serious *safety* problems, and individual may require constant supervision.

E. Increased arteriosclerosis may lead to mental illness (dementia and other cognitive disorders).

IV. Socialization

A. Few significant relationships are maintained; deaths of friends, family, and associates cause isolation.

B. Individual may be preoccupied with immediate bodily needs and personal comforts; the *gastrointestinal tract* frequently becomes the major focus.

C. Individuals see they can provide others with an example of wisdom and courage.

D. Individuals come to terms with themselves.

E. Individuals are concerned with own immortality.

F. Individuals come to terms with the process of dying and prepare for own death.

❑ Fluid-Gas Transport

Conditions Affecting Fluid Transport

I. **Hypertension:** sustained, elevated, systemic, arterial blood pressure; diastolic elevation more serious, reflecting pressure on arterial wall during resting phase of cardiac cycle (Table 2.1).

A. **Pathophysiology:** increased peripheral resistance leading to thickened arteriole walls and left ventricular hypertrophy.

B. **Risk factors:**
1. Black race (2:1).
2. Use of birth control pills.
3. Overweight.
4. Smoking.
5. Stress.
6. Excessive sodium intake.
7. Lack of activity.

C. **Classifications:**
1. *Primary* (essential): occurs in 90% of patients; etiology unknown; diastolic pressure is ≥90 mm Hg and other causes of hypertension are absent. Benign hypertension (diastolic pressure ≤120 mm Hg)

considered controllable; malignant hypertension (diastolic >140–150 mm Hg) uncontrollable.
2. *Secondary:* occurs in remaining 10%; usually renal, endocrine, neurogenic, and/or cardiac in origin.
3. *Labile* (prehypertensive): a fluctuating blood pressure; increases during stress, otherwise normal or near normal.

◆ D. **Assessment:**
1. *Subjective data*
a. Early morning headache, usually occipital.
b. Light-headedness, tinnitus.
c. Palpitations.
d. Fatigue, insomnia.
e. Forgetfulness, irritability.
f. Altered vision: white spots, blurring, or loss.
2. *Objective data*
a. Epistaxis (nosebleeds).
b. Elevated blood pressure: systolic >140 mm Hg, diastolic >90 mm Hg; narrowed pulse pressure.
c. Retinal changes; papilledema.
d. Shortness of breath on slight exertion.
e. Cardiac, cerebral, and renal changes.

◆ E. **Analysis/nursing diagnosis:**
1. *Altered peripheral tissue perfusion* related to increased peripheral resistance.
2. *Decreased cardiac output* related to ventricular hypertrophy.
3. *Risk for injury* related to altered vision.
4. *Risk for activity intolerance* related to inadequate oxygenation.
5. *Fatigue* related to poor perfusion.

◆ F. **Nursing care plan/implementation:**
1. Goal: *provide for physical and emotional rest.*
a. Rest periods before/after eating, visiting hours; avoid upsetting situations.
b. Give tranquilizers, sedatives, as ordered.
2. Goal: *provide for special safety needs.*
a. Monitor blood pressure: both arms; standing, sitting, lying positions.
b. Limit/prevent activities that increase pressure (anxiety, anger, frustration, upsetting visitors, fatigue).
c. Assist with ambulation; change position gradually to prevent dizziness and light-headedness (postural hypotension).
d. Monitor for electrolyte imbalance when on low-sodium diet, diuretic therapy; I&O to prevent fluid depletion and arrhythmias from potassium loss.
e. Observe for signs of hemorrhage, shock, and stroke, which may occur following surgery.
3. Goal: *health teaching* (patient and family).

■ **TABLE 2.1** **Imbalances in Blood Pressure: Comparative Assessment of Hypotension and Hypertension**

	Hypotension	Hypertension
Common causes		
	Angina pectoris	Essential hypertension
	Myocardial infarction	Iron deficiency anemia
	Acute and chronic pericarditis	Pernicious anemia
	Valvular defects	Arteriosclerosis obliterans
	Congestive heart failure	Polycythemia vera
Assessment		
Behavior	Anxiety, apprehension, decreasing mentation, confusion	Nervousness, mood swings, irritability, difficulty with memory, depression, confusion
Neurologic	Essentially noncontributory	Decreased vibratory sensations, increased/decreased reflexes, Babinski reflex, changes in coordination
Head/neck	Distended neck veins, worried expression	Bruits over carotids, distended neck veins, epistaxis, diplopia, ringing in ears, dull occipital headaches on arising
Skin	Pale, cool, moist	Dry, pale, glossy, flaky, cold; decreased or absent hair
GI	Anorexia, nausea, vomiting, constipation	Anorexia, flatulence, diarrhea, constipation
Respiratory	Dyspnea, orthopnea, paroxysmal nocturnal dyspnea, tachypnea, moist rales, cough	Dyspnea, orthopnea, crackles
Cardiovascular	Tires easily	Decreased exercise tolerance, weakness, palpitations
	Blood pressure—decreased systolic, decreased systolic/diastolic	Blood pressure—increased systolic, increased systolic and diastolic
	Pulse—increased/decreased, weak, thready, irregular, arrhythmias	Decreased or absent pedal pulses
Renal	Oliguria	Oliguria, nocturia, proteinuria
Extremities	Dependent edema	Tingling, numbness, or cold hands and feet, dependent edema, ulcers of legs or feet

a. Procedures to decrease anxiety; relaxation techniques, stress-management.
b. Side effects of hypotensive drugs: diuretics; adrenergic blockers; vasodilators, calcium channel blockers (faintness, nausea, vomiting, postural hypotension, sexual dysfunction). See Unit 4 for specific pharmacologic actions.
c. Weight control to reduce arterial pressure.
d. Restrictions: stimulants (tea, coffee, tobacco), sodium, calories, fat.
e. Life-style adjustments: daily exercise needed; reduce occupational and environmental stress; importance of rest.
f. Blood pressure measurement: daily, same conditions, position preference of physician.
g. Signs, symptoms, complications of disease (headache, confusion, visual changes, nausea/vomiting, convulsions).
h. Causes of intermittent hypotension: alcohol, hot weather, exercise, febrile illness, hot bath.

◆ **G. Evaluation/outcome criteria:**
  1. Blood pressure within normal range for age (diastolic <90 mm Hg)—stable.
  2. Minimal or no pathophysiologic or therapeutic complications (e.g., visual changes, CVA, drug side effects).
  3. Reduces weight to reasonable level for height, bone structure.
  4. Takes prescribed medications regularly, even when symptoms have resolved.
  5. Complies with restrictions: no smoking, restricted sodium, fat.
  6. Exercises regularly—program compatible with personal and health care goals.

II. Cardiac arrhythmias: any variation in normal rate, rhythm, or configuration of waves on ECG (Figure 2.1).
  A. Pathophysiology
    1. Dysfunction of SA node, atria, AV node, or ventricular conduction.
    2. Primary heart problem or secondary systemic problem.
  B. Risk factors
    1. Myocardial infarction.
    2. Drug toxicity.
    3. Stress.

■ FIGURE 2.1   Interpretation of normal cardiac cycle. (Modified from Holloway N. *Nursing the Critically Ill Adult*, [3rd ed.]. Menlo Park, CA: Addison-Wesley, 1988. Pp 270, 277.)

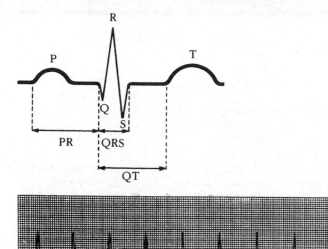

P wave	Atrial depolarization
QRS complex	Ventricular depolarization
T wave	Ventricular repolarization
PR interval	Time from start of atrial depolarization to start of ventricular depolarization (12–20 sec)
QRS interval	Total time for ventricular depolarization (6–10 sec)
QT interval	Total time for ventricular depolarization and repolarization
Rate/rhythm	60–100, regular
P-QRS ratio	1:1

Normal Sinus Rhythm

4. Cardiac surgery.
5. Hypoxia.
6. See also Table 2.2.

◆ **C. Assessment:** see Table 2.2 for specific arrhythmias.

◆ **D. Analysis/nursing diagnosis:**
1. *Decreased cardiac output* related to abnormal ventricular function.
2. *Altered tissue perfusion* related to inadequate cardiac functioning.
3. *Risk for injury* (death) related to improper cardiac function.
4. *Risk for activity intolerance* related to inadequate oxygenation.
5. *Anxiety* related to dependence, fear of death.

◆ **E. Nursing care plan/implementation:**
1. Goal: *provide for emotional and safety needs.*
   a. Document ECG tracing for presence of arrhythmia.
   b. Encourage discussion of fears, feelings.
   c. Bedrest; restricted activities; quiet environment; limit visitors.
   d. Oxygen, if ordered.
   e. Check vital signs frequently for shock, HF, drug toxicity.
   f. Prepare for cardiac emergency: CPR.
   g. Give cardiac medications; check lab tests for digitalis and potassium levels, to prevent drug toxicity.
2. Goal: *prevent thromboemboli.*

   a. Apply antiembolic stockings (TED hose).
   b. Give anticoagulants as ordered. (Check for bleeding—gums, urine; monitor lab tests—Lee White clotting time and partial thromboplastin time with heparin; prothrombin time with coumarin.)
   c. Encourage flexion-extension of feet.
3. Goal: *provide for physical and emotional needs with pacemaker insertion.*
   a. *General concerns*
      (1) Report excessive bleeding/infection at insertion site—hematoma may contribute to wound infection.
      (2) Encourage verbalization of feelings.
      (3) Report prolonged hiccoughs, which may indicate pacemaker failure.
      (4) Know pacing mode: fixed-rate or demand (most common).
   b. *Temporary pacemaker*
      (1) Limit excessive activity of extremity if antecubital insertion, to prevent displacement; subclavian insertion increases catheter stability.
      (2) Secure wires to chest to prevent tension on catheter.
      (3) Do *not* defibrillate over insertion site, to avoid electrical hazards.
      (4) Electrical safety (grounding; disconnect electric beds/call lights; use battery-operated equipment).
   c. *Permanent pacemaker*

■ **TABLE 2.2   Comparison of Selected Cardiac Dysrhythmias**

Dysrhythmia	Description	Etiology	Symptoms/ Consequences	Treatment
Dysrhythmias of Sinus Node				
Sinus dysrhythmia	Phasic shortening then lengthening of P-P and R-R interval	Respiratory variation in impulse initiation by SA node	Usually none	Usually none
Sinus tachycardia	P waves present followed by QRS Rhythm regular Heart rate 100–150 beats/min	Increased metabolic demands Decreased oxygen delivery, heart failure, shock, hemorrhage, anemia	May produce palpitations Prolonged episodes may lead to decreased cardiac output	Treat underlying cause Occasionally sedatives
Sinus bradycardia	P waves present followed by QRS Rhythm regular Heart rate <60 beats/ min	Physical fitness Parasympathetic stimulation (sleep) Brain lesions Sinus dysfunction Digitalis excess	Very low rates may cause decreased cardiac output: lightheadedness, faintness, chest pain	Atropine if cardiac output is decreased Pacemaker Treat underlying cause if necessary
Atrial Dysrhythmias				
Premature atrial beats	Early P wave QRS may or may not be normal Rhythm irregular	Stress, ischemia, atrial enlargement, caffeine, nicotine	May produce palpitations Frequent episodes may decrease cardiac output Is sign of chamber irritability	Sedation Quinidine May require no other treatment
Atrial tachycardia	P wave present (may merge into previous T wave), QRS usually normal, rapid heart rate usually >150 beats/min	Sympathetic stimulation, chemical stimuli (caffeine, nicotine), drug toxicity	Palpitations Possible anxiety	Usually none Prolonged episodes may require carotid artery pressure, vagal stimulation, verapamil, digitalis, or beta blockers
Atrial fibrillation	Rapid, irregular P waves (>350/min) Ventricular rhythm irregularly irregular Ventricular rate varies, may increase to 120–150/min if untreated	Rheumatic heart disease Mitral stenosis Atrial infarction Coronary atherosclerotic heart disease Hypertensive heart disease Thyrotoxicosis	Pulse deficit Decreased cardiac output if rate is rapid Promotes thrombus formation in atria	Digitalis Quinidine Cardioversion
Ventricular Dysrhythmias				
Premature ventricular beats (PVBs)	Early wide bizarre QRS, not associated with a P wave Rhythm irregular	Stress, acidosis, ventricular enlargement Electrolyte imbalance Myocardial infarction Digitalis toxicity Hypoxemia, hypercapnia	Same as for premature atrial beats	Procainamide Quinidine Disopyramide (Norpace) Lidocaine Mexiletine Oxygen Sodium bicarbonate Potassium Treat heart failure
Ventricular tachycardia	No P wave before QRS; QRS wide and bizarre; ventricular rate >100, usually 140–240	PVB striking during vulnerable period; hypoxemia; drug toxicity; electrolyte imbalance; bradycardia	Decreased cardiac output, hypotension, loss of consciousness, respiratory arrest	Lidocaine Procainamide Bretylium Mexiletine Cardioversion
Ventricular fibrillation	Chaotic electrical activity No recognizable QRS complex	Myocardial infarction Electrocution Freshwater drowning Drug toxicity	No cardiac output Absent pulse or respiration Cardiac arrest	Defibrillation Epinephrine Sodium bicarbonate Bretylium CPR

continued

■ **TABLE 2.2** *(Continued)*

Dysrhythmia	Description	Etiology	Symptoms/Consequences	Treatment
Ventricular Dysrhythmias (cont.)				
Ventricular standstill	Can be distinguished from ventricular fibrillation only by ECG P waves *may* be present No QRS "Straight line"	Myocardial infarction Chronic diseases of conducting system	Same as for ventricular fibrillation	CPR Pacemaker Intracardiac epinephrine Isoproterenol
Impulse Conduction Deficits				
First-degree atrioventricular (AV) block	PR interval prolonged, >0.20 sec	Rheumatic fever Digitalis toxicity Degenerative changes of coronary atherosclerotic heart disease Infections Decreased oxygen in AV node	Warns of impaired conduction	Usually none as long as it occurs as an isolated deficit
Bundle branch block	Same as normal sinus rhythm (NSR) except QRS duration > 0.10	Hypoxia, acute myocardial infarction, congestive heart failure, coronary atherosclerotic heart disease, pulmonary embolus, hypertension	Same as first-degree AV block	Usually none unless severe blockage of left posterior division (see text)
Second-degree AV blocks	P waves usually occur regularly at rates consistent with SA node initiation (not all P waves followed by QRS; PR interval may lengthen before nonconducted P wave or may be consistent; QRS may be widened)	Acute myocardial infarction	Serious dysrhythmia that may lead to decreased heart rate and cardiac output	May require temporary pacemaker
Complete third-degree AV block	Atria and ventricles beat independently P waves have no relation to QRS Ventricular rate may be as low as 20–40/min	Digitalis toxicity Infectious disease Coronary artery disease Myocardial infarction	Very low rates may cause decreased cardiac output: lightheadedness, faintness, chest pain	Pacemaker Isoproterenol to increase heart rate Epinephrine if isoproterenol ineffective

Source: Phipps W, Long B, Woods N, Cassmeyer V. (eds). *Medical-Surgical Nursing* (5th ed). St. Louis: Mosby, 1995.

(1) Limit activity of shoulder for 48–72 h with transvenous catheter to prevent dislodgement.
(2) Postinsertion ROM (passive) at least once per shift after 48 h to prevent frozen shoulder.
d. *Health teaching* following permanent pacemaker
  (1) Explain procedure: duration, equipment, purpose, type of pacemaker.
  (2) MedicAlert bracelet; pacemaker information card.
  (3) Daily pulse taking upon arising (report variation of ±5 beats).
  (4) Signs, symptoms of: *malfunction* (vertigo, syncope, dyspnea, slowed speech, confusion, fluid retention); *infection* (fever, heat, pain, skin breakdown at insertion site).
  (5) Restrictions: contact sports; electromagnetic interferences (few)—TV/radio transmitters, improperly functioning microwave ovens, certain cautery machines; may trigger airport metal-detector alarm.
◆ F. **Evaluation/outcome criteria:**
  1. Regular cardiac rhythm; monitors own radial pulse.
  2. No complications (e.g., pacemaker malfunction).
  3. Returns for regular follow-up of pacemaker function.
  4. Tolerates physical or sexual activity.

Adult

5. Wears identification bracelet; carries pace-maker identification card.

III. Cardiac arrest: sudden unexpected cessation of heartbeat and effective circulation leading to in-adequate perfusion and sudden death.

  A. Risk factors:
1. Myocardial infarction.
2. Multiple traumas.
3. Respiratory arrest.
4. Drowning.
5. Electric shock.
6. Drug reactions.

◆ **B. Assessment**—*objective data:*
1. Unresponsive to stimuli (i.e., verbal, pain-ful).
2. Absence of breathing, carotid pulse.
3. Pale or bluish: lips, fingernails, skin.
4. Pupils: dilated.

◆ **C. Analysis/nursing diagnosis:**
1. *Decreased cardiac output* related to heart failure.
2. *Impaired gas exchange* related to breath-lessness.
3. *Altered tissue perfusion* related to pulse-lessness.

◆ **D. Nursing care plan/implementation:**
1. Goal: *prevent irreversible cerebral anoxic damage:* initiate CPR within 4–6 min; continue until relieved; document assess-ment factors, effectiveness of actions; presence or absence of pulse at 1 min and every 4–5 min.
2. Goal: *establish effective circulation, respi-ration:* see Emergency Nursing Proce-dures, p. 212 for complete protocols.

◆ **E. Evaluation/outcome criteria:**
1. Carotid pulse present; check after 1 min and every few minutes thereafter.
2. Responds to verbal stimuli.
3. Pupils constrict in response to light.
4. Return of spontaneous respiration; ade-quate ventilation.

IV. Arteriosclerosis: loss of elasticity, thickening, hardening of arterial walls; common type—ath-erosclerosis. Arteriosclerosis precedes angina pectoris and myocardial infarction.

  A. Pathophysiology:
1. Atherosclerotic plaque, discrete lumpy thickening of arterial wall.
2. Narrows lumen, can occlude vessel.

  B. Risk factors:
1. Increased serum cholesterol (low-density lipids).
2. Hypertension.
3. Cigarette smoking.
4. Diabetes mellitus.

(See V. Angina pectoris, below, and VI. Myocardial in-farction, p. 56, for nursing implications.)

  V. Angina pectoris: transient paroxysmal epi-sodes of substernal or precordial pain.

    A. Pathophysiology:

1. Insufficient blood flow through coronary arteries.
2. Temporary myocardial ischemia.

  B. Risk factors:
1. Cardiovascular:
  a. Atherosclerosis.
  b. Thromboangiitis obliterans.
  c. Aortic regurgitation.
  d. Hypertension.
2. Hormonal:
  a. Hyperthyroidism.
  b. Diabetes mellitus.
3. Blood disorders:
  a. Anemia.
  b. Polycythemia vera.

◆ **C. Assessment:**
1. *Subjective data*
  a. Pain (Table 2.3).
    (1) *Type:* squeezing, pressing, burning.
    (2) *Location:* retrosternal, substernal, left of sternum, radiates to left arm.
    (3) *Duration:* short, usually 3–5 min, <30 min.
    (4) *Cause:* emotional stress, overeat-ing, physical exertion, exposure to cold.
    (5) *Relief:* rest, nitroglycerin.
  b. Dyspnea.
  c. Palpitations.
  d. Dizziness; faintness.
  e. Epigastric distress; indigestion; belch-ing.
2. *Objective data*
  a. Tachycardia.
  b. Pallor.
  c. Diaphoresis.

◆ **D. Analysis/nursing diagnosis:**
1. *Altered cardiopulmonary tissue perfusion* related to insufficient blood flow.
2. *Pain* related to myocardial ischemia.
3. *Activity intolerance* related to onset of pain.

◆ **E. Nursing care plan/implementation:**
1. Goal: *provide relief from pain.*
  a. Rest until pain subsides.
  b. Nitroglycerin or amyl nitrite, as or-dered.
  c. Identify precipitating factors: large meals, heavy exercise, stimulants (cof-fee, smoking), sex when fatigued, cold air.
  d. Vital signs; hypotension.
  e. Assist with ambulation; dizziness, flushing occur with nitroglycerin.
2. Goal: *provide emotional support.*
  a. Encourage verbalization of feelings, fears.
  b. Reassurance; positive self-concept.
  c. Acceptance of limitations.
3. Goal: *health teaching.*

■ TABLE 2.3 Comparison of Physical Causes of Chest Pain

Characteristic	Myocardial Infarction	Pericarditis	Gastric Disorders	Angina	Dissecting Aneurysm	Pulmonary Embolism
Onset	Gradual or sudden	Sudden	Gradual or sudden	Gradual or sudden	Abrupt, without prodromal symptoms	Gradual or sudden
Precipitating factors	Can occur at rest or after exercise or emotional stress	Breathing deeply, rotating trunk, recumbency, swallowing or yawning	Inflammation of stomach or esophagus; hypersecretion of gastric juices; some medications	Usually after physical exertion, emotional stress, eating, exposure to cold or defecation; unstable angina occurs at rest	Hypertension	Immobility or prolonged bedrest following surgery, trauma, hip fracture, HF, malignancy, oral contraceptives
Location	Substernal, anterior chest, or midline; rarely back; radiates to jaw or neck	Precordial; radiates to neck or left shoulder and arm	Xiphoid to umbilicus	Substernal, anterior chest; poorly localized	Correlates with site of intimal rupture; anterior chest or back; between shoulder blades	Pleural area, retrosternal area
Quality	Crushing, burning, stabbing, squeezing or vicelike	Pleuritic, sharp	Aching, burning, cramplike, gnawing	Squeezing, feeling of heavy pressure; burning	Sharp, tearing or ripping sensation	Sharp, stabbing
Intensity	Asymptomatic to severe; increases with time	Mild to severe	Mild to severe	Mild to moderate	Severe and unbearable; maximal from onset	Aggravated by breathing
Duration	30 min to 1–2 h; may wax and wane	Continuous	Periodic	Usually 2–10 min; average 3–5 min	Continuous; does not abate once started	Variable
Relief	Narcotics	Sitting up, leaning forward	Physical and emotional rest, food, antacids, H_2-receptor antagonists	Nitroglycerin, rest	Large, repeated doses of narcotics	O_2; sitting up; morphine
Associated symptoms	Nausea, fatigue, heartburn; peripheral pulses equal	Fever, dyspnea, nausea, anorexia, anxiety	Nausea, vomiting, dysphagia, anorexia, weight loss	Belching, indigestion, dizziness	Syncope, loss of sensations or pulses, oliguria; discrepancy between BP in arms; decrease in femoral or carotid pulse	Dyspnea, tachypnea, diaphoresis, hemoptysis, cough, apprehension

a. Pain: alleviation, differentiation of angina from myocardial infarction, precipitating factors (see Table 2.3).

b. Medication: frequency, expected effects (headache, flushing); carry fresh nitroglycerin; loses potency after 6 mo ("stings" under tongue when potent); may use nitroglycerin paste—instruct how to apply.

c. *Diet:* restricted calories if weight loss indicated; restricted fat, cholesterol, gas-producing foods; small, frequent meals.

d. Diagnostic tests if ordered (e.g., cardiac catheterization; see Unit 5).

e. Exercise: regular, graded, to promote coronary circulation.

f. Prepare for coronary bypass surgery, if necessary.

g. Behavior modification to assist with life-style changes, i.e., stress-reduction, stop smoking.

◆ **F. Evaluation/outcome criteria:**
1. Relief from pain.
2. Fewer attacks.
3. No myocardial infarction.
4. Alters life-style; complies with limitations.
5. No smoking.

VI. Myocardial infarction (MI): localized area of necrotic tissue in myocardium from cessation of blood flow; leading cause of death in North America.

A. Pathophysiology:
1. Coronary occlusion due to thrombosis, embolism, or hemorrhage adjacent to atherosclerotic plaque.
2. Insufficient blood flow from cardiac hypertrophy, hemorrhage, shock, or severe dehydration.

B. Risk factors:
1. Age (35–70 yr).
2. Men more than women until menopause.
3. Life-style.
4. Stress.
5. High-cholesterol diet (specifically low-density lipoproteins).
6. Chronic illness (diabetes, hypertension).

◆ **C. Assessment:**
1. *Subjective data*
   a. Pain (see Table 2.3).
      (1) *Type:* sudden, severe, crushing, heavy tightness.
      (2) *Location:* substernal; radiates to one or both arms, jaw, neck.
      (3) *Duration:* >30 min.
      (4) *Cause:* unrelated to exercise; frequently occurs when sleeping (REM stage).
      (5) *Relief:* oxygen, narcotics; *not* relieved by rest or nitroglycerin.
   b. Nausea.
   c. Shortness of breath.

d. Apprehension, fear of impending death.
e. History of cardiac disease (family); occupational stress.

2. *Objective data*
   a. Vital signs: shock; rapid (>100), thready pulse; fall in blood pressure; tachypnea, shallow respirations; elevated temperature within 24 h (100°–103°F).
   b. Skin: cyanotic, ashen or clammy; diaphoretic.
   c. Emotional: restless.
   d. Lab data: *increased*—WBC (12,000–15,000/μL), serum enzymes (CPK-MB, LDH, >LDH$_2$ "flipped LDH"); *changes*—ECG (elevated ST segment, inverted T wave, arrhythmia).

◆ **D. Analysis/nursing diagnosis:**
1. *Decreased cardiac output* related to myocardial damage.
2. *Impaired gas exchange* related to poor perfusion, shock.
3. *Pain* related to myocardial ischemia.
4. *Activity intolerance* related to pain or inadequate oxygenation.
5. *Fear* related to possibility of death.

◆ **E. Nursing care plan/implementation:**
1. Goal: *reduce pain, discomfort.*
   a. Narcotics—morphine, meperidine (Demerol) HCl; note response.
   b. Humidified oxygen; mouth care—oxygen is drying.
   c. *Position:* semi-Fowler's to improve ventilation.
2. Goal: *maintain adequate circulation.*
   a. Monitor vital signs and urine output; observe for cardiogenic shock.
   b. Monitor ECG for arrhythmias.
   c. Give medications as ordered: *antiarrhythmics*—lidocaine HCl, quinidine HCl, procainamide (Pronestyl), bretylium (Bretylol); propranolol (Inderal); verapamil; *anticoagulants*—heparin sodium, bishydroxycoumarin or dicoumarin; *thrombolytic agents*—streptokinase, tPA, APSAC/anistreplase (Eminase).
   d. Recognize heart failure: edema, cyanosis, dyspnea, cough, crackles.
   e. Check lab data—normal: serum enzymes (CPK 0–7 IU/L; LDH <115 IU/L; LDH$_2$ <LDH$_2$); blood gases (pH 7.35–7.45; CO$_2$ 35–45; Po$_2$ 80–100; HCO$_3$ 22–26); electrolytes (K$^+$ 3.5–5.0 mEq/L); clotting time (APTT 16–25 sec; PTT 30–45 sec; PT 11–15 sec).
   f. CVP—zero level at right atrium; fluctuates with respiration; normal range 5–15 cm H$_2$O; note trend; increases with heart failure.

▶ g. ROM of lower extremities; TED hose/antiembolic stockings.

3. Goal: *decrease oxygen demand/promote oxygenation.*
   a. O₂ as ordered.
   b. Activity: bedrest (24–48 h); planned rest periods; control visitors.
   c. *Position:* semi-Fowler's to facilitate lung expansion and decrease venous return.
   d. Anticipate needs of patient: call light, water.
   e. Assist with feeding, turning.
   f. Environment: quiet, comfortable.
   g. Reassurance; stay with anxious patient.
   h. Give medications as ordered: cardiotonics, calcium channel blockers, vasodilators, vasopressors.

4. Goal: *maintain fluid, electrolyte, nutritional status.*
   a. IV (keep vein open); CVP; vital signs; urine output—30 mL/h.
   b. Lab data within normal limits (Na⁺ 135–145 mEq/L; K⁺ 3.5–5.0 mEq/L).
   c. Monitor ECG—*hyperkalemia:* peaked T wave; *hypokalemia:* depressed T wave.
   d. *Diet:* progressive low calorie, low sodium, low cholesterol, low fat.

5. Goal: *facilitate fecal elimination.*
   a. Medications: stool softeners to prevent Valsalva (straining); mouth breathing during bowel movement; recognize complications of Valsalva—chest pain, cyanosis, diaphoresis, arrhythmias.
   b. Bedside commode if possible.

6. Goal: *provide emotional support.*
   a. Recognize fear of dying: denial, anger, withdrawal.
   b. Encourage expression of feelings, fears, concerns.
   c. Discuss rehabilitation, life-style changes: prevent cardiac-invalid syndrome by promoting self-care activities, independence.

7. Goal: *promote sexual functioning.*
   a. Encourage discussion of concerns re: activity, inadequacy, limitations, expectations—include partner (usually resume activity 5–8 wk following uncomplicated MI).
   b. Identify need for referral for sexual counseling.

8. Goal: *health teaching.*
   a. Diagnosis and treatment regimen.
   b. *Caution* about when to *avoid* sexual activity: following heavy meal, alcohol ingestion; when fatigued, tense, under stress; with unfamiliar partners; in extreme temperatures.
   c. Information about sexual activity: less fatiguing positions (side to side; noncardiac on top); vasodilators, if ordered, prior to intercourse; select comfortable, familiar environment.
   d. Available community resources for information, support groups (e.g., American Heart Association, Stop Smoking Clinics).
   e. Medications: administration, importance, untoward effects, pulse taking.
   f. Control risk factors: rest, diet, exercise, no smoking, weight control, stress-reduction techniques.
   g. Need for follow-up care for regulation of medications, evaluating risk factors.
   h. Prepare for coronary bypass if planned.

◆ F. **Evaluation/outcome criteria:**
   1. No complications: stable vital signs; relief of pain.
   2. Adheres to prescribed medication regimen, demonstrates knowledge about medications.
   3. Activity tolerance is increased, participates in program of progressive activity.
   4. Reduction or modification of risk factors. Plans to alter life-style (e.g., loses weight, quits smoking).

VII. Cardiac valvular defects: alteration in the structure of a valve; impede flow of blood or permit regurgitation.
   A. **Pathophysiology:**
      1. *Stenosis*—narrowing of valvular opening due to adherence, thickening, and rigidity of valve cusp.
      2. *Insufficiency* (incompetence)—incomplete closure of valve due to contraction of chordae tendineae, papillary muscles, or to calcification, scarring of leaflets.
      3. *Mitral stenosis*
         a. Most common residual cardiac lesion of rheumatic fever.
         b. Affects *women* <45 yr more often than men.
         c. Narrowing of mitral valve.
         d. Interferes with filling of left ventricle.
         e. Produces pulmonary hypertension, right-sided heart failure.
      4. *Mitral insufficiency* (incompetence)
         a. Leaking/regurgitation of blood back into left atrium.
         b. Results from rheumatic fever, bacterial endocarditis; less common.
         c. Affects *men* more often.
         d. Produces pulmonary congestion, right-sided heart failure.
      5. *Aortic stenosis*
         a. Fusion of valve flaps between left ventricle and aorta.
         b. Congenital or acquired from atherosclerosis or from rheumatic fever and bacterial endocarditis; seen in *men*

more often; pulmonary circulation congested, cardiac output decreased.
  6. *Aortic insufficiency*
     a. Incomplete closure of valve between left ventricle and aorta (regurgitation).
     b. Left ventricular failure leading to right-sided heart failure.
  B. Risk factors:
     1. Congenital abnormality.
     2. History of rheumatic fever.
     3. Atherosclerosis.
◆ **C. Assessment:** Table 2.4.
◆ **D. Analysis/nursing diagnosis:**
     1. *Decreased cardiac output* related to inadequate ventricular filling.
     2. *Fluid volume excess* related to compensatory response to decreased cardiac output.
     3. *Impaired gas exchange* related to pulmonary congestion.
     4. *Activity intolerance* related to impaired cardiac function.
     5. *Fatigue* related to poor oxygenation.
◆ **E. Nursing care plan/implementation:**
     1. Goal: *reduce cardiac workload.*
     2. Goal: *promote physical comfort and psychological support.*
     3. Goal: *prevent complications.*
     4. Goal: *prepare patient for surgery* (commissurotomy, valvuloplasty, or valvular replacement, depending on defect and severity of condition).

  5. See X. Cardiac surgery, p. 59, for specific nursing actions.
◆ **F. Evaluation/outcome criteria:**
     1. Relief of symptoms.
     2. Increase in activity level.
     3. No complications following surgery.
VIII. Cardiac catheterization: a diagnostic procedure to evaluate cardiac status. Introduces a catheter into the heart, blood vessels; analyzes blood samples for oxygen content, cardiac output, pulmonary blood flow; done prior to heart surgery; frequently combined with angiography to visualize coronary arteries; also provides access for specialized cardiac techniques (e.g., internal pacing and coronary angioplasty).
  A. Approaches
     1. *Right-heart* catheterization—venous approach (antecubital or femoral) → right atrium → right ventricle → pulmonary artery.
     2. *Left-heart* catheterization—retrograde approach: right brachial artery or percutaneous puncture of femoral artery → ascending aorta → left ventricle.
        a. Transseptal: femoral vein → right atrium → septum → left atrium → left ventricle.
        b. Angiography/arteriography: done during left-heart catheterization.
  B. Precatheterization
  ◆ 1. **Assessment:**

■ **TABLE 2.4 Comparison of Symptomatology for Valvular Defects**

Assessment	Mitral Stenosis	Mitral Insufficiency	Aortic Stenosis	Aortic Insufficiency
Subjective Data				
Fatigue	✔	✔	✔	✔
Shortness of breath	✔			
Orthopnea	✔		✔	✔
Paroxysmal nocturnal dyspnea	✔		✔	✔
Cough	✔	✔		
Dyspnea on exertion		✔	✔	✔
Palpitations		✔	✔	
Syncope on exertion			✔	
Angina			✔	✔
Weight loss		✔		
Objective Data				
Vital signs				
Blood pressure:				
Low or normal	✔	✔		
Normal or elevated			✔	✔
Pulse:				
Weak, irregular	✔	✔		
Rapid, "waterhammer"				✔
Respirations:				
Increased, shallow	✔			
Cyanosis	✔			
Jugular vein distention	✔			
Enlarged liver	✔		✔	
Dependent edema	✔		✔	
Murmur	✔	✔	✔	✔

a. *Subjective data*
   (1) Allergies: iodine, seafood.
   (2) Anxiety.
b. *Objective data*
   (1) Vital signs: baseline data.
   (2) Distal pulses: mark for reference after catheterization.

◆ 2. **Analysis/nursing diagnosis:**
   a. *Anxiety* related to fear of unknown.
   b. *Knowledge deficit* related to difficulty learning or limited exposure to information.

◆ 3. **Nursing care plan/implementation:**
   a. Goal: *provide for safety, comfort.*
      (1) Signed informed consent.
      (2) NPO (except for medications 6–8 h before).
      (3) Have patient urinate before going to lab.
      (4) Give sedatives, as ordered, 30 min before procedure (e.g., midazolam HCl [Versed]).
   b. Goal: *health teaching.*
      (1) Procedure: length (1–3 h).
      (2) Expectations (strapped to table for safety, must lie still, awake but mildly sedated).
      (3) Sensations (hot, flushed feeling in head with dye injection; thudding in chest from premature beats during catheter manipulation; desire to cough, particularly with right-heart angiography and contrast-medium injection).
      (4) Alert physician to unusual sensations (coolness, numbness, paresthesia).

C. **Postcatheterization**
◆ 1. **Assessment** (potential complications):
   a. *Subjective data*
      (1) Puncture site: increasing pain, tenderness.
      (2) Palpitations.
      (3) Affected extremity: tingling numbness, pain from hematoma or nerve damage.
   b. *Objective data*
      (1) Vital signs: shock, respiratory distress (related to pulmonary emboli, allergic reaction).
      (2) Puncture site: bleeding (hematoma).
      (3) ECG: arrhythmias, signs of MI.
      (4) Affected extremity: color, temperature, peripheral pulses.

◆ 2. **Analysis/nursing diagnosis:**
   a. *Decreased cardiac output* related to arrhythmias or MI.
   b. *Altered tissue perfusion* related to bleeding following procedure.
   c. *Pain* related to puncture site tenderness.

◆ 3. **Nursing care plan/implementation:**
   a. Goal: *prevent complications.*
      (1) Bedrest: 3–6 h; with femoral approach, *supine position,* 12–24 h on bedrest; encourage ankle flexion, extention, and rotation.
      (2) Vital signs: record q15min for 1 h, q30min for 3 h or until stable; check BP on opposite extremity.
      (3) Puncture site: observe for bleeding, swelling, inflammation, or tenderness; check pulse distal to insertion site to determine patency of artery; report complaints of coolness, numbness, or paresthesia in extremity.
      (4) ECG: monitor, document rhythm.
      (5) Give medications as ordered: sedatives; mild narcotics; antiarrhythmics.
   b. Goal: *provide emotional support.*
      (1) Explanations: brief, accurate; patient anxious to learn results of test.
      (2) Counseling: refer as indicated.
   c. Goal: *health teaching.*
      (1) Late complications: infection.
      (2) Prepare for surgery if indicated.
      (3) Follow-up medical care.

◆ 4. **Evaluation/outcome criteria:** no complications (e.g., cardiac arrest, hematoma at insertion site).

IX. **Percutaneous transluminal coronary angioplasty** (PTCA): a balloon-tipped catheter is threaded to site of coronary occlusion and inflated repeatedly until blood flow increases distal to the obstruction; a nonsurgical alternative to bypass surgery for coronary artery occlusion; recommended in patients with poorly controlled angina, mild or no symptoms, multiple- or single-vessel disease with a noncalcified, discrete, and proximal lesion that can be reached by the catheter; costs less and requires shorter hospitalization and rehabilitation period (see VIII. Cardiac catheterization, p. 58, for nursing process). **Athrectomy** may also be done; a cutter is positioned against the blockage and mechanically debrides the plaque. An **intravascular stent,** a coilspring tube, may be placed in the coronary artery, and the stent acts as a mechanical scaffold to reopen the blocked artery. The patient will receive anticoagulant and antiplatelet therapy following the procedure.

X. **Cardiac surgery:** done to alter the structure of the heart or vessels when congenital or acquired disorders interfere with cardiac functioning: septal defects; transposition of great vessels; tetralogy of Fallot; pulmonary/aortic stenosis; coronary artery bypass; valve replacement.

Cardiopulmonary bypass (open-heart surgery): blood from cardiac chambers and great vessels is diverted into a pump oxygenator; allows full visualization of heart during surgery; maintains perfusion and body functioning.

A. Preoperative

◆ 1. **Assessment:** see specific conditions for preoperative signs and symptoms, i.e., valvular defects, angina, MI; also see I. Preoperative preparation, p. 102. Establish complete baseline: daily weight; vital signs—integrity of all pulses, BP both arms; CVP or pulmonary artery pressures (*Swan-Ganz*); neurologic status; emotional status; nutritional and elimination patterns; lab values (urine, electrolytes, enzymes, coagulation studies); pulmonary function studies.

◆ 2. **Analysis/nursing diagnosis** (see also VI. Myocardial infarction, p. 56):
   a. *Decreased cardiac output* related to myocardial damage.
   b. *Activity intolerance* related to poor cardiac function.
   c. *Knowledge deficit* related to insufficient time for teaching.
   d. *Anxiety* related to fear of unknown.
   e. *Fear* related to possible death.
   f. *Spiritual distress* related to possible death.

◆ 3. **Nursing care plan/implementation:**
   a. Goal: *provide emotional and spiritual support.*
      (1) Arrange for religious consultation if desired.
      (2) Provide opportunity for family visit morning of surgery.
      (3) Encourage verbalization/questions: fear, depression, despair frequently occur.
   b. Goal: *health teaching.*
      (1) Diagnostic procedures, treatments, specifics for surgery (i.e., leg incision with use of saphenous vein in coronary bypass surgery).
      (2) Postoperative regimen: turn, cough, deep breathe, ROM, equipment used, medication for pain.
      (3) Tour ICU; meet personnel.
      (4) Alternative method of communication while intubated.

◆ 4. **Evaluation/outcome criteria:**
   a. Displays moderate anxiety level.
   b. Verbalizes/demonstrates postoperative expectations.
   c. Quits smoking before surgery.

B. Postoperative

◆ 1. **Assessment:**
   a. *Subjective data*
      (1) Pain.
      (2) Fatigue—sleep deprivation.
   b. *Objective data*
      (1) Neurologic: level of consciousness; pupillary reactions; movement of limbs (purposeful, spontaneous).
      (2) Respiratory: rate changes (increases occur with obstruction, pain; decreases occur with CO_2 retention); depth (shallow with pain, atelectasis); symmetry; skin *color;* patency/*drainage* from chest tubes; *sputum* (amount, color); endotracheal tube placement (bilateral breath sounds).
      (3) Cardiovascular:
         (a) BP—*hypotension* may indicate heart failure, tamponade, hemorrhage, arrhythmias, or thrombosis; *hypertension* may indicate anxiety, hypervolemia.
         (b) Pulse: radial, apical, pedal; rate (>100 may indicate shock, fever, hypoxia, arrhythmias); rhythm, quality.
         (c) CVP or Swan-Ganz (elevated in cardiac failure); temperature (normal postop: 98.6°–101.6°F oral).
      (4) GI: nausea, vomiting, distention.
      (5) Renal: urine—minimum output (30 mL/h); color; specific gravity (<1.010 occurs with *overhydration,* renal tubular damage; >1.020 present with *dehydration,* oliguria, blood in urine).

◆ 2. **Analysis/nursing diagnosis:**
   a. *Decreased cardiac output* related to decreased myocardial contractility or postoperative hypothermia.
   b. *Pain* related to incision.
   c. *Ineffective airway clearance* related to effects of general anesthesia.
   d. *Altered tissue perfusion* related to postoperative bleeding or thromboemboli.
   e. *Fluid volume deficit* related to blood loss.
   f. *Risk for infection* related to wound contamination.
   g. *Altered thought processes* related to anesthesia or stress.
   h. *Body image disturbance* related to incision or limitations.
   i. *Sleep pattern disturbance* related to ICU environment or pain.

◆ 3. **Nursing care plan/implementation:**
   a. Goal: *provide constant monitoring to prevent complications.*
      (1) Respiratory:
         (a) Observe for respiratory distress: restlessness, nasal flaring, Cheyne-Stokes, dusky/cyanotic; assisted or controlled ventilation via endotracheal tube common first 24 h; supplemental O_2 after extubation.
         (b) Suctioning; cough, deep breathe.

(c) Elevate head of bed.

(d) Position chest tube to facilitate drainage; mediastinal sump tube maintains patency—"milking" not necessary. See also chest tube care in Table 5.5, p. 306.

(2) *Cardiovascular:*

(a) Vital signs: BP >80–90 systolic; *CVP:* range 5–15 cm H_2O unless otherwise ordered; pulmonary artery line (Swan-Ganz): mean pressure 4–12 mm Hg; I&O: report <30 mL urine/h from indwelling urinary catheter.

(b) ECG; PVCs occur most frequently following aortic valve replacement and bypass surgery.

(c) Peripheral pulses if leg veins used for grafting.

(d) Activity: turn q2h; ROM; progressive, early ambulation.

(3) Inspect dressing for bleeding.

(4) Medications according to therapeutic directives—*cardiotonics* (digoxin); *coronary vasodilators* (nitrates); *antibiotics* (penicillin); *analgesics; anticoagulants* (with valve replacements); *antiarrhythmics* (quinidine, procainamide HCl [Pronestyl]).

b. Goal: *promote comfort, pain relief.*

(1) Medicate: Demerol or morphine sulfate, as severe pain lasts 2–3 d.

(2) Splint incision when moving or coughing.

(3) Mouth care: keep lips moist.

(4) *Position:* use pillows to prevent tension on chest tubes, incision.

c. Goal: *maintain fluid, electrolyte, nutritional balance.*

(1) I&O; urine specific gravity.

(2) Measure chest drainage—should not exceed 200 mL/h for first 4–6 h.

(3) Give fluids as ordered; maintain IV patency.

(4) *Diet:* clear fluids → solid food if no nausea, GI distention; sodium restricted, low fat.

d. Goal: *promote emotional adjustment.*

(1) Anticipate behavior disturbances (depression, disorientation often occur 3 d postop) related to medications, fear, sleep deprivation.

(2) Calm, oriented, supportive environment, as personalized as possible.

(3) Encourage verbalization of feelings (family and patient).

(4) Encourage independence to avoid cardiac-cripple role.

e. Goal: *health teaching.*

(1) Alterations in life-style; activity, diet, work.

(2) Available community resources for cardiac rehabilitation (e.g., American Heart Association, Mended Hearts).

(3) Drug regimen: purpose, side effects.

(4) Potential complications: dyspnea, pain, palpitations common postoperatively.

◆ 4. **Evaluation/outcome criteria:**

a. No complications; incision heals.

b. Activity level increases—no signs of overexertion (e.g., fatigue, dyspnea, pain).

c. Relief of symptoms.

d. Returns for follow-up medical care.

e. Takes prescribed medications; knows purposes and side effects.

XI. **Heart failure** (HF): inability of the heart to meet the peripheral circulatory demands of body; cardiac decompensation; combined right- and left-sided heart failure.

A. **Pathophysiology:** increased cardiac workload or decreased effective myocardial contractility → decreased cardiac output (forward effects). Left ventricular failure → pulmonary congestion; right atrial and right ventricular failure → systemic congestion → peripheral edema (backward effects). Compensatory mechanisms in HF include tachycardia, ventricular dilation, and hypertrophy of the myocardium; develop in 50–60% of heart disease patients.

B. **Risk factors:**

1. Decreased myocardial contractility:

a. Myocarditis.

b. MI.

c. Tachyarrhythmias.

d. Bacterial endocarditis.

e. Acute rheumatic fever.

2. Increased cardiac workload:

a. Elevated temperature.

b. Physical/emotional stress.

c. Anemia.

d. Hyperthyroidism (thyrotoxicosis).

e. Valvular defects.

◆ C. **Assessment:**

1. *Subjective data*

a. Shortness of breath.

(1) Orthopnea (sleeps on two or more pillows).

(2) Paroxysmal nocturnal dyspnea (sudden breathlessness during sleep).

(3) Dyspnea on exertion (climbing stairs).

b. Apprehension; anxiety; irritability.

c. Fatigue; weakness.
d. Reported weight gain; feeling of puffiness.

2. *Objective data*
   a. Vital signs:
      (1) BP: decreasing systolic; narrowing pulse pressure.
      (2) Pulse: pulsus alternans (alternating strong-weak-strong cardiac contraction), increased.
      (3) Respirations: crackles.
   b. Edema: dependent, pitting (1+ to 4+ mm).
   c. Liver: enlarged, tender.
   d. Neck veins: distended.
   e. Chest X ray:
      (1) Cardiac enlargement.
      (2) Dilated pulmonary vessels.
      (3) Diffuse interstitial lung edema.

◆ **D. Analysis/nursing diagnosis:**
1. *Decreased cardiac output* related to decreased myocardial contractility.
2. *Activity intolerance* related to generalized weakness and inadequate oxygenation.
3. *Fatigue* related to edema and poor oxygenation.
4. *Altered tissue perfusion* related to peripheral edema and inadequate blood flow.
5. *Fluid volume excess* related to compensatory mechanisms.
6. *Impaired gas exchange* related to pulmonary congestion.
7. *Anxiety* related to shortness of breath.
8. *Sleep pattern disturbance* related to paroxysmal nocturnal dyspnea.

◆ **E. Nursing care plan/implementation:**
1. Goal: *provide physical rest/reduce emotional stimuli.*
   a. *Position:* sitting or semi-Fowler's until tachycardia, dyspnea, edema resolved; change position frequently; pillows for support.
   b. Rest: planned periods; limit visitors, activity, noise.
   c. Support: stay with anxious patient; have supportive family member present; administer sedatives/tranquilizers as ordered.
   d. Warm fluids if appropriate.
2. Goal: *provide for relief of respiratory distress; reduce cardiac workload.*
   a. Oxygen: low flow rate; encourage deep breathing (5–10 min q2h); auscultate breath sounds for congestion, pulmonary edema.
   b. *Position:* head of bed 20–30 cm (8–10 in.) alleviates pulmonary congestion.
   c. Medications as ordered:
      (1) *Digitalis* preparations.
      (2) *Beta-adrenergics*—dobutamine, dopamine.

(3) *Diuretics*—thiazides, furosemide, ethacrynic acid.
(4) *Tranquilizers*—phenobarbital, diazepam (Valium), chlordiazepoxide (Librium) HCl.
(5) *Stool softeners* to avoid Valsalva maneuver.

3. Goal: *provide for special safety needs.*
   a. Skin care:
      (1) Inspect, massage, lubricate bony prominences.
      (2) Use foot cradle, heel protectors; sheepskin.
   b. Siderails up if hypoxic (disoriented).
   c. Vital signs: monitor for signs of fatigue, pulmonary emboli.
   d. ROM: active, passive; elastic stockings.
4. Goal: *maintain fluid and electrolyte balance, nutritional status.*
   a. Urine output: 30 mL/h minimum; estimate insensible loss in diaphoretic patient.
   b. Daily weight; same time, clothes, scale.
   c. IV: use microdrip to avoid circulatory overloading.
   d. *Diet:*
      (1) Low sodium as ordered.
      (2) Small, frequent feedings.
      (3) Discuss food preferences with patient.
5. Goal: *health teaching.*
   a. Diet restrictions; meal preparation.
   b. Activity restrictions, if any; planned rest periods.
   c. Medications: schedule, purpose, dosage, side effects (importance of daily pulse taking, daily weights, intake of *potassium*-containing foods).
   d. Available community resources for dietary assistance, weight reduction, exercise program.

◆ **F. Evaluation/outcome criteria:**
1. Increase in activity level tolerance—fatigue decreased.
2. No complications—pulmonary edema, respiratory distress.
3. Reduction in dependent edema.

XII. Pulmonary edema: sudden transudation of fluid from pulmonary capillaries into alveoli.
   A. Pathophysiology: increased pulmonary capillary permeability; increased hydrostatic pressure (pulmonary hypertension); and/or decreased blood colloidal osmotic pressure; fluid accumulation in alveoli → decreased compliance → decreased diffusion of gas → hypoxia, hypercapnea.
   B. Risk factors:
   1. Left-sided heart failure.
   2. Pulmonary embolism.
   3. Drug overdose.
   4. Smoke inhalation.
   5. CNS damage.

6. Fluid overload.
◆ **C. Assessment:**
1. *Subjective data*
   a. Anxiety.
   b. Restlessness at onset progressing to agitation.
   c. Stark fear.
   d. Intense dyspnea, orthopnea, fatigue.
2. *Objective data*
   a. Vital signs:
      (1) Pulse: tachycardia; gallop rhythm.
      (2) Respiration: tachypnea, moist, bubbling, wheezing.
      (3) Temperature: normal to subnormal.
   b. Skin: pale, cool, diaphoretic, cyanotic.
   c. Auscultation: crackles, wheezes.
   d. Cough: productive of large quantities of pink, frothy sputum.
   e. Right-sided heart failure: distended neck veins, peripheral edema, hepatomegaly, ascites.
   f. Mental status: restless, confused, stuporous.
◆ **D. Analysis/nursing diagnosis:**
1. *Decreased cardiac output* related to decreased myocardial contractility.
2. *Impaired gas exchange* related to pulmonary congestion.
3. *Altered tissue perfusion* related to inadequate blood flow.
4. *Anxiety,* severe, related to difficulty breathing.
5. *Fear* related to pulmonary congestion.
◆ **E. Nursing care plan/implementation:**
1. Goal: *promote physical, psychological relaxation measures to relieve anxiety.*
   a. Slow respirations: morphine sulfate, as ordered, to reduce respiratory rate, to sedate, and to produce vasodilation.
   b. Remain with patient.
   c. Encourage slow, deep breathing; assist with coughing.
   d. Work calmly, confidently, unhurriedly.
   e. Frequent rest periods.
2. Goal: *improve cardiac function, reduce venous return, relieve hypoxia.*
   ▶ a. O₂: 100%, preferably by demand valve to slow respiratory rate, provide uniform ventilation, reduce venous return, and inhibit "leaky capillary" syndrome.
   b. IV: D5W.
   c. Give aminophylline, as ordered, to lower venous pressure and increase cardiac output.
   d. *Position:* high Fowler's, extremities in dependent position, to reduce venous return and facilitate breathing.
   e. Medications as ordered: digitalis; diuretics—furosemide (Lasix); sympathomimetic agents—dobutamine (Dobutrex), dopamine; nitroglycerin.
   f. Vital signs; auscultate breath sounds.

g. *Diet:* low sodium; fluid restriction as ordered.
3. Goal: *health teaching* (include family or significant other).
   a. Medications.
      (1) Side effects.
      (2) Potassium supplements if indicated.
      (3) Pulse taking.
   b. Exercise; rest.
   c. *Diet:* low sodium.
   d. Signs of complications: edema; weight gain of 2–3 lb (0.9–1.4 kg) in a few days; dyspnea.
◆ **F. Evaluation/outcome criteria:**
1. No complications; vital signs stable; clear breath sounds.
2. No weight gain; weight loss if indicated.
3. Alert, oriented, calm.

XIII. Shock: a critically severe deficiency in nutrients, oxygen, and electrolytes delivered to body tissues, plus deficiency in removal of cellular wastes; results from cardiac failure, insufficient blood volume, and/or increased vascular bed size.
A. Types, pathophysiology, and risk factors:
1. *Hypovolemic* (hemorrhagic, hematogenic)—markedly decreased **volume** of blood (hemorrhage or plasma loss from intestinal obstruction, burns, physical trauma, or dehydration) → decreased venous return, cardiac output → decreased tissue perfusion.
2. *Cardiogenic*—failure of cardiac muscle **pump** (myocardial infarction) → generally decreased cardiac output → pulmonary congestion, hypoxia → inadequate circulation; high mortality.
3. *Distributive:*
   a. Neurogenic—massive **vasodilatation** from reduced vasomotor, vasoconstrictor tone (e.g., spinal shock, head injuries, anesthesia, pain); interruption of sympathetic nervous system; blood volume that is normal but inadequate for vessels → decreased venous return → tissue hypoxia.
   b. Vasogenic (anaphylactic, septic, endotoxic)—severe reaction to foreign protein (insect bites, drugs, toxic substances, aerobic, gram-negative organisms) → histamine release → **vasodilatation,** venous stasis → diminished venous return.
◆ **B. Assessment:** varies, depending on degree of shock (Table 2.5).
1. *Subjective data*
   a. Anxiety; restlessness.
   b. Dizziness; fainting.
   c. Thirst.
   d. Nausea.
2. *Objective data*

■ TABLE 2.5 Signs and Symptoms of Hypovolemic Shock

Blood Loss	Assessment Parameters
<800 mL	Usually none (equivalent to donating one unit of blood)
800–1500 mL (15–30%)	Anxiety and restlessness Pulse >100* Systolic pressure unchanged Diastolic pressure ↑ Urine output ↓
2000 mL (30–40%)	Pulse >120* Respirations >30 Systolic pressure ↓ Mental status ↓
>2500 mL (>40%)	Pulse >120* Respirations >30 Narrow pulse pressure (= systolic − diastolic) Cold, clammy skin

*In some cases of abdominal trauma, there is shock without a rapid pulse.
Adapted from Caroline NL. *Emergency Care in the Streets* (5th ed). Boston: Little, Brown, 1995. P 194.

a. Vital signs:
  (1) *BP*—hypotension (postural changes in early shock; systolic <70 mm Hg in late shock).
  (2) *Pulse*—tachycardia, thready; irregular (cardiogenic shock); could be slow if conduction system of heart damaged.
  (3) *Respirations*—increased depth, rate; wheezing (anaphylactic shock).
  (4) *Temperature*—decreased (elevated in septic shock).
b. Skin:
  (1) Pale (or mottled), cool, clammy (warm to touch in septic shock).
  (2) Urticaria (anaphylactic shock).
c. Level of consciousness: alert, oriented → unresponsive.
d. CVP:
  (1) *Below* 5 cm H$_2$O with hypovolemic shock.
  (2) *Above* 15 cm H$_2$O with cardiogenic, possibly septic shock.
e. Urine output: decreased (<30 mL/h).
f. Capillary refill: slowed (Figure 2.2).

◆ **C. Analysis/nursing diagnosis:**
1. *Altered tissue perfusion* related to vasoconstriction or decreased myocardial contractility.
2. *Impaired gas exchange* related to ventilation-perfusion imbalance.
3. *Decreased cardiac output* related to loss of circulating blood volume or diminished cardiac contractility.

■ FIGURE 2.2 Capillary refill test. Press on the fingernail (A) until it blanches. Then release the pressure (B). The skin under the nail should "pink up" within 2 seconds if the patient is normally perfused. (From Caroline NL. *Emergency Care in the Streets* (5th ed). Boston: Little, Brown, 1995.)

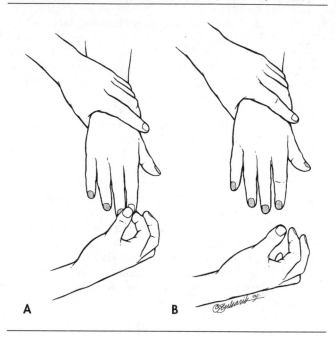

A   B

4. *Altered urinary elimination* related to decreased renal perfusion.
5. *Fluid volume deficit* related to blood loss.
6. *Anxiety* related to severity of condition.
7. *Risk for injury* related to death.
◆ **D. Nursing care plan/implementation:**
Goal: *promote venous return, circulatory perfusion.*
1. *Position:* foot of bed *elevated* 20 degrees (12–16 in.), knees straight, trunk horizontal, head slightly elevated; *avoid* Trendelenburg position.
2. Ventilation: monitor respiratory effort, loosen restrictive clothing; O$_2$ as ordered.
3. Fluids: maintain IV infusions; give blood, plasma expanders as ordered (exception—*stop* blood immediately in anaphylactic shock).
4. Vital signs:
  a. CVP (↓ with hypovolemia) arterial line, Swan-Ganz (↑ pulmonary artery wedge pressure indicating cardiac failure).
  b. Urine output (insert catheter for hourly output).
  c. Monitor ECG (↑ rate, arrhythmias).
5. Medications (depending on type of shock) as ordered:
  a. *Antihypotensives*—epinephrine (Adrenalin), norepinephrine (Levo-

phed), isoproterenol (Isuprel), dopamine (Intropin).
   b. *Antiarrhythmics.*
   c. *Cardiac glycosides.*
   d. *Adrenocorticoids.*
   e. *Antibiotics.*
   f. *Vasodilators* (nitroprusside).
   g. *Beta-adrenergics* (dobutamine).
6. Mechanical support: military antishock trousers (MAST) or pneumatic antishock garment (PASG); used to promote internal autotransfusion of blood from legs and abdomen to central circulation; at lower pressures may control bleeding and promote hemostasis; *do not* remove (deflate) suddenly to examine underlying areas or BP will drop precipitously; *compartment syndrome* may result with prolonged use and high pressure; controversial.

◆ **E. Evaluation/outcome criteria:**
   1. Vital signs stable, within normal limits.
   2. Alert, oriented.
   3. Urine output >30 mL/h.

XIV. Disseminated intravascular coagulation (DIC): diffuse or widespread coagulation initially within arterioles and capillaries leading to hemorrhage.
   A. Pathophysiology: activation of coagulation system from tissue injury → fibrin microthrombin form in brain, kidneys, lungs → microinfarcts, tissue necrosis → red blood cells, platelets, prothrombin, other clotting factors trapped, destroyed in process → excessive clotting → release of fibrin split products → inhibition of platelet clotting → bleeding.
   B. Risk factors:
      1. Obstetric complications.
      2. Neoplastic disease.
      3. Low perfusion states.
   ◆ **C. Assessment**—*objective data:*
      1. Skin, mucous membranes: petechiae, ecchymosis.
      2. Extremities (fingers, toes): cyanosis.
      3. Bleeding: venipuncture sites, wound, oral, rectal, vaginal.
      4. Urine output: oliguria → anuria.
      5. Level of consciousness: convulsions, coma.
      6. Lab data: *prolonged*—prothrombin time (PT) >15 sec; *decreased*—platelets, fibrinogen level.
   ◆ **D. Analysis/nursing diagnosis:**
      1. *Altered tissue perfusion* related to peripheral microthrombi.
      2. *Risk for injury* (death) related to bleeding.
      3. *Risk for impaired skin integrity* related to ischemia.
      4. *Altered urinary elimination* related to renal tubular necrosis.
   ◆ **E. Nursing care plan/implementation:** Goal: *prevent and detect further bleeding.*

1. Carry out nursing measures designed to alleviate underlying problem (e.g., shock, birth of fetus, surgery/irradiation for cancer).
2. Medications: heparin SO_4 IV, 1000 U/h, if ordered, to reverse abnormal clotting (controversial).
3. IVs: blood to lessen shock; platelets, cryoprecipitate, fresh plasma to restore clotting factors, fibrinogen.
4. Observe: vital signs, CVP (normal 5–15 mm Hg), PAP (normal 20–30 systolic and 8–12 diastolic), and intake and output for signs of shock or fluid overload from frequent infusions; specimens for occult blood (urine, stool).
5. Precautions: *Avoid* IM injections if possible; pressure 5 min to venipuncture sites; *no* rectal temperatures.

◆ **F. Evaluation/outcome criteria:**
   1. Clotting mechanism restored (increased platelets, normal PT).
   2. Renal function restored (urine output >30 mL/h).
   3. Circulation to fingers, toes; no cyanosis.
   4. No irreversible damage from renal, cerebral, cardiac, or adrenal hemorrhage.

XV. Pericarditis: inflammation of parietal and/or visceral pericardium; acute or chronic condition; may occur with or without effusion.
   A. Pathophysiology: fibrosis or accumulation of fluid in pericardium → compression of cardiac pumping → decreased cardiac output → increased systemic, pulmonic venous pressure.
   B. Risk factors:
      1. Bacterial, viral, and/or fungal infections.
      2. Tuberculosis.
      3. Collagen diseases.
      4. Uremia.
      5. Transmural MI.
      6. Trauma.
   ◆ **C. Assessment:**
      1. *Subjective data*
         a. Pain:
            (1) *Type*—sharp, moderate to severe.
            (2) *Location*—wide area of pericardium, may radiate; right arm, jaw/teeth.
            (3) *Precipitating factors*—movement, deep inspiration, swallowing.
         b. Chills; sweating.
         c. Apprehension; anxiety.
         d. Fatigue.
         e. Abdominal pain.
         f. Shortness of breath.
      2. *Objective data*
         a. Vital signs:
            (1) BP: decreased pulse pressure; pulsus paradoxus—abnormal drop in systemic BP of >8–10 mm Hg during inspiration.

(2) Pulse: tachycardia.
(3) Temperature: elevated; erratic course; low grade.
b. Pericardial friction rub.
c. Increased CVP; distended neck veins; dependent pitting edema; liver engorgement.
d. Restlessness.
e. Lab data: elevated ALT[SGOT], WBC; chest X ray—cardiac enlargement.

◆ **D. Analysis/nursing diagnosis:**
1. *Decreased cardiac output* related to impaired cardiac muscle contraction.
2. *Pain* related to pericardial inflammation.
3. *Anxiety* related to unknown outcome.
4. *Fatigue* related to inadequate oxygenation.
5. *Ineffective breathing pattern* related to discomfort during inspiration.

◆ **E. Nursing care plan/implementation:**
1. Goal: *promote physical and emotional comfort.*
   a. *Position:* semi-Fowler's (upright or sitting); bedrest.
   b. Vital signs: q2–4h and prn: apical and radial pulse; notify physician if heart sounds decrease in amplitude or if pulse pressure *narrows,* indicating cardiac tamponade; cooling measures as indicated.
   c. O$_2$ as ordered.
   d. Medications as ordered:
      (1) *Analgesics*—aspirin, morphine sulfate.
      (2) *Nonsteroidal anti-inflammatory agents.*
      (3) *Antibiotics.*
      (4) *Digitalis* and *diuretics,* if heart failure present.
   e. Assist with aspiration of pericardial sac (pericardiocentesis) if needed: medicate as ordered; elevate head 60 degrees; monitor ECG; have defibrillator and pacemaker available.
   f. Prepare for pericardectomy (excision of constricting pericardium) as ordered.
   g. Continual emotional support.
   h. Enhance effects of analgesics: positioning; turning; warm drinks.
   i. Monitor for *signs of cardiac tamponade:* tachycardia; tachypnea; hypotension; pallor; narrowed pulse pressure; pulsus paradoxus; distended neck veins.
2. Goal: *maintain fluid, electrolyte balance.*
   a. Parenteral fluids as ordered; strict I&O.
   b. Assist with feedings; *low-sodium* diet may be ordered.

◆ **F. Evaluation/outcome criteria:**
1. Relief of pain, dyspnea.
2. No complications (e.g., cardiac tamponade).
3. Return of normal cardiac functioning.

XVI. Arteriosclerosis obliterans: most common obstructive disorder of the arterial system (aorta, large and medium-size arteries); frequently involves the femoral artery.

A. Pathophysiology: fatty deposits in intimal, medial layer of arterial walls; plaque formation → narrowed arterial lumens; decreased distensibility → decreased blood flow; ischemic changes in tissues.

B. Risk factors:
1. Age (>50).
2. Sex (men).
3. Diabetes mellitus.
4. Hyperlipidemia—obesity.
5. Cigarette smoking.
6. Hypertension.
7. Polycythemia vera.

◆ **C. Assessment:**
1. *Subjective data*
   a. Pain:
      (1) *Type*—cramplike.
      (2) *Location*—foot, calf, thigh, buttocks.
      (3) *Duration*—variable, may be relieved by rest.
      (4) *Precipitating causes*—exercise (intermittent claudication), but occasionally may occur when at rest.
   b. Tingling, numbness in toes, feet.
   c. Persistent coldness of one or both lower extremities.
2. *Objective data*
   a. Lower extremities:
      (1) Pedal pulses—absent or diminished.
      (2) Skin—shiny, glossy, dry, cold, chalky white, decreased/absent hair, ulcers, gangrene.
   b. Lab data: increased serum cholesterol, triglycerides, CBC, platelets
   c. Angiography—indicates location, nature of occlusion.

◆ **D. Analysis/nursing diagnosis:**
1. *Altered tissue perfusion* related to peripheral vascular disease.
2. *Risk for activity intolerance* related to pain and sensory changes.
3. *Pain* related to ischemia.
4. *Risk for impaired skin integrity* related to poor circulation.
5. *Risk for injury* related to numbness of extremities.

◆ **E. Nursing care plan/implementation:**
1. Goal: *promote circulation; decrease discomfort.*
   a. *Position:* elevate head of bed on blocks (3–6 in.), as gravity aids perfusion to thighs, legs; elevating legs increases pain.
   b. Comfort: keep warm; avoid chilling or use of heating pads, which may burn skin; apply bed socks.

c. Circulation: check pedal pulses, skin color, temperature qid.

d. Medications:
   (1) *Vasodilators.*
   (2) *Anticoagulants*—heparin sodium, dicumarol, ASA.
   (3) *Antihyperlipidemics*—clofibrate, cholestyramine resin, nicotinic acid.

2. Goal: *prevent infection, injury.*
   a. Skin care: use bed cradle, sheepskin, heel pads; milk soap; dry thoroughly; lotion; do not massage, so as to prevent release of thrombus.
   b. Foot care: wear properly fitting shoes, slippers when out of bed; inspect for injury or pressure areas; nail care by podiatrist.
   c. *Diet:* high in vitamins B and C to improve cardiovascular functioning and skin integrity.

3. Goal: *health teaching.*
   a. Skin care; inspect daily.
   b. Activity: balance exercise, rest to increase collateral circulation; walk only until painful.
   c. Exercises: walking, Buerger-Allen exercises (gravity alternately fills and empties blood vessels).
   d. *Diet:* low in fat, high in vitamins B, C.
   e. Avoid smoking.
   f. Recognizes and reports signs of occlusion (e.g., pain, cramping, numbness in extremities, color changes—white or blue, temperature changes—cool to cold).

◆ **F. Evaluation/outcome criteria:**
   1. Decreased pain.
   2. Skin integrity preserved; no loss of limb.
   3. Quits smoking.
   4. Does exercises to increase collateral circulation.

XVII. Aneurysms (thoracic or abdominal aortic): localized or diffuse dilatations/outpouching of a vessel wall, usually an artery; exerts pressure on adjacent structures; affects primarily males over age 60; resected surgically, reconstructed with synthetic or vascular graft.

A. Risk factors:
   1. Atherosclerosis.
   2. Trauma.
   3. Syphilis.
   4. Congenital weakness.
   5. Local infection.

◆ **B. Assessment:**
   1. *Subjective data*
      a. Pain:
         (1) Constant, boring, neuralgic, intermittent—low back, abdominal.
         (2) Angina—sudden onset may mean rupture or dissection, which are **emergency** conditions.
      b. Dyspnea; orthopnea.
      c. Dysphagia.
   2. *Objective data*
      a. Vital signs:
         (1) Radial pulses differ.
         (2) Tachycardia.
         (3) Hypotension following rupture leading to shock.
      b. Pulsating mass: abdominal, chest wall pulsation; edema of chest wall (thoracic aneurysm); periumbilical (abdominal aneurysm); audible bruit over aorta.
      c. Cyanosis, mottled below level of aneurysm.
      d. Veins: dilated, superficial—neck, chest, arms.
      e. Cough: paroxysmal, brassy.
      f. Diaphoresis, pallor, fainting following rupture.
      g. Peripheral pulses:
         (1) Femoral present.
         (2) Pedal weak or absent.
      h. Stool bloody from irritation.

◆ **C. Analysis/nursing diagnosis:**
   1. *Altered peripheral tissue perfusion* related to distal arterial emboli.
   2. *Pain* related to pressure on lumbar nerves.
   3. *Anxiety* related to risk of rupture.

◆ **D. Nursing care plan/implementation:**
   1. Goal: *provide emergency care prior to surgery for dissection or rupture.*
      a. Vital signs: at least every 5 min (systolic BP <100 mm Hg and pulse >100 with rupture).
      b. IVs: may have 2–4 sites; lactated Ringer's may be ordered.
      c. Urine output: monitored every 15–30 min.
      d. O$_2$: usually via nasal prongs.
      e. Medications as ordered: antihypertensives to prevent extension of dissection.
      f. Transport to operating room quickly.
      g. See The Perioperative Experience, p. 102, for general preoperative care.
   2. Goal: *prevent complications postoperatively.*
      a. *Position:* initially flat in bed; avoid sharp flexion of hip and knee, which places pressure on femoral and popliteal arteries; turn gently side to side; note erythema on back from pooled blood.
      b. Vital signs: CVP; hourly peripheral pulses distal to graft site, including neurovascular check of lower extremities; absent pulses for 6–12 h indicates occlusion; check with Doppler blood flow detector.

c. Urine output: hourly from indwelling catheter.
   (1) Immediately report anuria or oliguria (<30 mL/h).
   (2) Check color for hematuria.
   (3) Monitor daily blood urea nitrogen (BUN) and creatinine.
d. Observe for *signs of atheroembolization* (patchy areas of ischemia); report change in color, motor ability, or sensation of lower extremities.
e. Observe for *signs of bowel ischemia* (decreased/absent bowel sounds, pain, guaiac-positive diarrhea, abdominal distention); may have nasogastric tube.
f. Measure abdominal girth; increase seen with graft leakage.
3. Goal: *promote comfort*.
   a. Position: alignment, comfort; prevent heel ulcers.
   b. Medication: narcotics.
4. Goal: *health teaching*.
   a. Minimize recurrence: avoid trauma, infection, smoking, high-cholesterol diet, obesity.
   b. Regular medical supervision.
◆ **E. Evaluation/outcome criteria:**
1. Surgical intervention before rupture.
2. No loss of renal function.

XVIII. Varicose veins: abnormally lengthened, tortuous, dilated superficial veins (saphenous); result of incompetent valves, especially in lower extremities; process is irreversible.
A. Pathophysiology: dilated vein → venous stasis → edema, fibrotic changes, pigmentation of skin, lowered resistance to trauma.
B. Risk factors:
1. Congenital defect of venous valves.
2. Trauma.
3. Deep-vein thrombosis.
4. Pregnancy.
5. Abdominal tumors.
6. Chronic disease (heart, liver).
7. Occupations requiring long periods of standing.
◆ **C. Assessment:**
1. *Subjective data*
   a. Dull aches; heaviness in legs.
   b. Pain; muscle cramping.
   c. Fatigue in lower extremities, increased with hot weather, high altitude, history of prolonged standing.
2. *Objective data*
   a. Nodular protrusions along veins.
   b. Edema.
   c. Diagnostic tests: Trendelenburg test; phlebography; Doppler flowmeter.
◆ **D. Analysis/nursing diagnosis:**
1. *Altered tissue perfusion* related to venous valve incompetence.

2. *Pain* related to edema and muscle cramping.
3. *Risk for activity intolerance* related to leg discomfort.
4. *Body image disturbance* related to disfigurement of leg.
◆ **E. Nursing care plan/implementation:**
1. Goal: *promote venous return from lower extremities*.
   a. Activity: walk every hour.
   b. Discourage prolonged sitting, standing, sitting with crossed legs.
   c. *Position:* elevate legs q2–3h; elastic stockings or Ace wraps.
2. Goal: *provide for safety*.
   a. Assist with early ambulation.
   b. Surgical asepsis with wounds, leg ulcers.
   c. Observe for hemorrhage—if occurs: elevate leg, apply pressure, notify physician.
   d. Observe for allergic reactions if sclerosing drugs used; have antihistamine available.
3. Goal: *health teaching*.
   a. Weight-reducing techniques, dietary approaches if indicated.
   b. Preventive measures: leg elevation; avoiding prolonged standing, sitting, high chairs, tight girdles, constrictive clothing; wear support hose.
   c. Expectations for Trendelenburg test.
     (1) While patient is lying down, elevate leg 65 degrees to empty veins.
     (2) Apply tourniquet high on upper thigh (do not constrict deep veins).
     (3) Patient stands with tourniquet in place.
     (4) Filling of veins is observed.
     (5) Normal response is slow filling from below in 20–30 sec, with no change in rate when tourniquet is removed.
     (6) Incompetent veins distend very quickly with back flow.
   d. Prepare for vein ligation and stripping.
◆ **F. Evaluation/outcome criteria:**
1. Relief or control of symptoms.
2. Activity without pain.

XIX. Vein ligation and stripping: surgical intervention for advancing varicosities, stasis ulcerations, and cosmetic needs of patient. Procedure involves ligation of the saphenous vein at the groin, where it joins the femoral vein; saphenous stripping from the groin to the ankle; legs are wrapped with a pressure bandage.
◆ **A.** See XVIII. Varicose veins, above, for assessment data and nursing diagnosis of the patient requiring surgery.

◆ **B. Nursing care plan/implementation:**

1. Goal: *prevent complications.*
   a. *Position:* elevate legs 18 out of 24 h above level of heart, for 1 wk.
   b. Activity:
      (1) Assist with early, frequent ambulation; medicate for pain before ambulation.
      (2) No chair sitting to prevent venous pooling, thrombus formation.
   c. Bleeding: check elastic bandages, dressings several times a day.
2. Goal: *health teaching* to prevent recurrence.
   a. Weight reduction.
   b. Avoid constricting garments.
   c. Change positions frequently.
   d. Wear support hose/stockings to enhance venous return.
   e. No crossing legs at knees.

◆ **C. Evaluation/outcome criteria:**

1. No complications—hemorrhage, infection, nerve damage, deep-vein thrombosis.
2. No recurrence of varicosities.
3. Adequate circulation to legs: strong pedal pulses.
4. Resumes daily activities; free of pain.

XX. Thrombophlebitis: formation of a blood clot in an inflamed vein, secondary to phlebitis or partial obstruction; may lead to venous insufficiency and pulmonary embolism.

A. Pathophysiology: endothelial inflammation → formation of platelet plug (blood clot) → slowing of blood flow → increase in procoagulants in local area → initiation of clotting mechanisms.

B. Risk factors:

1. Immobility.
2. Venous disease.
3. Prolonged sitting—knees bent.
4. Childbirth.
5. Hypercoagulability of blood.
6. Venous trauma (IVs).
7. Fractures.

◆ **C. Assessment:**

1. *Subjective data*
   a. Calf stiffness, soreness.
   b. Severe pain: walking, dorsiflexion of foot (*Homans' sign*).
2. *Objective data*
   a. Vein: redness, heat, hardness, threadiness.
   b. Limb: swollen, pale, cold.
   c. Vital signs: low-grade fever.

◆ **D. Analysis/nursing diagnosis:**

1. *Altered peripheral tissue perfusion* related to venous stasis.
2. *Pain* related to inflammation.
3. *Activity intolerance* related to leg pain.

◆ **E. Nursing care plan/implementation:**

1. Goal: *provide rest, comfort, and relief from pain.*
   a. Bedrest.
   b. *Position:* as ordered; usually extremity *elevated;* watch for pressure points.
   c. Apply warm, moist heat to affected area as prescribed (cold may also be ordered).
   d. Assess progress of affected area: swelling, pain, soreness, temperature, color.
   e. Administer analgesics as ordered.
2. Goal: *prevent complications.*
   a. Observe for signs of embolism (pain at site of embolism); allergic reaction (anaphylactic shock) with streptokinase.
   b. Precautions: *no* rubbing or massage of limb.
   c. Medications: anticoagulants (sodium heparin, coumarin); streptokinase (Varidase). (Table 2.6.)
   d. Bleeding: hematuria, epistaxis, ecchymosis.
   e. Skin care, to relieve increased redness/maceration from hot or cold applications.
   f. ROM: unaffected limb.
3. Goal: *health teaching.*
   a. Precautions: tight garters, girdles; sitting with legs crossed; oral contraceptives.
   b. Preventive measures: walking daily, swimming several times weekly if possible, wading, rest periods—with legs elevated, elastic stockings (may remove at bedtime).
   c. Medication side effects: anticoagulants—pink toothbrush, hematuria, easily bruised.
      (1) Carry MedicAlert card/bracelet.
      (2) Contraindicated drugs—aspirin, glutethimide (Doriden), chloramphenicol (Chloromycetin), neomycin, phenylbutazone (Butazolidin), barbiturates.
   d. Prepare for surgery (thrombectomy, vein ligation).

◆ **F. Evaluation/outcome criteria:**

1. No complications (e.g., embolism).
2. No recurrence of symptoms.
3. Free of pain—ambulates without discomfort.

XXI. Peripheral embolism: fragments of thrombi, globules of fat, clumps of tissue, calcified plaques, or air moves in the circulation and lodges in vessel, obstructing blood flow; thrombic emboli most common; may be venous or arterial.

Conditions Affecting Tissue Perfusion

I. Iron deficiency anemia (hypochromic microcytic anemia): inadequate production of red blood cells

■ TABLE 2.6   Nursing Responsibilities with Anticoagulant Therapy

	Heparin	Warfarin (Coumadin)
Monitor	PTT (25–38 sec) (2–3 times baseline)	PT (11–15 sec) (1½–2½ times baseline)
Inspect	Ecchymosis, bleeding gums, petechiae, hematuria	Bleeding, ecchymosis
Administer	With an infusion pump; never mix with other drugs; never aspirate; avoid massaging site	Same time every day; PO
Avoid	Salicylates and other anticoagulants, e.g., antacids, corticosteroids, penicillin, phenytoin	Same as heparin
Antidote	Protamine sulfate	Vitamin K

due to lack of heme (iron); common in infants, pregnant women, and premenopausal women.

A. **Pathophysiology:** decreased dietary intake, impaired absorption, or increased utilization of iron decreases the amount of iron bound to plasma transferrin and transported to bone marrow for hemoglobin synthesis; decreased hemoglobin in erythrocytes decreases amount of oxygen delivered to tissues.

B. **Risk factors:**
  1. *Excessive menstruation.*
  2. *Gastrointestinal bleeding*—peptic ulcer, hookworm, tumors.
  3. *Inadequate diet*—anorexia, fad diets, cultural practices.
  4. *Poor absorption*—stomach, small intestine disease.

◆ C. **Assessment:**
  1. *Subjective data*
    a. Fatigue: increasing.
    b. Headache.
    c. Change in appetite; difficulty swallowing due to pharyngeal edema/ulceration; heartburn.
    d. Shortness of breath on exercise.
    e. Extremities: numb, tingling.
    f. Flatulence.
    g. Menorrhagia.
  2. *Objective data*
    a. Vital signs:
      (1) *BP*—increased systolic, widened pulse pressure.
      (2) *Pulse*—tachycardia.
      (3) *Respirations*—tachypnea.
      (4) *Temperature*—normal or subnormal.
    b. Skin/mucous membranes: pale, dry.
    c. Sclera: pearly white.
    d. Nails: brittle, spoon-shaped, flattened.
    e. Lab data: *decreased*—hemoglobin (<10 g/dL blood), serum iron (<65 µg/dL blood); *increased* total iron-binding capacity.

◆ D. **Analysis/nursing diagnosis:**
  1. *Altered nutrition, less than body requirements,* related to inadequate iron absorption.

  2. *Altered tissue perfusion* related to reduction in red cells.
  3. *Risk for activity intolerance* related to profound weakness.
  4. *Impaired gas exchange* related to decreased oxygen-carrying capacity.

◆ E. **Nursing care plan/implementation:**
  1. Goal: *promote physical and mental equilibrium.*
    a. *Position:* optimal for respiratory excursion; deep breathing; turn frequently to prevent skin breakdown.
    b. Rest: balance with activity, as tolerated; assist with ambulation.
    c. Medication (hematinics):
      (1) Oral iron therapy (ferrous sulfate)—give *with* meals.
      (2) Intramuscular therapy (iron dextran)—use second needle for injection after withdrawal from ampule; use Z track method; inject 0.5 cc of air before withdrawing needle, to prevent tissue necrosis; use 2–3-in. needle; rotate sites; do *not* rub site or allow wearing of constricting garments after injection.
    d. Keep warm: *no* hot water bottles, heating pads, due to decreased sensitivity.
    e. *Diet:* high in protein, iron, vitamins (see Unit 3); assistance with feeding, if needed.
  2. Goal: *health teaching.*
    a. Dietary regimen.
    b. Iron therapy: explain purpose, dosage, side effects (black or green stools, constipation, diarrhea); take with meals.
    c. Activity: exercise to tolerance, with planned rest periods.

◆ F. **Evaluation/outcome criteria:**
  1. Hemoglobin level returns to normal range.
  2. Tolerates activity without fatigue.
  3. Selects foods appropriate for dietary regimen.

II. **Hemolytic anemia** (normocytic normochromic anemia): unknown factor causes antibodies to destroy the body's own erythrocytes (autoimmune);

may occur secondary to malignant lymphoma, ulcerative colitis, lupus erythematosus, or drug therapy; common in those over age 40.

A. Risk factors:
1. Malignant lymphoma.
2. Ulcerative colitis.
3. Lupus erythematosus.
4. Drug therapy.

◆ **B. Assessment:**
1. *Subjective data*
   a. Fatigue; physical weakness.
   b. Dizziness.
   c. Shortness of breath.
   d. Diaphoresis on slight exertion.
2. *Objective data*
   a. Skin: pallor, jaundice.
   b. Posture: drooping.
   c. Lab data:
   (1) Decreased hemoglobin.
   (2) Increased reticulocyte count.
   (3) Direct Coombs test positive.

◆ **C.** See I. Iron deficiency anemia, p. 69, for analysis, nursing care plan/implementation, and evaluation/outcome criteria.

III. Pernicious anemia (hyperchromic macrocytic anemia): lack of intrinsic factor found in gastric mucosa, which is necessary for vitamin B_{12} (extrinsic factor) absorption; slow developing, usually after age 50; may be an autoimmune disorder.

A. Pathophysiology: atrophy or surgical removal of glandular mucosa in fundus of stomach → degenerative changes in brain, spinal cord, and peripheral nerves from lack of vitamin B_{12}.

B. Risk factors:
1. Partial or complete gastric resection.
2. Prolonged iron deficiency.
3. Heredity.

◆ **C. Assessment:**
1. *Subjective data*
   a. Hands, feet: tingling, numbness.
   b. Weakness, fatigue.
   c. Sore tongue, anorexia.
   d. Difficulties with memory, balance.
   e. Irritability, mild depression.
   f. Shortness of breath.
   g. Palpitations.
2. *Objective data*
   a. Skin: pale, flabby, jaundiced.
   b. Sclera: icterus (yellow).
   c. Tongue: smooth, glossy, red, swollen.
   d. Vital signs:
      (1) *BP*—normal or elevated.
      (2) *Pulse*—tachycardia.
   e. Nervous system:
      (1) Decreased vibratory sense in lower extremities.
      (2) Loss of coordination.
      (3) *Babinski* present (flaring of toes with stimulation of sole of foot).
      (4) Positive *Romberg* (loses balance when eyes closed).
      (5) Increased or diminished reflexes.
   f. Lab data:
      (1) *Increased*—hemoglobin, bilirubin.
      (2) *Decreased*—RBCs, platelets, gastric secretions, Schilling test (radioactive vitamin B_{12} urine test).

◆ **D. Analysis/nursing diagnosis:**
1. *Altered nutrition, less than body requirements,* related to B_{12} deficiency.
2. *Impaired physical mobility* related to numbness of extremities.
3. *Fatigue* related to decreased oxygen-carrying capacity.
4. *Altered oral mucous membrane* related to changes in gastric mucosa.
5. *Altered thought processes* related to progressive neurologic degeneration.

◆ **E. Nursing care plan/implementation:**
1. Goal: *promote physical and emotional comfort.*
   a. Activity: bedrest or activity as tolerated—restrictions depend on neurologic or cardiac involvement.
   b. Comfort: keep extremities warm—light blankets, loose-fitting socks.
   c. Medication: vitamin B_{12} therapy as ordered.
   d. *Diet:*
      (1) Six small feedings.
      (2) Soft or pureed.
      (3) Organ meats, fish, eggs.
   e. Mouth care: before and after meals, to increase appetite and relieve mouth discomfort.
2. Goal: *health teaching.*
   a. Medication:
      (1) Lifelong therapy.
      (2) Injection techniques; rotation of sites.
   b. Diet.
   c. Rest; exercise to tolerance.

◆ **F. Evaluation/outcome criteria:**
1. No irreversible neurologic or cardiac complications.
2. Takes vitamin B_{12} for the rest of life—uses safe injection technique.
3. Returns for follow-up care.

IV. Polycythemia vera: abnormal increase in circulating red blood cells; considered to be a form of malignancy; occurs more frequently among middle-aged Jewish men.

A. Pathophysiology: unknown causes → massive increases of erythrocytes, myelocytes (bone marrow leukocytes), and thrombocytes → increased blood viscosity/volume and tissue/organ congestion; increased peripheral vascular resistance; intravascular thrombosis usually develops in middle age, particularly in Jewish men; in contrast, *secondary* polycythemia occurs as a compensatory response to tissue hypoxia associated with prolonged exposure to high altitude, chronic lung disease, and heart disease.

◆ **B. Assessment:**
   1. *Subjective data*
      a. Headache; dizziness; ringing in ears.
      b. Weakness; loss of interest.
      c. Feelings of abdominal fullness.
      d. Shortness of breath; orthopnea.
      e. Pruritus, especially after bathing.
      f. Pain: gouty-arthritic.
   2. *Objective data*
      a. Skin: mucosal erythema, ruddy complexion (reddish purple).
      b. Ecchymosis; gingival (gum) bleeding.
      c. Enlarged liver, spleen.
      d. Hypertension.
      e. Lab data:
         (1) *Increased*—hemoglobin, hematocrit, RBCs, leukocytes, platelets, uric acid.
         (2) *Decreased* bone marrow iron.

◆ **C. Analysis/nursing diagnosis:**
   1. *Altered tissue perfusion* related to capillary congestion.
   2. *Risk for injury* related to dizziness, weakness.
   3. *Fluid volume excess* related to mass production of red blood cells.
   4. *Risk for impaired skin integrity* related to pruritus.
   5. *Ineffective breathing pattern* related to shortness of breath, orthopnea.

◆ **D. Nursing care plan/implementation:**
   1. Goal: *promote comfort and prevent complications.*
      a. Observe for signs of bleeding, thrombosis—stools, urine, gums, skin, ecchymosis.
      b. Reduce occurrence: *avoid* prolonged sitting, knee gatch.
      c. Assist with ambulation.
      d. *Position:* elevate head of bed.
      e. Skin care: cool-water baths to decrease pruritus; may add bicarbonate of soda to water.
      f. Fluids: *force,* to reduce blood viscosity and promote urine excretion; 1500–2500 mL/24 h.
      g. *Diet:* avoid foods high in iron, to reduce RBC production.
      h. Assist with venesection (phlebotomy), as ordered.
   2. Goal: *health teaching.*
      a. *Diet:* foods to *avoid* (e.g., liver, egg yolks); fluids to be increased.
      b. Signs/symptoms of complications: infections, hemorrhage.
      c. *Avoid:* falls, bumps; hot baths/showers (worsens pruritus).
      d. Drugs: myelosuppressive agents (busulfan [Myleran], cyclophosphamide [Cy-

toxan], chlorambucil, radioactive phosphorus); purpose; side effects.
      e. Procedures: venesection (phlebotomy) if ordered.

◆ **E. Evaluation/outcome criteria:**
   1. Acceptance of chronic disease.
   2. Reports at prescribed intervals for follow-up.
   3. Remission: reduction of bone marrow activity, blood volume and viscosity (RBC <6,500,000/μL; Hgb <18; Hct <45%; WBC <10,000).
   4. No complications (e.g., thrombi, hemorrhage, gout, CHF, leukemia).

V. Leukemia (acute and chronic): a neoplastic disease involving the leukopoietic tissue in either the bone marrow or lymphoid areas; acute leukemia occurs in children, young adults, chronic forms occur in later adult life.
   A. Types
      1. Acute nonlymphocytic (ANLL)—formerly acute myelogenous leukemia (AML); seen generally in older age (>60 yr).
      2. Acute lymphocytic (ALL)—common in children 2–10 yr.
      3. Chronic lymphocytic (CLL)—generally affects the elderly.
      4. Chronic myelogenous (CML)—also known as chronic granulocytic leukemia (CGL); more likely to occur between 25 and 60 yr.
   B. Pathophysiology: displacement of normal marrow cells by proliferating leukemic cells (abnormal, immature leukocytes) → normochromic anemia, thrombocytopenia.
   C. Risk factors:
      1. Viruses.
      2. Genetic abnormalities.
      3. Exposure to chemicals.
      4. Radiation.
      5. Treatment for other types of cancer (e.g., alkylating agents).

◆ **D. Assessment:**
   1. *Subjective data*
      a. Fatigue, weakness.
      b. Anorexia, nausea.
      c. Pain: joints, bones (acute leukemia).
      d. Night sweats, weight loss, malaise.
   2. *Objective data*
      a. Skin: pallor due to anemia; jaundice.
      b. Fever: frequent infections; mouth ulcers.
      c. Bleeding: petechiae, purpura, ecchymosis, epistaxis, gingiva.
      d. Organ enlargement: spleen, liver.
      e. Enlarged lymph nodes; tenderness.
      f. Bone marrow aspiration: ↑ presence of blasts.
      g. Lab data:
         (1) WBC—15,000–500,000.
         (2) RBC—normal to severely decreased.
         (3) Hgb—low or normal.
         (4) Platelets—low to elevated.

◆ **E. Analysis/nursing diagnosis:**

1. *Risk for infection* related to immature or abnormal leukocytes.
2. *Activity intolerance* related to hypoxia and weakness.
3. *Fatigue* related to anemia.
4. *Altered tissue perfusion* related to anemia.
5. *Anxiety* related to diagnosis and treatment.
6. *Altered oral mucous membrane* related to susceptibility to infection.
7. *Fear* related to diagnosis.
8. *Ineffective individual or family coping* related to potentially fatal disease.

◆ **F. Nursing care plan/implementation:**

1. Goal: *prevent, control, and treat infection.*
   a. Protective isolation if indicated.
   b. Observe for early signs of infection:
      (1) Inflammation at injection sites.
      (2) Vital-sign changes.
      (3) Cough.
      (4) Obtain cultures.
   c. Give antibiotics as ordered.
   d. Mouth care: clean q2h, examine for new lesions, avoid trauma.
2. Goal: *assess and control bleeding, anemia.*
   a. Activity: restrict to prevent trauma.
   b. Observe for hemorrhage: vital signs; body orifices, stool, urine.
   c. Control localized bleeding: ice, pressure at least 3–4 min after needle sticks, positioning.
   d. Use soft-bristle or foam-rubber toothbrush to prevent gingival bleeding.
   e. Give blood/blood components as ordered; observe for transfusion reactions.
3. Goal: *provide rest, comfort, nutrition.*
   a. Activity: 8 h sleep; daily nap.
   b. Comfort measures: flotation mattress, bed cradle, sheepskin.
   c. Analgesics: without delay.
      (1) Mild pain (acetaminophen [Tylenol], propoxyphene HCl [Darvon] without aspirin).
      (2) Severe pain (codeine, meperidine HCl [Demerol]).
   d. *Diet:* bland.
      (1) High in protein, minerals, vitamins.
      (2) Low roughage.
      (3) Small, frequent feedings.
      (4) Favorite foods.
   e. Fluids: 3000–4000 mL/d.
4. Goal: *reduce side effects from therapeutic regimen.*
   a. Nausea: antiemetics, usually half-hour *before* chemotherapy.
   b. Increased uric acid level: force fluids.
   c. Stomatitis: antiseptic anesthetic mouthwashes.
   d. Rectal irritation: meticulous toileting, sitz baths, topical relief (e.g., Tucks).
5. Goal: *provide emotional/spiritual support.*
   a. Contact clergy if patient desires.
   b. Allow, encourage patient-initiated discussion of death (developmentally appropriate).
   c. Allow family to be involved in care.
   d. If death occurs, provide privacy, listening, sharing of grief for family.
6. Goal: *health teaching.*
   a. Prevent infection.
   b. Limit activity.
   c. Control bleeding.
   d. Reduce nausea.
   e. Mouth care.
   f. Chemotherapy: regimen; side effects.

◆ **G. Evaluation/outcome criteria:**

1. Alleviate symptoms; obtain remission.
2. Prevent complications (e.g., infection).
3. Ventilates emotions—accepts and deals with anger.
4. Experiences peaceful death (e.g., pain free).

VI. Idiopathic thrombocytopenic purpura (ITP): potentially fatal disorder characterized by spontaneous increase in platelet destruction; possible autoimmune response; remissions occur spontaneously or following splenectomy; in contrast, secondary thrombocytopenia (STP) is caused by viral infections, drug hypersensitivity (i.e., *quinidine, sulfonamides*), lupus, or bone marrow failure; treat cause.

◆ **A. Assessment:**

1. *Subjective data*
   a. Spontaneous skin hemorrhages—lower extremities.
   b. Menorrhagia.
   c. Epistaxis.
2. *Objective data*
   a. Bleeding: GI, urinary, nasal; following minor trauma, dental extractions.
   b. Petechiae; ecchymosis.
   c. Lab data:
      (1) *Decreased* platelets ($<100,000/mm^3$).
      (2) Increased bleeding time.
      (3) Tourniquet test—positive, demonstrating increased capillary fragility.

◆ **B. Analysis/nursing diagnosis:**

1. *Risk for injury* related to hemorrhage.
2. *Altered tissue perfusion* related to fragile capillaries.
3. *Impaired skin integrity* related to skin hemorrhages.

◆ **C. Nursing care plan/implementation:**

1. Goal: *prevent complications from bleeding tendencies.*
   a. Precautions:
      (1) Injections—use small-bore needles; rotate sites; apply direct pressure.
      (2) Avoid bumping, trauma.
      (3) Use swabs for mouth care.
   b. Observe for signs of bleeding, petechiae following blood pressure reading, ecchymosis, purpura.
   c. Administer steroids (e.g., prednisone) with ITP to increase platelet count; give

platelets for count below 20,000–30,000/
µL with STP.
2. Goal: *health teaching.*
   a. Avoid traumatic activities:
      (1) Contact sports.
      (2) Violent sneezing, coughing, nose blowing.
      (3) Straining at stool.
      (4) Heavy lifting.
   b. *Signs of decreased platelets*—petechiae, ecchymosis, gingival bleeding, hematuria, menorrhagia.
   c. Use MedicAlert tag/card.
   d. Precautions: self-medication; particularly avoid aspirin-containing drugs.
   e. Prepare for splenectomy if drug therapy unsuccessful (prednisone, cyclophosphamide, azathioprine [Imuran]).
◆ **D. Evaluation/outcome criteria:**
   1. Returns for follow-up.
   2. No complications (e.g., hemorrhage).
   3. Platelet count >200,000/µL.
   4. Skin remains intact.
   5. Resumes self-care activities.
VII. Splenectomy: removal of spleen following rupture due to acquired hemolytic anemia, trauma, tumor, or idiopathic thrombocytopenic purpura.
◆ **A. Analysis/nursing diagnosis:**
   1. *Risk for fluid volume deficit* related to hemorrhage.
   2. *Risk for infection* related to impaired immune response.
   3. *Pain* related to abdominal distention.
◆ **B. Nursing care plan/implementation:**
   1. Goal: *prepare for surgery.*
      a. Give whole blood, as ordered.
      b. Insert nasogastric tube to decrease postoperative abdominal distention, as ordered.
   2. Goal: *prevent postoperative complications.*
      a. Observe for:
         (1) *Hemorrhage*—bleeding tendency with thrombocytopenia due to decreased platelet count.
         (2) *Gastrointestinal distention*—removal of enlarged spleen may result in distended stomach and intestines, to fill void.
      b. Recognize 101°F temp as normal for 10 d.
      c. Incision: splint when coughing, to prevent high incidence of atelectasis, pneumonia with upper-abdominal incision.
   3. Goal: *health teaching.*
      a. Increased risk of infection postsplenectomy.
      b. Report signs of infection *immediately.*
◆ **C. Evaluation/outcome criteria:**
   1. No complications (e.g., respiratory, subphrenic abscess or hematoma, thromboemboli, infection).

2. Complete and permanent remission—occurs in 60–80% of patients.

Fluid and Electrolyte Imbalances

Imbalances in fluid and electrolytes may be due to changes in the total quantity of either substance (deficit or excess), protein deficiencies, and/or extracellular fluid volume shifts. Older patients and very young patients are particularly susceptible.

I. Fluid volume deficits: decreased quantities of fluid and electrolytes may be caused by *deficient intake* (poor dietary habits, anorexia, and nausea), *excessive output* (vomiting, nasogastric suction, and prolonged diarrhea), or *failure of regulatory mechanism.*
   A. Pathophysiology: water moves out of the cells to replace a significant water loss; cells eventually become unable to compensate for the lost fluid, and cellular dehydration begins, leading to circulatory collapse.
   B. Risk factors:
      1. No fluids available.
      2. Available fluids not drinkable.
      3. Inability to take fluids independently.
      4. No response to thirst; does not recognize the need for fluids.
      5. Inability to communicate need; does not speak same language.
      6. Aphasia.
      7. Weakness, comatose.
      8. Inability to swallow.
      9. Psychological alterations.
◆ **C. Assessment:**
      1. *Subjective data*
         a. Thirst.
         b. Behavioral changes: apprehension, apathy, lethargy, confusion, restlessness.
         c. Dizziness.
         d. Numbness and tingling of hands and feet.
         e. Anorexia and nausea.
         f. Abdominal cramps.
      2. *Objective data*
         a. Sudden weight loss of 5%.
         b. Vital signs:
            (1) *Decreased* BP; postural changes.
            (2) *Increased* temperature.
            (3) Irregular, weak, rapid pulse.
            (4) Increased rate and depth of respirations.
         c. Skin: cool and pale in absence of infection; decreased turgor.
         d. Urine: oliguria to anuria, high specific gravity.
         e. Eyes: soft, sunken.
         f. Tongue: furrows.
         g. Lab data:
            (1) Blood—increased hematocrit and BUN.
            (2) Urine—decreased 17-ketosteroids.

Adult

◆ **D. Analysis/nursing diagnosis:**
1. *Fluid volume deficit* related to inadequate fluid intake.

◆ **E. Nursing care plan/implementation:**
1. Goal: *restore fluid and electrolyte balance—*increase fluid intake to hydrate client.
   a. IVs as ordered; small, frequent drinks by mouth.
   b. Daily weights (same time of day) to monitor progress of fluid replacement.
   c. I&O, hourly outputs (when in acute state).
   d. *Avoid* hypertonic solutions (may cause fluid shift when compensatory mechanisms begin to function).
2. Goal: *promote comfort.*
   a. Frequent skin care (lack of hydration causes dry skin, which may increase risk for skin breakdown).
   b. *Position:* change every hour to relieve pressure.
   c. Medications as ordered: antiemetics, antidiarrheal.
3. Goal: *prevent physical injury.*
   a. Frequent mouth care (mucous membrane dries due to dehydration; therefore, patient is at risk for breaks in mucous membrane, halitosis).
   b. Monitor IV flow rate—observe for circulatory overload, pulmonary edema related to potential fluid shift when compensatory mechanisms begin, or patient is unable to tolerate rate of fluid replacement.
   c. Monitor vitals, including level of consciousness (decreasing BP and level of consciousness indicate continuation of fluid loss).
   d. Prepare for surgery if hemorrhage present (internal bleeding can only be relieved by surgical intervention).

◆ **F. Evaluation/outcome criteria:**
1. Mentally alert.
2. Moist, intact mucous membranes.
3. Urinary output approximately equal to intake.
4. No further weight loss.
5. Gradual weight gain.

II. Fluid volume excess: excessive quantities of fluid and electrolytes may be due to *increased ingestion,* tube feedings, intravenous infusions, multiple tap-water enemas, or a *failure of regulatory systems,* resulting in inability to excrete excesses.

A. Pathophysiology: hypo-osmolar water excess in extracellular compartment leads to intracellular water excess because the concentration of solutes in the intracellular fluid is greater than that in the extracellular fluid. Water moves to equalize concentration, causing swelling of the cells.

B. Risk factors:
1. Excessive intake of electrolyte-free fluids.

2. Increased secretion of ADH in response to stress, drugs, anesthetics.
3. Decreased or inadequate output of urine.
4. Psychogenic polydipsia.
5. Certain medical conditions: tuberculosis; encephalitis; meningitis; endocrine disturbances; tumors of lung, pancreas, duodenum.
6. Inadequate kidney function or kidney failure.

◆ **C. Assessment:**
1. *Subjective data*
   a. Behavioral changes: irritability, apathy, confusion, disorientation.
   b. Headache.
   c. Anorexia, nausea, cramping.
   d. Fatigue.
   e. Dyspnea.
2. *Objective data*
   a. Vital signs: elevated blood pressure.
   b. Skin: warm, moist; edema—eyelids, facial, dependent, pitting.
   c. Sudden weight gain of 5%.
   d. Pink, frothy sputum; productive.
   e. Urine: polyuria, nocturia.
   f. Lab data:
      (1) Blood—*decreasing* hematocrit, BUN.
      (2) Urine—*decreasing* specific gravity.

◆ **D. Analysis/nursing diagnosis:**
1. *Fluid volume excess* related to excessive fluid intake or decreased fluid output.

◆ **E. Nursing care plan/implementation:**
1. Goal: *maintain oxygen to all cells.*
   a. *Position:* semi-Fowler's or Fowler's to facilitate improved gas exchange.
   b. Vital signs: q4h.
   c. Fluid restriction.
   d. Possible rotating tourniquets as needed (especially for interstitial-to-plasma shift).
2. Goal: *promote excretion of excess fluid.*
   a. Medications as ordered: diuretics.
   b. If in kidney failure: may need dialysis; explain procedure.
   c. Assist patient during paracentesis, thoracentesis, phlebotomy.
      (1) Monitor vital signs to detect shock.
      (2) Prevent injury by monitoring sterile technique.
      (3) Prevent falling by stabilizing appropriate position during procedure.
      (4) Support patient psychologically.
3. Goal: *obtain/maintain fluid balance.*
   a. Daily weights; 1 kg = 1000 mL fluid.
   b. Measure: all edematous parts, abdominal girth, I&O.
   c. *Limit:* fluids by mouth, IVs, sodium.
   d. Strict monitoring of IV fluids.
4. Goal: *prevent tissue injury.*
   a. Skin and mouth care as needed.
   b. Evaluate feet for edema and discoloration when patient is out of bed.

c. Observe suture line on surgical patients (potential for evisceration due to excess fluid retention).

d. IV route preferred for parenteral medications; Z track if medications are to be given IM (otherwise injected liquid will escape through injection site).

5. Goal: *health teaching*.

a. Improve nutritional status with low-sodium diet.

b. Identify cause that put patient at risk for imbalance, methods to avoid this situation in the future.

c. Desired and side effects of diuretics and other prescribed medications.

d. Monitor urinary output, ankle edema, and report to health care manager when fluid retention is noticed.

e. Limit fluid intake when kidney/cardiac function impaired.

◆ **F. Evaluation/outcome criteria:**

1. Fluid balance obtained.

2. No respiratory, cardiac complications.

3. Vital signs within normal limits.

4. Urinary output improved, no evidence of edema.

III. Common electrolyte imbalances: electrolytes are taken into the body in foods and fluids; normally lost through sweat and urine. May also be lost through hemorrhage, vomiting, and diarrhea. Clinically important electrolytes are:

A. Sodium (Na^+): normal 135–145 mEq/L. Most prevalent cation in extracellular fluid. Controls osmotic pressure; essential for neuromuscular functioning and intracellular chemical reactions. Aids in maintenance of acid-base balance. Necessary for glucose to be transported into cells.

1. *Hyponatremia*—sodium deficit, resulting from either a sodium loss or water excess. Serum-sodium level below 135 mEq/L; symptoms usually do not occur until below 120 mEq/L unless rapid drop.

2. *Hypernatremia*—excess sodium in the blood, resulting from either high sodium intake, water loss, or low water intake. Serum-sodium level above 145 mEq/L.

B. Potassium (K^+): normal 3.5–5.0 mEq/L. Direct effect on excitability of nerves and muscles. Contributes to intracellular osmotic pressure and influences acid-base balance. Major cation of the cell. Required for storage of nitrogen as muscle protein.

1. *Hypokalemia*—potassium deficit related to dehydration, starvation, vomiting, diarrhea, diuretics. Serum-potassium level below 3.5 mEq/L; symptoms may not occur until below 2.5 mEq/L.

2. *Hyperkalemia*—potassium excess related to severe tissue damage, renal disease, excess administration of oral or IV potassium. Serum-potassium level above 5 mEq/L; symptoms usually occur when above 6.5 mEq/L.

C. Calcium (Ca^+): normal 4.5–5.5 mEq/L. Essential to muscle metabolism, cardiac function, and bone health. Controlled by parathyroid hormone; reciprocal relationship between calcium and phosphorus.

1. *Hypocalcemia*—loss of calcium related to inadequate intake, vitamin D deficiency, hypoparathyroidism, damage to the parathyroid gland, decreased absorption in the GI tract, excess loss through kidneys. Serum-calcium level below 4.5 mEq/L.

2. *Hypercalcemia*—calcium excess related to hyperparathyroidism, immobility, bone tumors, renal failure, excess intake of Ca^{2+} or Vitamin D. Serum-calcium level above 5.5 mEq/L.

D. Magnesium (Mg^{2+}): normal 1.5–2.5 mEq/L. Essential to cellular metabolism of carbohydrates and proteins.

1. *Hypomagnesemia*—magnesium deficit related to impaired absorption from GI tract, excess loss through kidneys, and prolonged periods of poor nutritional intake. Hypomagnesemia leads to neuromuscular irritability. Serum-magnesium level below 1.5 mEq/L.

2. *Hypermagnesemia*—magnesium excess related to renal insufficiency, overdose during replacement therapy, severe dehydration, repeated enemas with Mg^{2+} sulfate (epsom salts). Serum-magnesium level above 2.5 mEq/L.

◆ **E.** Table 2.7 provides assessment, analysis, nursing care plan/implementation, and evaluation/outcome criteria of the various electrolyte imbalances.

IV. Acid-base balance: concentration of hydrogen ions in extracellular fluid is determined by the ratio of bicarbonate to carbonic acid. The normal ratio is 20:1. Even when arterial blood gases are abnormal, if the ratio remains at 20:1, no imbalance will occur. Table 2.8 shows blood gas variations with acid-base imbalances.

A. Causes of blood gas abnormalities: Table 2.9.

B. Types of acid-base imbalance:

1. *Acidosis:* hydrogen ion concentration increases and pH decreases.

2. *Alkalosis:* hydrogen ion concentration decreases and pH increases.

3. *Metabolic imbalances: bicarbonate* is the problem. In primary conditions, the level of bicarbonate is directly *proportional* to pH.

a. *Metabolic acidosis:* excessive acid is produced or added to the body, bicarbonate is lost or acid is retained due to poorly functioning kidneys. Deficit of bicarbonate.

b. *Metabolic alkalosis:* excessive acid is lost or bicarbonate or alkali is retained. Excess of bicarbonate.

c. As compensatory mechanism, P_{CO_2} will be *low in metabolic acidosis,* as the body attempts to eliminate excess carbonic acid and elevate pH. P_{CO_2} will become *elevated in metabolic alkalosis.*

4. *Respiratory imbalances: carbonic acid* is the problem. In primary conditions, P_{CO_2} is inversely proportional to the pH.

a. *Respiratory acidosis:* pulmonary ventilation decreases, causing an elevation in the level of carbon dioxide or carbonic acid. Excess of P_{CO_2}.

b. *Respiratory alkalosis:* pulmonary ventilation increases, causing a decrease in the level of carbon dioxide or carbonic acid. Deficit of P_{CO_2}.

c. As a compensatory mechanism, the level of bicarbonate will *increase in respiratory acidosis* and *decrease in respiratory alkalosis.*

◆ **C. Assessment:** Table 2.10.

◆ **D. Analysis/nursing diagnosis:**

1. *Impaired gas exchange* related to hyperventilation.

2. *Ineffective breathing pattern* related to decreased thoracic movements.

3. *Ineffective airway clearance* related to retained secretions.

4. *Risk for injury* related to poorly functioning kidneys.

5. *Altered renal tissue perfusion* related to dehydration.

6. *Altered urinary elimination* related to renal failure.

7. *Fluid volume excess* related to altered kidney function.

8. *Fluid volume deficit* related to diarrhea or dehydration.

9. *Knowledge deficit* related to self-administration of antacid medications.

◆ **E. Nursing care plan/implementation:** see Table 2.10.

◆ **F. Evaluation/outcome criteria:** see Table 2.10.

Conditions Affecting Gas Transport

I. Pneumonia: acute inflammation of lungs with exudate accumulation in alveoli and other respiratory passages that interferes with ventilation process.

A. Types:

1. *Typical/classic pneumonia: pneumococcal;* related to diminished defense mechanisms, history of alcoholism, recent respiratory tract infection, viral influenza, increased age, and COPD.

2. *Atypical pneumonia:* related to contact with specific organisms.

a. *Mycoplasma pneumoniae* or *Legionella pneumophila,* if untreated, can lead to serious complications such as disseminated intravascular coagulation (DIC), thrombocytopenic purpura, renal failure, inflammations of the heart, neurologic disorders, or possible death.

b. *Pneumocystis carinii* in conjunction with AIDS.

3. *Aspiration pneumonia:*

a. *Noninfectious:* aspiration of fluids (gastric secretions, foods, liquids, tube feedings) into the airways.

b. *Bacterial aspiration pneumonia:* related to poor cough mechanisms due to anesthesia, coma (mixed flora of upper respiratory tract cause pneumonia).

4. *Hematogenous pneumonia bacterial infections:* related to spread of bacteria from the bloodstream.

B. Pathophysiology: caused by infectious or noninfectious agents, clotting of an exudate rich in fibrogen, consolidated lung tissue.

◆ **C. Assessment:**

1. *Subjective data*

a. Pain location: chest (affected side), referred to abdomen, shoulder, flank.

b. Irritability, restlessness.

c. Apprehensiveness.

d. Nausea, anorexia.

e. History of exposure.

2. *Objective data*

a. Cough

(1) Productive, rust (blood) or yellowish sputum (greenish with atypical pneumonia).

(2) Splinting of affected side when coughing.

b. Sudden increased fever, chills.

c. Nasal flaring, circumoral cyanosis.

d. Respiratory distress: tachypnea.

e. Auscultation

(1) Decreased breath sounds on *affected* side.

(2) Exaggerated breath sounds on *unaffected* side.

(3) Crackles, bronchial breath sounds.

(4) Dullness over consolidated area.

(5) Possible pleural friction rub.

f. Chest retraction (air hunger in infants).

g. Vomiting.

h. Facial herpes simplex.

i. Diagnostic studies:

(1) Chest X ray: haziness to consolidation.

(2) Sputum culture: specific organisms, usually pneumococcus.

j. Lab data:

(1) Blood culture: organism specific except when viral.

(2) WBC: leukocytosis.

(3) Sedimentation rate: elevated.

◆ **D. Analysis/nursing diagnosis:**

1. *Ineffective airway clearance* related to retained secretions.

Adult

■ **TABLE 2.7 • Electrolyte Imbalances**

Disorder and Related Condition	Assessment		Analysis/Nursing Diagnosis	Nursing Care Plan/Implementation	Evaluation/Outcome Criteria
	Subjective Data	Objective Data			
Hyponatremia Addison's disease Starvation GI suction Thiazide diuretics Excess water intake, enemas Fever Fluid shifts Ascites Burns Small-bowel obstruction Profuse perspiration	Apathy, apprehension, mental confusion, delirium Fatigue Vertigo, headache Anorexia, nausea Abdominal and muscle cramps	*Pulse:* rapid and weak *BP:* postural hypotension Shock, coma *GI:* weight loss, diarrhea, loss through NG tubes Muscle weakness	Diarrhea Fluid volume deficit Altered nutrition: less than body requirements Sensory/perceptual alteration (kinesthetic)	*Obtain normal sodium level:* identify cause of deficit, *increase sodium intake* PO (salty foods), IVs—hypertonic solutions *Prevent further sodium loss:* irrigate NG tubes with saline; hourly I&O to monitor kidney output *Prevent injury related to* shock, dizziness, decreased sensorium; dangle before ambulation *Skin care*	Na⁺ 135–145 mEq/L No complications of shock present Return of muscle strength Alert, oriented Limits intake of plain water
Hypernatremia High sodium intake Low water intake Diarrhea High fever with rapid respirations Impaired renal functions Acute tracheobronchitis	Lethargy Restlessness, agitation Confusion	*BP and temperature:* elevated *Neuromuscular:* diminished reflexes *Skin:* flushed; firm turgor *GI:* mucuous membrane dry, sticky *GU:* decreased output	Fluid volume deficit Fluid volume excess Altered nutrition: less than body requirements Sensory/perceptual alteration (kinesthetic)	*Obtain normal sodium level: decrease sodium intake* I&O to recognize signs and symptoms of complications, e.g., heart failure, pulmonary edema	Na⁺ 135–145 mEq/L No complaint of thirst Alert, oriented Relaxed in appearance Identifies high-sodium foods to avoid
Hypokalemia *Decreased intake:* Poor potassium food intake Excessive dieting Nausea Alcoholism IV fluids without added potassium *Increased loss:* GI suctioning, vomiting, diarrhea Ulcerative colitis Drainage: ostomy, fistulas Medications: potassium-losing diuretics, digoxin, cathartics Increased aldosterone production Renal disorders	Apathy, lethargy, fatigue, weakness Irritability, mental confusion Anorexia, nausea Leg cramps	*Muscles:* Weakness, paralysis, paresthesia, hyporeflexia *Respirations:* shallow to respiratory arrest *Cardiac:* decreased BP; elevated, weak, irregular pulse; arrhythmias *ECG:* low, flat T waves; prolonged ST segment; elevated U wave; potential arrest *GI:* vomiting, flatulence, constipation; decreased motility → distention → paralytic ileus *GU:* urine not concentrated; polyuria, nocturia; kidney damage *Speech*—slow	Decreased cardiac output Fatigue Altered cardiopulmonary tissue perfusion Ineffective breathing patterns Constipation Bathing/hygiene self-care deficit Impaired home maintenance management Sensory/perceptual alteration (gustatory)	*Replace lost potassium: increase potassium in diet* (see Unit 3); liquid PO potassium medications—dilute in juice to aid taste; give potassium only if kidneys functioning *Prevent injury to tissues:* prevent infiltration, pain, tissue damage *Prevent potassium loss:* irrigate NG tubes with saline, not water	K⁺ 3.5–5.0 mEq/L Identifies cause of imbalance Lists foods to include in diet Lists signs and symptoms of imbalance Return of muscle strength No cardiac arrhythmias

continued

Adult

Hyperkalemia				
Burns	Irritability	*Muscles:* paresthesia, flaccid muscle paralysis (later)	*Decreased cardiac output*	*Decrease amount of potassium in body; identify and treat cause of imbalance; give foods low in K^+; avoid drugs or IV fluids containing K^+*
Crushing injuries	Weakness, muscle cramps	*Cardiac:* irregular pulse; arrhythmias; bradycardia → asystole	*Altered urinary elimination*	*If kidney failure present, may need to prepare for dialysis*
Kidney disease	Nausea, intestinal cramps	*ECG:* high T waves; depressed ST segment; widened or absent P waves; ventricular fibrillation	*Activity intolerance*	
Excessive infusion or ingestion of K^+			*Ineffective breathing patterns*	
Adrenal insufficiency		*GI:* Explosive diarrhea; hyperactive bowel sounds	*Diarrhea*	
Mercurial poisoning		*Kidney:* scanty to no urine	*Impaired home maintenance management*	

K^+ 3.5–5.0 mEq/L.
No complications (e.g., arrhythmias, acidosis, respiratory failure)

Hypocalcemia				
Acute pancreatitis	Fatigue	Spasms: tonic muscles, carpopedal, laryngeal	*Pain*	*Prevent tetany (**medical emergency**):* calcium gluconate IV, 2.5–5.0 mL 10% solution; repeated q10min to maximum dose of 30 mL
Diarrhea	Tingling/numbness; fingers and circumoral	Grimacing: hyperirritable facial nerves	*Diarrhea*	*Prevent tissue injury due to hypoxia and sloughing; administer slowly; avoid infiltration*
Peritonitis	Abdominal cramps	Tetany → convulsions	*Altered nutrition: less than body requirements*	*Prevent injury related to medication administration. Caution:* drug interaction with carbonate, phosphate, digitalis; avoid hypercalcemia
Damage to parathyroid during thyroidectomy	Palpitations	Osteoporosis → fractures	*Risk for injury*	*In less acute condition:* increase calcium intake—calcium gluconate or lactate
Hypothyroidism		Arrhythmias → arrest	*Sensory/perceptual alteration (gustatory)*	
Burns		Dyspnea, laryngeal spasm		
Pregnancy and lactation		Diarrhea		
Low vitamin D intake				
Multiple blood transfusions				
Renal disorders				
Massive infection				

Calcium level 4.5–5.5 mEq/L
No signs of tetany
Absent *Trousseau's* and *Chvostek's* signs
Lists foods high in vitamin D and calcium

Adult

■ **TABLE 2.7** (Continued)

Disorder and Related Condition	Assessment		Analysis/Nursing Diagnosis	Nursing Care Plan/Implementation	Evaluation/Outcome Criteria
	Subjective Data	Objective Data			
Hypercalcemia Parathyroid glands: overactive, tumor Increased immobility Decreased renal function Bone cancer Increased vitamin D and calcium intake Milk-alkali syndrome—self-administration of antacids; increased milk in diet to relieve GI symptoms	*Pain*: flank, deep bone, shin splints Muscle weakness, fatigue Anorexia, nausea Headache Thirst → polyuria	Relaxed muscles Kidney stones Increased milk intake Constipation Dehydration Stupor → coma	*Decreased cardiac output* *Constipation* *Activity intolerance* *Altered urinary elimination* *Pain*	*Reduce calcium intake: decrease foods high in calcium*; identify cause of imbalance; give steroids, diuretics as ordered; isotonic saline IV *Prevent injury: prevent pathologic fractures* (e.g., advanced cancer); *prevent renal calculi by increasing fluid intake*	Calcium 4.5–5.5 mEq/L No pain reported No fractures/calculi seen on X-ray exam
Hypomagnesemia Impaired GI absorption Prolonged malnutrition or starvation Alcoholism Excess loss of magnesium through kidneys, related to increased aldosterone production Prolonged diarrhea Draining GI fistulas	Agitation Depression Confusion Paresthesia	*Muscles*: irritable, tremors, spasticity, tetany → convulsions Arrhythmias, tachycardia	*Risk for injury related to seizure activity* *Decreased cardiac output*	*Provide safety: prevent injury to disoriented patient*; administer magnesium salts PO or IV *Health teaching: diet—high-magnesium foods*, fruits, green vegetables, whole grain cereals, milk, meats, nuts	Serum magnesium level 1.5–2.5 mEq/L
Hypermagnesemia Renal failure Diabetic ketoacidosis Severe dehydration Antacid therapy	Drowsiness, lethargy	Loss of deep-tendon reflexes Hypotension Respiratory depression Cardiac arrest	*Ineffective breathing pattern* *Decreased cardiac output* *Fluid volume deficit* *Fluid volume excess* *Altered cardiopulmonary tissue perfusion*	*Obtain normal magnesium level: IV calcium*; fluids; possible dialysis	Magnesium 1.5–2.5 mEq/L No complications (e.g., respiratory depression, arrhythmias) Identifies magnesium-based antacids (e.g., Gelusil) Deep-tendon reflexes 2+

■ TABLE 2.8 Blood Gas Variations with Acid-Base Imbalances

Blood Gas Feature	Normal Value	Value with:			
		Respiratory Acidosis	Respiratory Alkalosis	Metabolic Acidosis	Metabolic Alkalosis
HCO₃ (bicarbonate)	22–26 mm Hg	Normal or ↑	Normal or ↓	↓	↑
PCO₂	35–45 mm Hg	↑	↓	Normal or ↓	Normal or ↑
(Carbonic acid*)	(1.05–1.35)	↑	↓	Normal or ↓	Normal or ↑
pH (hydrogen-ion concentration)	7.35–7.45	↓	↑	↓	↑

↑ = increased; ↓ = decreased.
*To obtain carbonic acid level, multiply PCO₂ value by 0.03.

■ TABLE 2.9 Causes of Blood Gas Abnormalities

Elevated PCO₂
(hypercarbia, hypercapnea)

Increased CO₂ production
1. Fever
2. Muscular exertion
3. Anaerobic metabolism
Decreased CO₂ elimination (hypoventilation)
1. Decreased tidal volume
   a. Pain (rib fractures, pleurisy)
   b. Weakness (myasthenia gravis)
   c. Paralysis (spinal cord injury, polio)
2. Decreased respiratory rate
   a. Head injury
   b. Depressant drugs
   c. Cerebrovascular accident (stroke)

Decreased PO₂
(hypoxemia, shunt)

Fluid in the alveoli
1. Pulmonary edema
2. Pneumonia
3. Near-drowning
4. Chest trauma
Collapsed alveoli (atelectasis)
1. Airway obstruction
   a. By the tongue
   b. By a foreign body
2. Failure to take deep breaths
   a. Pain (rib fracture, pleurisy)
   b. Paralysis of respiratory muscles (spinal cord injury, polio)
   c. Depression of the respiratory center (head injury, drug overdose)
3. Collapse of the whole lung (pneumothorax)
Other gases in the alveoli
1. Smoke inhalation
2. Inhalation of toxic chemicals
3. Carbon monoxide poisoning
Respiratory arrest

Source: Caroline NL. *Emergency Care in the Streets* (5th ed). Boston: Little, Brown, 1995. P 451.

2. *Activity intolerance* related to inflammatory process.
3. *Pain* related to continued coughing.
4. *Knowledge deficit* related to proper management of symptoms.
5. *Risk for fluid volume deficit* related to tachypnea.
◆ E. **Nursing care plan/implementation:**
   1. Goal: *promote adequate ventilation.*
      a. Deep breathe, cough.
      b. Remove respiratory secretions, suction prn.
      c. High humidity with or without oxygen therapy.
   ▶ d. Intermittent positive-pressure breathing (IPPB); incentive spirometry, chest physiotherapy, as ordered and needed to loosen secretions.
      e. Use of expectorants as ordered.
   2. Goal: *control infection.*
      a. Monitor vital signs; hypothermia for elevated temperature.
      b. Administer *antibiotics* as ordered to control infection—cephalexin (Keflex), cephalothin (Keflin), erythromycin, gentamicin sulfate (Garamycin), penicillin G. *Note:* need cultures *before* starting on antibiotics.
   3. Goal: *provide rest and comfort.*
      a. Planned rest periods.
      b. Adequate hydration by mouth, I&O.
      c. *Diet:* high carbohydrate, high protein to meet energy demands and assist in the healing process.
   4. Goal: *prevent potential complications.*
      a. Cross infection: use good handwashing technique.
      b. Hyperthermia: tepid baths, hypothermia blanket.
      c. Respiratory insufficiency and acidosis: clear airway, promote expectoration of secretions.
      d. Assess cardiac and respiratory function.
   5. Goal: *health teaching.*
      a. Proper disposal of tissues, cover mouth when coughing.
      b. Expected side effects of prescribed medications.
      c. Need for rest, limited interactions, increased caloric intake.
      d. Need to avoid future respiratory infections.
      e. Correct dosage of antibiotics and the importance of taking entire prescription at prescribed times (times evenly distributed throughout the 24-h period to maintain blood level of antibiotic) for increased effectiveness.

■ **TABLE 2.10   Acid-Base Imbalances**

Disorder and Related Conditions	Assessment		Nursing Care Plan/ Implementation	Evaluation/ Outcome Criteria
	Subjective Data	**Objective Data**		
Respiratory Acidosis COPD Emphysema Respiratory obstruction Atelectasis Damage to respiratory center Pneumonia Asthmatic attack Drug overdose	Headache Irritability Disorientation Weakness Dyspnea on exertion Nausea	Increased respirations Cyanosis Tachycardia Diaphoresis Dehydration Coma (CO_2 narcosis) Hyperventilation to compensate if no pulmonary pathology present ___ HCO_3 normal, P_{CO_2} elevated, pH <7.35	*Assist with normal breathing:* encourage coughing; suction airway; postural drainage; pursed-lip breathing; raise HOB *Protect from injury:* oxygen at 2 L; encourage fluids; avoid sedation; medications as ordered—bicarbonates, antibiotics, bronchial dilators, detergent *Health teaching:* identify cause, prevent future episodes; increase awareness regarding risk factors and early signs of impending imbalance; encourage compliance	Normal acid-base balance obtained Respiratory rate slows, <30 No signs of pulmonary infection (e.g., sputum colorless, breath sounds clear) Demonstrates breathing exercises (e.g., diaphragmatic breathing)
Metabolic Acidosis Diabetic ketoacidosis Hyperthyroidism Severe infections Lactic acidosis in shock Renal failure → uremia Prolonged starvation diet; low-protein diet Diarrhea, dehydration Hepatitis Burns	Headache Restlessness Apathy, weakness Disorientation Thirst Nausea, abdominal pain	Kussmaul's respirations: deep, rapid air hunger; ↑temperature Vomiting, diarrhea Dehydration Stupor → convulsions → coma ___ HCO_3 below normal P_{CO_2} normal, K^+ >5; pH < 7.35	*Restore normal metabolism:* correct underlying problem; sodium bicarbonate PO/IV; sodium lactate; fluid replacement, Ringer's solution; *diet:* high calorie *Prevent complications:* regular insulin for ketoacidosis; hourly outputs; prepare for dialysis if in kidney failure *Health teaching:* identify signs and symptoms of primary illness; prevent complications, cardiac arrest; diet instructions	Normal acid-base balance obtained No rebound respiratory alkalosis following therapy No tetany following return of normal pH Alert, oriented No signs of K^+ excess
Respiratory Alkalosis Hyperventilation—CO_2 loss Fever Metabolic acidosis Increased ICP, encephalitis Salicylate poisoning After intense exercise Hypoxia, high altitudes	Circumoral paresthesia Weakness Apprehension	Increased respirations Increased neuromuscular irritability; hyperreflexia, muscle twitching, tetany, positive Chvostek's sign Convulsions Unconsciousness Hypokalemia ___ HCO_3 normal, P_{CO_2} decreased, pH > 7.45	*Increase carbon dioxide level:* rebreathing into a paper bag; adjusting respirator for CO_2 retention and oxygen inspired *Prevent injury:* safety measures for those who are unconscious; hypothermia for elevated temperature *Health teaching:* recognize stressful events; counseling if problem is hysteria	Normal acid-base balance obtained Recognizes psychological and environmental factors causing condition Respiratory rate returns to normal limits No cardiac arrhythmias Alert, oriented

continued

■ **TABLE 2.10 Acid-Base Imbalances**

Disorder and Related Conditions	Assessment		Nursing Care Plan/ Implementation	Evaluation/ Outcome Criteria
	Subjective Data	Objective Data		
Metabolic Alkalosis Potassium deficiencies Vomiting GI suctioning Intestinal fistulas Inadequate electrolyte replacement Increased use of antacids Diuretic therapy, steroids Increased ingestion/ injection of bicarbonates	Lethargy Irritability Disorientation Nausea	*Respirations:* shallow; apnea, decreased thoracic movement; cyanosis *Pulse:* irregular → cardiac arrest Muscle twitching → tetany, convulsions Vomiting, diarrhea, paralytic ileus HCO_3 elevated above 26, Pco_2 normal, K^+ < 3.5, pH > 7.45	*Obtain, maintain acid-base balance:* irrigate NG tubes with saline; monitor I&O; IV saline, potassium added; isotonic solutions PO; monitor vital signs *Prevent physical injury:* monitor for potassium loss, side effects of medications *Health teaching:* increase sodium when loss expected; instructions regarding self-administration of medications (e.g., baking soda)	Normal acid-base balance obtained No signs of potassium deficit Respiratory rate 16–20 No arrhythmias—pulse regular Lists food sources high in potassium

◆ **F. Evaluation/outcome criteria:**
  1. Adheres to medication regimen.
  2. Has improved gas exchange as shown by improved pulmonary function tests.
  3. No acid-base or fluid imbalance: normal pH.
  4. Energy level increased.
  5. Sputum production decreased, normal color.
  6. Vital signs stable.
  7. Breath sounds clear.
  8. Cultures negative.
  9. Reports comfort level increased.
II. **Atelectasis:** collapsed alveoli in part or all of the lung.
  A. Pathophysiology: due to compression (tumor), airway obstruction, decreased surfactant production, or progressive regional hypoventilation.
  B. Risk factors:
  1. Shallow breathing due to pain, abdominal distention, narcotics, or sedatives.
  2. Decreased ciliary action due to anesthesia, smoking.
  3. Thickened secretions due to immobility, dehydration.
  4. Aspiration of foreign substances.
  5. Bronchospasms.
◆ **C. Assessment:**
  1. *Subjective data:* restlessness.
  2. *Objective data*
    a. Tachypnea.
    b. Tachycardia.
    c. Dullness on percussion.
    d. Absent bronchial breathing.
    e. Tactile fremitus in affected area.
  ⚑ f. X ray:
    (1) Patches of consolidation.
    (2) Elevated diaphragm.

    (3) Mediastinal shift.
◆ **D. Analysis/nursing diagnosis:**
  1. *Impaired gas exchange* related to shallow breathing.
  2. *Pain* related to collapse of lung.
  3. *Fear* related to altered respiratory status.
◆ **E. Nursing care plan/implementation:**
  1. Goal: *relieve hypoxia.*
    a. Frequent respiratory assessment.
    b. Respiratory hygiene measures, cough, deep breathe.
    c. Oxygen as ordered.
    d. Monitor effects of respiratory therapy, ventilators, breathing assistance measures to ensure proper gas exchange.
    e. *Position* on unaffected side to allow for lung expansion.
  2. Goal: *prevent complications.*
    a. Antibiotics as ordered.
    b. Sterile technique when tracheal bronchial suctioning to reduce risk of possible infection.
    c. Turn, cough, and deep breathe.
    d. Increase fluid intake to liquefy secretions.
  3. Goal: *health teaching.*
    a. Need to report signs and symptoms listed in assessment data for early recognition of problem.
    b. Importance of coughing and deep breathing to improve present condition and prevent further problems.
◆ **F. Evaluation/outcome criteria:**
  1. Lung expanded on X ray.
  2. Acid-base balance obtained and maintained.
  3. No pain on respiration.
  4. Activity level increased.

III. Pulmonary embolism: undissolved mass that travels in bloodstream and occludes a blood vessel; can be thromboemboli, fat, air, or catheter. Constitutes a **critical medical emergency.**

   A. Pathophysiology: obstructs blood flow to lung → increased pressure on pulmonary artery and reflex constriction of pulmonary blood vessels → poor pulmonary circulation → pulmonary infarction.

   B. Risk factors:
1. Thrombophlebitis.
2. Recent surgery.
3. Invasive procedures.
4. Immobility.
5. Obesity.
6. Myocardial infarction, heart failure.

◆ **C. Assessment:**
1. *Subjective data*
  a. Chest pain: substernal, localized; type—crushing, sharp, stabbing with respirations.
  b. Dyspnea.
  c. Restless, irritable, anxious.
  d. Sense of impending doom.
2. *Objective data*
  a. Respirations: either rapid, shallow or deep, gasping.
  b. Elevated temperature.
  c. Auscultation: friction rub, crackles; diminished breath sounds.
  d. Shock
    (1) Tachycardia.
    (2) Hypotension.
    (3) Skin: cold, clammy.
  e. Cough: hemoptysis.
  f. X ray: area of density.
  g. Lab data:
    (1) Decreased P_{CO_2}.
    (2) Elevated WBC.

◆ **D. Analysis/nursing diagnosis:**
1. *Ineffective breathing pattern* related to shallow respirations.
2. *Impaired gas exchange* related to dyspnea.
3. *Pain* related to decreased tissue perfusion.
4. *Altered peripheral tissue perfusion* related to occlusion of blood vessel.
5. *Fear* related to emergency condition.
6. *Anxiety* related to sense of impending doom.

◆ **E. Nursing care plan/implementation:**
1. Goal: *monitor for signs of respiratory distress.*
  a. Monitor blood coagulation studies, e.g., PTT.
  b. Ambulate as tolerated and indicated.
  c. Administer IVs, transfusions, and vasopressor medications.
  d. Fluids, by mouth, when able.
  e. Monitor signs: *Homans',* acidosis.
  f. Prepare for surgery if peripheral embolectomy indicated.

2. Goal: *health teaching.*
  a. Prevent further occurrence.
  b. Decrease stasis.
  c. If history of thrombophlebitis, avoid birth control pills.
  d. Need to continue medication.
  e. Follow-up care.

◆ **F. Evaluation/outcome criteria:**
1. No complications; no further incidence of emboli.
2. Respiratory rate returns to normal.
3. Coagulation studies within normal limits (PTT 25–38 sec).
4. Reports comfort achieved.

IV. Histoplasmosis: infection found mostly in central U.S. *Not transmitted from human to human but from dust and contaminated soil.* Progressive histoplasmosis, seen most frequently in middle-aged white males who have chronic obstructive pulmonary disease, is characterized by cavity formation, fibrosis, and emphysema.

   A. Pathophysiology: spores of *Histoplasma capsulatum* (from droppings of infected birds and bats) are inhaled, multiply, and cause fungal infections of respiratory tract. Leads to necrosis and healing by encapsulation.

◆ **B. Assessment:**
1. *Subjective data*
  a. Malaise.
  b. Chest pain, dyspnea.
2. *Objective data*
  a. Weight loss.
  b. Nonproductive cough.
  c. Fever.
  d. Positive skin test for histoplasmosis.
  e. Benign acute pneumonitis.
  f. Chest X ray: nodular infiltrate.
  g. Sputum culture shows *Histoplasma capsulatum.*
  h. Hepatomegaly, splenomegaly.

◆ **C. Analysis/nursing diagnosis:**
1. *Ineffective airway clearance* related to pneumonitis.
2. *Ineffective breathing pattern* related to dyspnea.
3. *Pain* related to infectious process.
4. *Risk for infection* related to repeated exposure to fungal spores.
5. *Impaired gas exchange* related to chronic pulmonary disease.
6. *Knowledge deficit* related to prevention of disease.

◆ **D. Nursing care plan/implementation:**
1. Goal: *relieve symptoms of the disease:*
  a. Administer medications as ordered.
    (1) Amphotericin B (IV) and ketoconazole.
      (a) Monitor for drug side effects: local phlebitis, renal toxicity, hypokalemia, anemia, anaphylaxis, bone marrow depression.

(b) Azotemia (presence of nitrogen-containing compounds in blood) is monitored by biweekly BUN or creatinine levels. BUN >40 or creatinine of 3.0 necessitates stopping amphotericin B until values return to within normal limits.

(2) Aspirin, diphenhydramine HCl [Benadryl], promethazine HCl [Phenergan], prochlorperazine [Compazine]: used to decrease systemic toxicity of chills, fever, aching, nausea, and vomiting.

2. Goal: *health teaching:*
   a. Desired effects and side effects of prescribed medications; importance of taking medications for entire course of therapy (usually from 2 wk to 3 mo).
   b. Importance of follow-up laboratory tests to monitor toxic effects of drug.
   c. Identify source of contamination if possible and avoid future contact if possible.
   d. Importance of deep breathing, pursed lip breathing, coughing (see VI. Emphysema, p. 86, for specific care).
   e. Signs and symptoms of chronic histoplasmosis, chronic obstructive pulmonary disease (COPD), drug toxicity, and drug side effects, as in (1)(a), p. 84.

◆ **E. Evaluation/outcome criteria:**
1. Complies with treatment plan.
2. Respiratory complications avoided.
3. Symptoms of illness decreased.
4. No further spread of disease.
5. Source of contamination identified and removed.

V. Tuberculosis: inflammatory, communicable disease that commonly attacks the lungs, although may occur in other body parts.
   A. Pathophysiology: exposure to causative organism (*Mycobacterium tuberculosis*) in the alveoli in susceptible individual leads to inflammation. Infection spreads by lymphatics to hilus; antibodies are released, leading to fibrosis, calcification, or inflammation. Exudate formation leads to caseous necrosis, then liquefication of caseous material leads to cavitation.
   B. Risk factors:
   1. Persons who have been exposed to tubercule bacillus.
   2. Persons who have diseases or therapies known to suppress the immune system.
   3. Immigrants from Latin America, Africa, Asia, and Oceania living in the U.S. for less than a year.
   4. Americans living in those regions for a prolonged time.
   5. Residents of overcrowded metropolitan cities.
   6. Men >65.
   7. Women between ages 25–44 and >65.

8. Children <5 yr.
◆ **C. Assessment:**
1. *Subjective data*
   a. Loss of appetite, weight loss.
   b. Weakness, loss of energy.
   c. Pain: knifelike, chest.
   d. Though patient may be symptom free, the disease is found on screening.
2. *Objective data*
   a. Night sweats.
   b. Fever: low grade, late afternoon.
   c. Pulse: increased.
   d. Respiratory assessment:
      (1) Productive cough, hemoptysis.
      (2) Respirations: normal, increased depth.
      (3) Asymmetric lung expansion.
      (4) Increased tactile fremitus.
      (5) Dullness to percussion.
      (6) Crackles following short cough.
   e. Diagnostic tests:
      (1) *Positive tuberculin test* (Mantoux—reaction to test begins approximately 12 h after administration with area of redness and a central area of induration. The peak time is 48 h. Determination of positive or negative is made. A reaction is positive when it measures 10 mm. Contacts reacting from 5–10 mm may need to be treated prophylactically).
      (2) *Sputum:* positive for acid fast (smear and culture).
      (3) X ray: infiltration cavitation.
   f. Lab data: blood: decreased RBC, increased sedimentation rate.

   g. Classification of tuberculosis:

Class	Description
0	No TB exposure, not infected.
1	TB exposure, no evidence of infection.
2	TB infection, no disease.
3	TB: current disease (persons with completed diagnostic evidence of TB—both a significant reaction to tuberculin skin test and clinical and/or X-ray evidence of disease).
4	TB: no current disease (persons with previous history of TB or with abnormal X-ray films but no significant tuberculin skin test reaction or clinical evidence).
5	TB: suspect (diagnosis pending) (used during diagnostic testing period of suspect persons, for no longer than a 3-mo period).

◆ **D. Analysis/nursing diagnosis:**
1. *Ineffective airway clearance* related to productive cough.

2. *Impaired gas exchange* related to asymmetric lung expansion.
3. *Pain* related to unresolved disease process.
4. *Body image disturbance* related to feelings about tuberculosis.
5. *Social isolation* related to fear of spreading infection.
6. *Knowledge deficit* related to medication regimen.

◆ **E.   Nursing care plan/implementation:**
1. Goal: *reduce spread of disease.*
   a. Administer medications: isoniazid (INH), rifampin—most commonly used.
   b. The following may need to take 300 mg of INH daily for 1 yr as prophylactic measure: positive skin test reactors, including contacts; persons who have diseases or are receiving therapies that affect the immune system; persons who have leukemia, lymphoma, or uncontrolled diabetes or who have had a gastrectomy.
   c. *Avoid direct contact with sputum.*
      (1) Use good handwashing technique after contact with patient, personal articles.
      (2) Have patient cover mouth and nose when coughing and sneezing, and use disposable tissues to collect sputum.
   d. *Provide good circulation of fresh air.* (Changes of air dilute the number of organisms. This plus chemotherapy provide protection needed to prevent spread of disease.)
   e. Implement respiratory isolation procedure (Table 2.11).
2. Goal: *promote nutrition.*
   a. *Increased protein, calories* to aid in tissue repair and healing.
   b. Small, frequent feedings.
   c. Increased fluids, to liquefy secretions so they can be expectorated.
3. Goal: *promote increased self-esteem.*

■ **TABLE 2.11   Respiratory Isolation**

When used:
For infectious diseases that are transmitted through droplet transmission (e.g., tuberculosis).
Precautions:
Isolate in private room (patients infected with same disease can be placed in same room).
Patient should wear mask if out of room for testing, etc.
Masks to be worn by personnel when working within 3 ft of patient.
Gowns not necessary.
Contaminated articles need to be labeled before being sent for decontamination.
Provide adequate ventilation in the patient's room.
Careful handwashing.

a. Encourage patient and family to express concerns regarding long-term illness and treatment protocol.
b. Explain methods of disease prevention, and encourage contacts to be tested and treated if necessary.
c. Encourage patient to maintain role in family while home treatment is ongoing and to return to work and social contacts as soon as it is determined safe for progress of treatment plan.
4. Goal: *health teaching.*
   a. Desired effects and side effects of medications:
      (1) *INH* may affect memory and ability to concentrate. May result in peripheral neuritis, hepatitis, rash, or fever.
      (2) *Streptomycin* may cause eighth cranial nerve damage and vestibular ototoxity, causing hearing loss; may cause labyrinth damage, manifested by vertigo and staggering; also may cause skin rashes, itching, and fever.
      (3) Important for patient to know that medication regimen must be adhered to for entire course of treatment.
      (4) Discontinuation of therapy may allow organism to flourish and make the disease more difficult to treat.
   b. Need for follow-up, long-term care, and contact identification.
   c. Importance of nutritious diet, rest, avoidance of respiratory infections.
   d. Identify community agencies for support and follow-up.
   e. Inform that this communicable disease must be reported.

◆ **F.   Evaluation/outcome criteria:**
1. Complies with medication regimen.
2. Lists desired effects and side effects of medications prescribed.
3. Gains weight, eats food high in protein and carbohydrates.
4. Sputum culture becomes negative.
5. Retains role in family.
6. No complications (i.e., no hemorrhage, bacillus not spread to others).

VI. Emphysema: chronic disease with excessive inflation of the air spaces distal to the terminal bronchioles, alveolar ducts, and alveoli; characterized by increased airway resistance and decreased diffusing capacity. Emphysema, asthma, and chronic bronchitis together constitute chronic obstructive pulmonary disease (COPD).

A.   Pathophysiology: increased airway resistance during expiration results in air trapping and hyperinflation → increased residual volumes. Increased dead space → unequal ventilation → perfusion of poorly ventilated alveoli → hypoxia and carbon dioxide retention (hypercapnia). Chronic hypercapnia reduces sensitivity of respiratory center; chemoreception in aortic arch and carotid sinus become principal regulators of respiratory drive (respond to hypoxia).

B. **Risk factors:**
  1. Smoking.
  2. Air pollution: fumes, dust.
  3. Antienzymes and alpha-1-antitrypsin deficiencies.
  4. Destruction of lung parenchyma.
  5. Family history and increased age.

◆ C. **Assessment:**
  1. *Subjective data*
    a. Weakness, lethargy.
    b. History of repeated respiratory infections.
    c. Long-term smoking.
    d. Irritability.
    e. Inability to accept medical diagnosis and treatment plan.
    f. Refusal to stop smoking.
  2. *Objective data*
    a. Increased BP, pulse.
    b. Dyspnea on exertion, dyspnea at rest.
    c. Nostrils: flaring.
    d. Cough: chronic, productive.
    e. Episodes of wheezing, rhonchi.
    f. Increased anterior-posterior diameter of chest (barrel chest).
    g. Use of accessory respiratory muscles, abdominal and neck.
    h. Asymmetric thoracic movements, decreased diaphragmatic excursion.
    i. *Position:* sits up, leans forward to compress abdomen and push up diaphragm, increasing intrathoracic pressure, producing more efficient expiration
    j. Pursed lips for greater expiratory breathing phase (pink puffer).
    k. Weight loss due to hypoxia.
    l. Skin: ruddy color, nail clubbing; when combined with bronchitis: cyanosis (blue bloater).
    m. Respiratory: early disease—alkalosis; late disease—acidosis, respiratory failure.
    n. Spontaneous pneumothorax.
    o. Cor pulmonale (emergency cardiac condition involving right ventricular failure due to increased pressure within pulmonary artery).
  ▲ p. X ray: hyperinflation of lung, flattened diaphragm.
  ▲ q. Pulmonary function tests:
    (1) Prolonged rapid, forced exhalation.
    (2) Decreased: vital capacity (<4000 mL); forced expiratory volume.
    (3) Increased: residual volume (may be 200%); total lung capacity.
    r. Lab data:
    (1) PO_2 <80 mm Hg, pH <7.35.
    (2) PCO_2 >45 mm Hg.

Note: In patients whose compensatory mechanisms are functioning, lab values may be out of the normal range, but if a 20:1 ratio of bicarbonate to carbonic acid is maintained, then appropriate acid-base balance also will be maintained. (Carbonic acid value can be obtained by multiplying the PCO_2 value by 0.003.)

◆ D. **Analysis/nursing diagnosis:**
  1. *Impaired gas exchange* related to thick pulmonary secretions.
  2. *Ineffective breathing pattern* related to hyperinflated alveoli.
  3. *Altered nutrition, less than body requirements,* related to weight loss due to hypoxia.
  4. *Activity intolerance* related to increased energy demands used for breathing.
  5. *Sleep pattern disturbance* related to changes in body positions necessary for breathing.
  6. *Anxiety* related to disease progression.

◆ E. **Nursing care plan/implementation:**
  1. Goal: *promote optimal ventilation.*
    a. Institute measures designed to decrease airway resistance and enhance gas exchange.
    b. *Position:* Fowler's or leaning forward to encourage expiratory phase.
  ▶ c. Oxygen with humidification, as ordered—no more than 2 L/min to prevent depression of hypoxic respiratory drive (see Oxygen Therapy in Unit 5, p. 301).
  ▶ d. Intermittent positive-pressure breathing (IPPB) with nebulization as ordered.
    e. Assisted ventilation.
  ▶ f. Postural drainage, chest physiotherapy.
    g. Medications, as ordered:
      (1) Bronchodilators to increase air flow through bronchial tree: aminophylline, theophylline, terbutaline, isoproterenol (Isuprel).
      (2) Antimicrobials to treat infection (determined by sputum cultures and sensitivity): tetracycline and ampicillin most common (condition deteriorates with respiratory infections).
      (3) Steroids used when bronchodilators are ineffective or for short-term therapy in acute episodes: prednisone, methylprednisolone sodium succinate (Solu-Medrol), dexamethasone (Decadron).
      (4) Expectorants (increase water intake to achieve desired effect): glyceryl guaiacolate (Robitussin).
      (5) Bronchial detergents/liquefying agents (Mucomyst).
  2. Goal: *employ comfort measures and support other body systems.*

a. Oral hygiene prn; frequently, patient is mouth breather.

b. Skin care: water bed, air mattress, foam pads to prevent skin breakdown.

▶ c. Active and passive ROM exercises to prevent thrombus formation; antiembolic stocking or woven elastic (Ace) bandages may be applied.

d. Increase activities to tolerance.

e. Adequate rest and sleep periods to prevent mental disturbances due to sleep deprivation and to reduce metabolic rate.

3. **Goal:** *improve nutritional intake.*

a. *High-protein, high-calorie diet* to prevent negative nitrogen balance.

b. Give small, frequent meals.

c. Supplement diet with high-calorie drinks.

d. *Push fluids* to 3000 mL/d, unless contraindicated—helps moisten secretions.

4. **Goal:** *provide emotional support for patient and family.*

a. Identify factors that increase anxiety:
   (1) Fears related to mechanical equipment.
   (2) Loss of body image.
   (3) Fear of dying.

b. Assist family coping:
   (1) Do not reinforce denial or encourage overconcern.
   (2) Give accurate, up-to-date information on patient's condition.
   (3) Be open to questioning.
   (4) Encourage patient-family communication.
   (5) Provide appropriate diversional activities.

5. **Goal:** *health teaching.*

a. Breathing exercises, such as pursed-lip breathing and diaphragmatic breathing.

b. Stress-management techniques.

c. Methods to stop smoking.

d. Importance of avoiding respiratory infections.

e. Desired effects and side effects of prescribed medications, possible interactions with over-the-counter drugs.

f. Purposes and techniques for effective bronchial hygiene therapy.

g. Rest/activity schedule that increases with ability.

h. Food selection for high-protein, high-calorie diet.

i. Importance of taking 2500–3000 mL fluid per d (unless contraindicated by another medical problem).

j. Importance of medical follow-up.

◆ **F. Evaluation/outcome criteria:**

1. Takes prescribed medication.

2. Participates in rest/activity schedule.

3. Improves nutritional intake, gains appropriate weight for body size.

4. No complications of respiratory failure, cor pulmonale.

5. No respiratory infections.

VII. Asthma: increased responsiveness of the trachea and bronchi to various stimuli, with difficulty in breathing; caused by narrowing of the airways. *Immunologic* asthma occurs in childhood and follows other allergic disease. *Nonimmunologic* asthma occurs in adulthood and is associated with history of recurrent respiratory tract infections.

A. Pathophysiology: bronchial smooth muscle constricts, bronchial secretions increase, mucosa swell, and there is a significant narrowing of air passages. Histamine is produced by the lung. Bronchospasm, production of large amounts of thick mucus, and inflammatory response all contribute to the respiratory obstruction.

1. *Immunologic,* or allergic, asthma in persons who are atopic (hypersensitivity state that is subject to hereditary influences); immunoglobulin E (IgE) usually elevated.

2. *Nonimmunologic,* or nonallergic, asthma in persons who have a history of repeated respiratory tract infections; age usually >35.

3. *Mixed,* combined immunologic and nonimmunologic; any age, allergen or nonspecific stimuli.

B. Risk factors:

1. History of allergies to identified or unidentified irritants; seasonal and environmental inhalants.

2. Recurrent respiratory infection.

3. Decreased ability to effectively cope with emotional stress.

◆ **C. Assessment:**

1. *Subjective data*

a. History: URI, rhinitis, allergies, family history of asthma.

b. Increasing tightness of the chest → dyspnea.

c. Anxiety, restlessness.

d. Attack history:
   (1) *Immunologic:* contact with allergen to which person is sensitive; seen most often in children and young adults.
   (2) *Nonimmunologic:* develops in adults >35; aggravated by infections of the sinuses and respiratory tract.

2. *Objective data*

a. Tachycardia, tachypnea.

b. Cough: dry, hacking, persistent.

c. Respiratory assessment: audible expiratory wheeze (also inspiratory) on auscultation, crackles, rib retraction, use of accessory muscles on inspiration.

  d. General appearance: pallor, cyanosis, diaphoresis, chronic barrel chest, elevated shoulders, flattened molar bones, narrow nose, prominent upper teeth, dark circles under eyes, distended neck veins, orthopnea.

  e. Expectoration of tenacious mucoid sputum.

  f. Diagnostic tests:

    (1) Vital capacity: reduced.

    (2) Forced expiratory volume: decreased.

    (3) Residual volume: increased.

  g. Lab data: Blood gases: elevated PCO_2; decrease PO_2, pH.

    Emergency Note: Persons severely affected may develop *status asthmaticus,* a life-threatening asthmatic attack in which symptoms of asthma continue and do not respond to usual treatment. Could lead to respiratory failure and hypoxemia.

D. Analysis/nursing diagnosis:

1. *Ineffective airway clearance* related to tachypnea.
2. *Impaired gas exchange* related to constricted bronchioles.
3. *Anxiety* related to breathlessness.
4. *Activity intolerance* related to persistent cough.
5. *Knowledge deficit* related to causal factors.

E. Nursing care plan/implementation:

1. Goal: *promote pulmonary ventilation.*
   a. *Position:* high Fowler's for comfort.
   b. Medications as ordered:
     (1) Bronchodilators and expectorants to improve ventilation (monitor for alterations in BP and tachycardia).
     (2) Antibiotics to control infection.
     (3) Steroids to reduce inflammatory response.
   c. Oxygen therapy with increased humidity as ordered.
   d. Frequent monitoring for respiratory distress.
   e. Rest periods and gradual increase in activity.
2. Goal: *facilitate expectoration.*
   a. High humidity.
   b. Increase fluid intake.
   c. Monitor for dehydration.
   d. Respiratory therapy: IPPB.
3. Goal: *health teaching to prevent further attack.*
   a. Identify and avoid allergen.
   b. Encourage medication compliance.
   c. Medication side effects, withdrawals.
   d. Postural drainage, percussion techniques to family.

  e. Breathing techniques to increase expiratory phase.
  f. Teach effective stress-management techniques.
  g. Recognition of precipitating factors.

F. Evaluation/outcome criteria:

1. No complications.
2. Has fewer attacks.
3. Takes prescribed medications, avoids infections.
4. Adjusts life-style.

VIII. Bronchitis: acute or chronic inflammation of bronchus resulting as a complication from colds and flu. *Acute bronchitis* is caused by an extension of upper-respiratory infection, such as a cold, and can be given to others. It can also result from an irritation from physical or chemical agents. *Chronic bronchitis* is characterized by hypersecretion of mucus and chronic cough for 3 mo a year for 2 consecutive years.

A. Pathophysiology: bronchial walls are infiltrated with lymphocytes and macrophages; lumen becomes obstructed due to decreased ciliary action and repeated bronchospasms. Hyperventilation of alveolar sacs occurs. Long-term condition results in respiratory acidosis, recurrent pneumonitis, emphysema, and cor pulmonale.

B. Risk factors:

1. Smoking.
2. Repeated respiratory infections.
3. History of living in area where there is much air pollution.

C. Assessment:

1. *Subjective data*
   a. History: recurrent, chronic cough, especially when arising in the morning.
   b. Anorexia.
2. *Objective data*
   a. Respiratory:
     (1) Shortness of breath.
     (2) Use of accessory muscles.
     (3) Cyanosis, dusky complexion (blue bloater).
     (4) Sputum: excessive, nonpurulent.
     (5) Vesicular and bronchovesicular breath sounds; wheezing.
   b. Weight loss.
   c. Fever.
   d. Pulmonary function tests:
     (1) Decreased forced expiratory volume.
     (2) PO_2 <90 mm Hg; PCO_2 >40 mm Hg.
   e. Lab data:
     (1) RBC: elevated to compensate for hypoxia (polycythemia).
     (2) WBC: elevated to fight infection.

D. Analysis/nursing diagnosis:

1. *Ineffective airway clearance* related to excessive sputum.

2. *Ineffective breathing pattern* related to need to use accessory muscles for breathing.
3. *Impaired gas exchange* related to shortness of breath.
4. *Activity intolerance* related to increased energy used for breathing.

◆ **E. Nursing care plan/implementation:**
  1. Goal: *assist in optimal respirations.*
    a. Increase fluid intake.
    ▶ b. IPPB, chest physiotherapy.
    c. Administer medications as ordered:
      (1) Bronchodilators.
      (2) Antibiotics.
      (3) Bronchial detergents, liquefying agents.
  2. Goal: *minimize bronchial irritation.*
    a. Avoid respiratory irritants—for example, smoke, dust, cold air, allergens.
    b. Environment: air-conditioned, increased humidity.
    c. Encourage nostril breathing rather than mouth breathing.
  3. Goal: *improve nutritional status.*
    a. *Diet:* soft, high-calorie.
    b. Small, frequent feedings.
  4. Goal: *prevent secondary infections.*
    a. Administer antibiotics as ordered.
    b. Avoid exposure to infections, crowds.
  5. Goal: *health teaching.*
    a. Avoid respiratory infections.
    b. Medications: desired effects and side effects.
    c. Methods to stop smoking.
    d. Rest and activity balance.
    e. Stress management.

◆ **F. Evaluation/outcome criteria:**
  1. Stops smoking.
  2. Acid-base balance maintained.
  3. Respiratory infections less frequent.

IX. Acute adult respiratory distress syndrome (ARDS) (formerly called by other names, including *shock lung*): noncardiogenic pulmonary infiltrations resulting in stiff, wet lungs and refractory hypoxemia in previously healthy adult. Acute hypoxemic respiratory failure without hypercapnea.

  A. Pathophysiology: damage to alveolar capillary membrane, increased vascular permeability to pulmonary edema, and impaired gas exchange; decreased surfactant production and potential atelectasis; severe hypoxia → death.

  B. Risk factors:
  1. Primary
    a. Shock, multiple trauma.
    b. Infections.
    c. Aspiration, inhalation of chemical toxins.
    d. Drug overdose.
    e. Disseminated intravascular coagulation (DIC).
    f. Emboli, especially fat emboli.

  2. Secondary
    a. Overaggressive fluid administration.
    b. Oxygen toxicity.

◆ **C. Assessment:**
  1. *Subjective data*
    a. Restlessness, anxiety.
    b. History of risk factors.
  2. *Objective data*
    a. Severe dyspnea → cyanosis (Table 2.12).
    b. Tachycardia.
    c. Hypotension.
    d. Hypoxemia, acidosis.
    e. Crackles.
    f. Death if untreated.

◆ **D. Analysis/nursing diagnosis:**
  1. *Anxiety* related to serious physical condition.
  2. *Ineffective breathing pattern* related to severe dyspnea.
  3. *Impaired gas exchange* related to alveolar damage.
  4. *Altered tissue perfusion* related to hypoxia.

◆ **E. Nursing care plan/implementation:**
  1. Goal: *assist in respirations.*
    a. May require mechanical ventilatory support to maintain respirations.
    b. May need to be transferred to ICU.
    c. May need oxygen to combat hypoxia.
    d. Suction prn.
    e. Monitor blood gas results to detect early signs of acidosis/alkalosis.
    f. If not on ventilator, assess vital signs and respiratory status every 15 min.
    g. Cough, deep breathe every hour.
    h. May need:
      (1) Chest percussion, vibration.
      (2) Postural drainage, suction.
      (3) Bronchodilator medications.
  2. Goal: *prevent complications.*
    a. Decrease anxiety and provide psychological care:
      (1) Maintain a calm atmosphere.
      (2) Encourage rest to conserve energy.
      (3) Emotional support.
    b. Obtain fluid balance:
      (1) Slow IV flow rate.
      (2) Diuretics: rapid acting, low dose.
    c. Monitor:
      (1) Pulmonary artery and capillary wedge pressure.
      (2) CVP (central venous pressure), cardiac output, peripheral perfusion.
      (3) I&O.
      (4) Assess for bleeding tendencies, potential for disseminated intravascular coagulation.
    d. Protect from infection:
      (1) Strict aseptic technique.
      (2) Antibiotic therapy.
    e. Provide physiologic support:
      (1) Maintain nutrition.
      (2) Skin care.

■ **TABLE 2.12 Differential Diagnosis of Dyspnea**

	Pulmonary Edema	COPD	Spontaneous Pneumothorax	Pulmonary Emboli	Asthma
Possible **history**	Symptoms of acute myocardial infarction "Water pills" Sudden weight gain Cough, watery sputum Orthopnea	Emphysema, bronchitis Heavy smoking Recent cold *Chronic* dyspnea "Breathing pills" or inhalers	Sudden, sharp chest pain *Sudden* dyspnea, brought on by strenuous exertion, coughing, air travel Patient often young, tall, thin	Sudden, sharp chest pain *Sudden* dyspnea Prolonged immobilization, recent surgery or trauma to lower extremities Thrombophlebitis Sickle cell anemia Birth control pills	Acute, episodic dyspnea Often younger patient Allergic history Relieved by shots in the past Cold or flu may have preceded attack
Possible **physical findings**	Distended neck veins Crackles S_3 gallop	↑ Anteroposterior diameter of chest Pursed-lip breathing Wheezing, crackles Prolonged expiratory phase of respiration Use of accessory muscles to breathe	↓ Breath sounds and ↑ resonance on side of collapsed lung Tracheal deviation	Tachypnea Tachycardia Hypotension Pleural rub Phlebitis in legs	Wheezing Hyperresonance If bronchospasm severe, chest may be silent

Source: Caroline NL. *Emergency Care in the Streets* (5th ed). Boston: Little, Brown, 1995. P 472.

3. Goal: *health teaching.*
   a. Briefly explain procedures as they are happening (emergency situation can frighten patient).
   b. Give rationale for follow-up care.
   c. Identify risk factors as appropriate for prevention of recurrence.
◆ **F. Evaluation/outcome criteria:**
   1. Patient survives and is alert.
   2. Skin warm to touch.
   3. Respiratory rate within normal limits.
   4. Lab values and pressures within normal limits.
   5. Urinary output >30 mL/h.
X. Pneumothorax: presence of air within the pleural cavity; occurs spontaneously or as a result of trauma.
   A. Types:
   1. *Closed:* rupture of a subpleural bulla, tuberculous focus, carcinoma, lung abscess, pulmonary infarction, severe coughing attack, or blunt trauma.
   2. *Open:* communication between atmosphere and pleural space because of opening in chest wall.
   3. *Tension:* positive pressure within chest cavity resulting from accumulated air that cannot escape during expiration. Leads to collapse of lung, mediastinal shift, and compression of the heart and great vessels.
   B. Pathophysiology: pressure builds up in the pleural space, lung on the affected side collapses, and the heart and mediastinum shift toward the unaffected lung.
◆ **C. Assessment:**
   1. *Subjective data*

   a. Pain
      (1) Sharp, aggravated by activity.
      (2) Location—chest; may be referred to shoulder, arm on affected side.
   b. Restlessness, anxiety.
   2. *Objective data*
      a. Dyspnea, cough.
      b. Cessation of normal movements on affected side.
      c. Absence of breath sounds on affected side.
      d. Pallor, cyanosis.
      e. Shock.
      f. Tracheal deviation to unaffected side.
      g. X ray; air in pleural space.
◆ **D. Analysis/nursing diagnosis:**
   1. *Ineffective breathing pattern* related to collapse of lung.
   2. *Impaired gas exchange* related to abnormal thoracic movement.
   3. *Pain* related to trauma to chest area.
   4. *Fear* related to emergency situation.
◆ **E. Nursing care plan/implementation:**
   1. Goal: *protect against injury during thoracentesis.*
      a. Provide sterile equipment.
      b. Explain procedure.
      c. Monitor vital signs for shock.
      d. Monitor for respiratory distress, mediastinal shift.
   2. Goal: *promote respirations.*
      a. *Position:* Fowler's.
      b. Oxygen therapy as ordered.
      c. Encourage slow breathing to improve gas exchange.

d. Careful administration of narcotics to prevent respiratory depression (avoid morphine).

▶ 3. Goal: *prepare patient for closed chest drainage, physically and psychologically.*
   a. Explain purpose of the procedure—to provide means for evacuation of air and fluid from pleural cavity; to reestablish negative pressure in pleural space; to promote lung reexpansion.
   b. Explain procedure and apparatus (see Chest tubes in Table 5.5).
   c. Cleanse skin at tube insertion site, place patient in sitting position, ensuring safety by having locked over-bed table for patient to lean on, or have a nurse stay with patient so appropriate position is maintained throughout the procedure.

4. Goal: *prevent complications with chest tubes.*
   a. Observe for and immediately report crepitations (air under skin, also called subcutaneous emphysema), labored or shallow breathing, tachypnea, cyanosis, tracheal deviation, or signs of hemorrhage.
   b. Monitor for signs of infection.
   c. Ensure that tubing stays intact.
   d. Monitor for proper tube function (*fluctuation or oscillation* of water in the tube located in the water bottle will occur with respirations; water level will rise in the tube when patient inhales or coughs; water level in tube will lower during exhalation). *If no bubbling in water,* check tubing for kinks or lack of patency. Manipulation of chest tube done only according to specific physician order.
   e. Monitor for air leaks (*continuous bubbling* of water in the bottle).
   f. Arm and shoulder ROM.

5. Goal: *health teaching.*
   a. How to prevent recurrence by avoiding overexertion; avoid holding breath.
   b. Signs and symptoms of condition.
   c. Methods to stop smoking.
   d. Encourage follow-up care.

◆ F. **Evaluation/outcome criteria:**
   1. No complications noted.
   2. Closed system remains intact until chest tubes are removed.
   3. Lung reexpands, breath sounds heard, pain diminished, symmetric thoracic movements.

XI. Hemothorax: *presence of blood* in pleural cavity related to trauma or ruptured aortic aneurysm. See X. Pneumothorax, p. 91, for assessment, analysis/nursing diagnosis, nursing care plan/implementation, and evaluation/outcome criteria; see also Table 2.13.

XII. Chest trauma
   Flail chest: multiple rib fractures resulting in instability of the chest wall, with subsequent paradoxical breathing (portion of lung under in-

jured chest wall moves in on inspiration while remaining lung expands; on expiration the injured portion of the chest wall expands while unaffected lung tissue contracts).
   Sucking chest wound: penetrating wound of chest wall with hemothorax and pneumothorax, resulting in lung collapse and mediastinal shift toward unaffected lung.

◆ A. **Assessment:**
   1. *Subjective data*
      a. Severe sudden, sharp pain.
      b. Dyspnea.
      c. Anxiety, restlessness, fear, weakness.
   2. *Objective data*
      a. Vital signs:
         (1) Pulse: tachycardia, weak.
         (2) BP: hypotension.
         (3) Respirations: shallow, decreased expiratory force, tachypnea, stridor, accessory muscle breathing.
      b. Skin color: cyanosis, pallor.
      c. Chest:
         (1) Asymmetric chest expansion (*paradoxical movement*).
         (2) Chest wound, rush of air through trauma site.
         (3) Crepitus over trauma site (from air escaping into surrounding tissues).
         (4) Lateral deviation of trachea, mediastinal shift.
      d. Pneumothorax: documented by absence of breath sounds, X-ray examination.
      e. Hemothorax: documented by needle aspiration by physician, X-ray examination.
      f. Shock; blood and fluid loss.
      g. Hemoptysis.
      h. Distended neck veins.

◆ B. **Analysis/nursing diagnosis:**
   1. *Ineffective airway clearance* related to shallow respirations.
   2. *Impaired gas exchange* related to asymmetric chest expansion.
   3. *Pain* related to chest trauma.
   4. *Fear* related to emergency situation.
   5. *Risk for trauma* related to fractured ribs.
   6. *Risk for infection* related to open chest wound.

◆ C. **Nursing care plan/implementation:**
   1. Goal: *restore adequate ventilation and prevent further air from entering pleural cavity:* **MEDICAL EMERGENCY.**
      a. In emergency situation: place air-occlusive dressing or hand over open wound as patient exhales forcefully against glottis (*Valsalva maneuver* helps expand collapsed lung by creating positive intrapulmonary pressures); or place patient's weight onto *affected* side. Administer oxygen.
      b. Assist with endotracheal tube insertion; patient will be placed on volume-

■ **TABLE 2.13 Differentiating among Tension Pneumothorax, Hemothorax, and Cardiac Tamponade**

	Tension Pneumothorax	Massive Hemothorax	Cardiac Tamponade
Presenting sign or symptom	Respiratory distress	Shock	Shock
Neck veins	Distended	Flat	Distended
Trachea	Deviated	Midline	Midline
Breath sounds	Decreased or absent on side of injury	Decreased or absent on side of injury	Equal on both sides
Percussion of chest	Hyperresonant on side of injury	Dull on side of injury	Normal
Heart sounds	Normal	Normal	Muffled

Source: Caroline NL. *Emergency Care in the Streets* (5th ed). Boston: Little, Brown, 1995. P 373.

controlled ventilator. (See discussion of ventilators under Oxygen Therapy, Unit 5.)

   c. Assist with thoracentesis and insertion of chest tubes with connection to water-seal drainage as ordered. (See Chest tubes section of Table 5.5.)

   d. Monitor vital signs to determine early shock.

   e. Monitor blood gases to determine early acid-base imbalances.

   f. Pain medications given with caution, so as not to depress respiratory center.

◆ **D. Evaluation/outcome criteria:**

   1. Respiratory status stabilizes, lung reexpands.

   2. Shock and hemorrhage are prevented.

   3. No further damage done to surrounding tissues.

   4. Pain is controlled.

XIII. Thoracic surgery: used for bronchogenic and lung carcinomas, lung abscesses, tuberculosis, bronchiectasis, emphysematous blebs, and benign tumors.

  A. Types:

   1. *Thoracotomy*—incision in the chest wall, pleura is entered, lung tissue examined, biopsy secured. *Chest tube is needed postoperatively.*

   2. *Lobectomy*—removal of a lobe of the lung. *Chest tube is needed postoperatively.*

   3. *Pneumonectomy*—removal of an entire lung. *No chest tube is needed postoperatively.*

◆ **B. Analysis/nursing diagnosis:**

   1. *Risk for injury* related to chest wound.

   2. *Impaired gas exchange* related to pain from surgical procedure.

   3. *Ineffective airway clearance* related to decreased willingness to cough due to pain.

   4. *Pain* related to surgical incision.

   5. *Impaired physical mobility* related to large surgical incision and chest tube drainage apparatus.

   6. *Knowledge deficit* related to importance of coughing and deep breathing to prevent complications.

◆ **C. Nursing care plan/implementation:**

   1. *Preoperative*

    a. Goal: *minimize pulmonary secretions.*

     (1) Humidify air to moisten secretions.

     (2) Use IPPB, as ordered, to improve ventilation.

     (3) Administer bronchodilators, expectorants, and antibiotics as ordered.

     (4) Use postural drainage, cupping, and vibration to mobilize secretions.

    b. Goal: *preoperative teaching.*

     (1) Teach patient to cough against a closed glottis to increase intrapulmonary pressure for improved expiratory phase.

     (2) Instruct in diaphragmatic breathing and coughing.

     (3) Encourage to stop smoking.

     (4) Instruct and supervise practice of postoperative arm exercises—flexion, abduction, and rotation of shoulder—to prevent ankylosis.

     (5) Explain postoperative use of chest tubes, IV, and oxygen therapy.

   2. *Postoperative*

    a. Goal: *maintain patent airway.*

     (1) Auscultate chest for breath sounds; report diminished or absent breath sounds on unaffected side (indicates decreased ventilation → respiratory embarrassment).

     (2) Turn, cough, and deep breathe, every 15 min to 1 h first 24 h and prn according to pulmonary congestion heard on auscultation.

    b. Goal: *promote gas exchange.*

     (1) Splint chest during coughing—support incision to help *cough up*

sputum (most important activity postoperatively).

  (2) *Position:* high Fowler's.

    (a) Turn patient who has had a *pneumonectomy* to *operative* side (avoid extreme lateral positioning and mediastinal shift) to allow unaffected lung expansion and drainage of secretions; can also be turned onto back.

    (b) Patient who has had a *lobectomy* or *thoracotomy* can be turned on *either* side or back because chest tubes will be in place.

  c. Goal: *reduce incisional stress and discomfort*—pad area around chest tube when turning on operative side to maintain tube patency and promote comfort.

  d. Goal: *prevent complications related to respiratory function.*

▶ (1) Maintain chest tubes to water-seal drainage system.

  (2) See Chest tubes section in Table 5.5.

  (3) Observe for *mediastinal shift* (trachea should always be midline; movement toward either side indicates shift).

    (a) Move patient onto back or toward opposite side.

    (b) **MEDICAL EMERGENCY:** Notify physician immediately.

  e. Goal: *maintain fluid and electrolyte balance.*

▶ (1) Administer parenteral infusion *slowly* (risk of pulmonary edema due to decrease in pulmonary vasculature with removal of lung lobe or whole lung).

  f. Goal: *postoperative teaching.*

▶ (1) Prevent ankylosis of shoulder— teach passive and active ROM exercises of operative arm.

  (2) Importance of early ambulation, as condition permits.

  (3) Importance of stopping smoking.

  (4) Dietary instructions—nutritious diet to aid in healing process.

  (5) Importance of deep breathing, coughing exercises, to prevent stasis of respiratory secretions.

  (6) Importance of *increased fluids* in diet to liquefy secretions.

  (7) Desired and side effects of prescribed medications.

  (8) Importance of rest, avoidance of heavy lifting and work during healing process.

  (9) Importance of follow-up care; give names of referral agencies where patient and family can obtain assistance.

  (10) Signs and symptoms of complications.

◆ **D. Evaluation/outcome criteria:**

1. Patient and/or significant other will be able to:

  a. Give rationale for activity restriction and demonstrate prescribed exercises.

  b. Identify name, dosage, side effects, and schedule of prescribed medications.

  c. State plans for necessary modifications in life-style, home.

  d. Identify support systems.

2. Wound heals without complications.

3. Obtains ROM in affected shoulder.

4. No complications of thoracotomy:

  a. *Respiratory*—pulmonary insufficiency, respiratory acidosis, pneumonitis, atelectasis, pulmonary edema.

  b. *Circulatory*—hemorrhage, hypovolemia, shock, myocardial infarction.

  c. *Mediastinal shift.*

  d. *Renal failure.*

  e. *Gastric distention.*

XIV. Tracheostomy: opening into trachea, temporary or permanent. *Rationale:* airway obstruction due to foreign body, edema, tumor, excessive tracheobronchial secretions, respiratory depression, decreased gaseous diffusion at alveolar membrane, or increased dead space (e.g., severe emphysema).

◆ **A. Analysis/nursing diagnosis:**

1. *Ineffective airway clearance* related to increased secretions and decreased ability to cough effectively.

2. *Ineffective breathing pattern* related to physical condition that necessitated tracheostomy.

3. *Impaired verbal communication* related to inability to speak when tracheostomy tube cuff inflated.

4. *Fear* related to need for specialized equipment to breathe.

◆ **B. Nursing care plan/implementation:**

1. **Preoperative**

  a. Goal: *relieve anxiety and fear.*

    (1) Explain purpose of procedure and equipment.

    (2) Demonstrate suctioning procedure.

    (3) Establish means of postoperative communication, e.g., paper and pencil, magic slate, picture cards, and call bell. Specialized tubes such as a fenestrated tracheostomy tube or a tracheostomy button allow the individual to talk when the external opening is plugged.

(4) Remain with patient as much as possible.
2. **Postoperative**
   a. Goal: *maintain patent airway* (Table 2.14).
   b. Goal: *alleviate apprehension.*
      (1) Remain with patient as much as possible.
      (2) Encourage patient to communicate feelings using preestablished communication system.
   c. Goal: *improve nutritional status.*
      (1) Provide nutritious foods/liquids the patient can swallow.
      (2) Give supplemental drinks to maintain necessary calories.
   d. Goal: *health teaching.*
      (1) Explain all procedures.
      (2) Teach alternative methods of communication (best if done before the tracheostomy if it is not an emergency situation).
      (3) Teach self-care of tracheostomy as soon as possible.
◆ **C. Evaluation/outcome criteria:**
   1. Airway patent.
   2. Acid-base balance maintained.
   3. No respiratory infection/obstruction.

■ **TABLE 2.14   Tracheostomy Suctioning Procedure**

1. Suction as necessary to facilitate respirations.
2. *Position:* semi-Fowler's to prevent forward flexion of neck, to facilitate respiration, to promote drainage, and to minimize edema.
3. Administer *mist* to tracheostomy since natural humidifying of oropharynx pathways has been eliminated.
4. Auscultate for moist, noisy respirations as nonproductive coughing may indicate need for suctioning.
5. Prevent hypoxia by administering *100% oxygen before suctioning* (unless contraindicated).
6. Use *strict aseptic technique* and sterile suctioning catheters with each aspiration; use sterile saline to clear catheter of secretions. Keep dominant hand gloved with sterile glove, nondominant hand with nonsterile glove to control thumb control of suction. Suction tracheostomy before nose or mouth.
7. *Do not apply suction when inserting* suction catheter to prevent injury to respiratory tract and prevent loss of oxygen.
8. If patient coughs during suctioning, gently remove catheter to permit ejection and suction of mucus.
9. Apply suction intermittently for *no longer* than 10 to 15 sec as prolonged suction decreases arterial oxygen concentrations. Do not suction for more than 3–5 min.
10. Cuff deflation: if high-volume, low-pressure cuffed tube is used, deflation not necessary. If other tracheostomy cuffed tube is used, deflate for 5 min every hour to prevent damage to trachea.
11. Use caution not to dislodge tube when changing dressing or ties that secure tube.

☐ Protective Functions

I. Burns: wounds caused by exposure to excessive heat, chemicals, fire, steam, radiation, or electricity; most often related to carelessness or ignorance; 10,000–12,000 deaths annually; survival best at ages 15–45 yr and in burns covering less than 20% of total body surface.

A. Pathophysiology:
1. *Emergent phase* (injury to 72 h): shock due to pain, fright, or terror → fatigue, failure of vasoconstrictor mechanisms → hypotension. Capillary dilatation, increased permeability → plasma loss to blisters, edema → hemo-concentration → hypovolemia → hypotension → decreased renal perfusion → renal shutdown.
2. *Acute phase* (3–5 d): interstitial-to-plasma-fluid shift → hemodilution → hypervolemia → heart failure → pulmonary edema.

◆ **B. Assessment:**
1. *Subjective data:* how the burn occurred.
2. *Objective data*
   a. Extent of body surface involved: *"rule of nines"*—head and both upper extremities, 9% each; front and back of trunk, 18% each; lower extremities, 18% each; and perineum, 1%. Requires adjustment for variation in size of head and lower extremities according to age.
   b. *Location*—facial, perineal, and hand and foot burns have potentially more complications and fatalities because of poor vascularization.
   c. *Depth* of burn (Table 2.15):
      (1) *First degree (superficial)*—epidermal tissue only; not serious unless large areas involved.
      (2) *Second degree (shallow or deep partial thickness)*—epidermal and dermal tissue; hospitalization required if over 25% of body surface involved (major burn).
      (3) *Third degree (full thickness)*—destruction of all skin layers; requires immediate hospitalization; involvement of 10% of body surface considered major burn.
      (4) *Fourth degree (deep penetrating)*—skin and structures underneath.
   d. Indications of airway burns, e.g., singed nasal hair, brassy cough, sooty expectoration, increased mortality; edema may occur in 1 h.
   e. Poorer prognosis—*infants,* due to immature immune system and effects of fluid loss; *elderly,* due to degenerative diseases and poor healing.
   f. Medical history—presence of hypertension, diabetes, alcohol abuse, or chronic

Adult

■ **TABLE 2.15   Burn Characteristics According to Depth of Injury**

Classification	Tissue Damage	Appearance	Pain	Clinical Course
Superficial (First degree)	Epidermis	Mild to fiery red erythema; no blisters	Very painful	Ordinarily heals in 3–7 d
Partial thickness; superficial or deep (Second degree)	Epidermis and dermis	*Superficial:* mottled, moist, pink or red; may or may not blanch with pressure; usually blisters *Deep:* dry	*Superficial:* extreme pain and hypersensitivity to touch *Deep:* may or may not be painful	Healing takes 10–18 d; if infection develops in deep burn, it converts to full thickness burn
Full thickness (Third degree)	All layers of skin and subcutaneous tissue	Charred, leathery or pale and dry	Usually absent	Heals only with grafting or scarring
*Fourth degree	All layers of skin, subcutaneous tissue, muscle, and bone	Black	Same as full thickness	Same as full thickness

*Used in some classification systems. May require several days after a severe burn to determine fourth degree.

obstructive pulmonary disease increases complication rate.

◆ **C. Analysis/nursing diagnosis:**
   1. *Impaired skin integrity* related to thermal injury.
   2. *Pain* (depending on type of burn) related to exposure of sensory receptors.
   3. *Fluid volume excess or deficit* related to hemodynamic changes.
   4. *Risk for infection* related to destruction of protective skin.
   5. *Impaired gas exchange* related to airway injury.
   6. *Body image disturbance* related to scarring, disfigurement.
   7. *Ineffective individual or family coping* related to traumatic experience.

◆ **D. Nursing care plan/implementation:**
   1. Goal: *alleviate pain, relieve shock, and maintain fluid and electrolyte balance.*
      a. Medications: give narcotic while physical exam is being completed and removing burned clothing.
      b. *Fluids:* IV therapy (see Unit 5); colloids, crystalloids, or 5% dextrose according to burn formula.
      c. Monitor hydration status:
         (1) Insert indwelling catheter.
         (2) Note color, odor, and amount of urine; report fixed specific gravity—may indicate kidney problems.
         (3) *Strict* intake and output.
         (4) Check hematocrit (normal: men >40%; women >37%).
         (5) Weigh daily.
      d. Soak: small burns may be soaked in cool saline.
   2. Goal: *prevent physical complications.*
      ▶ a. Vital signs: hourly; central venous pressure (CVP) for signs of shock or fluid overload.

   b. Assess respiratory function (particularly with head, neck burns); patent airway; breath sounds.
   c. Give medications as ordered—*tetanus booster; antibiotics* to prevent infection; *sedatives* and *analgesics; steroids; antipyretics*—avoid aspirin.
   d. *Isolation:* protective; *strict* surgical asepsis (handwashing, protective clothing).
   e. *Positioning:* turn q2h; prevent contractures—Stryker frame or circle bed if circumferential trunk burns present.
      (1) Head and neck burns—use pillows under shoulders only for hyperextension of neck.
      (2) Hand burns—use towel rolls or sandbags to align hands.
      (3) Upper-body burns—keep arms at 90-degree angle from body and slightly above shoulders.
      (4) Ankle and foot burns—allow feet to hang at 90-degree angle from ankles in prone position; use footboards to maintain angle in supine position; elevate to prevent edema.
      (5) Traction and splints to maintain positions.
      (6) ROM exercises according to therapy guidelines; usually several times per d; active exercises most beneficial.
   f. *Diet:* initially NPO; begin oral fluids after bowel sounds return; do *not* give ice chips or free water, as these may contribute to electrolyte imbalance; food as tolerated—high protein, high calorie for energy and tissue repair (promote positive nitrogen balance).
   g. Observe for:
      (1) *Curling's (stress) ulcer*—sudden drop in hemoglobin, melena (give antacids, cimetidine as ordered).

(2) Constriction due to *eschar* (circumferential or chest wall)—prepare for escharotomy (lengthwise incisions), painless procedure.

3. Goal: *promote emotional adjustment and provide supportive therapy.*
   a. Care by same personnel as much as possible, to develop rapport and trust.
   b. Involve patient in care plans.
   c. Answer questions clearly, accurately.
   d. Encourage family involvement and participation.
   e. Provide diversional activities and change furnishings or room adornments when possible, to prevent perceptual deprivation related to immobility.
   f. Point out signs of progress (e.g., decreased edema, healing) as patient and family tend to become discouraged and cannot see progress.
   g. Encourage self-care to highest level tolerated.
   h. Anticipate psychological changes:
      (1) *Acute period*—severe anxiety, mental confusion: orient to person, place, time; maintain eye contact; explain procedures.
      (2) *Intermediate period*—reactions associated with pain, dependency, depression, anger: give medications to decrease pain; explain procedures; use other patients as models; have open, nonjudgmental attitude; use consistent approaches to care; contract with patient regarding division of responsibilities; encourage self-care.
      (3) *Recuperative period*—grief process reactivated. Anxiety, depression, anger, bargaining, as patient tries to cope with altered body image, leaving security of hospital, finances. Encourage verbalization; refer to self-help group to assist adaptation.

4. Goal: *promote wound healing*—wound care:
   a. *Open method*—exposure of burns to drying effect of air; useful in burns of neck, face, trunk, and perineum; eliminates painful dressing changes; protective isolation may be required.
   b. *Closed method*—pressure dressings applied to burned areas, particularly extremities; changed 1–3 times/d; if ordered, give pain medication 30 min before change; tubbing facilitates removal.
   c. *Topical antimicrobial therapies* (Table 2.16).
   d. *Tubbing and debridement:*
      (1) Hydrotherapy—body temperature bath water; loosens dressings so they float off; soak 20–30 min; encourage

limb exercises; do not leave unattended; loss of body heat may occur, with chilling and poor perfusion resulting.
      (2) Removal of eschar (*debridement*)—done with forceps and curved scissors; medicate for pain before; use sterile technique; only loose eschar removed, to prevent bleeding; examine wound for infection, color change, decreased granulation—report changes immediately.
   e. Wound coverage, to decrease chances of infection:
      (1) Temporary wound dressings (Table 2.17).
      (2) *Autograft*—patient donates skin for wound coverage.
         (a) Types—free (unattached to donor site) and pedicle grafts (attached to donor site).
         (b) Procedure—general anesthesia; donor sites shaved and prepared; graft applied to granulation bed; face, hands, and arms grafted first.
         (c) *Post–skin-graft care:*
            ▶ (i) Roll graft with cotton-tipped applicator to remove excess exudate, maintaining dressings, and with aseptic technique using heat lamps to dry donor sites.
            (ii) Third to fifth d—graft takes on pink appearance if it has taken.
            ▶ (iii) Skeletal traction may be applied, to prevent contractures.
            (iv) Elastic bandages may be applied 6 mo to 1 yr, to prevent hypertrophic scarring.

5. Goal: *health teaching.*
   a. Mobility needs: exercise; physical therapy; splints, braces.
   b. Community resources: mental health practitioner or psychotherapist if needed for problems with self-image or sexual role; referrals as needed.
   c. Techniques to camouflage appearance: slacks, turtlenecks, long sleeves, wigs, makeup.

◆ **E. Evaluation/outcome criteria:**
   1. Return of vital signs to preburn levels.
   2. Minimal to no hypertrophic scarring.
   3. Free of infection; demonstrates wound care.
   4. Maintains functional mobility of limbs; no contractures.
   5. Adjusts to changes in body image; no depression.
   6. Regains independence; returns to work, social activities.

■ **TABLE 2.16   Topical Antimicrobials Used in Burn Care**

Agent	Advantages	Disadvantages	Nursing Implications
Silver sulfadiazine 1% (Silvadene)	Wide-spectrum antimicrobial Antifungal Nonstaining Relatively painless Usable without dressings No systemic metabolic abnormalities	Less eschar penetration than mafenide acetate (Sulfamylon) Decreased granulocyte formation; transient leukopenia Macular rash	Check for allergy to sulfa
Mafenide acetate (Sulfamylon) cream or solution	Eschar penetration Effective with *Pseudomonas* Topical of choice for electrical burns Suitable for open method of treatment (cream) Used for gram-negative organisms	Severe pain and burning sensation (lasts 30 min) Metabolic acidosis Carbonic anhydrase inhibitor Ineffective against fungi May cause hypersensitivity rash	Administer pretreatment analgesic Monitor for metabolic acidosis and hyperventilation Check for allergy to sulfa; observe for rash
Silver nitrate	Low cost Broad spectrum Effective with *Candida*	Continuous wet soaks Superficial penetration Black staining Stinging Electrolyte imbalances (low sodium, low chloride, low calcium, low potassium), alkalosis	Check serum electrolytes daily Rewet dressing q̄2h

■ **TABLE 2.17   Temporary Burn Dressings**

Example	Advantage	Disadvantage	Nursing Implications
Biologic Xenograft-pigskin	Promotes healing of clean wound; relieves pain; readily available; reduces water and heat loss	Easily digested by wound collagenase	Change q2–5d if over granulation tissue; overlap edges slightly; trim away when skin underneath has healed
Homograft-cadaver skin	Reduces water and heat loss; relieves pain; used with antimicrobial mesh; may be left in place for up to 8 d; debrides exudative wounds	May harbor disease	Observe for signs of infection
Amnion	Relieves pain; reduces water and heat loss; has bacteriostatic properties	Limited shelf life; requires special preparation for use	Change cover dressing q48h; leave on wound until it sloughs
Biosynthetic Biobrane	Protects from microbial penetration; decreases pain; promotes healing in partial-thickness burn	Not effective for preparing a granulation bed	Must be secured to skin with sutures, closure straps, tape, or staples; wrap with gauze; after 48 h, check for adherence; once adherence has occurred, may be left open to air; check for signs of infection

II. **Lyme disease:** a spirochetal illness (syndrome) carried by infected ticks; incidence greatest during May through August when outdoors and wearing fewer clothes; only a small percentage of people hospitalized.
   A. **Stages:**
      (I)   Rash at site of tick bite; bullseye or target pattern; may appear as hives or cellulitis; common in moist areas (groin, armpit, behind knees). Flulike symptoms may occur (joint pain, chills, fever).
      (II) If untreated, may progress to cardiac problems (10% of patients) or neurologic disturbances—Bell's palsy (10% of patients); occasionally meningitis, encephalitis, and eye damage may result.

(III) From 4 wk to a year after the tick bite, "arthritis" develops in half the patients. If untreated, chronic neurologic problems may develop.

◆ **B. Assessment** (depends on stage):

1. *Subjective data*
   a. Malaise (I).
   b. Headache (I).
   c. Joint, neck, or back pain (I and III).
   d. Weakness (II and III).
   e. Chest pain (II).
   f. Light-headedness (II).
   g. Numbness, pain in arms or legs (III).

2. *Objective data*
   a. Rash—erythema migrans (I).
   b. Dysrhythmias; heart block (II).
   c. Facial paralysis (II).
   d. Conjunctivitis, iritis, optic neuritis (II).
   e. Lab data: Lyme titer—elevated (II and III).
   f. Diagnostic tests: joint aspiration—fibrous exudate, WBCs, immune complexes; synovium biopsy—lymphocytic infiltrates.

◆ **C. Analysis/nursing diagnosis:**

1. *Anxiety* related to diagnosis.
2. *Pain* related to joint inflammation.
3. *Fatigue* related to viral illness.
4. *Impaired physical mobility* related to joint pain.
5. *Altered thought processes* related to neurologic deficit.
6. *Decreased cardiac output* related to dysrhythmias.
7. *Knowledge deficit* related to treatment and course of disease.

◆ **D. Nursing care plan/implementation:**

1. Goal: *minimize irreversible tissue damage and complications.*
   a. Medications: *Stage I*—oral antibiotics for 21 d (doxycycline and Pen V K); *Stages II and III*—intravenous antibiotics for 14 d (penicillin or ceftriaxone).
   b. If hospitalized, monitor vital signs q4h for increased temperature, signs of heart failure; check level of consciousness and cranial nerve functioning.
   c. Note treatment response: worsening of symptoms during first 24 h; redder rash, higher fever, greater pain (*Jarisch-Herxheimer reaction*).

2. Goal: *alleviate pain, promote comfort.*
   a. Medications: salicylates, nonsteroidal anti-inflammatory agents or other analgesic, as ordered; observe for side effects (GI irritation).
   b. Rest: give instructions on relaxation techniques; create a quiet environment.

3. Goal: *maintain physical and psychological well-being.*
   a. Activity: ROM at regular intervals; *medicate* for *pain* prior to exercise; encour-

age proper posture to reduce joint stress; rest periods between activities and treatments.
   b. Referral: occupational and/or physical therapy as appropriate.
   c. Reassurance: give psychological support; encourage discussion of feelings.

4. Goal: *health teaching.*
   a. Information on disease.
   b. Instructions for home IV antibiotics with heparin lock, if ordered.
   c. Side effects of antibiotics (drug specific); importance of completing therapy.
   d. Signs of disease recurrence (later stages of disease; less severe attacks).
   e. Preventing subsequent infections: wear proper clothing and tick repellent on clothing; conduct "tick checks" of self, children, and pets.

◆ **E. Evaluation/outcome criteria:**

1. Achieves reasonable comfort.
2. Regains normal physiologic and psychological functioning—no irreversible complications; vital signs within normal limits.
3. Resumes previous activity level; returns to work.
4. Adheres to follow-up care recommendations.
5. Knows ways to minimize risk of reinfection.

III. Rheumatoid arthritis: chronic, systemic, collagen, inflammatory disease; etiology unknown; may be autoimmune, viral, or genetic; affects primarily women 20–40 yr of age; present in 2–3% of total population; follows a course of exacerbations and remissions.

A. Pathophysiology: synovitis with edema → proliferation of various blood material (formation of pannus) → destruction and fibrosis of cartilage (fibrous ankylosis); calcification of fibrous tissue (osseous ankylosis).

◆ **B. Assessment:**

1. *Subjective data*
   a. Joints: pain; stiffness; swelling.
   b. Easily fatigues; malaise.
   c. Anorexia; weight loss.

2. *Objective data*
   a. Subcutaneous nodules over bony prominences.
   b. Bilateral symmetric involvement of joints: crepitation, creaking, grating.
   c. Deformities: contractures, muscle atrophy.
   d. Lab data: blood: *decreased*—RBCs; *increased*—WBCs (12,000–15,000), sedimentation rate (>20 mm/h), rheumatoid factor.

◆ **C. Analysis/nursing diagnosis:**

1. *Pain* related to joint destruction.
2. *Impaired physical mobility* related to joint contractures.
3. *Risk for injury* related to the inflammatory process.

4. *Body image disturbance* related to joint deformity.
5. *Self-care deficit* related to musculoskeletal impairment.
6. *Risk for activity intolerance* related to fatigue and stiffness.
7. *Altered nutrition, less than body requirements,* related to anorexia and weight loss.
8. *Self-esteem disturbance* related to chronic illness.

◆ **D. Nursing care plan/implementation:**
1. Goal: *prevent or correct deformities.*
   a. Activity:
      (1) Bedrest during exacerbations.
   ▶ (2) Daily ROM—active and passive exercises *even* in acute phase 5–10-min periods; avoid fatigue and persistent pain.
   💊 (3) Heat and/or pain medication before exercise.
   💊 b. Medications: *aspirin* (high dosages); *nonsteroidals; steroids; antacids* given for possible GI upset with ASA, steroids.
   c. *Fluids:* at least 1500 mL liquid daily to avoid renal calculi; milk for GI upset.
2. Goal: *health teaching.*
   a. Side effects of medications: tarry stools (GI bleeding); tinnitus (ASA).
   b. Psychosocial aspects: possible need for early retirement; financial hardship; loss of libido; unsatisfactory sexual relations.
   c. Prepare for joint repair or replacement if indicated.

◆ **E. Evaluation/outcome criteria:**
1. Remains as active as possible; limited loss of mobility; performs self-care activities.
2. No side effects from drug therapy (e.g., GI bleeding).
3. Copes with necessary life-style changes; complies with treatment regimen.

IV. Systemic lupus erythematosus (SLE): chronic inflammatory disease of connective tissue; may affect or involve any organ; vague etiology, but genetic factors, viruses, hormones, or drugs are being investigated; occurs primarily in women ages 18–35.

A. Pathophysiology: possible toxic effects from immune complexes deposited in tissue—fibrinoid necrosis of collagen in connective tissue, small arterial walls (kidneys and heart particularly) → cellular death, obstructed blood flow.

◆ **B. Assessment:**
1. *Subjective data*
   a. Pain: joints.
   b. Anorexia; weight loss.
   c. Photophobia; sensitivity to sun.
   d. Weakness.
   e. Nausea, vomiting.
2. *Objective data*
   a. Fever.

b. Rash: butterfly distribution across nose, cheeks.
c. Ulcerations: oral or nasopharyngeal.
d. Lab data:
   (1) Blood: *increased* LE cells; *decreased*—RBCs, WBCs, thrombocytes.
   (2) *Urine*—hematuria, proteinuria (nephritis).

◆ **C. Analysis/nursing diagnosis:**
1. *Risk for injury* related to possible autoimmune disorder.
2. *Pain* related to joint inflammation.
3. *Risk for activity intolerance* related to extreme fatigue, anemia.
4. *Impaired skin integrity* related to sunlight sensitivity and rashes.
5. *Altered nutrition, less than body requirements,* related to anorexia, nausea, vomiting.
6. *Altered oral mucous membrane* related to ulcerations.

◆ **D. Nursing care plan/implementation:**
1. Goal: *minimize or limit immune response and complications.*
   a. Activity: rest; 8–10 h sleep; unhurried environment; assist with stressful activities; ROM to prevent joint immobility and stiffness.
   b. Skin care: hygiene; topical steroid cream as ordered for inflammation, pruritus, scaling.
   c. Mouth care: several times daily if stomatitis present; *soft, bland, or liquid diet* to prevent irritation.
   d. *Diet:* low sodium if edematous; low protein with renal involvement.
   e. Observe for signs of complications:
      (1) *Cardiac* (tachycardia, tachypnea, dyspnea, orthopnea).
      (2) *GI* (diarrhea, abdominal pain, distention).
      (3) *Renal* (increased weight, oliguria, decreased specific gravity).
      (4) *Neurologic* (ptosis, ataxia).
      (5) *Hematologic* (malaise, weakness, chills, epitaxis); report immediately.
   💊 f. Medications, as ordered:
      (1) *Analgesics.*
      (2) *Anti-inflammatory* agents (aspirin, prednisone) and *immunosuppressive drugs* (azathioprine [Imuran], cyclophosphamide [Cytoxan]) to control inflammation.
      (3) *Antimalarials* for skin and joint manifestations.
2. Goal: *health teaching.*
   a. Disease process: diagnosis, prognosis, effects of treatment.
   b. *Avoid* precipitating factors:
      (1) Sun (aggravates skin lesions; thus, cover body as much as possible).

(2) Altering dosage of medications.
(3) Pregnancy needs medical clearance.
(4) Fatigue, stress.
(5) Infections.
  c. Medications: side effects of immunosuppressives and corticosteroids.
  d. Regular exercise: walking, swimming; but avoid fatigue.
  e. Wear MedicAlert bracelet.

◆ **E. Evaluation/outcome criteria:**
  1. Attains a state of remission.
  2. No organ involvement (e.g., cardiac, renal complications).
  3. Keeps active within limitations.
  4. Continues follow-up medical care—recognizes symptoms requiring immediate attention.

V. Acquired immune deficiency syndrome (AIDS): the terminal stage of the disease continuum caused by human immunodeficiency virus (HIV), a retrovirus; typically progresses from asymptomatic seronegative status to asymptomatic seropositive status to subclinical immune deficiency to lymphadenopathy (early AIDS) to AIDS-related complex (middle stage with combination of symptoms) to AIDS; hallmarks of HIV infection include opportunistic infections: *Pneumocystis carinii* pneumonia (PCP); cytomegalovirus (CMV); *Mycobacterium* tuberculosis; hepatitis B; herpes simplex or zoster; candidiasis; may take 7–10 yr before signs and symptoms occur.

  A. High-risk populations:
    1. Men, homosexual or bisexual (52%).
    2. Injection drug users (IDU) (25%).
    3. IDU/homosexual (5%).
    4. Hemophiliacs and multiple transfusion recipients (2%).
    5. Heterosexual (9%).
    6. Undetermined/other (7%).

  B. Pathophysiology: abnormal response to foreign antigen stimulation (acquired immunity) → deficiency in cell-mediated immunity—T lymphocytes, specifically helper cells (T4 cells) and hyperactivity of the humoral system (B cells).

◆ **C. Assessment:**
  1. *Subjective data*
    a. Fatigue: prolonged; associated with headache or light-headedness.
    b. Unexplained weight loss: >10%.
  2. *Objective data*
    a. Fever: prolonged or night sweats >2 wk.
    b. Lymphadenopathy.
    c. Skin or mucous membrane lesions: purplish-red, nodules (Kaposi's sarcoma).
    d. Cough: persistent, heavy, dry.
    e. Diarrhea: persistent.
    f. Tongue/mouth "thrush"; oral hairy leukoplakia.
    g. Diagnostic tests (with permission of patient): enzyme-linked immunosorbent assay (ELISA); Western blot test.

    h. Lab data: *Decreased*—CD4 (T4) lymphocytes, hematocrit, WBC, platelets. Seropositive—syphilis, hepatitis B; enzyme-linked immunosorbent assay (ELISA)—positive; Western blot test—positive (mean time for seroconversion is 6 wk after infection).

◆ **D. Analysis/nursing diagnosis:**
  1. *Risk for infection* related to immunocompromised state.
  2. *Fatigue* related to anemia.
  3. *Altered nutrition, less than body requirements,* related to anorexia.
  4. *Impaired skin integrity* related to nonhealing viral lesions, Kaposi's sarcoma.
  5. *Diarrhea* related to infection or parasites.
  6. *Risk for activity intolerance* related to shortness of breath.
  7. *Ineffective airway clearance* related to pneumonia.
  8. *Visual sensory/perception alteration* related to retinitis.
  9. *Risk for altered body temperature* (fever) related to opportunistic infections.
  10. *Social isolation* related to stigma attached to AIDS.
  11. *Powerlessness* related to inability to control disease progression.
  12. *Altered thought processes* related to dementia.
  13. *Ineffective individual coping* related to poor prognosis.
  14. *Risk for violence, self-directed,* related to anger, panic, or depression.

◆ **E. Nursing care plan/implementation:**
  1. Goal: *reduce risk of infection; slow disease progression.*
    a. Observe signs of opportunistic infections: weight loss, diarrhea, skin lesions, sore throat.
    b. Monitor vital signs (including temperature).
    c. Note secretions and excretions: changes in color, consistency, or odor indicating infection.
    d. *Diet:* monitor fluid and electrolytes; strict measurement; encourage adequate dietary intake (high calorie, high nutrient, low bulk); 5–10 times RDA for water-soluble vitamins (B complex, C); favorite foods from home; enteral feedings.
    e. *Protective isolation,* if indicated, for severe immunocompromise.
    f. Medications, as ordered: zidovudine (Retrovir), trimethoprim-sulfamethoxazole (Septra), acyclovir (Zovirax), and/or pentamidine; do not give at mealtime; may need antinauseants or antiemetics to control side effects.

2. Goal: *prevent the spread of disease.*
   a. Frequent handwashing, even after wearing gloves.
   b. *Avoid* exposure to blood, body fluids of patient; wear gloves, gowns; proper disposal of needles, IV catheters (Table 2.18).
3. Goal: *provide physical and psychological support.*
   a. Oral care: frequent.
   b. Cooling bath: 1:10 concentration of isopropyl alcohol in tepid water; avoid plastic-backed pads with night sweats.
   c. Encourage verbalization of fears, concerns without condemnation; may suffer loss of job, life-style, significant other.
   d. Determine status of support network: arrange contact with support group.
   e. Observe for severe emotional symptoms (suicidal tendencies).
   f. Address issues surrounding death to ensure quality of life: designation of durable power of attorney for health care; code blue status; reassurance of comfort and pain control.
4. Goal: *health teaching.*
   a. Avoidance of environmental sources of infection (kitty litter, bird cages, tub bathing).
   b. Precautions following discharge: risk-reducing behaviors; condoms (latex), limit number of sexual partners, avoid exposure to blood or semen during intercourse.
   c. Family counseling; availability of community resources.
   d. Information on disease progression and life span.
   e. Stress-reduction techniques: visualization, guided imagery, meditation.
   f. Expected side effects with drug therapy; importance of compliance.

◆ **F. Evaluation/outcome criteria:**
1. Relief of symptoms (e.g., afebrile, gains weight).
2. Resumes self-care activities; returns to work; improved quality of life.
3. Accepts diagnosis; participates in support group.
4. Progression of disease slows; improved survival probability.
5. Retains autonomy, self-worth.
6. Permitted to die with dignity.

The Perioperative Experience

I. Preoperative preparation

◆ **A. Assessment:**
1. *Subjective data*
   a. Understanding of proposed surgery—site, type, extent of hospitalization.
   b. Previous experiences with hospitalization.
   c. Concerns or feelings about surgery:
      (1) Exaggerated ideas of surgical risk, i.e., fear of colostomy when none is being considered.
      (2) Nature of anesthesia, i.e., fears of going to sleep and not waking up, saying or revealing things of a personal nature.
      (3) Degree of pain, i.e., may be incapacitating.
      (4) Misunderstandings regarding prognosis.
   d. Identification of significant others as a source of patient support and/or care responsibilities postdischarge.
2. *Objective data*
   a. Speech patterns indicating anxiety—repetition, changing topics, avoiding talking about feelings.
   b. Interactions with others—withdrawn or involved.
   c. Physical signs of anxiety, i.e., increased pulse, respirations; clammy palms, restlessness.
   d. Baseline physiologic status: vital signs; breath sounds; peripheral circulation; weight; hydration status (hematocrit, skin turgor, urine output); degree of mobility; muscle strength.

■ **TABLE 2.18   Universal Precautions**

■ **Wear gloves** whenever potential exposure to blood or other body fluids. Wear surgical latex gloves for performing venipunctures, for touching mucous membranes or nonintact skin, or whenever there is a possibility of exposure to blood or body fluids. **Change gloves** after contact with each patient. **Discard used gloves** immediately after use in an appropriate receptacle (e.g., a plastic bag with a "biohazard" label). **Wash your hands** immediately after you remove your gloves.

■ Use additional BARRIER PROTECTION (*mask, protective eyewear, face shield, gown*) during any procedure that is likely to generate splashes of blood or other body fluids.

■ **Wash your hands** or any other skin surfaces immediately and thoroughly if they become contaminated with blood or other body fluids. Use lots of soap and hot water to wash your hands.

■ Handle all **needles, intravenous equipment,** and **sharp instruments** with extreme care:
1. *Never* recap, remove, bend, or break needles after use or manipulate them in any other way by hand.
2. Dispose of syringes, needles, scalpel blades, and other sharp items in a puncture-resistant container kept within easy reach.

■ Although saliva has *not* been implicated in HIV transmission, it is preferable for health workers to use a pocket mask (with one-way valve) or bag-valve-mask for artificial ventilation. Such devices, therefore, should always be immediately accessible.

Source: Caroline NL. *Emergency Care in the Streets* (5th ed). Boston: Little, Brown, 1995. P 718.

◆ **B. Analysis/nursing diagnosis:**
1. *Anxiety* related to proposed surgery.
2. *Knowledge deficit* related to incomplete teaching or lack of understanding.
3. *Fear* related to threat of death or disfigurement.
4. *Risk for injury* related to surgical complications.
5. *Ineffective individual coping* related to anticipatory stress.

◆ **C. Nursing care plan/implementation:**
1. Goal: *reduce preoperative and intraoperative anxiety and prevent postoperative complications.*
   a. *Preoperative teaching:*
      (1) Provide information about hospital and nursing routines to reduce fear of unknown.
      (2) Explain purpose of diagnostic procedures to enhance ability to cooperate and tolerate procedure.
      (3) What will occur and what will be expected in the postoperative period:
         (a) Will return to room, recovery room, or intensive care unit.
         (b) Special equipment—monitors, tubes, suction equipment.
2. Goal: *instruct in exercises to reduce complications.*
   a. *Diaphragmatic breathing*—refers to flattening of diaphragm during inspiration, which results in enlargement of upper abdomen; during expiration the abdominal muscles are contracted, along with the diaphragm.
      (1) The patient should be in a *flat, semi-Fowler's,* or *side* position, with knees flexed and hands on the mid-abdomen.
      (2) Have the patient take a deep breath through nose and mouth, letting the abdomen rise.
      (3) Have patient exhale through nose and mouth, squeezing out all air by contracting the abdominal muscles.
      (4) Repeat 10–15 times, with a short rest after each five to prevent hyperventilation.
      (5) Inform patient that this exercise will be repeated 5–10 times every hour postoperatively.
   b. *Coughing*—helps clear chest of secretions and, although uncomfortable, will not harm incision site.
      (1) Have patient lean forward slightly from a sitting position, and place patient's hands over incisional site; this acts as a splint during coughing.
      (2) Have patient inhale and exhale several times.
      (3) Have patient inhale deeply and cough sharply 3 times as exhaling—

patient's mouth should be slightly open.
      (4) Tell patient to inhale again and to cough deeply once or twice.
   c. *Turning and leg exercises*—help prevent circulatory stasis, which may lead to thrombus formation and postoperative flatus, or "gas pains," as well as respiratory problems.
      (1) Tell patient to turn on one side with uppermost leg flexed; use siderails to facilitate the movement.
      (2) In a supine position, have patient bend the knee and lift the foot; this position should be held for a few seconds, then the leg should be extended and lowered; repeat 5 times, and do the same with the other leg.
      (3) Teach patient to move each foot through full ROM.
3. Goal: *reduce the number of bacteria on the skin to eliminate incision contamination.* **Skin preparation:**
   a. Prepare area of skin wider and longer than proposed incision in case a larger incision is necessary.
   b. Gently scrub with an antiseptic agent such as povidone-iodine (Betadine). Note possibility of allergy to iodine.
      (1) Hexachlorophene should be left on the skin for 5–10 min.
      (2) If benzalkonium (Zephiran) Cl solution is ordered, do *not* soap skin prior to use; soap reduces effectiveness of benzalkonium by causing it to precipitate.
   c. Use clean safety razor with a new blade if shaving ordered; shave against grain of hair shaft.
   d. Note any nicks, cuts, or irritations, potential infection sites.
   e. Depilatory creams: if ordered, leave on skin for 10 min, then wash off along with the hair; occasional side effect—transient rashes.
   f. Clipping of hair, rather than shaving or depilatories, may be ordered.
   g. Skin prep may be done in surgery.
4. Goal: *reduce the risk of vomiting and aspiration during anesthesia; prevent contamination of abdominal operative sites by fecal material.* **Gastrointestinal tract preparation:**
   a. No food or fluid at least 6–8 h prior to surgery.
   b. Remove food and water from bedside.
   c. Place NPO signs on bed or door.
   d. Inform kitchen and oncoming nursing staff that patient is NPO for surgery.
   e. Give IV infusions up to time of surgery if dehydrated or malnourished.

f. Enemas: two or three may be given the evening prior to surgery with intestinal, colon, or pelvic surgeries; 3 d of cleansing with large-intestine procedures.

g. Possible antibiotic therapy to reduce colonic flora with large-bowel surgery.

▶ h. Gastric or intestinal intubation may be inserted the evening prior to major abdominal surgery.
  (1) Types of tubes:
    (a) *Levin:* single lumen; sufficient to remove fluids and gas from stomach; suction may damage mucosa.
    (b) *Salem-sump:* large lumen; prevents tissue-wall adherence.
    (c) *Miller-Abbott:* long single or double lumen; required to remove the contents of jejunum or ileum.
  (2) Pressures: low setting with Levin and intestinal tubes; high setting with Salem-sump; excessive pressures will result in injury to mucosal lining of intestine or stomach.

5. Goal: *promote rest and facilitate reduction of apprehension.*
  a. Medications as ordered: on evening prior to surgery may give barbiturate—pentobarbital (Nembutal), secobarbital (Seconal).
  b. Quiet environment: eliminate noises, distractions.
  c. Position: reduce muscle tension.
  d. Back rub.

6. Goal: *protect from injury; ensure final preparation for surgery.* Day of surgery:
  a. Operative permit signed and on chart; physician responsible for obtaining informed consent.
  b. Shower or bathe.
    (1) Dress: hospital pajamas.
    (2) Remove: hair pins (cover hair); nail polish, to facilitate observation of peripheral circulation; jewelry (tape wedding bands securely); pierced earrings; contact lenses; dentures (store and give mouth care); give valuable personal items to family; chart disposition of items.
  c. Proper identification—check band for secureness and legibility.
  d. Vital signs—baseline data.
  e. Void, to prevent distention and possible injury to bladder.
  f. Give preoperative medication to ensure smooth induction and maintenance of anesthesia:
    (1) Administered 45–75 min before anesthetic induction.
    (2) Siderails up (client will begin to feel drowsy and light-headed).

(3) Expect complaint of dry mouth if atropine SO_4 given.
(4) Observe for side effects—morphine SO_4 and meperidine (Demerol) HCl may cause nausea and vomiting or drop in blood pressure.
(5) Quiet environment until transported to operating room.

g. Note completeness of chart:
  (1) Surgical checklist completed.
  (2) Vital signs recorded.
  (3) Routine laboratory reports present.
  (4) Preoperative medications given.
  (5) Significant patient observations.

h. Assist patient's family in finding proper waiting room.
  (1) Inform them that the surgeon will contact them after the procedure is over.
  (2) Explain length of time patient is expected to be in recovery room.
  (3) Prepare family for any special equipment or devices that may be needed to care for patient postoperatively—oxygen, monitoring equipment, ventilator, or blood transfusions.

II. **Intraoperative preparation**—anesthesia: blocks transmission of nerve impulses, suppresses reflexes, promotes muscle relaxation, and in some instances achieves reversible unconsciousness.

A. **Regional anesthesia**—purpose is to block pain reception and transmission in a specified area. Commonly used drugs are lidocaine HCl, tetracaine HCl, cocaine HCl, and procaine HCl. Types of regional anesthetics:

1. *Topical*—applied to mucous membranes or skin; drug anesthetizes the nerves immediately *below* the area. May be used for bronchoscopic or laryngoscopic examinations. *Side effects:* rare anaphylaxis.

2. *Local infiltration*—used for minor procedures; anesthetic drug is injected directly into the area to be incised, manipulated, or sutured. *Side effects:* rare anaphylaxis.

3. *Peripheral nerve block*—regional anesthesia is achieved by injecting drug into or around a nerve after it passes from vertebral column; procedure is named for nerve involved, such as brachial-plexus block. Requires a high degree of anatomic knowledge. *Side effects:* may be absorbed into bloodstream. Observe for signs of excitability, twitching, changes in vital signs, or respiratory difficulties.

4. *Field block*—a group of nerves is injected with anesthetic as the nerves branch from a major or main nerve trunk. May be used for dental procedures, plastic surgery. *Side effects:* rare.

5. *Epidural anesthesia*—anesthetizing drug is injected into the epidural space of vertebral canal; produces a bandlike anesthesia

around body. Frequently used in obstetrics. Rare complications.

6. *Spinal anesthesia*—anesthetizing drug is injected into the subarachnoid space and mixes with spinal fluid; drug acts on the nerves as they emerge from the spinal cord, thereby inhibiting conduction in the autonomic, sensory, and motor systems.
   a. *Advantages:* rapid onset; produces excellent muscle relaxation.
   b. Utilization: surgery on lower limbs, perineum, and lower abdomen.
   c. *Disadvantages:*
      (1) Loss of sensation below point of injection for 2–8 h—watch for signs of *bladder distention;* prevent injuries by maintaining alignment, keeping bedclothes straightened.
      (2) Patient awake during surgical procedure—avoid light or upsetting conversations.
      (3) Leakage of spinal fluid from puncture site—keep flat in bed for 8 h to prevent headache. Keep well hydrated to aid in spinal-fluid replacement.
      (4) Depression of vasomotor responses—frequent checks of vital signs.

7. *Intravenous regional anesthesia*—used in an extremity whose circulation has been interrupted by a tourniquet; the anesthetic is injected into vein, and blockage is presumed to be achieved from extravascular leakage of anesthetic near a major nerve trunk. Precautions as for peripheral nerve block.

B. General anesthesia—a reversible state in which the patient loses consciousness due to the inhibition of neuronal impulses in the brain by a variety of chemical agents; may be given intravenously, by inhalation, or rectally.
1. *Side effects:*
   a. Respiratory depression.
   b. Nausea, vomiting.
   c. Excitement.
   d. Restlessness.
   e. Laryngospasm.
   f. Hypotension.

◆ 2. **Nursing care plan/implementation**—
   Goal: *prevent hazardous drug interactions.*
   a. *Notify anesthesiologist* if patient is taking any of the following drugs:
      (1) *Antibiotics,* such as neomycin SO_4, streptomycin SO_4, polymyxin A and B SO_4, colistin SO_4, and kanamycin SO_4—when mixed with curariform muscle relaxant they interrupt nerve transmission and may cause *respiratory paralysis and apnea.*
      (2) *Antidepressants*—particularly MAO (monoamine oxidase) inhibitors,

which increase *hypotensive* effects of anesthetic agents.
      (3) *Diuretics*—particularly thiazide diuretics, which may induce *potassium depletion;* a potassium deficit may lead to *respiratory depression* during anesthesia.
      (4) *Antihypertensives,* such as reserpine, hydralazine, and methyldopa—*potentiate* the hypotensive effects of anesthetic agents.
      (5) *Anticoagulants,* such as heparin, warfarin (Coumadin)—increase bleeding times, which may result in excessive *blood loss* and/or hemorrhage.
      (6) *Aspirin*—decreases platelet aggregation and may result in increased *bleeding.*
      (7) *Steroids,* such as cortisone—anti-inflammatory effect may *delay* wound healing.
   b. *Stages of inhalation anesthesia and nursing goals:*
      (1) Stage I—extends from beginning of induction to loss of consciousness. Nursing goal: *reduce external stimuli,* as all movement and noises are exaggerated for the patient and can be highly distressing.
      (2) Stage II—extends from loss of consciousness to relaxation; stage of delirium and excitement. Nursing goal: *prevent injury* by assisting anesthesiologist to restrain patient if necessary; maintain a quiet, nonstimulating environment.
      (3) Stage III—extends from loss of lid reflex to cessation of voluntary respirations. Nursing goal: *reduce risk of untoward effects* by preparing the operative site, assisting with procedures, and observing for signs of complications.
      (4) Stage IV—indicates overdose and consists of respiratory arrest and vasomotor collapse due to medullary paralysis. Nursing goal: *promote restoration of ventilation and vasomotor tone* by assisting with cardiac arrest procedures and by administering cardiac stimulants or narcotic antagonists as ordered.

C. Muscle relaxants—given to supplement general anesthetic agents, i.e., curare, succinylcholine Cl (Anectine).
1. **Actions:**
   a. Facilitate endotracheal intubation.
   b. Relax abdominal muscles.
   c. Facilitate the administration of lower doses of potent general anesthetic.

◆ 2. **Nursing care plan/implementation:**

a. Goal: *observe for respiratory depression*—respiratory rate >30, shallow, quiet, use of accessory muscles.
b. Goal: *document observations.*

D. **Hypothermia**—a specialized procedure in which the patient's body temperature is lowered to 28°–30°C (82°–86°F).

1. Reduces tissue metabolism and oxygen requirements.
2. Used in heart surgery, brain surgery, and surgery on major blood vessels.
◆ 3. **Nursing care plan/implementation:**
   a. Goal: *prevent complications:*
      (1) Monitor vital signs for shock.
      (2) Note levels of consciousness.
      (3) Record intake and output accurately.
      (4) Maintain good body alignment; reposition to prevent edema, pressure, or discoloration of skin.
      (5) Maintain patent IV.
   b. Goal: *promote comfort.*
      (1) Apply blankets to rewarm and prevent shivering.
      (2) Mouth care.

◆ E. **Evaluation/outcome criteria:** complete reversal of anesthetic effects (e.g., spontaneous respirations, pupils react to light).

III. **Postoperative experience**
◆ A. **Assessment:**
   1. *Subjective data*
      a. Pain: location, onset, intensity.
      b. Nausea.
   2. *Objective data*
      a. Operative summary:
         (1) Type of operation performed.
         (2) Pathologic findings if known.
         (3) Anesthesia and medications received.
         (4) Problems during surgery that will affect recovery, i.e., arrhythmias, bleeding (estimated blood loss).
         (5) Fluids received: type, amount.
         (6) Need for drainage or suction apparatus.
      b. Observations:
         (1) Patency of airway.
         (2) Vital signs.
         (3) Skin color and dryness.
         (4) Level of consciousness.
         (5) Status of reflexes.
         (6) Dressings.
         (7) Type and rate of IV infusion and blood transfusion.
         (8) Tubes/drains: urinary, chest, Penrose, Hemovac; note color and amount of drainage.

◆ B. **Analysis/nursing diagnosis:**
   1. *Ineffective breathing pattern* related to general anesthesia.
   2. *Ineffective airway clearance* related to absent or weak cough.
   3. *Risk for aspiration* related to vomiting.

4. *Pain* related to surgical incision.
5. *Altered tissue perfusion* related to shock.
6. *Risk for fluid volume deficit* related to blood loss.
7. *Risk for injury* related to disorientation.
8. *Risk for infection* related to disruption of skin integrity.
9. *Urinary retention* related to anesthetic effects.
10. *Constipation* related to decreased peristalsis.

◆ C. **Nursing care plan/implementation**—*immediate postanesthesia nursing care:* refers to time following surgery that is usually spent in the recovery room (1–2 h).
   1. Goal: *promote a safe, quiet, nonstressful environment.*
      a. Siderails up at all times.
      b. Nurse in constant attendance.
   2. Goal: *promote lung expansion and gas exchange.*
   3. Goal: *Prevent aspiration and atelectasis.*
      a. *Position:* side or back, with head turned to side to prevent obstruction of airway by tongue; allows for drainage from mouth.
      b. Airway: leave the oropharyngeal or nasopharyngeal airway in place until patient awakens and begins to eject; gagging and vomiting may occur if not removed before pharyngeal reflex returns.
      c. After removal of airway: turn on side in a *lateral position;* support upper arm with pillow.
   ▶ d. Suction: remove excessive secretions from mouth and pharynx.
      e. Encourage coughing and deep breathing: aids in upward movement of secretions.
   ▶ f. Give humidified oxygen as necessary: reduces respiratory irritation and keeps bronchotracheal secretions soft and moist.
   ▶ g. Mechanical ventilation: Bird or Bennet respirators if needed (see Ventilators in Unit 5, p. 303).
   4. Goal: *promote and maintain cardiovascular function.*
      a. Vital signs, as ordered: usually q15min until stable.
         (1) Compare with preoperative vital signs.
         (2) Immediately report: systolic blood pressure that *drops 20* mm Hg or more, a pressure *below 80* mm Hg, or a pressure that continually drops 5–10 mm Hg over several readings; pulse rates *under 60* or *over 110* beats/min, or irregularities; respirations *over 30*/min; becoming shallow, quiet, slow; use of neck and dia-

phragm muscles (symptoms of *respiratory depression*).

b. Observe for other alterations in circulatory function—pallor; thready pulse; cold, moist skin; decreased urine output; restlessness.

(1) Immediately report to physician.

(2) Initiate oxygen therapy.

(3) Place patient in shock position unless contraindicated—feet elevated, legs straight, head *slightly* elevated to increase venous return.

c. Intravenous infusions: time, rate, orders for added medications.

▶ d. Monitor *blood transfusions* if ordered: observe for signs of *reaction* (chills, elevated temperature, urticaria, laryngeal edema, and wheezing). Table 2.19, p. 108, illustrates the nursing care plan/implementation.

e. If reaction occurs, immediately stop transfusion and notify physician. Send stat urine to lab.

5. Goal: *promote psychological equilibrium.*

a. Reassure on awakening—orient frequently.

b. Explain procedures even though patient does not appear alert.

c. Answer patient's questions briefly and accurately.

d. Maintain quiet, restful environment.

e. Comfort measures:

(1) Good body alignment.

(2) Support dependent extremities to avoid pressure areas and possible nerve damage.

(3) Check for constriction: dressings, clothing, bedding.

(4) Check IV sites frequently for patency and signs of infiltration (swelling, blanching, cool to touch).

6. Goal: *maintain proper function of tubes and apparatus.* (See Table 5.5).

D. General postoperative nursing care: refers to period of time from admission to the general nursing unit until anticipated recovery and discharge from the hospital. See Table 2.19 for a review of postoperative complications.

1. Goal: *promote lung expansion, gaseous exchange, and elimination of bronchotracheal secretions.*

a. Turn, cough, and deep breathe q2h.

▶ b. Use incentive spirometer as ordered to enable patient to observe depth of ventilation.

c. Administer nebulization as ordered to help mobilize secretions.

d. Encourage hydration to thin mucous secretions.

e. Assist in ambulation as soon as allowed.

2. Goal: *provide relief of pain.*

a. Assess type, location, intensity, and duration; possible causative factors, such as poor body alignment or restrictive bandages.

b. Observe and evaluate reaction to discomfort.

c. Utilize comfort measures, such as back rubs and proper ventilation, staying with patient and encouraging verbalization.

d. Reduce incidence of pain: change position frequently; support dependent extremities with pillows, sandbags, and footboards; keep bedding dry and straight.

e. Give analgesics or tranquilizers as ordered; assure patient that they will help.

f. Observe for desired and untoward effects of medication.

3. Goal: *promote adequate nutrition and fluid and electrolyte balance.*

a. Parenteral fluids, as ordered.

b. Monitor blood pressure, I&O to assess adequate, deficient, or excessive extracellular fluid volume.

c. *Diet:* liquid when nausea and vomiting stop and bowel sounds are established, progress as ordered.

4. Goal: *assist patient with elimination.*

a. Encourage voiding within 8–10 h after surgery.

(1) Allow patient to stand or use commode, if not contraindicated.

(2) Run tap water or soak feet in warm water to promote micturition.

(3) Catheterization if bladder is distended and conservative treatments have failed.

b. Maintain accurate I&O records.

c. Expect bowel function to return in 2–3 d.

5. Goal: *facilitate wound healing and prevent infection.*

a. Incision care: avoid pressure to enhance venous drainage and prevent edema.

b. Elevate injured extremities to reduce swelling and promote venous return.

c. Support or splint incision when coughing.

d. Check dressings q2h for drainage.

▶ e. Change dressings on draining wounds prn; aseptic technique; protective ointments to reduce skin irritation may be ordered.

f. Carefully observe wound suction (e.g., *Jackson-Pratt*), if applied, for kinking or twisting of the tubes.

6. Goal: *promote comfort and rest.*

a. Recognize factors that may cause restlessness—fear, anxiety, pain, oxygen lack, wet dressings.

■ **TABLE 2.19   Postoperative Complications**

Condition and Etiology	Assessment: Signs and Symptoms	Nursing Care Plan/ Implementation
Respiratory Complications—Most Common Are Atelectasis, Pneumonias (Lobar, Bronchial, and Hypostatic), and Pleuritis; Other Complications Are Hemothorax and Pneumothorax		
Atelectasis—undetected preoperative upper respiratory infections, aspiration of vomitus; irritation of the tracheobronchial tree with increased mucous secretions due to intubation and inhalation anesthesia, a history of heavy smoking or chronic obstructive pulmonary disease; severe postoperative pain or high abdominal or thoracic surgery, which inhibits deep breathing; and debilitation or old age, which lowers the patient's resistance	Dyspnea; ↑ temperature; absent or diminished breath sounds over affected area, asymmetric chest expansion, ↑ respirations and pulse rate; tracheal shift to affected side when severe; anxiety and restlessness	1. *Position:* unaffected side 2. Turn, cough, and deep breathe 3. Postural drainage 4. Nebulization 5. Force fluids if not contraindicated
Pneumonia—see *Atelectasis* for etiology	Rapid, shallow, painful respirations; crackles; diminished or absent breath sounds; asymmetric lung expansion; chills and fever; productive cough, rust-colored sputum; and circumoral and nailbed cyanosis	1. *Position* of comfort—semi- to high Fowler's 2. Force fluids to 3000 mL/d 3. Provide humidification of air and oxygen therapy 4. Oropharyngeal suction prn 5. Assist during coughing 6. Administer antibiotics and analgesics as ordered 7. *Diet:* high calorie, as tolerated 8. Cautious disposal of secretions; proper oral hygiene
Pleuritis—see *Atelectasis* for etiology	Knifelike chest pain on inspiration; intercostal tenderness; splinting of chest by patient; rapid, shallow respirations; pleural friction rub; ↑ temperature; malaise	1. *Position: affected* side to splint the chest 2. Manually splint patient's chest during cough 3. Apply binder or adhesive strapping as ordered 4. Administer analgesics as ordered
Hemothorax—chest surgery, gunshot or knife wounds, and multiple fractures of chest wall	Chest pain; increased respiratory rate; dyspnea, decreased or absent breath sounds; decreased blood pressure; tachycardia, and mediastinal shift may occur (heart, trachea, and esophagus great vessels are pushed toward unaffected side)	1. Observe vital signs closely for signs of shock and respiratory distress 2. Assist with thoracentesis (needle aspiration of fluid) 3. Assist with insertion of thoracostomy tube to closed-chest drainage (see care of water-sealed drainage system)
Pneumothorax, closed or tension—thoracentesis (needle nicks the lung), rupture of alveoli or bronchi due to accidental injury, and chronic obstructive lung disease	Marked dyspnea, sudden sharp chest pain, subcutaneous emphysema (air in chest wall tissue); cyanosis; tracheal shift to unaffected side; hyperresonance on percussion, decreased or absent breath sounds; increased respiratory rate, tachycardia; asymmetric chest expansion, feeling of pressure within chest; *mediastinal shift*—severe dyspnea and cyanosis, deviation of larynx and trachea toward unaffected side, deviation either medially or laterally of apex of heart, decreased blood pressure; distended neck veins; increased pulse and respirations	1. Remain with patient—keep as calm and quiet as possible 2. *Position:* high Fowler's (sitting) 3. Notify physician through another nurse, and have thoracentesis equipment brought to bedside 4. Administer oxygen as necessary 5. Take vital signs to evaluate respiratory and cardiac function 6. Assist with thoracentesis 7. Assist with initiation and maintenance of closed-chest drainage

continued

■ **TABLE 2.19** *(Continued)*

Condition and Etiology	Assessment: Signs and Symptoms	Nursing Care Plan/Implementation
Circulatory Complications—Shock, Thrombophlebitis, Pulmonary Embolism, and Disseminated Intravascular Coagulation		
Shock—hemorrhage, sepsis, decreased cardiac contractility (myocardial infarction, cardiac failure, tamponade), drug sensitivities, transfusion reactions, pulrmonary embolism and emotional reaction to pain or deep fear	Dizziness; fainting; restlessness; anxiety *BP:* ↓ or falling *Pulse:* weak, thready *Respirations:* ↑, shallow *Skin:* pale, cool, clammy, cyanotic ↓ temperature; oliguria; CVP <5 cm H_2O; thirst	1. *Position:* foot of bed raised 20 degrees, knees straight, trunk horizontal, head slightly elevated; *avoid* Trendelenburg's position 2. Administer blood transfusions, plasma expanders, and intravenous infusions as ordered; medications specific to type of shock 3. Check: vital signs, CVP, temperature 4. Insert urinary catheter to monitor hourly urine output 5. Administer oxygen as ordered
Thrombophlebitis—injury to vein wall by tight leg straps or leg holders during gynecologic surgery; hemoconcentration due to dehydration or fluid loss; stasis of blood in extremities due to postoperative circulatory depression	Calf pain or cramping, redness and swelling (the left leg is affected more frequently than the right); slight fever, chills; Homans' sign and tenderness over the anteromedian surface of thigh	1. Maintain complete bedrest, *avoiding positions* that restrict venous return 2. Apply elastic stockings or wrap legs from toes to groin with elastic bandages to prevent swelling and pooling of venous blood 3. Apply warm, moist soaks to area as ordered 4. Administer anticoagulants as ordered 5. Use bed cradle over affected limb 6. Provide active and passive ROM exercises in unaffected limb
Pulmonary embolism—obstruction of a pulmonary artery by a foreign body in bloodstream, usually a blood clot that has been dislodged from its original site	*Sudden,* severe stabbing chest pain; *severe* dyspnea; cyanosis; *rapid* pulse; anxiety and apprehension; pupillary dilatation; *profuse* diaphoresis; *loss* of consciousness	1. Administer oxygen and inhalants while patient is sitting upright 2. Maintain bedrest and frequent reassurance 3. Administer heparin sodium, as ordered 4. Administer analgesics, such as morphine SO_4, to reduce pain and apprehension
Wound Complications—Infection, Dehiscence, and Evisceration		
Wound infection—*obesity* or *undernutrition,* particularly protein and vitamin deficiencies; *decreased* antibody production in aged; *decreased* phagocytosis in newborn; metabolic disorder, such as diabetes mellitus, Cushing's syndrome, malignancies, and shock; breakdown in aseptic technique	Redness, tenderness, and heat in area of incision; wound drainage; ↑ temperature; ↑ pulse rate.	1. Assist in cleansing and irrigation of wound and insertion of a drain 2. Apply hot, wet dressings as ordered 3. Give antibiotics as ordered; observe responses
Wound dehiscence and evisceration—obesity and undernutrition, particularly protein and vitamin C deficiencies; immunosuppression; metabolic disorders; cancer; liver disease; common site is midline abdominal incision, frequently about 7 d postoperatively; precipitating factors include abdominal distention, vomiting, coughing, hiccups, and uncontrolled motor activity	Slow parting of wound edges with a gush of pinkish serous drainage; or rapid parting with coils of intestines escaping onto the abdominal wall; the latter accompanied by pain and often by vomiting	1. *Position:* bedrest, low Fowler's or horizontal position 2. Notify physician stat 3. Cover exposed coils of intestines with sterile towels or dressing and keep moist with sterile normal saline 4. Monitor vital signs frequently 5. Remain with patient, reassure that physician is coming 6. Prepare for physician's arrival; set up IV, suction equipment, and nasogastric tube; obtain sterile gown, mask, gloves, towels, and warmed normal saline 7. Notify surgery that patient will be returning to operating room

continued

■ **TABLE 2.19**   *(Continued)*

Condition and Etiology	Assessment: Signs and Symptoms	Nursing Care Plan/ Implementation
Urinary Complications—Retention and Infections		
Urinary retention—obstruction in bladder or urethra; neurologic disease; mechanical trauma as in childbirth or gynecologic surgery; psychological conditioning that inhibits voiding in bed; prolonged bedrest; pain with lower abdominal surgery	Inability to void *10–18* h postsurgery, despite adequate fluid replacement; palpable bladder, frequent voiding of small amounts of urine or dribbling; suprapubic pain	1. Assist patient to stand, or use bedside commode if not contraindicated 2. Provide privacy 3. Reduce tension, provide support 4. Use warm bedpan 5. Run tap water 6. Place patient's feet in warm water 7. Pour warm water over perineum 8. Catheterize if conservative measures fail
Urinary infections—urinary retention, bladder distention, repeated or prolonged catheterization	*Urinary:* burning and frequency *Pain:* low back or flank Pyuria, hematuria; ↑ temperature, chills; anorexia; positive urine culture	1. *Push fluids* to 3000 mL daily, unless contraindicated 2. *Avoid* stimulants such as caffeine 3. Give antibiotics, sulfonamides, or acidifying agents as ordered 4. Give perianal care after each bowel movement
Gastrointestinal Complications—Gastric Distention, Paralytic Ileus, and Intestinal Obstruction		
Gastric distention—depressed gastric motility due to sympathoadrenal stress response; idiosyncrasy to drugs; emotions, pain, shock; fluid and electrolyte imbalances	Feeling of fullness, hiccups, overflow vomiting of dark, foul-smelling liquid; severe retention leads to decreased blood pressure (due to pressure on vagus nerve) and other symptoms of shock syndrome	1. Report signs to physician *immediately* 2. Insert or assist in insertion of NG tube; attach to intermittent suction 3. Irrigate nasogastric tube with *saline* (water will deplete electrolytes and result in metabolic alkalosis) 4. Administer IV infusions with electrolytes as ordered
Paralytic ileus—see *Gastric distention*	Greatly decreased or absent bowel sounds, failure of either gas or feces to be passed by rectum; nausea and vomiting; abdominal tenderness and distention; fever; dehydration	1. Notify physician 2. Insert or assist with insertion of NG tube; attach to low, intermittent suction 3. Insert rectal tube 4. Administer IV infusion with electrolytes as ordered 5. Irrigate nasogastric tube with saline 6. Assist with insertion of Miller-Abbott tube if indicated 7. Administer medications to increase peristalsis as ordered
Intestinal obstruction—due to poorly functioning anastomosis, hernia, adhesions, fecal impaction	Severe, colicky abdominal pains, mild to severe abdominal distention, nausea and vomiting, anorexia and malaise; fever; lack of bowel movement; electrolyte imbalance; high-pitched tinkling bowel sounds	1. Assist with insertion of nasoenteric tube and attach to intermittent suction 2. Maintain IV infusions with electrolytes 3. Encourage nasal breathing to avoid air swallowing 4. Check abdomen for distention and bowel sounds every 2 h 5. Encourage verbalization 6. Plan rest periods for patient 7. Administer oral hygiene frequently
Transfusion Reactions—Allergic, Febrile, and Hemolytic		
Allergic and febrile reactions—unidentified antigen or antigens in donor blood or transfusion equipment; previous reaction to transfusions; small thrombi; bacteria; lysed red cells	Fever to 103°F, may have *sudden* onset; chills; itching; erythema; urticaria; nausea; vomiting; dyspnea and wheezing, occasionally	1. *Stop* transfusion and notify physician 2. Administer *antihistamines,* as ordered 3. Send stat urine to lab for analysis 4. Institute *cooling* measures if indicated 5. Maintain *strict* input and output records 6. Send remaining blood to lab for analysis, and order recipient blood sample for analysis

continued

■ **TABLE 2.19** *(Continued)*

Condition and Etiology	Assessment: Signs and Symptoms	Nursing Care Plan/ Implementation
Transfusion Reactions—Allergic, Febrile, and Hemolytic *(Continued)*		
Hemolytic reaction—infusion of incompatible blood (less common, more serious)	*Early* chills and fever; throbbing headache, feeling of burning in face; hypotension; tachycardia; chest, back, or flank pain; nausea, vomiting; feeling of doom; *later* spontaneous and diffuse bleeding; icterus; oliguria; anuria; hemoglobinuria	1. *Stop* infusion immediately; take vital signs and notify physician 2. Send patient blood sample and unused blood to lab for analysis 3. Send stat urine to lab 4. Save *all* urine for observation of discoloration 5. Administer parenteral infusions to combat shock, as ordered 6. Administer medications as ordered— *diuretics, sodium bicarbonate, hydrocortisone,* and *vasopressors*
Emotional Complications		
Emotional disturbances—grief associated with loss of body part or loss of body image; previous emotional problems; decreased sensory and perceptual input; sensory overload; fear and pain; decreased resistance to stress as a result of age, exhaustion, or debilitation	Restlessness, insomnia, depression, hallucinations, delusions, agitation, suicidal thoughts	1. Report symptoms to physician 2. Encourage verbalization of feelings; give realistic assurance 3. Orient to time and place as necessary 4. Provide safety measures, such as siderails 5. Keep room lit, to reduce incidence of visual hallucinations 6. Administer tranquilizers as ordered. 7. Use restraints as a *last* resort

b. Comfort measures: analgesics or barbiturates; apply oxygen as indicated; change positions; encourage deep breathing; massage back to reduce restlessness.

c. Allow rest periods between care-group activities.

d. Give antiemetic for relief of nausea and vomiting, as ordered.

e. Vigorous oral hygiene (brushing) to prevent "surgical mumps" or parotitis from preop atropine or general anesthesia.

7. Goal: *encourage early movement and ambulation to prevent complications of immobilization.*

a. Turn or reposition q2h.

b. ROM: passive and active exercises.

c. Encourage leg exercises.

d. Assist with standing or use of commode if allowed.

e. Encourage resumption of personal care as soon as possible.

f. Assist with ambulation in room as soon as allowed. Avoid chair sitting as it enhances venous pooling and may predispose to thrombophlebitis.

◆ **E. Evaluation/outcome criteria:**

1. Incision heals without infection.

2. No complications, i.e., atelectasis, pneumonia, thrombophlebitis.

3. Normal bowel and bladder functions resume.

4. Carries out activities of daily living, self-care.

5. Accepts possible limitations: dietary, activity, body image (e.g., no depression, complies with treatment regimen).

❑ Nutrition

I. **General nutritional deficiencies**

◆ A. **Assessment:**

1. *Subjective data*

a. Mental irritability or confusion.

b. History of poor dietary intake.

c. History of lack of adequate resources to provide adequate nutrition.

d. Lack of knowledge about proper diet, food selection, or preparation.

e. History of eating disorders.

f. Paresthesia (burning and tingling): hands and feet.

2. *Objective data*

a. *Appearance:* listless; *posture:* sagging shoulders, sunken chest, poor gait.

b. *Muscle:* weakness, fatigue, wasted appearance.

c. *GI:* indigestion, vomiting, enlarged liver, spleen.

d. *Cardiovascular:* tachycardia on minimal exertion; bradycardia at rest; enlarged heart, elevated BP.

e. *Hair:* brittle, dry, thin, sparse; lack of natural shine; color changes; can be easily plucked out.
f. *Skin:* dryness (xerosis), scaly, dyspigmentation, petechiae, lack of fat under skin.
g. *Mouth:*
  (1) *Teeth:* missing, abnormally placed, caries.
  (2) *Gums:* bleed easily, receding.
  (3) *Tongue:* swollen, sore.
  (4) *Lips:* red, swollen, angular fissures at corners.
h. *Eyes:* pale conjunctiva, corneal changes.
i. *Nails:* brittle, ridged.
j. *Nervous system:* abnormal reflexes.
k. Lab data: blood: *decreased* albumin, iron-binding capacity, lymphocyte, hemoglobin, and hematocrit.
l. Anthropometric measurements document nutritional deficiencies.

◆ **B. Analysis/nursing diagnosis:**
1. *Altered nutrition, less than body requirements,* related to poor dietary intake.
2. *Knowledge deficit* related to nutritional requirements.
3. *Altered health maintenance* related to inability to provide own nutritional care.
4. *Ineffective individual coping* related to eating disorders.
5. *Ineffective family coping, disabling,* related to inadequate resources or knowledge to provide appropriate family nutrition.

◆ **C. Nursing care plan/implementation:**
1. Goal: *prevent complications of specific deficiency.*
  a. Identify etiology of nutritional deficiency.
  b. Recognize signs of nutritional deficiencies (Table 2.20).

c. Identify foods high in deficient nutrient (see Unit 3).
d. Evaluate economic resources to purchase appropriate foods.
e. Identify community resources for assistance.
f. Monitor progress for potential additional illnesses.
2. Goal: *health teaching.*
  a. Effects of nutritional deficiencies on health.
  b. Foods to include in diet to avoid deficits.

◆ **D. Evaluation/outcome criteria:**
1. Complications do not occur.
2. Patient gains weight.
3. Patient selects appropriate foods to alleviate deficiency.

II. **Celiac disease** (nontropical sprue): gluten-induced intestinal disease affecting adults and children, characterized by inability to digest and utilize sugars, starches, and fats.
A. **Pathophysiology:** intolerance to the gliadin fraction of grains causing degeneration of the epithelial surface of the intestine, atrophy of the intestinal villi, and impaired absorption of essential nutrients.
B. **Risk factors:**
1. Possible genetic or familial factors.
2. Hypersensitivity response.
3. History of childhood celiac disease.

◆ **C. Assessment:**
1. *Subjective data:* family history.
2. *Objective data*
  a. Loss: weight, fat deposits, musculature.
  b. Anemia.
  c. Vitamin deficiencies.
  d. Abdomen distended with flatus.
  e. Stools: diarrhea, foul smelling, bulky, fatty, float in commode.

■ **TABLE 2.20 Common Mineral Deficiencies**

Mineral	Function	Deficiency Leads to
Calcium	Aids in formation and maintenance of bones and teeth; permits healthy nerve functioning and normal blood clotting	↑ neuromuscular irritability, impaired blood clotting
Phosphorus	Bone building	Rickets
Magnesium	Cellular metabolism of carbohydrates and protein	↓ cellular metabolism of carbohydrates and protein; tetany
Sodium	Fluid and electrolyte balance; acid-base balance; electro-chemical impulses of nerves and muscles	Fluid and electrolyte imbalance; ↓ muscle contraction
Potassium	Osmotic pressure and water balance	Fluid and electrolyte imbalance; ↓ cardiac and skeletal muscular contractility
Chloride	Fluid and electrolyte balance; acid-base balance; digestion	Fluid imbalances; alkalosis
Iron	Hemoglobin formation; cellular oxidation	Anemia
Iodine	Synthesis of thyroid hormone; overall body metabolism	Goiter
Zinc	Constituent of cell enzyme system; CO_2 carrier in RBC	↓ metabolism of protein and carbohydrates; delayed wound healing

f. History of acute attacks of fluid/electrolyte imbalances.

🔔 g. Diagnostic tests: small-bowel biopsy, stool for fat.

h. *Gluten-free* diet leads to remission of symptoms.

◆ **D. Analysis/nursing diagnosis:**

1. *Altered nutrition, less than body requirements,* related to inability to digest and utilize sugars, starches, and fats.

2. *Diarrhea* related to intestinal response to gluten in diet.

3. *Fluid volume deficit* related to loss through excessive diarrhea.

4. *Knowledge deficit* related to dietary restrictions to control symptoms.

◆ **E. Nursing care plan/implementation:**

1. Goal: *prevent weight loss.*

a. *Diet:* high in calories, protein, vitamins, and minerals, and gluten free.

   (1) Avoid wheat, rye, oats, barley.

   (2) All other foods permitted.

b. Daily weights to monitor weight changes.

2. Goal: *health teaching.*

a. Nature of disease.

b. Dietary restrictions and allowances.

c. Complications of noncompliance.

◆ **F. Evaluation/outcome criteria:**

1. No further weight loss.

2. Normal stools.

3. Fluid/electrolyte balance obtained and maintained.

III. Hepatitis: inflammation of the liver.

A. Pathophysiology:

1. Infection with either hepatitis A (infectious hepatitis), hepatitis B (serum hepatitis), non-A, non-B hepatitis (caused by at least two unidentified viruses), or delta hepatitis (infection caused by a defective RNA virus that requires HBV to multiply) → inflammation, necrosis, and regeneration of liver parenchyma. Hepatocellular injury impairs clearance of urobilinogen → elevated urinary urobilinogen; and, as injury increases → conjugated bilirubin not reaching the intestines → decreased urine and fecal urobilinogen → increased serum bilirubin → jaundice.

2. Failure of liver to detoxify products → increased toxic products of protein metabolism → gastritis and duodenitis.

B. Risk factors:

1. Exposure to virus.

2. Exposure to carriers of virus.

3. Exposure to hepatotoxins such as dry cleaning agents.

4. Nonimmunized.

◆ **C. Assessment:**

1. *Subjective data*

a. Anorexia, nausea.

b. Malaise, dull ache in upper right quadrant.

c. Repugnance to food, cigarette smoke, strong odors, alcohol.

d. Headache.

2. *Objective data*

a. Fever.

b. Liver: enlarged (hepatomegaly), tender, smooth.

c. Skin: icterus in sclera of eyes, jaundice; rash; pruritus; petechiae, bruises.

d. Urine: normal, dark.

e. Stool: normal, clay-colored, loose.

f. Vomiting, weight loss.

g. Lymph nodes: enlarged.

h. Lab data:

   (1) Blood—leukocytosis.

   (2) Increased AST[SGOT], ALT[SGPT], and bilirubin levels, alkaline phosphatase.

   (3) Urine—increased urobilinogen.

i. See also Table 2.21.

◆ **D. Analysis/nursing diagnosis:**

1. *Pain* related to inflammation of liver.

2. *Impaired skin integrity* related to pruritus.

3. *Activity intolerance* related to malaise.

4. *Risk for infection* to others related to incubation/infectious period.

5. *Altered nutrition, less than body requirements,* related to repugnance of food.

6. *Social isolation* related to isolation precautions.

◆ **E. Nursing care plan/implementation:**

1. Goal: *promote comfort.*

a. Bedrest to combat fatigue and reduce metabolic needs until hepatomegaly subsides; *semi-Fowler*'s or *supine* positioning.

b. Oral hygiene q1–2h to decrease nausea.

c. ROM exercises to maintain muscle strength.

d. *Measures to reduce pruritus:*

   (1) Mild, oil-based lotion to reduce itching.

   (2) Nails cut short, cotton gloves, long-sleeved clothing to prevent skin injury from scratching.

   (3) Environment: cool and dry.

   (4) Cool wet soaks to skin.

   (5) Diversional activities.

💊   (6) Medications as ordered:

      (a) Emollients to relieve dry skin.

      (b) Topical corticosteroids to reduce inflammation.

      (c) Antihistamines to reduce itch.

      (d) Tranquilizers and sedatives to allow rest and prevent exhaustion.

2. Goal: *prevent spread of infection to others.*

▶ a. Isolation according to type

   (1) *Infectious hepatitis A:*

■ TABLE 2.21   Etiology, Incidence, Epidemiologic, and Clinical Comparison of Hepatitis A, Hepatitis B, Hepatitis C, and Delta Hepatitis

	Infectious Hepatitis A	Serum Hepatitis B	Hepatitis C	Delta Hepatitis
Incubation	2–6 wk	4 wk–6 mo	Variable: 14–160 d; average, 50 d	Same as hepatitis B
Communicable	Until 7–9 d after jaundice occurs	Several months—as long as virus present in blood	As long as virus present in blood	As long as virus present in blood
Transmission	Fecal-oral; blood; sexual	Parenteral; sexual	Percutaneous, via contaminated blood, parenteral drug abuse; some fecal-oral forms	Parenteral; blood
Sources	Crowding; contaminated food, milk or water	Contaminated needles, syringes, surgical instruments	Persons who have received 15 or more blood transfusions; IV drug users; persons traveling to contaminated areas	Contaminated needles, syringes
Portal of entry	GI tract; asymptomatic carriers	Integumentary: blood plasma or transfusions	Blood	Integumentary: blood
HB antigen	Not present	Present	Not present	Present as with hepatitis B
Incidence	Sporadic epidemics; increased in children <15	Increased in ages 15–29, particularly in heroin addiction; occupational hazard for laboratory workers, nurses, physicians	All age groups; higher in adults because of exposure to risk factors	Same as hepatitis B
Immunity	*Preexposure:* immune globulin, 0.02 mL/kg *Postexposure:* within 2 wk of exposure, as above	*Preexposure:* hepatitis B vaccine *Postexposure:* immune globulin with high amounts of anti-HBs (HBIG); hepatitis B vaccine	None; immune globulin may be given	None
Prevention	Handwashing, use of gloves	Care when handling products contaminated by blood, use of gloves	Same as hepatitis B	Same as hepatitis B
Severity	Mild	Mild to moderate	Mild to moderate	Moderate to severe
Fever	Common	Uncommon	Uncommon	Uncommon
Nausea/vomiting	Common	Common	Common	Common

▶ (a) Enteric precautions (Table 2.22).
  (b) Private room preferred.
  (c) Gown/gloves for direct contact with feces.
  (d) Handwashing when indirect contact with feces.
(2) *Serum hepatitis B:* blood and body fluid precautions.
  (a) Needle/dressing precautions.
  (b) Private room not necessary.
  (c) Gown: only if enteric precautions also necessary.
  (d) Handwashing: use gloves when in direct contact with blood.
(3) *Hepatitis C:* blood and body fluid precautions.
  (a) Same as B, except when in countries with fecal-oral form,

■ TABLE 2.22   Enteric Precautions

1. Private room if the patient's hygiene is poor. In general, patients with the same infection *may share* a room.
2. Masks are *not* indicated.
3. Gowns are indicated if soiling is likely.
4. Gloves are indicated for touching infective material.
5. Hands must be washed before and after touching the patient or potentially contaminated articles.
6. Contaminated articles should be discarded or bagged and labeled.

then use hepatitis A precautions also.
(4) *Delta*
  (a) Same as hepatitis B.
◆ b. Passive immunity for contacts
  (1) *Infectious hepatitis A:* immune serum globulin (ISG).

(2) *Serum hepatitis B:* hepatitis serum globulin (HGIB) or ISG.

(3) *Hepatitis C:* prophylaxis not as effective; IG may be given.

(4) *Delta:* same as for hepatitis B.

c. Goal: *promote healing.*
  (1) *Diet* as tolerated:
    (a) NPO with parenteral infusions, when in acute stage.
    (b) High protein, high carbohydrate, low fat, offered in frequent small meals.
    (c) Push fluids, if not contraindicated; I&O.

d. Goal: *monitor for increase in disease process, failure to respond to prescribed treatment.*
  (1) Observe urine—dark due to presence of bile and stool, clay colored.
  (2) Observe sclera, lab tests for increasing jaundice.
  (3) Mental confusion, unusual somnolence may indicate decreased liver function.
  (4) Weigh daily—increase indicates fluid retention and possible ascites.

e. Goal: *health teaching.*
  (1) Diet and fluid intake to promote liver regeneration.
  (2) Importance of rest and limited activity to reduce metabolic workload of liver.
  (3) Personal hygiene practices to prevent contamination.
  (4) Avoid alcohol, blood donations, and contact with communicable infections.
  (5) Follow-up case referral; may take 6 mo for full recovery.
  (6) Teach contacts about available immunizations.

◆ F. **Evaluation/outcome criteria:**
  1. Tolerates food; nausea and vomiting decreased.
  2. Signs of infection/inflammation absent.
  3. No complications, hemorrhage, liver damage, ascites.
  4. No jaundice noted.

IV. **Pancreatitis:** inflammatory disease of the pancreas; caused by alcoholism or alcohol consumption, biliary tract disease, carcinoma, adenoma, infections, drugs, metabolic diseases, hypercalcemia, and trauma.

A. **Pathophysiology:** proteolytic enzymes within the pancreas are activated by endotoxins, exotoxins, ischemia, anoxia, or trauma. Pancreatic enzymes begin process of autodigestion of pancreas and surrounding tissues; also activate other enzymes that digest cellular membranes. Autodigestion leads to edema, hemorrhage, vascular damage, coagulation necrosis, and fat necrosis.

B. **Risk factors:**
  1. Obesity.
  2. Alcoholism.
  3. Biliary tract disease.
  4. Abdominal trauma.
  5. Surgery.
  6. Drugs.
  7. Metabolic problems.
  8. Intestinal disease.

◆ C. **Assessment:**
  1. *Subjective data*
    a. Pain:
      (1) Sudden onset; severe, widespread, constant, and incapacitating.
      (2) Location—epigastrium, right upper quadrant (RUQ) and left upper quadrant (LUQ) of abdomen; radiates to back, flanks, and substernal area.
    b. Nausea.
    c. History of risk factors.
    d. Dyspnea.
  2. *Objective data*
    a. *Elevated:* temperature, pulse, respirations, BP (unless in shock).
    b. Decreased breath sounds related to atelectasis/pleural effusion.
    c. Increased crackles, cyanosis.
    d. Hemorrhage, shock.
    e. Vomiting.
    f. Fluid and electrolyte imbalances, dehydration.
    g. Decreased bowel sounds; abdominal tenderness with guarding.
    h. Stools: bulky, pale, foul smelling.
    i. Skin: pale, moist, cold; may be jaundiced.
    j. Muscle rigidity.
    k. Supine position leads to increased pain.
    l. Lab data:
      (1) *Elevated:*
        (a) Amylase, serum, and urine.
        (b) Serum lipase, AST[SGOT].
        (c) Alkaline phosphatase.
        (d) Bilirubin, glucose; serum and urine.
        (e) Urine protein, WBC.
        (f) Leukocytes.
        (g) BUN.
      (2) *Decreased:*
        (a) Serum calcium.
        (b) Protein.

◆ D. **Analysis/nursing diagnosis:**
  1. *Altered nutrition, less than body requirements,* related to nausea and vomiting.
  2. *Pain* related to inflammatory and autodigestive processes of pancreas.
  3. *Fluid volume deficit* related to inflammation, decreased intake, and vomiting.
  4. *Ineffective breathing pattern* related to pain and pleural effusion.

5. *Knowledge deficit* related to risk factors and disease management.

◆ **E. Nursing care plan/implementation:**
1. Goal: *control pain.*
   a. Medications: analgesics—meperidine (not morphine or codeine due to spasmodic effect).
   b. *Position:* sitting with knees flexed.
2. Goal: *rest injured pancreas.*
   a. NPO.
   ▶ b. NG tube to low suction.
   c. Medications:
      (1) Antacids.
      (2) Antibiotics.
      (3) Antiemetics.
      (4) Antispasmotics.
3. Goal: *prevent fluid and electrolyte imbalance.*
   a. Monitor: vitals, CVP.
   b. IVs, fluids, blood, albumin, plasma.
4. Goal: *prevent respiratory and metabolic complications.*
   a. Cough, deep breathe, change position.
   b. Monitor: blood sugar as ordered.
   c. Monitor calcium levels: *Chvostek's* and *Trousseau's sign* positive when calcium deficit exists (see XVI. Thyroidectomy, p. 184, for description of tests).
5. Goal: *provide adequate nutrition.*
   a. *Low-fat diet.*
   b. Bland, small, frequent meals.
   c. Vitamin supplements.
   d. *Avoid* alcohol.
6. Goal: *prevent complications.*
   a. Monitor for signs of:
      (1) Peritonitis.
      (2) Bowel obstruction, perforation.
      (3) Respiratory complications.
      (4) Hypotension, shock.
      (5) DIC.
      (6) Hemorrhage from ulcers, varices.
      (7) Anemia.
      (8) Encephalopathy.
7. Goal: *health teaching.*
   a. Food selections for low-fat, bland diet.
   b. Necessity of vitamin therapy.
   c. Importance of avoiding alcohol.
   d. Signs and symptoms of recurrence.
   e. Importance of rest, to prevent relapse.
   f. Desired effects and side effects of prescribed medications:
      (1) Narcotics for pain.
      (2) Antiemetics for nausea and vomiting.
      (3) Pancreatic hormone and enzymes to replace enzymes not reaching duodenum.

◆ **F. Evaluation/outcome criteria:**
1. Pain is relieved.
2. No complications, e.g., peritonitis, respiratory.
3. States dietary allowances and restrictions.

4. Takes medications as ordered; states purposes, side effects.

V. Cirrhosis: chronic inflammation and fibrosis of the liver in which some liver cells (hepatocytes) undergo necrosis and others undergo proliferative regeneration.
   A. Pathophysiology: progressive destruction of hepatic cells → loss of normal metabolic function of the liver and formation of scar tissue. Regeneration and proliferation of fibrous tissue → obstruction of the portal vein → increased portal hypertension, ascites, liver failure, and eventual death.
   B. Risk factors:
   1. Alcohol abuse most common cause.
   2. Nutritional deficiency with decreased protein intake.
   3. Hepatotoxins.
   4. Virus.

◆ **C. Assessment:**
1. *Subjective data*
   a. Chronic feeling of malaise.
   b. Anorexia, nausea.
   c. Abdominal pain.
   d. Pruritus.
2. *Objective data*
   a. GI:
      (1) Malnutrition, weight loss.
      (2) Vomiting.
      (3) Flatulence.
      (4) Ascites.
      (5) Enlarged liver and spleen.
      (6) Glossitis.
      (7) Fetid breath (sweet, musty odor).
   b. Blood—coagulation defects, possible esophageal varicosities, portal hypertension, bleeding from gums and injection sites.
   c. Skin and hair—edema, jaundice, spider angioma, palmar erythema, decreased pubic and axillary hair.
   d. Reproductive—menstrual abnormalities, gynecomastia, testicular atrophy, impotence.
   e. Neurologic deficits, including memory loss, hepatic coma, decreased level of consciousness; flappy tremor, grimacing.
   f. Lab data:
      (1) *Decreased:* albumin, potassium, magnesium, BUN.
      (2) *Elevated:* prothrombin time, globulins, ammonia, AST[SGOT], BSP, alkaline phosphate, uric acid, blood sugar.

◆ **D. Analysis/nursing diagnosis:**
1. *Altered nutrition, less than body requirements,* related to decreased intake, nausea, and vomiting.
2. *Risk for injury* related to decreased prothrombin production.
3. *Activity intolerance* related to fatigue.

4. *Fatigue* related to anorexia and nutritional deficiencies.
5. *Self-esteem disturbance* related to physical body changes.
6. *Risk for impaired skin integrity* related to pruritus.

◆ **E. Nursing care plan/implementation:**
   1. Goal: *provide for special safety needs.*
      a. Monitor vitals (including neurologic) frequently for hemorrhage from esophageal varices (may have *Sengstaken-Blakemore* or *Linton* tube inserted).
      b. Prepare patient for *LeVeen shunt* surgery for portal hypertension as needed.
      c. Assist with *paracentesis* performed for ascites; monitor vitals to prevent shock during procedure.
   2. Goal: *relieve discomfort caused by complications.*
      a. *Position:* semi-Fowler's or Fowler's to decrease pressure on diaphragm due to ascites.
      b. Deep breathing q2h to prevent respiratory complications.
      c. Skin care, topical medications to relieve pruritus; nail care to decrease possibility of further skin injury.
      d. Frequent oral hygiene related to nausea, vomiting, and fetid breath.
   3. Goal: *improve fluid and electrolyte balance.*
      a. IV fluids and vitamins.
      b. I&O, hourly urines during acute attacks.
      c. Daily: girths, weights to monitor fluid balance.
      d. Diuretics as ordered to decrease edema.
      e. May receive serum albumin to promote adequate vascular volume, prevent azotemia and encephalopathy, and promote diuresis (observe carefully, as albumin could escape quickly through cell walls and cause increase in ascites).
   4. Goal: *promote optimum nutrition within dietary restrictions.*
      a. NPO during acute episodes.
      b. Small, frequent meals when able to eat.
      c. *Low protein* (to decrease the amount of nitrogenous materials in the intestines) and *sodium* (to decrease fluid retention).
      d. *Moderate carbohydrate* (to meet energy demands) and *fat* (to make diet more palatable to anorexic patients).
   5. Goal: *provide emotional support.*
      a. Quiet environment during acute episodes to decrease external stimuli.
      b. Identify community agencies for assistance for patient, e.g., Alcoholics Anonymous; for family, Alanon/Ala-teen.
   6. Goal: *health teaching.*
      a. Avoid alcohol, exposure to infections.
      b. Dietary allowances, restrictions (see Unit 3: Sodium-restricted diet, p. 243 and Purine-restricted diet, p. 245).

c. Drugs: names, purposes.
d. Signs, symptoms of disease, and complications.
e. Stress-management techniques.

◆ **F. Evaluation/outcome criteria:**
   1. No complications.
   2. Nutritional status improves; lists dietary restrictions.
   3. No alcohol consumption.
   4. Lists signs and symptoms of increased disease process and complications.
   5. Complies with discharge plan, becomes involved with an alcohol treatment program.

VI. Esophageal varices: life-threatening hemorrhage from tortuous dilated, thin-walled veins in submucosa of lower esophagus. May rupture when chemically or mechanically irritated or when pressure is increased because of sneezing, coughing, use of the Valsalva maneuver, or excessive exercise.

   A. Pathophysiology: portal hypertension related to cirrhosis of the liver → distended branches of the azygos and vena cava veins where they join the smaller vessels of the esophagus.

   B. Risk factors for hemorrhage:
   1. Exertion that increases abdominal pressure.
   2. Trauma from ingestion of coarse foods.
   3. Acid pepsin erosion.

◆ **C. Assessment:**
   1. *Subjective data*
      a. Fear.
      b. Dysphagia.
      c. History: alcohol ingestion, liver dysfunction.
   2. *Objective data*
      a. Hematemesis.
      b. Hemorrhage: sudden, often fatal.
      c. Decreased BP; increased pulse, respirations.
      d. Melena (occult blood in stool).

◆ **D. Analysis/nursing diagnosis:**
   1. *Fluid volume deficit* related to blood loss.
   2. *Risk for injury* related to hemorrhage.
   3. *Fear* related to massive blood loss.
   4. *Ineffective individual coping* related to complications of cirrhosis.

◆ **E. Nursing care plan/implementation:**
   1. Goal: *provide safety measures related to hemorrhage.*
      a. Recognize signs of shock; vitals q15min.
      b. Assist with insertion of *Sengstaken-Blakemore* or *Linton tube* (tube is large and uncomfortable for patient during insertion); explain procedure briefly to decrease fear and attempt to gain patient's cooperation.
      c. While tube in place, observe for respiratory distress; if present, *deflate the bal-*

loon by releasing pressure; do not cut the tube.

   d. Deflate the balloon as ordered to prevent necrosis.

▶ e. NG tube to low gastric suction; monitor for amount of bright red blood; irrigate only as ordered using tepid, *not* iced, solutions.

   f. Vitamin K as ordered to control bleeding.

2. Goal: *promote fluid balance.*
   a. IV fluids, expanders, blood.
   b. Fresh blood as ordered to avoid increased ammonia; aids in coagulation.

3. Goal: *prevent complications of hepatic coma.*
   a. Saline cathartics as ordered to remove old blood from GI tract.
   b. Antibiotics as ordered to prevent infection.

4. Goal: *provide emotional support.*
   a. Stay with patient.
   b. Calm atmosphere.

5. Goal: *health teaching.*
   a. Explain use of tube to patient and family.
   b. Bland diet instructions.
   c. Recognize signs of bleeding.
   d. *Avoid* straining at stool.
   e. *Avoid* aspirin because of increased bleeding tendency.

◆ **F. Evaluation/outcome criteria:**
1. Survives acute bleeding episode.
2. Further episodes prevented by avoiding irritants, especially alcohol.
3. Improves nutritional status.
4. Recognizes symptoms of complications, e.g., bleeding.
5. Demonstrates knowledge of medications by avoiding aspirin.

VII. Diaphragmatic hernia (hiatus hernia): protrusion of part of stomach through diaphragm and into thoracic cavity. *Types:* sliding (most common); paraesophageal "rolling."

  A. Pathophysiology: weakening of the musculature of the diaphragm, aggravated by increased intraabdominal pressure → protrusion of the abdominal organs through the esophageal hiatus → reflux of gastric contents → esophagitis.

  B. Risk factors:
1. Congenital abnormality.
2. Penetrating wound.
3. Age (middle-aged or elderly).
4. Women more than men.
5. Obesity.
6. Ascites.
7. Pregnancy.
8. History of constipation.

◆ **C. Assessment:**
1. *Subjective data*
   a. Pressure: substernal.

    b. Pain: epigastric, burning.
    c. Eructation, heartburn after eating.
    d. Dysphagia.
    e. Symptoms aggravated when recumbent.

2. *Objective data*
   a. Cough, dyspnea.
   b. Tachycardia, palpitations.
   c. Bleeding: hematemesis, melena, signs of anemia due to gastroesophageal irritation, ulceration, and bleeding.
   d. Diagnostic tests:
      (1) Chest X rays, showing protrusion of abdominal organs into thoracic cavity.
      (2) Barium swallow (upper GI) to show presence of hernia.

◆ **D. Analysis/nursing diagnosis:**
1. *Pain* related to irritation of lining of GI tract.
2. *Altered nutrition, less than body requirements,* related to dysphagia.
3. *Sleep pattern disturbance* related to increase in symptoms when recumbent.
4. *Risk for aspiration* related to reflux of gastric contents.
5. *Activity intolerance* related to dyspnea.
6. *Anxiety* related to palpitations.

◆ **E. Nursing care plan/implementation:**
1. *Presurgical*
   a. Goal: *promote relief of symptoms.*
      (1) *Diet:*
         (a) Small, frequent feedings of soft, bland foods, to reduce abdominal pressure and reflux.
         (b) Fluid when swallowing solids may push food into stomach; hot fluid may work best.
         (c) Avoid eating 2 h before bedtime.
         (d) High-protein, low-fat foods to decrease heartburn.
      (2) *Positioning:* head elevated to increase movement of food into stomach. Symptoms may decrease if head of bed at home is elevated on 8-in. blocks.
      (3) Weight reduction to decrease abdominal pressure.
      (4) Medications as ordered:
         (a) 30 mL antacid 1 h after meals and at bedtime.
         (b) Avoid anticholinergic drugs, which decrease gastric emptying.

2. *Postsurgical*
   a. Goal: *provide for postoperative safety needs.*
      (1) Respiratory: deep breathing, coughing, splint incision area.
   ▶ (2) *Nasogastric tube:* check patency

      (a) Drainage: should be small amount.

      (b) Color: dark brown 6–12 h after surgery, changing to greenish yellow.

      (c) Do *not* disturb tube placement to avoid traction on suture line.

    (3) *Position:* initially head of bed elevated slightly, then semi-Fowler's; turn side to side frequently, to prevent pressure on diaphragm.

    (4) Maintain closed chest drainage if indicated (see Table 5.5).

    (5) Check for return of bowel sounds.

  b. Goal: *promote comfort and maintain nutrition.*

    (1) IVs for hydration and electrolytes.

▶   (2) Initiate feeding through *gastrostomy* tube if present.

      (a) Usually attached to intermittent, low suction after surgery.

      (b) Aspirate gastric contents before feeding—delay if 75 mL or more is present; report these findings to physician.

      (c) Feed in *high-Fowler's* or sitting position; keep head elevated for 30 min after eating.

      (d) Warm feeding to room temperature; dilute with H_2O if too thick.

      (e) Give 50 mL H_2O before feeding; 200–500 mL feeding by gravity over 10–15 min; follow with 50 mL H_2O.

      (f) Give frequent mouth care.

  c. Goal: *health teaching.*

    (1) Avoid constricting clothing and activities that increase intraabdominal pressure, e.g., lifting, bending, straining at stool.

    (2) Weight reduction.

    (3) Dietary needs: small, frequent, soft, bland meals; chew thoroughly; upright position for at least 1 h after meals.

◆ **F. Evaluation/outcome criteria:**

  1. Relief from symptoms, comfortable.

  2. Receiving adequate, balanced nutrition.

  3. Describes dietary changes, recommended positioning, and activity limitations to prevent recurrence.

VIII. Peptic ulcer disease: circumscribed loss of mucosa, submucosa, or muscle layer of the gastrointestinal tract caused by a decreased resistance of gastric mucosa to acid-pepsin injury. *Peptic ulcer disease* is a chronic disease and may occur in the distal esophagus, stomach, upper duodenum, or jejunum. *Gastric ulcers,* located on the lesser curvature of stomach, are larger, deeper than duodenal ulcers and tend to become *malignant. Duodenal ulcers* are located on the first part of the duodenum; they are more common than gastric ulcers. *Stress ulcers,* an acute problem, occur after a major insult to the body.

A. Pathophysiology: failure of the body to regenerate mucous epithelium at a sufficient rate to counterbalance the damage to tissue during the breakdown of protein; decrease in the quantity and quality of the mucus; poor local mucosal blood flow, along with individual susceptibility to ulceration.

B. Risk factors:

  1. *Gastric ulcers*

    a. Decreased resistance to acid-pepsin injury.

    b. Gastritis.

    c. Increased histamine release → inflammatory reaction.

    d. Cigarette smoking, increased caffeine/alcohol use.

    e. Family history.

    f. Difficulty coping with high-stress environment.

    g. Ulcerogenic drugs that aggravate preexisting condition.

    h. Increased hydrogen ion back-diffusion.

    i. Age >50.

  2. *Duodenal ulcers*

    a. Elevated gastric acid secretory rate.

    b. Elevated gastric acid levels postprandially (after eating).

    c. Increased rate of gastric emptying → increased amount of acid into duodenum → irritation and breakdown of duodenal mucosa.

    d. Men more than women; possible influence of endocrine factors such as estrogen and adrenal steroids.

    e. Seasonal influence: spring and fall.

    f. Cigarette smoking; increased caffeine/alcohol use.

    g. Family history.

    h. Difficulty coping with high-stress environment.

    i. Ulcerogenic drugs that aggravate preexisting condition.

    j. Persons with blood type O.

    k. Age 25–50.

  3. *Stress ulcers*

    a. Severe trauma or major illness.

    b. Severe burns (*Curling's ulcer*); develop in 72 h with majority of persons with burns over more than 35% of their body surface.

    c. Head injuries or intracranial disease (*Cushing's ulcers*).

    d. Medications in large doses: corticosteroids, salicylates, ibuprofen, indomethacin, phenylbutazone (Butazolidin).

e. Shock.

f. Sepsis.

◆ **C. Assessment:**

1. *Subjective data*

    a. *Gastric ulcers*

    (1) Pain

       (a) Type: gnawing, aching, burning.

       (b) Location: epigastric, left of midline, localized.

       (c) Occurrence: period pain, often 2 h after eating.

       (d) Relief: antacids; may be aggravated, not relieved, by food.

    (2) Nausea.

    (3) History of risk factors as above.

    b. *Duodenal ulcers*

    (1) Pain

       (a) Type: gnawing, aching, burning, hungerlike, boring.

       (b) Location: right epigastric, localized; steady pain near midline of back may indicate perforation.

       (c) Occurrence: 1–3 h after eating, worse at end of day or during the night; initial attack occurs spring or fall; history of remissions and exacerbations.

       (d) Relief: food and/or antacids.

    (2) Nausea.

    (3) History of risk factors as above.

    c. *Stress ulcers*

    (1) Pain: often painless until serious complication (hemorrhage, perforation) occurs.

    (2) History of risk factors as above.

2. *Objective data*

    a. *Gastric ulcer*

    (1) Vomiting.

    (2) Melena (tarry stools).

    (3) Weight loss.

    🧪 (4) X ray (upper GI series) confirms "crater" (punched out appearance, clean base).

    🧪 (5) Endoscopy confirms presence of ulcer; biopsy for cytology.

    (6) Monitor for blood loss: CBC, stool for occult blood.

    b. *Duodenal ulcer*

    (1) Eructation.

    (2) Vomiting.

    (3) Regurgitation of sour liquid into back of mouth.

    (4) Constipation.

    🧪 (5) X ray (upper GI series) confirms ulcer craters and niches as well as outlet deformities; round or oval funnellike lesion extending into musculature.

    (6) Common complications: hemorrhage or perforation.

c. *Stress ulcer*

    (1) GI bleeding.

    (2) Multiple, superficial erosions affecting large area of gastric mucosa.

◆ **D. Analysis/nursing diagnosis** (all types):

1. *Pain* related to erosion of gastric lining.

2. *Ineffective individual coping* related to inability to change life-style.

3. *Altered nutrition, less than body requirements,* related to inadequate intake.

4. *Knowledge deficit* regarding preventive measures.

5. *Risk for injury* related to possible hemorrhage or perforation.

◆ **E. Nursing care plan/implementation** (all types):

1. Goal: *promote comfort.*

    💊 a. Medications as ordered to decrease pain (see 4. Goal: Health teaching); sedatives to decrease anxiety.

    🧪 b. Prepare for diagnostic tests.

    (1) X rays; upper GI series (barium swallow); lower GI (barium enema).

    (2) Endoscopy.

    (3) Gastric analysis, to determine amount of hydrochloric acid in GI tract.

2. Goal: *prevent/recognize signs of complications.*

    a. Monitor vitals for shock.

    b. Check stool for occult blood/hemorrhage.

    c. Palpate abdomen for perforation (rigid, boardlike); arterial bleeding.

3. Goal: *provide emotional support.*

    a. Stress-management techniques.

    b. Restful environment.

    c. Prepare for surgery, if necessary.

4. Goal: *health teaching.*

    💊 a. Medications:

    (1) Antacids: *give 1–3 h after meals and at bedtime* to decrease pain by lowering acidity; monitor for:

       (a) Diarrhea (seen most often with magnesium carbonate and magnesium oxide).

       (b) Constipation (seen most often with calcium carbonate or aluminum hydroxide).

       (c) Electrolyte imbalance (seen with systemic antacid, soda bicarbonate).

       (d) Best 1–3 h *after meals.*

       (e) Liquids more effective than tablets; if taking tablets, chew slowly.

    (2) Histamine antagonists: *given with meals/bedtimes* to block the action of histamine-stimulated gastric secretions (basal and stimulated); inhibits pepsin secretion and re-

duces the volume of gastric secretion.

  (a) Cimetidine (Tagamet) inhibits gastrin release, can be given PO, IV, or IM; cannot be given within 1 h of antacid therapy.

  (b) Ranitidine (Zantac) has greater reduction of acid secretion, longer duration, less frequent administration (bid vs qid), and fewer side effects than cimetidine.

 (3) Sucralfate (Carafate): *given 1 h before meals and at bedtime.*

  (a) Locally active topical agent that forms a protective coat on mucosa, prevents further digestive action of both acid and pepsin.

  (b) Must not be given within ½ h of antacids.

 (4) Anticholinergic *when used, given before meals* to decrease gastric acid secretion and delay gastric emptying.

 (5) Important: *avoid aspirin* (could increase bleeding possibility).

 b. *Diet:*

  (1) *Avoid*

   (a) Stress at mealtimes.

   (b) Milk (increases gastric acid production).

   (c) Substances that cause pain.

   (d) Coffee with or without caffeine.

   (e) Foods or liquids containing caffeine.

   (f) Alcohol.

   (g) Tobacco.

  (2) *Plan:*

   (a) Small, frequent meals (to prevent exacerbation of symptoms related to an empty stomach).

   (b) Weight control.

 c. Complications—signs and symptoms:

  (1) Gastric ulcers may be premalignant.

  (2) Perforation.

  (3) Hemorrhage.

  (4) Obstruction.

 d. Life-style changes:

  (1) Decrease:

   (a) Smoking.

   (b) Noise.

   (c) Rush.

   (d) Confusion.

  (2) Increase:

   (a) Communications.

   (b) Mental/physical rest.

   (c) Compliance with medical regimen.

◆ **F. Evaluation/outcome criteria:**

 1. Remains on specified diet.

 2. Takes prescribed medications.

 3. Pain decreases.

 4. No complications.

 5. States signs and symptoms of complications.

 6. Participates in stress-reduction activities.

IX. Gastric surgery: performed when ulcer medical regimen is unsuccessful, ulcer is determined to be precancerous, or complications are present.

 A. Types:

  1. *Subtotal gastrectomy:* removal of a portion of the stomach.

  2. *Total gastrectomy:* removal of the entire stomach.

  3. *Antrectomy:* removal of entire antrum (lower) portion of the stomach.

  4. *Pyloroplasty:* repair of the pyloric opening of the stomach.

  5. *Vagotomy:* interruption of the impulses carried by the vagus nerve, which results in reduction of gastric secretions and decreased physical activity of the stomach (being done less often).

  6. Combination of vagotomy and gastrectomy.

◆ **B. Analysis/nursing diagnosis:**

 1. *Pain* related to surgical incision.

 2. *Ineffective breathing pattern* related to high surgical incision.

 3. *Risk for trauma* related to possible complications postgastrectomy.

 4. *Knowledge deficit* related to inability to manage ulcer disease on medical regimen.

 5. *Fear* related to possible precancerous lesion.

 6. *Ineffective individual coping* related to risk factors influencing peptic ulcer disease.

◆ **C. Nursing care plan/implementation:**

 1. Goal: *promote comfort in the postoperative period.*

  a. Analgesics: to relieve pain and allow patient to cough, deep breathe to prevent pulmonary complications.

  b. *Position:* semi-Fowler's to aid in breathing.

 2. Goal: *promote wound healing.*

  a. Keep dressings dry.

 ▶ b. *NG tube* to low intermittent suction (Levine) or low continuous (Salem-sump).

   (1) Check drainage from NG tube; normally bloody first 2–3 h postsurgery, then brown to dark green.

   (2) Excessive bright red blood drainage: take vital signs; report: vital signs, color and volume of drainage to MD immediately.

   (3) Irrigate *gently* with saline in amount ordered; do **not** irrigate against resistance; may not be done in early postop period.

Adult

(4) Tape securely to face, but prevent obstructed vision.

(5) Frequent mouth and nostril care.

3. Goal: *promote adequate nutrition and hydration.*

a. Administer parenteral fluids as ordered.

b. Accurate I&O.

▶ c. Check bowel sounds, at least q4h; NPO 1–3 days; bowel sounds normally return 24–36 h; oral fluids as ordered when bowel sounds present—usually 30 mL, then small feedings, then bland liquids to soft diet.

d. Observe for nausea and vomiting due to suture line edema, food intake (too much, too fast).

4. Goal: *prevent complications.*

a. Check dressing q4h for bleeding.

b. Vitamin B$_{12}$ and iron replacement as ordered to avoid pernicious anemia or iron deficiency anemia.

c. Avoid dumping syndrome.

◆ **D. Evaluation/outcome criteria:**

1. Hemorrhage, dumping syndrome avoided.

2. Healing begins.

3. Adjust life-style to prevent recurrence/marginal ulcer.

X. **Dumping syndrome:** hypoglycemic-type episode; occurs postoperatively after gastric resection (may also occur post vagotomy, antrectomy, or gastroenterostomy), when food and fluids that are more hyperosmolar than the jejunal secretions pass *quickly* into jejunum, producing fluid shifts from bloodstream to jejunum. This is a mild problem for about 20% of patients and will disappear in a few months to a year. Symptoms cause serious problem for about 7% of the patients. This discomfort may occur during a meal or up to 30 min after the meal and last from 20–60 min. The reaction is greatest after the ingestion of sugar.

◆ **A. Assessment:**

1. *Subjective data*

a. Feeling of fullness, weakness, faintness.

b. Palpitations.

c. Nausea.

d. Discomfort during or after eating.

2. *Objective data*

a. Diaphoresis.

b. Diarrhea.

c. Fainting.

d. Symptoms of hypoglycemia.

◆ **B. Analysis/nursing diagnosis:**

1. *Altered nutrition, more than body requirements,* related to body's inability to properly digest high-carbohydrate, high-sodium foods.

2. *Diarrhea* related to food passing into jejunum too quickly.

3. *Risk for injury* related to hypoglycemia.

4. *Knowledge deficit* related to dietary restrictions.

◆ **C. Nursing care plan/implementation:**

1. Goal: *health teaching.*

a. *Include:*

(1) *Increased fat, protein* to delay emptying.

(2) Rest after meals.

(3) Small, frequent meals.

(4) Fluids *between* meals.

b. *Avoid:*

(1) Foods high in *salt, carbohydrate.*

(2) Large meals.

(3) Stress at mealtime.

(4) Fluids at mealtime.

◆ **D. Evaluation/outcome criteria:**

1. No complications.

2. Patient heals.

3. No further ulcers.

4. Incorporates health teaching into life-style and prevents syndrome.

XI. **Total parenteral nutrition:** provide nutrition through a central venous line to patients who are in a catabolic state; are malnourished and cannot tolerate food by mouth; are in negative nitrogen balance; or have conditions that interfere with protein ingestion, digestion, and absorption, e.g., Crohn's disease, major burns, and side effects of radiation therapy of abdomen.

A. Types of solutions:

1. Hydrolyzed proteins (Hyprotein, Amigen).

2. Synthetic amino acids (Freamine).

3. Usual components:

a. 3–8% amino acid.

b. 10–25% glucose.

c. Multivitamins.

d. Electrolytes.

4. Supplements that can be added:

a. Fructose.

b. Alcohol.

c. Minerals: iron, copper, calcium.

d. Trace elements: iodine, zinc, magnesium.

e. Vitamins: A, B, C.

f. Androgen hormone therapy.

g. Insulin.

B. Administration:

1. Dosage varies with clinical condition; 1 liter q5–8h; rate of flow must be constant.

2. Solution prepared under laminar flow hood (usually in pharmacy); solution must be *refrigerated;* when refrigerated, expires in 24 h; once removed from refrigerator, expires in 12 h.

3. Incompatible with many antibiotics; check with pharmacy.

4. Route: catheter inserted in a large vein (e.g., subclavian) by physician; placement confirmed by X ray before beginning infusion (Figure 2.3).

5. *Side effects:*

a. Hyperosmolar coma.

b. Hyperglycemia >130.

c. Septicemia.

d. Thrombosis/sclerosis of vein.

■ **FIGURE 2.3   Hyperalimentation. A. Patient with subclavian hyperalimentation line. B. Gauze dressing. C. Taping hyperalimentation line.**

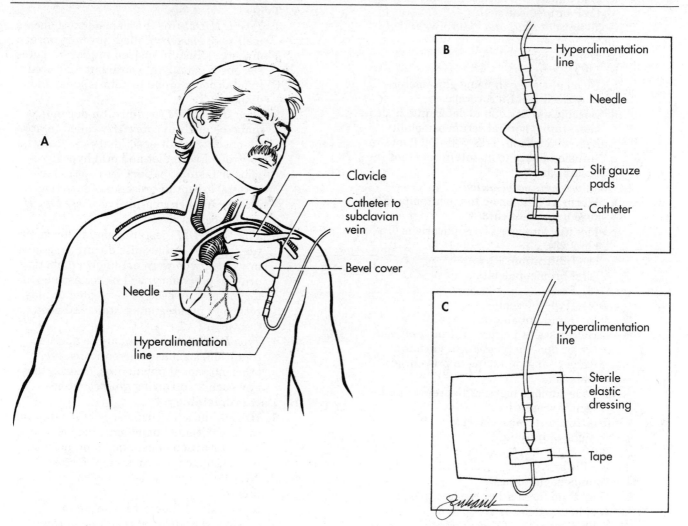

e. Air embolus.
f. Pneumothorax.
6. Prolonged use: >10 d, fat needed; intralipids piggybacked close to insertion site; do not give through filter; observe for hypersensitivity (e.g., tachypnea, tachycardia, nausea, urticaria).

◆ **C. Analysis/nursing diagnosis:**
1. *Fluid volume excess, potential,* related to inability to tolerate amount and consistency of solution.
2. *Fluid volume deficit* related to state of malnutrition.
3. *Risk for injury* related to possible complications.
4. *Altered nutrition, more or less than body requirements,* related to ability to tolerate parenteral nutrition.

◆ **D. Nursing care plan/implementation:**
1. Goal: *prevent infection.*
   a. Dressing change:

(1) Strict aseptic technique.
(2) Nurse and patient wear mask during dressing change.
(3) Cleanse skin with solution as ordered:
   (a) Acetone to defat the skin, destroy the bacterial wall.
   (b) Iodine 1% solution as antiseptic agent.
(4) Dressing changed q48–72h; transparent polyurethane dressings may be changed weekly.
(5) Mark with nurse's initials, date and time of change.
(6) Air occlusive dressing.
   b. Attach final filter on tubing set-up, to prevent air embolism.
   c. Solution: change q12h to prevent infection.
   d. Culture wound and catheter tip if signs of infection appear.

  e. Monitor temperature q4h.
  f. Use lumen line for feeding only (not for CVP or medications).
2. Goal: *prevent fluid and electrolyte imbalance.*
  a. Daily weights.
  b. I&O.
  c. Blood glucose q4h using glucometer; may need insulin coverage.
  d. Specific gravity q8h to determine hydration status; normal serum osmolality 275–295 mOsm, TPN 600–1400 mOsm.
  e. Infusion pump to maintain constant infusion rate.
3. Goal: *prevent complications.*
  a. Warm TPN solution to room temperature to prevent chills.
  b. Monitor for signs of complications (Table 2.23).
    (1) Infiltration.
    (2) Thrombophlebitis.
    (3) Fever.
    (4) Hyperglycemia.
    (5) Fluid imbalance.
  c. Have patient perform *Valsalva maneuver,* or apply a plastic-coated clamp when changing tubing to prevent air embolism.
  d. Tape tubings together to prevent accidental separation.
◆ E. **Evaluation/outcome criteria:**
1. No signs of infection.
2. Blood sugar <130 mg/100 mL.
3. Specific gravity between 1.010 and 1.020.
4. Wounds begin to heal.
5. Weight: no further loss, begins to gain.

XII. Diabetes: heterogeneous group of diseases involving the disruption of the metabolism of car-bohydrates, fats, and protein. If uncontrolled, serious vascular and neurologic changes occur.

A. Types:
1. *Type I: IDDM* (insulin-dependent diabetes mellitus): *formerly* called "juvenile-onset diabetes." Insulin needed to prevent ketosis; onset usually in youth but may occur in adulthood; prone to ketosis, unstable diabetes.
2. *Type II: NIDDM* (non-insulin-dependent diabetes mellitus): *formerly* called "maturity-onset or adult-onset diabetes." May be controlled with diet and oral hypoglycemics or insulin; patient less apt to have ketosis, except in presence of infection. May be further classified as *obese type II* or *nonobese type II.*
3. *Type III: GDM* (gestational diabetes mellitus): glucose intolerance during pregnancy in women who were not known diabetics prior to pregnancy; will be reclassified after birth; may need to be treated or may return to prepregnancy state and need no treatment.
4. *Type IV:* diabetes secondary to another condition, such as pancreatic disease, other hormonal imbalances, or drug therapy such as involving glucocorticoids.

B. Pathophysiology:
1. IDDM—absolute deficiency of insulin due to destruction of pancreatic beta cells by the interaction of genetic, immunologic, hereditary, or environmental factors.
2. NIDDM—relative deficiency of insulin due to:
  a. An islet cell defect resulting in a slowed or delayed response in the re-

■ **TABLE 2.23   Complications Associated with Total Parenteral Nutrition**

Problem	Nursing Intervention
Infection	
Local infection (pain, redness, edema)	Sterile dressings; administer antibiotics as ordered; general
Generalized, systemic infection (elevated temperature, WBC)	comfort measures
Arterial Puncture	
Artery is punctured instead of vein	Needle is withdrawn and pressure is applied
Physician aspirates bright red blood that is pulsating strongly	
Air Embolus	
Air enters venous system during catheter insertion or tubing changes; or catheter/tubing pull apart	Stat ABGs, chest X ray, ECG
Chest pain, dizziness, cyanosis, confusion	Connect catheter to sterile syringe, and aspirate air
	Clean catheter tip, connect to new tubing
	Place patient on left side with head lowered (left Trendelenburg prevents air from going into pulmonary artery)
	Prevention: have patient perform Valsalva maneuver or use plastic-coated clamp on catheter at insertion or tubing changes
Catheter Embolus	
Catheter must be checked for placement by X ray and observed when removed to be sure it is intact	Careful observation of catheter
	Monitor for signs of distress
Pneumothorax	
If needle punctures pleura, patient reports dyspnea, chest pain	May seal off or may need chest tubes

lease of insulin to a glucose load; or

b. Reduction in the number of insulin receptors from continuously elevated insulin levels; or

c. A postreceptor defect; or

d. A major peripheral resistance to insulin induced by hyperglycemia. These factors lead to deprivation of insulin-dependent cells → a marked decrease in the cellular rate of glucose uptake, and therefore elevated blood glucose.

C. Risk factors:

1. Obesity.
2. Family history of diabetes.
3. Elderly.
4. Women whose babies at birth weighed more than 9 lb.
5. History of autoimmune disease.

◆ **D. Assessment:**

1. *Subjective data*
   a. *Eyes:* blurry vision.
   b. *Skin:* pruritus vulvae.
   c. *Neuromuscular:* paresthesia, peripheral neuropathy, lethargy, weakness, fatigue, increased irritability.
   d. *GI:* polydipsia (increased thirst).
   e. *Reproductive:* impotence.

2. *Objective data*
   a. *Genitourinary:* polyuria, glycosuria, nocturia (nocturnal enuresis in children).
   b. *Vital signs:*
      (1) Pulse and temperature normal or elevated.
      (2) BP normal or decreased, unless complications present.
      (3) Respirations, increased rate and depth (Kussmaul's respirations).
   c. *GI:*
      (1) Polyphagia, dehydration.
      (2) Weight loss, failure to gain weight.
      (3) Acetone breath.
   d. *Skin:* cuts heal slowly; frequent infections, foot ulcers, vaginitis.
   e. *Neuromuscular:* loss of strength, peripheral neuropathy.
   f. Lab data:
      (1) *Elevated:*
         (a) Blood sugar >115 mg/dL fasting or >160 1–2 h after eating.
         (b) Glucose tolerance test.
         (c) Glycosuria (>170 mg/100 mL).
         (d) Potassium (>5) and chloride (>145).
         (e) Hemoglobin A_{1c} > 7%.
      (2) *Decreased:*
         (a) pH (<7.4).
         (b) P_{CO_2} (<32).
   g. Long-term pathologic considerations:
      (1) *Cataract formation and retinopathy:* thickened capillary basement

membrane, changes in vascularization and hemorrhage, due to chronic hyperglycemia.

(2) *Nephropathy:* due to glomerulosclerosis, arteriosclerosis of renal artery and pyelonephritis, progressive uremia.

(3) *Neuropathy:* due to reduced tissue perfusion; affecting motor, sensory, voluntary, and autonomic functions.

(4) *Arteriosclerosis:* due to lesions of the intimal wall.

(5) *Cardiac:* angina, coronary insufficiency, myocardial infarction.

(6) *Vascular changes:* occlusions, intermittent claudication, loss of peripheral pulses, arteriosclerosis.

◆ **E. Analysis/nursing diagnosis:**

1. *Altered nutrition, less than body requirements,* related to inability to metabolize nutrients and weight loss.
2. *Altered nutrition, more than body requirements,* related to excessive glucose intake.
3. *Risk for injury* related to complications of uncontrolled diabetes.
4. *Body image disturbance* related to long-term illness.
5. *Knowledge deficit* related to management of long-term illness.
6. *Ineffective individual coping* related to inability to follow diet/medication regimen.
7. *Sexual dysfunction* related to impotence of diabetes and treatment.

◆ **F. Nursing care plan/implementation:**

1. Goal: *obtain and maintain normal sugar balance.*
   a. Monitor: vital signs; blood glucose before meals, at bedtime, and as symptoms demand (urine testing for glucose levels is *not* as accurate as capillary blood testing).
   b. Medications: oral hypoglycemics or insulin, as ordered.
   c. *Diet,* as ordered.
      (1) Carbohydrate, 50–60%; protein, 20%; fats, 30% (saturated fats limited to 10%, unsaturated fats, 90%).
      (2) Calorie reduction in obese adults; enough calories to promote normal growth and development for children or nonobese adults.
      (3) Limit refined sugars.
      (4) Add vitamins, minerals as needed for well-balanced diet.
   d. Monitor for signs of acute or chronic complications.

2. Goal: *health teaching.*
   a. *Diet:* foods allowed, restricted, substitutions.

b. Medications: administration techniques, importance of utilizing room-temperature insulin, and rotating injection sites to prevent tissue damage.

c. Desired and side effects of prescribed insulin type; onset, peak, and duration of action of prescribed insulin.

d. Blood glucose testing techniques.

e. Signs of complications (Table 2.24).

f. Importance of health maintenance:
   (1) Infection prevention, especially foot and nail care.
   (2) Routine checkups.
   (3) Maintain stable balance of glucose by carefully monitoring glucose level and making necessary adjustments in diet and activity level; seeking medical attention when unable to maintain balance; regular exercise program.

◆ **G. Evaluation/outcome criteria:**
   1. Optimal blood-glucose levels achieved.
   2. Ideal weight maintained.
   3. Adequate hydration.
   4. Carries out self-care activities; blood or urine testing, foot care, exchange diets, medication administration, exercise.
   5. Recognizes and treats hyper- or hypoglycemic reactions.
   6. Seeks medical assistance appropriately.

XIII. Hyperglycemic hyperosmolar nonketotic coma (HHNC): profound hyperglycemia and dehydration without ketosis or ketoacidosis; seen in non-insulin-dependent diabetics; brought on by infection or illness. The patient is *critically ill.*

A. Pathophysiology: hyperglycemia greater than 1000 mg/dL causes osmotic diuresis, depletion of extracellular fluid, and hyperosmolarity related to infection or another stressor as the precipitating factor. Patient unable to replace fluid deficits with oral intake.

B. Risk factors:
   1. Old age.
   2. History of non-insulin-dependent diabetes.
   3. Infections: pneumonia, pyelonephritis, pancreatitis, gram-negative infections.
   4. Kidney failure: uremia and peritoneal dialysis.
   5. Shock:
      a. Lactic acidosis related to bicarbonate deficit.
      b. Myocardial infarction.
   6. Hemorrhage:
      a. GI.
      b. Subdural.
      c. Arterial thrombosis.
   7. Medications:
      a. Diuretics.
      b. Glucocorticoids.

◆ **C. Assessment:**
   1. *Subjective data*
      a. Confusion.
      b. Lethargy.
   2. *Objective data*
      a. Nystagmus.
      b. Dehydration.
      c. Aphasia.
      d. Nuchal rigidity.
      e. Hyperreflexia.
      f. Lab data:
         (1) Blood-glucose level 1000 mg/dL.
         (2) Serum sodium and chloride—normal to elevated.
         (3) BUN >60 mg/dL (higher than in ketoacidosis because of more severe gluconeogenesis and dehydration).
         (4) Arterial pH—slightly depressed.

◆ **D. Analysis/nursing diagnosis:**
   1. *Risk for injury* related to hyperglycemia.
   2. *Altered renal peripheral tissue perfusion* related to vascular collapse.
   3. *Ineffective airway clearance* related to coma.

◆ **E. Nursing care plan/implementation:**
   1. Goal: *promote fluid and electrolyte balance.*
      a. IVs: fluids and electrolytes, saline solution used initially to combat dehydration. Lab values will determine fluid replacement.
      b. Monitor I&O because of the high volume of fluid replaced in the critical stage of this condition.
      c. Administer nursing care for problem that precipitated this serious condition.
      d. Food by mouth when client is able.
   2. Goal: *prevent complications.*
      a. Administer *regular* insulin (initial dose usually 5–15 U) and food, as ordered.
      b. Uncontrolled condition leads to cardiovascular disease, renal failure, blindness, and diabetic gangrene.

◆ **F. Evaluation/outcome criteria:**
   1. Blood sugar returns to normal level of 80–120 mg/dL.
   2. Patient is alert to time, place, and person.
   3. Primary medical problem resolved.
   4. Patient recognizes and reports signs of imbalance.

XIV. Cholecystitis/cholelithiasis: inflammation of gallbladder due to bacterial infection, presence of cholelithiasis (stones, cholesterol, calcium, or bile in the gallbladder), or choledocholithiasis (stone in the common bile duct) and/or obstruction. Acute cholecystitis is abrupt in onset, but the patient usually has a history of several at-

■ TABLE 2.24   Comparison of Diabetic Complications

	Hypoglycemia	**Ketoacidosis**
Pathophysiology	Major metabolic complication when too little food or too large dose of insulin or hypoglycemic agents administered; interferes with oxygen consumption of nervous tissue	Major metabolic complication in which there is insufficient insulin for metabolism of carbohydrates, fats, and proteins; seen most frequently with patients who are insulin dependent; precipitated in the known diabetic by stressors (such as infection, trauma, major illness) that increase insulin needs
Risk factors	Too little food Emotional or added stress Vomiting or diarrhea Added exercise	Insufficient insulin or oral hypoglycemics Noncompliance with dietary instructions Major illness/infections Therapy with steroid administration Trauma, surgery Elevated blood sugar: >200 mg/100 mL
Assessment	**Behavioral change:** *Subjective data*—nervous, irritable, anxious, confused, disoriented *Objective data*—abrupt mood changes, psychosis **Visual:** *Subjective data*—blurred vision, diplopia *Objective data*—dilated pupils **Skin:** *Objective data*—diaphoresis, **pale,** cool, clammy, goose bumps (piloerection), tenting **Vitals:** *Objective data*—tachycardia; palpitations, thready **Gastrointestinal:** *Subjective data*—hunger, nausea *Objective data*—diarrhea, vomiting **Neurologic:** *Subjective data*—headache; lips/tongue: tingling, numbness *Objective data*—fainting, yawning; speech: incoherent; convulsions; coma **Musculoskeletal:** *Subjective data*—weak, fatigue *Objective data*—trembling Blood sugar: <80 mg/100 mL	**Behavioral change:** *Subjective data*—irritable, confused *Objective data*—drowsy **Visual:** *Objective data*—eyeballs: soft, sunken **Skin:** *Objective data*—loss of turgor, **flushed face,** pruritus vulvae **Vitals:** *Objective data*—respirations-Kussmaul's Breath: fruity; BP: hypovolemic shock **Gastrointestinal:** *Subjective data*—increased thirst and hunger, abdominal pain, nausea *Objective data*—vomiting, diarrhea, dry mucous membrane; lips, tongue: red, parched **Neurologic:** *Subjective data*—headache; irritability; confusion; lethargy, weakness **Musculoskeletal:** *Subjective data*—fatigue; general malaise. **Renal:** *Objective data*—polyuria Blood sugar: >130 mg/100 mL
Analysis/nursing diagnosis	*Risk for injury* related to deficit of needed glucose *Knowledge deficit* related to proper dietary intake or proper insulin dosage *Altered nutrition, less than body requirements,* related to glucose deficiency	*Risk for injury* related to glucose imbalance *Knowledge deficit* related to proper balance of diet and insulin dosage
Nursing care plan/ implementation	Goal: *provide adequate glucose to reverse hypoglycemia:* administer simple sugar stat, PO or IV, glucose paste absorbed in mucous membrane; monitor blood sugar levels: identify events leading to complication Goal: *health teaching:* how to prevent further episodes (see Diabetes, Health teaching, p. 125); importance of careful monitoring of balance between glucose levels and insulin dosage	Goal: *promote normal balance of food and insulin:* **regular** insulin as ordered; IV saline, as ordered; bicarbonate and electrolyte replacements, as ordered; potassium replacements once therapy begins and urine output is adequate Goal: *health teaching:* diet instructions; desired effects and side effects of prescribed insulin or hypoglycemic agent (onset, peak, and duration of action); importance of recognizing signs of imbalance
Evaluation/ outcome criteria	Adheres to diet and correct insulin dosage Adjusts dosage when activity is increased Glucose level 80–120 mg/L	Serious complications avoided Accepts prescribed diet Takes medication (correct dose and time) Glucose level 80–120 mg/dL

tacks of fatty-food intolerance. Patient with chronic cholecystitis has a history of several attacks of moderate severity and has usually learned to avoid fatty foods to decrease symptoms.

A. Pathophysiology: calculi from increased concentration of bile salts, pigments, or cholesterol due to metabolic or hemolytic disorders, biliary stasis → precipitation of salts into stones, or inflammation causing bile constituents to become altered.

B. Risk factors:
1. Women.
2. Obesity.
3. Pregnancy.
4. Cirrhosis of the liver.
5. Diabetes.

◆ **C. Assessment:**
1. *Subjective data*
   a. Pain:
      (1) Type—severe colic, radiating to back under the scapula and to the right shoulder.
      (2) Positive *Murphy's sign*—a sign of gallbladder disease consisting of pain on taking a deep breath when pressure is placed over the location of the gallbladder.
      (3) Location—right upper quadrant, epigastric area, flank (Figure 2.4).
      (4) Duration—spasm of duct attempting to dislodge stone lasts until dislodged or relieved by medication, or sometimes by vomiting.
   b. GI—anorexia, nausea, feeling of fullness, indigestion, intolerance of fatty foods.
2. *Objective data*
   a. GI—belching, vomiting, clay-colored stools.
   b. Vital signs—increased pulse, fever.
   c. Skin—chills, jaundice.
   d. Urine—dark amber.
   e. Lab data—*elevated:*
      (1) WBC.
      (2) Alkaline phosphatase.
      (3) Serum amylase, lipase.
      (4) AST[SGOT].
      (5) Bilirubin.

◆ **D. Analysis/nursing diagnosis:**
1. *Pain* related to obstruction of bile duct due to cholelithiasis.
2. *Altered nutrition, more than body requirements,* related to fatty foods.
3. *Altered nutrition, less than body requirements,* related to hesitancy to eat due to anorexia and nausea.
4. *Risk for fluid volume deficit* related to episodes of vomiting.
5. *Knowledge deficit* related to fat-free diet.

◆ **E. Nursing care plan/implementation:**
1. Nonsurgical interventions:
   a. Goal: *promote comfort.*
      (1) Medications as ordered: meperidine, antibiotics, antispasmodics, electrolytes.
      (2) *Avoid* morphine due to spasmodic effect.
      ▶ (3) NG tube to low suction.
      (4) *Diet:* fat free when able to tolerate food.
   b. Goal: *health teaching.*
      (1) Signs, symptoms, and complications of disease.
      (2) Fat-free diet.
      (3) Desired effects and side effects of prescribed medications.
      (4) Prepare for possible removal of gallbladder (cholecystectomy) if conservative treatment unsuccessful.
2. Surgical interventions:
   a. *Preoperative*—Goal: *prevent injury:* see I. Preoperative preparation, p. 102.
   b. *Postoperative*—Goal: *promote comfort* (see also III. Postoperative experience, p. 106).
      (1) Promote tube drainage.
         (a) NG tube to low suction.
         ▶ (b) *T-tube* to closed-gravity drainage, to preserve patency of edematous common duct and ensure bile drainage; usual amount 500–1000 mL/24 h; dark brown drainage.
         (c) Provide enough tubing to allow turning without tension.
         (d) Empty and record bile drainage q8h.
      (2) *Position:* low to semi-Fowler's to facilitate T-tube drainage.
      (3) Dressing: dry to protect skin (as bile excoriates skin).
      (4) Clamp T-tube as ordered.
         (a) Observe for abdominal distention, pain, nausea, chills, or fever.
         (b) Unclamp tube and notify MD if symptoms appear.
   c. Goal: *prevent complications.*
      (1) IV fluids with vitamins.
      (2) Cough, turn, and deep breathe (prone to respiratory complication because of high incision).
      (3) Early ambulation to prevent vascular complications and aid in expelling flatus.
      (4) Monitor for jaundice: skin, sclera, urine, stools.

■ **FIGURE 2.4**   **Possible causes of abdominal pain according to location. (From Caroline NL.** *Emergency Care in the Streets* **[5th ed]. Boston: Little, Brown, 1995. P 641.)**

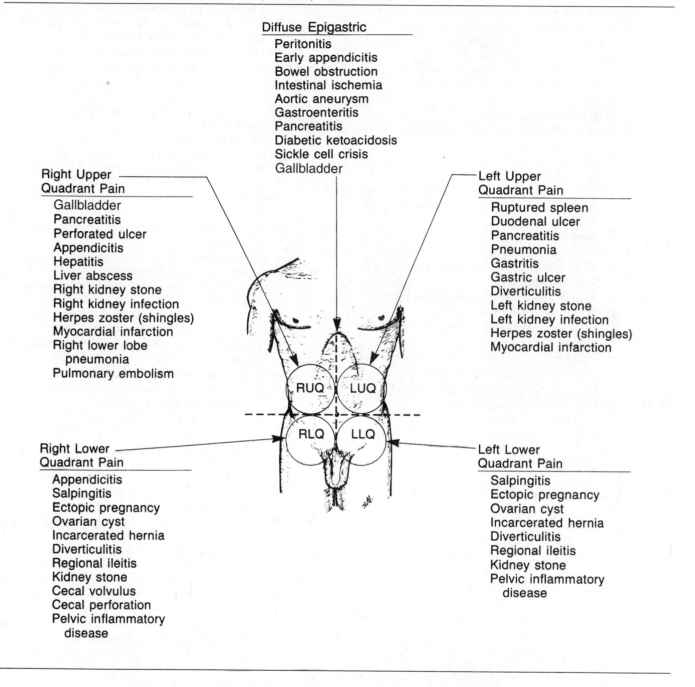

Diffuse Epigastric
Peritonitis
Early appendicitis
Bowel obstruction
Intestinal ischemia
Aortic aneurysm
Gastroenteritis
Pancreatitis
Diabetic ketoacidosis
Sickle cell crisis
Gallbladder

Right Upper
Quadrant Pain
Gallbladder
Pancreatitis
Perforated ulcer
Appendicitis
Hepatitis
Liver abscess
Right kidney stone
Right kidney infection
Herpes zoster (shingles)
Myocardial infarction
Right lower lobe
   pneumonia
Pulmonary embolism

Left Upper
Quadrant Pain
Ruptured spleen
Duodenal ulcer
Pancreatitis
Pneumonia
Gastritis
Gastric ulcer
Diverticulitis
Left kidney stone
Left kidney infection
Herpes zoster (shingles)
Myocardial infarction

Right Lower
Quadrant Pain
Appendicitis
Salpingitis
Ectopic pregnancy
Ovarian cyst
Incarcerated hernia
Diverticulitis
Regional ileitis
Kidney stone
Cecal volvulus
Cecal perforation
Pelvic inflammatory
   disease

Left Lower
Quadrant Pain
Salpingitis
Ectopic pregnancy
Ovarian cyst
Incarcerated hernia
Diverticulitis
Regional ileitis
Kidney stone
Pelvic inflammatory
   disease

RUQ   LUQ
RLQ   LLQ

    (5) Monitor for signs of hemorrhage, infection.
  d. Goal: *health teaching.*
    (1) Diet: fat free for 6 wk.
    (2) Signs of complications of food intolerance, pain, infection, hemorrhage.
◆ **F.** **Evaluation/outcome criteria:**
  1. No complications.
  2. Able to tolerate food.
  3. Plans follow-up care.
  4. Possible weight reduction.

❏ Elimination

Conditions Affecting Bowel Elimination

I. **Appendicitis:** obstruction of appendiceal lumen and subsequent bacterial invasion of appendiceal wall; acute emergency.
  A. **Pathophysiology:** when obstruction is partial or mild, inflammation begins in mucosa with slight appendiceal swelling, accompanied by periumbilical pain. As the inflammatory pro-

cess escalates and/or obstruction becomes more complete, appendix becomes more swollen, lumen fills with pus, mucosal ulceration begins. When inflammation extends to peritoneal surface, pain is referred to right lower abdominal quadrant. *Danger:* rigidity over the entire abdomen is usually indicative of ruptured appendix; patient then prone to peritonitis.

B. Risk factors:
1. Men more than women.
2. Most frequently seen between 10 and 30 yr old.

◆ **C. Assessment:**
1. *Subjective data*
   a. Pain: generalized, then right lower quadrant at McBurney's point, with rebound tenderness.
   b. Anorexia, nausea.
2. *Objective data*
   a. Vital signs: elevated temperature, shallow respirations.
   b. Either diarrhea or constipation.
   c. Vomiting, fetid breath odor.
   d. Splinting of abdominal muscles, flexion of knees onto abdomen.
   e. Lab data:
      (1) WBC elevated (>10,000).
      (2) Neutrophil count elevated (>75%).

◆ **D. Analysis/nursing diagnosis:**
1. *Pain* related to inflammation of appendix.
2. *Risk for trauma* related to ruptured appendix.
3. *Knowledge deficit* related to possible surgery.

◆ **E. Nursing care plan/implementation:**
1. Goal: *promote comfort.*
   a. *Preoperative:*
      (1) Explain procedures.
      (2) Assist with diagnostic workup.
   b. *Postoperative:*
      (1) Relieve pain related to surgical incision.
      (2) Prevent infection: wound care, dressing technique.
      (3) Prevent dehydration: IVs, I&O, fluids to solids by mouth as tolerated.
      (4) Promote ambulation to prevent postoperative complications.

◆ **F. Evaluation/outcome criteria:**
1. No infection.
2. Tolerates fluid; bowel sounds return.
3. Heals with no complications.

II. Hernia: protrusion of the intestine through a weak portion of the abdominal wall.
   A. Types:
   1. *Reducible:* visceral contents return to their normal position, either spontaneously or by manipulation.
   2. *Irreducible, or incarcerated:* contents cannot be returned to normal position.

3. *Strangulated:* blood supply to the structure within the hernia sac becomes occluded (usually a loop of bowel).
4. Most common hernias: umbilical, femoral, inguinal, incisional, and hiatus.

B. Pathophysiology: weakness in the wall may be either congenital or acquired. Herniation occurs when there is an increase in intraabdominal pressure from coughing, lifting, crying, straining, obesity, or pregnancy.

◆ **C. Assessment:**
1. *Subjective data*
   a. Pain, discomfort.
   b. History of feeling a lump.
2. *Objective data*
   a. Soft lump, especially when straining or coughing.
   b. Sometimes alteration in normal bowel pattern.
   c. Swelling.

◆ **D. Analysis/nursing diagnosis:**
1. *Activity intolerance* related to pain and discomfort.
2. *Risk for trauma* related to lack of circulation to affected area of bowel.
3. *Pain* related to protrusion of intestine into hernia sac.

◆ **E. Nursing care plan/implementation:**
1. Goal: *prevent postoperative complications.*
   a. Monitor bowel sounds.
   b. Prevent postoperative scrotal swelling with inguinal hernia by applying ice and support to scrotum.
2. Goal: *health teaching.*
   a. Prevent recurrence with correct body mechanics.
   b. Gradual increase in exercise.

◆ **F. Evaluation/outcome criteria:** healing occurs with no further hernia occurrence.

III. Diverticulosis: a *diverticulum* is a small pouch or sac composed of mucous membrane that has protruded through the muscular wall of the intestine. The presence of several of these is called *diverticulosis.* Inflammation of the diverticula is called *diverticulitis.*
   A. Pathophysiology: weakening in a localized area of muscular wall of the colon (especially the sigmoid colon), accompanied by increased intraluminal pressure.
   B. Risk factors:
   1. Diverticulosis
      a. Age: seldom before 35; 60% incidence in older adults.
      b. History of constipation.
      c. Diet history: low in vegetable fiber, high in carbohydrate.
   2. Diverticulitis: highest incidence between ages 50 and 60.

◆ **C. Assessment:**
1. *Subjective data:* pain: cramplike; left lower quadrant of abdomen.
2. *Objective data:*

a. Constipation or diarrhea, flatulence.
b. Fever.
c. Rectal bleeding.
🝪 d. Diagnostic procedures:
  (1) Palpation reveals tender colonic mass.
  (2) Barium enema (done only in absence of inflammation) reveals presence of diverticula.
  (3) Sigmoidoscopy.

◆ **D. Analysis/nursing diagnosis:**
  1. *Constipation* related to dietary intake.
  2. *Pain* related to inflammatory process of intestines.
  3. *Risk for fluid volume deficit,* related to episodes of diarrhea or bleeding.
  4. *Risk for injury* related to bleeding.
  5. *Knowledge deficit* related to prevention of constipation.

◆ **E. Nursing care plan/implementation:**
  1. Goal: *bowel rest during acute episodes.*
    a. *Diet:* soft, liquid.
    b. Fluids, IVs if oral intake not adequate.
    c. Pain medications, as ordered.
    d. Monitor stools for signs of bleeding.
  2. Goal: *promote normal bowel elimination.*
    a. *Diet:* bland, high in vegetable fiber if no inflammation.
      (1) *Include:* fruits, vegetables, wholegrain cereal, unprocessed bran.
      (2) *Avoid:* foods difficult to digest (corn, nuts).
    b. Bulk-forming agents as ordered: methylcellulose, psyllium.
    c. Monitor: abdominal distention, acute bowel symptoms.
  3. Goal: *health teaching.*
    a. Methods to avoid constipation.
    b. Foods to include/avoid in diet.
    c. Relaxation techniques.
    d. Signs and symptoms of complications of chronic inflammation, abscess, obstruction, fistulas, perforation, or hemorrhage.

◆ **F. Evaluation/outcome criteria:**
  1. Inflammation decreases.
  2. Bowel movements return to normal.
  3. Pain decreases.
  4. No complications of perforation, fistulas, or abscesses noted.

IV. Ulcerative colitis: inflammation of mucosa and submucosa of the distal colorectal area. Inflammation leads to ulceration with bleeding. Involved areas are continuous. Disease is characterized by remissions and exacerbations.
  A. Pathophysiology: specific physiologic response to emotional trauma. Edema and hyperemia of colonic mucous membrane → superficial bleeding with increased peristalsis, shallow ulcerations, abscesses; bowel wall thins and shortens and becomes at risk for perforation. Increased rate of flow of liquid il-

eal contents → decreased water absorption and diarrhea.
  B. Risk factors:
    1. Highest occurrence in young adults (20–40 yr of age).
    2. Genetic predisposition: higher in whites, Jews.
    3. Autoimmune response.
    4. Infections.
    5. More common in urban areas (upper-middle incomes and higher educational levels).
    6. May be influenced by smoking.
    7. Exacerbations often related to stressful event.

◆ **C. Assessment:**
  1. *Subjective data*
    a. Urgency to defecate, particularly when standing (tenesmus).
    b. Loss of appetite, nausea.
    c. Coliclike stomach pain.
    d. History of intolerance to dairy products.
    e. Emotional depression.
  2. *Objective data*
    a. *Diarrhea:* 10–20 stools/d; can be chronic or intermittent, episodic or continual; stools contain blood, mucus, and pus.
    b. Weight loss and malnutrition, dehydration.
    c. Fever.
    d. Lab data: *decreased:* RBC, potassium, sodium, calcium, bicarbonate related to excessive diarrhea.
    e. Lymphadenitis.
  🝪 f. Diagnostic tests:
      (1) Sigmoidoscopy for visualization of lesions.
      (2) Barium enema.

◆ **D. Analysis/nursing diagnosis:**
  1. *Diarrhea* related to increased flow rate of ileal contents.
  2. *Self-esteem disturbance* related to progression of disease and increased number and odor of stools.
  3. *Pain* related to inflammatory process.
  4. *Fluid volume deficit* related to frequent episodes of diarrhea.
  5. *Knowledge deficit* related to methods to control symptoms.
  6. *Social isolation* related to continual diarrhea episodes.

◆ **E. Nursing care plan/implementation:**
  1. Goal: *reduce psychological stress.*
    a. Provide quiet environment.
    b. Encourage verbalization of concerns.
  2. Goal: *relieve discomfort.*
    a. Administer medications as ordered.
      (1) Sedatives and tranquilizers to *promote rest and comfort.*
      (2) Absorbents, kaolin-pectin (Kaopectate).
      (3) Anticholinergics and antispasmotics *to relieve cramping and diarrhea,*

e.g., atropine sulfate, phenobarbital, atropine sulfate–diphenoxylate HCl (Lomotil).

 (4) Antimicrobial agents to *relieve bacterial overgrowth* in bowel and *limit secondary infection.*

 (5) Steroids to *relieve inflammation and produce remission.*

 (6) Potassium supplements to *relieve deficiencies.*

3. Goal: *health teaching.*

 a. *Diet:*

  (1) *Avoid:* coarse-residue, high-fiber foods, e.g., raw fruits and vegetables, whole milk, cold beverages (because of inflammation).

  (2) *Include:* bland, high-protein, high-vitamin, high-mineral, high-calorie foods.

  (3) Parenteral hyperalimentation for severely ill.

  (4) Force fluids by mouth.

4. Goal: *prepare for surgery if medical regimen unsuccessful.*

 a. Possible surgical procedures:

  (1) Permanent ileostomy.

  (2) Continent ileostomy (*Kock pouch*).

  (3) Total colectomy, anastomosis with rectum.

  (4) Total colectomy, anastomosis with anal sphincter.

◆ **F. Evaluation/outcome criteria:**

1. Fluid balance is obtained and maintained.
2. Alterations in life-style managed.
3. Stress-management techniques successful.
4. Complications such as fistulas, obstruction, perforation, and peritonitis are avoided.
5. Patient is prepared for surgery if medical regimen is unsuccessful or complications develop.

V. Crohn's disease: a chronic, progressive inflammatory disease usually affecting the terminal ileum.

 A. Pathophysiology: *one of two conditions called "inflammatory bowel disease"* (ulcerative colitis is the other) that affects all layers of the ileum and/or the colon, causing patchy shallow, longitudinal mucosal ulcers; possible correlation with autoimmune disease and adenocarcinoma of the bowel.

 B. Risk factors:

1. Age: 15–20, 55–60.
2. White, especially Jewish.
3. Familial predisposition.
4. Possible virus involvement.
5. Possible psychosomatic involvement.
6. Possible hormonal or dietary influences.

◆ **C. Assessment** (See IV. Ulcerative colitis, p. 131, for analysis/nursing diagnosis, nursing care plan/implementation, and evaluation/outcome criteria):

1. *Subjective data*

 a. Abdominal pain.

b. Anorexia.

c. Nausea.

d. Malaise.

e. History of isolated, intermittent, or recurrent attacks.

2. *Objective data*

 a. Diarrhea.

 b. Weight loss, vomiting.

 c. Fever, signs of infection.

 d. Fluid/electrolyte imbalances.

 e. Malnutrition, malabsorption.

 f. Occult blood in feces.

VI. Intestinal obstruction: blockage in movement of intestinal contents through small or large intestine.

 A. Pathophysiology:

1. *Mechanical causes*—physical impediments to passage of intestinal contents, e.g., adhesions, hernias, neoplasms, inflammatory bowel diseases, foreign bodies, fecal impactions, congenital or radiational strictures, intussusception, or volvulus.

2. *Paralytic causes*—passageway remains open, but peristalsis ceases, e.g., after abdominal surgery, abdominal trauma, hypokalemia, myocardial infarction, pneumonia, spinal injuries, peritonitis, or vascular insufficiency.

◆ **B. Assessment:**

1. *Subjective data:* pain related to

 a. *Proximal loop obstruction:* upper abdominal, sharp, cramping, intermittent pain.

 b. *Distal loop obstruction:* poorly localized, cramping pain.

2. *Objective data*

 a. Bowel sounds: initially loud, high pitched; then when smooth muscle atony occurs, bowel sound absent.

 b. Increased peristalsis above level of obstruction in attempt to move intestinal contents through the obstructed area.

 c. Obstipation (no passage of gas or stool through obstructed portion of bowel; no reabsorption of fluids).

 d. Distention.

 e. Vomiting:

  (1) *Proximal loop obstruction:* profuse nonfecal vomiting.

  (2) *Distal loop obstruction:* less frequent fecal-type vomiting.

 f. Urinary output: decreased.

 g. Temperature: elevated; tachycardia; hypotension → shock if untreated.

 h. Dehydration, hemoconcentration, hypovolemia.

 i. Lab data:

  (1) Leukocytosis.

  (2) *Decreased:* sodium (<138), potassium (<3.5).

  (3) *Increased:* pH (>7.45), bicarbonates (>26 mm), BUN (>18 mg/dL).

◆ **C. Analysis/nursing diagnosis:**
1. *Fluid volume deficit* related to vomiting.
2. *Pain* related to increased peristalsis above the level of obstruction.
3. *Altered nutrition, less than body requirements,* related to vomiting.
4. *Risk for trauma* related to potential perforation.

◆ **D. Nursing care plan/implementation:**
1. Goal: *obtain and maintain fluid balance.*
   ▶ a. Nursing care of patient with nasogastric tube (see Table 5.5):
      (1) *Miller-Abbott tube:* dual lumen, balloon inflated with air after insertion.
      (2) *Cantor tube:* has mercury in distal sac, which helps move tube to point of obstruction.
         Caution: do not tape either tube to face until tube reaches point of obstruction.
   b. Nothing by mouth, IV therapy, strict I&O.
   c. Take daily weights (early morning), monitor CVP for hydration status.
   d. Monitor abdominal girth for signs of distention and urinary output for signs of retention or shock.
2. Goal: *relieve pain and nausea.*
   a. Medications as ordered:
      (1) Analgesics, antiemetics.
      (2) If problem is paralytic: medical treatment includes neostigmine *to stimulate peristalsis.*
   b. Observe for bowel sounds, flatus (tape intestinal tube to face once peristalsis begins).
   c. Skin and frequent mouth care.
3. Goal: *prevent respiratory complications.*
   a. Encourage coughing and deep breathing.
   b. *Semi-Fowler's* or position of comfort.
4. Goal: *Postoperative nursing care* (if treated surgically): see III. Postoperative experience, p. 106.

◆ **E. Evaluation/outcome criteria:**
1. Fluid balance obtained and maintained.
2. Shock is prevented.
3. Obstruction is resolved.
4. Pain is decreased.
5. Fluids tolerated by mouth.
6. Complications such as perforation and peritonitis avoided.

VII. Fecal diversion—*stomas:* performed because of disease or trauma; may be temporary or permanent.
   A. Types (Table 2.25):
   1. *Temporary*—fecal stream rerouted to allow GI tract to heal or to provide outlet for stool when obstructed.
   2. *Permanent*—intestine cannot be reconnected. Rectum and anal sphincter removed (abdominal perineal resection).

Often performed for cancer of the colon and/or rectum.

◆ **B. Analysis/nursing diagnosis:**
1. *Bowel incontinence* related to lack of sphincter in newly formed stoma.
2. *Altered health maintenance* related to knowledge of ostomy care.
3. *Body image disturbance* related to stoma.
4. *Fluid volume deficit* related to increased output through stoma.

◆ **C. Nursing care plan/implementation:**
1. *Preoperative period*
   a. Goal: *prepare bowel for surgery.*
      (1) Administer neomycin as ordered to reduce colonic bacteria.
      (2) Administer cathartics, enemas as ordered to cleanse the bowel of feces.
      (3) Administer *low-residue or liquid diet* as ordered.
   b. Goal: *relieve anxiety and assist in adjustment to surgery.*
      (1) Provide accurate, brief, and reassuring explanations of procedures; allow time for questions.
      (2) Have enterostomal nurse visit to discuss ostomy management and placement of stoma appliance.
      (3) Offer opportunity for a visit with an Ostomy Association Visitor.
   c. Goal: *health teaching.*
      (1) Determine knowledge of surgery and potential impact.
      (2) Begin teaching regarding ostomy.
2. *Postoperative period*
   a. Goal: *maintain fluid balance.*
      (1) Monitor I&O as large volume of fluid is lost through stoma.
      (2) Administer IV fluids as ordered.
      (3) Monitor losses through NG tube.
   b. Goal: *prevent other postoperative complications.*
      (1) Monitor for signs of intestinal obstruction.
      (2) Maintain sterility when changing dressings; avoid fecal contamination of incision.
      (3) Observe appearance of stoma; rosy pink, raised.
   ◆ c. Goal: *initiate ostomy care.*
      (1) Protect skin around stoma: use commercial preparation to toughen skin and use protective barrier wafer (Stomahesive) or paste (Karaya or substitute) to keep drainage (which can cause excoriation) off the skin.
      (2) Keep skin around stoma clean and dry; empty appliance frequently. Check for drainage in appliance at least twice during each shift. If

■ **TABLE 2.25   Comparison of Ileostomy and Colostomy**

	Ileostomy	Colostomy
Procedure	Surgical formation of a fistula, or stoma, between the abdominal wall and *ileum;* continent ileostomy (*Kock* pouch) may be constructed	Surgical formation of an artificial opening between the surface of the abdominal wall and *colon* *Single barrel*—only one loop of bowel is opened to the abdominal surface *Double barrel*—two loops of bowel, a proximal and distal portion, are open to the abdominal wall; feces will be expelled from the proximal loop, mucus will be expelled from the distal loop; patient may expel some excreta from rectum as well
Reasons performed	Unresponsive ulcerative colitis: complications of ulcerative colitis, e.g., hemorrhage, carcinoma (suspected)	*Single barrel:* colon or rectal cancer *Double barrel:* relieve obstruction
Results	Permanent stoma	*Single barrel:* permanent stoma *Double barrel:* temporary stoma
Discharge	Green liquid, nonodorous	Consistency of feces dependent on diet and portion of the bowel used as the stoma; from brown odorous liquid to normal stool consistency
Nursing care	See VII. Fecal diversion, p. 133	See Tables 5.6 and 5.7, and VII. Fecal diversion, p. 133

drainage present (diarrhea-type stool):

(a) Unclip the bottom of bag.

(b) Drain into bedpan.

(c) Use a squeeze-type bottle filled with warm water to rinse inside of appliance.

(d) Clean off clamp, if soiled.

(e) Put a few drops of deodorant in appliance if not odorproof.

(f) Fasten bottom of appliance securely (fold bag over clamp 2–3 times before closing).

(g) Check for leakage under appliance every 2–4 h.

(3) Change appliance when drainage leaks around seal, or approximately every 2–3 d. Initially, size of stoma will be large due to edema. Pouch opening should be slightly larger than stoma so it will not constrict. Stoma will need to be measured for each change until swelling subsides to ensure appropriate fit.

(a) Gather equipment: gloves, skin prep packet, colostomy appliance measured to fit stoma properly (use stoma measuring guide), skin barrier, warm water and soap, face cloth/towel, plastic bag for disposal of old equipment.

(b) Remove old appliance carefully, pulling from area with least drainage to area with most drainage.

(c) Wash skin area (not stoma) with soap and water. Be careful not to irritate skin, put soap on stoma, irritate stoma; do not put anything dry onto stoma. Remember: bowel is very fragile; working near bowel increases peristalsis so that feces and flatulence may be expelled.

(d) Observe skin area for potential breakdown.

(e) Use packet of skin prep on the skin around the stoma. Do not put this solution onto stoma, as it will cause irritation. Allow skin prep solution to dry on skin before applying colostomy appliance.

(f) Apply skin barrier you have measured and cut to size.

(g) Put appliance on so that bottom of appliance is easily accessible for emptying (e.g., if patient is *out* of bed most of the time, put the bottom facing the feet; if patient is *in* bed most of the time, have bottom face the side). Picture frame the adhesive portion of the appliance with 1-in. tape.

(h) Put a few drops of deodorant in appliance if not odorproof.

(i) Use clamp to fasten bottom of appliance.

(j) Talk to patient (or communicate in best way possible during and after procedure). THIS

IS A VERY DIFFICULT AL-
TERATION IN BODY IMAGE.
    (k) Good handwashing technique.
    (4) Use deodorizing drops in appliance
    and provide adequate room ventila-
    tion to decrease odors. *Caution:* de-
    odorizing drops must be safe for
    mucous membranes. No pinholes in
    pouch.
    (5) If continent ileostomy, a *Kock
    pouch,* has been constructed, the
    patient does not have to wear an
    external pouch. The stool is stored
    intraabdominally. The patient
    drains the pouch several times
    daily, when there is a feeling of
    fullness, using a catheter. The
    stoma is flat and on the right side
    of the abdomen.
  d. Goal: *promote psychological comfort.*
    (1) Support patient and family—ac-
    cept feelings and behavior.
    (2) Recognize that such a procedure
    may initiate the grieving process.
  e. Goal: *health teaching.*
    (1) Self-management skills related to
    ostomy appliance, skin care, and ir-
    rigation, if indicated (Table 2.26).
    (2) *Diet:* adjustments to control charac-
    ter of feces; avoid foods that in-
    crease flatulence.
    (3) Signs of complications of infection,
    obstruction, or electrolyte imbal-
    ance.
    (4) Community referral for follow-up
    care.
◆ **D. Evaluation/outcome criteria:**
    1. Demonstrates self-care skill for indepen-
    dent living.
    2. Makes dietary adjustments.
    3. Ostomy functions well.
    4. Adjusts to alteration in bowel elimination
    pattern.
VIII. Hemorrhoids: enlarged vein in mucous mem-
    brane of rectum.

■ **TABLE 2.26 Colostomy Irrigation**

1. Assemble all equipment for irrigation and appliance change.
2. Remove and discard old pouch.
3. Clean the peristomal skin.
4. Apply the irrigating sleeve; place in toilet or bedpan.
5. Fill container with 500–1000 mL. of warm water, *never* more
   than 1000 mL. Clear air from tubing. Insert lubricated tubing
   2–4 in. into stoma. Do not force. Hold container about 18 in.
   above stoma. Infuse gently over 7–10 min.
6. Allow stool to empty into toilet. Evacuation usually occurs in
   20–25 min.
7. If no return after irrigation, ambulate, gently massage
   abdomen, or give patient a warm drink.
8. Once complete, remove the sleeve, and follow guidelines for
   applying appliance.

A. Pathophysiology: venous congestion and
    interference with venous return from hem-
    orrhoidal veins → increase in pelvic pres-
    sure, swelling, and distortion.
B. Risk factors:
    1. Straining to expel constipated stool.
    2. Pregnancy.
    3. Intraabdominal or pelvic masses.
    4. Interference with portal circulation.
    5. Prolonged standing or sitting.
    6. History of low-fiber, high-carbohydrate
    diet, which contributes to constipation.
    7. Family history of hemorrhoids.
    8. Enlarged prostate.
◆ **C. Assessment:**
    1. *Subjective data:* discomfort, anal pruri-
    tus, pain.
    2. *Objective data*
      a. Bleeding, especially on defecation.
      b. Narrowing of stool.
      c. Grapelike clusters around anus (pink,
      red, or blue).
      d. Diagnosis:
        (1) Visualization for *external* hemor-
        rhoids.
        (2) Digital exam or proctoscopy for *in-
        ternal* hemorrhoids.
◆ **D. Analysis/nursing diagnosis:**
    1. *Pain* related to defecation.
    2. *Constipation* related to dietary habits
    and pain at time of defecation.
    3. *Knowledge deficit* related to foods to pre-
    vent constipation.
◆ **E. Nursing care plan/implementation:**
    1. Goal: *reduce anal discomfort.*
      a. Sitz baths, as ordered; perineal care to
      prevent infection.
      b. Hot or cold compresses as ordered to
      reduce inflammation and pruritus.
      c. Topical medications as ordered:
        (1) Anti-inflammatory: hydrocortisone
        cream.
        (2) Astringents: witch hazel–impreg-
        nated pads.
        (3) Topical anesthetics: dibucaine
        (Nupercaine).
    2. Goal: *prevent complications related to
    surgery.*
      a. Encourage postoperative ambulation.
      b. Pain relief until packing removed.
      c. Monitor for: bleeding, infection, pul-
      monary emboli, phlebitis.
      d. Facilitate bowel evacuation: stool soft-
      eners, laxatives, suppositories, oil ene-
      mas as ordered.
      e. Monitor for syncope/vertigo during
      first postoperative bowel movement.
      f. *Diet:*
        (1) Low residue (postoperative)—un-
        til healing has begun.
        (2) High fiber to prevent constipation
        after healing.

g. Increase fluid intake.

3. Goal: *health teaching*—methods to avoid constipation.

◆ **F. Evaluation/outcome criteria:**
1. No complications.
2. Patient has bowel movement.
3. Incorporates knowledge of correct foods into life-style.

Conditions Affecting Urinary Elimination

I. **Pyelonephritis (PN):** acute or chronic inflammation due to bacterial infection of the parenchyma and renal pelvis; 95% of cases caused by gram-negative enteric bacilli (*Escherichia coli*); occurs more frequently in young women and older men.

 A. **Pathophysiology:** inflammation of renal medulla or lining of the renal pelvis → nephron destruction; hypertrophy of nephrons needed to maintain urine output → impaired sodium reabsorption (salt wasting); inability to concentrate urine; progressive renal failure; hypertension (two-thirds of all cases).

 B. **Risk factors:**
 1. Obstruction.
 2. Hypertension.
 3. Hypokalemia.
 4. Diabetes mellitus.
 5. Pregnancy.
 6. Catheterization.

◆ C. **Assessment:**
 1. *Subjective data*
 a. *Pain:* flank—one or both sides; back; dysuria; headache.
 b. *Loss of appetite;* weight loss.
 c. *Night sweats;* chills.
 d. *Urination:* frequency, urgency.
 2. *Objective data*
 a. Fever.
 b. Lab data:
 (1) *Blood*—polymorphonuclear leukocytosis >11,000.
 (2) *Urine*—leukocytosis, hematuria, white blood cell casts, proteinuria (<3 g in 24 h), positive cultures; specific gravity—normal or increased with acute PN, decreased with chronic PN; cloudy; foul smelling.
 c. Intravenous pyelogram (IVP)—may manifest structural changes.

◆ D. **Analysis/nursing diagnosis:**
 1. *Altered urinary elimination* related to kidney disease.
 2. *Pain* related to dysuria and kidney damage.
 3. *Altered nutrition, less than body requirements,* related to impaired sodium reabsorption and protein loss.

4. *Risk for fluid volume* excess related to renal failure.

◆ E. **Nursing care plan/implementation:**
 1. Goal: *combat infection, prevent recurrence, alleviate symptoms.*
 a. Medications:
 (1) *Antibiotics, urinary antiseptics* and/or sulfonamides appropriate for causative organism; also reduce pain.
 (2) *Analgesics* for pain—phenazopyridine (Pyridium); stronger if calculi present.
 (3) *Antipyretics* for fever—acetaminophen (Tylenol).
 b. *Fluids:* 1500–2000 mL/d to flush kidneys, relieve dysuria, reduce fever, prevent dehydration.
 c. Observe hydration status: I&O (output minimum 1500 mL/24 h); daily weight; urine—check each voiding for protein, blood, specific gravity; vital signs q4h to monitor for hypertension, tachycardia; skin turgor.
 d. Hygiene: meticulous perineal care; cleanse with soap and water; antimicrobial ointment may be used around urinary meatus with retention catheter.
 e. Cooling measures: tepid sponging.
 f. *Diet:* sufficient calories and protein to prevent malnutrition; sodium supplement as ordered.
 2. Goal: *promote physical and emotional rest.*
 a. Activity: bedrest or as tolerated—depends on whether anemia or fever is present; encourage activities of daily living as tolerated.
 b. Emotional support: encourage expression of fears (possible renal failure, dialysis); provide diversional activities; include family in care; answer questions.
 3. Goal: *health teaching.*
 a. Medications: take regularly to maintain blood level; side effects.
 b. Personal care: perineal hygiene; avoid urethral contamination; avoid tub baths.
 c. Possible recurrence with pregnancy.
 d. Monitoring daily weight.

◆ F. **Evaluation/outcome criteria:**
 1. Normal renal function (minimum 1500 mL urine/24 h).
 2. Blood pressure within normal range.
 3. No recurrence of symptoms.

II. **Acute glomerulonephritis:** see Unit 8, p. 529.
III. **Acute renal failure:** broadly defined as rapid onset of oliguria accompanied by a rising BUN and serum creatinine; usually reversible.

 A. **Pathophysiology:** acute renal ischemia → tubular necrosis → decreased urine output. *Oliguric phase* (<400 mL/24 h)—waste products are retained → metabolic acidosis → water and electrolyte imbalances → anemia. *Recovery phase*—diuresis → dilute urine → rapid depletion of sodium, chloride, and water → dehydration.

B. Types and risk factors:

1. *Prerenal*—due to factors outside of kidney; usually circulatory collapse—hemorrhage, severe dehydration, myocardial infarction, shock, vascular obstruction.

2. *Intrinsic renal*—parenchymal disease from ischemia or nephrotoxic damage; nephrotoxic agents—poisons, such as carbon tetrachloride; heavy metals (arsenic, mercury); antibiotics (kanamycin SO_4, neomycin SO_4); incompatible blood transfusion; alcohol myopathies; acute renal disease—acute glomerulonephritis, acute pyelonephritis.

3. *Postrenal*—obstruction in collecting system; renal or bladder calculi; tumors of bladder, prostate, or renal pelvis; gynecologic or urologic surgery in which ureters are accidentally ligated.

◆ **C. Assessment:**

1. *Subjective data*
   a. Sudden decrease or cessation of urine output (<400 mL/24 h).
   b. Anorexia, nausea, vomiting from azotemia.
   c. Sudden weight gain from fluid accumulation.
   d. Headache.

2. *Objective data*
   a. Vital signs (vary according to cause and severity):
      (1) *BP*—usually elevated.
      (2) *Pulse*—tachycardia, irregularities.
      (3) *Respirations*—increased rate, depth, crackles.
   b. Neurologic: decreasing mentation, unresponsive to verbal or painful stimuli, psychoses, convulsions.
   c. Halitosis; cracked mucous membranes.
   d. Skin: dry, rashes, purpura, itchy, pale.
   e. Lab data:
      (1) Blood: *increased*—potassium, BUN, creatinine, WBC; *decreased*—pH, bicarbonate, hematocrit, hemoglobin.
      (2) Urine: *decreased*—volume, specific gravity (↓ 1.010); *increased*—protein, casts, red and white blood cells, sodium.

◆ **D. Analysis/nursing diagnosis:**

1. *Altered urinary elimination* related to kidney malfunction.
2. *Fluid volume excess* related to decreased urine output.
3. *Altered nutrition, less than body requirements,* related to anorexia.
4. *Altered oral mucous membrane* related to stomatitis.

5. *Altered thought processes* related to uremia.

◆ **E. Nursing care plan/implementation:**

1. Goal: *maintain fluid and electrolyte balance and nutrition.*
   a. Monitor: daily weight (should not vary more than ±1 lb); vital signs—include CVP
      blood chemistries (BUN 6–20 mg/dL; creatinine 0.6–1.5 mg/dL).
   b. *Fluids:* IV as ordered; blood: plasma, packed cells, electrolyte solutions to replace losses; restricted to 400 mL/24 h if hypertension present or during oliguric phase to prevent fluid overload.
   c. *Diet,* as tolerated: high carbohydrate, low protein, may be low potassium and low sodium; hypertonic glucose (TPN) if oral feedings not tolerated; intravenous L-amino acids and glucose.
   d. Control hyperkalemia: infusions of hypertonic glucose and insulin to force potassium into cells; calcium gluconate (IV) to reduce myocardial irritability from K^+; sodium bicarbonate (IV) to correct acidosis; polystyrene sodium sulfonate (Kayexalate) or other exchange resins, orally or rectally (enema), to remove excess K^+; peritoneal or hemodialysis.
   e. Medications—*diuretics* (mannitol, furosemide [Lasix]).

2. Goal: *use assessment and comfort measures to reduce occurrence of complications.*
   a. Respiratory: monitor rate, depth, breath sounds, arterial blood gases; encourage deep breathing, coughing, turning; use incentive spirometer or nebulizer as indicated.
   b. Frequent oral care to prevent stomatitis.
   c. Observe for signs of:
      (1) *Infection*—elevated temperature, localized redness, swelling, heat, or drainage.
      (2) *Bleeding*—stools, gums, venipuncture sites.

3. Goal: *maintain continual emotional support.*
   a. Same caregivers, consistency in procedures.
   b. Give opportunities to express concerns, fears.
   c. Allow family interactions.

4. Goal: *health teaching.*
   a. Preparation for dialysis (indications: uremia, uncontrolled hyperkalemia, or acidosis).
   b. Dietary restrictions: low sodium, fluid restriction.
   c. Disease process; treatment regimen.

Adult

◆ **F. Evaluation/outcome criteria:**
1. Return of kidney function—normal creatinine level (<1.5 mg/dL), urine output.
2. Resumes normal life pattern (about 3 mo after onset).

IV. Chronic renal failure: as a result of progressive destruction of kidney tissue, the kidneys are no longer able to maintain their homeostatic functions; considered irreversible.

A. Pathophysiology: destruction of glomeruli → reduced glomerular filtration rate → retention of metabolic waste products; decreased urine output; severe fluid, electrolyte, acid-base imbalances → uremia. Clinical picture includes:
1. Ammonia in skin and alimentary tract by bacterial interaction with urea → inflammation of mucous membranes.
2. Retention of phosphate → decreased serum calcium → muscle spasms, tetany, and increased parathormone release → demineralization of bone.
3. Failure of tubular mechanisms to regulate blood bicarbonate → metabolic acidosis → hyperventilation.
4. Urea osmotic diuresis → flushing effect on tubules → decreased reabsorption of sodium → sodium depletion.
5. Waste product retention → depressed bone marrow function → decreased circulating RBCs → renal tissue hypoxia → decreased erythropoietin production → further depression of bone marrow → anemia.

B. Risk factors:
1. Polycystic kidney disease.
2. Chronic glomerulonephritis.
3. Chronic urinary obstruction, ureteral stricture, calculi, neoplasms.
4. Chronic pyelonephritis.
5. Severe hypertension.
6. Congenital or acquired renal artery stenosis.
7. Systemic lupus erythematosus.

◆ **C. Assessment:**
1. *Subjective data:* excessive fatigue, weakness.
2. *Objective data*
   a. Skin: bronze-colored, uremic frost.
   b. Ammonia breath.
   c. Also see III. Acute renal failure, p. 136; symptoms gradual in onset.

◆ **D. Analysis/nursing diagnosis:**
1. In addition to the following, see III. Acute renal failure, p. 136.
2. *Fatigue* related to severe anemia.
3. *Risk for impaired skin integrity* related to pruritus.
4. *Ineffective individual coping* related to chronic illness.
5. *Body image disturbance* related to need for dialysis.
6. *Noncompliance* related to denial of illness.

◆ **E. Nursing care plan/implementation:**
1. Goal: *maintain fluid/electrolyte balance and nutrition.* (Also see III. Acute renal failure, p. 136.)
   a. *Diet:* low sodium; foods high in calcium, vitamin B complex, vitamins C and D, and iron (to reduce edema, replace deficits, and promote absorption of nutrients).
   b. Medications: calcium carbonate; supplemental vitamins if deficient; electrolyte modifier (aluminum hydroxide [Alu-cap., Amphogel]).
   c. I&O; intake should be no more than 600–800 mL more than previous day's output to prevent fluid retention.
2. Goal: *employ comfort measures that reduce distress and support physical function.*
   a. Activity: bedrest; facilitate ventilation; turn, cough, deep breathe q2h; ROM—active and passive, to prevent thrombi.
   b. Hygiene: mouth care to prevent stomatitis and reduce discomfort from mouth ulcers; perineal care.
   c. Skin care: soothing lotions to reduce pruritus.
   d. Encourage communication of concerns.
3. Goal: *health teaching.*
   a. Dietary restrictions: no added salt when cooking; change cooking water in vegetables during process to decrease potassium; read food labels to avoid Na^+ and K^+.
   b. Importance of daily weight: same scale, time, clothing.
   c. Prepare for dialysis; transplantation.

F. Evaluation/outcome criteria:
1. Acceptance of chronic illness (no indication of indiscretions, destructive behavior, suicidal tendency).
2. Compliance with dietary restriction—no signs of protein excess (e.g., nausea, vomiting) or fluid/sodium excess (e.g., edema, weight gain).

V. Dialysis: diffusion of solute through a semipermeable membrane that separates two solutions; direction of diffusion depends on concentration of solute in each solution; rate and efficiency depend on concentration gradient, temperature of solution, pore size of membrane, and molecular size; two methods available (Table 2.27).

A. Indications: acute poisonings; acute or chronic renal failure; hepatic coma; metabolic acidosis; extensive burns with azotemia.

B. Goals
1. *Reduce level of nitrogenous waste.*
2. *Correct acidosis, reverse electrolyte imbalances, remove excess fluid.*

C. *Hemodialysis:* circulation of patient's blood through a compartment formed of a semipermeable membrane (cellophane or cuprophane) surrounded by dialysate fluid.

■ **TABLE 2.27 Comparison of Hemodialysis and Peritoneal Dialysis**

	Hemodialysis	**Peritoneal Dialysis**
Process	Rapid—uses either external AV shunt (acute renal failure) or internal AV fistula (chronic renal failure); typical treatment is 3–4 h 3 d/wk; also used for barbiturate overdoses to remove toxic agent quickly	Intermittent—up to 24–72 h for hospitalized patients; outpatients 10–14 h 3–4 times a week; dwell time 30–45 min for manual dialysis or 10–20 min for automatic cycler; either rigid stylet catheter or surgically inserted soft catheter; advantage for patients who cannot tolerate rapid fluid and electrolyte changes Continuous—four cycles in 24 h; dwell time is 4–5 h during the day and 8 h overnight; no need for machinery, electricity, or water source; surgically inserted soft catheter; closely resembles normal renal function
Vascular access	Required	Not necessary; therefore suitable for patients with vascular problems
Heparinization	Required; systemic or regional	Little or no heparin necessary; therefore suitable for patients with bleeding problems
Complications (other than fluid and electrolyte imbalances, which are common to all)	Dialysis disequilibrium syndrome (preventable) Mechanical dysfunctions of dialyzer	Peritonitis Hypoalbuminemia Bowel or bladder perforation Plugged or dislodged catheter

1. Types of dialyzers
   a. Coil type.
   b. Parallel plate.
   c. Capillary.
2. Types of venous access for hemodialysis
   a. External shunt (Figure 2.5).
      (1) Cannula is placed in a large vein and a large artery that approximate each other.
      (2) External shunts, which provide easy and painless access to bloodstream, are prone to infection and clotting and cause erosion of the skin around the insertion area.
         (a) Daily cleansing and application of a sterile dressing.
         (b) Prevention of physical trauma and avoidance of some activities, such as swimming.
   b. Arteriovenous fistulas (Figure 2.6).
      (1) Large artery and vein are sewn together (anastomosed) below the surface of the skin.
      (2) Purpose is to create one blood vessel for withdrawing and returning blood.
      (3) *Advantages:* greater activity range than AV shunt and no protective asepsis.
      (4) *Disadvantage:* necessity of two venipunctures with each dialysis.
3. Complications during hemodialysis
   a. *Disequilibrium syndrome*—rapid removal of urea from blood → reverse osmosis, with water moving into brain cells → cerebral edema → possible headache, nausea, vomiting, confusion, and convulsions; usually occurs with initial dialysis

   treatments; shorter dialysis time and slower rate minimizes.
   b. *Hypotension*—results from excessive ultrafiltration or excessive antihypertensive medications.
   c. *Hypertension*—results from volume overload (water and/or sodium), causing disequilibrium syndrome or anxiety.
   d. *Transfusion reactions* (see Unit 5).
   e. *Arrhythmias*—due to hypotension, fluid overload, or rapid removal of potassium.
   f. *Psychological problems*
      (1) Patients react in varying ways to dependence on hemodialysis.
      (2) Nurse needs to identify patient reactions and defense mechanisms and to employ supportive behaviors, i.e., include patient in care; continual repetition and reinforcement; do not interpret patient's behavior—for example, do not say, "You're being hostile" or "You're acting like a child"; answer questions honestly regarding quality and length of life with dialysis and/or transplantation; encourage independence as much as possible.
D. *Intermittent peritoneal dialysis:* involves introduction of a dialysate solution into the abdomen, where the peritoneum acts as the semipermeable membrane between the solution and blood in abdominal vessels. *Procedures:*
1. Area around umbilicus is prepared, anesthetized with local anesthetic, and a catheter is inserted into the peritoneal cavity through a trocar; the catheter is then sutured into place to prevent displacement.

■ **FIGURE 2.5   AV shunt (cannulae). (Adapted and used by permission of Ann Holmes, RN, Head Nurse, West Contra Costa Dialysis Clinic, San Pablo, CA.)**

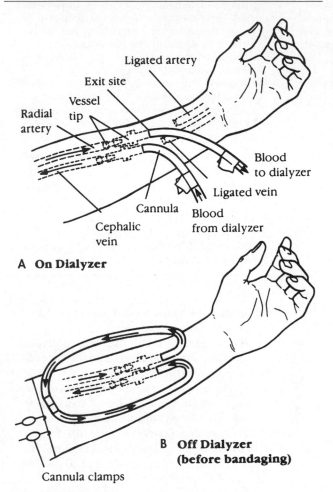

A   On Dialyzer

B   Off Dialyzer (before bandaging)

■ **FIGURE 2.6   AV fistula. (Adapted and used by permission of Ann Holmes, RN, Head Nurse, West Contra Costa Dialysis Clinic, San Pablo, CA.)**

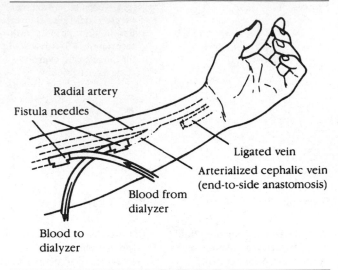

2. Warmed dialysate is then allowed to flow into the peritoneal cavity. Inflow time: 5–10 min; 2 liters of solution are used in each cycle in the adult; solutions contain glucose, Na$^+$, Ca^{2+}, Mg^{2+}, K$^+$, Cl$^-$, and lactate or acetate.

3. When solution bottle is empty, dwell time (exchange time) begins. *Dwell time:* 10–20 min with automatic, 30–45 min with manual; processes of diffusion, osmosis, and filtration begin to move waste products from bloodstream into peritoneal cavity.

4. Draining of the dialysate begins with the unclamping of the outflow clamp. *Outflow time:* usually 20 min; returns <2 liters usually result from incomplete peritoneal emptying; turn side to side to increase return; 30 cycles in 24 h is ideal.

E. *Continuous ambulatory peritoneal dialysis* (CAPD): functions on the same principles as peritoneal dialysis, yet allows greater freedom

and independence for dialysis patients. *Procedure:*

1. Dialysis solution is infused into peritoneum three times daily and once prior to bedtime.

2. *Dwell time*—5 h for each daily exchange, and overnight for the fourth (8 h).

3. Indwelling peritoneal catheter is connected to solution bag at all times—serves to fill and drain peritoneum; concealed in cloth pouch, strapped to the body during dwell time; patient can move about doing usual activities.

VI. **Kidney transplantation:** placement of a donor kidney (from sibling, parent, cadaver) into the iliac fossa of a recipient and the anastomosis of its ureter to the bladder of the recipient; indicated in end-stage renal disease.

A. Criteria for recipient: irreversible kidney function; under 55 yr of age; patent and functional lower urinary tract; and good surgical risk, free of serious cardiovascular complications. *Contraindicated* in metastatic carcinoma and oxalosis (excessive oxalate in urine).

B. Donor selection
   1. Sibling or parent—survival rate of kidney is greater; preferred for transplantation.
   2. Cadaver—greater rate of rejection following transplantation, although majority of transplantations are with cadaver kidneys.

C. Bilateral nephrectomy: necessary for patients with rapidly progressive glomerulonephritis, malignant hypertension, or chronic kidney infections; prevents complications in transplanted kidney (see VII. Nephrectomy for nursing care, p. 142).

◆ D. **Analysis/nursing diagnosis:**

1. *Altered urinary elimination* related to kidney failure.
2. *Fear* related to potential transplant rejection.
3. *Risk for infection* related to immunosuppression.
4. *Body image disturbance* related to immunosuppression.

◆ **E. Nursing care plan/implementation:**
1. *Preoperative*
   a. Goal: *promote physical and emotional adjustment.*
      (1) Informed consent.
      (2) Lab work completed—histocompatibility, CBC, urinalysis, blood type and crossmatch.
      (3) Skin preparation.
   b. Goal: *encourage expression of feelings:* origin of donor, fear of complications, rejection.
   c. Goal: *minimize risk of organ rejection:* give medications: begin immunosuppression (azathioprine, corticosteroids, cyclosporine); anti-infectives if ordered.
   d. Goal: *health teaching.*
      (1) Nature of surgery; placement of kidney.
      (2) Postoperative expectations: deep breathing, coughing, turning, early ambulation; reverse isolation.
      (3) Medications: immunosuppressive therapy: purpose, effect.
2. *Postoperative*
   a. Goal: *promote uncomplicated recovery of recipient.*
      (1) Vital signs; CVP; I&O—may see large amounts urine (3–20 L) in early postoperative period from sodium diuresis, or kidney may not work for a week or more and dialysis will be needed within 24–48 h.
      ▶ (2) *Isolation:* strict reverse isolation with immunosuppression; wear face mask when out of room.
      (3) *Position:* back to unoperative side; semi-Fowler's to promote gas exchange.
      ▶ (4) Indwelling catheter care: characteristics of urine—report gross hematuria, heavy sediment; clots; perineal care.
      (5) Activity: ambulate 24 h after surgery; avoid prolonged sitting.
      (6) *Weigh daily.*
      ▶ (7) Medications: immunosuppressives; analgesics as ordered.
      (8) Drains: irrigate *only* on physician order; *meticulous* catheter care.
      (9) *Diet:* regular; liberal amounts of protein; *restrict* fluids, sodium, potassium *only if* oliguric.

   b. Goal: *observe for signs of rejection*—most dangerous complication. Three classifications:
      (1) Hyperacute—occurs with 5–10 min up to 48 h after transplantation (RARE).
      (2) Acute—occurs within 6 wk; most common 3 mo.
      (3) Chronic—occurs several months to years.
   Assessment:
      (a) *Subjective data*
          (i) Lethargy, anorexia.
          (ii) Tenderness over graft site.
      (b) *Objective data*
          (i) Lab data: Urine: *decreased*—output, creatinine clearance, sodium; *increased*—protein. Blood: *increased*—BUN, creatinine.
          (ii) Rapid weight gain.
          (iii) Vital signs: BP, temperature—elevated.
   c. Goal: *Maintain immunosuppressive therapy.*
      (1) Azathioprine (Imuran)—an antimetabolite that interferes with cellular division. *Side effects:*
          (a) Gastrointestinal bleeding (give PO form with food).
          (b) Bone marrow depression; leukopenia; anemia.
          (c) Development of malignant neoplasms.
          (d) Infection.
          (e) Liver damage.
      (2) Prednisone—believed to affect lymphocyte production by inhibiting nucleic acid synthesis: anti-inflammatory action helps prevent tissue damage if rejection occurs. *Side effects:*
          (a) Stress ulcer with bleeding (give with food).
          (b) Decreased glucose tolerance (hyperglycemia).
          (c) Muscle weakness.
          (d) Osteoporosis.
          (e) Moon facies.
          (f) Acne and striae.
          (g) Depression and hallucinations.
      (3) Cyclosporine (cyclosporin A)—a polypeptide antibiotic used to prevent rejection of kidney, liver, or heart allografts; PO dose given with room temperature chocolate milk or OJ in a glass dispenser. *Side effects:*
          (a) Nephrotoxicity (increased BUN, creatinine).
          (b) Hypertension.
          (c) Tremor.
          (d) Hirsutism, gingival hyperplasia.

(e) *GI*—nausea, vomiting, anorexia, diarrhea, abdominal pain.

(f) *Infections*—pneumonia, septicemia, abscesses, wound.

(4) Additional drugs may include cyclophosphamide (Cytoxan), methylprednisolone, antilymphocyte globulin (ALG), and anti-T-lymphocyte monoclonal antibody (OKT3).

d. Goal: *health teaching.*
  (1) Signs of rejection (see goal b. above).
  (2) Drugs: side effects of immunosuppression (see goal c. above).
  (3) Self-care activities: temperature, blood pressure, I&O, urine specimen collection.
  (4) Avoidance of infection.
  (5) See also goals of care, III. Postoperative experience, p. 107.

◆ **F. Evaluation/outcome criteria:**
  1. No signs of rejection (e.g., weight gain, oliguria).
  2. No depression.
  3. Patient resumes role responsibilities.

VII. Nephrectomy: removal of kidney through flank, retroperitoneal, abdominal, thoracic, or thoracic-abdominal approach; indicated with malignant tumors, severe trauma, or under certain conditions before renal transplantation (see VI. Kidney transplantation, p. 140).

◆ **A. Analysis/nursing diagnosis:**
  1. *Pain* related to surgical incision.
  2. *Risk for infection* related to wound contamination.
  3. *Risk for aspiration* related to vomiting.
  4. *Constipation* related to paralytic ileus.
  5. *Anxiety* related to possible loss of function in remaining kidney.
  6. *Dysfunctional grieving* related to perceived loss.

◆ **B. Nursing care plan/implementation:**
  1. *Preoperative:* Goal: *optimize physical and psychological functioning* (see I. Preoperative preparation, p. 102).
  2. *Postoperative:* Goal: *promote comfort and prevent complications.*
    a. Observe for signs of:
      (1) *Paralytic ileus*—abdominal distention, absent bowel sounds, vomiting (common complication following renal surgery).
      (2) *Hemorrhage.*
    b. Fluid balance: daily weight—maintain within 2% of preoperative level.

◆ **C. Evaluation/outcome criteria:**
  1. No complications (e.g., hemorrhage, paralytic ileus, wound infection).
  2. Acceptance of loss of kidney.

VIII. Renal calculi (urolithiasis): formation of calculi (stones) in renal calyces or pelvis that pass to lower regions of urinary tract—ureters, bladder, or urethra; occurs after age 30, with greatest incidence in *men,* particularly over age 50.

A. Pathophysiology: organic crystals form (75% of stones contain calcium) → obstruction, infection; increased backward pressure in kidney → hydronephrosis → atrophy, fibrosis of renal tubules.

B. Risk factors:
  1. Changes in urine pH and concentration from readily precipitable, crystalline materials—sulfonamides, uric acid, calcium salts.
  2. Urinary tract infection.
  3. Indwelling Foley catheter.
  4. Vitamin A deficiency.

◆ **C. Assessment** (depends on size, shape, location of stone):
  1. *Subjective data*
    a. Pain: occasional, dull, in loin or back when stones are in calyces or renal pelvis; *excruciating* in flank area (renal colic), radiating to groin when stones are ureteral.
    b. Nausea associated with pain.
  2. *Objective data*
    a. Pallor, sweating, syncope, shock, and vomiting due to pain.
    b. Palpable kidney mass with hydronephrosis.
    c. Fever and pyuria with infection.
    d. Lab data:
      (1) Urinalysis: abnormal—pH (acidic or alkaline); RBCs (injury); WBCs (infection); increased—specific gravity; casts; crystals; other organic substances, depending on type of stone (i.e., uric acid, calcium); positive culture.
      (2) Blood: *increased* calcium, phosphorus, total protein, alkaline phosphatase, creatinine, uric acid, BUN.
    e. Diagnostic tests:
      (1) IVP: reveals nonopaque stones, degree of obstruction.
      (2) X ray; radiopaque stones seen.
      (3) Ultrasound may also be used.

◆ **D. Analysis/nursing diagnosis:**
  1. *Pain* related to passage of stone.
  2. *Altered urinary elimination* related to potential obstruction.
  3. *Urinary retention* related to obstruction of urethra.

◆ **E. Nursing care plan/implementation:**
  1. Goal: *reduce pain and prevent complications.*
    a. Medication: *narcotics, antiemetics, antibiotics.*
    b. Fluids: 3–4 L/d; IVs if nauseated, vomiting.

c. Activity: ambulate to promote passage of stone, except bedrest during acute attack (colic).

d. Reduce spasms: warm soaks to affected flank.

e. Observe for signs of:
   (1) *Obstruction*—decreased urinary output, increased flank pain.
   (2) *Passage of stone*—cessation of pain; filter urine with gauze.

f. Monitor: hydration status—I&O, daily weight; vital signs—particularly temperature for sign of infection; urine—color, odor.

2. Goal: *health teaching.*
   a. Importance of fluids: minimum 3000 mL/d; 2 glasses during night.
   b. *Diet:* modify according to stone type.
      (1) *Uric acid stones*—low purine.
      (2) *Calcium oxalate and calcium phosphate stones*—low calcium phosphorus and oxalate (e.g., tea, cocoa, cola, beans, spinach, acidic fruits).
      (3) *Cystine stones*—low protein.
   c. *Acid-ash diet* with: calcium oxalate and calcium phosphate stones, magnesium and ammonium phosphate stones.
   d. *Alkaline-ash diet* with: calcium oxalate, uric acid, and cystine stones (see Common Therapeutic Diets in Unit 3, p. 243).
   e. Signs of urinary infection: dysuria, frequency, hematuria; seek immediate treatment.
   f. Prepare for removal if indicated; 60–80% of patients will have lithotripsy done; cystoscopy or ureterolithotomy may also be ordered; nephrectomy in *extreme cases.*

◆ F. **Evaluation/outcome criteria:**
   1. Relief from pain.
   2. No signs of urinary obstruction (e.g., increased flank pain, decreased urine output).
   3. No recurrence of lithiasis (adheres to diet and fluid regimen).

IX. **Extracorporeal lithotripsy:** a noninvasive mechanical procedure used to break up renal calculi so they can pass spontaneously, in most cases. The trunk of the patient is submerged in water. In addition to being strapped to a frame, the patient may also be sedated, as the procedure takes 30–45 min, and remaining still is important. An underwater electrode generates shock waves that fragment the stone so it can be excreted in the urine a few days after the procedure. A degree of renal colic may occur requiring antispasmodics. Nursing measures should encourage ambulation and promote diuresis through forcing fluids.

X. **Prostatic hypertrophy** (prostatism): malfunction of the urinary tract resulting from a lesion (benign or malignant) of the prostate gland.

A. **Pathophysiology:** prostate enlarges, bulges upward, blocks flow of urine from bladder into urethra → obstruction → hydroureter, hydronephrosis.

B. **Risk factors:**
   1. Benign
      a. Changes in estrogen and androgen levels.
      b. Men >50.
   2. Malignant
      a. Genetic tendency.
      b. Hormonal factors (e.g., late puberty, higher fertility).
      c. Diet (high fat).
      d. Chemical carcinogens (fertilizer, rubber, cadmium batteries).

◆ C. **Assessment:**
   1. *Subjective data—urination:*
      a. Difficulty starting stream.
      b. Smaller, less forceful.
      c. Dribbling.
      d. Frequency.
      e. Urgency.
      f. Nocturia.
      g. Retention (incomplete emptying).
      h. Inability to void after ingestion of alcohol or exposure to cold.
   2. *Objective data*
      a. Catheterization for residual urine: 25–50 mL after voiding.
      b. Enlarged prostate on rectal exam.
      c. Lab data:
         (1) Urine—*increased* RBC, WBC.
         (2) Blood—*increased* creatinine.

◆ D. **Analysis/nursing diagnosis:**
   1. *Urinary retention* related to incomplete emptying.
   2. *Altered urinary elimination* related to obstruction.
   3. *Urinary incontinence* related to urgency, pressure.
   4. *Anxiety* related to potential surgery.
   5. *Body image disturbance* related to threat to male identity.

◆ E. **Nursing care plan/implementation:**
   1. Goal: *relieve urinary retention.*
      a. Catheterization: release maximum of 1000 mL initially; *avoid* bladder decompression, which results in hypotension, bladder spasms, ruptured blood vessels in bladder; empty 200 mL every 5 min.
   ▶ b. Patency: irrigate intermittently or continually, as ordered.
      c. *Fluids:* minimum 2000 mL/24 h.
   2. Goal: *health teaching.*
      a. Preparation for surgery (cystostomy, prostatectomy):
         (1) Expectations—indwelling catheter (will feel urge to void).

(2) *Avoid* pulling on catheter (this increases bleeding and clots).

(3) Bladder spasms common 24–48 h after surgery, particularly with TUR and suprapubic approaches.

(4) Threatening nature of procedure (possibility of impotence with perineal prostatectomy).

b. See also I. Preoperative preparation, p. 102.

XI. Prostatectomy: surgical procedure to relieve urinary retention and frequency caused by benign prostatic hypertrophy or cancer of the prostate.

A. Types

1. *Transurethral resection (TUR)*—removal of obstructive prostatic tissue surrounding urethra by an electric wire (resectoscope) introduced through the urethra; hypertrophy may recur, and TUR repeated.

2. *Suprapubic*—low midline incision is made directly over the bladder; bladder is opened and large mass of prostatic tissue is removed through incision in urethral mucosa.

3. *Retropubic*—removal of hypertrophied prostatic tissue high in pelvic area through a low abdominal incision; bladder is not opened.

4. *Perineal*—removal of prostatic tissue low in pelvic area is accomplished through an incision made between the scrotum and the rectum; usually results in impotency.

◆ **B. Nursing care plan/implementation:**

1. *Preoperative:* see X. Prostatic hypertrophy, p. 143.

2. *Postoperative*

a. Goal: *promote optimal bladder function and comfort.*

(1) Urinary drainage: sterile closed-gravity system—maintain external traction as ordered.

(2) Reinforce purposes, sensations to expect.

(3) Bladder irrigation to control bleeding, keep clots from forming.

▶ (4) Suprapubic catheter care (suprapubic prostatectomy)—closed-gravity drainage system; observe character, amount, flow of drainage.

(5) *After removal:*
(a) Observe for urinary drainage q4h for 24 h.
(b) Skin care.
(c) Report excessive drainage to physician.

(6) Dressings: keep dry, clean; reinforce if necessary (may need to change suprapubic dressing if urinary drainage); notify physician of *excessive bleeding.*

(7) Observe for signs of:
(a) *Bladder distention*—distinct mound over pubis, slow drop in collecting bottle; irrigate catheter as ordered.
(b) *Increased bleeding*—bright red drainage and clots; cool, clammy, pale skin; and increased pulse rate.

b. Goal: *assist in rehabilitation.* Emotional support: *fears* of incontinence, loss of male identity, impotence.

c. Goal: *health teaching.*

(1) Expectations: mild incontinence, dribbling for a while (several months) after surgery; need to void as soon as urge is felt; push fluids.

(2) Exercises: perineal 1–2 d after surgery—buttocks are tightened for a count of ten, 20–50 times daily.

(3) *Avoid:*
(a) Long auto trips, vigorous exercise, heavy lifting, and sexual intercourse for about 3 wk or until medical permission, as this may increase tendency to bleed.
(b) Alcoholic beverages for 1 mo, as this may cause burning on urination.
(c) Tub baths, as this increases chance of infection.

▬▶ (4) Medications: stool softeners or mild cathartics to decrease straining.

◆ **C. Evaluation/outcome criteria:**

1. Relief of symptoms.

2. No complications (e.g., hemorrhage, impotence).

XII. Urinary diversion (*ileal conduit*): implantation of ureters into a portion of the terminal ileum, with formation of a stoma; common method for urinary diversion; also known as *Bricker's procedure.*

A. Indications:

1. Congenital anomalies of bladder.

2. Neurogenic bladder.

3. Mechanical obstruction to urine flow (e.g., bladder cancer).

4. Severe cystitis.

5. Trauma to lower urinary tract.

◆ **B. Analysis/nursing diagnosis:**

1. *Altered urinary elimination* related to surgical diversion.

2. *Risk for impaired skin integrity* related to leakage of urine.

3. *Risk for infection* related to contamination of stoma.

4. *Constipation* related to absence of peristalsis.

5. *Body image disturbance* related to stoma.

◆ **C. Nursing care plan/implementation:**

1. *Preoperative:* optimal bowel and stoma-site preparation.

a. *Diet:* nonresidue several days before surgery.

▬▶ b. Medications:

(1) Neomycin (for bowel sterilization).

(2) Cathartics, enemas.

c. Site selection: appliance faceplate must bond securely; avoid areas of pressure from clothing (waistline); usual site is right or left lower abdominal quadrant.

d. See also I. Preoperative preparation, p. 102.

2. *Postoperative*

a. Goal: *present complications and promote comfort.*

(1) Observe for signs of:

(a) *Paralytic ileus* (common complication)—keep NG tube patent.

(b) *Stoma necrosis*—dusky or cyanotic color (**emergency** situation).

(2) Skin care: check for leakage around ostomy bag.

(3) See III. Postoperative experience, p. 107.

b. Goal: *health teaching.*

(1) Self-care activities:

(a) *Peristomal skin care*—prevent irritation, breakdown; proper cleansing—soap and water; adhesive remover, if needed.

(b) *Appliance application and emptying;* do not remove each day; change appliance every 4–5 d or when leaking.

(c) *Odor control*—dilute urine, acid-ash diet, hygiene, avoid asparagus, tomatoes; mucus normal.

(d) *Use of night drainage system* if necessary for uninterrupted sleep.

(2) Signs of *complications:* change in urine color, clarity, quantity, smell; stomal color change.

◆ **D. Evaluation/outcome criteria:**

1. Acceptance of new body image.

2. Regains independence.

3. Demonstrates confidence in management of self-care activities.

❑ Sensory/Perceptual Functions

I. Laryngectomy (radical neck dissection): removal of entire larynx, lymph nodes, sternomastoid muscle, and jugular vein for cancer of the larynx that extends beyond the vocal cords. Permanent tracheostomy; new methods of speech will have to be learned.

Partial laryngectomy: removal of lesion on larynx. Patient will be able to speak after operation, but quality of voice may be altered.

◆ **A. Assessment:**

1. *Subjective data*

a. Feeling of lump in throat.

b. Pain: Adam's apple; may radiate to ear.

c. Dysphagia.

2. *Objective data*

a. Hoarseness: persistent, progressive.

b. Lymphadenopathy: cervical.

c. Breath odor: foul.

◆ **B. Analysis/nursing diagnosis:**

1. *Impaired verbal communication* related to removal of larynx.

2. *Body image disturbance* related to radical neck dissection.

3. *Ineffective airway clearance* related to copious amounts of mucus.

4. *Fear* related to diagnosis of cancer.

5. *Impaired swallowing* related to edema.

6. *Impaired social interaction* related to altered speech.

◆ **C. Nursing care plan/implementation:**

1. *Preoperative*

a. Goal: *provide emotional support and optimal physical preparation.*

(1) Encourage verbalization of fears; answer all questions honestly, particularly about having no voice after surgery.

(2) Visit from person with laryngectomy (contact International Association of Laryngectomees).

b. Goal: *health teaching.*

(1) Prepare for tracheostomy.

(2) Other means to speak (esophageal "burp" speech).

2. *Postoperative*

a. Goal: *maintain patent airway and prevent aspiration.*

(1) *Position:* semi-Fowler's, preventing forward flexion of neck to reduce edema and keep airway open.

(2) Observe for hypoxia:

(a) *Early signs:* increased respiratory and pulse rates, apprehension, restlessness.

(b) *Late signs:* dyspnea, cyanosis; swallowing difficulties—patient should chew food well and swallow with water.

(3) *Laryngectomy* tube care:

(a) Observe for stridor (coarse, high-pitched inspiratory sound)—**report immediately.**

(b) Have extra laryngectomy tube at bedside.

▶ (c) Suction with sterile equipment; instill 2–3 mL sterile saline into stoma to loosen secretions.

b. Goal: *promote optimal physical and psychological function.*

(1) Frequent mouth care.

▶ (2) Dressings: may be pressure-type; note color and amount of drainage; reinforce as ordered.

▶ (3) *Tubes:* Hemovac (Figure 2.7); expect 80–120 mL serosanguineous drainage first postoperative day; drainage should decrease daily; observe patency.

(4) Post-Hemovac removal—observe: skin flaps down, adherent to underlying tissue; may have to "roll" flaps to prevent drainage buildup.

(5) Use surgical asepsis.

(6) Answer call bell *immediately;* use preestablished means of communication.

(7) Reexplain all procedures while giving care.

(8) Support head when lifting.

c. Goal: *health teaching.*

(1) Speech rehabilitation as soon as esophageal suture is healed.

(a) Information on laryngeal speech (International Association of Laryngectomees, American Cancer Society, American Speech and Hearing Association).

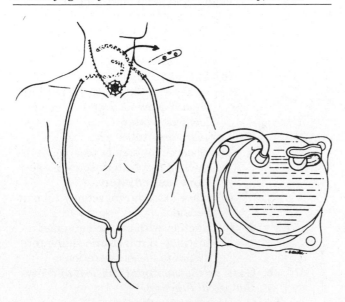

■ **FIGURE 2.7   Hemovac apparatus for constant closed suction. In this system of wound drainage, suction is maintained by a plastic container with a spring inside that tries to force apart the lids and thereby produces suction that is transmitted through the plastic tubing. The neck skin is pulled down tight, and no external dressing is required. The container serves as both suction source and receptacle for blood. It is emptied as required, and drainage tubes are left in the neck for 3 days. (From DeWeese DD, Saunders WH. *Textbook of Otolaryngoloty* (6th ed). St. Louis: Mosby, 1987.)**

(b) Esophageal speech best learned in speech clinic—learn to burp column of air needed for speech; new voice sounds are natural but hoarse.

▶ (2) *Stoma* care:

(a) Cover with scarf or shirt of a porous material (material substitutes for nasal passage—warms and filters out particles).

(b) Use source of humidification ("mister" or commercial humidifier).

(c) Caution while bathing or showering, to decrease likelihood of aspiration.

(d) Swimming and boating permitted only with snorkel device.

(e) Procedure for suctioning if cough ineffective.

(3) Simple ROM of neck; how to support head.

(4) Possible *contraindications:* use of talcum powder, tissues.

◆ D. **Evaluation/outcome criteria:**

1. No surgical complications (e.g., airway obstruction, infection, hemorrhage).
2. Learns alternative speech 60–90 d after surgery.
3. Demonstrates proper stoma care.
4. Resumes productive life-style (work, family).
5. Normal response to change in body image (e.g., anger, grief, denial).

II. **Aphasia:** impaired ability to understand or use commonly accepted words or symbols; interferes with ability to speak, write, and/or read; usually occurs with right-sided hemiplegia with a cerebrovascular accident.

A. **Types and pathophysiology:**

1. *Receptive (sensory)*—lesion usually Wernicke's area of temporal lobe; difficulty understanding spoken word (*auditory* aphasia) or written word (*visual* aphasia).
2. *Expressive (motor)*—lesion usually in Broca's area of frontal lobe; difficulty expressing thoughts in speech or writing (*motor* aphasia).

B. **Risk factors:**

1. Vascular disease of the brain (cerebral vascular accident).
2. Alzheimer's disease.
3. Sickle cell anemia.

◆ C. **Analysis/nursing diagnosis:**

1. *Impaired verbal communication* related to cerebral cortex disorder.
2. *Powerlessness* related to inability to express needs/concerns.
3. *Impaired social interaction* related to difficulty communicating.

◆ D. **Nursing care plan/implementation:** Goal: *assist with communication.*

1. Assess comprehension: use simple requests; write questions or use picture cards.
2. Stand on patient's unaffected side (stay within patient's visual field).
3. Talk slowly, clearly; do not shout or "talk down" (there is no intellectual impairment).
4. Use short, simple phrases, repeat words; ask questions needing one-word answers.
5. Use alternative ways to communicate; hand gestures, picture cards.
6. Avoid frustration for patient: do not force patient to repeat words; allow ample time to respond; anticipate needs.
7. Respond to patient's speech; if not understood, tell patient; encourage patient to use other words.
8. Reinforce techniques taught by speech therapist.
9. Maintain one-way communication: receptive aphasia does not always accompany expressive aphasia.

◆ **E. Evaluation/outcome criteria:**
1. Communication reestablished.
2. Minimal frustration exhibited.
3. Participates in speech therapy.

III. **Meniere's disease:** chronic, recurrent disorder of inner ear; attacks of vertigo, tinnitus, and vestibular dysfunction; lasts 30 min to full day; usually no pain or loss of consciousness.

   A. Pathophysiology: associated with excessive dilatation of cochlear duct (unilateral) from overproduction or decreased absorption of endolymph → progressive sensorineural loss.

   B. Risk factors:
   1. Emotional or endocrine disturbance (diabetes mellitus).
   2. Spasms of internal auditory artery.
   3. Head trauma.
   4. Allergic reaction.
   5. High salt intake.
   6. Smoking.
   7. Ear infections.

◆ **C. Assessment:**
   1. *Subjective data*
      a. Tinnitus.
      b. Headache.
      c. True vertigo; sudden attacks; room appears to spin.
      d. Depression; irritability; withdrawal.
      e. Nausea on sudden head motion.
   2. *Objective data*
      a. Impaired hearing, especially *low* tones.
      b. Change in gait; lack of coordination.
      c. Vomiting with sudden head motion.
      d. Nystagmus—during attacks.
      e. Diagnostic test: caloric (cold water in ear canal)—may precipitate attack; audiometry—loss of hearing.

◆ **D. Analysis/nursing diagnosis:**
   1. *Risk for injury* related to vertigo, lack of coordination.

2. *Auditory sensory/perceptual alteration* related to progressive hearing loss.
3. *Anxiety* related to uncertainty of treatment.
4. *Risk for activity intolerance* related to sudden onset of vertigo.
5. *Sleep pattern disturbance* related to tinnitus.
6. *Ineffective individual coping* related to chronic disorder.

◆ **E. Nursing care plan/implementation:**
   1. Goal: *provide safety and comfort during attacks.*
      a. Activity: bedrest during attack; siderails up; lower to chair or floor if attack occurs while standing; assist with ambulation (sudden dizziness common).
      b. *Position:* recumbent; affected ear uppermost usually.
      c. Identify prodromal symptoms (aura, ear pressure, increased tinnitus).
      d. Call bell within reach.
   2. Goal: *minimize occurrence of attacks.*
      a. Give medications as ordered:
         (1) *Diuretics* (chlorothiazide [Diuril], acetazolamide [Diamox]) to decrease endolymphatic fluids.
         (2) *Antihistamines* (dimenhydrinate [Dramamine], diphenhydramine HCl [Benadryl]) to inhibit tissue edema.
         (3) *Vasodilators* (nicotinic acid) to control vasospasms.
         (4) *Antiemetics and antivertigo agents* (diazepam [Valium], meclizine HCl [Antivert]).
      b. *Diet:* low sodium; limited fluids to reduce endolymphatic pressure.
      c. Avoid precipitating stimuli: bright, glaring lights; noise; sudden jarring; turning head or eyes (stand in front of patient when talking).
   3. Goal: *health teaching.*
      a. No smoking (causes vasospasm) or alcoholic beverages (fluid retention, contraindicated with medications).
      b. Management of symptoms: play radio to mask tinnitus, particularly at night.
      c. Keep medication available at all times.
      d. Prepare for surgery if indicated (labyrinthectomy if hearing gone or endolymphatic sac decompression to preserve hearing).

◆ **F. Evaluation/outcome criteria:**
   1. Decreased frequency of attacks.
   2. Complies with treatment regimen and restrictions (e.g., low-sodium diet, no smoking).
   3. Hearing preserved.

IV. **Otosclerosis:** insidious, progressive deafness; most common cause of conductive deafness; cause unknown.

A. **Pathophysiology:** formation of new spongy bone in labyrinth → fixation of stapes → prevention of sound transmission through ossicles to inner ear fluids.

B. **Risk factors:**
1. Heredity.
2. Females, puberty to 45 yr.

◆ C. **Assessment:**
1. *Subjective data*
   a. Tinnitus.
   b. Difficulty hearing—gradual loss in both ears.
2. Diagnostic tests:
   a. *Rinne* (tuning fork placed over mastoid bone)—reduced sound conduction by air and intensified by bone.
   b. *Weber* (tuning fork placed on top of head)—increased sound conduction to affected ear.
   c. *Audiometry*—diminished hearing ability.

◆ D. **Analysis/nursing diagnosis:**
1. *Auditory sensory/perceptual alteration* related to hearing loss.
2. *Body image disturbance* related to aid.
3. *Ineffective individual coping* related to grief reaction to loss.
4. *Impaired social interaction* related to hearing loss.

◆ E. **Nursing care plan/implementation, evaluation/outcome criteria:** see V. Stapedectomy, below.

V. **Stapedectomy:** removal of the stapes and replacing it with a prosthesis (steel wire, Teflon piston, or polyethylene); treatment for deafness due to otosclerosis, which fixes the stapes, preventing it from oscillating and transmitting vibrations to the fluids in the inner ear.

◆ A. **Analysis/nursing diagnosis:**
1. *Sensory/perceptual alteration* related to edema and ear packing.
2. See The Perioperative Experience, p. 102, for diagnoses relating to surgery.

◆ B. **Nursing care plan/implementation:**
1. *Preoperative:* health teaching.
   a. Important to keep head in position ordered by physician postoperatively.
   b. *Avoid:* sneezing, blowing nose, vomiting, coughing—all of which increase pressure in eustachian tubes.
   c. Breathing exercises.
2. *Postoperative*
   a. Goal: *promote physical and psychological equilibrium.*
      (1) *Position:* as ordered by physician—varies according to preference; side-rails up as vertigo is common.
      (2) Activity: assist with ambulation; avoid rapid turning, which might increase vertigo.
      (3) Dressings: check frequently; may change cotton pledget in outer ear.

(4) Give medications as ordered:
   (a) *Antiemetics.*
   (b) *Analgesics.*
   (c) *Antibiotics.*
(5) Reassurance: reduction in hearing is normal; hearing may *not* immediately improve after surgery.
b. Goal: *health teaching.*
   (1) Ear care: keep covered outdoors; keep outer ear plug clean, dry, and changed.
   (2) *Avoid:*
      (a) Washing hair for 2 wk.
      (b) Swimming for 6 wk.
      (c) Air travel for 6 mo.
      (d) Individuals with upper respiratory infections.
      (e) Heavy lifting or straining.

◆ C. **Evaluation/outcome criteria:**
1. Hearing improves—evaluate 1 mo postoperatively (may require hearing aid).
2. Returns to work (usually 2 wk after surgery).
3. Continues medical supervision.

VI. **Deafness:** (1) *Hard of hearing*—slight or moderate hearing loss that is serviceable for activities of daily living. (2) *Deaf*—hearing is nonfunctional for activities of daily living.

A. **Risk factors:**
1. *Conductive* hearing losses (transmission deafness):
   a. Impacted cerumen (wax).
   b. Foreign body in external auditory canal.
   c. Defects (thickening, scarring) of eardrum.
   d. Otosclerosis of ossicles.
2. *Sensory* hearing losses (perceptive or nerve deafness):
   a. Arteriosclerosis.
   b. Infectious diseases (mumps, measles, meningitis).
   c. Drug toxicities (quinine, streptomycin, neomycin SO_4).
   d. Tumors.
   e. Head traumas.
   f. High-intensity noises.

◆ B. **Assessment**—*objective data:*
1. Inattentive or strained facial expression.
2. Excessive loudness or softness of speech.
3. Frequent need to clarify content of conversation or inappropriate responses.
4. Tilting of head while listening.
5. Lack of response when others speak.

◆ C. **Analysis/nursing diagnosis:**
1. *Auditory sensory/perceptual alteration* related to loss of hearing.
2. *Impaired social interaction* related to deafness.

◆ D. **Nursing care plan/implementation:**
1. Goal: *maximize hearing ability and provide emotional support.*

a. Gain person's attention before speaking; avoid startling.

b. Provide adequate lighting so person can see you when you are speaking.

c. Look at the person when speaking.

d. Use nonverbal cues to enhance communication, e.g., writing, hand gestures, pointing.

e. Speak slowly, distinctly; do not shout (excessive loudness distorts voice).

f. If person doesn't understand, use different words; write it down.

g. Use alternative communication system:
   (1) Speech (lip) reading.
   (2) Sign language.
   (3) Hearing aid.
   (4) Paper and pencil.
   (5) Flash cards.

h. Supportive, nonstressful environment.

2. Goal: *health teaching.*

a. Prepare for evaluative studies—audiogram.

b. Appropriate community resources: National Association of Hearing and Speech Agencies for *counseling* services; National Association for the Deaf to assist with *employment, education, legislation;* Alexander Graham Bell Association for the Deaf, Inc., serves as *information* center for those working with the deaf; American Hearing Society provides educational information, employment services, *social clubs.*

c. Use of hearing aid: care; testing; carry spare battery at all times.

d. Safety precautions: when crossing street, driving.

◆ **E. Evaluation/outcome criteria:**

1. Method of communication established.

2. Achieves independence (use of Dogs for Deaf, special telephones, visual signals).

3. Copes with life-style changes (minimal depression, anger, hostility).

VII. Glaucoma (acute and chronic): increased intraocular pressure; affects 2% of population >40 yr.

A. Pathophysiology:

1. *Acute (closed-angle)*—impaired passage of aqueous humor into the circular canal of Schlemm due to closure of the angle between the cornea and the iris. *Medical emergency; requires surgery.*

2. *Chronic (open-angle)*—local obstruction of aqueous humor between the anterior chamber and the canal. *Most common; treated with medication* (miotics, carbonic anhydrase inhibitors).

3. Untreated: imbalance between rate of secretion of intraocular fluids and rate of absorption of aqueous humor → increased aqueous humor pressures → decreased peripheral vision → corneal edema → halos and blurring of vision → blindness.

B. Risk factors—unknown, but associated with:

1. Emotional disturbances.
2. Hereditary factors.
3. Allergies.
4. Vasomotor disturbances.

◆ **C. Assessment:**

1. *Subjective data*
   a. *Acute* (closed-angle):
      (1) Pain: severe, in and around eyes.
      (2) Headache.
      (3) Rainbow halos around lights.
      (4) Blurring of vision.
      (5) Nausea, vomiting.
   b. *Chronic* (open-angle):
      (1) Eyes tire easily.
      (2) Loss of peripheral vision.

2. *Objective data*
   a. Corneal edema.
   b. Decreased peripheral vision.
   c. Increased cupping of optic disc.
   d. Tonometry—pressures >22 mm Hg.
   e. Pupils: dilated.
   f. Redness of eye.

◆ **D. Analysis/nursing diagnosis:**

1. *Visual sensory/perceptual alterations* related to increased intraocular pressure.

2. *Pain* related to sudden increase in intraocular pressure.

3. *Risk for injury* related to blindness.

4. *Impaired physical mobility* related to impaired vision.

◆ **E. Nursing care plan/implementation:**

1. Goal: *reduce intraocular pressure.*
   a. Activity: bedrest.
   b. *Position:* semi-Fowler's.
   c. Medications as ordered:
      (1) *Miotics* (pilocarpine, carbachol).
      (2) *Carbonic anhydrase inhibitors* (acetazolamide [Diamox]).
      (3) *Anticholinesterase* (demecarium bromide [Humorsol]) to facilitate outflow of aqueous humor.
      (4) *Ophthalmic* (timolol) to decrease intraocular pressure.

2. Goal: *provide emotional support.*
   a. Place personal objects within field of vision.
   b. Assist with activities.
   c. Encourage verbalization of concerns, fears of blindness, loss of independence.

3. Goal: *health teaching.*
   a. *Prevent* increased intraocular pressure by avoiding:
      (1) Anger, excitement, worry.
      (2) Constrictive clothing.
      (3) Heavy lifting.
      (4) Excessive *fluid* intake.
      (5) Atropine or other mydriatics.
      (6) Straining at stool.
      (7) Eye strain.

Adult

b. Relaxation techniques; stress-management if indicated.
c. Prepare for surgical intervention, if ordered: laser trabeculoplasty, trabeculectomy (filtering).
d. Medications: purpose, dosage, frequency; eye-drop installation; have extra bottle in case of breakage or loss.
e. Activity: moderate exercise—walking.
f. Safety measures: eye protection (shield or glasses); MedicAlert band or tag; avoid driving 1–2 h after instilling miotics.
g. Community resources as necessary.

◆ **F. Evaluation/outcome criteria:**
1. Eyesight preserved if possible.
2. Intraocular pressure lowered (<22 mm Hg).
3. Continues medical supervision for life—reports reappearance of symptoms immediately.

VIII. Cataract: developmental or degenerative opacification of the crystalline lens.
   A. Risk factors:
   1. Aging.
   2. Trauma.
   3. Toxins.
   4. Congenital defect.

◆ **B. Assessment:**
1. *Subjective data*—vision: blurring, loss of acuity (see best in low-lit conditions); distortion; diplopia; photophobia.
2. *Objective data*
   a. Blindness: unilateral or bilateral (particularly in congenital cataracts).
   b. Loss of red reflex: gray opacity of lens.

◆ **C. Analysis/nursing diagnosis:**
1. *Visual sensory/perceptual alterations* related to opacity of lens.
2. *Risk for injury* related to accidents.
3. *Social isolation* related to impaired vision.

IX. Cataract removal: removal of opacified lens because of loss of vision; extracapsular cataract extraction followed by intraocular lens (IOL) insertion is procedure of choice.

◆ **A. Nursing care plan/implementation:**
1. *Preoperative*
   a. Goal: *prepare for surgery.* Antibiotic drops or ointment, mydriatic eye drops as ordered; note dilation of pupils; avoid glaring lights; usually done under local anesthetic with sedation.
   b. Goal: *health teaching.* Postoperative expectations: do not rub, touch, or squeeze eyes shut after surgery; eye patches will be on; assistance will be given for needs; overnight hospitalization not required unless complications occur; mild iritis usually occurs.
2. *Postoperative*

   a. Goal: *reduce stress on the sutures and prevent hemorrhage.*
      (1) Activity: ambulate as ordered, usually soon after surgery; generally discharged 5–6 h after surgery.
      (2) *Position:* flat or low Fowler's; on back or turn to *nonoperative* side, as turning to operative side increases pressure.
      (3) *Avoid* activities that increase intraocular pressure: straining at stool, vomiting, coughing, brushing teeth, brushing hair, shaving, lifting objects over 20 lb, *bending,* or *stooping;* wear glasses or shaded lens during day, eyeshield at night.
      (4) Provide: mouthwash, hair care, personal items within easy reach, "step-in" slippers.
   b. Goal: *promote psychological well-being.* With elderly, frequent contacts to prevent sensory deprivation.
   c. Goal: *health teaching.*
      (1) If prescriptive glasses are used (aphakic glasses), explain about magnification, perceptual distortion, blind areas in peripheral vision; guide through activities with glasses; need to look through central portion of lens and turn head to side when looking to the side to decrease distortion.
      (2) Eye care: instillation of eye drops (mydriatics and carbonic anhydrase inhibitors to prevent glaucoma and adhesions if IOL not inserted; with IOL steroid-antibiotic used); eye shield at night to prevent injury for 1 mo.
      (3) Signs/symptoms of: *infection* (redness, pain, edema, drainage); iris *prolapse* (bulging or pear-shaped pupil); *hemorrhage* (sharp eye pain, half-moon of blood).
      (4) *Avoid:* heavy lifting; potential eye trauma.

◆ **B. Evaluation/outcome criteria:**
1. Vision restored.
2. No complications (e.g., severe eye pain, hemorrhage).
3. Performs self-care activities (e.g., instills eye drops).
4. Returns for follow-up ophthalmology care—recognizes symptoms requiring immediate attention.

X. Retinal detachment: separation of retina from choroid.
   A. Risk factors:
   1. Trauma.
   2. Degeneration.

◆ **B. Assessment:**
1. *Subjective data*

a. Flashes of light before eyes.
b. Vision: blurred, sooty (sudden onset); sensation of floating particles; blank areas of vision.

2. *Objective data*—ophthalmic exam: retina is grayish in area of tear; bright red, horseshoe-shaped tear.

◆ **C. Analysis/nursing diagnosis:**
1. *Visual sensory/perceptual alteration* related to blurred vision.
2. *Anxiety* related to potential loss of vision.
3. *Risk for injury* related to blindness.

◆ **D. Nursing care plan/implementation:**
1. *Preoperative*
   a. Goal: *reduce anxiety and prevent further detachment.*
   (1) Encourage verbalization of feelings; answer all questions; reinforce physician's explanation of surgical procedures.
   (2) Activity: bedrest; eyes usually covered to promote rest and maintain normal position of retina; siderails up.
   (3) *Position:* according to location of retinal tear; involved area of eye should be in a dependent position.
   (4) Give medications as ordered: *cycloplegic* or *mydriatics* to dilate pupils widely and decrease intraocular movement.
   (5) Relaxing diversion: conversation, music.
   b. Goal: *health teaching.* Prepare for surgical intervention:
   (1) *Cryotherapy*—supercooled probe is applied to the sclera, causing a scar, which pulls the choroid and retina together.
   (2) *Laser photocoagulation*—a beam of intense light from a carbon arc is directed through the dilated pupil onto the retina; seals hole if retina not detached.
   (3) *Scleral buckling*—the sclera is resected or shortened to enhance the contact between the choroid and retina.
   (4) *Banding or encirclement*—silicone band or strap is placed under the extraocular muscles around the globe.
2. *Postoperative*
   a. Goal: *reduce intraocular stress and prevent hemorrhage.*
   (1) *Position:* flat or low Fowler's; sandbags may be used to position head; turn to nonoperative side if allowed, retinal tear dependent; special positions may be prone, side-lying, or sitting with face down on table.

(2) Activity: bedrest; decrease intraocular pressure by not stooping, bending, or prone positioning.
(3) Give medications as ordered:
   (a) *Mydriatics.*
   (b) *Antibiotics.*
   (c) *Corticosteroids* to reduce eye movements, inflammation, and prevent infection.
(4) ROM—isometric, passive; elastic stockings to avoid thrombus related to immobility.
   b. Goal: *support coping mechanisms.*
   (1) Plan all care with patient.
   (2) Encourage verbalization of feelings, fears.
   (3) Encourage family interaction.
   (4) Diversional activities.
   c. Goal: *health teaching.*
   (1) Eye care: eye patch or shield at night to prevent touching of the eye while asleep; dark glasses; avoid rubbing, squeezing eyes.
   (2) Limitations: no reading for 3 wk, no physical exertion for 6 wk.
   (3) Medications: dosage, frequency, purpose, side effects: avoid nonprescription medications.
   (4) Signs of redetachment: flashes of light, increase in "floaters," blurred vision.

◆ **E. Evaluation/outcome criteria:**
1. Vision restored.
2. No further detachment—recognizes signs and symptoms.
3. No injury occurs—accepts limitations.

XI. Blindness: legally defined as vision less than 20/200 with the use of corrective lenses, or a visual field of no greater than 20 degrees; greatest incidence after 65 yr.

A. Risk factors:
1. Glaucoma.
2. Cataracts.
3. Diabetic retinopathy.
4. Atherosclerosis.
5. Trauma.

◆ **B. Analysis/nursing diagnosis:**
1. *Visual sensory/perceptual alteration* related to blindness.
2. *Impaired social interaction* related to loss of sight.
3. *Risk for injury* related to visual impairment.
4. *Self-care deficit* related to visual loss.

◆ **C. Nursing care plan/implementation:**
1. Goal: *promote independence and provide emotional support.*
   a. Familiarize with surroundings; encourage use of touch.
   b. Establish communication lines; answer questions.

c. Deal with feelings of loss, overprotectiveness by family members.
d. Provide diversional activities: radio, CDs, talking books, tapes.
e. Encourage self-care activities; allow voicing of frustrations when activity is not done to satisfaction (spilling or misplacing something), to decrease anger and discouragement.

2. Goal: *facilitate activities of daily living.*
   a. *Eating:*
      (1) Establish routine placement for table pieces, e.g., plate, glass.
      (2) Help person mentally visualize the plate as a clock or compass (e.g., "3 o'clock" or "east").
      (3) Take person's hand and guide the fingertips to establish spatial relationship.
   b. *Walking:*
      (1) Have person hold your forearm: walk a half step in front.
      (2) Tell the person when approaching stairs, curb, incline.
   c. *Talking:*
      (1) Speak when approaching person; tell them before you touch them.
      (2) Tell them who you are and what you will be doing.
      (3) Do not avoid words such as "see" or discussing the appearance of things.

3. Goal: *health teaching.*
   a. Accident prevention in the home.
   b. Community resources
      (1) Voluntary agencies:
         (a) American Foundation for the Blind—provides catalogs of devices for visually handicapped.
         (b) National Society for the Prevention of Blindness—comprehensive educational programs and research.
         (c) Recording for the Blind, Inc.—provides recorded educational books on free loan.
         (d) Lion's Club.
         (e) Catholic charities.
         (f) Salvation Army.
      (2) Government agencies;
         (a) Social and Rehabilitation Service—counseling and placement services.
         (b) Veterans Administration—screening and pensions.
         (c) State Welfare Department, Division for the Blind—vocational.

◆ **D. Evaluation/outcome criteria:**
   1. Acceptance of disability—participates in self-care activities, remains socially involved.
   2. Regains independence with rehabilitation.

XII. Traumatic injuries to the brain
   A. Types:
      1. *Concussion*—transient disorder due to injury in which there is brief loss of consciousness due to paralysis of neuronal function; recovery is usually total.
      2. *Contusion*—structural alteration of brain tissue characterized by extravasation of blood cells (bruising); injury may occur on side of impact or on opposite side (when cranial contents shift forcibly within the skull with impact).
      3. *Laceration*—tearing of brain tissue or blood vessels due to a sharp bone fragment or object or tearing force.
      4. *Hematomas*
         a. *Subdural*—blood from ruptured or torn vein collects between arachnoid and dura; may be acute, subacute, or chronic.
         b. *Extradural* (epidural)—blood clot located between dura and inner surface of skull; most often from tearing of middle meningeal artery; **emergency** condition.

   B. Pathophysiology of impaired CNS functioning:
      1. Depressed neuronal activity in reticular activating system → depressed *consciousness* (Table 2.28).
      2. Depressed neuronal functioning in lower brain stem and spinal cord → depression of reflex activity → decreased eye movements, unequal pupils → decreased response to light stimuli → widely dilated and fixed *pupils.*
      3. Depression of respiratory center → altered respiratory pattern → decreased rate → *respiratory arrest.*

■ **TABLE 2.28 Levels of Consciousness**

Stage	Characteristics
Alertness	Aware of time and place
Automatism	Aware of time and place but demonstrates abnormality of mood (euphoria to irritability)
Confusion	Inability to think and speak in coherent manner; responds to verbal requests but is unaware of time and place
Delirium	Restlessness and violent activity; may not comply with verbal instructions
Stupor	Quiet and uncommunicative; may appear conscious—sits or lies with glazed look; unable to respond to verbal instructions; bladder and rectal incontinence may occur
Semicoma	Unresponsive to verbal instructions but responds to vigorous or painful stimuli
Coma	Unresponsive to vigorous or painful stimuli

C. **Risk factors:** accidents—automobile, industrial and home, motorcycle, military.

◆ D. **Assessment:**
   1. *Subjective data*
      a. Headache.
      b. Dizziness, loss of balance.
      c. Double vision.
      d. Nausea.
   2. *Objective data*
      a. Laceration or abrasion around face or head.
      b. Drainage from ears or nose.
      c. Projectile vomiting, hematemesis.
      d. Vital signs indicating increased intracranial pressure (see XIII. Increased intracranial pressure, p. 153).
      e. Neurologic exam:
         (1) *Altered level of consciousness*; a numerical assessment, such as the Glasgow Coma Scale (Table 2.29), may be used. The lower the score, the poorer the prognosis, generally.
         (2) Pupils—equal, round, react to light, *or* unequal, dilated, unresponsive to light.
         (3) Extremities—paresis or paralysis.
         (4) Reflexes—hypo- or hypertonia; *Babinski* present (flaring of great toe when sole is stroked).

◆ E. **Analysis/nursing diagnosis:**
   1. *Altered thought processes* related to brain trauma.
   2. *Sensory/perceptual alteration* related to depressed neuronal activity.
   3. *Risk for injury* related to impaired CNS functioning.
   4. *Risk for aspiration* related to respiratory depression.
   5. *Self-care deficit* related to altered level of consciousness.
   6. *Risk for disuse syndrome* related to paresis or paralysis.

■ **TABLE 2.29   Glasgow Coma Scale**

Best eye-opening response	Purposeful and spontaneous
	To voice
	To pain
	No response
	Untestable
Best verbal response	Oriented
	Disoriented
	Inappropriate words
	Incomprehensible sounds
	No response
	Untestable
Best motor response	Obeys commands
	Localizes pain
	Withdraws to pain
	Flexion to pain
	Extension to pain
	No response
	Untestable

◆ F. **Nursing care plan/implementation:**
   1. Goal: *sustain vital functions and minimize or prevent complications.*
      ▶ a. Patent airway: endotracheal tube or tracheostomy may be ordered.
      ▶ b. Oxygen: as ordered (as hypoxia increases cerebral edema).
      c. *Position:* semiprone or prone (coma position) with head level to prevent aspiration (*keep off back*); turn side to side to prevent stasis in lungs.
      d. Vital signs as ordered.
      e. Neurologic check: pupils, level of consciousness, muscle strength; report changes.
      f. Seizure precautions: padded siderails.
      g. Medications as ordered:
         (1) *Steroids* (dexamethasone [Decadron]).
         (2) *Anticonvulsants* (phenytoin [Dilantin], phenobarbital).
         (3) *Analgesics* (**morphine contraindicated**).
      h. Cooling measures or hypothermia for elevated temperature.
      i. Assist with diagnostic tests:
         (1) Lumbar puncture (contraindicated with increased intracranial pressure).
         (2) Electroencephalogram (EEG).
      j. *Diet:* NPO for 24 h, progressing to clear liquids if awake.
      k. Fluids: IVs; nasogastric tube feedings; I&O.
      l. Monitor blood chemistries: sodium imbalance common with head injuries.
   2. Goal: *provide emotional support and use comfort measures.*
      a. Comfort: skin care, oral hygiene; sheepskins; wrinkle-free linen.
      b. Eyes: lubricate q4h with artificial tears if periocular edema present.
      c. ROM—passive, active; physical therapy as tolerated.
      d. Avoid restraints.
      e. Encourage verbalization of concerns about changes in body image, limitations.
      f. Encourage family communication.

◆ G. **Evaluation/outcome criteria:**
   1. Alert, oriented—no residual effects (e.g., cognitive processes intact).
   2. No signs of increased intracranial pressure (e.g., decreased respirations, increased systolic pressure with widening pulse pressure, bradycardia).
   3. No paralysis—regains motor/sensory function.
   4. Resumes self-care activities.

XIII. Increased intracranial pressure (ICP): intracranial hypertension associated with altered states of consciousness.

A. **Pathophysiology:** increases in intracranial blood volume, cerebrospinal fluid, and/or brain tissue mass → increased intracranial pressure → impaired neural impulse transmission → cellular anoxia, atrophy.

B. **Risk factors:**
1. Congenital anomalies (hydrocephalus).
2. Space-occupying lesions (abscesses or tumors).
3. Trauma (hematomas or skull fractures).
4. Circulatory problems (aneurysms, emboli).
5. Inflammation (meningitis, encephalitis).

◆ C. **Assessment:**
1. *Subjective data*
   a. Headache.
   b. Nausea.
2. *Objective data*
   a. Changes in level of consciousness.
   b. Pupillary changes—unequal, dilated, and unresponsive to light (late sign).
   c. Vital signs—changes are variable.
      (1) Blood pressure—gradual or rapid elevation, widened pulse pressure.
      (2) Pulse—bradycardia, tachycardia; significant sign is *slowing of pulse as blood pressure rises.*
      (3) Respirations—pattern changes (*Cheyne-Stokes,* apneusis, *Biot's*), deep and sonorous.
      (4) Temperature—moderate elevation.
   d. Projectile vomiting.

◆ D. **Analysis/nursing diagnosis:**
1. *Altered cerebral tissue perfusion* related to increased intracranial pressure.
2. *Altered thought processes* related to cerebral anoxia.
3. *Ineffective breathing pattern* related to compression of respiratory center.
4. *Risk for aspiration* related to unconsciousness.
5. *Self-care deficit* related to altered level of consciousness.
6. *Impaired physical mobility* related to abnormal motor responses.

◆ E. **Nursing care plan/implementation:** *promote adequate oxygenation and limit further impairment.*
1. Vital signs: report changes **at once.**
2. Patent airway: keep alkalotic, to prevent increased intracranial pressure from elevated CO_2; hyperventilate if necessary.
3. Give medications as ordered:
   a. *Hyperosmolar diuretics* (mannitol, urea) to reduce brain swelling.
   b. *Steroids* (dexamethasone [Decadron]) for anti-inflammatory action.
   c. *Antacids* or H_2 antagonist to prevent stress ulcer.
4. *Position:* head of bed elevated 30 degrees.
5. Fluids: *restrict;* strict I&O.

6. Cooling measures to reduce temperature, as fever increases ICP.
7. Prepare for surgical intervention (see XIV. Craniotomy, below).

◆ F. **Evaluation/outcome criteria:**
1. No irreversible brain damage—regains consciousness.
2. Resumes self-care activities.

XIV. **Craniotomy:** excision of a part of the skull (burr hole to several centimeters) for exploratory purpose and biopsy; to remove neoplasms, evacuate hematomas or excess fluid, control hemorrhage, repair skull fractures, remove scar tissue, repair or excise aneurysms, and drain abscesses; produces minimal neurologic deficit.

◆ A. **Analysis/nursing diagnosis:**
1. *Altered cerebral tissue perfusion* related to edema.
2. *Altered thought processes* related to disorientation.
3. *Self-care deficit* related to continued neurologic impairment.
4. Also see nursing diagnosis for XII. Traumatic injuries to the brain, XIII. Increased intracranial pressure, and The Perioperative Experience, p. 102.

◆ B. **Nursing care plan/implementation:**
1. *Preoperative*
   a. Goal: *obtain baseline measures.*
      (1) Vital signs.
      (2) Level of consciousness.
      (3) Mental, emotional status.
      (4) Pupillary reactions.
      (5) Motor strength and functioning.
   b. Goal: *provide psychological support:* listen; give accurate, brief explanations.
   c. Goal: *prepare for surgery.*
      (1) Cut hair; shave scalp (may be done in surgery).
      (2) Cover scalp with clean towel.
      (3) Enema and/or cathartics as ordered.
      (4) Insert indwelling Foley catheter as ordered.
2. *Postoperative:*
   a. Goal: *prevent complications and limit further impairment.*
      (1) Vital signs (*indications of complications*):
         (a) Decreased blood pressure—*shock.*
         (b) Widened pulse pressure—*increased ICP.*
         (c) Respiratory failure—*compression* of medullary *respiratory* centers.
         (d) Hyperthermia—disturbance of heat-regulating mechanism; *infection.*
      (2) Neurologic:

(a) Pupils—ipsilateral dilation (increased ICP), visual disturbances.

(b) Altered level of consciousness.

(c) Altered cognitive or emotional status—disorientation common.

(d) Motor function and strength—hypertonia, hypotonia, seizures.

(3) Blood gases, to monitor adequacy of ventilation.

(4) Dressings: check frequently; aseptic technique; reinforce as necessary.

(5) Observe for:

(a) CSF leakage (glucose-positive drainage from nose, mouth, ears)—*report immediately.*

(b) Periorbital edema—apply light ice compresses as necessary—remove crusts from eyelids.

(6) Check integrity of seventh cranial nerve (facial)—incomplete closure of eyelids.

(7) *Position:*

(a) *Supratentorial surgery* (cerebrum)—*semi-Fowler's* (30-degree elevation); may *not* lie on operative side.

(b) *Infratentorial* (brain stem, cerebellum)—*flat* in bed (prone); may turn to either side but *not* onto back.

(8) Fluids: NPO for 24–48 h.

(9) Medications as ordered:

(a) *Osmotic diuretics* (mannitol).

(b) *Corticosteroids* (dexamethasone [Decadron]).

(c) *Mild analgesics* (do not mask neurologic or respiratory depression).

(10) Orient frequently to person, time, place—to reduce restlessness, confusion.

(11) Siderails up for safety.

(12) Avoid restraints (may increase agitation and ICP).

(13) Ice bags to head to reduce headache.

(14) Activity: assist with ambulation.

b. Goal: *provide optimal supportive care.*

(1) Cover scalp once dressings are removed (scarves, wigs).

(2) Deal realistically with neurologic deficits—facilitate acceptance, adjustment, independence.

c. Goal: *health teaching.*

(1) Prepare for physical, occupational, and/or speech therapy, as needed.

(2) Activities of daily living.

◆ C. Evaluation/outcome criteria:

1. Regains consciousness—is alert, oriented.

2. Resumes self-care activities within limits of neurologic deficits.

XV. Epilepsy: seizure disorder characterized by sudden transient aberration of brain function; associated with motor, sensory, autonomic, or psychic disturbances.

A. **Seizure:** involuntary muscular contraction and disturbances of consciousness from abnormal electrical activity.

B. **Risk factors:**

1. Brain injury.

2. Infection (meningitis, encephalitis).

3. Water and electrolyte disturbances.

4. Hypoglycemia.

5. Tumors.

6. Vascular disorders (hypoxia or hypocapnia).

C. **Generalized seizures:**

1. *Tonic-clonic* (grand mal) seizures:

a. **Pathophysiology:** increased excitability of a neuron → possible activation of adjacent neurons → synchronous discharge of impulses → vigorous involuntary sustained muscle spasms (*tonic* contractions). Onset of neuronal fatigue → intermittent muscle spasms (*clonic* contractions) → cessation of muscle spasms → fatigue.

◆ b. **Assessment:**

(1) *Subjective data*—aura: flash of light; peculiar smell, sound; feelings of fear; euphoria.

(2) *Objective data*

(a) *Convulsive stage*—tonic and clonic muscle spasms, loss of consciousness, breathholding, frothing at mouth, biting of tongue, urinary or fecal incontinence; lasts 2–5 min.

(b) *Postconvulsion*—headache, fatigue (postictal sleep), malaise, nausea, vomiting, sore muscles, choking on secretions, aspiration.

2. *Absence* (petit mal) seizures:

a. **Pathophysiology:** unknown etiology, momentary loss of consciousness (10–20 sec); usually no recollection of seizure; resumes previously performed action.

◆ b. **Assessment**—*objective data*

(1) Fixation of gaze; blank facial expression.

(2) Flickering of eyelids.

(3) Jerking of facial muscle or arm.

3. *Minor motor* seizures:

a. *Myoclonic*—involuntary jerking contraction of major muscles; may throw person to the floor.

b. *Akinetic*—momentary loss of muscle movement.

c. *Atonic*—total loss of muscle tone; person falls to the floor.

D. Partial (focal) seizures:

1. *Partial motor:* arises from region in motor cortex (posterior frontal lobe); most commonly begins in upper extremities, spreading to face and lower extremity (jacksonian march); noting progression is important in identifying area of cortex involved.

2. *Partial sensory:* sensory symptoms occur with partial seizure activity; varies with region in brain; transient.

3. *Partial complex* (psychomotor): arises out of anterior temporal lobe; frequently begins with an aura; characteristic feature is automatism (lip smacking, chewing, patting body, picking at clothes); lasts from 2–3 min to 15 min; do not restrain.

◆ **E. Analysis/nursing diagnosis:**

1. *Risk for injury* related to convulsive disorder.

2. *Anxiety* related to sudden loss of consciousness.

3. *Self-esteem disturbance* related to chronic illness.

4. *Impaired social interaction* related to self-consciousness.

◆ **F. Nursing care plan/implementation** (generalized seizures):

1. Goal: *prevent injury* during *seizure.*

a. Do not force jaws open during convulsion.

b. Do not restrict limbs—protect from injury; place something soft under head (towel, jacket, hands).

c. Loosen constrictive clothing.

d. Note time, level of consciousness, type and duration of seizure.

2. Goal: *postseizure care:*

a. *Turn on side* to drain saliva and facilitate breathing.

b. Suction as necessary.

c. Orient to time and place.

d. Oral hygiene if tongue or cheek injured.

e. Check vital signs, pupils, level of consciousness.

3. Goal: *prevent or reduce recurrences of seizure activity.*

a. Encourage patient to identify precipitating factors.

b. Moderation in diet and exercise.

c. Medications as ordered: phenytoin (Dilantin); phenobarbital; carbamazepine (Tegretol); primidone (Mysoline); trimethadione (Tridione)—petit mal only.

4. Goal: *health teaching.*

a. Medications:

(1) Actions, side effects (apathy, ataxia, hyperplasia of gums).

(2) Complications with sudden withdrawal (status epilepticus).

b. Attitude toward life and treatment; adhere to medication program.

c. Clarify misconceptions, fears—especially about insanity, bad genes.

d. Maintain activities, interests—*except* no driving until seizure free for period of time specified by state Department of Motor Vehicles.

e. *Avoid:* stress; lack of sleep; emotional upset; alcohol.

f. Relaxation techniques; stress-management.

g. Use MedicAlert band or tag.

h. Appropriate community resources.

◆ **G. Evaluation/outcome criteria:**

1. Avoids precipitating stimuli—achieves seizure control.

2. Complies with medication regimen.

3. Retains independence.

XVI. **Transient ischemic attacks** (TIAs): temporary, complete, or relatively complete cessation of cerebral blood flow to a localized area of brain, producing symptoms ranging from weakness and numbness to monocular blindness; an important precursor to cerebral vascular accident (CVA). Surgical intervention includes *carotid endarterectomy;* most common postoperative cranial nerve damage causes vocal cord paralysis or difficulty managing saliva and tongue deviation (CN VII, X, XI, XII); usually temporary; stroke may also occur.

XVII. **Cerebral vascular accident** (CVA): brain lesions resulting from damage to blood vessels supplying brain.

A. Pathophysiology: reduced or interrupted blood flow → interruption of nerve impulses down corticospinal tract → decreased or absent voluntary movement on one side of the body (fine movements are more affected than coarse movements); later, autonomous reflex activity → spasticity and rigidity of muscles.

B. Risk factors:

1. Cerebral thrombosis (most common), embolism, hemorrhage.

2. Prior ischemic episodes (TIAs).

3. Hypertension.

4. Oral contraceptives.

5. Emotional stress.

6. Family history.

7. Age.

8. Diabetes mellitus.

◆ **C. Assessment:**

1. *Subjective data*

a. Weakness; sudden or gradual loss of movement of extremities on one side.

b. Difficulty forming words.

c. Difficulty swallowing (dysphagia).

d. Nausea, vomiting.

e. History of TIAs.

2. *Objective data*
   a. Vital signs:
      (1) BP—elevated; widened pulse pressure.
      (2) Temperature—elevated.
      (3) Pulse—normal, slow.
      (4) Respirations—tachypnea, altered pattern; deep; sonorous.
   b. Neurologic:
      (1) Altered level of consciousness.
      (2) Pupils—unequal; vision—homonymous hemianopia.
      (3) Ptosis of eyelid, drooping mouth.
      (4) Paresis or paralysis (hemiplegia).
      (5) Loss of sensation and reflexes.
      (6) Incontinence of urine or feces.
      (7) Aphasia (see p. 146).

◆ **D. Analysis/nursing diagnosis:**
   1. *Impaired physical mobility* related to hemiplegia.
   2. *Impaired swallowing* related to paralysis.
   3. *Impaired verbal communication* related to aphasia.
   4. *Risk for aspiration* related to unconsciousness.
   5. *Sensory/perceptual alterations* related to altered cerebral blood flow, visual field blindness.
   6. *Altered thought processes* related to cerebral edema.
   7. *Self-care deficit* related to paresis or paralysis.
   8. *Body image disturbance* related to hemiplegia.
   9. *Total incontinence* related to interruption of normal nerve transmission.
   10. *Impaired social interaction* related to aphasia or neurologic deficit.
   11. *Risk for impaired skin integrity* related to immobility.
   12. Unilateral neglect related to cerebral damage.

◆ **E. Nursing care plan/implementation:**
   1. Goal: *reduce cerebral anoxia.*
      a. Patent airway:
      ▶ (1) Oxygen therapy as ordered; suctioning to prevent aspiration.
         (2) Turn, cough, deep breathe q2h due to high incidence of pneumonia.
      b. Activity: bedrest; progressing to out of bed as tolerated.
      c. *Position:*
         (1) Maximize ventilation.
         (2) Support with pillows when on side; use hand rolls and arm slings as ordered.
   2. Goal: *promote cardiovascular function and maintain cerebral perfusion.*
      a. Vital signs; neurologic checks.
      b. Medications as ordered:

      (1) *Antihypertensives* to prevent rupture.
      (2) *Anticoagulants* to prevent thrombus.
   c. *Fluids:* IVs to prevent hemoconcentration; I&O; weigh daily.
   d. ROM exercises to prevent contractures, muscle atrophy, phlebitis.
   e. Skin care and position changes to prevent decubiti.
   3. Goal: *provide for emotional relaxation.*
      a. Identify grief reaction to changes in body image.
      b. Encourage expression of feelings, concerns.
   4. Goal: *patient safety.*
      a. Identify existence of *homonymous hemianopia* (visual field blindness) and *agnosia* (disturbance in sensory information).
      b. Use siderails and assist as needed.
      c. Remind to walk slowly, take adequate rest periods, ensure good lighting, look where patient is going.
   5. Goal: *health teaching.*
      a. Exercise routines.
      b. Diet: self-feeding, but assist as needed.
      c. Resumption of self-care activities.
      d. Use of supportive devices; transfer techniques.

◆ **F. Evaluation/outcome criteria:**
   1. No complications (e.g., pneumonia).
   2. Regains functional independence—resumes self-care activities.
   3. Return of control over body functions (e.g., bowel, bladder, speech).

XVIII. **Bacterial meningitis** (see Unit 8, p. 532).
XIX. **Encephalitis:** inflammation of the brain and its coverings, which usually results in a lengthy coma.
   A. Pathophysiology: brain tissue injury → release of enzymes that increase vascular dilatation, capillary permeability → edema formation → increased intracranial pressure → depression of CNS function.
   B. Risk factors:
      1. Syphilis.
      2. Lead or arsenic poisoning.
      3. Carbon monoxide.
      4. Typhoid fever.
      5. Measles; chickenpox.
      6. Viruses.
   ◆ **C. Assessment:**
      1. *Subjective data*
         a. Headache—severe.
         b. Fever—sudden.
         c. Nausea, vomiting.
         d. Sensitivity to light (photophobia).
         e. Difficulty concentrating.
      2. *Objective data*
         a. Altered level of consciousness.

b. Nuchal rigidity.
c. Tremors; facial weakness.
d. Nystagmus.
e. Elevated temperature.
⚗ f. Diagnostic test: lumbar puncture—fluid cloudy; increased neutrophils, protein.
g. Lab data: blood—slight to moderate leukocytosis (about 14,000).

◆ **D. Analysis/nursing diagnosis:**
1. *Self-care deficit* related to altered level of consciousness.
2. *Risk for injury* related to coma.
3. *Sensory/perceptual alteration* related to brain tissue injury.
4. *Altered thought processes* related to increased intracranial pressure.

◆ **E. Nursing care plan/implementation:**
1. Goal: *support physical and emotional relaxation.*
   a. Vital signs; neurologic signs as ordered.
   b. Seizure precautions.
   c. *Position:* to maintain patent airway; prevent contractures; ROM.
   ▣ d. Medications as ordered:
      (1) Analgesics for pain.
      (2) Antipyretics for fever.
      (3) Sedatives for agitation.
      (4) Anticonvulsants for seizures.
      (5) Antibiotics for infection.
      (6) Osmotic diuretics (mannitol) to reduce cerebral edema.
   e. No isolation.
2. Goal: *health teaching:* self-care activities with residual motor and speech deficits; physical therapy.

◆ **F. Evaluation/outcome criteria:**
1. Regains consciousness; is alert, oriented.
2. Performs self-care activities with minimal assistance.

❏ Comfort, Rest, Activity, and Mobility

I. Pain
A. Types of pain:
1. *Superficial somatic tissues*—skin, subcutaneous or fibrous tissue, and ligaments have pain receptors, and thus pain is localized.
2. *Deep somatic tissues and viscera*—may be diffuse and radiating pain because these do not have direct connection with sensory-discriminative system.
3. *Neurogenic pain*—results from damage to peripheral or central nervous system; any sensation may be perceived as pain due to abnormal processing of afferent impulses or paroxysmal activity.

4. *Psychogenic pain*—due to fantasies and psychological need for injury or punishment (called conversion).

B. Components of pain experience—pain related to:
1. *Stimuli*—sources: chemical, ischemic, mechanical trauma, extremes of heat/cold.
2. *Perception*—viewed with fear by children, can be altered by level of consciousness, interpreted and influenced by previous and current experience, is more severe when alone at night or immobilized.
3. *Response*—variations in physiologic, cultural, and learned responses; anxiety is created; pain seen as justified punishment; pain as means for attention-getting.

◆ **C. Assessment:**
1. *Subjective data*
   a. *Site*—medial, lateral, proximal, distal.
   b. *Strength:*
      (1) Certain tissues are more sensitive.
      (2) Change in intensity.
      (3) Based on expectations.
      (4) Affected by distraction or concentration, state of consciousness.
      (5) Described as slight, medium, severe, excruciating.
   c. *Quality*—aching, burning, crushing, dull, piercing, shifting, throbbing, tingling.
   d. *Antecedent factors*—physical exertion, eating, extreme temperatures, physical and emotional stressors (fear, for example).
   e. *Previous experience*—influences reaction to pain.
   f. *Behavioral clues*—demanding, worried, irritable, restless, difficult to distract, sleepless.
2. *Objective data*
   a. *Verbal clues*—moaning, groaning, crying.
   b. *Nonverbal clues*—clenching teeth, grimacing, splinting of body parts, body position, knees drawn up, involuntary reflex movements, tossing/turning, rhythmic rubbing movements, voice pitch and speed, eyes shut.
   c. *Physical clues*—breathing irregularities, abdominal distention, skin color changes, skin temperature changes, excessive salivation, perspiration.
   d. *Time/duration*—onset, duration, recurrence, interval, last occurrence.

◆ **D. Analysis/nursing diagnosis:**
1. *Pain,* acute or chronic, related to specific patient condition.
2. *Activity intolerance* related to discomfort.
3. *Sleep pattern disturbance* related to pain.
4. *Fatigue* related to state of discomfort or emotional stress.
5. *Ineffective individual coping* related to chronic pain.

◆ **E. Nursing care plan/implementation:**

1. Goal: *provide relief of pain.*
   a. Assess level of pain; ask patient to rate on scale of 0–10 (0 = no pain; 10 = worst pain) (Table 2.30).
   b. Determine cause and try nursing *comfort* measures *before* giving drugs:
      (1) *Environmental factors:* noise, light, odors, motion.
      (2) *Physiologic needs:* elimination, hunger, thirst, fatigue, circulatory impairment, muscle tension, ventilation, pressure on nerves.
      (3) *Emotional:* fear of unknown, helplessness, loneliness (especially at night).
   c. Determine pain reactions; explore meaning of "pain" (how much, when, how long, where, why, what it feels like).
   d. *Relieve:* anger, anxiety, boredom, loneliness.
   e. Report **sudden, severe, new** pain; pain **not** relieved by medications or comfort measures; pain associated with **casts or traction.**
   f. *Remove pain stimulus:*
      (1) Administer pain medication (e.g., analgesic, antispasmodic) at appropriate time intervals; do not withhold due to overestimated danger of addiction.
      (2) Avoid cold (to reduce immediate tissue reaction to trauma).
      (3) Apply heat (to relieve ischemia).
      (4) Change activity (e.g., restrict activity in cardiac pain).
      (5) Change, loosen dressing.
      (6) Comfort (e.g., smooth wrinkled sheets, change wet dressing).
      (7) Give food (e.g., for ulcer).
   g. *Reduce pain-receptor reaction.*
      (1) Ointment (use as coating).
      (2) Local anesthetics.

      (3) Padding (of bony prominences).
   h. Assist with medical/surgical interventions to *block pain-impulse transmission:*
      (1) Injection of local anesthetic into nerve (e.g., dental).
      (2) Chordotomy—sever anterolateral spinal cord nerve tracts.
      (3) Electrical stimulation—transcutaneous (skin surface), percutaneous (peripheral nerve).
      (4) Peripheral nerve implant—electrode to major sensory nerve.
      (5) Dorsal column stimulator—electrode to dorsal column.
   i. *Avoid causes of inadequate pain control:*
      (1) Incorrect assessment.
      (2) Insufficient knowledge of pharmacologic effects.
      (3) Personal attitudes, e.g., concern for addiction.
      (4) Fear of respiratory depression.
      (5) Reluctance to accept subjective data.
   j. *Document response to pain-relief measures.*
2. Goal: *alter pain perception* by raising pain threshold.
   a. *Distraction,* e.g., TV (cerebral cortical activity blocks impulses from thalamus).
   b. *Analgesics*—give *prior* to occurrence of severe pain; give routinely for chronic/terminal pain.
   c. *Hypnosis*—assess appropriateness for use for psychogenic pain and for anesthesia; needs to be open to suggestion.
   d. *Acupuncture*—assess emotional readiness and belief in it.
3. Goal: *alter interpretation and response to pain.*
   a. Administer narcotics—result: no longer sees pain as disturbing.
   b. Administer hypnotics—result: changes perception and decreases reaction.
   c. Help patient obtain interpersonal satisfaction from ways other than attention received when in pain.
4. Goal: *promote patient control of pain and analgesia: patient-controlled analgesia* (PCA), an analgesia administration system designed to maintain optimal serum analgesia levels, safely delivers intermittent bolus doses of a narcotic analgesic; preset to maximum hourly dose.
   a. *Advantages:* decreased patient anxiety; improved pulmonary function; fewer side effects.
   b. *Limitations:* requires an indwelling intravenous line; analgesia targets central pain, may not relieve peripheral discomfort; cost of PCA unit.
5. Goal: *health teaching.*
   a. Explain causes of pain and how to describe pain.

■ **TABLE 2.30   PQRST Format for Assessing Pain**

P What **P**rovokes the pain? Did something in particular bring it on? Does anything make it worse? Does anything make it better?

Q What is the **Q**uality of the pain? Dull? Sharp? Cutting? Throbbing? Crushing? Squeezing?

R Does the pain **R**adiate to any other area, or does it stay in one place?

S What is the **S**everity of the pain? Ask the patient to grade it on a scale of 0 (no pain) to 10 (worst pain).

T What is the **T**iming of the pain? When did it start? What has happened to it over time (gotten worse? gotten better?)? If there are associated symptoms, what is their relative timing (e.g., did the pain come on before or after the nausea?)?

Source: Caroline NL. *Emergency Care in the Streets* (5th ed). Boston: Little, Brown, 1995.

b. Explain that it is acceptable to admit existence of pain.

c. Relaxation exercises.

d. Biofeedback methods of pain perception and control.

e. Proper medication administration, when necessary, for self-care.

◆ **F. Evaluation/outcome criteria:**

1. Verbalizes comfort; awareness of pain decreased.

2. Knows source of pain; how to reduce stimulus and perception.

3. Uses alternative measures for pain relief.

4. Able to cope with pain, e.g., remains active, relaxed appearance; verbal and nonverbal clues of pain absent.

II. Immobility: impaired physical mobility or limitation of physical movement may be accompanied by a number of complications that can involve any or all of the major systems of the body. Regardless of the cause of immobilization, there are a number of conditions that arise primarily as a complication of immobility. These are discussed in Table 2.31.

A. Types of immobility:

1. *Physical*—physical restriction due to limitation in movement or physiologic processes (e.g., breathing).

2. *Intellectual*—lack of action due to lack of knowledge (e.g., mental retardation, brain damage).

3. *Emotional*—immobilized when highly stressed (e.g., after loss of loved person or diagnosis of terminal illness).

4. *Social*—decreased social interaction due to separation from family when hospitalized or when alone, as in old age.

B. Risk factors:

1. Pain, trauma, injury.

2. Loss of body function or body part.

3. Chronic disease.

4. Emotional, mental illness; neglect.

5. Malnutrition.

6. Bedrest, traction, surgery, medications.

◆ **C. Assessment:**

1. *Subjective data: psychological/social effects* of immobility:

a. Decreased motivation to learn; decreased retention.

b. Decreased problem-solving abilities.

c. Diminished drives; decreased hunger.

d. Changes in body image, self-concept.

e. Exaggerated emotional reactions, inappropriate to situation or person; aggression, apathy, withdrawal.

f. Deterioration of time perception.

g. Fear, anxiety, worthlessness related to change in role activities, e.g., when no longer employed.

2. *Objective data: physical effects* of immobility:

a. Cardiovascular

(1) Orthostatic hypotension.

(2) Increased cardiac load.

(3) Thrombus formation.

b. Gastrointestinal

(1) Anorexia.

(2) Diarrhea.

(3) Constipation.

c. Metabolic

(1) Tissue atrophy and protein catabolism.

(2) BMR reduced.

(3) Fluid/electrolyte imbalances.

d. Musculoskeletal

(1) Demineralization (osteoporosis).

(2) Contractures and atrophy.

(3) Skin breakdown.

e. Respiratory

(1) Decreased respiratory movement.

(2) Accumulation of secretions in respiratory tract.

(3) O_2/CO_2 ratio imbalance.

f. Urinary

(1) Calculi.

(2) Bladder distention, stasis.

(3) Infection.

(4) Frequency.

◆ **D. Analysis/nursing diagnosis:**

1. *Impaired physical mobility* related to specific patient condition.

2. *Impaired skin integrity* related to physical immobilization.

3. *Urinary retention* related to incomplete emptying of bladder.

4. *Constipation* related to inactivity.

5. *Risk for disuse syndrome* related to lack of range of motion.

6. *Bathing/hygiene self-care deficit* related to musculoskeletal impairment.

7. *Sensory/perceptual alteration* related to complications of immobility.

8. *Body image disturbance* related to physical limitations.

◆ **E. Nursing care plan/implementation:**

1. Goal: *prevent physical, psychological hazards.*

a. Apply nursing measures to promote venous flow, muscle strength, endurance, joint mobility, skin integrity.

b. Assess and counteract *psychological* impact of immobility (e.g., feelings of helplessness, hopelessness, powerlessness).

c. Help maintain accurate sensory processing to prevent and lessen *sensory disturbances.*

d. Help adapt to *altered body image* due to increased dependency, sensory deprivation, and changes in status and power that accompany immobility.

e. Offer counseling when sexual expression is impaired.

2. Goal: *health teaching:* how to prevent physical problems related to immobility (e.g., anticonstipation diet, range of motion, skin

care); teach activities while immobile that encourage independence and provide sensory stimulation.

◆ **F. Evaluation/outcome criteria:**
1. Minimal contractures, skin breakdown, muscle atrophy or loss of strength.
2. Interest in self and environment; positive self-image.
3. Returns to optimal level of physical activity.

III. Fractures: disruptions in the continuity of bone as the result of trauma or various disease processes, such as Cushing's syndrome, that weaken the bone structure.

A. Types:
1. *Open or compound*—fractured bone extends *through skin* and mucous membranes; increased potential for infection.
2. *Closed or simple*—fractured bone *does not* protrude through skin.
3. *Complete*—fracture extends through *entire bone*, disrupting the periosteum on both sides of the bone, producing two or more fragments.
4. *Incomplete*—fracture extends *only part way* through bone; bone continuity is not totally interrupted.
5. *Greenstick* or *willow-hickory stick*—fracture of *one side of bone; other side merely bends;* usually seen only in children.
6. *Impacted or telescoped*—fracture in which bone fragments are *forcibly driven into* other or adjacent bone structures.
7. *Comminuted*—fracture having *more than one* fracture line and with bone fragment broken into *several pieces.*
8. *Depressed*—fracture in which bone or bone fragments are driven *inward,* as in skull or facial fractures.

B. Methods used to reduce/immobilize fractures: reduction or setting of the bone—restores bone alignment as nearly as possible.
1. *Closed reduction*—manual traction or manipulation. Usually done under general anesthesia to reduce pain and muscle spasm. Maintenance of reduction and immobilization is accomplished by casting (fiberglass or plaster of Paris).
2. *Open reduction*—operative procedure utilized to achieve bone alignment; pins, wire, nails, or rods may be used to secure bone fragments in position; prosthetic implants may also be used.
3. *Traction reduction*—force is applied in two directions, to obtain alignment and to reduce or eliminate muscle spasm. Used for fractures of long bones. May be:
   a. Continuous—used with fractures or dislocations of bones or joints.
   b. Intermittent—used to reduce flexion contractures or lessen pain and muscle spasm.
   c. Applied as follows:
      (1) *Skin*—traction applied to skin by using a commercial foam-rubber Buck's traction splint or by using adhesive, plastic, or a moleskin strip bound to the extremity by elastic bandage; exerts indirect traction on bone or muscles (e.g., *Buck's* extension, *Bryant's, Russell's*, pelvic). (Figure 2.8, parts a–d, p. 167.)
      (2) *Skeletal*—direct traction applied to bone using pins (*Steinman*), wires (*Kirschner*). Pin is inserted through the bone in or close to the involved area and usually protrudes through skin on both sides of the extremity. Skeletal traction for fractured vertebrae accomplished with tongs (*Crutchfield* tongs, *Gardner-Wells* tongs).
   d. Specific types of traction
      (1) *Cervical*—direct traction applied to cervical vertebrae using a head halter or *Crutchfield, Gardner-Wells,* or *Vinke* tongs that are inserted into the skull (see Figure 2.8, parts e and f). Traction is increased with weights until vertebrae move into position and alignment is regained. After reduction is obtained, weights are decreased to the amount needed to maintain reduction. *Weight amount is prescribed by physician.*
      (2) *Balanced suspension*—countertraction produced by a force other than patient's body weight; extremity is suspended in a traction apparatus that maintains the line of traction despite changes in the patient's position (e.g., *Russell's* leg traction, *Thomas'* splint with *Pearson's* attachment). See Figure 2.8, parts c and g.
      (3) *Running*—traction that exerts a pull in one plane; countertraction is supplied by the weight of the patient's body or can be increased through use of weights and pulleys in the opposite direction (e.g., *Buck's* extension, *Russell's* traction). See Figure 2.8, parts a and c.
      (4) *Halo*—an apparatus that employs both a plastic and metal frame; molded frame extends from the axilla to iliac crest and houses a metal frame. The struts of the frame extend to skull and attach to round metal (halo) device. The halo is attached to skull by four pins—two located anterolaterally and two located posterolaterally. They are inserted into external cortex of the cranium (see Figure 2.8, part h).

■ TABLE 2.31 Complications of Immobilization

Disorder	Pathophysiology	Assessment	Analysis/Nursing Diagnosis	Nursing Care Plan/Implementation	Evaluation/Outcome Criteria
Orthostatic hypotension	A decrease in BP >30/15 caused by failure of vasomotor responses to compensate for change from a recumbent to an upright position	*Subjective data:* weakness; dizziness. *Objective data:* decreased BP >30/15 measured 2 min after moving from a supine to a sitting or standing position; loss of muscle tone and strength; patient may faint	*Decreased cardiac output* related to orthostatic hypotension. *Risk for injury* related to vertigo. *Activity intolerance,* potential, related to dizziness	*Prevent trauma due to sudden decrease in BP.* 1. Change position gradually 2. Elastic stockings 3. Leg exercises 4. Dangle before getting up 5. Tilt table 6. Sitting and lying BP 7. Monitoring side effects of drugs. *Health teaching* 1. Explains signs and symptoms to patient 2. Encourage patient to dangle before standing 3. Encourage slow movement from sitting to standing 4. Exercises to maintain muscle tone	Patient tolerates increased activity. No trauma occurs. BP remains within normal limits
Cardiac overload	When the body is recumbent, some of the total blood volume that would be in the legs due to gravity is redistributed to other parts of the body, thereby increasing the circulating volume and increasing the workload of the heart; heart rate, which is decreased because blood is prevented from entering the thoracic vessels by pressure from the Valsalva maneuver, increases when normal breathing resumes	*Subjective data:* fear; apprehension. *Objective data:* Valsalva maneuver (pressure against the closed glottis when breath is held) 10–20 times/h, when trying to move in bed; tachycardia; decreased exercise tolerance	*Risk for injury* related to increased workload of heart. *Activity intolerance* related to increased workload of heart. *Fear* related to tachycardia	*Prevent injury and further ischemic damage to cardiac tissue by decreasing workload of heart.* 1. Out of bed in chair when possible 2. *Semirecumbent position* when in bed; pillows between legs when side-lying 3. Exercises: passive and active ROM, isometric 4. Encourage participation in self-care 5. Turn every 2 h, dangle 6. *Avoid* Valsalva, fatigue 7. Minimize constipation 8. Encourage slow, deep breathing when moving in bed. *Health teaching* 1. Exhale while turning, don't hold breath 2. Measures to conserve energy	No complications noted. Patient tolerates increased activity. Heart rate within normal limit
Thrombus formation	Mass of blood constituents formed in the heart or blood vessels due to pooling of blood from lack of activity; increased viscosity related to dehydration or possible external pressure	*Subjective data:* discomfort over involved vessel. *Objective data:* increased RBC; venous stasis; hypercoagulability	*Altered peripheral tissue perfusion* related to obstructed vessel. *Risk for injury* related to emboli	*Prevent injury by reducing risk factors and venous stasis* 1. *Position:* change q12h 2. Do not gatch bed (causes pressure against leg vessels) 3. Increase fluid intake 4. Monitor coagulation lab values 5. *Medications:* anticoagulation therapy, as prescribed for patients at risk (immobilized, trauma, low pelvic surgery)	No thromboemboli. *Note:* if *Homans'* sign present (discomfort behind knee on forced dorsiflexion of the foot), see nursing care for patient with thromboemboli, p. 69

continued

Adult

Assessment	Nursing diagnosis	Plan/Implementation	Evaluation/outcome
		6. Ambulate as soon as possible *Health teaching* 1. How to recognize signs of thrombophlebitis/thromboemboli 2. Leg exercise program to strengthen muscles for improved tone, to prevent pooling of blood in vessels 3. Precautions necessary when on anticoagulation therapy 4. Side effects of anticoagulation therapy (bleeding from gums, body fluids, obvious bleeding)	No respiratory complications or excess secretions noted
Respiratory congestion related to decreased respiratory movements Decreased thoracic movement due to restriction against bed or chair, lack of position change, restrictive clothing or binders/bandages, or abdominal distention *Subjective data:* dyspnea; pain *Objective data:* trauma; immobilization of thorax or abdomen, due to position in bed; inability to cough or deep breathe; abdominal distention	*Ineffective breathing pattern* related to splinting to reduce pain *Ineffective airway clearance* related to retained secretions *Impaired physical mobility* related to trauma	*Prevent complications related to respiratory status* 1. Maintain a clear airway, assist with ventilation prn 2. Remove or minimize causes of dyspnea 3. Conserve patient's energy (periods of rest and activity—patient able to cough more effectively when rested) 4. Incentive spirometry *Promote comfort* 1. Maintain hydration and nutrition. 2. *Position:* change q2h; out of bed in chair when possible (chest expansion greater when sitting in chair) *Health teaching* 1. Methods to allay anxieties precipitated by dyspnea 2. Effective breathing and coughing exercises	No respiratory complications Patient coughs and removes secretions
Respiratory congestion related to pooled secretions Inability of cilia to move normal secretions out of bronchial tree due to ineffective coughing, lack of thoracic expansion, or effects of medications *Subjective data:* dyspnea; pain *Objective data:* dehydration; drugs—anticholinergic, CNS depressants, anesthesia; inadequate coughing; stationary position	*Ineffective airway clearance* related to pooled secretions *Impaired gas exchange* related to ineffective coughing	*Prevent atelectasis, infection, stasis of air and secretions in lungs* 1. Maintain patent airway; cough; suction; change position 2. See nursing care plan for Respiratory congestion related to decreased respiratory movements, above *Health teaching* 1. Effective coughing techniques 2. Importance of adequate hydration	

Adult

■ TABLE 2.31 *(Continued)*

Disorder	Pathophysiology	Assessment	Analysis/Nursing Diagnosis	Nursing Care Plan/Implementation	Evaluation/Outcome Criteria
Oxygen–carbon dioxide imbalance	Imbalance in oxygen and carbon dioxide levels related to pulmonary congestion, ineffective breathing patterns, trauma, or effects of medications	*Subjective data:* confusion, irritable, restless, dyspnea *Objective data:* hypoxia, hypercapnia, cyanosis	*Impaired gas exchange related to immobilization*	*Promote improved respirations* 1. Change position frequently 2. Increase humidification 3. Monitor side effects of administered medication, especially narcotics, barbiturates 4. See nursing care plan for Respiratory congestion related to decreased respiratory movements, p. 163	No respiratory complications Respiratory rate and depth are adequate for maintaining balance of oxygen and carbon dioxide
Malnutrition of immobilized adult	Lack of adequate dietary intake to maintain healthy tissue related to lack of food; lack of knowledge about food; problems with ingestion, digestion, or absorption; or psychosocial factors that influence patient's motivation to eat	*Subjective data:* anorexia, nausea; diet history validating lack of adequate nutritional intake; mental irritability *Objective data:* 1. Recent weight loss of >10% 2. Decreased: healing ability, GI motility, absorption, secretion of digestive enzymes 3. Appearance: listlessness, muscle weakness; posture—sagging shoulders, sunken chest 4. Anthropometric data (measurement of size, weight, and body proportions) <85% of standard 5. Cardiovascular: tachycardia (>100) on minimal exertion; bradycardia at rest 6. Hair: brittle, dry, thin 7. Skin: dry, scaly 8. Lack of financial resources: sociocultural influences 9. Decreased blood values: serum albumin, iron-binding capacity, lymphocyte levels, hemocrit, and hemoglobin	*Altered nutrition, less than body requirements,* related to decreased appetite *Knowledge deficit* related to nutrition requirements	*Improved nutritional intake* to maintain basal metabolism requirements and replace losses from catabolism 1. Provide balanced or prescribed diet, soft or ground food if cannot chew or is edentulous 2. Increase fluid intake 3. Attain/maintain normal weight 4. Feed, assist with feeding, or place foods within patient's reach *Promote comfort* 1. Mouth care: to facilitate mastication of food→improved digestion and absorption 2. Relieve constipation (see nursing care plan for Constipation, p. 165) 3. Observe for stomatitis, bleeding, changes in skin texture, color 4. Medications: monitor nausea and vomiting side effects of prescribed medications; administer antiemetics as ordered to control nausea and vomiting 5. Ambulate to alleviate flatulence and distention 6. Alleviate pain and discomfort by distractions, increased social interactions, pleasant environment, backrubs, and administration of prn pain medications, as ordered *Health teaching* 1. Diet and elimination 2. See Unit 3 for foods *high in protein and carbohydrate*	No complications Patient obtains/maintains normal weight No tissue breakdown

Condition	Definition	Assessment	Nursing diagnosis	Plan/implementation	Evaluation
Constipation	Waste material in the bowel is too hard to pass easily; or bowel movements are so infrequent that patient has discomfort	*Subjective data:* discomfort, pain, distress, and pressure in the rectum; reported decrease in normal elimination pattern *Objective data:* immobilization; hard-formed stool, possible palpable impaction; decreased bowel sounds; bowel elimination less frequent than usual	*Constipation* related to decreased water and fiber intake *Knowledge deficit* related to dietary and exercise requirements to prevent constipation	*Promote normal pattern of bowel elimination* 1. Administer: stool softeners or bulk cathartics as ordered; oil retention, soap suds enemas as ordered 2. Encourage change of position and activity as tolerated 3. Provide *high-bulk* diet 4. *Increase fluid* intake 5. Provide for privacy 6. Encourage regular time for evacuation *Health teaching* 1. Dietary instructions regarding increased fiber 2. Exercise program as tolerated 3. Increase fluids	Patient has normal bowel elimination pattern No impactions Increases fluid and fiber in diet
Osteoporosis	Metabolic bone disorder in which there is a generalized loss of bone density due to an imbalance between formation and bone resorption; immobilization can cause calcium losses of 200–300 mg/d	*Subjective data:* backache *Objective data:* demineralization of bone seen on X ray; kyphosis; spontaneous fracture of bone	*Pain* related to bone fractures or body structural changes	*Prevent injury related to decreased bone strength* 1. *Position:* correct body alignment, firm mattress 2. Encourages self-care activities: plan maximum activity allowed by physical condition; muscle exercises against resistance as tolerated 3. Rest/activity pattern: encourage ROM exercise; *avoid* fatigue 4. Weight-bearing positions, tilt table 5. *Diet:* high protein, high vitamin C, calcium rich 6. Increase fluids to prevent renal calculi (calcium from bones could cause kidney stones) *Health teaching* 1. Dietary instructions, foods to include for high-protein, high-vitamin C, high-calcium diet 2. Exercise program 3. Signs and symptoms of renal calculi	No fractures No renal calculi Incorporates dietary improvements in daily menu selection Participates in exercise program on a regular basis
Contractures	Abnormal shortening of muscle tissue, rendering the muscle highly resistant to stretching; related to lack of active or passive ROM, or improper support and	*Subjective data:* pain *Objective data:* muscles—fixed, shortened, decreased tone; resistance of muscles to stretch; decreased ROM in affected limb	*Impaired physical mobility* related to muscle weakness and contractures *Pain* related to injury *Self-care deficit* related to immobility	*Prevent deformities* 1. Active and/or passive ROM 2. *Positioning:* functional, correct alignment 3. Footboard to prevent footdrop 4. *Avoid* knee gatch	ROM maintained No deformities noted

continued

Adult

■ TABLE 2.31 *(Continued)*

Disorder	Pathophysiology	Assessment	Analysis/Nursing Diagnosis	Nursing Care Plan/Implementation	Evaluation/Outcome Criteria
Contractures *continued*	positioning of joints affected by arthritis or injury			*Health teaching* 1. Importance of ROM exercises 2. Correct anatomic positions	No skin breakdown
Skin breakdown	Presence of risk factors that could lead to skin breakdown, such as immobility, inadequate nutrition, lack of position changes	*Subjective data:* fatigue; pain; inability to turn on own *Objective data:* interruption of skin integrity, especially over ears, occiput, heels, sacrum, scrotum, elbows, trochanter, ischium, scapular; immobilization; malnutrition	*Impaired skin integrity* related to lack of frequent position change	*Prevent skin breakdown* 1. Change position q1–2h and prn, out of bed when possible 2. Protect from infection 3. Increase *dietary* intake: protein, carbohydrates 4. Increase *fluids* Assess for / reduce contributing factors known to cause decubitus ulcers: incontinence, stationary position, malnutrition, obesity, sensory deficits, emotional disturbances, paralysis *Promote healing* 1. Wash gently, pat dry—to avoid skin abrasion 2. Clean, dry, wrinkle-free bed linens and pads 3. Massage skin with lotion that does *not contain alcohol* (alcohol dries skin) 4. Protect with wafer barrier, alternating mattress, sheepskin pads, protectors, flotation devices 5. No "doughnuts" or rubber rings (interfere with circulation of tissue within center of ring)	
Urinary stasis	Immobility leads to inability to completely empty the bladder, which increases risk for urinary tract infection and renal calculi	*Subjective data:* pain, due to infection or renal calculi *Objective data:* difficulty in urinating due to position or lack of privacy; infection related to catheter insertion or stasis of urine; hematuria	*Altered urinary elimination* related to inability to empty bladder	*Prevent urinary infections, stasis, or renal calculi* 1. Increase activity as allowed 2. Check for distended bladder 3. Increase fluids, I&O 4. *Diet:* acid ash to increase acidity, thereby preventing infection 5. *Avoid* catheterization; use intermittent catheterization instead of Foley whenever possible or *Crede maneuver* to empty bladder (manual exertion of pressure on the bladder to force urine out) 6. Bladder training	No urinary infections or evidence of renal calculi; bladder emptied, no urinary stasis

■ **FIGURE 2.8** **Types of traction. A. Buck's extension.** Skin traction applied to the medial and lateral aspects of an extremity with adhesive foam, moleskin, or use of "Buck's boot." **B. Bryant's traction.** Vertical suspension skin traction in which child's pelvis is elevated from the bed. **C. Russell's traction.** Skin traction composed of Buck's extension on the foreleg, three pulleys at the bottom, and a sling under the knee. Affords more freedom of movement than Buck's. **D. Pelvic traction.** Skin traction applied to the lumbosacral region by means of a pelvic belt. **E. Head halter.** Cervical traction applied to the head by means of a halter under the chin. **F. Crutchfield tongs.** Cervical traction using tongs into the skull. **G. Thomas' splint.** Full-leg splint that keeps the leg fully extended and the long bones in alignment. Pressure is on the ischium and perineal area. May be used with skin or skeletal traction. **H. Halo vest assembly.** Applied in operating room. Patient will usually be ambulatory 24 hours after application. (From Saxton DF, et al. *The Addison-Wesley Manual of Nursing Practice.* Menlo Park, CA: Addison-Wesley, 1983.)

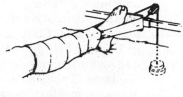

A

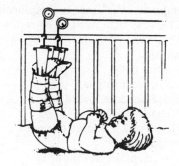

B

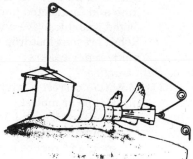

C

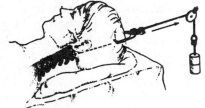

D

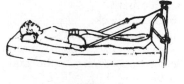

E

F

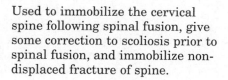

G

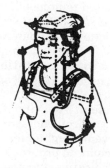

H

Used to immobilize the cervical spine following spinal fusion, give some correction to scoliosis prior to spinal fusion, and immobilize non-displaced fracture of spine.

4. *Immobilization*—maintains reduction and promotes healing of bone fragments. Achieved by:
   a. *External fixation*
      (1) Casts—types:

(a) *Spica*—applied to immobilize hip or shoulder joints.
(b) Body cast—applied to trunk.
(c) Arm or leg cast—joints above and below site included in cast.
(2) Splints, continuous traction.
(3) External fixation devices (Charnley)—multiple pins/rods through limb above and below fracture site, attached to external metal supports. Patient able to become ambulatory.
b. *Internal fixation*—pins, wires, nails, rods. See VI. Total hip replacement, p. 175, and VII. Total knee replacement, p. 177.

◆ **C. Assessment:**
1. *Subjective data*
   a. Pain, tenderness.
   b. Tingling, numbness.
   c. Nausea.
   d. History of traumatic event.
2. *Objective data*
   a. Function: abnormal or lost.
   b. Deformities.
   c. Ecchymosis, increased heat over injured part.
   d. Localized edema.
   e. Muscle spasm.
   f. Crepitation (grating sensations heard or felt as bone fragments rub against each other).
   g. Signs of shock.
   h. Indicators of anxiety.
   i. X ray: *fracture*—positive interruption of bone; *dislocation*—abnormal position of bone.

◆ **D. Analysis/nursing diagnosis:**
1. *Pain* related to interruption in bone.
2. *Impaired physical mobility* related to fracture/treatment modality.
3. *Risk for injury* related to complications of fractures.
4. *Knowledge deficit* regarding cast care, crutch walking, traction.
5. *Constipation* related to immobilization.
6. *Risk for impaired skin integrity* related to immobility or friction from materials used to immobilize the fracture during healing.

◆ **E. Nursing care plan/implementation:**
1. Goal: *promote healing and prevent complications of fractures* (Table 2.32).
   a. *Diet:* high protein, iron, vitamins, to improve tissue repair; moderate carbohydrates to prevent weight gain; no increase in calcium, to prevent kidney stones (decalcification and demineralization occur when patient is immobilized).
   b. Encourage *increased fluid intake,* to prevent kidney stones.
   c. Prevent or correct constipation through *increasing bulk foods, fruits, and fruit juices,* or utilizing prescribed stool softeners, laxatives, or cathartics as necessary.
   d. Provide activities to reduce perceptual deprivation—reading, handcrafts, music, special interests/hobbies that can be done while maintaining correct position for healing.
2. Goal: *prevent injury or trauma in relation to:*
▶ a. *Fracture care*
   (1) Maintain affected part in optimum alignment.
   (2) Maintain skin integrity; check all bony prominences for evidence of pressure q4h and prn, depending on amount of pressure.
   (3) Monitor: circulation in, sensation of, and motion of (CSM) affected part q15min for first 4 h; q1h until 24 h; q4h and prn, depending on amount of edema. (Table 2.33).
   (4) Maintain mobility in unaffected limb and unaffected joints of affected limb by active and passive ROM; prevent footdrop by using ankle-top sneakers.
▶ b. *Skin traction*
   (1) Maintain correct alignment:
      (a) If tape or moleskin is used, shave extremity and apply benzoin to improve adherence of strip and reduce itching.
      (b) Check apparatus for slippage, bunching, and replace prn.
   (2) Prevent tissue injury:
      (a) Check all bony prominences for evidence of pressure: q15min for first 4 h; q1h until 24 h, q4h and prn, depending on amount of edema.
      (b) Nonadhesive traction may be removed q8h to check skin (e.g., Bryant's).
▶ c. *Skeletal traction*
   (1) Maintain affected part in optimum alignment:
      (a) Ropes on pulleys.
      (b) Weights hang free.
      (c) Elevate head of bed as prescribed.
      (d) Check knots routinely.
   (2) Maintain skin integrity:
      (a) Frequent skin care.
      (b) Keep bedlinens free of crumbs and wrinkles.
   (3) Prevent infection: special skin care to pin insertion site tid. Keep area around pins clean and dry. Utilize prescribed solution for cleansing.

(4) Monitor: circulation, sensation, motion of affected part (see a. Fracture care, p. 168).

(5) Maintain mobility in unaffected limb and unaffected joints; prevent footdrop of affected limb.

► d. *Running traction*

(1) Keep well centered in bed.

(2) *Elevate head of bed only* to point of countertraction.

(3) *No* turning from side to side—will cause rubbing of bony fragments.

(4) Check distal circulation frequently.

(5) Frequent back care to prevent skin breakdown.

(6) Fracture bed pan for toileting.

(7) *Avoid* excessive padding of splints in groin area to prevent tissue trauma.

► e. *Balanced suspension traction:*

(1) Maintain alignment and countertraction:

   (a) Ropes on pulleys.

   (b) Weights hang free.

   (c) Elevate head of bed as prescribed.

   (d) Check knots routinely.

(2) May move patient, but turn only slightly (no more than 30 degrees to *unaffected* side).

(3) Heel of affected leg must remain free of the bed.

(4) *20-degree angle* between thigh and bed.

(5) Check for pressure from sling to popliteal area.

(6) Provide foot support to prevent footdrop.

(7) Maintain *abduction* of extremity.

(8) Check for signs of infection at pin insertion sites; cleanse tid as ordered.

(9) If tape or moleskin is used, shave extremity and apply benzoin to improve adherence of strip and reduce itching.

► f. *Cervical traction:*

(1) May be placed on specialized bed, e.g., Stryker frame.

(2) *Position:* maintain body alignment.

(3) Keep tongs free from bed, and keep weights hanging freely to allow traction to function properly.

g. *Halo traction:*

(1) Several times a day, check screws to the head and screws that hold the upper portion of the frame, to determine correct position.

(2) Pin sites cleansed tid with bacteriostatic solution to prevent infection.

(3) Monitor for signs of infection.

(4) *Position* as any other patient in body cast, except no pressure to rest on halo—pillows may be placed under abdomen and chest when patient is prone.

(5) Institute ROM exercises to prevent contractures.

(6) Turn frequently to prevent development of pressure areas.

(7) Allow patient to verbalize about having screws placed in skull.

(8) Postapplication nursing care same as pin insertion for other traction.

► h. *External fixation devices:*

(1) Pin care same as for skeletal traction.

(2) Teach clothing adjustment.

(3) Teach to adjust for size of apparatus.

i. *Internal fixation devices:*

(1) Monitor for signs of infection/allergic reaction to materials used for maintenance of reduction (drainage, pain, increased temperature).

(2) Position as ordered to prevent dislocation.

► j. *Casts:*

(1) Support drying cast on firm pillow; avoid finger imprints on cast.

(2) *Elevate* limb to reduce edema.

(3) Prevent complications of fractures as listed.

(4) Closely monitor: *circulation* (blanching, swelling, decreased temperature); *sensation* (absence of feeling or pain or burning); and *motion* (inability to move digits of affected limb).

(5) **Be prepared to notify MD or cut cast if circulatory impairment occurs.**

(6) Protect skin integrity: avoid pressure of edges of cast; petal prn.

(7) Monitor for signs of infection if skin integrity impaired.

3. Goal: *provide care related to ambulation with crutches.*

► a. See Teaching Crutch Walking (Table 2.34).

b. Measure crutches correctly (Table 2.35).

(1) Subtract 16 in. from total height; top of crutch should be 2 in. below the axilla.

(2) Complete extension of the elbows should be possible without pressure of axilla bar into the axilla.

(3) Handgrip should be adjusted so that complete wrist extension is possible.

(4) Instruct in correct body alignment:

   (a) Head erect.

   (b) Back straight.

■ TABLE 2.32   Complications of Fractures

Complication	Assessment	Analysis/Nursing Diagnosis	Nursing Care Plan/Implementation	Evaluation/Outcome Criteria
Shock (see p. 63)				
Thrombophlebitis (see p. 69)				
Fat emboli: serious, potentially life-threatening complication in which pressure changes in interior of fracture force molecules of fat from marrow into systemic circulation; may cause problems in respiratory or nervous system; seen most frequently on third day after multiple fractures, fractures of long bones, or comminuted fracture	*Subjective data:* dyspnea, severe chest pain; confusion, agitation; decrease in level of consciousness; numbness; feeling faint; history of diabetes, obesity *Objective data:* cyanosis; pupillary changes; muscle twitching; petechiae—chest, buccal cavity, axilla, conjunctiva, soft palate; extremities—pallor, cold; shock; vomiting	*Risk for injury* related to fat emboli *Altered tissue perfusion* related to fat emboli	1. *Position:* high Fowler's to relieve respiratory symptoms 2. Administer oxygen stat, to relieve anoxia and reduce surface tension of fat globules 3. Institute respiratory support measures, as ordered—IPPB, respiratory assistive devices: **be prepared for CPR** in event of respiratory failure 4. Monitor vital signs, cardiac monitor, q15min during acute episode and prn (shock/cardiac failure possible) 5. Obtain baseline data and monitor level of consciousness, neurologic signs q15 min during acute episode and prn (neurologic involvement possible) 6. Administer parenteral fluids, as ordered: IV alcohol, blood and fluid replacements 7. Administer medications as ordered: corticosteroids; digitalis; aminophylline; heparin sodium 8. **DO NOT RUB ANY LEG CRAMPS, BUT REPORT IMMEDIATELY**	Patient alert Pain relieved Respiratory, cardiac, and neurologic statuses have no permanent damage
Nerve compression: pressure on nerve in affected area from edema, dislocation of bone, or immobilization apparatus; if pressure not relieved, permanent paralysis can result	*Subjective data:* discomfort, pain, referred pain; burning, tingling, "stinging sensation"; numbness, altered sensation, inability to distinguish touch *Objective data:* limited movement; muscle weakness; paralysis; reflexes—diminished, irritable, or absent; color changes related to impaired circulation	*Pain* related to pressure on nerve *Potential for physical injury* related to pressure on nerve *Impaired tissue perfusion* related to impaired circulation *Impaired physical mobility* related to joint contracture, numbness	1. Monitor for potential signs q1h for first 48 h; neurovascular assessment q12h and prn as condition indicates (circulation, sensation, motion—CSM) 2. *Elevate* affected limb; flex hand or foot of affected extremity; passive and active ROM exercises 3. **Be prepared to cut cast or remove constrictions if signs of impairment present** 4. Begin active ROM exercises to unaffected extremities 5. Use footboard to prevent footdrop 6. Encourage use of trapeze if applicable 7. Isometric exercises, as ordered 8. Ambulation, weight bearing as ordered, support casts	Sensation, motor function are normal No complications noted
Avascular necrosis/circulatory impairment: interference with normal circulation to affected area due to interruption of blood vessel, pres-	*Subjective data:* tenderness; pain, especially on passive motion *Objective data:* edema, swelling in affected area; decreased	*Risk for altered peripheral tissue perfusion,* related to vessel damage	1. Monitor for potential signs q1h for first 48 h; blanching, coolness, edema; palpate pulse above and below injury, report absent or major discrepancies stat 2. *Elevate* affected limb to decrease edema	Circulation adequate to limb, to prevent tissue damage

Assessment	Nursing diagnosis	Nursing care plan/implementation	Evaluation/outcome criteria
sure on the vessel from dislocation, edema, or immobilization devices; results of impaired circulation lead to discomfort and, if not corrected, necrosis of tissue and bone due to lack of oxygen supply color, temperature, mobility; bleeding from wound		3. Report to physician if signs persist 4. Be prepared to assist with bivalving of casts, or cut cast to relieve pressure 5. Monitor size of drainage stains on casts; measure accurately and report if size increases	No infection or heals with no serious complications
Infection *Subjective data:* pain *Objective data:* elevated temperature and pulse; erythema—discoloration of surrounding skin; edema—sudden, local induration; drainage—thin, watery, foul-smelling exudate; crepitus (may be indicative of gas gangrene); with cast—warm area, foul smell	*Risk for injury* related to tissue destruction *Altered peripheral tissue perfusion* related to swelling	1. Monitor vital signs, drainage 2. Ensure patient has had prophylactic tetanus toxoid 3. May have prophylactic antibiotics ordered if wound was contaminated at time of injury 4. Instruct patient *not* to touch open wound, pin sites or put anything inside cast (could interrupt skin interity and become potential source of infection)	
Delayed union/nonunion: failure of bone to heal within normal time related to lack of use, inadequate circulation, other complicating medical conditions such as diabetes or poor nutrition *Subjective data:* pain *Objective data:* lack of callus formation on X ray; poor alignment	*Risk for injury* related to poor healing of bone fracture *Impaired physical mobility* related to lower-limb fractures *Dressing/grooming, bathing/hygiene, self-care deficit* related to upper-limb fracture	1. Maintain immobilization and alignment of affected limb 2. Maintain adequate nutrition 3. *Avoid* trauma to affected limb 4. Monitor for circulatory or infection complication 5. Dietary instructions regarding foods containing *calcium* and *protein* necessary for bone healing	Bone heals No complications noted Pain decreased Ambulation and self-care return to preinjury status
Skin breakdown (related to cast) *Subjective data:* pain *Objective data:* temperature and pulse elevated; erythema; edema—cast edges, exposed distal portion of limb, limb area within cast; drainage and foul odor from break in skin, may be under cast and stain through or exit at ends of cast; crepitus (crackling sound could indicate gas gangrene); hyperactive reflexes	*Impaired skin integrity* related to cast trauma	1. If open wound: verify tetanus administration; monitor site through cast window, change dressing daily and prn 2. Apply lotion or cornstarch to exposed skin (no powder) 3. Petal tape edges of cast to reduce irritation 4. Inspect skin for irritation, edema, odor, drainage—q2h initially, then q3h 5. Instruct patient not to place any object under cast as skin abrasions may lead to decubitus ulcers 6. Promote drying of cast by leaving it uncovered and exposed to air for 48 h; use no plastic 7. Prevent indenting casts with fingertips or hard surface: place on pillows; use palms of hands when positioning affected limb 8. *Avoid* excessive padding of Thomas splint in groin area—padding traps moisture, skin breakdown	No skin breakdown

continued

Adult

■ **TABLE 2.32** *(Continued)*

Complication	Assessment	Analysis/Nursing Diagnosis	Nursing Care Plan/Implementation	Evaluation/Outcome Criteria
Duodenal distress (with spica cast): spica cast incorporates the trunk and affected limb and can cause respiratory or abdominal distress when edema is present under the cast or cast is too tight to allow for normal body functions	*Subjective data:* anorexia, nausea, abdominal pain *Objective data:* duodenal distress, vomiting, distention, cast too tight	*Ineffective breathing pattern* related to pressure from cast *Pain* related to abdominal distress from pressure *Fear* related to cast constriction	1. Place on firm mattress; use bed boards if necessary to reduce muscle spasm 2. Maintain warmth by covering uncasted areas 3. *Avoid* turning for first 8 h; when turning: use enough personnel to log-roll; do not use bar between legs while turning device; support chest with pillows 4. Monitor for signs of respiratory distress: increased respirations, apprehension 5. Monitor for signs of duodenal distress: vomiting, distention; *if these signs occur:* place in prone position; have cast bivalved; may need NG tube; monitor for fluid imbalance 6. Protect cast with nonabsorbent material during elimination	Complications avoided or detected early enough to prevent serious damage

■ **TABLE 2.33 Assessing Neurovascular Status in an Injured Limb**

- Assessing *circulation* to the limb
  1. Warmth and color
  2. Capillary refill
  3. Peripheral pulse(s)
- Assessing *nerve supply* to the limb
  1. Upper extremities
     a. Sensory: pinprick over fingertips, dorsum of hand
     b. Motor: dorsiflexion and palmar flexion of wrist
  2. Lower extremities
     a. Sensory: pinprick over heel and dorsum of foot
     b. Motor: dorsiflexion and plantar flexion of foot

Source: Caroline NL. *Emergency Care in the Street* (5th ed.), Boston: Little, Brown, 1995.

■ **TABLE 2.34 Teaching Crutch Walking**

A. When only *one* leg can bear weight:
  1. *Swing-to gait:* crutches forward; swing body to crutches
     a. Move both crutches forward
     b. Move both legs to meet the crutches
     c. Continue pattern
  2. *Swing-through gait:* crutches forward; swing body through crutches
     a. Move both crutches forward
     b. Move both legs farther ahead than crutches
     c. Continue pattern
  3. *Three-point gait:* crutches and affected extremity forward; swing forward, placing nonaffected foot ahead or between crutches
     a. Both crutches and affected limb move at same time
     b. Move both crutches and affected leg (e.g., left) ahead 6 in.
     c. Move unaffected leg (e.g., right) to same place as left and crutches
     d. Continue pattern
B. When *both* legs can move separately and bear some weight:
  1. *Four-point gait:* right crutch forward, left foot forward; swing weight to right side while bringing left crutch forward, then right foot forward; gait simulates normal walking
     a. Move right crutch forward 4–6 in.
     b. Move left foot forward same distance as right crutch
     c. Move left crutch forward ahead of left foot
     d. Move right foot forward to meet right crutch
     e. Continue pattern
  2. *Two-point gait:* as four-point gait but faster; one crutch and opposite leg moving forward at same time
     a. Opposite crutch and limb move together
     b. Move right crutch and left leg ahead 6 in.
     c. Move left crutch and right leg ahead
     d. Continue pattern
C. When patient is *unable* to walk: *tripod* gait: crutches forward at a wide distance; drag legs to point just behind crutches, balance, and repeat

            (c) Chest forward.
            (d) Feet 6–8 in. apart, wide base for support.
        4. Goal: *provide safety measures related to possible complications following fracture* (see Table 2.32).

■ **TABLE 2.35 Measuring Crutches Correctly**

1. Have patient lie on a flat surface. Measure from anterior fold of axilla to 4 in. lateral to heel.
2. Have patient stand. Measure from 1–2 in. below axilla to 2 in. in front of and 6 in. to the side of the foot.
3. Hand placement on bar of crutch: have patient stand upright, support body weight with hand on bar (not putting weight on axilla). Elbow flexion should be 30 degrees.
4. Slightly pad the shoulder rests of the crutches for general comfort.
5. Make sure there are nonskid rubber tips on the crutches.

        5. Goal: *health teaching.*
           a. Explain and show apparatus before application, if possible.
           b. Pin care at least once daily to prevent granulation and cellulitis.
           c. Correct position for rest/sleep and prevention of injury with halo traction—no pressure on halo.
           d. Purpose of cast: to immobilize, to support body tissues, to prevent or correct deformities.
           e. Teach signs and symptoms of complications to report related to cast care (i.e., numbness, odor, crack/break in cast; extremity cold, bluish).
           f. Isometric exercises for use with affected joint.
        ▶ g. *Safety measures with crutches:*
              (1) Weight bearing on hands, not axilla.
              (2) Position crutches 4 in. to side and 4 in. to front.
              (3) Use short strides, looking ahead, not at feet.
              (4) Prevent injury: if patient begins to fall, throw crutches to side to prevent falling on them; body should be relaxed.
              (5) Check for environmental hazards: rugs, water spills.
   ◆ **F. Evaluation/outcome criteria:**
        1. No injury or complications related to apparatus or immobilization (e.g., infection, tissue injury, altered circulation/sensation, dislocation).
        2. Bone remains in correct alignment and begins to heal.
        3. Demonstrates elevated limb position to relieve edema with casted extremity.
        4. Lists complications related to circulation and/or neurologic impairment and infection.
        5. Begins to use affected part.
        6. Demonstrates correct technique for ambulation with crutches—no pressure on axilla, utilizes strength of arms and wrists.
        7. No falls while using crutches.
IV. Compartment syndrome: an accumulation of fluid in the muscle compartment, resulting in an increase in pressure that reduces blood flow to the

tissues. Can lead to neuromuscular deficit, amputation, and death.

A. Risk factors:
1. Fractures.
2. Burns.
3. Crushing injuries.
4. Restrictive bandages.
5. Cast.
6. Prolonged lithotomy positioning.

B. Pathophysiology: inability of the fascia surrounding the muscle group to expand to accommodate the increased volume of fluid → compartment pressure increases → venous flow impaired → arterial flow continues, increasing capillary pressure → fluid pushed into the extravascular space → intracompartment pressure further increased → prolonged or severe ischemia → muscle and nerve cells destroyed, contracture, loss of function, necrotic tissue, infection, release of potassium, hydrogen, and myoglobin into bloodstream.

◆ **C. Assessment:**
1. *Subjective data*
    a. Severe, unrelenting pain, unrelieved by narcotics and associated with passive stretching of muscle.
    b. Paresthesias.
2. *Objective data*
    a. Edema; tense skin over limb.
    b. Paralysis.
    c. Decreased or absent pulses.
    d. Poor capillary refill.
    e. Limb temperature change (colder).
    f. Ankle-arm pressure index (API) decreased; 0.4 indicates ischemia (see Unit 5, Doppler ultrasonography, p. 294).
    g. Urine output—decreased (developing acute tubular necrosis); reddish-brown color.

◆ **D. Analysis/nursing diagnosis:**
1. *Pain* related to tissue swelling and ischemia.
2. *Risk for injury* related to neuromuscular deficits.
3. *Impaired physical mobility* related to contracture and loss of function.
4. *Risk for infection* related to tissue necrosis.
5. *Altered urinary elimination* related to acute tubular necrosis from myoglobin accumulation.
6. *Body image disturbance* related to limb disfigurement.

◆ **E. Nursing care plan/implementation:**
1. Goal: *recognize early indications of ischemia.*
    a. Assess neurovascular status frequently (q1h): skin temperature, capillary refill, peripheral pulses, mobility, and sensation.
    b. Listen to patient complaints; report suspected complications.
    c. Report nonrelief of pain with narcotics.

    d. Recognize unrelenting pain with passive muscle stretching.
2. Goal: *prevent complications.*
    a. *Elevate* injured extremity initially; if ischemia suspected, keep extremity at heart level to prevent compensatory increase in blood flow.
    b. Avoid tight bandages, splints, or casts.
    c. Monitor intravenous infusion for signs of infiltration.
    d. Prepare patient for fasciotomy (incision of skin and fascia to release tight compartment).

◆ **F. Evaluation/outcome criteria:**
1. Relief from pain; normal perfusion restored.
2. Neurovascular status within normal limits.
3. Retains function of limb; no contractures or infection.
4. Compartment pressure returns to normal (<20 mm Hg.).
5. No systemic complications (e.g., normal cardiac and renal function, acid-base balance within normal limits).

V. Osteoarthritis: joint disorder characterized by degeneration of articular cartilage and formation of bony outgrowths at edges of weight-bearing joints.

A. Pathophysiology: excessive friction combined with risk factors → thinning of articular cartilage, narrowing of joint space, and loss of joint stability; cartilage erodes, producing shallow pits on articular surface and exposing bone in joint space. Bone responds by becoming denser and harder.

B. Risk factors:
1. Aging (>50).
2. Rheumatoid arthritis.
3. Arteriosclerosis.
4. Obesity.
5. Trauma.
6. Family history.

◆ **C. Assessment:**
1. *Subjective data*
    a. Pain; tender joints.
    b. Fatigability, malaise.
    c. Anorexia.
    d. Cold intolerance.
    e. Extremities: numb, tingling.
2. *Objective data*
    a. Joints
        (1) Enlarged.
        (2) Stiff, limited movement.
        (3) Swelling, redness, and heat around affected joint.
        (4) Shiny stretched skin over and around joint.
        (5) Subcutaneous nodules.
    b. Weight loss.
    c. Fever.
    d. Crepitation (creaking or grating of joints).
    e. Deformities, contractures.

f. Cold, clammy extremities.

g. Lab data: decreased Hgb, elevated WBC.

h. Diagnostic tests: X ray, thermography, arthroscopy.

◆ **D. Analysis/nursing diagnosis:**

1. *Pain* related to friction of bones in joints.
2. *Bathing/hygiene self-care deficit* related to decreased mobility of involved joints.
3. *Risk for injury* related to fatigability.
4. *Impaired physical mobility* related to stiff, limited movement.
5. *Impaired home maintenance management* related to contractures.

◆ **E. Nursing care plan/implementation:**

1. Goal: *promote comfort: reduce pain, spasms, inflammation, swelling.*
   a. Medications as prescribed:
      (1) Anti-inflammatory agents: aspirin (Ecotrin), ibuprofen (Motrin), indomethacin (Indocin), corticosteroids.
      (2) Antimalarials: chloroquine (Aralen), HCl/hydroxychoroquine (Plaquenil), to relieve symptoms.
   b. Heat to reduce muscle spasm.
   c. Cold to reduce swelling and pain.
   d. Prevent contractures:
      (1) Exercise.
      (2) Bedrest on firm mattress during attacks.
      (3) Splints to maintain proper alignment.
   e. *Elevate* extremity to reduce swelling.
   f. Rest.
   g. Assistive devices to decrease weight bearing of affected joints (canes, walkers).
2. Goal: *health teaching to promote independence.*
   a. Encourage self-care with assistive devices for ADL.
   b. Activity, as tolerated, with ambulation-assistive devices.
   c. Scheduled rest periods.
   d. Correct body posture and body mechanics.
3. Goal: *provide for emotional needs.*
   a. Accept feelings of frustration regarding long-term debilitating disorder.
   b. Provide diversional activities appropriate for age and physical condition to promote comfort and satisfaction.

◆ **F. Evaluation/outcome criteria:**

1. Remains independent as long as possible.
2. No contractures.
3. States comfort has improved.
4. Uses methods that are successful in pain control.

VI. Total hip replacement: femoral head and acetabulum are replaced by a prosthesis, which is cemented into the bone with plastic cement. Performed to replace a joint with limited and painful function due to bony alkalosis and deformity, caused by degenerative joint disease. Goal of the surgery: restore or improve mobilization of hip joint and prevent complications of extended immobilization.

A. Risk factors:

1. Rheumatoid arthritis.
2. Osteoarthritis.
3. Complications of femoral neck fractures (Table 2.36).
4. Congenital hip disease.

◆ **B. Analysis/nursing diagnosis:**

1. *Risk for injury* related to implant surgery.
2. *Knowledge deficit* regarding joint replacement surgery.
3. *Impaired physical mobility* related to major hip surgery.
4. *Pain* related to surgical incision.
5. *Risk for impaired skin integrity* related to immobility.

◆ **C. Nursing care plan/implementation:**

1. *Preoperative*
   a. Goal: *prevent thrombophlebitis or pulmonary emboli.*
      (1) Antiembolic stockings.
      (2) Increase fluid intake.
   b. Goal: *prevent infection:* antibiotics as ordered, given prophylactically.
   c. Goal: *health teaching.*
      (1) *Isometric exercises*—gluteal, abdominal, and quadricep setting, dorsiflexion and plantar flexion of the feet.
      (2) Use of trapeze.
      (3) Explain position of operative leg and hip postoperatively to prevent *adduction* and flexion.
      (4) Transfer techniques—bed to chair and chair to crutches; dangle at bedside first time out of bed.
      (5) Assist patient with skin scrubs with antibacterial soap.
2. *Postoperative*
   a. Goal: *prevent respiratory complications.*
      (1) Turn, cough, and deep breathe.
      (2) Incentive spirometry.
   b. Goal: *prevent complications of shock or infection.*
      (1) Check dressings for drainage q1h for first 4 h; then q4h and prn; may have Hemovac or other drainage tubes inserted in wound to keep dressing dry.
      (2) Monitor I&O and vital signs hourly for 4 h, then q4h and prn.
   c. Goal: *prevent contractures, muscle atrophy:* initiate exercises as soon as allowed; isometric quadriceps, dorsiflexion and plantar flexion of foot, and flexion and extension of the ankle.
   d. Goal: *promote early ambulation and movement.*

Adult

■ **TABLE 2.36** **Types of Hip Fractures**

	Assessment	Treatment	Complications
Femoral neck (intracapsular)	History of slight trauma Pain in groin and hip Pain with hip movement Usually occurs in women >60 Lateral rotation and shortening of leg with minimal deformity	Femoral head replacement with prosthesis, threaded pins Occasionally, primary total hip replacement	Avascular necrosis of femoral head Nonunion Pin complications Dislocation of prosthesis
Intertrochanteric (extracapsular)	History of direct trauma over trochanter Severe pain Tenderness over trochanter Usually women 60–85 or younger women with osteoporosis External rotation and shortening of leg with obvious deformity Loss of hip motion	Open reduction: internal fixation with nail, pin, compression plate with screw	Shortening of the leg Traumatic arthritis Pin migration; bending or breaking of pin Fracture impaction Loss of reduction Delayed union or nonunion of bone
Subtrochanteric (extracapsular)	History of direct trauma of great force Proximal leg pain Usually women >60 External rotation and shortening of leg with some deformity Large hematoma	Open reduction: internal fixation with intramedullary nail, sliding nail plates, and other fixed plates Closed reduction with nail insertion Closed intramedullary device (nail)	Shortening of the leg; metal fatigue Lateral displacement of proximal fragment Metal fatigue

Source: Dunajcik L. The hip: Nursing fracture patients to full recovery. *RN* 52(4):1989; 57.

(1) Use trapeze.

(2) Transfer technique (pivot on unaffected leg); crutches/walker.

(3) Initiate progressive ambulation as ordered; ensure maximum extension of leg when walking.

(4) Administer anticoagulation therapy as ordered prophylactically to prevent thromboemboli.

(5) Recognize early side effects of medications and report appropriately.

e. Goal: *prevent constipation.*
   (1) Increase fluid intake.
   (2) Use fracture bed pan.

f. Goal: *prevent dislocation of prosthesis.*
   (1) Maintain *abduction* of the affected joint (prevent external rotation); elevate head of bed, turn according to physician's order. When turning to unaffected side, turn with abduction pillow between legs to maintain abduction.

   ▶ (2) Buck's extension or Russell's traction may be applied (temporary skin traction).

   (3) Plaster booties with an abduction bar may be used.

   (4) Wedge Charnley (triangle-shaped) pillow to *maintain abduction* between knees and lower legs.

   (5) Provide periods throughout day when patient lies flat in bed to *prevent hip flexion* and strengthen hip muscles.

   (6) Report signs of dislocation: *anteriorly*—knee flexes, leg turns outward, leg looks longer than other, femur head may be felt in groin area; *posteriorly*—leg turns inward, appears shorter than other, greater trochanter elevated.

g. Goal: *promote comfort.*
   (1) Initiate skin care; monitor pressure points for redness; back care q2h.
   (2) Alternating pressure mattress; sheepskin when sitting in chair.

h. Goal: *health teaching.*
   (1) Exercise program with written list of activity restrictions.
   (2) Methods to prevent hip adduction.
   (3) *Avoid* sitting for more than 1 h: stand, stretch, and walk frequently to prevent hip flexion contractures.
   (4) Advise *not to exceed 90 degrees of hip flexion* (dislocation can occur, particularly with posterior incisions); avoid low chairs.
   (5) Teach altered methods of usual self-care activities to prevent hip dislocation—e.g., *avoid:* bending from waist to tie shoes, sitting up straight in a low chair, using a low toilet seat.
   (6) *Avoid* crossing legs, driving a car for 6 wk.

(7) Wear support hose for 6 wk to enhance venous return and avoid thrombus formation.

◆ **D. Evaluation/outcome criteria:**
1. Participates in postoperative nursing care plan to prevent complications.
2. Reports pain has decreased.
3. Ambulates with assistive devices.
4. Complications of immobility avoided.
5. Able to resume self-care activities.

VII. Total knee replacement: both sides of the joint are replaced by metal or plastic implants.

◆ **A. Analysis:** see VI. Total hip replacement, p. 175.

◆ **B. Nursing plan/implementation:**
1. See VI. Total hip replacement, p. 175.
2. Goal: *to achieve active flexion beyond 70 degrees.*
   a. *Immediately postop:* may have continuous passive motion (CPM) device for flexion/extension of affected knee. Maximum flexion 90 degrees.
   ▶ b. Monitor drainage in *Hemovac* (q15min for first 4 h, q1h until 24 h; q4h and prn while Hemovac in place).
   💊 c. Analgesics as ordered for pain.
   d. While dressings are still on: quadriceps-setting exercises for approximately 5 d (consult with physical therapist for specific instructions).
   e. After dressings removed: active flexion exercises.
   f. Avoid pressure on heel.

◆ **C. Evaluation/outcome criteria:**
1. No complications of infection, hemorrhage noted.
2. ROM of knee increases with exercises.

VIII. Amputation: surgical removal of a limb due to trauma or circulatory impairment (gangrene). The amount of tissue amputated is determined by the severity of disease or trauma and the ability of the remaining tissue to heal.

A. Risk factors:
1. Artherosclerosis obliterans.
2. Uncontrolled diabetes mellitus.
3. Malignancy.
4. Extensive and intractable infection.
5. Result of severe trauma.

◆ **B. Assessment:** *preoperative*
1. *Subjective data:* pain in affected part.
2. *Objective data*
   a. Soft-tissue damage.
   b. Partial or complete severance of a body part.
   c. Lack of peripheral pulses.
   d. Skin color changes, pallor → cyanosis → gangrene.
   e. Infection, hemorrhage, or shock.

◆ **C. Analysis/nursing diagnosis:**
1. *Impaired physical mobility* related to lower-limb amputation.

2. *Body image disturbance* related to loss of body part.
3. *Pain* related to interruption of nerve pathways.
4. *Anxiety* related to potential change in life-style.
5. *Knowledge deficit* related to rehabilitation goals.

◆ **D. Nursing care plan/implementation:**
1. Goal: *prepare for surgery, physically and emotionally.*
   a. Validate that patient and family are aware that amputation of body part is planned.
   b. Validate that informed consent is signed.
   c. Allow time for grieving.
   d. If time allows, prepare patient for postoperative phase, e.g., teach arm-strengthening exercises if lower limb is to be amputated; teach altered methods of ambulation.
   e. Provide time to discuss feelings.
   f. Prepare surgical site to decrease possibility of infection (e.g., shave, scrub as ordered).
   g. Discuss postoperative expectations.
2. Goal: *promote healing postoperatively.*
   ▶ a. Monitor respiratory status q1–4h and prn: rate, depth of respiration; auscultate for signs of congestion; and question patient about chest pain (pulmonary emboli common complication).
   b. Monitor for hemorrhage; keep tourniquet at bedside.
   💊 c. Medicate for pain as ordered—patient may have phantom pain.
   d. Support stump on pillow for first 24 h; **remove pillow** after 24 h to prevent contracture.
   e. *Position: turn patient onto stomach* to prevent hip contracture.
   f. ROM exercises for joint above amputation to prevent joint immobilization; strengthening exercises for arms, nonaffected limbs, abdominal muscles.
   ▶ g. *Stump care:*
      (1) Early postoperative dressings changed prn.
      (2) As incision heals, bandage is applied in cone shape to prepare stump for prosthesis.
      (3) Inspect for blisters, redness, abrasions.
      (4) Remove stump sock daily and prn.
   h. Assist in rehabilitation program.

◆ **E. Evaluation/outcome criteria:**
1. Begins rehabilitation program.
2. No hemorrhage, infection.
3. Adjusts to altered body image.

IX. Gout: disorder of purine metabolism; genetic disease believed to be transmitted by a dominant gene, characterized by recurrent attacks of acute pain and swelling of one joint (usually the great toe).

A. Pathophysiology: urate crystals and infiltrating leukocytes appear to damage the intracellular phagolysosomes, resulting in leakage of lysomal enzymes into the synovial fluid, causing tissue damage and joint inflammation.

B. Risk factors:
1. Men.
2. Age (>50).
3. Genetic/familial tendency.
4. Prolonged hyperuricemia (elevated serum uric acid).

◆ **C. Assessment:**
1. *Subjective data*
   a. Pain: excruciating.
   b. Fatigue.
   c. Anorexia.
2. *Objective data*
   a. Joint: erythema (redness), hot, swollen, difficult to move; skin stretched and shiny over joint.
   b. Subcutaneous nodules, trophi (deposits of nonsodium urate) on hands and feet.
   c. Weight loss.
   d. Fever.
   e. Sensory changes, with cold intolerance.
   f. Lab data:
      (1) Serum uric acid: increased significantly (6.5/100 mL in females, 7.5/100 mL in males) in chronic gout; only slightly increased in acute gout.
      (2) WBC: 12,000–15,000/μL.
      (3) Erythrocyte sedimentation rate: >20 mm.
      (4) 24-h urinary uric acid: slightly elevated.
      (5) Proteinuria (chronic gout).
      (6) Axotemia (presence of nitrogen-containing compounds in blood) in chronic gout.

◆ **D. Analysis/nursing diagnosis:**
1. *Pain* related to inflammation and swelling of affected joint.
2. *Impaired physical mobility* related to pain.
3. *Knowledge deficit* related to diet restrictions and increased fluid needs.
4. *Altered urinary elimination* related to kidney damage.

◆ **E. Nursing care plan/implementation:**
1. Goal: *decrease discomfort.*
   a. Administer antigout medications as ordered:
      (1) Treatment of acute attacks: colchicine, phenylbutazone (Butazolidin), indomethacin (Indocin), allopurinol (Zyloprim).
      (2) Preventive therapy: probenecid (Benemid), sulfinpyrazone (Anturane).

   b. Absolute rest of affected joint → gradual increase in activities, to prevent complications of immobilization; at the same time, rest for comfort.
2. Goal: *prevent kidney damage.*
   a. Increase fluid intake to 2000–3000 mL/d.
   b. Monitor urinary output.
3. Goal: *health teaching.*
   a. Need for *low-purine diet* during acute attack (see VII. Purine-restricted diet, Common Therapeutic Diets, Unit 3, p. 245).
   b. Importance of *increased fluid in diet.*
   c. Signs and symptoms of increased disease.
   d. Dosage and side effects of prescribed medications.

◆ **F. Evaluation/outcome criteria:**
1. Swelling decreased.
2. Discomfort alleviated.
3. Mobility returned to status prior to attack.
4. Lab values return to normal.

X. Herniated/ruptured disk (ruptured nucleus pulposus): strain or injury to a weakened cartilage between vertebrae can result in herniation of the nucleus, causing pressure on nerve roots in spinal canal, pain, and disability.

A. Pathophysiology: pulpy substance of disk interior (nucleus pulposus) bulges or ruptures through the outer annulus fibrosus → irritation and pressure on nerve endings in the spinal ligaments → muscle spasm and distortion of the joints of vertebral arches.

B. Risk factors:
1. Strain as result of poor body mechanics.
2. Trauma.
3. History of back injuries.

◆ **C. Assessment:**
1. *Lumbar injuries* (90% of herniations):
   a. *Subjective data*
      (1) Pain: low back, radiating to buttocks, posterior thigh, and calf; relieved by recumbency; aggravated by sneezing, coughing, and flexion; sciatic pain continues even when back pain subsides.
      (2) Numbness, tingling.
   b. *Objective data*
      (1) Muscle weakness—leg and foot.
      (2) Inability to flex leg.
      (3) Sensory loss, leg and foot.
      (4) Alterations in posture: leans to side, unable to stand up straight.
      (5) Edema: leg and foot.
      (6) Positive *Lasègue's sign:* straight leg raising with hip flexed and knee extended will produce sciatic pain.
2. *Cervical injuries* (10% of herniations):
   a. *Subjective data*

(1) Pain—upper extremities, radiating to hands and fingers; aggravated by coughing, sneezing, and straining.
(2) Tingling, burning sensation in upper extremities and back of neck.
b. *Objective data*
(1) Upper extremities: weakness and atrophy.
(2) Neck: restricted movement.
(3) Diagnostic tests for both lumbar and cervical injuries.
  (a) Spine X rays.
  (b) CAT scan.
  (c) MRI.
  (d) Myelography (less preferred than CAT scan or MRI).
  (e) Electromyography.
  (f) Neurologic exam: special attention to sensory status, including pain, touch, and temperature identification, and to motor status, including strength, gait, and reflexes.

◆ **D. Analysis/nursing diagnosis:**
1. *Pain* related to pressure on nerve roots.
2. *Fear* related to disease progression and/or potential surgery.
3. *Knowledge deficit* related to correct body mechanics.
4. *Impaired physical mobility* related to continued pain.
5. *Sleep pattern disturbance* related to difficulty finding comfortable position.

◆ **E. Nursing care plan/implementation:**
1. Goal: *relieve pain and promote comfort.*
  a. Bedrest with bedboard.
  b. *Position*—avoid twisting.
    (1) *Lumbar disk: William's* (head elevated 30 degrees, knee gatch elevated to flatten the lumbosacral curve).
    (2) *Cervical:* low Fowler's.
  c. Medications as ordered:
    (1) Analgesics.
    (2) Muscle relaxants.
    (3) Anti-inflammatory.
    (4) Stool softeners.
  d. Moist heat.
  e. Fracture bedpan.
  f. Gradual increase in activity.
  g. Brace application for support.
  h. Traction application prn for comfort.
  i. Prepare for surgery if medical regime unsuccessful.
2. Goal: *health teaching.*
  a. Correct body mechanics, keep back straight.
  b. Exercise program as symptoms decrease.

F. Evaluation/outcome criteria:
1. Reports pain decreased.

2. Mobility increased, normal body posture attained.

XI. Laminectomy: excision of dorsal arch of vertebrae with or without spinal fusion of two or more vertebrae with a bone graft from iliac crest, to stabilize spine.

◆ **A. Analysis/nursing diagnosis:**
1. *Pain* related to edema of surgical procedure.
2. *Impaired physical mobility* related to pain and discomfort resulting from surgery.

◆ **B. Nursing care plan/implementation:**
1. Goal: *relieve anxiety.*
  a. Answer questions, explain routines.
  b. See The Perioperative Experience, p. 102.
2. Goal: *prevent injury postoperatively.*
  a. Monitor vital signs:
    (1) Neurologic signs, e.g., check sensation and motor strength of limbs.
    (2) Respiratory status (risk for respiratory depression with cervical laminectomy).
  b. Monitor I&O (urinary retention common, especially with cervical laminectomy); may need catheterization. Encourage fluids.
  c. Monitor bowel sounds (paralytic ileus common with lumbar laminectomy).
  d. Monitor dressing for possible bleeding.
  e. Bed *position* as ordered:
    (1) *For lumbar laminectomy: head of bed flat;* supine with slight flexion of legs; with pillow between knees for turning and side-lying position.
    (2) *For cervical laminectomy: head of bed elevated,* neck immobilized with collar or sand bags.
  f. Encourage deep breathing to prevent respiratory complications.
  g. Prevent strain or flexion at surgical site: log-rolling with spinal fusion.
3. Goal: *promote comfort.*
  a. Administer analgesics as sciatic-type pain continues after lumbar surgery (arm pain after cervical surgery), due to edema from trauma of surgery.
4. Goal: *prepare for early discharge.*
  a. Patients having microsurgery for repair of herniated disk will usually be discharged from the hospital 1 d postoperative; teaching regarding allowed and restricted activities must be done early.
5. Goal: *health teaching.*
  a. How to *turn and move* from side to side in one motion, *sit up,* and *get out of bed without twisting spine;* to get out of bed: raise head of bed while in side-lying position, then put feet over edge of bed, and stand.
  b. Proper positioning and *ambulation* techniques.

c. Correct posture, *body mechanics,* activities to prevent further injury; increase activities according to tolerance.
d. Physiotherapy; encourage compliance for full rehabilitation.

◆ **C. Evaluation/outcome criteria:**
1. No respiratory, bowel, bladder complications noted.
   a. Lung sounds clear.
   b. Bowel sounds present; able to pass gas and feces.
   c. Urinary output adequate.
2. Regains mobility.
3. Comfort level increases: reports leg and back pain decreased.
4. Demonstrates protective positioning and ambulation techniques.

XII. Spinal cord injuries: trauma from hyperextension, hyperflexion, axial compression, lateral flexion, or shearing of the spine.

A. Types:
1. *C-1 and C-2 injury level*—resulting deficit:
   a. Phrenic nerve involvement.
   b. Diaphragmatic paralysis.
   c. Respiratory difficulties (require permanent ventilatory support).
   d. Possible quadriplegia.
   e. Possible death.
2. *C-4 through T-1 injury level*—resulting deficit: quadriplegia.
3. *Thoracic-lumbar injury level*—resulting deficit: paraplegia.

B. Pathophysiology: trauma → vertebral dislocation or fractures → cord trauma, compression or severance of the cord.

C. Risk factors:
1. Motor vehicle accidents.
2. Diving, surfing, contact sports.
3. Falls.
4. Gunshot wounds.

◆ **D. Assessment:**
1. *Subjective data*
   a. Pain at the level of injury.
   b. Numbness/weakness, loss of sensation below level of injury.
   c. Psychological distress related to severity of injury and its effects.
2. *Objective data*
   a. Symptoms depend on extent of injury to spinal cord/spinal nerves.
   b. Paralysis: motor, sphincter.
      (1) Initially a period of *flaccid paralysis* and loss of reflexes, called spinal or neural shock.
      (2) *Incomplete injuries* may lead to loss of voluntary movement and sensory deficits below injury level (symptoms vary depending on injury).
      (3) *Complete injury* leads to loss of function and all voluntary movement below level of injury.
   c. Respiratory distress.

d. Alterations in temperature control.
e. Alterations in bowel and bladder function.
f. Involved muscles become spastic and hyperreflexic within days or weeks.

◆ **E. Analysis/nursing diagnosis:**
1. *Ineffective breathing patterns* related to high-level injury.
2. *Impaired physical mobility* related to injuries affecting lower limbs.
3. *Fear* related to uncertain future health status.
4. *Anxiety* related to loss of control over own activities of daily living.
5. *Bathing/hygiene self-care deficit* related to injuries above T-1.
6. *Impaired home maintenance management* related to quadriplegia and possibly paraplegia.
7. *Risk for altered body temperature* related to absence of sweating below level of injury.
8. *Risk for injury* related to equipment necessary for daily activities.
9. *Tactile sensory/perceptual alterations* related to injury level.
10. *Body image disturbance* related to permanent change in physical status.

◆ **F. Nursing care plan/implementation:**
1. Goal: *maintain patent airway.*
   a. Suction, cough, tracheostomy care, prn.
   b. Oxygen, ventilator care.
   c. Monitor blood gas levels.
2. Goal: *prevent further damage.*
   a. Immobilize spine.
   b. Firm mattress, *Stryker frame, Foster frame, CircO-electric* bed, traction, casts, braces (see III. Fractures, p. 161).
   c. Skeletal traction via tongs: Crutchfield, Gardner-Wells (see III. Fractures, p. 161).
   d. Halo traction (see III. Fractures, p. 161).
3. Goal: *relieve edema:* anti-inflammatory medications, corticosteroids.
4. Goal: *relieve discomfort:* analgesics, sedatives, muscle relaxants.
5. Goal: *promote comfort:*
   a. Maintain fluid intake: PO/IV, I&O.
   b. Increase nutritional intake.
   c. Prevent contractures and decubiti.
   d. Assist patient to deal with psychosocial issues, e.g., role changes.
   e. Begin rehabilitation plan.
6. Goal: *prevent complications.*
   a. Monitor for spinal shock during initial phase of injury (see XIII. Spinal shock, p. 181).
   b. Monitor for hyperreflexia with severed spinal cord injuries (see XIV. Autonomic hyperreflexia, p. 181).

7. Goal: *health teaching*.
  a. Self-care techniques for highest level of independence; include significant others in teaching.
  b. How to use ambulation assistive devices (battery-operated wheelchair controlled by mouthpiece or hand controls, depending on level of paralysis).
  c. Identify community resources for follow-up care and career counseling.
  d. Signs and symptoms of autonomic hyperreflexia (see Section XIV, p. 182).
  e. Methods to prevent skin breakdown, infections of respiratory, urinary tract.
  f. Bowel, bladder program.

◆ **G. Evaluation/outcome criteria:**
  1. Complications avoided.
  2. Accomplishes self-care to greatest level for injury.
  3. Participates in rehabilitation plan.
  4. Grieves over loss and begins to integrate self into society.

XIII. Spinal shock: temporary flaccid paralysis and areflexia following a severe injury to the spinal cord.

  A. Pathophysiology: squeezing or shearing of the spinal cord due to fractures or dislocation of vertebrae; interruption of sensory tracts; loss of conscious sensation; interruption of motor tracts; loss of voluntary movement; loss of facilitation; loss of reflex activity; loss of muscle tone; loss of stretch reflexes, leading to bowel and bladder retention. If injury between T-1 and L-2, leads to loss of sympathetic tone and decrease in blood pressure. Afferent impulses are unable to ascend from below the injured site to the brain, and efferent impulses are unable to descend to points below the site.

  B. Risk factors:
  1. Automobile/motorcycle accidents.
  2. Athletic accidents, e.g., diving in shallow water.
  3. Gunshot wounds.

◆ **C. Assessment:**
  1. *Subjective data*
    a. Loss of sensation below level of injury.
    b. Inability to move extremities.
    c. Pain at level of injury.
  2. *Objective data*
    a. Neurologic exam:
      (1) *Absent:* pinprick, pressure, and vibratory sensations below level of injury; reflexes below level of injury.
      (2) Muscles: flaccid.
    b. Vital signs
      (1) BP decreased (loss of vasomotor tone below level of injury).
      (2) Bradycardia.
      (3) Elevated temperature.

      (4) Respirations: may be depressed; possible respiratory failure if diaphragm involved.
    c. Absence of sweating below level of injury.
    d. Urinary retention.
    e. Abdominal distention: retention of feces, paralytic ileus.
    f. Skin: cold, clammy.

◆ **D. Analysis/nursing diagnosis:**
  1. *Decreased cardiac output* related to loss of vasomotor tone below level of injury.
  2. *Ineffective breathing pattern* related to injuries involving diaphragm.
  3. *Impaired physical mobility* related to loss of voluntary movement of limbs.
  4. *Urinary retention* related to loss of stretch reflexes.
  5. *Fear* related to serious physical condition.
  6. *Risk for injury* related to potential organ damage if shock continues.

◆ **E. Nursing care plan/implementation:**
  1. Goal: *prevent injury related to shock*.
  ▶ a. Maintain patent airway: intubation and mechanical ventilation may be necessary with cervical spinal injuries due to involvement of diaphragm.
    b. Monitor vital signs; *profound hypotension* and bradycardia are most dangerous aspects of spinal shock.
    c. Administer blood/IV fluids as ordered.
    d. Nutrition and hydration:
      (1) NPO in acute stage: maintain nutrition by IV infusions as ordered.
      (2) When allowed to eat: *high-protein, high-calorie, high-vitamin diet*.
    e. Maintain proper *position* to prevent further injury.
      (1) Backboard is necessary to transport from place of injury.
      (2) Support head in neutral alignment and prevent flexion.
      (3) Skeletal traction will be applied once diagnosis is made.
    f. Monitor urinary output q1h; may have Foley catheter while in shock; later intermittent catheterization will be used as needed.
    g. Relieve bowel distention; use lubricant containing anesthetic, as necessary, when checking for or removing impaction.

◆ **F. Evaluation/outcome criteria:**
  1. Complications are avoided.
  2. Body functions are maintained.

XIV. Autonomic hyperreflexia (autonomic dysreflexia): a group of symptoms in which many spinal cord autonomic responses are activated simultaneously. This may occur when cord lesions are *above the sixth thoracic* vertebra; it is *most* *commonly* seen with cervical spinal cord injuries; may occur up to 6 yr after injury.

A. Pathophysiology: pathologic reflex condition, which is an acute **medical emergency** characterized by extreme hypertension and exaggerated autonomic responses to stimuli; primarily seen with cervical and high thoracic cord lesions.

B. Risk factors:
1. Distention of bladder or rectum.
2. Stimulation of skin, e.g., decubitus ulcers, wrinkled clothing.
3. Stimulation of pain receptors.

◆ **C. Assessment:**
1. *Subjective data*
   a. Severe headache.
   b. Blurred vision.
   c. Nausea.
   d. Restlessness.
   e. Feels flushed.
2. *Objective data*
   a. Severe hypertension (may reach 300 mm Hg).
   b. Bradycardia (30–40/min).
   c. Profuse diaphoresis.
   d. Flushing of skin above level of injury.
   e. Pale skin below level of injury.
   f. Pilomotor spasm (goose flesh).
   g. Nasal congestion.
   h. Distended bladder, bowel.
   i. Skin breakdown.

◆ **D. Analysis/nursing diagnosis:**
1. *Dysreflexia* related to high spinal cord injury.
2. *Risk for injury* related to complications of hypertension, CVA.
3. *Visual sensory/perceptual alteration* related to blurred vision.
4. *Urinary retention* related to inability to empty bladder due to spinal injury.
5. *Constipation* related to inability to establish successful bowel training program.
6. *Impaired skin integrity* related to immobility.

◆ **E. Nursing plan/implementation:**
1. Goal: *decrease symptoms to prevent serious side effects.*
   a. *Elevate head of bed;* this lowers BP in persons with high spinal cord injuries.
   b. Identify and correct source of stimulation if possible; notify physician.
   c. Monitor vital signs (BP) q15min and prn; uncontrolled hypertension can lead to CVA, blindness, death.
   d. Give medications as ordered: nitrates, nifedipine (Procardia), or hydralazine (Apresoline).
▶ 2. Goal: *maintain patency of catheter.*
   a. Monitor output; palpate for distended bladder.
   b. Check for tubing kinks; irrigate catheter prn.

   c. Insert new catheter *immediately* if blocked.
   d. Culture if infection suspected.
3. Goal: *promote regular bowel elimination.*
▶ a. Bowel training program.
   b. Administer suppository/enemas/laxatives as ordered and prn.
   c. When checking for and/or removing impaction, first use anesthetic ointment (e.g., dibucaine [Nupercainal] ointment) to decrease irritation.
4. Goal: *prevent decubitus ulcers.*
   a. Meticulous skin care.
   b. *Position change* q1–2h.
   c. Flotation pads, alternating pressure mattress on bed and wheelchair.
5. Goal: *health teaching.*
   a. How to recognize risk factors that could initiate this condition.
   b. Methods to prevent situations that increase risk, e.g., bowel program, bladder program, skin care, position change schedule.

◆ **F. Evaluation/outcome criteria:**
1. BP remains within normal limits.
2. No complications occur.

XV. Hyperthyroidism (also called *Thyrotoxicosis; Graves' disease*): spectrum of symptoms of accelerated metabolism caused by excessive amounts of circulating thyroid hormone.

A. Pathophysiology: diffuse hyperplasia of thyroid gland → overproduction of thyroid hormone and increased blood serum levels. Hormone stimulates mitochondria to increase energy for cellular activities and heat production. As metabolic rate increases, fat reserves are utilized, despite increased appetite and food intake. Cardiac output is increased to meet increased tissue metabolic needs, and peripheral vasodilation occurs in response to increased heat production. Neuromuscular hyperactivity → accentuation of reflexes, anxiety, and increased alimentary tract mobility. Graves' disease is caused by stimulation of the gland by immunoglobulins of the IgG class.

B. Risk factors:
1. Possible autoimmune response resulting in increase of a gamma globulin called *long-acting thyroid stimulator* (LATS).
2. Occurs in third and fourth decade.
3. Affects women more than men.
4. Emotional trauma, infection, increased stress.
5. Overdose of medications used to treat hypothyroidism.
6. Use of certain weight-loss products.

◆ **C. Assessment:**
1. *Subjective data*
   a. Nervousness, mood swings.
   b. Palpitations.
   c. Heat intolerance.

d. Dyspnea.
e. Weakness.
2. *Objective data*
   a. Eyes: exophthalmos, characteristic stare, lid lag.
   b. Skin:
      (1) Warm, moist, velvety.
      (2) Increased sweating, melanin pigmentation.
      (3) Pretibial edema with thickened skin and hyperpigmentation.
   c. Weight loss *despite* increased appetite.
   d. Muscle: weakness, tremors, hyperkinesia.
   e. Vital signs: BP—increased systolic pressure, widened pulse pressure; tachycardia.
   f. Goiter: thyroid gland noticeable and palpable.
   g. Abnormal menstruation.
   h. Frequent bowel movements.
   i. Activity pattern: overactivity leads to fatigue, which leads to depression, which stimulates patient into overactivity, and pattern continues.
      Danger: total exhaustion.
   j. Lab data:
      (1) *Elevated:* serum T_4 (> 11 µg/100 mL), free T_4 or free T_4 index, T_3 level ($> 35\%$) and free T_3 level.
      (2) *Elevated:* thyroid uptake of radioiodine (RAIU).
      (3) *Elevated:* metabolic rate (BMR).
      (4) *Decreased:* WBC caused by decreased granulocytosis (< 4500).

◆ **D. Analysis/nursing diagnosis:**
   1. *Altered nutrition, less than body requirements,* related to elevated basal metabolic rate.
   2. *Risk for injury* related to exophthalmos and tremors.
   3. *Activity intolerance* related to fatigue from overactivity.
   4. *Fatigue* related to overactivity.
   5. *Anxiety* related to tachycardia.
   6. *Sleep pattern disturbance* related to excessive amounts of circulating thyroid hormone.

◆ **E. Nursing care plan/implementation:**
   1. Goal: *protect from stress:* private room, restrict visitors, quiet environment.
   2. Goal: *promote physical and emotional equilibrium.*
      a. Environment: quiet, cool, well ventilated.
      b. Eye care:
         (1) Sunglasses to protect from photophobia, dust, wind.
         (2) Protective drops (methylcellulose) to soothe exposed cornea.
      c. *Diet:*
         (1) High: calorie, protein, vitamin B.
         (2) 6 meals/d, as needed.
         (3) Weigh daily.
         (4) Avoid stimulants (coffee, tea, colas, tobacco).
   3. Goal: *prevent complications.*
      a. Medications as ordered:
         (1) Propylthiouracil to block thyroid synthesis; hyperthyroidism returns when therapy is stopped.
         (2) Methimazole (Tapazole).
         (3) Iodine preparations: used in combination with above medications when hyperthyroidism not well controlled; saturated solution of potassium iodide (SSKI) or Lugol's solution; more palatable if diluted with water, milk, or juice; give through a straw to prevent staining teeth. Takes 2–4 wk before results are evident.
         (4) Propranolol to relieve tachycardia, tremors, and anxiety.
      b. Monitor for *thyroid storm (crisis)—* **medical emergency:** acute episode of thyroid overactivity caused when increased amounts of thyroid hormone are released into the bloodstream and metabolism is markedly increased.
         ◆ (1) **Risk factors** for thyroid storm: patient with uncontrolled hyperthyroidism (usually Graves' disease) who undergoes severe sudden stress, such as:
            (a) Infection.
            (b) Surgery.
            (c) Beginning labor to give birth.
            (d) Taking inadequate antithyroid medications before thyroidectomy.
         (2) *Subjective data*—thyroid storm:
            (a) Apprehension.
            (b) Restlessness.
         (3) *Objective data*—thyroid storm:
            (a) Vital signs: elevated temperature (106°F), hypotension, extreme tachycardia.
            (b) Marked respiratory distress, pulmonary edema.
            (c) Weakness and delirium.
            (d) **If untreated, patient could die of heart failure.**
         (4) Medications—thyroid storm:
            (a) Propylthiouracil or methimazole (Tapazole) to decrease synthesis of thyroid hormone.
            (b) Sodium iodide IV; Lugol's solution orally.
            (c) Propranolol (Inderal) to slow heart rate.
            (d) Aspirin to decrease temperature.
            (e) Steroids to combat crisis.

(f) Diuretics, digitalis to treat congestive heart failure.
4. Goal: *health teaching.*
   a. Stress-reduction techniques.
   b. Importance of medications, their desired and side effects.
   c. Methods to protect eyes from environmental damage.
   d. Signs and symptoms of thyroid storm (p. 183).
5. Goal: *prepare for additional treatment as needed.*
   a. *Radioactive iodine therapy:* [131]I, a radioactive isotope of iodine to decrease thyroid activity.
      (1) [131]I dissolved in water and given by mouth.
      (2) Hospitalization necessary only when large dose is administered.
      (3) Minimal precautions needed for usual dose.
         (a) Sleep alone for several nights.
         (b) Flush toilet several times after use.
      (4) Effectiveness of therapy seen in 2–3 wk; single dose controls 90% of patients.
      (5) Monitor for signs of hypothyroidism.
   b. Surgery: see XVI. Thyroidectomy.

◆ F. **Evaluation/outcome criteria:**
   1. Complications avoided.
   2. Compliance with medical regime.
   3. No further weight loss.
   4. Able to obtain adequate sleep.

XVI. **Thyroidectomy:** partial removal of thyroid gland (for hyperthyroidism) or total removal (for malignancy of thyroid).
   A. **Risk factor:** unsuccessful medical treatment of hyperthyroidism.
   ◆ B. **Analysis/nursing diagnosis:**
      1. *Risk for injury* related to possible trauma to parathyroid gland during surgery.
      2. *Ineffective breathing pattern* related to neck incision.
      3. *Pain* related to surgical incision.
      4. *Altered nutrition, less than body requirements,* related to difficulty in swallowing because of neck incision.
      5. *Impaired verbal communication* related to possible trauma of nerve during surgery.
      6. *Risk for altered body temperature* related to thyroid storm.
   ◆ C. **Nursing care plan/implementation:** *prepare for surgery* (see I. Preoperative preparation, p. 102). *Postoperative:*
      1. Goal: *promote physical and emotional equilibrium.*
         a. *Position:* semi-Fowler's to reduce edema.

b. Immobilize head with pillows/sandbags.
   c. Support head during position changes to avoid stress on sutures, prevent flexion or hyperextension of neck.
2. Goal: *prevent complications of hypocalcemia and tetany,* due to accidental trauma to parathyroid gland during surgery; signs of tetany indicate necessity of *calcium gluconate IV.*
   a. Check *Chvostek's sign*—tapping face in front of ear produces spasm of facial muscles.
   b. Check *Trousseau's sign*—compression of upper arm (usually with BP cuff) elicits carpal (wrist) spasm.
   c. Monitor for respiratory distress (due to laryngeal nerve injury, edema, bleeding); keep tracheostomy set/suction equipment at bedside.
   d. Monitor for elevated temperature, indicative of *thyroid storm* (see objective assessment data for thyroid storm, above).
   e. Monitor vital signs, check dressing and beneath head, shoulders for bleeding q1h and prn for 24 h; *hemorrhage* is possible complication; if swallowing is difficult, loosen dressing. If patient still complains of tightness when dressing is loosened, look for further signs of hemorrhage.
   f. Check voice postoperatively as soon as responsive after anesthesia and every hour (assessing possible *laryngeal nerve damage*); crowing voice sound indicates laryngeal nerves on both sides have been injured, *respiratory distress possible.*
      (1) Avoid unnecessary talking to lessen hoarseness.
      (2) Provide alternative means of communication.
3. Goal: *promote comfort measures.*
   a. Narcotics as ordered.
   b. Offer iced fluids.
   c. Ambulation and soft diet, as tolerated.
4. Goal: *health teaching.*
   a. How to support neck to prevent pressure on suture line: place both hands behind neck when moving head or coughing.
   b. Signs of hypothyroidism; needs supplemental thyroid hormone if total thyroidectomy.
   c. Signs and symptoms of hemorrhage and respiratory distress.
   d. Importance of adequate rest and nutritious diet.
   e. Importance of voice rest in early recuperative period.

◆ D. **Evaluation/outcome criteria:**

1. No respiratory distress, hemorrhage, laryngeal damage, tetany.
2. Preoperative symptoms relieved.
3. Normal range of neck motion obtained.
4. States signs and symptoms of possible complications.

XVII. Hypothyroidism (myxedema): deficiency of circulating thyroid hormone; often associated with the end result of *Hashimoto's thyroiditis* and *Graves' disease*.

  A. Pathophysiology: atrophy, destruction of gland by endogenous antibodies or inadequate pituitary thyrotropin production → insidious slowing of body processes, personality changes, and generalized, interstitial nonpitting (mucinous) edema—myxedema; pronounced involvement in systems with high protein turnover (e.g., cardiac, GI, reproductive, hematopoietic).

  B. Risk factors:
1. Total thyroidectomy; inadequate replacement therapy.
2. Inherited autosomal recessive genes.
3. Hypophyseal failure.
4. Dietary iodine deficiencies.
5. Radiation of thyroid gland.
6. Overtreatment of hyperthyroidism.

  ◆ **C. Assessment:**
1. *Subjective data*
  a. Weakness, fatigue, lethargy.
  b. Headache.
  c. Slow memory, psychotic behavior.
  d. Loss of interest in sexual activity.
2. *Objective data*
  a. Depressed basal metabolism rate (BMR).
  b. Cardiomegaly, bradycardia, hypotension, anemia.
  c. Menorrhagia, amenorrhea, infertility.
  d. Dry skin, brittle nails, coarse hair, hair loss.
  e. Slow speech, hoarseness, thickened tongue.
  f. Weight gain: edema, generalized interstitial; peripheral nonpitting; periorbital puffiness.
  g. Intolerance to cold.
  h. Hypersensitive to narcotics and barbiturates.

  ◆ **D. Analysis/nursing diagnosis:**
1. *Risk for injury* related to hypersensitivity to drugs.
2. *Altered nutrition, more than body requirements,* related to decreased BMR.
3. *Activity intolerance* related to fatigue.
4. *Constipation* related to decreased peristalsis.
5. *Decreased cardiac output* related to hypotension and bradycardia.
6. *Risk for impaired skin integrity* related to dry skin and edema.
7. *Social isolation* related to lethargy.

◆ **E. Nursing care plan/implementation:**
1. Goal: *provide for comfort and safety.*
  a. Monitor for infection or trauma; may precipitate *myxedema coma,* which is manifested by: unresponsiveness, bradycardia, hypoventilation, hypothermia, and hypotension.
  b. Provide warmth; prevent heat loss and vascular collapse.
  c. Administer thyroid medications as ordered: levothyroxine (Synthroid)—most common drug used; liothyronine sodium (Cytomel); dosage adjusted according to symptoms.
2. Goal: *health teaching.*
  a. *Diet:* low calorie, high protein.
  b. Signs and symptoms of hypothyroidism and hyperthyroidism.
  c. Life-long medications, dosage, desired and side effects.
  d. Medication dosage adjustment: take ⅓–½ usual dose of narcotics and barbituates.
  e. Stress-management techniques.
  f. Exercise program.

◆ **F. Evaluation/outcome criteria:**
1. No complications noted. Most common complications: atherosclerotic coronary heart disease, acute organic psychosis, and myxedema coma.
2. Dietary instructions followed.
3. Medication regime followed.
4. Thyroid hormone balance obtained and maintained.

XVIII. Cushing's disease: overactivity of adrenal gland leading to prolonged elevated plasma concentration of adrenal steroids.

  A. Pathophysiology:
1. Excess glucocorticoid production, leading to:
  a. *Increased* gluconeogenesis → raised serum-glucose levels → glucose in urine, increased fat deposits in face and trunk.
  b. *Decreased* amino acids → protein deficiencies, muscle wasting, poor antibody response, and lack of collagen.

  B. Risk factors:
1. Adrenal hyperplasia.
2. Excessive hypothalamic stimulation.
3. Tumors: adrenal, hypophyseal, pituitary, bronchogenic, or gallbladder.
4. Excessive steroid therapy.

  ◆ **C. Assessment:**
1. *Subjective data*
  a. Headache, backache.
  b. Weakness, decreased work capacity.
  c. Mood swings.
2. *Objective data*
  a. Hypertension, weight gain, pitting edema.

b. Characteristic fat deposits, supra-clavicular (buffalo hump).

c. Pendulous abdomen, purple striae, easy bruising.

d. Moon face, acne.

e. Hirsutism: face, arms, legs.

f. Hyperpigmentation.

g. Menstrual changes.

h. Impotence.

i. Lab data:

(1) Urine: elevated 17-ketosteroids (> 12 mg/24 h) and glucose (> 120 mg/dL).

(2) Plasma: elevated 17-hydroxycor-tico-steroids, cortisol (> 10 μg/dL). Cortisol does not decrease during the day as it should.

(3) Serum: *elevated*—glucose, RBC, WBC; *diminished*—potassium, chlorides, eosinophils, lympho-cytes.

j. X rays and scans to determine tu-mors/metastasis.

◆ **D. Analysis/nursing diagnosis:**

1. *Body image disturbance* related to changes in physical appearance.

2. *Activity intolerance* related to backache and weakness.

3. *Risk for injury* related to infection and bleeding.

4. *Knowledge deficit* related to manage-ment of disease.

5. *Pain* related to headache.

◆ **E. Nursing care plan/implementation.**

1. Goal: *promote comfort.*

a. Assist with preparation of diagnostic workup.

b. Explain procedures.

c. Protect from trauma.

2. Goal: *prevent complications;* monitor for:

a. Fluid balance—I&O, daily weights.

b. Glucose metabolism—blood, urine for sugar and acetone.

c. Hypertension—vital signs.

d. Infection—skin care, urinary tract; check temperature.

e. Mood swings—observe behavior.

3. Goal: *health teaching.*

a. *Diet: increased* protein, potassium; *decreased* calories, sodium.

b. Medications:

(1) Cytotoxic agents: aminogluteth-imide (Cytadren), trilostane (Modrastane), mitotane (Lyso-dren)—decrease cortisol produc-tion.

(2) Replacement hormones as needed.

c. Signs and symptoms of increased disease as noted in assessment.

d. Preparation for adrenalectomy if medical regime unsuccessful.

◆ **F. Evaluation/outcome criteria:**

1. Symptoms controlled by medication.

2. No complications—adrenal steroids within normal limits.

3. If adrenalectomy necessary, see follow-ing section.

XIX. **Adrenalectomy:** surgical removal of adrenal glands because of tumors or uncontrolled over-activity; also bilateral adrenalectomy may be performed to control metastatic breast or pros-tate cancer.

A. Risk factors:

1. Pheochromocytoma.

2. Adrenal hyperplasia.

3. Cushing's syndrome.

4. Metastasis of prostate or breast can-cer.

5. Adrenal cortex or medulla tumors.

◆ **B. Assessment:**

1. *Objective data:* validated evidence of:

a. Benign lesion (unilateral adrenalec-tomy) or malignant tumor (bilateral adrenalectomy).

b. Adrenal hyperfunction that cannot be managed medically.

c. Bilateral excision for metastasis of breast and sometimes metastasis of prostate carcinoma.

◆ **C. Analysis/nursing diagnosis:**

1. *Knowledge deficit* related to planned sur-gery.

2. *Risk for physical injury* related to hor-mone imbalance.

3. *Decreased cardiac output* (potential) re-lated to possible hypotensive state result-ing from surgery.

4. *Risk for infection* related to decreased normal resistance.

5. *Altered health maintenance* related to need for self-administration of steroid medications, orally or by injection.

◆ **D. Nursing care plan/implementation:**

1. Goal: *preoperative: reduce risk of postop-erative complications.*

a. Prescribed steroid therapy given 1 wk before surgery, is gradually decreased; will be given again postoperatively.

b. Antihypertensive drugs are discontin-ued as surgery may result in severe hypotension.

c. Sedation as ordered.

d. General preoperative measures (see p. 102).

2. Goal: *postoperative: promote hormonal balance.*

a. Administer hydrocortisone parenteral therapy as ordered; rate indicated by fluid and electrolyte balance, blood sugar, and blood pressure.

b. Monitor for signs of *addisonian crisis* (see p. 188).

3. Goal: *prevent postoperative complications.*
   a. Monitor vital signs until stability is regained; if on *vasopressor* drugs such as metaraminol (Aramine):
      (1) Maintain flow rate as ordered.
      (2) Monitor BP q5–15 min, notify physician of significant elevations in BP (dose needs to be decreased) or drop in BP (dose needs to be increased). *Note:* readings that are normotensive for some may be hypotensive for patients who have been hypertensive.
   b. NPO—attach nasogastric tube to intermittent suction; abdominal distention is common side effect of this surgery.
   c. Respiratory care:
      (1) Turn, cough, and deep breathe.
      (2) Splint flank incision when coughing.
      (3) Administer narcotics to reduce pain and allow patient to cough; flank incision is close to diaphragm, making coughing very painful.
      (4) Auscultate breath sounds q2h; decreased or absent sounds could indicate pneumothorax.
      (5) Sudden chest pain and dyspnea should be reported *immediately,* as spontaneous pneumothorax can occur.
   d. *Position:* flat or semi-Fowler's.
   e. Mouth care.
   f. Monitor dressings for bleeding; reinforce prn.
   g. Ambulation, as ordered.
      (1) Check BP q15min when ambulation is first attempted.
      (2) Place elastic stockings on lower extremities to enhance stability of vascular system.
   h. *Diet*—once NG tube removed, diet as tolerated.
4. Goal: *health teaching.*
   a. *Signs and symptoms of adrenal crisis:*
      (1) Pulse: rapid, weak, or thready.
      (2) Temperature: elevated.
      (3) Severe weakness and hypotension.
      (4) Headache.
      (5) Convulsions, coma.
   b. Importance of maintaining steroid therapy schedule to ensure therapeutic serum level.
   c. Weigh daily.
   d. Monitor blood-glucose levels daily.
   e. Report undesirable side effects of steroid therapy or adrenal crisis to physician.

f. *Avoid* persons with infections, due to decreased resistance.
g. Daily schedule: include adequate rest, moderate exercise, good nutrition.

◆ **E. Evaluation/outcome criteria:**
1. Adrenal crisis avoided.
   a. Vitals within normal limits.
   b. No neurologic deficits noted.
2. Healing progresses: no signs of infection or wound complications.
3. Adjust to alterations in physical status.
   a. Complies with medication regime.
   b. Avoids infections.
   c. Incorporates good nutrition, periods of rest and activity into daily schedule.

XX. **Addison's disease:** chronic primary adrenal cortical insufficiency.
   A. Pathophysiology:
   1. Atrophy of adrenal gland is most common cause of adrenal insufficiency; manifested by *decreased* adrenal cortical secretions.
      a. Deficiency in mineralocorticoid secretion (*aldosterone*) → increased sodium excretion → dehydration → hypotension → decreased cardiac output and resulting decrease in heart size.
      b. Deficiency in glucocorticoid secretion (*cortisol*) → decrease in gluconeogenesis → hypoglycemia and liver glycogen deficiency, emotional disturbances, diminished resistance to stress. Cortisol deficiency → failure to inhibit anterior pituitary secretion of ACTH and melanocyte-stimulating hormone → increased levels of ACTH and hyperpigmentation.
      c. Deficiency in androgen hormone → less axillary and pubic hair in women (testes supply adequate sex hormone in men, so no symptoms are produced).
   B. Risk factors:
   1. Autoimmune processes.
   2. Infection.
   3. Malignancy.
   4. Vascular obstruction.
   5. Bleeding.
   6. Environmental hazards.
   7. Congenital defects.
   8. Bilateral adrenalectomy.
   ◆ **C. Assessment:**
   1. *Subjective data*
      a. Muscle weakness, fatigue, lethargy.
      b. Dizziness, fainting.
      c. Nausea, food idiosyncrasies, anorexia.
      d. Abdominal pain/cramps.
   2. *Objective data*
      a. Vital signs: decreased BP, orthostatic hypotension, widened pulse pressure.
      b. Pulse—increased, collapsing, irregular.
      c. Temperature—subnormal.
      d. Vomiting and diarrhea.
      e. Tremors.

f. Skin: poor turgor, excessive pigmentation (bronze tone).

g. Lab data:
   (1) Blood:
      (a) *Decreased:* sodium (< 135 mEq/L); glucose (< 60 mg/dL), chloride (< 98 mEq/L), bicarbonate (< 23 mEq/L).
      (b) *Increased:* hematocrit, potassium (> 5 mEq/L).
   (2) Urine: *decreased* (or absent) 17-ketosteroids, 17-hydroxycorticosteroids (< 4 mg/24 h).

◆ **D. Analysis/nursing diagnosis:**
1. *Fluid volume deficit* related to decreased sodium.
2. *Altered renal tissue perfusion* related to hypotension.
3. *Decreased cardiac output* related to aldosterone deficiency.
4. *Risk for infection* related to cortisol deficiency.
5. *Activity intolerance* related to muscle weakness and fatigue.
6. *Altered nutrition, less than body requirements,* related to nausea, anorexia, and vomiting.

◆ **E. Nursing care plan/implementation:**
1. Goal: *decrease stress.*
   a. Environment: quiet, nondemanding schedule.
   b. Anticipate events where extra resources will be necessary.
2. Goal: *promote adequate nutrition.*
   a. *Diet: acute phase*—high sodium, low potassium; *nonacute phase*—increase carbohydrates and protein.
   b. *Fluids:* force, to balance fluid losses; monitor I&O, daily weights.
   c. Administer life-long exogenous replacement therapy as ordered:
      (1) Glucocorticoids—prednisone, hydrocortisone.
      (2) Mineralocorticoids—fludrocortisone (Florinef).
3. Goal: *health teaching.*
   a. Take medications *with* food or milk.
   b. May need antacid therapy to prevent GI disturbances.
   c. Side effects of steroid therapy.
   d. *Avoid* stress; may need adjustment in medication dosage when stress is increased.
   e. Signs and symptoms of *addisonian crisis:* very serious condition characterized by severe hypotension, shock, coma, and vasomotor collapse related to strenuous activity, infection, stress, omission of prescribed medications. **If untreated, could quickly lead to death.**

4. Goal: *prevent serious complications if addisonian crisis evident.*
   a. Complete bedrest; avoid stimuli.
   b. High dose of hydrocortisone IV or cortisone IM.
   c. Treat shock—IV saline.
   d. I&O, vital signs q15min to 1 h or prn until crisis passes.

◆ **F. Evaluation/outcome criteria:**
1. No complications occur.
2. Medication regimen followed, is adequate for patient's needs.
3. Adequate nutrition and fluid balance obtained.

XXI. **Multiple sclerosis:** progressive neurologic disease, common in northern climates, characterized by demyelination of brain and spinal cord leading to degenerative neurologic function.

A. Pathophysiology: multiple foci (patches) of nerve degeneration throughout brain, spinal cord, optic nerve, and cerebrum cause nerve impulses to be interrupted (blocked) or distorted (slowed); chronic remitting and relapsing disease; cause unknown. Exacerbations aggravated by fatigue, chilling, and emotional distress.

B. Risk factors:
1. Northern climate.
2. Onset age: 20–40 yr.
3. Affects men and women equally.

◆ **C. Assessment:**
1. *Subjective data*
   a. Extremities: weak, numb, decreased sensation.
   b. Emotional instability, apathy, irritability, mood swings, fatigue.
   c. Eyes: diplopia (double vision), spots before eyes (scotomas), potential blindness.
   d. Difficulty in swallowing.
2. *Objective data*
   a. Nystagmus (involuntary rhythmic movements of eyeball) and decreased visual acuity.
   b. Inappropriate outbursts of laughing or crying (sometimes related to ingestion of hot food).
   c. Disorders of speech.
   d. Susceptible to infections.
   e. Tremors to severe muscle spasms and contractures.
   f. Changes in muscular coordination; *gait:* ataxic, spastic.
   g. Changes in bowel habits, e.g., constipation.
   h. Urinary frequency and urgency.
   i. Incontinence, urine and feces.
   j. Lab tests: cerebrospinal fluid has presence of gamma globulin, IgG.

◆ **D. Analysis/nursing diagnosis:**
1. *Impaired physical mobility* related to changes in muscular coordination.

2. *Self-esteem disturbance* related to chronic, debilitating disease.
3. *Altered health maintenance* related to spasms and contractures.
4. *Risk for impaired skin integrity* related to contractures.
5. *Constipation* related to immobility.
6. *Impaired swallowing* related to tremors.
7. *Visual sensory/perceptual alteration* related to nystagmus and decreased visual acuity.

◆ **E. Nursing care plan/implementation:**
1. Goal: *maintain normal routine as long as possible.*
   a. Maintain mobility—encourage walking as tolerated; active and passive ROM; splints to decrease spasticity.
   b. Avoid fatigue, infections.
   c. Frequent position changes to prevent skin breakdown and contractures; *position at night:* prone to minimize flexor spasms of knees and hips.
   ▶ d. Bowel/bladder training program to minimize incontinence.
   e. Avoid stressful situations.
2. Goal: *decrease symptoms*—medications as ordered:
   a. Baclofen (Lioresal) for alleviating spasticity: 5 mg 3 times daily increased by 5 mg every 3 d; not to exceed 80 mg/d (20 mg 4 times/d). Optimal effect between 40 and 80 mg; sudden withdrawal of medication may cause hallucinations and rebound spasticity.
   b. Steroids during exacerbations.
   c. Diazepam (Valium), dantrolene (Dantrium) to relieve muscle spasm.
   d. Carbamazepine (Tegretol), phenytoin (Dilantin), or amitriptyline HCl (Elavil) for dysesthesias or neuralgia.
3. Goal: *health teaching to prevent complications.*
   a. Signs and symptoms of disease; measures to prevent exacerbations.
   b. Teach to monitor respiratory status to prevent infections.
   c. Importance of physical therapy to prevent contractures.
   d. Possible counseling or community support group for assistance in accepting long-term condition.
   e. Teach special skin care to prevent decubitus ulcers.
   f. Teach use of assistive devices to maintain independence.

◆ **F. Evaluation/outcome criteria:**
1. Establishes daily routine; adjusts to altered life-style.
2. Injuries prevented; no falls.
3. Urinary and bowel routines established; incontinence decreased.

4. Infections avoided.
5. Symptoms minimized by medications.

XXII. Myasthenia gravis: neuromuscular disease characterized by weakness and easy fatigability of facial, oculomotor, pharyngeal, and respiratory muscles.

A. Pathophysiology: inadequate acetylcholine or excessive or altered cholinesterase, leading to impaired transmission of nerve impulses to muscles at myoneural junction.

B. Risk factors:
1. Possible autoimmune reaction.
2. Thymus tumor.
3. Ages 20–40 yr: affects women more than men.
4. Older age groups: affects men and women equally.

◆ **C. Assessment:**
1. *Subjective data*
   a. Diplopia (double vision).
   b. Severe generalized fatigue.
2. *Objective data*
   a. Muscle weakness: hands and arms affected first.
   b. Ptosis (drooping of eyelids), expressionless facies.
   c. Hypersensitivity to narcotics, barbiturates, tranquilizers.
   d. Abnormal speech pattern, with high-pitched nasal voice.
   e. Difficulty chewing/swallowing food.
   f. Decreased ability to cough and deep breathe, vital capacity.
   ⚗ g. Positive Tensilon test (administration of edrophonium chloride, 10 mg IV, produces relief of symptoms within 30 sec).
   ⚗ h. Positive Prostigmin test (1.5 mg subcutaneous neostigmine methylsulfate produces relief of symptoms within 15 min, increased muscle strength within 30 min).

◆ **D. Analysis/nursing diagnosis:**
1. *Ineffective breathing patterns* related to weakness.
2. *Risk for injury* related to muscle weakness.
3. *Activity intolerance* related to severe fatigue.
4. *Bathing/dressing self-care deficit* related to progressive disease.
5. *Impaired physical mobility* related to decrease in strength.
6. *Anxiety* related to physical symptoms and disease progression.
7. *Knowledge deficit* related to medication administration and expected effectiveness.

◆ **E. Nursing care plan/implementation:**
1. Goal: *promote comfort.*
   a. Passive and active ROM, as tolerated, to increase strength.

b. Mouth care: before and after meals.

c. *Diet:* as tolerated, soft, pureed, or tube feedings.

d. Skin care to prevent decubiti.

e. Eye care: remove crusts; patch affected eye prn.

f. Monitor respiratory status—suction airway prn.

2. Goal: *decrease symptoms.*

a. Administer medications as ordered:

(1) Anticholinesterase (neostigmine [Prostigmin], pyridostigmine) to elevate concentration of acetylcholine at myoneural junction.

(2) Give *before* meals to aid in chewing, *with* milk or food to decrease GI symptoms; may be given parenterally.

3. Goal: *prevent complications.*

a. Respiratory assistance if breathing pattern not adequate.

b. Monitor for choking/increased oral secretion.

c. **Avoid:** narcotics, barbiturates, tranquilizers.

4. Goal: *promote increased self-concept.*

a. Encourage independence when appropriate.

b. Encourage communications; provide alternative methods when speech pattern impaired.

5. Goal: *health teaching.*

a. Medication information:

(1) Adjust dosage to maintain muscle strength.

(2) Medication must be taken at prescribed time to avoid:

(a) *Myasthenic crisis* (too little medication).

(b) *Cholinergic crisis* (too much medication).

b. *Signs and symptoms of crisis:* dyspnea, severe muscle weakness, respiratory distress, difficulty in swallowing.

c. Importance of avoiding upper respiratory infections.

d. Determine methods to conserve energy, to maintain independence as long as possible, while avoiding overexertion.

e. Refer to Myasthenia Gravis Foundation and other community agencies for assistance in reintegration into the community and plans for follow-up care.

◆ F. **Evaluation/outcome criteria:**

1. Independence maintained as long as possible.

2. Respiratory arrest avoided.

3. Infection avoided.

4. Medication regimen followed and crisis avoided.

XXIII. **Parkinson's disease:** progressive disease of the brain occurring in later life; characterized by stiffness of muscles and by tremors.

A. **Pathophysiology:** depigmentation of the substantia nigra of basal ganglia → decreased dopamine (neurotransmitter necessary for proper muscle movement) → decreased and slowed voluntary movement, wooden facies, and difficulty initiating ambulation. Decreased inhibitions of alpha-motoneurons → increased muscle tone → rigidity of both flexor and extensor muscles and tremors at rest.

B. **Risk factors:**

1. Occurs at ages 50–60.

2. Affects men and women equally.

3. Cause unknown; possibly connected to arteriosclerosis or viral infection.

4. Drug-induced parkinsonian syndromes have been linked to:

a. Phenothiazines.

b. Reserpine (Serpasil).

c. Butyrophenones (haloperidol).

◆ C. **Assessment:**

1. *Subjective data*

a. Insomnia.

b. Depression.

c. Defects in judgment, emotional instability; intelligence not impaired.

2. *Objective data*

a. Limbs, shoulders: stiff, offer resistance to passive ROM.

b. Loss of coordination, muscular weakness with rigidity.

c. Shuffling gait: difficulty in initiating, then propulsive, trunk bent forward.

d. Tremors: pill-rolling of fingers, to and fro head movements.

e. Loss of postural reflexes.

f. Weight loss, constipation.

g. Difficulty in maintaining social interactions because of impaired speech, lack of facial affect, drooling.

h. Facies: wide-eyed, eye blinking, decreased facial expression, akinesia (abnormal absence of movement).

i. Excessive salivation, drooling.

j. Speech: slowed, slurred; judgment defective; intelligence intact.

k. Heat intolerance.

◆ D. **Analysis/nursing diagnosis:**

1. *Impaired physical mobility* related to loss of coordination.

2. *Altered health maintenance* related to defective judgment.

3. *Risk for injury* related to altered gait.

4. *Dressing/grooming self-care deficit* related to muscular rigidity.

5. *Sleep pattern disturbance* related to insomnia.

6. *Body image disturbance* related to tremors and drooling.
7. *Social isolation* related to altered physical appearance.
8. *Altered nutrition, less than body requirements,* related to lack of appetite.
9. *Impaired swallowing* related to excessive drooling.
10. *Constipation* related to dietary changes.

◆ **E. Nursing care plan/implementation:**
1. Goal: *promote maintenance of daily activities.*
   a. ROM exercises, skin care, physical therapy.
   b. Encourage ambulation; discourage sitting for long periods.
   c. Assist with meals—*high protein, high calorie; soft diet;* small, frequent feedings; encourage increased fluids.
   d. Encourage compliance with medication regimen:
      (1) Dopamine agonists:
         (a) Levodopa: given in increasing doses until symptoms are relieved; given *with food* to decrease GI symptoms. *Side effects:* nausea, vomiting, anorexia, postural hypotension, mental changes, cardiac arrhythmias. Levodopa assists in restoring striated dopamine deficiency.
         (b) Sinemet (carbidopa and levodopa): limits the metabolism of levodopa peripherally and provides more levodopa for the brain.
      (2) Anticholinergics: effective in lessening muscle rigidity.
      (3) Antihistamines: exert mild central anticholinergic properties.
2. Goal: *protect from injury.*
   a. Monitor BP, side effects of medications, e.g., orthostatic hypotension.
   b. Monitor for GI disturbances.
   c. *Avoid* pyridoxine (vitamin B$_6$): cancels effect of levodopa.
   d. Levodopa *contraindicated* with:
      (1) Glaucoma (causes increased intraocular pressure).
      (2) Monoamine oxidase (MAO) inhibitors (causes possible hypertensive crisis).
3. Goal: *health teaching.*
   a. Teach patient and family about medications: dosage range, side effects, not discontinuing medications abruptly.

b. Exercise program to maintain ROM and normal body posture; also to get adequate rest to prevent fatigue.
c. *Dietary adjustment and precautions* regarding cutting food in small pieces to prevent choking, taking fluid with food for easier swallowing.
d. Importance of adding *roughage* to *diet* to prevent constipation.
e. Assist patient and family to adjust to this chronic debilitating illness.

◆ **F. Evaluation/outcome criteria:**
1. Activity level maintained.
2. Symptoms relieved by medications; no drug interactions.
3. Complications avoided.

XXIV. Amyotrophic lateral sclerosis (ALS; Lou Gehrig's disease): progressive degeneration of motor neurons within the brain and/or spinal cord, leading to death within 5–10 yr, usually from respiratory or bulbar paralysis.

A. Pathophysiology: myelin sheaths destroyed, replaced by scar tissue; involves lateral tracts of spinal cord, eventually medulla and ventral tracts.

B. Risk factors:
1. Affects men more than women.
2. Usually in middle age.
3. Viral infection possible causal agent.
4. Possible familial or genetic component.

◆ **C. Assessment:**
1. *Subjective data*
   a. Early symptoms: fatigue, awkwardness.
   b. Dysphagia, dysarthria.
   c. Alert, no sensory loss.
2. *Objective data*
   a. Symptoms depend on which motor neurons affected.
   b. Decreased fine finger movement.
   c. Progressive muscular weakness, atrophy.
   d. Spasticity of flexor muscles; one side of body becomes more involved than other.
   e. Progressive respiratory difficulties → diaphragmatic paralysis.
   f. Progressive disability of upper and lower extremities.
   g. Tongue fasciculations.

◆ **D. Analysis/nursing diagnosis:**
1. *Ineffective airway clearance* related to difficulty in coughing.
2. *Ineffective breathing pattern* related to progressive respiratory difficulties and eventually respiratory paralysis.
3. *Altered health maintenance* related to inability to perform self-care activities.
4. *Impaired physical mobility* related to progressive muscular weakness.

5. *Bathing/hygiene and dressing/grooming self-care deficit* related to neuromuscular impairment.
6. *Powerlessness* related to life-style of progressive physical helplessness.
7. *Impaired swallowing* related to disease progression.

◆ **E. Nursing care plan/implementation:**
1. Goal: *maintain independence as long as possible.*
   a. Assistance with ADL; splints, prosthetic devices to support weak limbs and maintain mobility.
   b. Skin care to prevent decubiti.
   c. *Soft/liquid diet* to aid in swallowing, prevent choking; suction prn; *head of bed elevated* when eating.
   ▶ d. Respiratory assistance as needed; ventilators as disease progresses and diaphragm becomes involved.
   e. Arrange long-term care arrangements if home maintenance no longer feasible.
   f. Emotional support, when patient is alert; continue involving patient in decisions regarding care.
2. Goal: *health teaching.*
   a. Skin care to prevent decubitus ulcer.
   b. Explain ramifications of disease so patient and family can make decisions regarding future care, whether patient will remain at home as disease progresses or enter a long-term care facility.
   c. How to use suction apparatus to clear airway.
   d. Care of nasogastric or gastrostomy feeding tube.

◆ **F. Evaluation/outcome criteria:**
1. Obtains physical and emotional support.
2. Complications avoided in early stage of disease.
3. Remains in control of ADL as long as possible.
4. Skin breakdown avoided.
5. Peaceful death.

❑ Cancer

I. The cancer patient: Cancer is a multisystem stressor. Regardless of the specific type of cancer, certain aspects of the disease and of nursing care are the same. The following principles apply universally and should be referred to when studying individual kinds of cancer.

A. Pathophysiology: result of altered cellular mechanisms. Several theories about causation, but current thinking is multiple causation. Alterations result in a progressive, uncontrolled multiplication of cells, with selective ability to invade and metastasize.

B. Risk factors:
1. Heredity, e.g., retinoblastoma.
2. Familial susceptibility, e.g., breast.
3. Acquired diseases, e.g., ulcerative colitis.
4. Virus, e.g., Burkitt's tumor.
5. Environmental factors:
   a. Tobacco.
   b. Alcohol.
   c. Radiation.
   d. Occupational hazards.
   e. Drugs, e.g., immunosuppressive, cytotoxic.
6. Age.
7. Air pollution.
8. Diet, e.g., high animal protein.
9. Chronic irritation.
10. Precancerous lesions, e.g., gastric ulcers.
11. Stress.

◆ **C. Assessment:**
1. Specific symptoms depend on the anatomic and functional characteristics of the organ or structure involved.
2. Mechanical effects:
   a. *Pressure*—tumors growing in confined areas such as bone produce pain early, whereas tumors growing in expandable areas such as the abdomen may be undetected for some time.
   b. *Obstruction*—tumors that compress tubular structures such as the esophagus, bronchi, or lymph channels may cause symptoms such as swallowing difficulties, shortness of breath, edema. Symptoms depend on location of tumor and on the particular organ or structure receiving pressure.
   c. *Interruptions of blood supply*—compression of blood vessels or diversion of blood supply may cause necrosis or ulceration or may precipitate hemorrhage.
3. Systemic effects:
   a. Anorexia, weakness, weight loss.
   b. Metabolic disturbances—malabsorption syndrome.
   c. Fluid and electrolyte imbalances.
   d. Hormonal imbalances—increased antidiuretic hormone (ADH), adrenocorticotropic hormone (ACTH), thyrotropin (TSH), or parathyroid hormone (PTH).
   ⚗ e. Diagnostic tests:
      (1) *Biopsy*—excision of part of tumor mass.
      (2) *Needle biopsy*—aspiration of cells from subcutaneous masses or organs such as liver.
      (3) *Exfoliative cytology*—scraping of any endothelium (cervix, mucous membranes) and applying to slide.
      (4) *X rays*—detect tumor growth in GI, respiratory, and renal systems.
      (5) *Endoscopy*—visualization of body cavity through endoscope.

(6) *Computerized axial tomography*—visualization of a body part whereby layers of tissue can be seen utilizing the very narrow beams of this type of X-ray equipment.

(7) *Magnetic resonance imaging (MRI) scan*—a scanning device using a magnetic field for visualization.

f. Lab data:
  (1) *Blood and urine tests*—refer to Appendix A for normal values.
  (2) *Alkaline phosphates*—greatly increased in osteogenic carcinoma (> 92 U/L).
  (3) *Calcium*—elevated in multiple myeloma bone metastases (> 10.5 mg/dL).
  (4) *Sodium*—decreased in bronchogenic carcinoma (< 135 mEq/L).
  (5) *Potassium*—decreased in extensive liver carcinoma (< 3.5 mEq/L).
  (6) *Serum gastrin*—measures gastric secretions. Decreased in gastric carcinoma. Normal value 40–150 pg/mL.
  (7) *Neutrophilic leukocytosis*—tumors.
  (8) *Eosinophilic leukocytosis*—brain tumors, Hodgkin's disease.
  (9) *Lymphocytosis*—chronic lymphocytic anemia.

◆ **D. Analysis/nursing diagnosis:**
  1. *Pain* related to diagnostic procedures, pressure, obstruction, interruption of blood supply, or potential side effects of drugs.
  2. *Anxiety* related to fear of diagnosis or disease progression, treatment, and its known or expected side effects.
  3. *Altered nutrition, less than body requirements,* related to anorexia.
  4. *Risk for injury* related to radioactive contamination of excreta.
  5. *Body image disturbance* related to loss of body parts, change in appearance as a result of therapy.
  6. *Powerlessness* related to diagnosis and own perception of its meaning.
  7. *Self-esteem disturbance* related to impact of cancer diagnosis.
  8. *Risk for infection* related to immunosuppression from radiation and chemotherapy.
  9. *Altered urinary elimination* related to dehydration.
  10. *Risk for injury* related to normal tissue damage from radiation source.
  11. *Fluid volume deficit* related to nausea and vomiting.
  12. *Diarrhea* related to radiation of bowel.
  13. *Constipation* related to dehydration.

◆ **E. Nursing care plan/implementation**—general care of the cancer patient:
  1. Goal: *promote psychosocial comfort.* (See also Unit 6.)

a. Assist with diagnostic workup by providing psychological support and information about diagnostic tests, diagnosis, and treatment options.

b. Reduce anxiety by listening, making referrals for special problems (peer support groups, self-help groups such as Reach to Recovery), supplying information, or correcting misinformation, as appropriate.

c. Stress-management techniques (see Orientation, Unit 1).

d. Nursing management related to depressed patient (see Unit 6).

2. Goal: *minimize effects of complications.*
  a. Anorexia/anemia:
    (1) *Decrease anemia* by:
      (a) Providing well-balanced, *iron-rich, small, frequent* meals.
      (b) Administering supplemental vitamins and iron as ordered.
      (c) Administering packed cells as ordered.
      (d) Maintaining hyperalimentation as ordered.
    (2) *Enhance nutrition* by providing nutritional supplements and a *diet high in protein;* necessary because of increased metabolism related to metastatic process. *Consult* with dietitian for suggestions of best food for individual patient.
  b. Hemorrhage: monitor platelet count and maintain platelet infusions as ordered. Teach patient to monitor for any signs of bleeding.
  c. Infection: observe for signs of sepsis (changes in vital signs, temperature of skin, mentation, urinary output or pain); monitor laboratory values; administer antibiotics as ordered.
  d. Pain and discomfort: alleviate by frequent position changes, diversions, conversations, imagery, relaxation, back rubs, and narcotics as ordered.
  e. Assist in adjusting to altered body image by encouraging expression of fears and concerns. Don't ignore patient's questions, and give honest answers: be available.

3. Goal: *general health teaching.*
  a. Self-care skills to maintain independence; e.g., patient who has a colostomy should know how to manage the colostomy before going home.
  b. Importance of follow-up care and routine physical examinations to monitor for general health and possible signs of further disease.
  c. Dietary instructions, adjustments necessary to maintain nutrition during and after treatment.

Adult

d. Health maintenance programs: teach hazards of the use of tobacco and alcohol. *Avoid* high-fat, low-roughage diet.

e. Risk factors: family history, stress, age, diet, occupation, environment.

F. General surgical intervention: surgery may be *curative* (when the lesion is localized or with minimal metastases to the lymph nodes) or *palliative* (to decrease symptomatology). (Also see The Perioperative Experience, p. 102, and specific types of cancer, following.)

◆ 1. **Nursing care plan/implementation—** *preoperative:*

a. Goal: *prevent respiratory complications.*
(1) Coughing and deep-breathing techniques.
(2) No smoking for 1 wk prior to surgery.

b. Goal: *counteract nutritional deficiencies.*
(1) *Diet:*
(a) High protein, high carbohydrate for tissue repair.
(b) Vitamin and mineral supplements.
(c) Hyperalimentation as ordered.
(2) Blood transfusions may be needed if counts are low.

c. Goal: *reduce apprehension.*
(1) Clarify postoperative expectations.
(2) Explain care of ostomies or tubes.
(3) Answer patient's questions honestly.

2. *Postoperative*

a. Goal: *prevent complications.*
(1) Monitor respiratory status and hemodynamic status.
▶ (2) Wound care; active and passive exercises as allowed; respiratory hygiene; coughing, deep breathing, and turning; fluids (see III. Postoperative experience, p. 106).

b. Goal: *alleviate pain and discomfort.*
(1) Encourage early ambulation, depending on surgical procedure.
(2) Administer prescribed medications as needed.
(3) Administer stool softeners and enemas as ordered.

c. Goal: *health teaching.*
(1) Involve patient, significant others, and family members in rehabilitation program.
(2) Prepare for further therapies, such as radiation or chemotherapy.
(3) Support groups, as appropriate: Reach to Recovery, Ostomy Associates, Laryngectomy Association.
(4) Develop skills to deal with disease progression if cure not realistic or metastasis evident (see J. Palliative care, p. 198).

G. Chemotherapy: used as single treatment or in combination with surgery and radiation, for early or advanced diseases. Antineoplastic agents' primary mode of action involves interfering with the supply and utilization of building blocks of nucleic acids as well as interfering with intact molecules of DNA or RNA, which are needed for replication and growth. Bone marrow, hair follicles, and the gastrointestinal tract are three areas of the body in which cells are actively dividing; this is why most side effects are related to these areas of the body.

1. *Types:* alkylating agents, antimetabolites, antitumor antibiotics, plant alkaloids, enzymes, hormones. See Unit 4, Table 4.6.

2. *Major problem:* lacks specificity, thus affecting normal as well as malignant cells.

3. *Major side effects:* bone marrow depression, stomatitis, nausea and vomiting, gastrointestinal ulcerations, diarrhea, and alopecia (Table 2.37).

4. *Routes of administration:* oral, intramuscular, intravenous (*Hickman catheter*), subclavian lines, porta caths, peripheral, intra-arterial (may have infusion pump for continuous or intermittent flow rate), intracavity (e.g., bladder through cystoscopy). (See p. 299 for information about administration of IV chemotherapeutic agents.)

◆ 5. **Nursing care plan/implementation:**

a. Goal: *assist with treatment of specific side effects.*

(1) *Nausea and vomiting*—antiemetic drugs as ordered and scheduled; small, frequent, *high-calorie, high-potassium, high-protein* meals; include milk and milk products when tolerated for *increased calcium;* carbonated drinks; frequent mouth care; antacid therapy as ordered; rest after meals; *avoid* food odors during preparation of meals; pleasant environment during meals; appropriate distractions; IV therapy; nasogastric tube for control of severe nausea or as route for tube feeding if unable to take food by mouth; hyperalimentation.

(2) *Diarrhea—low-residue diet; increased potassium;* increased fluids; atropine SO$_4$–diphenoxylate HCl (Lomotil) or kaolin-pectin (Kaopectate) as ordered; avoid hot or cold foods/liquids.

(3) *Stomatitis* (painful mouth)—soft toothbrushes or sponges (toothettes); mouth care q2–4h; viscous lidocaine HCl (Xylocaine) as ordered before meals. Oral salt and soda mouth rinses; *avoid* commercial mouthwashes that contain high level of alcohol, which could be very irritating to mucous membranes. *Avoid* hot

■ **TABLE 2.37 Common Toxicities of Antineoplastic Agents**

	Nausea and Vomiting	Mucositis	Diarrhea	Skin Reactions	Lung	Neurologic
Antimetabolites						
Cytosine arabinoside	0	0	+	0	+	0
	+ +	+	+ +	Alopecia	0	0
	+ + +	+	+ +	Alopecia	0	Cerebellar
Fludarabine	+	0	0	0	0	0
5-Fluorouracil	0	+	+	Phlebitis	0	Cerebellar
	0	+ + +	+ + +	Phlebitis	0	Cerebellar
	0	+	+	Hand-foot syndrome	0	0
	0	+	+ + +	Hand-foot syndrome	0	0
Methotrexate	+	+ +	+ +	Dermatitis	+	0
with leucovorin	+ + +	+ + +	+ + +	Dermatitis	+	0
2-Deoxycoformycin	+	0	0	Erythema	0	Lethargy, coma
6-Mercaptopurine	+	0	0	Rash	0	0
Thioguanine	+	+	0	0	0	0
2-Chlorodeoxyadenosine	+	0	0	0	0	0
Alkylating agents						
Busulfan	0	+	0	Hyperpigmentation	0	0
Chlorambucil	0	0	0	0	+	0
Cyclophosphamide	+	0	0	0	+	0
	+ +	+	0	Alopecia	+	0
	+ + +	+ + +	+ + +	Alopecia	+	0
DTIC	+ + +	0	0	0	0	0
Ifosfamide	+ + +	0	0	Alopecia	0	Encephalopathy
Mechlorethamine	+ + +	+	+	Alopecia, rash	0	0
Melphalan	0	0	0	0	0	0
Nitrosoureas						
Carmustine (BCNU)	+ + +	0	0	0	+	0
Lemustine (CCNU)	+	0	0	0	0	0
Streptozocin	+ + +	0	0	0	0	0
Thiotepa	+ +	+ + +	+ + +	Alopecia, rash	0	0
Tumor antimicrobials						
Bleomycin	0	0	0	Erythema	+	0
Dactinomycin	+ +	+ +	0	Alopecia, rash	0	0
Daunorubicin	+ +	+	+	Alopecia, vesicant	0	0
Doxurubicin	+ +	+	+	Alopecia, vesicant	0	0
Idarubicin	+ +	+	+	Alopecia, vesicant	0	0
Mitomycin C	+	+	0	Vesicant	+	0
Mitoxantrone	+	+	+	Alopecia, vesicant	0	0
Plant alkaloids						
Etoposide	0	0	0	0	0	0
Vinblastine	+	+	0	Alopecia, vesicant	0	+
Vincristine	0	0	0	Vesicant	0	+ + Neuropathy
Taxol	+	0	0	Alopecia	0	Neuropathy
Other agents						
Carboplatin	+ +	0	0	0	0	0
Cisplatin	+ + +	0	0	0	0	+
Hydroxyurea	0	0	0	Skin atrophy	0	0
L-Asparaginase	0	0	0	0	0	Encephalopathy
Procarbazine	+	0	0	Rash	0	Encephalopathy

0, none; +, mild; + +, moderate; + + +, severe.
Source: Adapted from Ewald G, McKenzie C (eds). *Manual of Medical Therapeutics.* Boston: Little, Brown, 1995.

foods/liquids; bland foods; cool temperatures; remove dentures if sores are under dentures; moisten lips with petroleum jelly.

(4) *Skin care*—monitor: wounds that do not heal, infections (patient receives frequent sticks for blood tests and therapy); *avoid* sunlight; use sunblock, especially if receiving doxorubicin (Adriamycin).

(5) *Alopecia*—ice caps during therapy or tourniquet around forehead for 20

min before, during, and after infusion of a few drugs (as ordered by physician); be gentle when combing or lightly brushing hair; use wigs, night caps, scarves; provide frequent linen changes. Advise patient to have hair cut short prior to treatment with drugs known to cause alopecia (bleomycin, cyclophosphamide, dactinomycin, daunomycin hydrochloride, doxorubicin hydrochloride, 5-fluorouracil, ICRF-159, hydroxyurea, methotrexate, mitomycin, VP 16-213, and vincristine).

b. Goal: *health teaching.*
(1) Orient patient and family to purpose of proposed drug regimen and anticipated side effects.
(2) Advise that frequent checks on hematologic status will be necessary (patient will receive frequent IV sticks, lab tests).
(3) Advise patient/family on increased risk for infection (avoid uncontrolled crowds and individuals with upper respiratory tract infections or childhood diseases).
(4) Monitor injection site for signs of extravasation (infiltration) (site must be changed if leakage suspected, and guidelines to neutralize must be followed according to drug protocol).

6. *Nursing precautions with chemotherapy*
a. Nurse should wear gloves and mask when preparing chemotherapy drugs for administration.
b. Drugs are toxic substance, and nurses must take every precaution to handle them with care.
c. When expelling air bubbles from syringes, care must be taken that the drugs are not sprayed into the atmosphere.
d. Contaminated needles and syringes should be disposed of intact (to prevent aerosol generation) in plastic-lined box and incinerated. Disposable equipment should be used whenever possible.
e. If skin becomes contaminated with a drug, wash under running water.
f. Nurses should know the half-life and excretion route of the drugs being administered and take the special precautions necessary. For example, while the drug is actively being excreted, use gloves when touching patient, stool, urine, dressings, vomitus, etc.
g. Nurses who are in the early phase of pregnancy should exercise caution when caring for the patient receiving chemotherapeutic agents.

H. Radiation therapy: used in high doses to kill cancer cells, or palliatively for pain relief. *Side effects of radiation therapy* depend on site of therapy (side effects are variable in each individual): nausea, vomiting, stomatitis, esophagitis, dry mouth, diarrhea, depression of bone marrow, suppression of immune response, decreased life span, and sterility.

1. **External radiation:** cobalt or linear accelerator machine.
a. *Procedure:* daily treatments, Monday through Friday, for prescribed number of times according to size and location of tumor (length of treatment schedule is usually 4–6 wk). Patient remains alone in room during treatment. (Nurse, therapist, family members cannot stay in room with patient due to radiation exposure during treatment.) Patient instructed to lie still so exactly same area irradiated each treatment. Marks (tattoos or via permanent-ink markers) are made on skin to delineate area of treatment; marks must not be removed during entire treatment course.
◆ b. **Nursing care plan/implementation:**
(1) Goal: *prevent tissue breakdown.*
(a) Do not wash off site-identification marks (tattoos cannot be removed); dosage area is carefully calculated and must be exact for each treatment.
(b) Assess skin daily and teach patient to do same (most radiation therapy is done on outpatient basis, so patient needs skills to manage independently).
(c) Keep skin dry; cornstarch usually the only topical application allowed:
(d) *Contraindications:*
(i) Talcum powders, due to potential radiation dosage alteration.
(ii) Lotions, due to increased moistening of skin.
(e) Reduce skin friction by *avoiding* constricting bedclothes or clothing and by using electric shaver.
(f) Dress areas of skin breakdown with non-adherent dressing and paper tape.
(2) Goal: *decrease side effects of therapy.*
(a) Provide meticulous oral hygiene.
(b) If diarrhea occurs, may need IV infusions, antidiarrheal medications; monitor bowel movements, possible adhesions from surgery and radiation treatments.
(c) Monitor vital signs, particularly respiratory function, and BP (sloughing of tissues puts patient at risk for hemorrhage).

(d) Monitor hematologic status—bone marrow depression can cause fatal toxicosis and sepsis.

(e) Institute *reverse isolation* as necessary to prevent infections (reverse isolation usually instituted if < 50% neutrophils).

(3) Goal: *health teaching.*

(a) Instruct patient to *avoid:*

(i) Strong sunlight; must wear sunblock lotion, protective clothing over radiation site.

(ii) Extremes in temperature to the area (hot-water bottles, ice caps).

(iii) Synthetic, nonporous clothes or tight constrictive clothing over area.

(iv) Eating 2–3 h before treatment and 2 h after, to decrease nausea; give small, frequent meals high in protein and carbohydrates and low in residue.

(v) Strong alcohol-base mouthwash; use daily salt and soda mouthwash.

(vi) Fatigue, an overwhelming problem. Need to pace themselves, nap; may need someone to drive them to therapy; can continue with usual activities as tolerated.

(vii) Crowds and persons with upper respiratory infections or any other infections.

(b) Provide appropriate birth control information for patients of childbearing age.

2. **Internal radiation: sealed** (radium, iridium, cesium)

a. Used for localized masses, e.g., mouth, cervix, breast, testes. Due to exposure from radiation source, precautions must be taken while it is in place. Health care personnel and family must adhere to *principles of time, distance, and shielding to decrease exposure* (*shortest* amount of time possible, stay as *far away* from the source of radiation, and wear *protective* lead apron, gloves). If source of radiation accidentally falls out, it should be picked up only with *forceps.* Radiation officer should be notified immediately. Patient should be in private room, and bed should be in the center of the room, if possible, to protect others. Unless the walls are lead lined, radiation will penetrate them; placing the bed in *center of room* will decrease exposure. Once the source of radiation has been removed, there is no exposure from patient, excretions, or linens.

◆ b. **Nursing care plan/implementation:**

▶ (1) Goal: *assist with cervical radium implantation* (cervical radium is used here as the most common example of internal radiation source).

(a) *Prior to insertion*—give douche, enema, perineal prep; insert Foley, as ordered.

(b) *After implantation*—check position of applicator q24h.

(i) Keep patient on bedrest in *flat position* to avoid displacing applicator (may turn to side for eating).

(ii) Notify physician if temperature elevates, nausea or/and vomiting occur (indicates radiation reaction or infection).

(iii) *After removal* of implant (48–144 h)—bathe, douche, and remove catheter as ordered.

(2) Goal: *health teaching.*

(a) Explain that nursing care will be limited to essential activities in postinsertion period.

(b) Signs and symptoms of complications so patient can notify staff if something unusual happens (bleeding, radiation source falls out, fever, etc.).

◆ c. **Nursing precautions for sealed internal radiation**

(1) **Never handle radium directly**—if applicators should accidentally be removed, pick up applicator by strings with long-handled forceps and **notify radiation officer.**

(2) Linen must remain in patient's room and not be sent to laundry until source of radiation has been accounted for and returned to its container.

(3) **Time, distance, and shielding** are factors that increase or decrease potential effects on personnel. Need to minimize exposure of nursing staff, patient's family, and other health professionals. Nurses who may be pregnant should not care for patients with radiation because of possible damage to the unborn fetus due to radiation exposure.

3. **Internal radiation: unsealed** (radioisotope/radionuclide)

a. Source of radiation is given orally or intravenously or instilled into a cavity as a liquid.

◆ b. **Nursing care plan/implementation:**
   Goal: *reduce radiation exposure of others.*
   (1) Isolate patient and tag room with radioactivity symbol.
   (2) *Rotate* personnel to avoid overexposure (principles of time, distance, and shielding). Staff should use good handwashing technique. Patient should be in a room with running water. (Nurse who may be pregnant should not care for patient while radiation source still active.)
   (3) Encourage family to maintain telephone contact or use intercom, to decrease exposure to others.
   (4) Plan independent diversional activities.

c. *Specific nursing precautions* (post in chart, on patient's door).

◆ (1) *Radioactive iodine* (^{131}I): half-life 8.1 d; excreted in urine, saliva, perspiration, vomitus, feces.
   (a) Wear gloves and isolation gowns when handling patient, excreta, or dressings directly.
   (b) Collect paper plates, eating utensils, dressings, and linen in impermeable bags; label and dispose according to agency protocol.
   (c) Collect excreta in shielded container and send to lab daily to monitor excretion rate and disposal.

(2) *Radioactive phosphorus* (^{32}P): half-life 14 d; injected into cavity or given IV or orally.
   (a) If injected into cavity, turn patient q10–15min for 2 h to ensure distribution.
   (b) No radiation hazard unless leakage from instillation site or from patient's excreta, which are collected in lead-lined containers and brought to the radioisotope laboratory for disposal. Linen is collected in container, marked *radioactive,* and brought to the radioisotope lab for special handling.
   (c) Seepage will stain linens blue; wear gloves when handling contaminated linens, dressings. Excreta disposed of as in (b) above.

(3) *Radioactive gold* (^{198}Au): half-life 2.7 d; usually injected into pleural or abdominal cavity.
   (a) May seep from instillation site or drainage tubes in cavity; stains purple.
   (b) Turn patient q15min for 2 h, as in (2)(a) above.

   (c) Same precautions regarding handling excreta as in (1)(a) and (2)(b) above.

◆ 4. **Precautions for nurses**
   a. Use *principles of time, distance,* and *shielding* when caring for patients who are having active radiation therapy treatments.
   b. Nurses who may be pregnant should *not* accept an assignment caring for patients who have active radiation in place.
   c. *Always* use gloves, gowns to protect skin and clothing.
   d. Wear detection badge to determine exposure to energy source.

I. Immunotherapy: it has been hypothesized that clinical malignancy may occur as a result of failure of the immunologic surveillance system of the body to fight off cancer cells as they develop. The goal of immunotherapy is to immunize patients against their own tumors.
   1. *Nonspecific* immunotherapy—encourages a host-immune response by use of an unrelated agent. *BCG* (bacillus Calmette-Guérin) vaccine and *Corynebacterium parvum* are the two agents used for this type of immunotherapy.
   2. *Specific* immunotherapy—uses substances that are antigenically related to the tumor that stimulate a specific host-immune response.
   3. *Side effects*—malaise, chills, nausea, vomiting, diarrhea; local reaction at site of injection, such as pruritus, scabbing.

◆ 4. **Nursing care plan/implementation:**
   a. Goal: *decrease discomfort associated with side effects of therapy.*
      (1) Identify measures to lessen symptoms of side effects (see E. Nursing care plan/implementation—general care of the cancer patient, previously, p. 193).
      (2) Know type of immunotherapy being used, adverse and desirable effects of therapy.
      (3) Administer fluids, encourage rest.
      (4) Administer acetaminophen as ordered to decrease flulike symptoms.
      (5) Administer antiemetics as ordered for nausea.
      (6) Monitor for respiratory distress.
      (7) Administer analgesics as ordered for pain.
   b. Goal: *health teaching.*
      (1) Comfort measures to decrease side effects of therapy.
      (2) Expected and side effects of therapy.
      (3) Investigational nature of therapy.
      (4) Care of site of administration.
      (5) Answer questions honestly.

J. Palliative care: When treatment has been ineffective in control of the disease, the nurse must plan palliative, terminal care. Cure is not possible for such patients in an advanced phase of malignancy. Symptoms increase in severity; patients and family have many special problems.

1. General problems of terminal cancer patient:
   a. *Cachexia:* progressive weakness, wasting, and weight loss.
   b. *Anemia:* leukopenia, thrombocytopenia, hemorrhage.
   c. *Gastrointestinal disturbances:* anorexia, constipation.
   d. *Tissue breakdown* leading to decubiti, seeping wounds.
   e. *Urine:* retention, incontinence, renal calculi, tumor obstruction of ureters.
   f. *Hypercalcemia* occurs in 10–30% of patients.
   g. *Pain* due to tumor growth, obstruction, vertebral compression, or secondarily to complications, e.g., decubiti, stiffened joints, stomatitis. Also neuropathy, due to prolonged use of neurotoxic chemotherapeutic agents such as vincristine.
   h. *Fatigue:* major and debilitating problem.

◆ 2. **Nursing care plan/implementation:**
   a. Goal: *make patient as comfortable as possible;* involve nursing staff, family, support personnel, clergy, volunteers, support groups, hospice, etc.
      (1) *Nutrition:* obtain nutritional consultation; *high-calorie, high-protein diet;* small, frequent meals; blenderized or strained; commercial nutritional supplements (Ensure, Vivonex, Sustagen).
      (2) Prevent tissue breakdown and vascular complications: frequent turning, massage, air mattress, active and passive ROM exercises.
      (3) GI tract disturbances: observe for toxic reactions to therapy, particularly vomiting and diarrhea; administer medications: antiemetics, antidiarrheal agents as ordered.
      (4) Relieve pain.
         (a) Use supportive measures such as massage, relaxation techniques, imagery, and drugs for pain relief; administer codeine, fentanyl, aspirin–oxycodone HCl (Percodan), pentazocine (Talwin), morphine, methadone, as ordered.
         (b) Monitor for side effects of narcotics, depressed respiratory status, constipation, anorexia.
   b. Goal: *assist patient to maintain self-esteem and identity.*
      (1) Encourage self-care.
      (2) Spend time with patient; isolation is a great fear for the dying patient.
   c. Goal: *assist patient with psychological adjustment*—see nursing care for grieving patients, dying patients (see Unit 6).

◆ K. **Evaluation/outcome criteria:**
   1. Tolerates treatment modality—complications of surgery are avoided; tolerates chemotherapy; completes radiation therapy.
   2. Side effects of treatment are managed by effective nursing care and health teaching.
   3. Maintains good nutritional status.
   4. Uses effective coping mechanisms or seeks appropriate assistance to deal with psychosocial concerns.
   5. Makes choices for follow-up care based on accurate information.
   6. Finds methods to control pain and minimize discomfort.
   7. Dignity maintained until and/or during death.

II. **Lung cancer**
   A. **Pathophysiology:** *squamous cell carcinoma:* undifferentiated, pleomorphic in appearance; accounts for 45–60% of all lung cancer; *small-cell (oat-cell) carcinoma:* small, dark cells located between cells of mucosal surfaces; characterized by early metastasis and poor prognosis; *large-cell (giant-cell) carcinoma:* located in the peripheral areas of the lung, has poor prognosis; *adenocarcinoma:* found in men and women; not necessarily related to smoking.
   B. **Risk factors:**
      1. Heavy cigarette smoking, 20-yr smoking history.
      2. Exposure to certain industrial substances, such as asbestos.
      3. Increased incidence in women during the last decade of life.

◆ C. **Assessment:**
   1. *Subjective data*
      a. Dyspnea.
      b. Pain: on swallowing; dull and poorly localized chest pain, referred to shoulders.
      c. Anorexia.
      d. History of cigarette smoking over a period of years; recurrent respiratory infections with chills and fever, especially pneumonia or bronchitis.
   2. *Objective data*
      a. Wheezing; dry to productive persistent cough; hemoptysis.
      b. Weight loss.
      c. Positive diagnosis: cytology report of cells from bronchoscopy.
      d. Chest pain.
      e. Signs of metastasis.
   D. Annual incidence: 152,000 new cases; 139,000 estimated deaths.

◆ E. **Analysis/nursing diagnosis:**
   1. *Ineffective breathing pattern* related to pain.
   2. *Impaired gas exchange* related to tumor growth.

Adult

Adult

3. *Pain* related to disease progressing.
4. *Fear* related to uncertain future.
5. *Powerlessness* related to inability to control symptoms.
6. *Knowledge deficit* related to disease and treatment.

◆ **F. Nursing care plan/implementation:**
1. Goal: *make patient aware of diagnosis and treatment options.*
   a. Allow time to talk and to discuss diagnosis.
   b. Patient makes informed decision regarding treatment.
2. Goal: *prevent complications related to surgery* for patient who is diagnosed early and for whom surgery is an option: wedge or segmental resection, lobectomy, or pneumonectomy are usual procedures.
   a. See Nursing care plan/implementation for the patient having thoracic surgery, p. 93.
   b. Monitor vital signs, including accurate respiratory assessment for respiratory congestion, blood loss, infection.
   c. Assist patient to deep breathe, cough, change position.
3. Goal: *assist patient to cope with alternative therapies* when surgery is deemed not possible.
   a. *Radiation:* megavoltage X ray, cobalt—usual form of radiation. (See Nursing care plan/implementation for the patient having radiation therapy, p. 196.)
   b. *Chemotherapy*
      (1) Cyclophosphamide (Cytoxan), doxorubicin (Adriamycin), CCNU, methotrexate, vincristine sulfate (Oncovin) are the usual drugs given for lung cancer.
      (2) See Nursing care plan/implementation for the patient having chemotherapy, p. 194.
4. Goal: *health teaching.*
   a. Encourage patient to stop smoking to offer best possible air exchange.
   b. Encourage *high-protein, high-calorie diet* to counteract weight loss.
   c. *Force fluids,* to liquefy secretions so they can be expectorated.
   d. Encourage adequate rest and activity to prevent problems of immobility.
   e. Desired effects and side effects of medications prescribed for therapy and pain relief.
   f. Coping mechanisms for maximal comfort and advanced disease (see J. Palliative care, p. 198).

◆ **G. Evaluation/outcome criteria:**
1. Copes with disease and treatment.
2. Side effects of treatment are minimized by proper nursing management.
3. Acid-base balance is maintained by careful management of respiratory problems.

4. Patient is aware of the seriousness of the disease.

III. Colon and rectal cancer
A. Risk factors:
1. Males, middle age, personal or family history of colon and rectal cancer, personal or family history of polyps in the rectum or colon, ulcerative colitis.
2. Diet high in beef and low in fiber.
3. *Gardner's syndrome* (multiple colonic adenomatous polyps, osteomas of the mandible or skull, multiple epidermoid cysts, or soft-tissue tumors of the skin).

B. Annual incidence: 147,000 new cases, 61,500 estimated deaths.

◆ **C. Assessment:**
1. *Subjective data*
   a. Change in bowel habits.
   b. Anorexia.
   c. Weakness.
   d. Abdominal cramping or vague discomfort with or without pain.
2. *Objective data*
   a. Diarrhea (pencillike or ribbon-shaped feces) or constipation.
   b. Weight loss.
   c. Rectal bleeding; anemia.
   d. Chills, fever.
   e. Digital exam reveals palpable mass if lesion is in ascending or descending colon.
   f. Signs of intestinal obstruction: obstipation, distention, pain, vomiting, fecal oozing.
   g. Diagnostic tests:
      (1) Digital examination.
      (2) Slides of stool specimen, for occult blood.
      (3) Proctoscopy.
      (4) Sigmoidoscopy.
      (5) Barium enema.
   h. Lab data: occult blood, blood serotonin increased, carcinoembryonic antigen (CEA); positive radioimmunoassay of serum or plasma indicates presence of carcinoma or adenocarcinoma of colon; positive results after resection indicates return of tumor.

◆ **D. Analysis/nursing diagnosis:**
1. *Constipation or diarrhea* related to presence of mass.
2. *Altered health maintenance* related to care of stoma.
3. *Sexual dysfunction* related to possible nerve damage during radical surgery.
4. *Body image disturbance* related to colostomy.

◆ **E. Nursing care plan/implementation** (see also E. Nursing care plan/implementation—general care of the cancer patient, p. 193).
1. *Radiation:* to reduce tumor or for palliation.

2. *Chemotherapy:* to reduce tumor mass and metastatic lesions.
   a. Antitumor antibiotics—mitomycin C, doxorubicin hydrochloride (Adriamycin).
   b. Aklylating agents—methyl-CCNU.
   c. Antimetabolites—5-fluorouracil (5-FU).
   d. Steroids and analgesics for symptomatic relief.
3. Prepare patient for surgery (colostomy) if necessary.

◆ **F. Evaluation/outcome criteria:**
1. Return of peristalsis and formed stool following resection and anastomosis.
2. Adjusts to alteration in bowel elimination route following abdominoperineal resection (e.g., no depression, resumes life-style).
3. Demonstrates self-care skills with colostomy.
4. Makes dietary adjustments that affect elimination as indicated.
5. Identifies alternative methods of expressing sexuality, if needed.

IV. Breast cancer
A. Risk factors:
1. Women > age 50.
2. Family history of breast cancer.
3. Never bore children, or bore first child after age 30.
4. Had breast cancer in other breast.
5. Menarche before age 11.
6. Menopause after age 50.
7. Excessive animal fat in diet.
8. Exposure to endogenous estrogens.

B. Annual incidence: 135,900 new cases; 42,300 estimated deaths.

◆ **C. Assessment:**
1. *Subjective data*
   a. Burning, itching of nipple.
   b. Reported painless lump.
2. *Objective data*
   a. Firm, nontender lump or mass.
   b. Asymmetry of breast.
   c. Nipple—retraction, discharge.
   d. Alteration in breast skin—redness, dimpling, ulceration.
   e. Palpation reveals lump.
   f. Diagnostic tests: mammography, needle biopsy, excisional biopsy—level of estrogen-receptor protein predicts response to hormonal manipulation of metastatic disease and may represent a prognostic indicator for primary cancer; carcinoembryonic antigen useful for patient with metastatic disease of the breast.

◆ **D. Analysis/nursing diagnosis:**
1. *Risk for injury* related to surgical intervention.
2. *Body image disturbance* related to effects of surgery, radiation, or chemotherapy.
3. *Altered sexuality patterns* related to loss of breast.

◆ **E. Nursing care plan/implementation** (see also E. Nursing care plan/implementation—general care of the cancer patient, p. 193).
1. Goal: *assist through treatment protocol.*
   a. *Radiation*—primary treatment modality; adjunctive, external, or implantation to primary lesion site or notes.
   b. *Chemotherapy*
      (1) Cytotoxic agents to destroy tumor and control metastasis.
      (2) Alkylating agents: cyclophosphamide (Cytoxan).
      (3) Antitumor antibiotics: doxorubicin (Adriamycin).
      (4) Antimetabolites: fluorouracil (5-FU); methotrexate (Amethopterine, MTX).
      (5) Plant alkaloids: vincristine sulfate (Oncovin).
      (6) Hormones to control metastasis, provide palliation: androgens, fluoxymesterone (Halotestin), testosterone (Teslac).
      (7) Antiestrogens: tamoxifen citrate (Nolvadex).
      (8) Cortisols: cortisone, prednisolone (Delta-Cortef), prednisolone acetate (Meticortelone), prednisone (Deltasone, Deltra).
      (9) Estrogens: diethylstilbesterol.
   c. *Surgery*
      (1) *Preoperative*
         (a) Goal: *prepare for surgery—types:*
            (i) *Lumpectomy* (with or without radiation)—used when lesion is small; section of breast is removed (often accompanied by radiation therapy and then radium interstitial implant).
            (ii) *Simple mastectomy*—breast removed, no alteration in nodes.
            (iii) *Modified radical mastectomy*—breast, some axillary nodes, subcutaneous tissue removed; pectoralis minor muscle removed.
            (iv) *Radical mastectomy*—breast, axillary nodes, and pectoralis major and minor muscles removed.
            (v) Reconstructive surgery—done at time of initial mastectomy or (most often) later, when other adjuvant therapy has been completed.
         (b) Goal: *promote comfort.*
            (i) Allow patient and family to express fears, feelings.

(ii) Provide correct information about diagnostic tests, operative procedure, postoperative expectations.

(2) *Postoperative*

(a) Goal: *facilitate healing.*

(i) Observe pressure dressings for bleeding; will appear under axilla and toward the back.

(ii) Report if dressing becomes saturated; reinforce dressing as needed; monitor drainage from Hemovac or suction pump.

(iii) *Position:* semi-Fowler's to facilitate venous and lymphatic drainage; use pillows to elevate affected arm above right atrium, to prevent edema if nodes removed.

(b) Goal: *prevent complications.*

(i) Monitor vital signs for shock.

(ii) Use gloves when emptying drainage.

(iii) Maintain joint mobility—flexion and extension of fingers, elbow, shoulder.

(iv) ROM as ordered to prevent ankylosis.

(v) If skin graft done, check donor site and limit exercises.

(c) Goal: *facilitate rehabilitation.*

(i) Encourage patient, significant others, and family to look at incision.

(ii) Involve patient in incisional care, as tolerated.

(iii) Refer to Reach to Recovery program of the American Cancer Society Breast Reconstructive Volunteers.

(iv) Exercise program, hydrotherapy for postmastectomy patients, to reduce lymphedema.

(d) Goal: *health teaching.*

(i) How to avoid injury to affected area; how to prevent lymphedema.

(ii) Exercises to gain full ROM.

(iii) Availability of prosthesis, reconstructive surgery.

(iv) Correct breast self-examination (BSE) technique (is at risk for breast cancer in remaining breast) (Figure 2.9). Best time for exam: premenopausal women, seventh day of cycle; postmeno-

pausal women, same day each month.

◆ **F. Evaluation/outcome criteria:**

1. Identifies feelings regarding loss.
2. Demonstrates postmastectomy exercises.
3. Gives rationale for avoiding fatigue and avoiding constricting garments on affected arm; necessity for avoiding injury (cuts, bruises, burns) while carrying out activities of daily living.
4. Describes signs and symptoms of infection.
5. Demonstrates correct BSE technique.

V. Uterine cancer (endometrial): originates from epithelial tissues of the endometrium; second only to cervical cancer as cause of pelvic cancer. Slow growing; metastasizes late; responsive to therapy with early diagnosis; Pap test not as effective—more effective to have endometrial tissue sample (Tables 2.38 and 2.39). Table 2.40 discusses cervical cancer.

A. Risk factors:

1. History of infertility (nulliparity).
2. Failure of ovulation.
3. Prolonged estrogen therapy.
4. Obesity.
5. Menopause after age 52.
6. Diabetes.

B. Annual incidence: 46,900 new cases; 10,000 estimated deaths.

◆ **C. Assessment:**

1. *Subjective data*
   a. History of risk factor(s).
   b. Pain (late symptom).
2. *Objective data*
   a. Obese.
   b. Abnormal cells obtained from aspiration of endocervix or endometrial washings.
   c. Postmenopausal uterine bleeding.
   d. Abnormal menses; intermenstrual or unusual discharge.

◆ **D. Analysis/nursing diagnosis:**

1. *Pain* related to surgery.
2. *Risk for injury* related to surgery.
3. *Body image disturbance* related to loss of uterus.

◆ **E. Nursing care plan/implementation** (see also care of the cancer patient, p. 193):

1. Goal: *assist patient through treatment protocol.*
   a. *Radiation*—external and/or internal with poor surgical risk patient.
   b. *Chemotherapy*—to reduce tumors and produce remission of metastasis. Antineoplastic drugs: dacarbazine (DTIC), doxorubicin (Adriamycin), medroxyprogesterone acetate (Provera), megestrol acetate (Megace).
2. Goal: *prepare patient for surgery—types:*
   a. *Subtotal hysterectomy:* removal of the uterus; cervical stump remains.

■ **FIGURE 2.9**   Breast self-examination. A. Examine breasts during bath or shower since flat fingers glide easily over wet skin. Use right hand to examine left breast and vice versa. B. Sit or stand before a mirror. Inspect breasts with hands at sides, then raised overhead. Look for changes in contour or dimpling of skin. C. Place hands on hips and press down firmly to flex chest muscles. D. Lie down with one hand under head and pillow or folded towel under that scapula. E. Palpate that breast with the other hand using concentric circle method. It usually takes three circles to cover all breast tissue. Include the tail of the breast and the axilla. Repeat with other breast. F. End in a sitting postion. Palpate the areola areas of both breasts, and inspect and squeeze nipples to check for discharge.

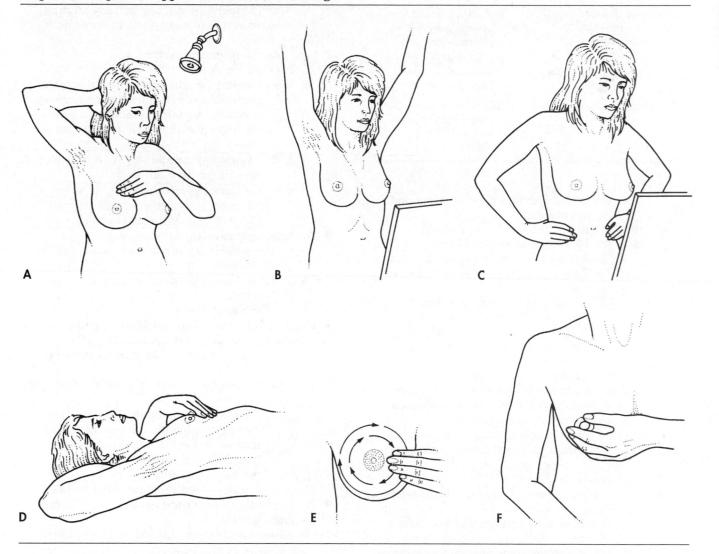

■ **TABLE 2.38   Papanicolaou-Smear Classes**

Class		Recommended Actions
I	Normal	
II	Atypical cells, nonmalignant	Treat vaginal infections; repeat Pap smears
III	Suspicious cells	Biopsy; dilatation & curettage
IV	Abnormal cells; suspicious of malignancy	Biopsy; dilatation & curettage; conization
V	Malignant cells present	See Table 2.39

  b. *Total hysterectomy:* removal of entire uterus, including cervix (abdominally—approximately 70%—or vaginally).
  c. *Total hysterectomy with bilateral salpingo-oophorectomy:* removal of entire uterus, fallopian tubes, and ovaries.
3. Goal: *reduce anxiety and depression:* allow for expression of feelings, concerns about femininity, role, relationships.
4. Goal: *prevent postoperative complications.*
▶ a. Catheter care—temporary bladder atony may be present as a result of edema or nerve trauma, especially when vaginal approach is used.

■ **TABLE 2.39** Uterine Cancer: Recommended Treatment, by Stage of Invasion

Stage of Invasion	Recommended Treatment
0 (In situ) Atypical hyperplasia	Cryosurgery, conization
I Uterus is of normal size	Hysterectomy
II Uterus slightly enlarged, but tumor is undifferentiated	Radiation implant, X ray; hysterectomy 4–6 wk postradiation
III Uterus enlarged, tumor extends outside uterus	Radiation implant, total hysterectomy 4–6 wk postradiation
IV Advanced metastatic disease	Radiation, chemotherapy; progestin therapy to reduce pulmonary lesions

b. Observe for abdominal distention and hemorrhage:
(1) Auscultate for bowel sounds.
(2) Measure abdominal girth.
(3) Utilize rectal tube to decrease flatus.
c. *Decrease pelvic congestion* and prevent venous stasis.
(1) *Avoid* high Fowler's position.
(2) Antiembolic stockings as ordered.
(3) Institute passive leg exercises.
(4) Apply abdominal support as ordered.
(5) Encourage early ambulation.
5. Goal: *support coping mechanisms* to prevent psychosocial response of depression: allow for verbalization of feelings.
6. Goal: *health teaching* to prevent complications of hemorrhage, infection, thromboemboli.
a. *Avoid:*
(1) Douching or coitus until advised by physician.
(2) Strenuous activity and work, for 2 mo.
(3) Sitting for long time and wearing constrictive clothing, which tend to increase pelvic congestion.
b. Explain hormonal replacement if applicable; correct dosage, desired and side effects of prescribed medications.
c. Explain:
(1) Menstruation will no longer occur.
(2) Importance of reporting symptoms, e.g., fever, increased or bloody vaginal discharge, and hot flashes.
◆ **F. Evaluation/outcome criteria:**
1. Adjusts to altered body image.
2. No complications—hemorrhage, shock, infection, thrombophlebitis.
VI. Prostate cancer
A. Risk factors:

1. Men > age 50.
2. Familial history.
3. Geographic distribution, environmental (e.g., industrial exposure to cadmium).
B. Annual incidence: 99,000 new cases; 29,000 estimated deaths.
◆ **C. Assessment:**
1. *Subjective data*
a. Difficulty in starting urinary stream.
b. Pain due to metastasis in lower back, hip.
c. Symptoms of cystitis.
2. *Objective data*
a. Urinary: smaller, less forceful stream; terminal dribbling; frequency, urgency, nocturia; *retention* (inability to void after ingestion of alcohol or exposure to cold).
b. Cystoscopy, needle biopsy, or specimen reveals positive cancer cells.
c. Lab data: *elevated:*
(1) prostate-specific antigen.
(2) prostatic acid phosphatase.
◆ **D. Analysis/nursing diagnosis:**
1. *Altered urinary elimination* related to incontinence.
2. *Altered sexuality pattern* related to nerve damage.
3. *Body image disturbance* related to surgery.
◆ **E. Nursing care plan/implementation** (see also care of the cancer patient, p. 193).
1. Goal: *assist patient through treatment protocol.*
a. *Radiation*—alone or in conjunction with surgery.
b. *Chemotherapy*—analgesics, antispasmotics, antibiotics, adrenocortical hormones, and cytotoxic drugs in conjunction with orchiectomy, to limit production of androgens.
c. *Surgery*—see Prostatectomy, p. 144.
◆ **F. Evaluation/outcome criteria:** see Prostatectomy, p. 144.
VII. Bladder cancer: The bladder is most common site of urinary tract cancer.
A. Risk factors:
1. Contact with certain dyes.
2. Cigarette smoking.
3. Excessive coffee intake.
4. Prolonged use of analgesics with phenacetin.
5. Three times more common in males.
B. Annual incidence: 46,000 new cases; 10,400 estimated deaths.
◆ **C. Assessment:**
1. *Subjective data*
a. Frequency, urgency.
b. Pain: flank, pelvic; dysuria.
2. *Objective data*
a. Painless hematuria (initially).
b. Diagnostic tests:

■ **TABLE 2.40 International System of Staging for Cervical Carcinoma**

Stage	Location	Prognosis	Treatment
0	In situ	Highly curable	Conization
I	Cervix	Cure rate decreases as stage progresses	Radiation
II	Cervix to upper vagina		Radiation
III	Cervix to pelvic wall or lower third of vagina		Surgeries: 1. Panhysterectomy, wide vaginal excision with removal of lymph nodes; ileal conduit
IV	Cervix to true pelvis, bladder, or rectum		2. Pelvic exenteration: a. Anterior: removal of vagina and bladder; ileal conduit b. Posterior: removal of rectum and vagina; colostomy c. Total: both anterior and posterior 3. Chemotherapy

(1) Cytoscopy, intravenous pyelogram *(IVP)*—mass or obstruction.
(2) Bladder biopsy, urine cytology—malignant cells.
c. Lab data: urinalysis—increased RBC (>4.8/μL—men); (>4.3/μL—women); erythrocytes (>30 mg/dL).

◆ **D. Analysis/nursing diagnosis:**
1. *Risk for injury* related to surgical intervention.
2. *Altered urinary elimination* related to surgery.

◆ **E. Nursing care plan/implementation** (see also care of the cancer patient, p. 193).
1. Goal: *assist patient through treatment protocol.*
   a. *Radiation*—cobalt, radioisotopes, radon seeds; often before surgery to slow tumor growth.
   b. *Chemotherapy*
      (1) Antitumor antibiotics: doxorubicin hydrochloride (Adriamycin).
      (2) Antimetabolites: 5-fluorouracil (5-FU).
      (3) Alkylating agents: thiotepa.
      (4) Sedatives, antispasmodics.
2. Goal: *prepare patient for surgery*—types:
   a. *Transurethral fulguration or excision:* used for small tumors with minimal tissue involvement.
   b. *Segmental resection:* up to half the bladder may be resected.
   c. *Cystectomy with urinary diversion:* complete removal of the bladder; performed when disease appears curable.
3. Goal: *assist with acceptance of diagnosis and treatment.*
4. Goal: *prevent complication during postoperative period.*
   a. *Transurethral fulguration or excision:*
      (1) Monitor for clots, bleeding, spasms.
      (2) Maintain patency of Foley catheter.
   b. *Urinary diversion with stoma:*
      (1) Protect skin, ensure proper fit of appliance—because constantly wet with urine (see also Ileal conduit, p. 144, and ostomies and stoma care, p. 133).
      (2) Prevent infection by increasing *acidity* of urine and increasing *fluid* intake.
      (3) Health teaching.
         (a) Self-care of stoma and appliance.
         (b) Expected and side effects of medications.
         (c) Importance of follow-up visits for early detection of metastasis.

◆ **F. Evaluation/outcome criteria:**
1. Accepts treatment plan.
2. Utilizes prescribed measures to decrease side effects of surgery, radiation, chemotherapy.
3. Plans follow-up visits for further evaluation.
4. Maintains dignity.

VIII. Laryngeal cancer
   A. Risk factors:
   1. Eight times more common in men.
   2. Occurs most often after age 60.
   3. Cigarette smoking.
   4. Alcohol.
   5. Chronic laryngitis, vocal abuse.
   6. Family predisposition to cancer.
   B. Annual incidence: 12,200 new cases; 3,800 estimated deaths.
   ◆ **C. Assessment:**
   1. *Subjective data*
      a. Dysphagia—pain in area of Adam's apple; radiates to ear.
      b. Dyspnea.
   2. *Objective data*
      a. Persistent hoarseness.

Adult

■ **TABLE 2.41 Selected Cancer Problems**

	Assessment		Risk Factors	Annual Incidence	Specific Treatment
	Subjective Data	**Objective Data**			
Gastrointestinal Tract					
Oral cancer	Difficulty chewing, swallowing, moving tongue or jaws; history of heavy smoking, drinking, or chewing tobacco	Sore that bleeds and does not heal; persistent red or white patch; diagnosis by biopsy; early detection: dental checks	Heavy smoking and drinking; user of chewing tobacco, men > age 40 (affects twice as many men as women)	30,200 new cases; 9050 estimated deaths	*Surgery,* with reconstructive surgery useful for cure and palliatively (see care of cancer patient having surgery, p. 193). *Radiation* using simulated computer localization to avoid destruction of normal tissue (see care of patient having radiation therapy, p. 196).
Esophageal cancer	Dysphagia—difficulty in swallowing; discomfort described as lump in throat, pressure in chest, pain; fatigue, lethargy, apathy, depression; anorexia	Weight loss; regurgitation, vomiting; diagnostic tests—*barium swallow, esophagoscopy; biopsy*	Over age 50, alcoholism, use of tobacco; increasing risk in nonwhite females, in people with achalasia (inability to relax lower esophagus with swallowing) or hiatal hernias	9800 new cases; 9200 estimated deaths	*Surgery:* resection with anastomosis, or removal with gastrostomy *Radiation:* best form of therapy *Chemotherapy:* antineoplastic drugs ineffective; medications to reduce symptoms of pain, discomfort, and anxiety; see nursing care plan/implementation for patient with cancer (p. 193); having radiation therapy (p. 196); having chemotherapy (p. 194); having surgery (p. 194)
Stomach cancer	Vague feeling of fullness, pressure, or epigastric pain following ingestion of food; anorexia, nausea, intolerance of meat; malaise	Eructation, regurgitation, vomiting; melena, hematemesis, anemia; jaundice, diarrhea, ascites; big belly, upper gastric area; often palpable mass	Men, lower socioeconomic classes, colder climates, early exposure to dietary carcinogens, blood group A, pernicious anemia, atrophic achlorhydric gastritis	24,800 new cases; 14,400 estimated deaths	*Surgery:* gastrectomy (see gastric surgery, p. 121, for nursing care). *Radiation:* not as useful because dosage needed would cause side effects unlikely to be tolerated by patient *Chemotherapy* alone or in conjunction with surgery: antitumor antibiotics, antimetabolites, nitrosureas, hematinics (see nursing care plan for patient having chemotherapy, p. 194)
Pancreatic cancer	Anorexia, nausea; pain in upper abdomen, radiating to back; dyspnea	Jaundice, vomiting, weight loss; determination of solid mass in area of pancreas by *computed tomographic scanning and ultrasound;* tissue identification by thin needle *percutaneous biopsy*	Excessive use of alcohol; exposure to dry cleaning chemicals, gasoline; coffee and decaffeinated coffee; possibly diabetes and chronic pancreatitis	27,000 new cases; 24,500 estimated deaths	*Surgery:* removal (must then have supplemental pancreatic enzymes, some patients become insulin-dependent diabetics) or bypass to relieve obstruction (see nursing care plan/implementation for patient with diabetes, p. 125) *Chemotherapy:* pain relief, antiemetics, insulin, pancrelipase, 5-FU, cytoxan, methotrexate, vincristine, mitomycin-C (see nursing care plan/implementation for patient having chemotherapy, p. 194)

continued

Adult

	Signs and symptoms	Risk factors	Incidence	Treatment
Gastrointestinal Tract (Continued)				
Pancreatic cancer *(Continued)*				*Radiation:* intraoperative high dose to pancreatic tumors with external high beam; palliative radiation therapy for pain (see nursing care plan/implementation for patient having radiation therapy, p. 196); see nursing care plan/implementation for patient with cancer, (p. 193)
Skin				
Skin cancer: basal cell	Reported painless lesion	Scaly plaques, papules that ulcerate; pale, waxy, pearly nodule or red, sharply outlined patch; unusual skin condition, change in size or color, or other darkly pigmented growth or mole	500,000 new cases; 7800 estimated deaths; 27,300 of these are malignant melanoma	*Surgery:* electrodesiccation (dehydration of tissue by use of needle electrode); cryosurgery (destruction of tissue by application of extreme cold) (see care of cancer patient, p. 193) *Radiation therapy* (see care of patient having radiation therapy, p. 196) *Prevention:* avoid sun from 10–3; use protective clothing, sunblock lotion
Nervous System				
Brain	*Headache:* steady, intermittent, severe (may be intensified by physical activity); nausea; lethargy, easy fatigability; forgetfulness, disorientation, impaired judgment; visual disturbances; blackouts	Vomiting, may be projectile; sight loss, auditory changes; signs of increased intracranial pressure; seizures; *diagnostic studies*—CT scan, arteriography, cytology of cerebrospinal fluid; paresthesia; behavior changes	None known for primary tumors; brain is common site for metastasis	14,700 new cases (brain and spinal cord); 10,900 estimated deaths	*Surgery:* craniotomy with excision of lesion; ventricular shunt to allow for drainage of fluid (see nursing care plan/implementation for craniotomy, p. 154; see nursing care plan/implementation for patient with cancer, p. 193) *Radiation:* cobalt (local or entire CNS); total brain radiation causes alopecia, which may be permanent (see nursing care plan/implementation for patient having radiation therapy, p. 196); could be used alone, with surgery, or with chemotherapy *Chemotherapy:* antineoplastic alkylating agents; nitrosureas (cross blood-brain barrier to reduce tumor)—carmustine (BCNU), lomustine (CCNU), semustine (methyl-CCNU); cerebral diuretics to reduce edema; anticonvulsants; analgesics; sedatives (see nursing care plan/implementation for patient having chemotherapy, p. 194)

Adult

■ **TABLE 2.41** (*Continued*)

	Assessment		Risk Factors	Annual Incidence	Specific Treatment
	Subjective Data	Objective Data			

Endocrine

Thyroid cancer

Subjective Data	Objective Data	Risk Factors	Annual Incidence	Specific Treatment
Painless nodule; dysphagia; difficulty breathing	Enlarged thyroid, thyroid nodule; palpable thyroid, lymph nodes; hoarseness; hypofunctional nodule seen on *isotopic imaging scanning; needle biopsy* for cytology studies	Radiation in childhood	11,000 new cases; 1100 estimated deaths	*Surgery:* total thyroidectomy, possible radical neck dissection (see *Thyroidectomy*, p. 184) *Radiation:* external, or with radioactive iodine (^{131}I) (see care of patient having radiation therapy, p. 196) *Chemotherapy:* chlorambucil, doxorubicin, vincristine (Leukeran, Adriamycin, Oncovin, respectively) (see care of patient having chemotherapy, p. 194)

Blood and Lymph Tissues

Hodgkin's disease

Subjective Data	Objective Data	Risk Factors	Annual Incidence	Specific Treatment
Fatigue; generalized pruritis; anorexia	Painless enlargement of lymph nodes, especially in cervical area; fever, night sweats; hepato-splenomegaly; anemia; peak age of incidence, 15–35; diagnostic tests—biopsy shows presence of *Reed-Sternberg cells; X rays, scans, laparotomy*	For young adults from 15–35 yr old, not clearly defined, some relationship to socioeconomic status; male-female ratio is 1.5:1; increased frequency among whites	7400 new cases; 1500 estimated deaths	*Staging and treatment:* *Stage I*—involvement of a single node or a single node region; excision of lesion, and total nodal radiation (see care of patient having radiation therapy, p. 196) *Stage II*—involvement of two or more lymph node regions on same side of diaphragm; excision of lesion and radiation (see care of patient having radiation therapy, p. 196) *Stage III*—involvement of lymph node regions on both sides of the diaphragm, which may include the spleen; combination of radiation and chemotherapy *Stage IV*—involvement of one or more extralymphatic organs or tissues, with or without lymphatic involvement; treated with chemotherapy alone, radiation therapy alone, or both Presence or absence of symptoms of night sweats, significant fever, and weight loss; treated with *chemotherapy,* MOPP protocol—Mustargen (mechlorethamine HCl, alkylating agent), Oncovin (vincristine, plant alkaloid), procarbazine (antineoplastic); prednisone (corticosteroid) (see care of patient having chemotherapy, p. 194)

Type	Signs/Symptoms	Lab/Diagnostic Findings	Predisposing/Epidemiology	Incidence	Treatment
Multiple myeloma	Weakness; history of frequent infections, especially pneumonias; severe bone pain on motion; neurologic symptoms, paralysis	Fractures of long bones; deformity of—sternum, ribs, vertebrae, pelvis; hepatosplenomegaly; renal calculi, renal insufficiency; anemia and bleeding tendencies; elevated uric acid	Exposure to ionizing irradiation; middle-aged or older females	11,600 new cases; 8200 estimated deaths	*Radiation therapy:* for some lesions (see nursing care plan/implementation for patients having radiation therapy, p. 196) *Surgery:* relieve spinal cord compression; orthopedic procedures to relieve or support bone problems (see nursing care plan/implementation for patients with internal fixation for fractures, p. 168; patient with spinal cord injuries when paralysis occurs, p. 180) *Chemotherapy:* alkylating agents; antitumor antibiotics; plant alkaloids; hormones—melphalan and prednisone (see nursing care plan/implementation for patients having chemotherapy, p. 194)
Urinary Organs Kidney cancer	Anorexia, nausea; fatigue; abdominal or flank pain	Painless, gross hematuria; firm, nontender, palpable kidney; vomiting and weight loss; *complications*—hypertension, nephrotic syndrome, lung metastasis; *lab and diagnostic tests:* IVP, urinalysis—presence of red cells and albumin; CBC—decrease in red cells and leukocytes, *reduction* in serum albumin, *elevation* of alpha globulin	More common among men than women, whites than blacks; radiation exposure, possible familial influence; common site of metastasis from lung, breast	22,500 new cases; 9600 estimated deaths	*Surgery:* nephrectomy (see pre/postoperative nursing care, p. 102) *Radiation:* local and irradiation of metastatic sites when tumor is radiosensitive (see nursing care plan/implementation for patient having radiation therapy, p. 196) *Chemotherapy:* plant alkaloids—vincristine (Oncovin); antitumor antibiotics—dactinomycin (Actinomycin D), doxorubicin (Adriamycin); alkylating agents—cyclophosphamide (Cytoxan) (see nursing care plan/implementation for patient having chemotherapy, p. 194)
Genital Organs Testicular cancer	Aching or dragging sensation in groin, usually painless	Gynecomastia; enlargement, swelling, lump, hardening of testes; early diagnosis in young adult male; early diagnosis—monthly testicular self-exam; See Figure 2.10, p. 211	Second most common malignancy among men between 25 and 40; possibly exposure to chemical carcinogens; trauma, orchitis; gonadal dysgenesis; cryptorchidism (undescended testicles)	5600 new cases; 350 estimated deaths; 95–100% 5-yr survival rate for early-detected nonmetastasized lesions	*Surgery:* orchiectomy (see nursing care plan/implementation for the pre- and postop patient, p. 102) *Radiation:* see nursing care plan/implementation for patient having radiation therapy, p. 196 *Chemotherapy:* chlorambucil (Leukeran), methotrexate, steroids (see nursing care plan/implementation for patient having chemotherapy, p. 194)

continued

■ **TABLE 2.41   Selected Cancer Problems**

| | Assessment | | | | |
	Subjective Data	Objective Data	Risk Factors	Annual Incidence	Specific Treatment
Cervical cancer	Vague pelvic or low back discomfort, pressure, or pain	Intermenstrual, postcoital, or postmenopausal bleeding; vaginal discharge—serosanguineous and malodorous hypermenorrhea; abdominal distention with urinary frequency; abnormal Pap test (see Table 2.38); recommended guidelines by American Cancer Society: *Pap test* annually; after 3 consecutive normal tests, MD may recommend less frequent testing; pelvic/uterine exam every 3 yr	Early age at first intercourse; multiple sex partners; low socioeconomic status; exposure to herpes virus 2	12,900 new cases; 7000 estimated deaths	*Staging* (See Table 2.40, p. 205): *Stage 0*—carcinoma in situ; no distinct tumor observable; stage may last for 8–10 yr; cure rate 100% following treatment of wedge or cone resection of cervix during childbearing years, or simple hysterectomy *Stage I*—malignant cells infiltrate cervical mucosa; lesion bleeds easily; cure rate 80% with treatment of hysterectomy *Stage II*—neoplasm spreads through cervical muscular layers, involves upper third of vaginal mucosa; cure rate 50% with treatment of radical hysterectomy *Stage III*—neoplasm involves lower third of vagina; cure rate 25% with pelvic exoneration *Stage IV*—involves metastasis to bladder, rectum, and surrounding tissues; considered incurable *Radiation:* external and/or internal, in conjunction with surgery or alone, depending on stage of disease or condition of patient (see nursing care plan/implementation for patient having radiation therapy, p. 196) *Chemotherapy:* progestin, antineoplastics, megestrol (Megace), medroxyprogesterone (Curretab, Provera); alkylating agents—dacarbazine (DTIC).

■ **FIGURE 2.10** **Testicular self-examination. A. Grasp testis with both hands; palpate gently between thumb and fingers. B. Abnormal lumps or irregularities are reported to physician.**

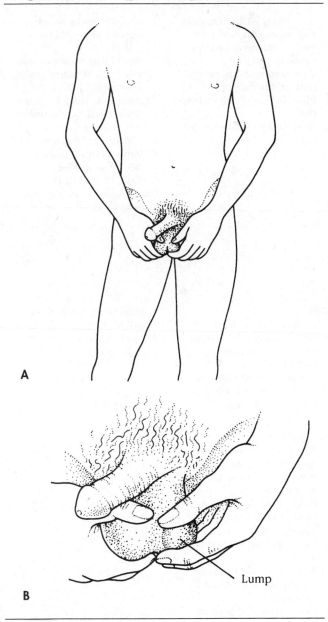

A

B

Lump

  b. Cough and hemoptysis.
  c. Enlarged cervical nodes.
  d. General debility and weight loss.
  e. Foul breath.
  🜭 f. Diagnosis made by history, laryngoscopy with biopsy and microscopic study of cells.
◆ **D. Analysis/nursing diagnosis:**
  1. *Impaired verbal communication* related to removal of larynx.
  2. *Body image disturbance* related to radical surgery.
  3. *Ineffective airway clearance* related to increased secretions through tracheoctomy.
◆ **E. Nursing care plan/implementation** (see also care of the cancer patient, p. 193): treatment primarily surgical (laryngectomy—see p. 145); radiation therapy may also be indicated.
◆ **F. Evaluation/outcome criteria:** see Laryngectomy, p. 146.
IX. Additional types of cancer—Table 2.41.

❏ Emergency Nursing Procedures

  I. Purpose—to initiate assessment and intervention procedures that will speed total care of the patient toward a successful outcome.
  II. Emergency nursing procedures for adults are detailed in Table 2.42.
  III. Legal issues in the emergency room—see Unit 9.

Adult

Adult

■ **TABLE 2.42 Nursing Care of the Adult in Medical and Surgical Emergencies**

Condition	Assessment: Signs and Symptoms	Prehospitalization Nursing Care	In-Hospital Nursing Care
Cardiovascular Emergencies			
Myocardial infarction—ischemia and necrosis of cardiac muscle secondary to insufficient or obstructed coronary blood flow	*Prehospital:* *Chest pain:* viselike choking, unrelieved by rest or nitroglycerin *Skin:* ashen, cold, clammy *Vital signs:* pulse—rapid, weak, thready; increased rate and depth of respirations; dyspnea *Behavior:* restless, anxious *In hospital:* *C/V:* blood pressure and pulse pressure decreased *Heart sounds:* soft; S_3 may be present *Respirations:* fine basilar rales *Lab:* ECG consistent with tissue necrosis (Q waves) and injury (ST-segment elevation); serum enzymes elevated	1. If coronary suspected, call physician, paramedic service, or emergency ambulance 2. Calm and reassure patient that help is coming 3. Place in semi-Fowler's position 4. Keep patient warm but not hot	1. Rapidly assess hemodynamic and respiratory status 2. Start IV as ordered—usually 5% D/W per microdrip to establish lifeline for emergency drug treatment 3. Draw blood for electrolytes, enzymes, as ordered 4. Place on cardiac monitor 5. Relieve pain—morphine SO_4 IV as needed 6. Take 12-lead ECG Once patient is stable, transfer to CCU
Cardiac arrest—cardiac stenosis or ventricular fibrillation secondary to rapid administration or overdose of anesthetics or narcotic drugs, obstruction of the respiratory tract (mucus, vomitus, foreign body), acute anxiety, cardiac disease, dehydration, shock, electric shock, or emboli	Cyanosis, gasping *Respirations:* rapid, shallow, absent *Pulse:* weak, thready, >120, absent Muscle twitching *Pupils:* dilated *Skin:* cold, clammy Loss of consciousness	*CPR* 1. *Position:* flat on back 2. Shake vigorously—establish unresponsiveness 3. Call for help 4. Tilt head back (chin lift) 5. Check for breathing—listen at mouth, look at chest, feel with cheek *No breathing* 1. Kneel close to head; place hand on forehead, bringing lower jaw forward and opening airway 2. Pinch nostrils shut and blow two full breaths into patient's mouth 3. Lips must form airtight seal 4. Watch chest for adequate expansion; clear throat if indicated 5. Check pulse—if present, breathe into mouth every 5 sec	1. If monitored, note rhythm; call for help and note time 2. Countershock if rhythm is ventricular fibrillation or ventricular tachycardia 3. If countershock unsuccessful, begin CPR, as in prehospital care

continued

■ **TABLE 2.42** *(Continued)*

Condition	Assessment: Signs and Symptoms	Prehospitalization Nursing Care	In-Hospital Nursing Care
		No heartbeat *Two-person CPR:* 80 chest compressions per minute, with one breath between every 5 compressions *One-person CPR:* 80 chest compressions per minute, with two quick breaths between every 15 compressions Check pulse at neck after 1 min and every few minutes thereafter Check pupils to determine effectiveness of CPR—should begin to constrict *If heartbeat returns:* Assist respiration and monitor pulse; continue CPR until help arrives	*Two-person rescue* *First person:* begins CPR as described in prehospital care *Second person:* 1. Pages arrest team 2. Brings defibrillator to bedside and countershocks, if indicated by rhythm 3. Brings emergency cart to bedside 4. Suctions airway, if indicated due to vomitus or secretions 5. Bags patient with 100% O_2 6. Assists with intubation when arrest team arrives 7. Establishes intravenous line if one is not available
Shock—cellular hypoxia and impairment of cellular function secondary to trauma, hemorrhage, fright, dehydration, cardiac insufficiency, allergic reactions, septicemia, impairment of nervous system, poisons	*Early shock* *Sensorium:* conscious, apprehensive, and restless; some slurring of speech *Pupils:* dull but reactive to light *Pulse:* rate <140/min; amplitude full to mildly decreased *Blood pressure:* normal to slightly decreased *Neck veins:* normal to slightly flat in supine position; may be full in septic shock or grossly distended in cardiogenic shock *Skin:* cool, clammy, pale *Respirations:* rapid, shallow *GI:* nausea, vomiting, thirst *Renal:* urine output 20–40 mL/h	1. Check breathing—clear airway if necessary; if no breathing, give artificial respirations; if breathing is irregular or labored, raise head and shoulders 2. Control bleeding by placing pressure on the wound or at pressure points (proximal artery) 3. Make comfortable and reassure 4. Cover lightly to prevent heat loss, but don't bundle up 5. If neck or spine injury is suspected—do *not* move, unless victim in danger of more injury	1. Check vital signs rapidly—pulse, pupils, respirations 2. Check airway; clear if necessary; PO_2 should be maintained above 60 mm Hg; elevated PCO_2 indicates need for intubation and ventilatory assistance 3. Control gross bleeding 4. Prepare for insertion of intravenous line and central lines—if abdominal injuries present 5. Peripheral line should be placed in upper extremity if fluids being lost in abdomen
		If patient unconscious or has wounds of the lower face and jaw—place on *side* to promote drainage of fluids; position patient on *back* unless otherwise indicated	1. Draw blood for specimens: Hgb, Hct, CBC, glucose, CO_2, sodium amylase, BUN, K^+; type and crossmatch, blood gases, enzymes, prothrombin times 2. Prepare infusion of 5% D/NS *unless* hypernatremia suspected; dextran if blood loss

continued

■ **TABLE 2.42** *(Continued)*

Condition	Assessment: Signs and Symptoms	Prehospitalization Nursing Care	In-Hospital Nursing Care
	Severe or late shock *Sensorium:* confused, disoriented, apathetic, unresponsive; slow, slurred speech, often incoherent *Pupils:* dilating, dilated, slow or nonreactive to light *Pulse:* rate >150/min, thready, weak *Blood pressure:* 80 mm Hg or unobtainable *Neck veins:* flat in a supine position—no filling; full to distended in septic or cardiogenic shock *Skin:* cold, clammy, mottled; circumoral cyanosis, dusky, cyanotic *Eyes:* sunken—vacant expression *Renal:* urine output <20 mL/h	1. *Raise* feet 6–8 in. unless patient has head or chest injuries; if victim becomes less comfortable, lower feet 2. If patient complains of thirst, do *not* give fluids unless you are more than 6 h away from professional medical help; under *no* conditions give water to patients who are unconscious, having seizures or vomiting, appearing to need general anesthetic, or with a stomach, chest, or skull injury 3. Be calm and confident; reassure patient help is on the way	1. Assess and intervene as above; then obtain information as to onset and past history 2. Catheterize and monitor patient urine output as ordered 3. Take 12-lead ECG 4. Insert nasogastric tube and assess aspirate for volume, color, and blood; save specimen if poison or drug overdose suspected 5. *If CVP low*—infuse 200–300 mL over 5–10 min *If CVP rises* sharply, fluid restriction necessary; if remains low, hypovolemia present 6. *If patient febrile*—blood cultures and wound cultures will be ordered 7. *If urine output* scanty or absent—give mannitol as ordered
Respiratory Emergencies *Choking*—obstruction of airway secondary to aspiration of a foreign object	Gasping, wheezing; looks panicky, but can still breathe, talk, cough Cough: weak, ineffective; breathing sounds like high-pitched crowing; color—white, gray, blue Difficulty speaking; clutches throat	Do not interfere; watch closely; call for assistance *Victim standing, sitting and conscious:* Perform *Heimlich maneuver:* stand behind victim, wrap arms around waist, place fist against abdomen, and with your other hand, press it into the victim's abdomen with a quick upward thrust until the obstruction is relieved or the victim becomes unconscious	As in prehospital care; do *not* slap on back
		Victim lying down: Roll the victim onto his or her back; straddle the victim's thighs; place heel of hand in the middle of abdomen; place other hand on top of the first; stiffen arms and deliver 6–10 abdominal thrusts	As in prehospital care

continued

■ TABLE 2.42   (Continued)

Condition	Assessment: Signs and Symptoms	Prehospitalization Nursing Care	In-Hospital Nursing Care
		Unconscious victim: Try to ventilate; if unsuccessful, deliver abdominal thrusts using technique described above; probe mouth for foreign objects; keep repeating above procedure until ventilation occurs; as victim becomes more deprived of air, muscles will relax and maneuvers that were previously unsuccessful will begin to work; when successful in removing obstruction, give two breaths; check pulse; start CPR if indicated On *obese or pregnant* victims—use chest thrusts instead of abdominal thrusts *You are victim and alone:* Place your two fists for abdominal thrusts; bend over back of chair, sink, etc. and exert hard, repeated pressure on abdomen to force object up; push fingers down your throat to encourage regurgitation	As in prehospital care; when probing mouth for foreign object, turn head to side, unless patient has neck injury; in event of neck injury, raise the arm opposite you and roll the head and shoulders as a unit, so that head ends up supported on the arm
Acute respiratory failure—sudden onset of an abnormally low P_{O_2} (<60 mm Hg) and/or high P_{CO_2} (>60 mm Hg) secondary to lung disease or trauma, peripheral or central nervous system depression, cardiac failure, severe obesity, airway obstruction, environmental abnormality	*Hypoxia* *Sensorium:* acute apprehension *Respiration:* dyspnea; shallow, rapid respirations *Skin:* circumoral cyanosis; pale, dusky skin and nailbeds *C/V:* slight hypertension and tachycardia, or hypotension and bradycardia *Hypercardia* *Sensorium:* decreasing mentation; headache *Skin:* flushed, warm, moist *C/V:* hypertension; tachycardia	If you suspect respiratory distress, call physician; calm and reassure patient; place in a chair or semisitting position; keep warm but not hot; phone for ambulance; if respirations cease or patient becomes unconscious, clear airway and commence respiratory resuscitation; check pulse: initiate CPR if necessary; continue resuscitation until help arrives	Check patient's ability to speak; maintain airway by placing in *high Fowler's position;* check vital signs: BP, pulse rate and rhythm, temperature, skin color, rate and depth of respirations Prepare for intubation if: 1. Patient has flail chest 2. Patient is comatose without gag reflex 3. Has respiratory arrest Maintain mouth to mouth until intubation 4. P_{CO_2} > 55 mm Hg 5. P_{O_2} < 60 mm Hg 6. F_IO_2 > 50% using nasal cannula, catheter, or mask 7. Respiratory rate >36 *After intubation:* 1. Check bilateral lung sounds 2. Observe for symmetric lung expansion 3. Maintain humidified oxygen at lowest F_IO_2 possible to achieve P_{O_2} of 60 mm Hg

continued

■ **TABLE 2.42** *(Continued)*

Condition	Assessment: Signs and Symptoms	Prehospitalization Nursing Care	In-Hospital Nursing Care
			Improve ventilation (decreased P_{CO_2}) by: 1. Liquefying secretions—oral and parenteral fluids; if intubated, frequent instillations of normal saline or sodium bicarbonate 2. Frequent suctioning 3. IPPB indicated if tidal volume ↓ 4. Chest physiotherapy Administer *drugs* as ordered: sympathomimetics, xanthines, antibiotics, and steroids Monitor: arterial blood gases, electrolytes, Hct, Hb, and WBC *Do not:* 1. Administer sedatives 2. Correct acid-base problems without monitoring electrolytes 3. Overcorrect P_{CO_2} 4. Leave patient alone while oxygen therapy is initiated Once patient is stable, transfer to ICU

Near-drowning—asphyxiation or partial asphyxiation due to immersion or submersion in a fluid or liquid medium	*Conscious victim:*
	Acute anxiety, panic; increased rate of respirations
	Pale, dusky skin
	Unconscious victim:
	Shallow or no respirations
	Weak or no pulse
	If victim not breathing, as soon as you have firm support begin mouth-to-mouth resuscitation
	Tilt head back, bring jaw forward, pinch nostril shut, give two quick breaths
		Conscious victim:
		1. Try to talk victim out of panic so can find footing and way to shore
		2. Utilize devices such as poles, rings, clothing to extend to victim; do not let panicked victim grab you; do not attempt swimming rescue unless specially trained
		3. If you suspect head or neck injury—handle carefully, floating victim back to shore with body and head as straight as possible; do not turn head or bend back
			Nonsymptomatic neardrowning victim:
			1. Draw blood for arterial blood gases with patient breathing room air
			2. PA and lateral chest X ray
			3. Auscultate lungs
			4. Admit to hospital for further evaluation if:
			  &boxed;a. $P_{O_2} < 80$ mm Hg
			  b. pH < 7.35&boxed;
			  c. Pulmonary infiltrates present, or auscultation reveals crackles
			  d. Victim inhaled fluids containing: chlorine, hydrocarbons, sewage, or hypotonic or fresh water

continued

■ **TABLE 2.42**   *(Continued)*

Condition	Assessment: Signs and Symptoms	Prehospitalization Nursing Care	In-Hospital Nursing Care

		On shore:
		1. Check breathing
		2. Lay victim flat on back; cover and keep warm
		3. Calm and reassure victim
		4. Do not give food or water
		5. Get to medical assistance as soon as possible
		6. *If unconscious and not breathing,* begin sequence for CPR; compress water from abdomen *only* if interfering with ventilation attempts
		7. *If airway obstructed,* reposition head; attempt to ventilate; perform 6–10 abdominal thrusts; sweep mouth deeply; attempt to ventilate; repeat until successful
		8. Once ventilation established, check pulse; if absent, begin chest compressions as in CPR, one-person or two-person rescue
		9. Continue CPR until victim revives or help arrives
		10. If victim revives, cover and keep warm; reassure victim help is on the way
		11. Rescue personnel can further assist emergency room personnel by:
		  a. Documenting prehospital resuscitation methods used
		  b. Immobilizing victims suspected of cervical spine injuries
		  c. Utilizing a sterile container to take a sample of immersion fluid
		  d. Taking on-scene arterial blood gas sample for later analysis
			Symptomatic near-drowning victim:
			1. Provide basic or advanced cardiac life support
			2. Provide clear airway and adequate ventilation by:
			  a. Suctioning airway
			  b. Inserting artificial airway and attaching it to ventilator as indicated
			  c. Inserting nasogastric tube to suction to minimize aspiration of vomitus
			3. Monitor ECG continuously
			4. Start IV infusion 5% D/W at keep-open rate for *fresh water near-drowning;* 5% D/NS in *salt water near-drowning*
			5. Assist with insertion of *CVP* and *Swan-Ganz* catheter to guide subsequent infusion rates
			6. Administer drugs as ordered: anticonvulsants; steroids, antibiotics, stimulants, antiarrhythmics
			7. Provide rewarming if hypothermia present
			8. Insert *Foley* to assess kidney output as fresh water near-drowning causes renal tubular necrosis due to RBC hemolysis
			9. Transfer to ICU when stabilized

continued

■ **TABLE 2.42**   *(Continued)*

Condition	Assessment: Signs and Symptoms	Prehospitalization Nursing Care	In-Hospital Nursing Care
Systemic Injuries *Multiple traumas*	*Sensorium:* alert; disoriented, stuporous, comatose *Respirations:* increased rate, depth; shallow; asymmetric; parodoxical breathing; mediastinal shift; gasping, blowing *C/V:* signs of shock (see pp. 213, 214) *Abdomen:* contusions; pain; abrasions; open wounds; rigidity; increasing distention *Skeletal system:* pain; swelling; deformity; inappropriate or no movement *Neurologic:* pupils round, equal, react to light; ipsilateral dilatation and unresponsive; fixed and dilated bilaterally Bilateral movement and sensation in all extremities Progressive contralateral weakness Loss of voluntary motor function See *Sensorium* above for level of consciousness	1. *Don't* move patient unless you must, to prevent further injury; send for help 2. Check breathing—give mouth-to-mouth resuscitation if indicated 3. Check for bleeding 4. Control bleeding by applying pressure on wound or on pressure points (artery proximal to wound) 5. Use tourniquet *only* if above pressure techniques fail to stop severe bleeding 6. Check for shock (pulse, pupils, skin color) and other injuries 7. Fractures: keep open-fracture area clean 8. Stop bleeding, observe for shock 9. Do not try to set bone 10. If patient must be moved—splint broken bones with splints that extend past the limb joints; tie splints on snugly but not so tight as to cut off circulation 11. Check peripheral pulses 12. If head or back injury suspected—keep body straight; move only with help 13. Reassure patient that help is on the way	1. Assess vital functions 2. Establish airway; ventilate with Ambu-bag, volume-cycled ventilator 3. Draw arterial blood gases 4. Control bleeding 5. Support circulation by closed chest massage 6. Prepare infusions of dextran, blood, crystalloids 7. Assess for other injuries: head injuries—suspect cervical neck injury with all head injuries 8. Place sandbags to immobilize head and neck 9. Do *mini-neurologic exam:* level of consciousness, pupils, bilateral movement, and sensation 10. Get history—time of injury; any loss of consciousness; any drug ingestion 11. Stop bleeding on or about head 12. Apply ice to contusions and hematomas 13. Check for bleeding from nose, pharynx, ears 14. Check for cerebrospinal fluid from ears or nose 15. Assist with spinal tap if ordered 16. Keep accurate I&O 17. Protect from injury if restless; seizures: orient to time, place, person 18. Administer steroids, diuretics, as ordered 19. *Check for signs of increasing intracranial pressure:* slowing pulse and respiration, widened pulse pressure, decreasing mentation
Spinal injuries			1. Assess and support vital functions as above 2. Immobilize—no flexion or extension allowed 3. *If in respiratory distress*—nasotracheal intubation or tracheostomy to avoid hyperextending neck

continued

■ **TABLE 2.42** *(Continued)*

Condition	Assessment: Signs and Symptoms	Prehospitalization Nursing Care	In-Hospital Nursing Care
			4. *Check for level of injury and function,* asking patient to: 　a. Lift elbow to shoulder height (C-5) 　b. Bend elbow (C-6) 　c. Straighten elbow (C-7) 　d. Grip your hand (C8–T1) 　e. Lift leg (L-3) 　f. Straighten knee (L-4, L-5) 　g. Wiggle toes (L-5) 　h. Push toes down (S-1) 5. *If patient comatose:* 　a. Rub sternum with knuckles 　b. If all extremities move, severe injury unlikely 　c. If one side moves and other does not, potential hemiplegia 　d. If arms move and legs don't, lower spinal cord injury 6. Administer steroids as ordered 7. Assist with application of skull tongs—*Vinke* or *Crutchfield* 8. Maintain IV infusions 9. Insert *Foley* as indicated 10. Assist with dressing of open wounds
Chest injuries			1. Note color and pattern of respirations, position of trachea 2. Auscultate lungs and palpate chest for: crepitus, pain, tenderness, and position of trachea 3. Chest tubes if pneumothorax or hemothorax present 4. Place gauze soaked in petroleum jelly over open pneumothorax (sucking chest wound) to seal hole and decrease respiratory distress 5. Assist with tracheostomy if indicated

continued

Adult

■ **TABLE 2.42** *(Continued)*

Condition	Assessment: Signs and Symptoms	Prehospitalization Nursing Care	In-Hospital Nursing Care
Abdominal injuries			1. Observe for rigidity 2. Check for hematuria 3. Auscultate for bowel sounds 4. Assist with paracentesis to confirm bleeding in abdominal cavity 5. Prepare for exploratory laparotomy 6. Insert nasogastric tube—to detect presence of UGI bleeding 7. Monitor vital signs *If organs protruding:* 1. *Flex* patient's knees 2. Cover intestines with sterile towel soaked in saline 3. Do not attempt to replace organs
Fractures			1. Administer tetanus toxoid as ordered 2. Observe for pain, peripheral pulses, pallor, loss of sensation and/or movement 3. Assist with wound cleansing, casting, X rays, reduction 4. Prepare for surgery if indicated 5. Monitor vital signs
Burns—tissue trauma secondary to scalding fluid or flame, chemicals, or electricity	*Superficial (first degree):* Erythema and tenderness Usually sunburn	Relieve pain by applying cold, wet towel or cold water (not iced)	1. Cleanse thoroughly with mild detergent and water 2. Apply gauze or sterile towel 3. Administer sedatives and narcotics as ordered 4. Arrange for follow-up care, or prepare for admission if burn ambulatory care impractical

	Partial thickness (second degree):
	Swelling, blisters; moisture due to escaping plasma
		1. Douse with cold water until pain relieved
		2. Blot skin dry and cover with clean towel
		3. Do *not* break blisters, remove pieces of skin, or apply antiseptic ointments
		4. If arm or leg burned, keep *elevated*
		5. Seek medical attention if *second-degree* burns:
		  a. Cover 15% of body surface in adult
		  b. Cover 10% of body surface in children
		  c. Involve hands, feet, or face
			1. Check tetanus immunization status
			2. Administer sedatives or narcotics as ordered
			3. Assess respiratory and hemodynamic status; oxygen or ventilatory assist as indicated, intravenous infusions as ordered to combat shock
			4. Remove all clothing from burn area
			5. Using *aseptic technique*, cleanse burns with antiseptic followed by soap and water, and irrigate with normal saline

continued

■ **TABLE 2.42** *(Continued)*

Condition	Assessment: Signs and Symptoms	Prehospitalization Nursing Care	In-Hospital Nursing Care

	Full thickness (third degree): White, charred areas	1. *Don't* remove charred clothing
		2. Cover burned area with clean towel, sheet
		3. *Elevate* burned extremi5ties
		4. Apply cold pack to hand, face, or feet
		5. Sit up patient with face or chest wound to assist respirations
		6. Maintain airway
		7. Observe for shock
		8. *Do not:*
		  a. Put ice water on burns or immerse wounds in ice water—may increase shock
		  b. Apply ointments
		9. Calm and reassure victim
		10. Get medical help promptly
		11. *If* patient conscious, not vomiting, and medical assistance is more than 6 h away: may give sips of weak solution of salt, soda, and water
			1. Do not break blebs or attempt debridement
			2. Assist with application of dressings as ordered
			3. Maintain frequent checks of vital signs, urine output
			4. Provide psychological support—explain procedures, orient, etc.
			5. Assist with application of splints as ordered
			6. Administer tetanus immune globulin or toxoid as ordered
			7. Assist with transfer to hospital unit

	Fourth degree: Black	Same as full thickness.	
	Chemical burns	1. Flush with copious amounts of water 2. Get rid of clothing over burned area	1. Flush with copious amounts of water 2. Administer sedation or narcotics as ordered
	Burns of the eye: Acid	1. Flush eye with water for at least 15 min 2. Pour water from inside to outside of eye to avoid contaminating unaffected eye 3. Cover—seek medical attention at once	1. Irrigate with water; *never* use neutralizing solution 2. Instill 0.5% tetracaine as ordered 3. Apply patch
	Alkali (laundry detergent or cleaning solvent)	1. Don't allow a patient to rub eye 2. Flush eye with water for at least 30 min 3. Cover—seek medical attention at once	As above for acid
Abdominal Emergencies *Aortic aneurysm*—rupture or dissection	Primarily males > age 60 Sudden onset of excruciating pain: abdominal, lumbosacral, groin, or rectal Orthopnea, dyspnea Fainting, hypotension; if dissecting, marked hypertension may be present Palpable, tender, pulsating mass in umbilical area Femoral pulse present; dorsalis pedes—weak or absent	1. Notify physician 2. Lay patient flat, or raise head if in respiratory distress 3. Cover—keep warm but not hot 4. Institute shock measures as above 5. Calm; reassure that help is on the way	1. Assess respiratory and hemodynamic status 2. Institute shock measures (see pp. 213, 214) if indicated 3. Evaluate and compare peripheral pulses 4. Assist with X rays 5. Assist with emergency preoperative treatment

continued

■ **TABLE 2.42**   *(Continued)*

Condition	Assessment: Signs and Symptoms	Prehospitalization Nursing Care	In-Hospital Nursing Care

Blunt injuries—Spleen	Left upper quadrant pain, tenderness and moderate rigidity; left shoulder pain (*Kehr's sign*)
	Hypotension; weak, thready pulse; increased respirations (shock)
		1. Lay patient *flat*
		2. Institute shock measures (see pp. 213, 214)
			1. Assess respiratory and hemodynamic status
			  a. Maintain airway and ventilation as indicated
			  b. Institute infusions of colloids and/or crystalloids as ordered
			  c. Insert both CVP and arterial monitoring lines
			  d. Insert Foley catheter
			2. Prepare for splenectomy

Eye and Ear Emergencies *Chemical burns*	See *Burns*	See *Burns*	See *Burns*
Blunt injuries secondary to flying missiles, e.g., balls, striking face against car dashboard	Decreased visual acuity, diplopia, blood in anterior chamber Pain, conjunctiva reddened, edema of eyelids	1. Prevent victim from rubbing eye 2. Cover with patch to protect eye 3. Seek medical help immediately	1. Test visual acuity of each eye using *Snellen* or *Jaeger* chart 2. Assist with *fluorescein* administration—to facilitate identifying breaks in cornea
Sharp ocular trauma—secondary to small or larger foreign bodies	History of feelings as if something were hitting eye Pain, tearing, reddened conjunctiva Blurring of vision Foreign object may be visible	1. Keep victim from rubbing eye 2. Cover very lightly—do not apply pressure	1. Check visual acuity in both eyes 2. Check pupils 3. Instill 1% tetracaine HCl as ordered to relieve pain 4. Administer antibiotic drops or ointment as ordered 5. Apply eye patch 6. Provide instructions for subsequent care and follow-up

Foreign bodies in ears—beans, peas, candy, foxtails, insects	Decreased hearing; pulling, poking at ear and ear canal; buzzing, discomfort	1. Do *not* attempt to remove object
		2. Seek medical assistance
			1. Inspect ear canal
			2. Assist with sedating children—restraint may be necessary
			3. Assist with procedures to remove object:
			  a. Forceps or curved probe for *foxtails, irregularly shaped* objects
			  b. 10F or 12F catheter with tip cut squarely off and attached to suction to remove *round* object
			4. Irrigate external auditory canal to flush out *insects,* materials that do not absorb water; do *not* irrigate if danger of perforation

❏ Questions

Select the one best answer for each question.

1. Nursing preparations for a gastroscopy procedure include:
   1. Holding the patient NPO for 24 hours before the procedure.
   2. Having an operative or procedure permit signed.
   3. Reassuring the patient that gastroscopy is not an uncomfortable procedure, though he or she will need to lie quietly.
   4. Removing dentures and administering pain medication prior to the procedure.

2. Which nursing action is the *first* priority during a generalized tonic-clonic seizure episode?
   1. Observe and record all events that occur prior to, during, and after the seizure.
   2. Maintain a patent airway by turning the head to the side.
   3. Protect the patient from injury.
   4. Monitor vital signs, with special attention directed to respiratory status.

3. Which nursing intervention would be the most beneficial in preparing the patient psychologically for ileostomy surgery?
   1. Include the patient's family in preoperative teaching sessions.
   2. Encourage the patient to express his or her concerns and to ask questions regarding the management of the ileostomy.
   3. Thorough, brief explanation of all preoperative and postoperative procedures.
   4. Have a member of an "ostomy club" visit the patient.

4. Which of the following indicates circulatory constriction in the patient with a newly applied long leg cast?
   1. Tingling and numbness of toes.
   2. Inability to move toes.
   3. Blanching or cyanosis of toes.
   4. Complaints of pressure or tightness of the cast.

5. Paralytic ileus is described by the nurse as:
   1. Edema of the intestinal mucosa.
   2. Acute dilatation of the colon.
   3. Absent, diminished, or uncoordinated autonomic stimulation of peristalsis.
   4. High, tinkling bowel sounds over the area of obstruction.

6. The doctor has ordered ambulation on crutches, with no weight bearing on the affected limb. An appropriate crutch gait for the nurse to teach the patient would be:
   1. Two-point gait.
   2. Three-point gait.
   3. Four-point gait.
   4. Tripod gait.

7. Nursing preparation for an upper GI series includes:
   1. NPO for 24 hours before the procedure.
   2. Administering an enema or cathartic to enhance visualization.
   3. Discouraging the patient from smoking the morning of the procedure because smoking can stimulate gastric motility.
   4. Instructing the patient that the test involves insertion of a rubber gastroscopy tube.

8. Burns are classified according to the depth of tissue destruction. The nurse would recognize a deep partial-thickness burn because the burn:
   1. Involves the epidermis only.
   2. Extends to the dermis and is very painful.
   3. Extends to subcutaneous tissues and is rarely painful.
   4. Extends to muscle and bone and is very painful.

9. The nurse's best explanation of the basic emotional issue underlying or contributing to the development of ulcers would be:
   1. Anxiety neurosis.
   2. Dependence-independence conflict.
   3. Repressed anger and hostility.
   4. Compulsive time orientation.

10. Which patient problem relating to altered nutrition is a consequence of impaired physical mobility?
    1. Increased appetite.
    2. Decreased protein catabolism.
    3. Increased carbohydrate needs.
    4. Increased secretion of digestive enzymes.

11. The signs and symptoms of open-angle glaucoma are related to:
    1. An imbalance between the rate of secretion of intraocular fluids and the rate of absorption of aqueous humor.
    2. A degenerative disease characterized by narrowing of the arterioles of the retina and areas of ischemia.
    3. An infectious process that causes clouding and scarring of the cornea.
    4. A dysfunction of aging in which the retina of the eye buckles from inadequate fluid pressures.

12. Patients suffering from dumping syndrome should be advised by the nurse to:
    1. Drink liquids between meals.
    2. Drink liquids only with meals.
    3. Drink liquids any time they want.
    4. Restrict fluid intake to 1200 mL/d.

13. Urinary output is closely assessed after nephrectomy. Which assessment finding is an early indicator of fluid retention in the postoperative period?
    1. Increased specific gravity of urine.
    2. Daily weight gain of 2 lb or more.
    3. A urinary output of 50 mL/h.
    4. Periorbital edema.

14. Which statement by the nurse accurately describes the Miller-Abbott tube?
    1. A double-lumen tube, with one lumen leading to the inflatable balloon and the other lumen used for aspiration.
    2. A plastic or rubber tube with holes near its tip facilitating withdrawal of fluids from the stomach.
    3. A single-lumen, saline-, air-, or water-weighted tube approximately 6 feet long.
    4. A 10-foot-long rubber tube with a saline, air, or water bag at its end.

15.

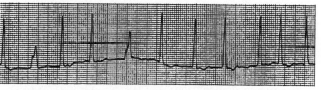

The correct interpretation of the above arrhythmia is:
   1. Sinus rhythm with multifocal premature ventricular contractions (PVCs).
   2. Atrial fibrillation with unifocal PVCs.
   3. Sinus tachycardia with unifocal PVCs.
   4. Second-degree atrioventricular block with unifocal PVCs.

16. If treatment with thyroid hormone is effective, the nurse should expect:

1. Diuresis, a decrease in pulse rate, and an increase in blood pressure.
2. Diuresis, a widening pulse pressure, and an increase in both temperature and respiratory rate.
3. Increased pulse rate, decreased respiratory rate, and decreased puffiness.
4. Weight loss, increased diastolic blood pressure, and decreased pulse rate.

17. A patient was admitted to the hospital due to deep partial-thickness burns of the left leg and thigh. The nurse would expect this patient's serum-sodium level to be within normal limits at the time of admission because:
    1. The pituitary has increased ADH release.
    2. Vascular fluid losses due to exudate and edema formation have resulted in hemoconcentration.
    3. Sodium has diffused from disrupted cells into the vascular compartment.
    4. Increased serum potassium depressed aldosterone secretion by the adrenal cortex.

18. Nursing actions for patients with Addison's disease include:
    1. Providing a low-sodium diet.
    2. Restriction of fluids to 1500 mL/d.
    3. Administering insulin-replacement therapy.
    4. Reducing physical and emotional stress.

19. The nurse explains to a patient that a vagotomy is done in conjunction with a subtotal gastrectomy because the vagus nerve:
    1. Stimulates increased gastric motility.
    2. Decreases gastric motility, thereby preventing the movement of HCl out of the stomach.
    3. Stimulates both increased gastric secretion and gastric motility.
    4. Stimulates decreased gastric secretion, thereby increasing nausea and vomiting.

20. In planning care for a patient with hyperkalemia, the nurse knows that the treatment of choice to reduce hyperkalemia is:
    1. Morphine sulfate.
    2. Sodium polystyrene sulfonate (Kayexalate).
    3. Insulin and 50% glucose solution.
    4. Synthetic aldosterone.

21. Understanding that prolonged immobilization could lead to decubitus ulcers, the nurse plans interventions to prevent alterations in skin integrity. Which would be the *least* appropriate intervention?
    1. Use of a bed cradle.
    2. Giving backrubs with alcohol.
    3. Encouraging a high-protein diet.
    4. Frequent assessment of the skin.

22. The nurse knows that the physiologic response to the stress of extensive burns may result in the following complication in the postburn period:
    1. Curling's ulcer due to elevated serum cortisol.
    2. Positive nitrogen balance due to mobilization of body proteins.
    3. Decreased hematocrit due to red-blood-cell agglutination by epinephrine.
    4. Hypo- and hyperthermia due to failure of hypothalamic temperature regulators.

23.

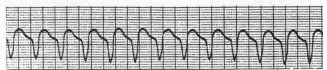

The nurse knows that the arrhythmia shown above, if untreated, is most likely to:
1. Progress to ventricular fibrillation.
2. Increase the blood pressure suddenly.
3. Intensify chest pain from a myocardial infarction (MI).
4. Cause no observable change in the patient.

24. Several hours after a long leg cast has been applied, the nurse notices that the patient's toes have become edematous. The physician decides to bivalve the cast. The nurse explains to the patient that this procedure:
    1. Requires recasting after 24 hours.
    2. Includes splitting and spreading the cast down the middle to relieve constriction.
    3. Includes splitting and spreading the cast on each side and cutting the underlying padding.
    4. Should be followed by placing the patient's leg in a dependent position.

25. Which statement would the nurse include in teaching regarding nasogastric tubes?
    1. Nasogastric tubes should be irrigated with sterile water.
    2. Patient should be in a sitting position with head slightly flexed for tube insertion.
    3. When resistance is met while irrigating a nasogastric tube, pressure should be increased to complete that irrigation, and the physician should be notified at the completion.
    4. Ice chips can be taken as often as desired to promote comfort in the throat.

26. To correctly instill pilocarpine in a patient's eyes, the nurse should gently pull down the lower lid of the eye and instill the drops:
    1. Directly on the central surface of the cornea.
    2. On the inner canthus of the eye.
    3. Into the conjunctival sac.
    4. Directly on the dilated pupil.

27. The nurse anticipates that the backbone of treatment for patients with myasthenia gravis will be:
    1. Adrenergic drugs.
    2. Anticholinergic drugs.
    3. Anticholinesterase drugs.
    4. Cholinergic drugs.

28. A patient's burns were treated by the closed method. The burned left leg was cleaned and the left ankle debrided. Mafenide 1% (Sulfamylon) was applied, and the leg was wrapped in fine mesh gauze. Nursing measures when this approach is used include:
    1. Cleansing of the wound daily and maintenance of strict isolation to prevent air contamination.
    2. Cleansing of the wound daily, or more often if needed, and application of new dressings using clean technique.
    3. Cleansing the wound one or more times each day and application of new dressing using sterile technique.
    4. Cleansing of the wound daily and utilization of heat lamps to help maintain normal body temperature.

29. The nurse tells a postoperative gastrectomy patient that dumping syndrome is a significant problem for:
    1. 70–80% of patients having gastrectomies.
    2. 50% of patients having gastrectomies.
    3. 25% of patients having gastrectomies.
    4. 5–10% of patients having gastrectomies.

30. The nurse knows that, in contrast to patients with hypothyroidism, patients with hyperthyroidism have:
    1. Increased serum cholesterol.
    2. Increased basal metabolic rate and serum T_3 and T_4.
    3. Increased serum TSH (thyroid-stimulating hormone).
    4. Increased menstrual volume.

Adult

31. Pilocarpine is the drug of choice in the treatment of open-angle glaucoma. The expected outcome following administration would be:
    1. Blocked action of cholinesterase at the cholinergic nerve endings, and therefore increased pupil size.
    2. Constricted pupil and therefore widened outflow channels and increased flow of aqueous fluid.
    3. Impaired vision from decreased aqueous humor production.
    4. Constriction of aqueous veins and therefore decreased venous pooling in the eye.

32. Hyponatremia may develop in burn patients due to:
    1. Displacement of sodium in edema fluids and loss through denuded areas of skin.
    2. Increased aldosterone secretion.
    3. Inadequate fluid replacement.
    4. Metabolic acidosis.

33. A patient has had a partial gastrectomy, vagotomy, and gastrojejunostomy. Which complication would the nurse primarily anticipate in this patient's postoperative period?
    1. Thrombophlebitis from decreased mobility.
    2. Abdominal distention due to air swallowing.
    3. Atelectasis due to shallow breathing.
    4. Urinary retention due to prolonged use of anticholinergic medications.

34. The nurse tells a postoperative gastrectomy patient that the nasogastric tube will be removed:
    1. Standardly on the fourth postoperative day.
    2. When bowel sounds are established and the patient has passed flatus or stool.
    3. Thirty-six hours after the cessation of bloody drainage.
    4. After 2 days of alternate clamping and unclamping of the tube.

35. A burn patient is to receive fluid replacement therapy. Besides assessing size and depth of the burn, which physical parameters are also important baseline data for fluid replacement therapy?
    1. Age, sex, and vital signs.
    2. Age, weight, vital signs, and skin turgor.
    3. Vital signs, level of mentation, and urine output.
    4. Vital signs and quantity and specific gravity of urine.

36. The nurse is to administer the drug of choice for long-term control of generalized tonic-clonic seizures. This drug is:
    1. Phenobarbital.
    2. Diazepam (Valium).
    3. Diphenylhydantoin (Dilantin) sodium.
    4. Trimethadione (Tridione).

37. An angiogram was performed using a catheter inserted into the left femoral artery. Which nursing action is the *first* priority following this procedure?
    1. Monitoring vital signs until stable.
    2. Frequently checking the puncture site for fresh bleeding, swelling, or increasing tenderness.
    3. Measuring the quantity and specific gravity of urinary output.
    4. Checking the peripheral pulses distal to the femoral puncture site.

38. Which replacement fluid will the nurse *least* often be expected to administer to a burn patient within the first 24 hours postburn?
    1. Ringer's lactate.
    2. Whole blood.
    3. Dextran.
    4. Dextrose and water.

39. The nurse must observe for which imbalance to occur with prolonged nasogastric suctioning?
    1. Hypernatremia.
    2. Hyperkalemia.
    3. Metabolic alkalosis.
    4. Hypoproteinemia.

40. After left nephrectomy, a patient has a large flank incision. In order to facilitate deep breathing and coughing, the nurse should:
    1. Have the patient lie on the unaffected side.
    2. Coordinate breathing and coughing exercises with administration of analgesics.
    3. Maintain the patient in high Fowler's position.
    4. Push fluid administration to loosen respiratory secretions.

41. The postoperative nephrectomy patient should be closely observed by the nurse for:
    1. Hemorrhage.
    2. Hyperkalemia.
    3. Respiratory alkalosis and tetany.
    4. Polyuria.

42. Two days postoperatively, a patient who has had an ileostomy begins to refuse care and repeatedly says to the staff, "Leave me alone, I just want to sleep." What would be the first nursing action?
    1. Provide accurate, brief, and reassuring explanations of all procedures.
    2. Encourage ambulation in the hall with other patients.
    3. Invite a member of an "ostomy club" to visit the patient.
    4. Encourage the patient to verbalize his or her feelings, fears, and questions.

43. Before insertion of a Miller-Abbott tube, the balloon is tested for patency and capacity and then deflated. Which nursing measure will ease the insertion of the nasoenteric tube?
    1. Chilling the tube before insertion.
    2. Administering a sedative to reduce anxiety.
    3. Warming the tube before insertion.
    4. Positioning the patient in low Fowler's position.

44. Small, frequent feedings of which type of diet would the nurse recommend for patients experiencing dumping syndrome?
    1. Low-protein, high-fat, low-carbohydrate diet.
    2. High-protein, high-fat, high-carbohydrate diet.
    3. High-protein, high-fat, low-carbohydrate diet.
    4. Low-protein, low-fat, high-carbohydrate diet.

45. The nurse recognizes that myasthenia gravis is:
    1. An upper motor neuron lesion.
    2. A lower motor neuron lesion.
    3. A combined upper and lower motor neuron lesion.
    4. A genetic dysfunction.

46. The mouth care measure that should be used with caution by the nurse when a patient has a nasogastric tube is:
    1. Regularly brushing teeth and tongue with soft brush.
    2. Sucking on ice chips to relieve dryness.
    3. Occasionally rinsing mouth with a nonastringent substance and massaging gums.
    4. Application of lemon juice and glycerine swabs to the lips.

47. The nurse can expect hyperkalemia to develop following burn damage because there is:
    1. Increased exudate formation at the burn site.
    2. Disruption of cell membrane integrity, allowing intracellular electrolytes to diffuse into the vascular compartment.

3. Decreased aldosterone secretion, increasing sodium excretion, and retention of potassium.
4. Hyperbilirubinemia secondary to red blood cell destruction.

48. Two days before discharge post left nephrectomy, a patient expressed renewed concern over the ability to continue many of his or her activities with only one kidney. The nurse responds:
    1. "You seem depressed. Actually you are very lucky, since the pathology reports indicate your tumor was encapsulated."
    2. "Lots of people do quite well with only one kidney."
    3. "Would you like me to call the doctor so you two can discuss it?"
    4. "I can understand your concern, but your remaining kidney is sufficient to maintain normal renal functions."

49. A patient is admitted to the orthopedic unit with a long leg cast, used to immobilize a transverse fracture of the right tibia and fibula. The cast is damp, and the patient is complaining that it feels very hot. The nurse should:
    1. Explain to the patient that the cast will feel hot for several hours as the moisture evaporates and the cast hardens.
    2. Recognize that this is a sign of excessive pressure on the soft tissues and notify the physician.
    3. Tell the patient not to worry, as this is a common complaint.
    4. Administer meperidine (Demerol) HCl, 50 mg IM, to relieve discomfort.

50. Diagnosis of myasthenia gravis is frequently based on the patient's response to an intravenous injection of edrophonium (Tensilon). If the patient responds positively to this drug, the nurse should expect:
    1. Exacerbation of symptomatology.
    2. Relief of ptosis but not of weakness in other facial muscles.
    3. A prompt and dramatic increase in muscle strength.
    4. A slight increase in muscle strength that is countered by an increase in muscle fatigability.

51. Assessment of the intraocular pressure as measured by tonometry would be normal if the value is in the range:
    1. 5–10 mm Hg.
    2. 12–22 mm Hg.
    3. 10–20 cm H_2O.
    4. 20–30 mm Hg.

52. On the morning of discharge, a patient who had an emergency abdominal hysterectomy is found sitting with her back to the door, staring out the window. She says that she no longer feels like a real woman. The nurse's response should be to:
    1. Ask her if she would like her diazepam (Valium).
    2. Notify the physician.
    3. Ask, "Can you tell me what makes you feel that way?"
    4. Reassure her that this is a common reaction.

53. Which behavior is *least* likely to be included in the nursing assessment of a burned patient during the recovery period?
    1. Anxiety with mild confusion.
    2. Desperation and panic.
    3. Withdrawal and depression.
    4. Dependency and regression.

54. Forty-eight hours after a nephrectomy, a patient complains of increasing nausea and abdominal pressure. The nurse's *first* nursing action is to:
    1. Change the patient's position to relieve abdominal pressure.

2. Auscultate bowel sounds.
3. Insert a rectal tube to relieve flatus.
4. Administer morphine SO_4, 6 mg, as ordered for the relief of discomfort.

55. Which instruction would be *inappropriate* when teaching a patient to use crutches?
    1. Utilize axilla to help carry weight.
    2. Use short strides to maintain maximum mobility.
    3. Keep feet 6–8 inches apart to provide a wide base for support.
    4. If the patient should begin to fall, throw crutches to the side to prevent falling on them.

56. The nurse explains that epileptic seizures or convulsions result from:
    1. Excessive exercise with lactic acid accumulation.
    2. Excessive, simultaneous, disordered neuronal discharge.
    3. Excessive cerebral metabolism, with local K^+ increased.
    4. Excessive circulating cerebrospinal fluid increasing cerebral pressures.

57. What nursing action best facilitates the passage of the nasoenteric tube from the stomach through the pylorus and into the duodenum?
    1. Gently advancing the tube 1–4 inches at regular time intervals.
    2. Positioning the patient on the right side for 2 hours after insertion.
    3. Maintaining strict bedrest and avoiding all unnecessary movement.
    4. Positioning the patient in a flat supine position.

58. During the initial stage of burns, a primary fluid imbalance occurs. The nurse knows that there has been a shift of fluids from:
    1. The cell to the interstitial space.
    2. The interstitial space into the cell.
    3. The interstitial space to the plasma.
    4. The plasma to the interstitial space.

59. Bedrest is ordered for a patient with chronic glaucoma during a period of acute distress, because activity tends to increase intraocular pressure. Which activity of daily living should this patient be instructed to avoid?
    1. Watching television.
    2. Brushing teeth and hair.
    3. Self-feeding.
    4. Passive range-of-motion exercises.

60. Nursing implications with diphenylhydantoin given during treatment of status epilepticus include giving the intravenous injection slowly and in small increments to prevent:
    1. Respiratory depression and/or arrest.
    2. Vasodepression and circulatory shock.
    3. Irritation and/or necrosis of the vein and surrounding tissue.
    4. Vasomotor stimulation, with a sudden, malignant increase in blood pressure.

61. The nurse would be alerted to a sudden increase in intraocular pressure if the patient with open-angle glaucoma complained of:
    1. Generalized decrease in peripheral vision over the past year.
    2. Difficulty with close vision.
    3. Increasing discomfort in the left eye with radiation to the forehead and left temple.
    4. Halos around lights.

62. The nurse will usually ambulate a postgastrectomy patient beginning:

1. The day after surgery.
2. Three to 4 days after surgery.
3. After 4 days bedrest.
4. Immediately upon awakening from anesthesia.

63. If "cholinergic crisis" is demonstrated in a patient who has myasthenia gravis, all anticholinesterase drugs are withdrawn. To reduce symptoms, which of the following drugs should the nurse be prepared to give?
   1. Atropine.
   2. Ephedrine sulfate.
   3. Potassium chloride.
   4. Neostigmine bromide.

64. Equally important as the depth of tissue destruction in determining severity of burns is the total body surface involved. The nurse would anticipate potential fluid and electrolyte problems when burns:
   1. Are superficial partial thickness and cover 20% of the body surface.
   2. Are deep partial thickness and cover 15% of the body surface.
   3. Are full thickness and cover 10% of the body surface.
   4. Are fourth degree and cover 5% of the body surface.

65. Patient teaching about glaucoma should include a comparison of the two types. Open-angle, or chronic, glaucoma differs from closed-angle, or acute, glaucoma in that:
   1. Open-angle glaucoma occurs less frequently than closed-angle glaucoma.
   2. Open-angle glaucoma's symptomatology includes pain, severe headache, nausea, and vomiting; closed-angle glaucoma has a slow, silent, and generally painless onset.
   3. The obstruction to aqueous flow in open-angle glaucoma generally occurs somewhere in Schlemm's canal or aqueous veins. It does not narrow or close the angle of the anterior chamber, as in closed-angle glaucoma.
   4. Open-angle glaucoma rarely occurs in families; however, there is a hereditary predisposition for closed-angle glaucoma.

66. The adequacy of fluid volume replacement in the early postburn period is best reflected by:
   1. Blood pressure, pulse rates, and daily weights.
   2. Quantity of urinary output and vital signs.
   3. Hemoglobin and hematocrit levels.
   4. Serum-electrolyte levels and urinary output.

67. Which aspect of open-angle glaucoma and its medical treatment is the *most frequent* cause of patient noncompliance?
   1. Loss of mobility due to severe driving restrictions.
   2. The painful and insidious progression of this type of glaucoma.
   3. Decreased light and near-vision accommodation due to miotic effects of pilocarpine.
   4. The frequent nausea and vomiting accompanying use of miotic drugs.

68. Which would the nurse expect to see with the dumping syndrome?
   1. Feeling of hunger.
   2. Constipation.
   3. Increased strength.
   4. Diaphoresis.

69. The nurse observes a patient in the orthopedic clinic using a long pencil to scratch the skin under the cast. The nurse should:
   1. Ask the physician for an oral medication order to relieve itching.

2. Explain to the patient that scratching under the cast should be avoided, as it may break the skin and cause an infection.
   3. Assist the patient by gently rolling the casted leg in the palmar surfaces of the nurse's hands.
   4. Take the pencil away from the patient.

70. The *best* explanation for the nurse to offer to a patient and family would be that myasthenia gravis is a:
   1. Degenerative dysfunction of the basal ganglia.
   2. Transmission dysfunction at the myoneural junction.
   3. Hypertrophic reaction in the anterior motor neurons of the spinal cord.
   4. Hereditary condition of cranial nerves VII, IX, and X.

71. Fifty-four hours after a patient sustained deep partial-thickness burns of the left leg and thigh, the patient's urine output increased from 1000 to 2300 mL/24 h. Laboratory values were as follows: serum sodium, 136 mEq/L; serum potassium, 4 mEq/L; and hematocrit, 34%. The nurse knows that the changes in the patient's urinary output and lab studies indicate:
   1. Beginning of the interstitial-to-plasma fluid shift phase of burns.
   2. Kidney failure.
   3. Circulatory overload due to rapid IV infusion rate.
   4. Hyponatremia.

72. A nursing care plan includes observing for the most common patient problems arising from the use of pyridostigmine (Mestinon) and neostiginine bromide (Prostigmin) which include:
   1. Gastric distress—nausea, anorexia, diarrhea.
   2. Elimination problems—urinary retention.
   3. Central nervous system excitation—flushing, irritability.
   4. Cardiac arrhythmias—palpitations, PVCs.

73. Before discharge a postoperative gastrectomy patient asks the nurse pointedly, "How long will it be before I can eat three meals a day like the rest of my family?" The nurse responds:
   1. "Eating six meals a day can be a bother, can't it?"
   2. "Some patients can tolerate three meals a day by the time they leave the hospital. Maybe it will be a little longer for you."
   3. "You will probably have to eat six meals a day for the rest of your life."
   4. "It varies from patient to patient, but generally in 6–12 months most patients can return to their previous meal patterns."

74. The nurse would be correct in saying that two common causes of primary hypothyroidism are:
   1. Destruction of thyroid tissue by radioactive iodine during therapy for hyperthyroidism, and spontaneous atrophy due to autoimmune response.
   2. Spontaneous atrophy due to autoimmune response, and surgical removal of the thyroid gland.
   3. Surgical removal of the thyroid gland, and tumors of the pituitary gland that decrease the amount of circulating thyroxine.
   4. Tumors of the pituitary gland and/or large doses of antithyroid drugs.

75. In order to take full advantage of the effects of pyridostigmine bromide and neostigmine bromide in reducing dysphagia related to myasthenia gravis, the nurse should plan to give the medications before meals. How long before?
   1. 2 hours.
   2. 45–60 minutes.
   3. 20–30 minutes.
   4. 10–15 minutes.

76. A patient recuperating from burns is withdrawn and depressed. The nurse can expect this patient to exhibit such psychological reactions during the recuperative stage because of:
1. Pain and immobility.
2. Changes in body image.
3. Financial concerns.
4. Anger.

77. Because medications have been increased for a patient with myasthenia gravis, it is important that the nurse observe for signs of "cholinergic crisis." These include:
1. Dilated pupils, profuse diaphoresis, and trembling.
2. Constricted pupils, hypersalivation, and hypotension.
3. Dilated pupils, nausea, and tachycardia.
4. Constricted pupils, dry mucous membranes, and bradycardia.

78. The nursing assessment of a patient recently diagnosed with hypothyroidism will likely reveal the most common clinical manifestations of hypothyroidism, which are:
1. Increased body temperature, tachycardia, and fatigue.
2. Decreased exercise tolerance and facial and pitting edema.
3. Increased sluggishness, increased cold intolerance, and puffy eyelids, hands, and feet.
4. Decreased facial expression, diarrhea, and weight gain.

79. In contrast to hypothyroidism, hyperthyroidism is due to excessive levels of thyroxine in the plasma. Clinical data gathered by the nurse indicating this endocrine dysfunction would include:
1. Systolic hypertension and heat intolerance.
2. Diastolic hypertension and widened pulse pressure.
3. Heat intolerance and weight gain.
4. Emotional hyperexcitability and anorexia.

80. Which statement by the nurse about myasthenia gravis is accurate?
1. Thymectomies rarely produce remissions in myasthenia gravis.
2. Myasthenia gravis is an acute illness that progresses rapidly.
3. Myasthenia gravis has increased muscle strength as a major symptom.
4. Myasthenia gravis may be an autoimmune disease.

81. Which nursing intervention would be included in the preoperative period for a patient who will have a partial gastrectomy, vagotomy, and gastrojejunostomy?
1. Insertion of a nasogastric tube on the morning of surgery.
2. Administration of diazepam (Valium), 4 mg, with 4 oz water 1 hour before surgery.
3. Detailed description of the possible complications that could happen postoperatively.
4. Instructions to avoid taking pain medication too frequently in the first 2 postoperative days to avoid drug dependency.

82. Both Cushing's syndrome and Addison's disease are due to dysfunction of the adrenal cortex. In order to plan for the care of a patient with Cushing's syndrome, the nurse should know that the primary pathology is:
1. Increased cortisol secretion.
2. Increased epinephrine secretion.
3. Decreased aldosterone secretion.
4. Decreased ACTH secretion.

83. Because cortisol is a glucocorticoid, the nurse should expect:
1. Hypoglycemia due to increased insulin production.
2. Skeletal-muscle wasting because glucocorticoids promote protein and fat mobilization.
3. Dependent edema and severe hypokalemia due to abnormal aldosterone secretion.
4. Discoloration or hyperpigmentation of the skin due to increased pituitary secretion of ACTH.

84. In Addison's disease, glucocorticoids, mineralocorticoids, and androgenic hormones are all reduced. Therefore, in contrast to Cushing's syndrome, the nurse should expect to find:
1. Hypotension, weight loss, and physical and mental exhaustion.
2. Hypertension, moon facies, and masculinization in females.
3. Hypotension, hyperglycemia, and weight gain.
4. Hypertension, male impotency, and menstrual disturbances.

85. Iron deficiency anemia is best described as:
1. Hypochromic microcytic.
2. Hyperchromic macrocytic.
3. Hyperchromic microcytic.
4. Hypochromic macrocytic.

86. The nurse should expect that a patient's emotional responses to acute rheumatoid arthritis would primarily depend on the patient's:
1. Self-concept, body image, and usual affective coping strategies.
2. Relationship with the patient's mother.
3. Usual affective or palliative coping strategies only.
4. Economic status and work history.

87. Since aldosterone is the major mineralocorticoid secreted by the adrenal cortex, which fluid and electrolyte imbalance should the nurse anticipate with decreased secretion of this hormone?
1. Hyperkalemia.
2. Hypernatremia.
3. Hypervolemia.
4. Hypercalcemia.

88. The care plan for a burned patient includes observing for side effects of mafenide 1% (Sulfamylon), such as:
1. Severe electrolyte disturbances.
2. Metabolic acidosis.
3. Metabolic alkalosis.
4. Staining of linen.

89. A patient complains of not having had a bowel movement since being admitted 2 days ago for multiple fractures of both lower legs. The patient is on bedrest and skeletal traction. Which intervention would be the *most* appropriate nursing action?
1. Administer an enema.
2. Put the patient on the bedpan every 2 hours.
3. Ensure maximum fluid intake (3000 mL/d).
4. Perform range-of-motion exercises to all extremities.

90. Which cardinal sign heralds the onset of thyroid storm?
1. Fever.
2. Tachycardia.
3. Hypertension.
4. Tremulousness.

91. The nurse would recognize drainage of blood from the nasogastric tube after gastrectomy surgery as abnormal if:
1. It continued for 4–6 hours.
2. It continued for a period longer than 12 hours.
3. It turned greenish yellow in less than 24 hours.
4. It was dark red in the immediate postoperative period.

92. Fluid therapy postburn may necessitate as much as 7 liters of fluid in 24 hours for a 70-kg individual. Using a

15-gtt/ml administration set, the drops per minute that the nurse would set to deliver this volume would be:
1. 48 gtt/min.
2. 75 gtt/min.
3. 60 gtt/min.
4. 90 gtt/min.

93. The nurse anticipates that osteoporosis may result from prolonged immobilization because of:
1. Lack of weight bearing, which decreases osteoblastic activity.
2. Decreased dietary calcium intake.
3. Deposition of excess calcium phosphate salts.
4. Lack of weight bearing, which increases bone formation.

94.

The appropriate nursing response to the above arrhythmia would be to:
1. Administer a bolus of lidocaine, 50 mg IV.
2. Limit patient activity while the arrhythmia is present.
3. Hold digoxin until atrioventricular node depression reverses.
4. Do nothing, particularly with no symptoms.

95. The nurse knows that in a patient who has deep partial- or full-thickness burns, the hematocrit is reduced due to:
1. Lack of erythropoietin factor.
2. Hemodilution and volume overload.
3. Metabolic acidosis.
4. Hypoalbuminemia.

96. Following gastrectomy surgery the nurse must observe for signs of pernicious anemia, which may be a problem after gastrectomy because:
1. The extrinsic factor is produced in the stomach.
2. The extrinsic factor is absorbed in the antral portion of the stomach.
3. The intrinsic factor is produced in the stomach.
4. Decreased hydrochloric acid production inhibits vitamin B_{12} reabsorption.

97. Which nursing intervention can aid in reducing the gastric side effects of pyridostigmine bromide (Mestinon) and neostigmine bromide (Prostigmin)?
1. Give with milk, soda crackers, or antacids.
2. Push fluids and encourage ambulation.
3. Keep room cool and discourage visitors.
4. Encourage food high in potassium.

98. The nurse would recognize a generalized tonic-clonic seizure if which of the following occurred?
1. Brief, abrupt loss of consciousness lasting 10–20 seconds.
2. Loss of consciousness for several minutes, with sustained and intermittent contractions of all motor muscle groups.
3. Sustained and intermittent contractions of selected motor groups in a somewhat confined area.
4. Twitching of facial muscles.

❏ Answers/Rationale

1. (2) All permits must be signed before the procedure. Patients are NPO 6–8 hours, not 24 hours (No. 1). Gastroscopy is an uncomfortable procedure; to mislead the patient by saying it isn't uncomfortable (No. 3) can only increase anxiety and discomfort during the procedure. This procedure involves the passage of a long tube into the stomach, with a lighted, mirrored lens that permits direct visualization of the stomach mucosa. The patient must lie quietly during insertion of the tube to prevent perforation of the esophagus. Usually sedatives, not pain medications (No. 4), are given prior to the procedure. **IMP,4,SECE**

2. (3) The first priority is to protect the patient from injury. Do not restrain the patient's arms or legs, but make sure he or she does not hit anything. Protect the head with the nurse's hand, a towel, or jacket. During the initial tonic phase, the patient usually stops breathing for up to a minute. There is no cause for alarm, as spontaneous breathing will, in most patients, return with no harm. In the absence of breathing, airway patency by this position change (No. 2) is *not* the *first* priority. Muscle contraction will prevent "positioning" of the head. A padded tongue blade, once indicated during a seizure, is also no longer used. **Nos. 1 and 4** are appropriate nursing actions *after* the seizure has ended. **PL,2,SECE**

3. (2) Although all of these interventions are appropriate in the preoperative period, research indicates that the *best* postoperative outcomes are related to the patient's reduced preoperative anxiety levels. Patients who deny apprehension and refuse information, as well as those who are highly anxious and who are unable to ask and/or assimilate information, have the most difficult post-surgical course. Patients who are able to express their concerns and who are given emotional support as well as accurate, brief explanations tend to have less pain and fewer postoperative complications. **Nos. 1, 3, and 4** do not address the patient's need to verbalize concerns. **PL,7,PsI**

4. (3) Signs of *circulatory* constriction include blanching (delayed capillary refill) and cyanosis, swelling of the toes, pain that is out of proportion for the type of fracture, and temperature changes. Tingling and numbness (No. 1), loss of movement (No. 2), and constant pain (No. 4) are symptoms associated with constriction or pressure on a peripheral nerve. **AS,6,PhI**

5. (3) Paralytic ileus is characterized by diminished, absent, or uncoordinated bowel sounds due to inappropriate or absent autonomic nervous system (vagal) stimulation of the intestinal tract. Paralytic ileus may occur due to anesthetic interruption of autonomic outflow or hypokalemia. Edema of the intestinal mucosa (No. 1) is usually found with inflammation or ulcerative colitis. Acute dilatation of the colon (No. 2) and high, tinkling bowel sounds (No. 4) are associated with large-bowel obstruction. **AN,8,PhI**

6. (2) The three-point gait is appropriate when weight bearing is not allowed on the affected limb. The swing-to and swing-through crutch gaits may also be used when only one leg can be used for weight bearing. **Nos. 1 and 3** are utilized when weight bearing is allowed on both

---

Key to codes following rationales Nursing process: **AS,** Assessment; **AN,** Analysis; **PL,** Plan; **IMP,** Implementation; **EV,** Evaluation. Category of human function: **1,** Protective; **2,** Sensory-perceptual; **3,** Comfort, Rest, Activity, and Mobility; **4,** Nutrition; **5,** Growth and Development; **6,** Fluid-Gas Transport; **7,** Psycho-Social-Cultural; **8,** Elimination. Client need: **SECE,** Safe, Effective Care Environment; **PhI,** Physiologic Integrity; **PsI,** Psychosocial Integrity; **HPM,** Health Promotion/Maintenance. See appendices for full explanation.

feet. **No. 4**, the tripod gait, is utilized when the patient has little or no sensation or movement (paralysis) in the lower limbs. **PL,3,PhI**

7. **(3)** Patients are NPO and encouraged not to smoke or take medications the morning of an upper GI series. Patients are NPO for 6–8 hours, not 24 hours **(No. 1)**. Enemas and/or cathartics **(No. 2)** are *not* administered before an upper GI series; however, they are given *after* the series, to aid in the elimination of the barium. The test involves an X ray, using a barium swallow as contrast medium. Gastroscopy **(No. 4)** is the direct visualization of the stomach. **IMP,4,SECE**

8. **(2)** Deep partial-thickness burns involve both the epidermis and some of the dermis. They have a pink-red appearance and are characterized by moisture or blisters. Deep partial-thickness burns are very painful, as nerve endings remain and may be exposed to the air. A superficial partial-thickness burn involves only the epidermis **(No. 1)**. An example is sunburn: the skin is usually red and dry. In full-thickness burns, subcutaneous tissue, muscle, and even bone are also involved **(Nos. 3 and 4)**. Typically, a full-thickness burn is white, gray, or charred in color and is dry and leathery in appearance. Nerve endings have been destroyed, so the area is painless. **AN,1,PhI**

9. **(2)** Some authorities believe that the basic psychosomatic issue underlying the development of ulcers is an unresolved dependence-independence conflict. This conflict frequently prevents the patient from accepting a dependent role, even on a temporary basis. However, the unresolved dependency wish that many of these people have frequently results in irritable, angry behavior when treatments aren't exactly on time. Other psychosomatic research has linked anxiety and neurotic behavior **(No. 1)** with the occurrence of angina pectoris; repressed anger and hostility **(No. 3)** with the development of rheumatoid arthritis; and compulsive time orientation **(No. 4)** (type A personality) with onset of myocardial infarction. **AN,7,PsI**

10. **(3)** Increased carbohydrates are needed for healing and tissue repair. Anorexia, *not increased appetite* **(No. 1)**, is a problem. Increased, *not decreased* protein catabolism is present **(No. 2)**. Digestive enzyme secretion is decreased, *not increased* **(No. 4)**. **AN,4,PhI**

11. **(1)** Glaucoma is defined as an imbalance between the rate of secretion of intraocular fluids and the rate of their absorption. Glaucoma may be acute/closed-angle (obstruction of the angle between the cornea and iris) or chronic/open-angle (obstruction occurs proximal or distal to the angle). It is characterized by increased intraocular pressures. Narrowing of the arterioles and retinal ischemia **(No. 2)** are the result of prolonged hypertension. Clouding of the cornea **(No. 3)** is not seen in glaucoma. Buckling of the retina **(No. 4)** is associated with retinal detachment. **AN,2,PhI**

12. **(1)** Patients experiencing dumping syndrome should be advised to ingest liquids between meals rather than with meals **(No. 2)** or at any time they desire **(No. 3)**. Taking fluids between meals allows for adequate hydration, reduces the amount of bulk ingested with meals, and aids in preventing rapid gastric emptying. Six small meals rather than three large meals, as well as resting after eating, are also measures used to prevent the occurrence of symptoms, which usually disappear over time. There is no need to restrict the quantity of fluids **(No. 4)**, just the timing. **PL,4,PhI**

13. **(2)** Daily weights are taken following nephrectomy. Daily increases of 2 lb or more is indicative of fluid re-

tention and should be reported to the physician. Intake and output records may also reflect this imbalance. Increased specific gravity of urine **(No. 1)** indicates that the patient is underhydrated rather than overhydrated. A urinary output of 50 mL/h **(No. 3)** is the desired minimum following renal surgery. Periorbital edema **(No. 4)** is a *later* sign of excess fluid retention. **AS,8,PhI**

14. **(1)** The Miller-Abbott tube is a double-lumen tube, with one lumen leading to the inflatable balloon and the other lumen utilized for aspiration of intestinal contents. **No. 2** is an example of a Levin tube, used for gastric suction. **No. 3** is an example of a Harris tube, and **No. 4**, a Cantor tube, both utilized for intestinal decompression, like the Miller-Abbott. **IMP,8,SECE**

15. **(2)** The narrow QRS complexes are normal, within 0.12 second, but there are no regular P waves for each QRS. The baseline appears "wavy" and the rhythm is "regularly irregular," which describes atrial fibrillation. The second and fifth QRS complexes are wide and bizarre but alike, indicating a unifocal origin. **No. 1** is incorrect because there is not one P wave for every QRS, and the multifocal PVCs would look different in configuration. Even though the rate is 100, **No. 3** is incorrect because the impulse is not originating from the SA node, which is necessary for a sinus rhythm. **No. 4** is incorrect because atrial tachycardia is more rapid and regular, and though the P waves are difficult to see, they are present. Also, the PVCs are unifocal, not multifocal, in origin. **AN,6,SECE**

16. **(2)** If treatment with thyroid hormone is effective, there should be an overall increase in metabolic rate and a decrease in fluid retention, that is, increased blood pressure, pulse rate, pulse pressure, temperature, and rate and depth of respirations. As a result of improved renal blood flow, glomerular filtration and urine output should also increase, thus reducing the weight gain due to fluid retention. **Nos. 1, 3, and 4** are incorrect because each contains at least one outcome that is not consistent with improved status. **EV,3,PhI**

17. **(2)** Aldosterone secretion by the adrenal cortex is stimulated by decreases in cardiac output. Aldosterone acts to conserve sodium in the kidney tubules, passively increasing water reabsorption and improving fluid volume balance. Normally, if the patient had only a water loss, he or she would also be hypernatremic because of this mechanism. However, in burns the patient's hypovolemia (hemoconcentration) is due to both fluid and electrolyte loss in edema fluids as well as through the denuded areas of skin. **No. 1** is not the best answer because, although ADH is being released, its action has not at this time prevented hemoconcentration. **No. 3** is incorrect because very little sodium is released due to cellular disruption. Sodium is the main cation of the extracellular fluid. **No. 4** is incorrect because increased serum-potassium levels stimulate the release of aldosterone. **AN,6,PhI**

18. **(4)** Since the patient's ability to react to stress is decreased, maintaining a quiet environment becomes a nursing priority. Dehydration is a common problem in Addison's disease, so close observation of the patient's hydration level is crucial. To promote optimal hydration and sodium intake, fluid intake is increased, particularly fluids containing electrolytes, such as broths, carbonated beverages, and juices. **No. 1** is incorrect because it limits sodium. **No. 2** is incorrect because it limits fluids. Daily weights and intake and output records are essential for monitoring fluid balance. Drug therapy in Addison's disease is directed toward oral re-

placement of adrenocorticosteroids such as cortisone, prednisone, and fludrohydrocortisone (Florinef). Insulin **(No. 3)** is not required. **IMP,3,PhI**

19. **(3)** The vagus nerve stimulates both an increase in hydrochloric acid secretion and gastric motility. Vagotomy not only decreases hydrochloric acid secretion but also alters the motility of the stomach and intestines; this may result in a sensation of fullness after meals, eructation, and abdominal distention. **No. 1** is incomplete. **Nos. 2 and 4** are the reverse of effects of vagal action. **AN,4,SECE**

20. **(3)** Potassium is transported back into the cells along with glucose; therefore the administration of insulin and glucose will facilitate the movement of potassium back into the cell. Sodium polystyrene sulfonate (Kayexalate) **(No. 2)** is a resin that attacks and binds potassium. It may be given either orally or as an enema; however, its use would not be indicated in this case unless more conservative means were unsuccessful. Morphine sulfate **(No. 1)** and synthetic aldosterone **(No. 4)** are not indicated for the management of hyperkalemia. **PL,6,SECE**

21. **(2)** Alcohol is extremely drying and contributes to skin breakdown. An emollient lotion should be used. Bed cradles **(No. 1)** keep the pressure of bed clothing off pressure points. High-protein diet **(No. 3)** aids in the healing process. Assessment of skin **(No. 4)** is vital, to recognize any red areas. **PL,1,SECE**

22. **(1)** The hypovolemia and shock that accompany burns greatly increase the body's stress response. Increased serum levels of norepinephrine, epinephrine, and aldosterone facilitate venous return and thus assist in maintaining cardiac output and blood pressure. The pituitary is also stimulated in the stress response to increase circulating levels of ADH (decreases water output) and cortisol. Increased levels of the latter hormone are implicated in the development of Curling's ulcer (stress ulcer), which may develop in patients of all ages and with both minor and major burns. Generally, H_2 antagonists and antacids are used to reduce its occurrence. **No. 2** is incorrect because negative iron balance occurs due to protein mobilization for healing. Patients with burns are given high-protein, high-calorie meals as well as supplemental vitamins to promote wound healing. **No. 3** is incorrect because hemolysis of red blood cells and decreased hematocrit are primarily due to the injury itself rather than to epinephrine agglutination. In thermal burns, up to 40% of the red blood cell mass may be hemolyzed. Hypothermia is a problem in the postburn period but is the result of the loss of skin areas; hence **No. 4** is incorrect. The patient treated by the open or exposed method of burn therapy is particularly susceptible to chilling. Increased thermostat settings and radiant heat lamps may be employed to aid in maintaining normal body temperature. **AN,1,PhI**

23. **(1)** Ventricular tachycardia occurs most commonly in patients with acute MI and coronary artery disease. Of immediate significance to the patient, if untreated, are the hemodynamic dysfunction, a drop in blood pressure rather than an increase **(No. 2)**, and the possibility of progressing to ventricular fibrillation. **No. 3** is incorrect because if pain does result it will be angina, not MI pain. **No. 4** is incorrect because ventricular tachycardia is potentially life threatening and requires intervention. **AN,6,PhI**

24. **(3)** Bivalving the cast involves full-length splitting of the cast on each side. The underlying padding is also cut, as blood-soaked padding shrinks and can also cause circulatory constriction. After the cast is cut, it is spread sufficiently to relieve constriction. This procedure does not disturb reduction of the bone. The cast is then reapplied **(No. 1)** *after* the swelling has gone down. **No. 2** is the technique used when the cast is removed. The patient's limb should always be elevated **(No. 4)** following bivalving, as the underlying condition (edema and swelling) is best relieved by elevation of the limb, ice packs, and isometric exercises. **IMP,3,SECE**

25. **(2)** The tube will be inserted with greater ease if the patient is sitting up with head slightly flexed. The tube should be lubricated and will be passed into the stomach with greater accuracy if the patient is given water to drink through a straw; at the same time that the patient is swallowing, the tube is advanced. **No. 1** is not correct because the tube should be irrigated with saline, *not* water, to prevent electrolyte imbalances. **No. 3** is not correct because pressure must *not* be utilized during irrigation. If resistance is met, the physician should be notified immediately. Ice chips **(No. 4)** should be used *sparingly, not* as often as desired, to prevent electrolyte imbalances from excessive hypotonic water ingestion. **IMP,4,SECE**

26. **(3)** Eye drops should be instilled into the conjunctival sac to prevent medication from hitting the sensitive cornea. The patient should then be instructed to close the eye, but not squeeze shut, so that the medication can be distributed evenly over the eye. **Nos. 1 and 4** are incorrect because instillation on these structures would increase corneal irritation. **No. 2** is incorrect because drops instilled into the inner canthus are likely to run down the outer aspects of the nose or be absorbed systemically through the tear duct. **IMP,2,SECE**

27. **(3)** The main treatment for patients with myasthenia gravis is anticholinesterase drugs. These drugs increase the response of muscles to nerve impulses and improve muscle strength by inhibiting the rapid removal of acetylcholine from the myoneural junction. **No. 1** is partially correct, in that adrenergic drugs such as ephedrine sulfate are administered to improve muscle tone but these drugs do not inhibit cholinesterase at the myoneural junction. Likewise, anticholinergic drugs **(No. 2)** such as atropine are also utilized in the treatment of myasthenia, primarily to reduce the incidence of side effects of the anticholinesterase drugs and to reverse their effect if "cholinergic crisis" occurs. Cholinergic drugs **(No. 4)** are not indicated in the treatment of myasthenia gravis. **PL,3,PhI**

28. **(3)** Patients with burns limited to an extremity are generally treated by a closed method; that is, wounds are covered with a layer of sterile, fine mesh gauze impregnated with an antibacterial agent such as mafenide 1%. Wounds are cleansed one or more times per day, and dressings are reapplied using strict sterile technique. Patients treated by the closed or semiopen method do not have to be isolated **(No. 1)**. Patients treated by the open method (wounds completely exposed to the air) require strict isolation to prevent infection. The open method is usually used for minor burns, areas difficult to dress (burns of trunk, perineum), or new skin grafts. **No. 2** is incorrect because sterile technique must be used. Heat lamp **(No. 4)** is incorrect because the wound is covered in the closed method. **IMP,1,SECE**

29. **(4)** While 70–80% of patients having subtotal gastrectomies may experience some symptoms of dumping syndrome, it is a significant problem for only a small percentage (5–10%). The term *dumping* is used because the symptoms are believed to be due to the rapid emptying of the gastric contents into the small intestine. This pro-

duces gastric distention, and some authorities believe that large amounts of extracellular fluid then enter the intestines to dilute the hypertonic stomach contents. The subsequent lowering of the blood volume produces shocklike symptoms, such as weakness, diaphoresis, faintness, and palpitations. **Nos. 1, 2, and 3** are incorrect percentages. **AN,4,PhI**

30. **(2)** Patients with hyperthyroidism have an increased BMR (basal metabolic rate) as well as increased T_3 and T_4. Increased serum cholesterol **(No. 1)**, increased TSH **(No. 3)**, and increased menstrual volume **(No. 4)** are findings consistent with hypothyroidism. Menstruation in hyperthyroidism characteristically is decreased in volume. Cycle lengths may be shortened or prolonged, but eventually amenorrhea develops. **AN,3,PhI**

31. **(2)** Pilocarpine constricts the pupil by causing contraction of the ciliary muscles, thus widening the outflow channels and increasing aqueous flow. **No. 1** is incorrect because pilocarpine is a parasympathomimetic; that is, it mimics the action of acetylcholine at cholinergic nerve endings, thus decreasing pupil size. **No. 3** is incorrect, in that diuretics such as acetazolamide (Diamox), which is a carbonic anhydrase inhibitor, are used to decrease aqueous production. **No. 4** does not describe the actions of any medication utilized in glaucoma therapy. **EV,2,PhI**

32. **(1)** Hyponatremia or decreased serum sodium may develop in burn patients because sodium tends to move with water into edema fluids as well as into denuded areas of skin. **Nos. 2 and 4** are incorrect because both these mechanisms tend to increase sodium reabsorption by the kidney tubules. Inadequate fluid replacement **(No. 3)** would tend to mask hyponatremia because of hemoconcentration. **AN,6,PhI**

33. **(3)** Patients with high abdominal incisions are prone to atelectasis following surgery because they tend to breathe shallowly to prevent incisional pain. However, the nurse must also institute measures to prevent thrombophlebitis **(No. 1)**, wound infection, and dehiscence. Abdominal distention due to air swallowing **(No. 2)** is unlikely because the patient has a nasogastric tube in place. Urinary retention after surgery **(No. 4)** is generally due to the effects of anesthesia on the autonomic nervous system rather than to the residual effects of anticholinergic medications. **EV,6,PhI**

34. **(2)** The nasogastric tube is removed after bowel sounds have been reestablished (generally around the third day) and after the patient has passed flatus or stool. **Nos. 1 and 3** are incorrect because they do not include the return of bowel sounds. Before removal, the tube is frequently clamped for a 2–4-hour period—not 2 days **(No. 4)**—to test the patient's tolerance. Gastric residue is measured after this period. If it is more than 100 mL, the nasogastric tube is left in place. Likewise, if the patient experiences any pain, nausea, vomiting, or distention during this period, the tube is left in. If no symptoms occur and there is a minimal amount of gastric residue, the tube is removed. **EV,8,SECE**

35. **(2)** Age is important baseline information because IV infusion rates to maintain appropriate quantity and specific gravity of urinary output differ, for example, 10–20 mL/h for infants versus 50–70 mL/h for adults. Weight is significant if the Evans or Brooke formula is used for fluid replacement therapy. Both these formulas utilize both the size of the burn and the weight of the patient to calculate the amount of fluid to be replaced. Vital signs and skin turgor are both important measures of the degree or extent of hypovolemia. As dehydration develops, skin turgor becomes poor, mucous membranes dry, and the eyeballs feel soft. Likewise, the pulse may become thready and the blood pressure may decrease. Size (weight), as discussed, not sex, would determine therapy **(No. 1)**. Level of mentation **(No. 3)** is less helpful in this particular situation because of the fear, pain, and acute anxiety experienced by some patients. Quantity and specific gravity of urine output **(No. 4)** are important in assessing the adequacy of fluid replacement rather than as part of the initial assessment. **AS,6,PhI**

36. **(3)** Dilantin (phenytoin, diphenylhydantoin) is consistently found to be effective against most types of seizures except absence seizures. Its precise action is unknown, but it appears to stabilize cell membranes by altering intracellular sodium concentrations. Plasma levels of the drug are checked frequently to avoid toxicity and to determine effective dosage. Side effects include gastritis and nervousness, and at toxic levels the drug may cause ataxia. Phenobarbital **(No. 1)** is also used *in conjunction* with diphenylhydantoin. Diazepam **(No. 2)** may be used as *adjunct* therapy in seizure disorders. Trimethadione **(No. 4)** is used in the control of absence seizures. **IMP,2,PhI**

37. **(2)** After arterial punctures, the *first* nursing priority is to observe for bleeding or hematoma formation, particularly in the first 4 hours after the procedure. Vital signs **(No. 1)** are monitored. The specific gravity and urinary output **(No. 3)** are monitored, but this is *not as significant* as observing the puncture site. The peripheral pulse distal to the puncture site **(No. 4)** is also monitored. Because of the size of the vessel, bleeding can quickly cause volume depletion and shock. **AN,6,SECE**

38. **(2)** With the exception of the Evans formula, whole blood is administered to burn patients *only when the hematocrit begins to manifest red blood cell loss*. Several fluid formulas have been developed to serve as a guideline for fluid replacement in the burn patient. The *Evans* formula is the oldest and is based on both the size of the wound and the patient's weight. Colloids (blood, dextran, plasma) and crystalloids (electrolyte solutions) *are* administered during the first 48 hours. The *Brooke* formula is quite similar, except that blood is not given until the hematocrit level has fallen and the need is demonstrated. The *Parkland* formula is based on the premise that volume expansion is dependent on the rate of infusion rather than the type of replacement. During the first 24 hours, fluid volume *is* replaced with electrolyte solutions (Ringer's lactate) only **(No. 1)**. Colloids are used only if urine output is not maintained **(No. 3)**. During the second 24 hours, dextrose and water **(No. 4)** are used to maintain fluid volume. **PL,6,SECE**

39. **(3)** Removal of gastric secretions incurs the *loss* of sodium, potassium, and hydrochloric acid ions. The loss of these ions may lead not only to metabolic alkalosis ($\downarrow$ H^+) but also to hypokalemia. **Nos. 1 and 2** are incorrect because hypernatremia and hyperkalemia indicate an *excess* in sodium and potassium ions. Hypoproteinemia **(No. 4)** occurs with liver dysfunctions and is *not* a side effect of nasogastric suctioning. **AN,4,PhI**

40. **(2)** Because the flank incision in nephrectomy is directly below the diaphragm, deep breathing is painful. Additionally, there is a greater incisional pull each time the person moves than there is with abdominal surgery. Incisional pain following nephrectomy generally requires analgesic administration every 3–4 hours for 24–48 hours after surgery. Therefore turning, coughing, and deep-breathing exercises should be planned to maximize the analgesic effects. The patient may be on either side,

as long as drainage tubes are not kinked and gravity flow is uninhibited (**No. 1**). A low Fowler's or semi-Fowler's position is generally more comfortable for the patient and of sufficient height to encourage gravity flow from drainage tubes (**No. 3**). Fluid administration is directed toward maintaining *blood* volume and *urinary* output (**No. 4**). **PL,6,SECE**

41. (1) Hemorrhage may follow nephrectomy because of the difficulty in securing ligatures in the short renal-artery stump. It may occur on the day of surgery or 8–12 days postoperatively, when normal tissue sloughing occurs with healing. Dressing and urine are observed for bright red bleeding, vital signs are monitored, and the patient is continually observed for any other indications of shock. Hyperkalemia (**No. 2**), tetany (**No. 3**), and polyuria (**No. 4**) are not common complications after nephrectomy. **AS,6,PhI**

42. (4) It is important to recognize that the loss of anatomic integrity initiates a grieving process. Allowing the patient to express feelings of depression, apathy, or disinterest indicates that such feelings are acceptable and not uncommon. **No. 1** is always appropriate and should be consistently carried out; however, in the situation depicted it would *follow* the verbalization of feelings. **Nos. 2 and 3** are also alternatives the nurse may wish to employ *after* assessing the patient's major concerns. **IMP,7,PsI**

43. (1) Chilling the tube before insertion assists in relieving some of the nasal discomfort. Water-soluble lubricants along with viscous lidocaine (Xylocaine) may also be used. However, since mercury is instilled into the balloon of the Miller-Abbott tube after insertion, it is usually only lightly lubricated before insertion. The patient may be administered a sedative (**No. 2**) on physician's orders to reduce apprehension during insertion. Warming the tube (**No. 3**) has no advantages. The patient is usually positioned (**No. 4**) in high Fowler's position during insertion to aid in swallowing the tube. **IMP,8,SECE**

44. (3) The symptoms of dumping syndrome are most likely to occur following the ingestion of large amounts of sugars or carbohydrates. Therefore a diet that is high in protein and fats and low in carbohydrates is recommended, to reduce symptomatology and to provide the patient with essential energy requirements. **Nos. 1 and 4** are incorrect because they do not supply sufficient protein for energy and tissue repair. High protein intake is essential after surgery and most prolonged illnesses for rebuilding tissue. **Nos. 2 and 4** are incorrect because they list high carbohydrates. **PL,4,PhI**

45. (2) Since the dysfunction in myasthenia gravis occurs at the myoneural junction, it is considered a lower motor neuron lesion. Upper motor neuron lesions (**No. 1**) involve cranial neurons and their axons in the spinal cord. Combined lesions (**No. 3**) generally occur with spinal injury when axons of cranial neurons are destroyed, resulting in hyperreflexia and increased muscle tone below the level of the lesion and destruction of motor neurons at the level of the injury, which in turn leads to hyporeflexia, decreased muscle tone, and muscle atrophy in those muscles normally innervated by these neurons. Myasthenia gravis is not an inherited disorder (**No. 4**). Recent evidence suggests an autoimmune basis. **AN,3,PhI**

46. (2) The patient should be cautioned to limit the number of ice cubes he or she sucks on because the nasogastric suction will remove not only the increased water ingested from the melted cubes but also essential electrolytes. **Nos. 1, 3, and 4** are appropriate mouth care measures for a patient who has a nasogastric tube. **IMP,1,SECE**

47. (2) Hyperkalemia (excesses in serum potassium) occurs in burns due to three separate mechanisms: (a) cellular injury resulting in the movement of potassium from the intracellular space into the extracellular space; (b) decreased glomerular filtration and urine output preventing excretion of increased serum potassium; and (c) inadequate tissue metabolism resulting in increased hydrogen ion formation (metabolic acidosis). In the kidney tubules, hydrogen and potassium ions are exchanged for sodium ions. In metabolic acidosis, more hydrogen ions are excreted than potassium ions. Exudate formation *itself does not* significantly affect serum-potassium levels (**No. 1**). During physical and emotional stress, aldosterone levels are *increased,* thereby *lowering* serum potassium (**No. 3**). Hyperbilirubinemia *itself does not* affect potassium concentration (**No. 4**), though red blood cell destruction probably increases the amount of circulating potassium, as potassium is the major intracellular cation. **EV,6,PhI**

48. (4) Recognizing the patient's concern is essential both in maintaining rapport and in keeping the lines of communication open. Having done this, the nurse can then assure the patient that one kidney is sufficient to handle renal functions. This statement can then be followed by other discharge instructions, such as the need for adequate fluid intake, avoiding infections, and untoward signs that the patient needs to observe for. **Nos. 1, 2, and 3** do not recognize the patient's concern or facilitate open communication. **IMP,7,PsI**

49. (1) A freshly applied cast generates heat as moisture evaporates and the cast hardens. To facilitate drying, keep it exposed to the air. Do not use plastic covers or Chux on pillows to elevate the limb, as these tend to slow drying. **No. 2** is incorrect; signs of increased pressure are numbness and tingling, pain, and loss of movement. **No. 3** is an inappropriate response to the question because it also fails to recognize the patient's cognitive needs. **No. 4** does not take into account that discomfort and apprehension can be reduced if the patient understands what is to be expected. **IMP,3,PhI**

50. (3) Edrophonium (Tensilon) is a short-acting anticholinesterase compound. A positive Tensilon test result (a prompt and dramatic increase in muscle strength) is consistent with the diagnosis of myasthenia gravis. **No. 1** is incorrect because an exacerbation of symptoms would indicate another cause for the muscle dysfunction. **No. 2** is partially correct: ptosis is relieved, but so is sagging of the other facial muscles. **No. 4** is incorrect because the increase in muscle strength is accompanied by *decreased* fatigability as long as the drug continues to circulate. **EV,3,PhI**

51. (2) The normal range of intraocular pressures is 12–22 mm Hg. **No. 1** is below the range of normal pressures and may occur in hypovolemia (soft eyeballs) or dehydration. **No. 3** is incorrect because ocular pressures are measured in millimeters of mercury. **No. 4** is incorrect because pressures above 22 mm Hg are considered elevated. **EV,2,PhI**

52. (3) It is not uncommon for a patient to feel that she will no longer be able to fulfill her role and needs as a woman following a hysterectomy. Verbalization of feelings allows the nurse to assess the patient's coping mechanisms and encourages the patient to deal with her emotional response. **No. 3** is an open-ended question that allows the patient room to respond. **Nos. 1 and 2**

avoid the problem initially. **No. 2** may be appropriate if, after talking to the patient, the nurse assesses that her responses represent a more significant or deep-seated problem. **No. 4** would be appropriate *after* the patient has aired her feelings. **IMP,7,PsI**

53. **(2)** Desperation and panic may strike while the injury is occurring but rarely occur during the recovery period. During the acute stage of burn recovery, anxiety is common due to the stress and pain of injury and dressing changes. Anxiety decreases the individual's ability to perceive situations realistically, which may result in an altered mental state **(No. 1)**. During the intermediate phase of burn recovery, patients may react to continued pain, changes in body image, and financial stress with various psychological responses, ranging from withdrawal and depression **(No. 3)** to acting out anger by refusing to cooperate with the medical regimen and by dependency **(No. 4)**. **AS,7,PsI**

54. **(2)** Though nausea may occur following the administration of narcotics, if it is accompanied by the absence of bowel sounds and upper abdominal distention, gastric or small-intestine dilatation should be suspected and the nurse's findings reported to the physician. Changing the patient's position **(No. 1)** and insertion of a rectal tube **(No. 3)** are not helpful if peristalsis is not present (bowel sounds). Administering morphine **(No. 4)** is not indicated until the source of the patient's discomfort is diagnosed. **IMP,8,SECE**

55. **(1)** In the use of crutches, all weight bearing should be on the hands. Constant pressure in the axilla from weight bearing can lead to damage of the brachial plexus nerves and produce crutch paralysis. **Nos. 2, 3, and 4** *are appropriate* instructions to give to the patient preparing for crutch walking. **IMP,3,PhI**

56. **(2)** Epileptic seizures or convulsions are the result of excessive, simultaneous, disordered neuronal discharge in the brain. This dysrhythmic electrical discharge may be focal (jacksonian seizure) or widely dispersed (grand mal seizures). **Nos. 3 and 4** are incorrect because theories for the initiation of these convulsions vary from decreased intracellular K^+ to decreased cerebral spinal fluid to alteration in neuronal defenses due to trauma, toxins, or inflammation. Depending on existing potential in the individual, **No. 1** may be a precipitating factor. **AN,2,PhI**

57. **(2)** After the tube has been inserted into the stomach, its movement into the duodenum is first facilitated by having the patient lie on the right side for 2 hours, then on the back with head elevated for 2 hours, and finally on the left side for 2 hours. After the tube has passed the pylorus (this is usually checked by X ray), ambulating the patient will help move the tube to the point of obstruction. After positioning and ambulation, the physician or the nurse may advance the tube 1–4 inches at specified time intervals **(No. 1)** to provide slack for peristaltic action. Remaining quiet or flat in bed **(Nos. 3 and 4)** will not facilitate the advancement of the tube either through the pylorus or through the small intestine. **IMP,8,SECE**

58. **(4)** The hypovolemia that occurs in the initial stage of burns is the result of fluid lost from denuded areas of skin and edema in and around the burned surface area. Edema formation is due to a shift of plasma fluids to the interstitial space. **Nos. 1, 2, and 3** are incorrect because when tissues are burned, a change in the permeability of both tissue and capillary membranes occurs. This change as well as increased vasodilation result in a shift of excessively large amounts of extracellular fluid (electrolytes and proteins) into the burned area. Most of this

fluid loss occurs deep in the wound, where fluid moves into the deeper tissue. Burns of a highly vascular area (muscle, face) are believed to cause more severe fluid volume shifts than comparable burns to other areas of the body. **AN,6,PhI**

59. **(2)** Vigorous activities such as brushing the teeth and brushing the hair are generally discouraged during periods of acute distress. These activities tend to increase aqueous production and therefore pressures because they activate sympathetic nervous system stimulation of the vasculature. Quiet activities such as watching TV **(No. 1)**, moderate reading, self-feeding **(No. 3)**, and passive range-of-motion exercises **(No. 4)** *are* encouraged. **IMP,2,HPM**

60. **(2)** Diphenylhydantoin (phenytoin, Dilantin) must be injected IV slowly and in small increments to prevent vasodepression and circulatory collapse. Respiratory depression **(No. 1)** is generally associated with morphine sulfate. Adrenergic (alpha) drugs such as norepinephrine bitartrate (Levophed) may cause vein and tissue necrosis **(No. 3)** and have only rarely caused sudden malignant increases in blood pressure **(No. 4)**. **IMP,2,SECE**

61. **(3)** Generally the patient with chronic, or open-angle, glaucoma has few complaints of intense symptomatology. The usual onset of this condition is slow, silent, and painless. However, some patients do experience prodromal symptoms, such as aching and discomfort around the eye, disturbed accommodation to darkness, and blurring of peripheral vision **(No. 1)**. Any complaint of pain or increasing discomfort with radiation to the forehead and temporal area is a grave sign of a sudden increase in pressure. Difficulty with close vision **(No. 2)** is not characteristic of glaucoma. Halos around lights **(No. 4)** occur less commonly. **EV,2,PhI**

62. **(1)** Patients are ambulated as soon as possible to prevent the complications of bedrest; generally ambulation can begin as soon as 24 hours after surgery. In some instances, as when the patient is severely debilitated or has complications due to ulcer perforation, bedrest may be prolonged, as in **Nos. 2 and 3**. If this is the case, the nurse will need to observe closely for signs of complications (atelectasis, thrombophlebitis, etc.) and institute measures to prevent them. The patient is rarely if ever gotten up immediately after awakening, as in **No. 4**. **PL,3,SECE**

63. **(1)** In cholinergic crisis, all anticholinesterase drugs are withdrawn and atropine (an anticholinergic drug) is given in 2-mg doses IV every hour until signs of atropine toxicity develop (dry mouth, blurred vision, tachycardia, rash or flushing of the skin, and elevated temperature). **Nos. 2, 3, and 4** are incorrect because they do not act to decrease cholinergic responses. Ephedrine **(No. 2)** is utilized in myasthenia gravis to increase muscle tone; potassium chloride **(No. 3)** is utilized to increase serum K^+ because it is believed that adequate serum-potassium levels potentiate the effects of cholinergic drugs; and neostigmine bromide **(No. 4)** is an anticholinesterase that acts to improve cholinergic transmission of impulses at the myoneural junction. **IMP,3,SECE**

64. **(3)** Critical burns are classified as deep partial-thickness over 30% of the body and/or full thickness over 10% of the body. Extensive burns involving the face, hands, and feet or those associated with respiratory injuries are also considered critical. The most frequently used method of calculating the extent of a burn is called the "rule of nines." While this method is fairly simple to apply, it is somewhat inaccurate. This is particularly true when it is applied to children because allowances are

not made for the proportional differences in head size and extremity size between children and adults. Hence superficial partial-thickness burns (**No. 1**) are not serious unless large areas are involved and the patient is very young or old. Deep partial-thickness burns (**No. 2**) are classified as a major burn if over 25% of the body is involved. The fourth-degree burn classification is not routinely used (**No. 4**). **EV,1,PhI**

65. (**3**) In chronic, or open-angle glaucoma, the obstruction to aqueous outflow is due to degenerative changes in either the trabeculum, Schlemm's canal, or the aqueous veins. Closed-angle glaucoma is characterized by obstruction of aqueous outflow due to narrowing of the angle between the anterior chamber and the root of the iris. The other answers are incorrect because chronic, or open-angle, glaucoma occurs more frequently than closed-angle (**No. 1**), is characterized by slow, insidious, painless onset *rather than* the acute symptoms of closed-angle glaucoma (**No. 2**), and *is* certainly familial, if not hereditary (**No. 4**). Due to this latter characteristic, family members of patients with open-angle glaucoma should be encouraged to have their intraocular pressures assessed annually, particularly past age 40. **AN,2,PhI**

66. (**2**) Although each of the listed measures can be used to assess the adequacy of the fluid replacement, hourly urine outputs and vital signs provide significant information on fluid balance in the acute burn period. Decreased urine output, increased pulse rate, and restlessness are early signs of inadequate fluid replacement. Increases in blood pressure, pulse, respirations, and urine output are early signs of circulatory overload. Changes in daily weights provide accurate data over the long run and are extremely important in monitoring fluid volumes in patients on diuretic therapy, such as patients with congestive heart failure or cirrhosis. **Nos. 1, 3, and 4** are *not* the *best* indicators. **EV,6,PhI**

67. (**3**) The most frequent cause of noncompliance to the medical treatment of chronic, or open-angle, glaucoma is the miotic effects of pilocarpine. Pupillary constriction impedes normal accommodation, making night driving difficult and hazardous, reducing the patient's ability to read for extended periods, and making participation in games with fast-moving objects impossible. **No. 1** is incorrect because *daytime* driving is *not* restricted. **No. 2** is incorrect because this process is painless. The fact that the process is painless and insidious may in fact increase patients' noncompliance because they do not usually experience any adverse reactions if they do not instill their eyedrops. Nausea and vomiting are *rare* toxic effects of pilocarpine and are usually very mild; hence **No. 4** is incorrect. **EV,2,PhI**

68. (**4**) Profuse perspiration, diaphoresis, is one of a group of symptoms that happens 5–30 minutes after a high-carbohydrate meal or when liquid is taken with the meal. This is caused by entrance of food into the jejunum before it has had a chance to begin the digestive process. Other symptoms include a feeling of fullness, *not* hunger (**No. 1**); diarrhea, *not* constipation (**No. 2**); and weakness, *not* increased strength (**No. 3**). **EV,4,PhI**

69. (**2**) It is not safe to insert any foreign object under a cast, as the skin may break and become infected. Scratching also disturbs the padded surface under the cast, causing it to become wrinkled, which may lead to skin irritation and breakdown. Itching under the cast can be relieved by directing air (from a blower) under the cast. Oral medication is not generally effective in relieving this type of skin irritation (**No. 1**). Rolling the

cast (**No. 3**) while the patient scratched would only increase the risk of skin damage. Taking the pencil from the patient (**No. 4**) would deny his or her ability both to understand the rationale and to take responsibility for actions. **IMP,3,SECE**

70. (**2**) The primary dysfunction in myasthenia gravis occurs at the myoneural junction (the synapse between the end of a myelinated nerve fiber and a skeletal muscle fiber). Normally, acetylcholine is secreted by the nerve ending, which acts on the muscle fiber membrane by increasing its permeability to sodium. If sufficient sodium enters the muscle fiber membrane, an action potential is promulgated and causes the muscle fiber to contract. To enable the muscle fiber to repolarize, the acetylcholine in the synaptic junction is destroyed by cholinesterase. In myasthenia gravis, these normal impulses are blocked at the myoneural junction. **No. 1** is incorrect because degeneration of the basal ganglia results in increased muscle tone, as occurs with *Parkinson's disease*. **No. 3** is incorrect because increased stimulation of muscle fibers by anterior motor neurons would also increase muscle contractions. **No. 4** is *partially* correct, in that there does seem to be a familial tendency toward the development of myasthenia; however, if myasthenia is generalized, it usually affects not only facial and mastication muscles but also ocular movement (diplopia and ptosis) as well as muscles of the neck, trunk (respirations), and limbs. **IMP,3,PhI**

71. (**1**) The diuretic stage of burns occurs 48–72 hours after injury. The fluid shift is just the opposite of that in the initial stage. Fluids, electrolytes, and proteins may move very rapidly from the interstitial space back into the vascular compartment. Unless renal damage has occurred and there is no indication (**No. 2**), diuresis ensues, due to the increased blood volume and renal blood flow. Serum electrolytes and hematocrit are decreased due to hemodilution. If urine output is insufficient at this time, symptoms of circulatory overload and cardiac failure will occur. There are *no data to support* **No. 3**. The sodium value is within *normal* limits (**No. 4**). **AN,8,PhI**

72. (**1**) The most common side effects of pyridostigmine (Mestinon) and neostigmine bromide (Prostigmin) include anorexia, nausea, diarrhea, and abdominal cramps. These symptoms are due to increased gastrointestinal secretions, smooth-muscle contractions (peristalsis), and irritation of the gastric mucosa. **No. 2** is incorrect because increased cholinergic discharge increases bladder tone and contraction, thus *facilitating* voiding. **Nos. 3 and 4** are incorrect because the symptoms listed are consistent with increased adrenergic, *not* cholinergic, discharge or stimulation. **AS,4,PhI**

73. (**4**) In response to direct questioning by the patient, the nurse needs to provide brief, accurate information. Some patients who have had gastrectomies are able to tolerate three meals a day before discharge from the hospital. However, for the majority of patients, it takes 6/014001/ months before their surgically reduced stomach has stretched enough to accommodate a larger meal. **No. 1** is incorrect because it is an open-ended response designed to elicit additional information. **No. 2** is correct as far as it goes, but still doesn't answer the patient's question. If the nurse does not know the answer to a question, he or she should admit it but try to get the information. **No. 3** is incorrect because it gives inaccurate information. **IMP,4,PsI**

74. (**1**) The most common cause of hypothyroidism today is excess thyroid tissue destruction due to radioactive io-

dine therapy for hyperthyroidism. Spontaneous hypothyroidism is believed due to an autoimmune response. Several studies have revealed a high incidence of antibodies for thyroid antigen in patients with spontaneous atrophy (**No. 2**). Other, *less common* causes include surgical removal (**No. 3**), Hashimoto's thyroiditis, overuse of antithyroid drugs (**No. 4**), and pituitary tumors or insufficiency that decrease the circulating levels of TSH (thyroid-stimulating hormone). **AN,3,PhI**

75. (3) In order to take full advantage of the effects of anticholinesterase drugs, they should generally be scheduled 20–30 minutes before eating. **Nos. 1 and 2** are not totally incorrect, in that these drugs generally act over a 3-hour period; however, peak action occurs quickly, and patients with dysphagia need time to eat, chew, and swallow during meals. Rushing at meals causes unnecessary fatigue. **No. 4** may not allow enough time for the drug to take effect. **PL,3,SECE**

76. (2) Body image changes are the most frequent basis for psychological responses during the recuperative phase. This is particularly true if the patient is young or has sustained facial or neck burns. Also, self-esteem is often lowered. The patient needs to be encouraged to talk about the perceived changes between what he or she was, and is now. Sessions with a psychiatric nurse specialist may be helpful. Occasionally individual and/or group therapy is indicated. Pain and immobility (**No. 1**) create problems in the *acute* phase of burns. Financial concerns (**No. 3**) may affect responses during the recuperative phase, but they are *not* a significant concern for all patients. Anger (**No. 4**) may be a response during *each phase* as the patient reacts to various real and imagined losses. **EV,7,PsI**

77. (2) Signs of "cholinergic crisis" include pupils constricted to <2 mm, severe diarrhea, nausea, vomiting, hypersalivation, lacrimation, pallor, and hypotension. Bradycardia may occur but is uncommon. In severe cases, confusion progressing to coma may occur due to blockage of cerebral synapses. **Nos. 1 and 3** are symptoms related to increased *adrenergic* discharge. **No. 4** is only partially correct. **AS,2,PhI**

78. (3) A deficiency of thyroid hormone causes widespread metabolic changes. Alterations in fluid and electrolyte balance due to increased capillary permeability lead to fluid retention that results in edema, particularly of the eyelids, hands, and feet. **No. 1** is incorrect because the lowered metabolic rate decreases cellular oxygen consumption; as a result, the heart rate, pulse pressure, and blood pressure are *reduced*. **No. 2** is incorrect because there is eyelid edema, *not* facial edema. The basal metabolic rate is reduced, causing symptoms of anorexia, constipation, and intolerance to cold due to a lowered body temperature. **No. 4** is incorrect because it includes diarrhea. Reduced cerebral blood flow affects both perception and coordination and results in symptoms of lethargy, generalized weakness, and slowing of both intellectual and motor functions. **AS,3 PhI**

79. (1) The patient with hyperthyroidism has an increased metabolic rate due to excess serum thyroxine leading to symptoms of systolic hypertension, heat intolerance, widened pulse pressure, and emotional excitability. **No. 2** is incorrect because the diastolic blood pressure reduces due to decreased peripheral resistance. Weight loss (not gain, as in **No. 3**) occurs because of increased catabolism despite an increase in appetite. Anorexia in **No. 4** is incorrect because the patient has increased appetite. **AS,3,PhI**

80. (4) Myasthenia gravis is a rare disease of unknown cause but is suspected to have autoimmune characteris-

tics. **No. 1** is not correct because thymectomy has *often* resulted in remission or improvement (in approximately 70% of patients), not rarely. **No. 2** is not correct because myasthenia gravis runs a *chronic* and progressive, not acute and rapid course. One of the major symptoms is muscle weakness, *not* increased strength (**No. 3**). **AN,3,PhI**

81. (1) A nasogastric tube will be inserted early on the surgical day. **No. 2** is not correct because the patient will not be allowed anything by mouth; all medications will be administered by injection in the immediate preoperative period. **No. 3** is not correct because, although it is important for the physician to explain possible complications when obtaining permission to perform the surgery, the timing is inappropriate for any lengthy descriptions of possible complications. **No. 4** is not a good choice because the patient should be *encouraged*, not discouraged, to take an appropriate amount of pain medications so he or she will be able to cough, turn, and deep breathe to avoid respiratory complications. **PL,1,SECE**

82. (1) The primary pathology in Cushing's syndrome is increased serum cortisol, which acts to accelerate the rate of gluconeogenesis in the body, thus mobilizing stored fats and proteins. Serum glucose is increased, stimulating insulin secretion by the pancreas and resulting in abnormalities in fat metabolism and deposition. Weight gain is common; the torso enlarges and fat pads develop on the back of the neck and in the cheeks, giving the patient the characteristic "buffalo hump" and "moon facies." Increased epinephrine secretion (**No. 2**) is associated with pheochromocytoma. Increased aldosterone (**No. 3**) is associated with primary aldosteronism. Decreased ACTH secretion (**No. 4**) is associated with dysfunctions of the pituitary gland. **AN,3,PhI**

83. (2) Lassitude and muscle weakness are early clinical signs of Cushing's syndrome. Catabolism from gluconeogenesis occasionally results in a marked decrease in skeletal mass and the patient's extremities may appear wasted. **No. 1** is incorrect because gluconeogenesis from excess cortisol secretion results in hyperglycemia. **No. 3** is partially correct: hypersecretion of aldosterone in Cushing's disease is rare; however, large quantities of cortisol tend to increase sodium and water retention and potassium excretion. Edema and hypokalemia occur only in severe cases. Discoloration and hyperpigmentation (**No. 4**) occur with adrenal insufficiency. **EV,3,PhI**

84. (1) Signs and symptoms of Addison's disease include hypotension, hypoglycemia, muscular weakness, fatigue, weight loss, hyperkalemia, and depression. These symptoms are primarily due to disturbances in sodium, water, and potassium imbalances that cause severe dehydration. **No. 2** includes symptoms of Cushing's syndrome. **No. 3** is incorrect because hyperglycemia and weight gain are consistent also with Cushing's syndrome. **No. 4** also includes symptoms of Cushing's syndrome. **AS,3,PhI**

85. (1) Iron deficiency anemia is characterized by a decrease in red blood cell color due to a decrease in iron (hypochromic) and an increase in immature red blood cells (microcytic). **No. 2** describes the red blood cells in pernicious anemia. **Nos. 3 and 4** describe no particular conditions. **AN,6,PhI**

86. (1) In assessing any patient's emotional responses, the nurse should first assess the patient's ego strength, body image, and coping abilities for life situations in general. The manner in which the patient views himself or herself will greatly affect attitudes toward disease and emotional response. If the patient normally denies or represses threatening information or situations, desirable

outcomes may be difficult to achieve. The evidence of recent research indicates that social supports are extremely important in maintaining health. The relationship between the patient and the patient's mother (**No. 2**) should be assessed. However, if the patient has a strong self-image, the issues between mother and adult child should be resolvable either alone or with objective outside help. **No. 3** is incomplete. Economic status and work history (**No. 4**), depending on their value to the patient, may not be important determinants of emotional response. **AN,7,PsI**

87. **(1)** The primary fluid and electrolyte imbalances in Addison's disease are hyponatremia, hypovolemia, and hyperkalemia. These imbalances are caused by decreased aldosterone secretion. **Nos. 2 and 3** are incorrect because they occur with excessive secretion of this hormone. Calcium levels are not affected by this condition (**No. 4**). **EV,6,PhI**

88. **(2)** Mafenide 1% (Sulfamylon) is a white antibacterial ointment applied once or twice daily. Besides causing pain on application, this medication is a carbonic anhydrase inhibitor that interferes with the kidney's ability to excrete hydrogen ions and thus may cause metabolic acidosis, not metabolic alkosis (**No. 3**). Patients who are treated with mafenide 1% need to have their acid-base balance monitored by blood gas determinations. Clinical signs of metabolic acidosis are increased rate and depth of respirations. *Silver nitrate* causes black discoloration of linens, and its hypotonicity causes electrolyte imbalances (**Nos. 1 and 4**). Patients treated with silver nitrate will need supplemental sodium, potassium, and chloride. **EV,1,SECE**

89. **(3)** The best early intervention would be to increase fluid intake because constipation is common when activity is decreased or usual routines have been interrupted. **No. 1** is incorrect because this may not be necessary and also needs a doctor's order. **No. 2** is incorrect because this is a great deal of exertion when the patient is not expressing an urge to defecate. Although activity usually helps bowel evacuation, it would be impossible to exercise extremities that have unhealed fractures (**No. 4**). **IMP,8,PhI**

90. **(1)** Thyroid storm may be precipitated by a number of stresses, such as infection, real or threatened loss of a loved one, or thyroid surgery undertaken before the patient was prepared adequately with antithyroid drugs. A change heralding thyroid storm is a fever: the patient's temperature may rise as high as 106°F (41°C). **Nos. 2, 3, and 4** are symptoms of hyperthyroidism and become exaggerated during thyroid storm. Without treatment, the patient progresses from delirium to coma; death ensues as the result of heart failure. **AS,3,PhI**

91. **(2)** Bloody drainage from the nasogastric tube more than 12 hours after surgery should be considered unusual and reported to the surgeon. Prolonged bleeding may be indicative of a slow bleeder, a blood dyscrasia, or problems with incisional closure. Any of these may increase blood loss and lead to shock. **Nos. 1, 3, and 4** are incorrect because they are *normal* findings in the *early* postgastrectomy period. **EV,6,PhI**

92. **(2)** Calculating the correct rate requires computation of the hourly volume (290 cc) and the minute volume (5 cc), and then multiplying the rate, in cc/min, by the drop factor (15 gtt/cc). (The hourly and minute volumes have been rounded to the nearest whole number.) **Nos. 1 and 3** are not fast enough to deliver this large a volume in the prescribed period. **No. 4** is too rapid. A quick method of computing the drip rate is to use the first two numbers in the 24-hour fluid volume, i.e., 7000 cc in 24 hours = 70 gtt/min. This shortcut may be useful when initially starting an infusion, before mathematically calculating the rate. Use only with 15 gtt/cc factor. **IMP,6,PhI**

93. **(1)** Osteoblastic activity (bone growth) needs the stress and strain of weight bearing to be proportional to osteoclastic activity (bone breakdown). When the patient is immobilized for an extended period of time, bone breakdown takes place. Although dietary intake is important, it is not recommended that there be an increase in calcium intake (**No. 2**) due to the potential for kidney stones as a result of immobilization. Osteoporosis is related to a *deficit* of calcium, not excess (**No. 3**). Bone growth is dependent on weight bearing, not lack of it (**No. 4**). **AN,3,PhI**

94. **(4)** Sinus arrhythmia is the most frequent arrhythmia and occurs as a normal phenomenon, often related to the respiratory cycle. **No. 1** is incorrect because lidocaine is used to treat life-threatening ventricular arrhythmias. **No. 2** is incorrect because exercise, which increases the heart rate, will abolish the arrhythmia, so rest or limited activity is not indicated. **No. 3** is incorrect because the arrhythmia originates in the sinoatrial node, not in the atrioventricular node, and digoxin is the treatment for atrial arrhythmias. **EV,6,SECE**

95. **(2)** Hematocrit is reduced due to hemodilution and volume overload resulting from the interstitial-to-plasma fluid shift. Erythropoietin factor (**No. 1**) is produced by the kidneys and would only be reduced if there were kidney failure. Metabolic acidosis (**No. 3**) does increase red blood cell fragility, but it is not applicable in this situation. Hypoalbuminemia (**No. 4**) causes loss of oncotic pressures in the vascular compartment. The primary effect of this phenomenon is movement of fluid from the vascular compartment to the interstitial space, the outcome of which is hemoconcentration. **AN,6,PhI**

96. **(3)** Pernicious anemia may occur following subtotal gastrectomy (when large portions of the stomach are removed) due to the loss of tissue that produces the intrinsic factor. Loss of this factor necessitates the parenteral administration of vitamin B_{12}, the extrinsic factor. **No. 1** is incorrect because the extrinsic factor is found in food. **Nos. 2 and 4** are incorrect because it is the loss of intrinsic factor that results in the malabsorption of vitamin B_{12}. **EV,4,PhI**

97. **(1)** The gastric distress that occurs as a side effect of these medications can be reduced by administering the drugs along with milk, soda crackers, or antacids. The nursing actions in **No. 2** are consistent with *elimination* problems (urinary retention); those in **No. 3** are consistent with *central nervous system* excitation (flushing, irritability); and the action in **No. 4** is consistent with *cardiac arrhythmias* (palpitations, PVCs). **IMP,4,PhI**

98. **(2)** Generalized tonic-clonic (grand mal) seizures are characterized by auras preceding the convulsive spasms of all muscle groups, loss of consciousness, and loss of sphincter control. Brief, abrupt loss of consciousness, with a characteristic "blank stare," is indicative of *absence (petit mal) seizures* (**No. 1**). *Focal or partial seizures* usually involve only a portion of the brain and reflect the area of the brain activated by abnormal discharge (such as tonic and clonic contractions of the large muscles in an arm or leg) (**No. 3**). Localized twitching of facial muscles, especially of the angle of the mouth, or within a finger or toe, is characteristic of a *jacksonian seizure* (**No. 4**). **AS,2,PhI**

Review of Nutrition

❏ Nutrition during Pregnancy and Lactation

Table 3.1.

I. **Milk group**—important for calcium, protein of high biologic value, and other vitamins and minerals.
   A. *Pregnancy*—three to four servings.
   B. *Lactation*—four to five servings.
   C. *Count as one serving*—1 cup milk; ½ cup undiluted evaporated milk; ¼ cup dry milk; 1¼ cups cottage cheese; 2 cups low-fat cottage cheese; 1½ oz cheddar or Swiss cheese; or 1½ cups ice cream.

II. **Meat, poultry, fish, dry beans, nuts, and eggs group**—important for protein, iron, and many B vitamins.
   A. *Pregnancy*—three servings.
   B. *Lactation*—three servings.
   C. *Count as one serving*—½ cup cooked dry beans, 1 egg, or 1½ tbsp peanut butter is equivalent to 1 oz meat; use peanut butter or nuts rarely to avoid excessive fat intake; limit eggs to reduce cholesterol intake; trim fat from meat, and remove skin from poultry.

III. **Vegetable and fruit group**—vitamins and minerals (especially A and C) and roughage.
   A. *Vegetables*
      1. *Pregnancy*—three to five servings.
      2. *Lactation*—three to five servings.
      3. *Count as one serving*—1 cup raw leafy greens, ½ cup of others.
   B. *Fruits*
      1. *Pregnancy*—two to four servings.
      2. *Lactation*—two to four servings.
      3. *Count as one serving*—½ medium grapefruit; 1 medium apple, banana, or orange; ¾ cup fruit juice.

   C. *Good sources (vitamin C)*—citrus, cantaloupe, mango, papaya, strawberries, broccoli, and green and red bell peppers.
   D. *Fair sources (vitamin C)*—tomatoes, honeydew melon, asparagus tips, raw cabbage, collards, kale, mustard greens, potatoes (white and sweet), spinach, and turnip greens.
   E. *Good sources (vitamin A)*—dark-green or deep-yellow vegetables and a few fruits (apricots, broccoli, pumpkin, sweet potato, spinach, cantaloupe, carrots, and winter squash).
   F. *Good sources of folic acid*—dark-green foliage-type vegetables.

IV. **Bread and cereal group**—good for thiamine, iron, niacin, and other vitamins and minerals.
   A. *Pregnancy*—six to 11 servings.
   B. *Lactation*—six to 11 servings.
   C. *Count as one serving*—1 slice bread, 1 oz ready-to-eat cereal, ½–¾ cup cooked cereal, cornmeal, grits, macaroni, noodles, rice, or spaghetti.

V. **Note:** use dark-green leafy and deep-yellow vegetables often; eat dry beans and peas often; count ½ cup cooked dry beans or peas as a serving of vegetables or 1 oz from meat group.

❏ Nutritional Needs of the Newborn

I. Calories—108 kcal/kg/d.
II. Protein—2.2 g/kg/d (1 g protein = 1 oz milk).
III. Fluids—3.5 oz/kg/24 h.
IV. Vitamin D—400 IU daily for bottle-fed babies after week 2.
V. Fluoride—0.25 mg daily regardless of content in local water supply.

■ **TABLE 3.1   Nutrient Needs during Pregnancy**

Nutrient	Maternal Need	Fetal Need	Food Source
Protein	Maternal tissue growth: uterus, breasts, blood volume, storage	Rapid fetal growth	Milk and milk products; animal meats—muscle, organs; grains, legumes; eggs
Calories	Increased BMR	Primary energy source for growth of fetus	Carbohydrates: 4 kcal/g Proteins: 4 kcal/g Fats: 9 kcal/g
Minerals			
Calcium (and phosphorus)	Increase in maternal Ca^{2+} metabolism	Skeleton and tooth formation	Milk and milk products, especially Swiss cheese*
Iron	Increase in RBC mass Prevent anemia Decrease infection risk	Liver storage (especially in third trimester)	Organ meats—liver, animal meat; egg yolk; whole or enriched grains; green leafy vegetables; nuts
Vitamins			
A	Tissue growth	Cell development—tissue and bone growth and tooth bud formation	Butter, cream, fortified margarine; green and yellow vegetables
Bs	Coenzyme in many metabolic processes	Coenzyme in many metabolic processes	Animal meats, organ meats; milk and cheese; beans, peas, nuts; enriched grains
Folic acid	Meet increased metabolic demands in pregnancy Production of blood products	Meet increased metabolic demands, including production of cell nucleus material	Liver; deep-green, leafy vegetables
C	Tissue formation and integrity Increase iron absorption	Tissue formation and integrity	Citrus fruit, berries, melons; peppers; green, leafy vegetables; broccoli; potatoes
D	Absorption Ca^{2+}, phosphorus	Mineralization of bone tissue and tooth buds	Fortified milk and margarine
E	Tissue growth; cell wall integrity; RBC integrity	Tissue growth; cell integrity; RBC integrity	Widely distributed: meat, milk, eggs, grains, leafy vegetables

*Swiss cheese contains twice the amount of calcium as 8 oz of whole milk but only 0.09 as much lactose; therefore, it is a good source for those with lactose intolerance. Tofu (soybean cake) also is high in calcium, and contains *no* lactose.

❑ Pediatric Nutrition

Table 3.2.

❑ Ethnic Food Patterns

Tables 3.3 and 3.4.

❑ Common Vitamins and Related Deficiencies

Table 3.5.

❑ Nutritional Needs of the Elderly

I. *Calories*—1500–2000 kcal/d to maintain ideal weight; 15–20% of calories from protein sources.

II. *High fiber*—prevent or alleviate constipation and dependence on laxatives.

III. *Sodium*—3–4 g/d according to cardiac and renal status.

IV. *Fats*—limit to help retard the development of cancer, atherosclerosis, obesity, and other diseases.

V. *Fluids*—6–8 glasses/d.

VI. Common deficiencies: calories, calcium, folic acid, thiamine, vitamins A and D, zinc.

VII. Factors contributing to food preferences:
   A. Physical ability to prepare, shop for, and eat food.
   B. Income.
   C. Availability of food if dependent on others.
   D. Food intolerances.

VIII. Table 3.6 provides interventions for common eating problems in the elderly.

■ TABLE 3.2 Median Heights and Weights and Recommended Energy Intake

Category	Age (yr) or Condition	Weight		Height		REE[a] (kcal/d)	Average Energy Allowance (kcal)[b]		
		kg	lb	cm	in.		Multiples of REE	Per kg	Per day[c]
Infants	0.0–0.5	6	13	60	24	320		108	650
	0.5–1.0	9	20	71	28	500		98	850
Children	1–3	13	29	90	35	740		102	1300
	4–6	20	44	112	44	950		90	1800
	7–10	28	62	132	52	1130		70	2000
Males	11–14	45	99	157	62	1440	1.70	55	2500
	15–18	66	145	176	69	1760	1.67	45	3000
	19–24	72	160	177	70	1780	1.67	40	2900
	25–50	79	174	176	70	1800	1.60	37	2900
	51+	77	170	173	68	1530	1.50	30	2300
Females	11–14	46	101	157	62	1310	1.67	47	2200
	15–18	55	120	163	64	1370	1.60	40	2200
	19–24	58	128	164	65	1350	1.60	38	2200
	25–50	63	138	163	64	1380	1.55	36	2200
	51+	65	143	160	63	1280	1.50	30	1900
Pregnant	1st trimester								+0
	2nd trimester								+300
	3rd trimester								+300
Lactating	1st 6 mo								+500
	2nd 6 mo								+500

[a]Resting energy expenditure.
[b]In the range of light to moderate activity, the coefficient of variation is ±20%.
[c]Figure is rounded.
The data in this table have been assembled from the observed median heights and weights of children together with desirable weights for adults for the mean heights of men (70 in.) and women (64 in.) between the ages of 18 and 34 yr as surveyed in the U.S. population (HEW/NCHS data). The energy allowances for the young adults are for men and women doing light work. The allowances for the two older age groups represent mean energy needs over these age spans, allowing for a 2% decrease in basal (resting) metabolic rate per decade and a reduction in activity of 200 kcal/d for men and women between 51 and 75 yr of age, 500 kcal for men over 75, and 400 kcal for women over 75. The customary range of daily energy output for adults is based on a variation in energy needs of ±400 kcal at any one age, emphasizing the wide range of energy intakes appropriate for any group of people. Energy allowances for children through age 18 are based on medium energy intakes of children these ages followed in longitudinal growth studies.
Source: Food and Nutrition Board, National Research Council. *Recommended Dietary Allowances* (10th ed). Washington, DC: National Academy of Sciences, 1989.

❑ Religious Considerations in Meal Planning

I. Orthodox Jews
   A. Kosher meat and poultry.
   B. No shellfish or pork products.
   C. Milk and dairy products cannot be consumed with meat or poultry; requires separate utensils.
II. Conservative and Reform Jews: dietary practices may vary from religious laws.
III. Muslims: no pork or alcohol.
IV. Hindus: vegetarians (cows are sacred).
V. Seventh-Day Adventists
   A. Vegetarianism is common (lacto-ovo).
   B. No shellfish or pork products.
   C. Avoid stimulants (coffee, tea, other caffeine sources).
   D. No alcohol.
VI. Mormons: no coffee, tea, or alcohol.

❑ Special Diets

I. **Low-carbohydrate diet**—ketogenic: low carbohydrate, high fat; *dumping syndrome:* low carbohydrate, high fat, high protein.
II. **Gluten-free diet**—elimination of all foods made from oats, barley, wheat, and rye; used for celiac disease.
III. **High-protein diet**—lean meat, cheese, and green vegetables.
   A. Nephrotic syndrome (may also be on low-sodium diet).
   B. Acute leukemia (combined with high-calorie and soft-food diets).
   C. Neoplastic disease.
IV. **Low-protein diet**
   A. Usually accompanied by high-carbohydrate diet and normal fats and calories.
   B. Renal failure, uremia, anuria, acute glomerulonephritis.
V. **Low-sodium diet**
   A. Heart failure.
   B. Nephrotic syndrome.

Nutrition

■ **TABLE 3.3   Ethnic Food Patterns**

Ethnic Group	Cultural Food Patterns	Dietary Excesses or Omissions
Mexican (native)	Basic sources of protein—dry beans, flan, cheese, many meats, fish, eggs Chili peppers and many deep-green and yellow vegetables Fruits include zapote, guava, papaya, mango, citrus Tortillas (corn, flour); sweet bread; fideo; tacos, burritos, enchiladas	*Limited* meats, milk, and milk products Some are using flour tortillas more than the more nutritious corn tortillas *Excessive* use of lard (manteca), sugar Tendency to boil vegetables for long periods of time
Filipino (Spanish-Chinese influence)	Most meats, eggs, nuts, legumes Many different kinds of vegetables Large amounts of rice and cereals	May *limit* meat, milk, and milk products (the latter may be due to lactose intolerance) Tend to prewash rice Tend to fry many foods
Chinese (mostly Cantonese)	Cheese, soybean curd (tofu), many meats, chicken and pigeon eggs, nuts, legumes Many different vegetables, leaves, bamboo sprouts Rice and rice-flour products; wheat, corn, millet seed; green tea Mixtures of fish, pork, and chicken with vegetables—bamboo shoots, broccoli, cabbage, onions, mushrooms, pea pods	Tendency among some immigrants to use *excess* grease in cooking May be *low* in protein, milk, and milk products (the latter may be due to lactose intolerance) Often wash rice before cooking Large amounts of soy and oyster sauces, both of which are *high in salt*
Puerto Rican	Milk with coffee Pork, poultry, eggs, dried fish; beans (habichuelas) Viandas (starchy vegetables; starchy ripe fruits) Avocados, okra, eggplant, sweet yams Rice, cornmeal	Utilize *large* amounts of lard for cooking *Limited* use of milk and milk products *Limited* amounts of pork and poultry
Black American	Milk with coffee Pork, poultry, eggs, dried fish; beans (habichuelas) Viandas (starchy vegetables; starchy ripe fruits) Avocados, okra, eggplant, sweet yams Rice, cornmeal Cereals (including grits, hominy, hot breads) Molasses (dark molasses is especially good source of calcium, iron, vitamins B_1 and B_2, and niacin)	*Limited* use of milk group (lactose intolerance) Extensive use of frying, "smothering," simmering for cooking *Large* amounts of fat: salt pork, bacon drippings, lard, gravies May have *limited* use of citrus and enriched breads
Middle Eastern (Greek, Syrian, Armenian)	Yogurt Predominantly lamb, nuts, dried peas, beans, lentils Deep-green leaves and vegetables; dried fruits Dark breads and cracked wheat	Tend to use *excessive* sweeteners, lamb fat, olive oil Tend to fry meats and vegetables *Insufficient* milk and milk products (almost no butter—use olive oil, which has no nutritive value except for calories) Deficiency in fresh fruits
Middle European (Polish)	Many milk products Pork, chicken Root vegetables (potatoes), cabbage, fruits Wheat products Sausages, smoked and cured meats, noodles, dumplings, bread, cream with coffee	Tend to use *excessive* sweets and to overcook vegetables *Limited* amounts of fruits (citrus), raw vegetables, and meats
Native American (American Indian—much variation)	If "Americanized," use milk and milk products Variety of meats: game, fowl, fish; nuts, seeds, legumes Variety of vegetables, some wild Variety of fruits, some wild, rose hips; roots Variety of breads, including tortillas, cornmeal, rice	*Nutrition-related problems:* obesity, diabetes, dental problems, iron deficiency anemia; alcoholism *Limited* quantities of high-protein foods depending on availability (flocks) and economic situation *Excessive* use of sugar
Italian	Staples are pasta with sauces; bread; eggs; cheese; tomatoes and vegetables such as artichokes, eggplant, greens, and zucchini Only small amount of meat is used	*Limited* use of whole grains *Insufficient* servings from milk group Tendency to overcook vegetables Enjoy sweets

■ TABLE 3.4　Hot-Cold Theory of Disease Treatment*

Hot Diseases or Conditions	Cold Diseases or Conditions	Hot Foods	Cold Foods	Hot Medicines and Herbs	Cold Medicines and Herbs
Infections	Cancer	Chocolate	Fresh vegetables	Penicillin	Bicarbonate of soda
Kidney diseases	Earache	Cheese	Tropical fruits	Aspirin	Milk of magnesia
Diarrhea	Rheumatism	Temperate-zone	Dairy products	Castor oil	Sage
Rashes and other	Tuberculosis	fruits	Low-prestige meats	Cod liver oil	Linden
skin eruptions	Common cold	Chili peppers	(goat, fish,	Iron preparations	Orange flower
Sore throat	Headache	Cereal grains	chicken)	Vitamins	water
Warts	Paralysis	Goat milk	Honey	Anise	
Constipation	Stomach cramps	High-prestige	Raisins	Cinnamon	
Ulcers	Teething	meats (beef,	Bottled milk	Garlic	
Liver complaints	Menstrual period	water fowl,	Barley water	Mint	
	Joint pain	mutton)	Cod	Ginger root	
	Malaria	Oils		Tobacco	
	Pneumonia	Hard liquor			
		Aromatic beverages			
		Coffee			
		Onions			
		Peas			
		Eggs			

*A Latin American, particularly Puerto Rican, approach to treating diseases. A "hot" disease is treated with "cold" treatments (foods, medicines) and vice versa.
Source: Reprinted with permission from Wilson HS, Kneisl CR. *Psychiatric Nursing* (2nd ed). Menlo Park, CA: Addison-Wesley, 1983. P 774.

C. Acute glomerulonephritis (varies with degree of oliguria).

❏ Common Therapeutic Diets

I. **Clear-liquid diet**
  A. *Purpose:* relieve thirst and help maintain fluid balance.
  B. *Use:* postsurgically and following acute vomiting or diarrhea.
  C. *Foods allowed:* carbonated beverages; coffee (caffeinated and decaffeinated); tea; fruit-flavored drinks; strained fruit juices; clear, flavored gelatins; broth, consommé; sugar; popsicles; commercially prepared clear liquids; and hard candy.
  D. *Foods avoided:* milk and milk products, fruit juices with pulp, and fruit.

II. **Full-liquid diet**
  A. *Purpose:* provide an adequately nutritious diet for patients who cannot chew or who are too ill to do so.
  B. *Use:* acute infection with fever, gastrointestinal upsets, after surgery as a progression from *clear liquids.*
  C. *Foods allowed:* clear liquids, milk drinks, cooked cereals, custards, ice cream, sherbets, eggnog, all strained fruit juices, vegetable juices, creamed vegetable soups, puddings, mashed potatoes, instant breakfast drinks, yogurt, mild cheese sauce or pureed meat, and seasonings.
  D. *Foods avoided:* nuts, seeds, coconut, fruit, jam, and marmalade.

III. **Soft diet**
  A. *Purpose:* provide adequate nutrition for those who have trouble chewing.
  B. *Use:* patients with no teeth or ill-fitting dentures; transition from full-liquid to general diet; and for those who cannot tolerate highly seasoned, fried, or raw foods following acute infections or gastrointestinal disturbances, such as gastric ulcer or cholelithiasis.
  C. *Foods allowed:* very tender minced, ground, baked, broiled, roasted, stewed, or creamed beef, lamb, veal, liver, poultry, or fish; crisp bacon or sweetbreads; cooked vegetables; pasta; all fruit juices; soft raw fruits; soft breads and cereals; all desserts that are soft; and cheeses.
  D. *Foods avoided:* coarse whole-grain cereals and breads; nuts; raisins; coconut; fruits with small seeds; fried foods; high-fat gravies or sauces; spicy salad dressings; pickled meat, fish, or poultry; strong cheeses; brown or wild rice; raw vegetables as well as lima beans and corn; spices such as horseradish, mustard, and catsup; and popcorn.

IV. **Sodium-restricted diet**
  A. *Purpose:* reduce sodium content in the tissues and promote excretion of water.
  B. *Use:* heart failure, hypertension, renal disease, cirrhosis, toxemia of pregnancy, and cortisone therapy.
  C. *Modifications:* mildly restrictive 2-g sodium diet to extremely restricted 200-mg sodium diet.

■ **TABLE 3.5   Physiologic Functions and Deficiency Syndromes of Common Vitamins**

Nutrient	Functions	Signs of Deficiency
Fat-Soluble Vitamins		
Vitamin A	Essential for formation and maintenance of epithelial cells; essential for normal function of the retina and the synthesis of rhodopsin (visual purple)	Night blindness; xerosis and softening of the cornea; dry, bumpy skin
Vitamin D	Necessary for absorption and metabolism of calcium and phosphorus; important for the formation of normal teeth and bones	Rickets in children; osteomalacia in adults
Vitamin E	Antioxidant that protects red blood cells from hemolysis; utilized in epithelial tissue maintenance and prostaglandin synthesis	Increased hemolysis of red blood cells, macrocytic anemia, increased capillary fragility
Vitamin K	Essential for the formation of prothrombin and other clotting factors by the liver	Hypoprothrombinemia; hemorrhagic disease in newborns
Water-Soluble Vitamins		
Vitamin C	Essential for the formation of collagen; promotes healing of wounds and fractures; reduces susceptibility to infections; promotes the absorption of iron; necessary for the conversion of folic acid to folinic acid, tryptophan to serotonin, and cholesterol to bile salts; may play a role in resistance to certain types of cancer	Scurvy—petechiae and ecchymoses, joint pain, delayed wound healing, gingivitis, bleeding gums, loss of teeth
Vitamin B_1 (thiamine)	Coenzyme in carbohydrate metabolism; essential for normal nerve function	Beriberi—peripheral neuropathy, muscle cramping, paresthesias, muscle degeneration, and heart failure
Vitamin B_2 (riboflavin)	Coenzyme in cellular metabolism and respiration; essential for healthy eyes	Red conjunctivae; fissures at corners of mouth, around nose and ears, and on tongue; magenta tongue
Vitamin B_3 (niacin)	Coenzyme in the metabolism of carbohydrates and amino acids; essential for the synthesis of fatty acids and cholesterol and the conversion of phenylalanine to tyrosine	Pellagra—cracks in skin and lips; red lesions of hands, feet, face, and neck; dementia
Vitamin B_6 (pyridoxine)	Coenzyme in protein metabolism and several other enzymatic reactions; necessary for the formation of norepinephrine, epinephrine, tyramine, dopamine, and serotonin	Seborrheic dermatitis, cheilosis, peripheral neuritis, and convulsions
Vitamin B_9 (folic acid)	Essential for DNA synthesis and normal maturation of red blood cells	Megaloblastic and macrocytic anemia; reduced platelet levels
Vitamin B_{12} (cyanocobalamin)	Coenzyme in protein metabolism; essential for red blood cell formation and maintenance of myelin sheaths of nerves	Pernicious anemia, progressive neuropathy owing to demyelination

Source: Shlafer M, Marieb E. *The Nurse, Pharmacology and Drug Therapy.* Menlo Park, CA: Addison-Wesley, 1989.

    D. *Foods avoided:* table salt; all commercial soups, including bouillon; gravy, catsup, mustard, meat sauces, and soy sauce; buttermilk, ice cream, and sherbet; sodas; beet greens, carrots, celery, chard, sauerkraut, and spinach; *all canned* vegetables; frozen peas; all baked products containing salt, baking powder, or baking soda; potato chips and popcorn; fresh or canned shellfish; all cheeses; smoked or commercially prepared meats; salted butter or margarine; bacon; olives; and commercially prepared salad dressings.

V. Renal diet

    A. *Purpose:* control protein, potassium, sodium, and fluid levels in body.

    B. *Use:* acute and chronic renal failure, hemodialysis.

    C. *Foods allowed:* high-biologic proteins such as meat, fowl, fish, cheese, and dairy products—range between 20 and 60 mg/d. Potassium is usually limited to 40 mEq/d. Vegetables such as cabbage, cucumber, and peas are lowest in potassium. Sodium is restricted to 500 mg/d. See IV. Sodium-restricted diet, p. 243. Fluid intake is restricted to the daily urine volume plus 500 mL, which represents insensible water loss. Fluid intake measures water in fruit, vegetables, milk, and meat.

    D. *Foods avoided:* cereals, bread, macaroni, noodles, spaghetti, avocados, kidney beans,

■ **TABLE 3.6** **Dietary Interventions for Eating Problems of the Elderly**

Problem	Rationale	Dietary Interventions
Difficulty chewing	Missing or ill-fitting dentures	Provide liquid, semisolid, mashed, or chopped foods as tolerated
Difficulty swallowing	Paralysis related to stroke	Thickened and gelled liquids are usually better tolerated than thin liquids; baby food can be used as a nutritious thickener
		Avoid overuse of puréed foods because of the negative connotations associated with it
Lack of appetite	Depression	Offer small, frequent meals
	Acute or chronic disease	Solicit food preferences
	Loss of sense of smell and taste	Allow plenty of time to eat
	Side effect of medication	Because appetite is usually greatest in the morning, emphasize a nutritious breakfast
	Loneliness	
	Early satiety	Encourage group eating
Impaired ability to feed self	Poor vision	Describe the meal and how it is arranged on the plate
	Arthritis of the hands; stroke	Assist the patient by opening packages of bread and crackers, buttering bread and vegetables, cutting meat, and opening milk cartons
		Assess the patient's ability to grasp utensils and guide food to the mouth
		Refer the patient to an occupational therapist to evaluate the need for assistive devices or retraining

Source: Dudek S. *Nutrition Handbook for Nursing Practice,* 2nd ed. Philadelphia: Lippincott, 1993. P 340. Reprinted by permission of J.B. Lippincott Company.

potato chips, raw fruit, yams, soybeans, nuts, gingerbread, apricots, bananas, figs, grapefruit, oranges, percolated coffee, Coca-Cola, Orange Crush, sport drinks, and breakfast drinks such as Tang or Awake.

VI. High-protein, high-carbohydrate diet

A. *Purpose:* corrects large protein losses and raises the level of blood albumin. May be modified to include low-fat, low-sodium, and low-cholesterol diets.

B. *Use:* burns, hepatitis, cirrhosis, pregnancy, hyperthyroidism, mononucleosis, protein deficiency due to poor eating habits, geriatric patients with poor food intake, nephritis, nephrosis, and liver and gallbladder disorders.

C. *Foods allowed:* general diet with added protein. In adults, high-protein diets usually contain 135–150 g protein.

D. *Foods avoided:* restrictions depend on modifications added to the diet. These modifications are determined by the patient's condition.

VII. Purine-restricted diet

A. *Purpose:* designed to reduce the amount of consumed uric acid–producing foods.

B. *Use:* high uric acid retention, uric acid renal stones, and gout.

C. *Foods allowed:* general diet plus 2–3 quarts of liquid daily.

D. *Foods avoided:* cheese containing spices or nuts, fried eggs, meat, liver, seafood, lentils, dried peas and beans, broth, bouillon, gravies, oatmeal and whole wheats, pasta, noodles, and alcoholic beverages. *Limited* quantities of meat, fish, and seafood allowed.

VIII. Bland diet

A. *Purpose:* provision of a diet low in fiber, roughage, mechanical irritants, and chemical stimulants.

B. *Use:* ulcers (gastric and duodenal), gastritis, hyperchlorhydria, functional GI disorders, gastric atony, diarrhea, spastic constipation, biliary indigestion, and hiatus hernia.

C. *Foods allowed:* varied to meet individual needs and food tolerances.

D. *Foods avoided:* fried foods, including eggs, meat, fish, and seafood; cheese with added nuts or spices; commercially prepared luncheon meats; cured meats such as ham; gravies and sauces; raw vegetables; potato skins; fruit juices with pulp; figs; raisins; fresh fruits; whole wheats; rye bread; bran cereals; rich pastries; pies; chocolate; jams with seeds; nuts; seasoned dressings; caffeinated coffee; strong tea; cocoa; alcoholic and carbonated beverages; and pepper.

IX. Low-fat, cholesterol-restricted diet

A. *Purpose:* reduce hyperlipidemia, provide dietary treatment for malabsorption syndromes and patients having acute intolerance for fats.

B. *Use:* hyperlipidemia, atherosclerosis, pancreatitis, cystic fibrosis, sprue, gastrectomy, massive resection of the small intestine, and cholecystitis.

C. *Foods allowed:* nonfat milk; low-carbohydrate, low-fat vegetables; most fruits; breads; pastas; cornmeal; lean meats; unsaturated fats such as corn oil; desserts made without whole milk; and unsweetened carbonated beverages.

D. *Foods avoided:* whole milk and whole-milk or cream products, avocados, olives, commercially prepared baked goods such as donuts and muffins, poultry skin, highly marbled meats, shellfish, fish canned in oil, nuts, coconut, commercially prepared meats, butter, ordinary margarines, olive oil, lard, pudding made with whole milk, ice cream, candies with chocolate, cream, sauces, gravies, and commercially fried foods.

X. Diabetic diet

A. *Purpose:* maintain blood glucose as near normal as possible; prevent or delay onset of diabetic complications.

B. *Use:* diabetes mellitus.

C. *Foods allowed:* composed of 50–60% carbohydrates, 25–30% fats, and 12–20% protein. Foods are divided into groups from which exchanges can be made. Coffee, tea, broth, bouillon, spices, and flavorings can be used as desired. Exchange groups include milk, vegetables, fruit, starch/bread (includes starchy vegetables), meat (divided into lean, medium fat, and high fat), and fat exchanges. The number of exchanges allowed from each group is dependent on the total number of calories allowed. Nonnutritive sweeteners (aspartame) if desired. Nutritive sweeteners (sorbitol) in moderation with controlled, normal-weight diabetics.

D. *Foods avoided:* concentrated sweets or regular soft drinks.

XI. Acid and alkaline ash diet

A. *Purpose:* furnish a well-balanced diet in which the total acid ash is greater than the total alkaline ash each day.

B. *Use:* retard the formation of renal calculi. The type of diet chosen depends on laboratory analysis of the stones.

C. *Acid and alkaline ash food groups:*
1. *Acid ash:* meat, whole grains, eggs, cheese, cranberries, prunes, plums.
2. *Alkaline ash:* milk, vegetables, fruit (except cranberries, prunes, and plums).
3. *Neutral:* sugars, fats, beverages (coffee and tea).

D. *Foods allowed:* all the patient wants of the following.
1. Breads: any, preferably whole grain; crackers; rolls.
2. Cereals: any, preferably whole grain.
3. Desserts: angel food or sunshine cake; cookies made without baking powder or soda; cornstarch pudding, cranberry desserts, custards, gelatin desserts, ice cream, sherbet, plum or prune desserts; rice or tapioca pudding.
4. Fats: any, such as butter, margarine, salad dressings, Crisco, Spry, lard, salad oils, olive oil, etc.
5. Fruits: cranberries, plums, prunes.

6. Meat, eggs, cheese: any meat, fish, or fowl, two servings daily; at least one egg daily.
7. Potato substitutes: corn, hominy, lentils, macaroni, noodles, rice, spaghetti, vermicelli.
8. Soup: broth as desired; other soups from foods allowed.
9. Sweets: cranberry or plum jelly; sugar; plain sugar candy.
10. Miscellaneous: cream sauce, gravy, peanut butter, peanuts, popcorn, salt, spices, vinegar, walnuts.

E. *Restricted foods:* no more than the amount allowed each day.
1. Milk: 1 pint daily (may be used in other ways than as beverage).
2. Cream: ⅓ cup or less daily.
3. Fruits: one serving of fruit daily (in addition to the prunes, plums, and cranberries); certain fruits listed under *Foods avoided,* below, are *not allowed at any time.*
4. Vegetables, including potatoes: two servings daily; certain vegetables listed under *Foods avoided,* below, are *not allowed at any time.*

F. *Foods avoided:*
1. Carbonated beverages, such as ginger ale, cola, root beer.
2. Cakes or cookies made with baking powder or soda.
3. Fruits: dried apricots, bananas, dates, figs, raisins, rhubarb.
4. Vegetables: dried beans, beet greens, dandelion greens, carrots, chard, lima beans.
5. Sweets; chocolate or candies other than those listed under *Foods allowed,* above; syrups.
6. Miscellaneous: other nuts, olives, pickles.

XII. High-fiber diet

A. *Purpose:* soften stool; exercise digestive tract muscles; speed passage of food through digestive tract to prevent exposure to cancer-causing agents in food; lower blood lipids; prevent sharp rise in blood glucose after eating.

B. *Use:* diabetes, hyperlipidemia, constipation, diverticulosis, anticarcinogenic (colon).

C. *Foods allowed:* recommended intake about 6 g crude fiber daily: all bran cereals; watermelon, prunes, dried peaches, apple with skin; parsnips, peas, brussels sprouts; sunflower seeds.

XIII. Low-residue (low-fiber) diet

A. *Purpose:* reduce stool bulk and slow transit time.

B. *Use:* bowel inflammation during acute diverticulitis or ulcerative colitis, preparation for bowel surgery, esophageal and intestinal stenosis.

C. *Foods allowed:* eggs; ground or well-cooked tender meat, fish, poultry; milk; mild cheeses; strained fruit juice (except prune); cooked or canned apples, apricots, peaches, pears; ripe bananas; strained vegetable juice; canned, cooked, or strained asparagus, beets, green beans, pumpkin, acorn squash, spinach; white bread; refined cereals (Cream of Wheat).

❏ Food List for Ready Reference in Menu Planning

I. High-cholesterol foods—over 50 mg/100-g portion: beef, butter, cheese, egg yolks, fish, kidney, liver, pork, veal.

II. High-sodium foods—over 500 mg/100-g portion: bacon—cured, Canadian; baking powder; beef—corned, cooked, canned, dried, creamed; biscuits, baking powder; bouillon cubes; bran, added sugar and malt; bran flakes with thiamine; raisins; breads—wheat, French, rye, white, whole wheat; butter, cheese—cheddar, Parmesan, Swiss, pasteurized American; cocoa; cookies, gingersnaps; cornflakes; cornbread; crackers—graham, saltines; margarine; milk—dry, skim; mustard; oat products; olives—green, ripe; peanut butter; pickles, dill; popcorn with oil and salt; salad dressing—blue cheese, Roquefort, French, Thousand Island; sausages—bologna, frankfurters; soy sauce; tomato catsup; tuna in oil.

III. High-potassium foods—more than 400 mg/100-g portion: almonds; bacon, Canadian; baking powder, low-sodium; beans—white, lima; beef, hamburger; fruits, fruit juices; bran with sugar and malt; cake—fruitcake, gingerbread; cashew nuts; chicken, light meat; cocoa; coffee, instant; cookies, gingersnaps; dates; garlic; milk—dry, skim, powdered; peanuts, roasted; peanut butter; peas; pecans; potatoes, boiled in skin; scallops; tea, instant; tomato puree; turkey, light meat; veal; walnuts, black; yeast, brewer's.

IV. Foods high in B vitamins
   A. *Thiamine:* pork, dried beans, dried peas, liver, lamb, veal, nuts, peas.
   B. *Riboflavin:* liver, poultry, milk, yogurt, whole-grain cereals, beef, oysters, tongue, fish, cottage cheese, veal.
   C. *Niacin:* liver, fish, poultry, peanut butter, whole grains and enriched breads, lamb, veal, beef, pork.

V. Foods high in vitamin C: oranges, strawberries, dark-green leafy vegetables, potatoes, grapefruit, tomato, cabbage, broccoli, melon, liver.

VI. Foods high in iron, calcium, and residue
   A. *Iron:* breads—brown, corn, ginger; fish, tuna; poultry; organ meats; whole-grain cereals; shellfish; egg yolk; fruits—apples, berries; dried fruits—dates, prunes, apricots, peaches, raisins; vegetables—dark-green leafy, potatoes, tomatoes, rhubarb, squash; molasses; dried beans and peas; peanut butter; brown sugar; noodles; rice.
   B. *Calcium:* milk—dry, skim, whole, evaporated, buttermilk; cheese—American, Swiss, hard; kale; turnip greens; mustard greens; collards; tofu.
   C. *Residue:* whole-grain cereals—oatmeal, bran, shredded wheat; breads—whole wheat, cracked wheat, rye, bran muffins; vegetables—lettuce, spinach, Swiss chard, raw carrots, raw celery, corn, cauliflower, eggplant, sauerkraut, cabbage; fruits—bananas, figs, apricots, oranges.

VII. Foods to be used in low-protein and low-carbohydrate diets
   A. *Low protein**: milk—buttermilk, reconstituted evaporated, low-sodium, skim, and dry; meat—chicken, lamb, turkey, beef (lean), veal; fish—sole, flounder, haddock, perch; cheese—cheddar, American, Swiss, cottage; eggs; fruits—apples, grapes, pears, pineapple; vegetables—cabbage, cucumbers, lettuce, tomatoes; cereals—cornflakes, puffed rice, puffed wheat, farina, rolled oats.
   B. *Low carbohydrate:* all meats; cheese—hard, soft, cottage; eggs; shellfish—oysters, shrimp; fats—bacon, butter, French dressing, salad oil, mayonnaise, margarine; vegetables—asparagus, green beans, beet greens, broccoli, brussels sprouts, cabbage, celery, cauliflower, cucumber, lettuce, green pepper, spinach, squash, tomatoes; fruits—avocados, strawberries, cantaloupe, lemons, rhubarb.

VIII. Food guide pyramid—guide to daily food selection (Figure 3.1).
   A. *Fats, oils:* use sparingly.
   B. *Milk group:* two to three servings.
   C. *Meat group:* two to three servings.
   D. *Fruit group:* two to four servings.
   E. *Vegetable group:* three to five servings.
   F. *Bread/cereal group:* six to 11 servings.

❏ Questions

Select the one best answer for each question.

1. A diabetic patient states she is a "peanut butter freak." Which exchange would be equivalent to 2 tbsp peanut butter?
   1. 8 oz whole milk.
   2. 2 tbsp butter.
   3. ¼ cup cottage cheese.
   4. 2 tbsp cream cheese.
2. A patient is placed on an 1800-calorie diabetic diet; a typical lunch would include two meat exchanges, two bread exchanges, one vegetable exchange, one fruit exchange,

---

*These proteins are allowed in various amounts in controlled-protein diets for *renal decompensation*.

■ **FIGURE 3.1   Food guide pyramid—guide to daily food choices. US Department of Agriculture.**

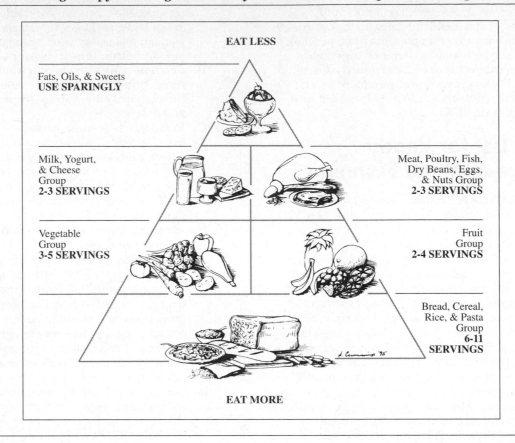

EAT LESS

Fats, Oils, & Sweets
USE SPARINGLY

Milk, Yogurt,
& Cheese
Group
2-3 SERVINGS

Meat, Poultry, Fish,
Dry Beans, Eggs,
& Nuts Group
2-3 SERVINGS

Vegetable
Group
3-5 SERVINGS

Fruit
Group
2-4 SERVINGS

Bread, Cereal,
Rice, & Pasta
Group
**6-11
SERVINGS**

EAT MORE

one fat exchange, and one milk exchange. Given these allowances, which would be inappropriate for this patient to consume at a birthday luncheon?
1. A piece of plain sponge cake.
2. An 8-oz glass of Coca-Cola.
3. A taco (tortilla, meat, cheddar cheese, lettuce).
4. Avocado and orange salad.

3. A patient has been placed on a high-protein diet. Which food would the nurse suggest this patient select?
1. Rice (1 cup).
2. Eggnog (8 oz).
3. Cheddar cheese (1 oz).
4. Broccoli (1 cup).

4. Which food would the nurse recommend be *avoided* by a patient experiencing dumping syndrome?
1. Liver and bacon.
2. Orange and avocado salad.
3. Creamed chicken.
4. Glazed donuts and coffee.

5. Dietary restriction of protein in chronic renal failure is used to prevent the accumulation of nitrogenous wastes and resulting azotemia. Which food containing amino acids would be allowed in a diet for a patient with chronic renal failure?
1. Roast beef.
2. Milk and eggs.
3. Chicken and turkey.
4. Shellfish.

6. Which food may be more likely to cause discomfort in a patient with cholecystitis?
1. Whole milk.

2. Cottage cheese.
3. Whole-grain breads.
4. Eggs.

7. Which food should the nurse advise a colostomy patient to *avoid?*
1. Carbonated drinks.
2. Fresh-cooked green beans.
3. Liver and bacon.
4. Cooked cereals.

8. A patient is a 30-year-old gravida 3 para 2 who is 4 weeks pregnant. She has been a vegetarian for 8 years. She eats no eggs or dairy products (vegan vegetarian). When assessing the adequacy of this patient's diet, to which food group would the nurse pay particular attention?
1. Grains.
2. Protein foods.
3. Vitamin C–rich foods.
4. Fruits and vegetables.

9. A patient is a 17-year-old primigravida. At 30 weeks' gestation she is diagnosed with an iron deficiency anemia. The patient takes her iron and vitamin supplements sporadically due to unacceptable GI side effects but eats many foods high in iron. In planning diet teaching, which nutrient will the nurse emphasize to promote heme production?
1. Niacin.
2. Vitamin A.
3. Vitamin D.
4. Folic acid.

❏ Answers/Rationale

1. (3) A diabetic's diet is most often based on an exchange system. Foodstuffs in this system are divided into six types. Foods from within each list can be substituted for another in the same list because they have approximately the same food value. Peanut butter is in the meat exchange list, as is cottage cheese, and therefore these can be substituted for one another. Whole milk **(No. 1)** is on the milk exchange list. Butter and cream cheese **(Nos. 2 and 4)** are considered to be fats. **IMP,4,PhI**

2. (2) Given the patient's food allowances, all these foods **(Nos. 1, 3, and 4)** would be allowed except for the Coca-Cola. All concentrated sweets and regular soft drinks are contraindicated on a diabetic diet. **PL,4,PhI**

3. (2) Eggs and milk are two sources of protein with the highest biologic values (high-quality proteins). Eggnog (8 oz) contains 15 g protein. Rice **(No. 1)** contains 4 g, cheddar cheese **(No. 3)** 7 g, and broccoli **(No. 4)** 5 g. Meat, fish, and legumes contain more protein than does eggnog, but their percent of protein utilization is lower, making them almost equal in value to eggnog. **IMP,4,PhI**

4. (4) Concentrated sugars and carbohydrates should be avoided by these patients. Likewise, fluid ingestion with meals or snacks should also be avoided to prevent rapid emptying of the stomach. **Nos. 1, 2, and 3** are examples of high-protein, high-fat, low-carbohydrate foods, which are appropriate. **PL,4,PhI**

Key to codes following rationales Nursing process: **AS,** Assessment; **AN,** Analysis; **PL,** Plan; **IMP,** Implementation; **EV,** Evaluation. Category of human function: **1,** Protective; **2,** Sensory-perceptual; **3,** Comfort, Rest, Activity, and Mobility; **4,** Nutrition; **5,** Growth and Development; **6,** Fluid-Gas Transport; **7,** Psychosocial-Cultural; **8,** Elimination. Client need: **SECE,** Safe, Effective Care Environment; **PhI,** Physiologic Integrity; **PsI,** Psychosocial Integrity; **HPM,** Health Promotion/Maintenance. See appendices for full explanation.

5. (2) The diet for patients with chronic renal failure is restricted in total amount of protein and amino acid content. Eggs and milk are generally included in the diet because they contain all the essential amino acids. Meats from animals **(No. 1)**, fowl **(No. 3)**, and fish **(No. 4)** are restricted due to their sulfur-containing, nonessential amino acids. **PL,4,PhI**

6. (1) Whole milk has a high fat content, so a patient with cholecystitis is generally advised to switch to low-fat or skim milk. Cottage cheese **(No. 2)**, whole-grain breads **(No. 3)**, and eggs **(No. 4)** are allowed in a low-fat diet, though eggs may be limited to four per week. **IMP,4,PhI**

7. (1) Carbonated drinks, cabbage, sauerkraut, and nuts tend to increase flatulence, and most patients feel uncomfortable passing flatus into the colostomy bag, as it causes it to inflate. Onions, cheese, and fish may cause odorous drainage. Generally the initial diet following a colostomy is a low-fiber diet for several weeks. As the diet is increased, the individual patient can determine more accurately which foods cause constipation, diarrhea, flatus, or dyspepsia. **Nos. 2, 3, and 4** are not troublesome to most such patients. **PL,4,PhI**

8. (2) Vegetarians who omit dairy foods may be unable to meet the requirement for an additional 30 g protein per day over their nonpregnant needs. **No. 1** is incorrect because individuals who have been vegetarians for some time usually have evolved diets adequate in grain intake. **Nos. 3 and 4** are incorrect because individuals who are vegan vegetarians usually ingest a wide variety of fruits and vegetables to meet pregnancy requirements for vitamin C, fiber, and other nutrients. **AS,4,PhI**

9. (4) Folic acid (folacin) is essential for increased heme production for hemoglobin and prevention of megaloblastic anemia. **No. 1** is incorrect because niacin has no direct or indirect role in erythropoiesis or heme production. **No. 2** is incorrect because vitamin A is essential for fetal bone growth and tooth development. **No. 3** is incorrect because vitamin D is essential for mineralization of bone tissue and calcium and phosphorus absorption. **PL,4,PhI**

Nutrition

Review of Pharmacology

❏ Guidelines for Administering Medications to Infants and Children

I. Developmental considerations
A. Be honest. Do not bribe or threaten child to obtain cooperation.
B. When administering medication, do so in the least traumatic manner possible.
C. Describe any sensations child may expect to experience, e.g., "pinch" of needle during IM.
D. Explain how child can "help" nurse, e.g., "Lie as still as you can."
E. Tell child that it's OK to cry; provide privacy.
F. Offer support, praise, and encouragement during and after giving medication.
G. Allow child opportunity for age-appropriate therapeutic play to work through feelings and experiences, to clarify any misconceptions, and to teach child more effective coping strategies.

II. Safety considerations
A. Be absolutely sure dose you are giving is both safe (check recommended mg/kg) and accurate (have another nurse check your calculations). Remember: dose should generally be smaller than adult dose.
B. Check identification band or ask parent or another nurse for child's first and last name.
C. Restrain child to avoid injury while giving medication; a second person is often required to help hold child.

III. Oral medications
A. Use syringe without needle to draw up medication.
B. *Position:* upright or semireclining.
C. Place tip of syringe along the side of infant's tongue, and give medication slowly, in small amounts, allowing infant to swallow. Medicine cups can be used for older infants and children. **Never** pinch infant or child's nostrils to force him or her to open mouth.
D. When giving tablets or capsules (that are **not** enteric coated), crush and mix into smallest possible amount of food or liquid to ensure that child takes entire dose. Do not mix with essential food or liquid (e.g., milk); select an "optional" food, such as applesauce.

IV. Ophthalmic installations
A. *Position:* supine or sitting with head extended.
B. For eye drops: hold dropper 1–2 cm above middle of conjunctival sac.
C. For eye ointment: squeeze 2 cm of ointment from tube onto conjunctival sac.
D. After giving drops or ointment, encourage child to keep eyes closed briefly, to maximize contact with eyes. Child should be asked to look in all directions (with eyes closed) to enhance even distribution of medication.
E. Whenever possible, administer eye ointments at nap time or bedtime, due to possible blurred vision.

V. Otic installations
A. *Position:* head to side so that affected ear is uppermost.
B. For child **under** 3 yr of age: pull pinna gently **down** and back.
C. For child 3 yr of age and **over:** pull pinna gently **up** and back.
D. After administering ear drops, encourage child to remain with head to side with affected ear uppermost, to maximize contact with entire external canal to reach eardrum.

Gentle massage of area in front of ear will facilitate entry of ear drops into canal.

E. If ear drops are kept in refrigerator, allow to warm to room temperature before instilling.

VI. Dermatologic installations

A. Remember: young child's skin is more permeable; therefore there is increased risk for medication absorption and resultant systemic effects; monitor for systemic effects.

B. Apply thin layer of cream or ointment, and confine it to portions of skin where it is essential.

VII. Rectal medication

A. Prepare child emotionally and physically; rectal route is invasive and embarrassing, particularly for children.

B. *Position:* side-lying with upper leg flexed.

C. Lubricate rounded end of suppository and insert past anal sphincter with gloved fingertip (wear gloves when inserting rectal medication).

D. Remove fingertip but hold child's buttocks gently together until child no longer strains or indicates urge to expel medication.

VIII. Intramuscular medication

A. Because the infant or child is much smaller physically than an adult, the nurse should select a shorter needle, generally ⅝ in. (infant) to 1 in. (child).

B. Preferred injection sites are on the thigh: vastus lateralis—lateral aspect; rectus femoris—anterior aspect. The deltoid muscle, though small, provides easy access and can be used in children with adequate muscle mass.

C. **Avoid** posterior gluteal muscle in children under age 4.

D. Because of vast differences in size, muscle mass, and subcutaneous tissue, it is especially important to note bony prominences as landmarks for intramuscular injections.

E. Have a second adult present to help restrain the child.

F. Once the nurse has told the child he or she is to receive an injection, the procedure should be carried out as quickly and skillfully as possible.

❏ Psychopharmacology: Common Psychotropic Drugs

I. Antipsychotics

A. Phenothiazines (perchlorperazine [Compazine], promazine HCl [Sparine], chlorpromazine HCl [Thorazine], thioridazine [Mellaril], trifluoperazine HCl [Stelazine], perphenazine [Trilafor], triflupromazine HCl [Vespirin], fluphenazine [Prolixin] enanthate).

B. Butyrophenones (haloperidol [Italdol, Serenace], droperidol/fentanyl citrate [Innovar]).

C. Thioxanthenes (chlorprothixene [Taractan], thiothixene [Navane])—chemically related to phenothiazines, with similar therapeutic effects.

1. *Use*—acute and chronic psychoses; most useful in cases of disorganization of thought or behavior; to decrease panic, fear, hostility, restlessness, aggression, and withdrawal.

◆ 2. **Assessment**—*side effects:*

a. *Hypersensitivity* effects

(1) *Blood dyscrasia*—agranulocytosis, leukopenia, granulocytopenia.

(2) *Skin reactions*—photosensitivity, dermatitis, flushing, blue-gray skin.

(3) Obstructive *jaundice.*

b. *Extrapyramidal symptoms (EPS)* affecting voluntary movement and skeletal muscles

(1) *Parkinsonism*—tremors, cogwheel rigidity, shuffling gait, pill-rolling, masklike facies, salivation, and difficulty starting muscular movement (dyskinesia).

(2) *Dystonia*—limb and neck spasms (torticollis), extensive rigidity of back muscles (opisthotonus), oculogyric crisis, speech and swallowing difficulties, and protrusion of tongue.

(3) *Akathisia*—motor restlessness, pacing, foot tapping, inner tremulousness, and agitation.

(4) *Tardive dyskinesia (TD)*—excessive blinking; vermiform tongue movement; stereotyped, abnormal, involuntary sucking, chewing, licking, and pursing movements of tongue and mouth; grimacing, blinking, frowning, rocking.

(a) *Cause*—long-term use of high doses of antipsychotic drugs.

(b) *Predisposing factors*—age, women, OBS; history of ECT or use of tricyclics or anti-Parkinson drugs.

c. *Potentiates* central nervous system depressants.

d. *Orthostatic hypotension* (less with butyrophenones).

e. *Anticholinergic effects* (atropinelike)— dry mouth, stuffy nose, blurred vision, urinary retention, and constipation.

f. Ocular changes (lens and corneal opacity).

◆ 3. **Nursing care plan/implementation:**

a. Goal: *anticipate, observe for, and check for side effects.*

(1) Protect the person's skin from sunburn when outside.

(2) For hypotension: take BP and have person lie down for 30 min, especially after an injection.

(3) Watch for signs of blood dyscrasia: sore throat, fever, malaise.

(4) Observe for symptoms of *hypo-* or *hyperthermic* reaction due to effect on heat-regulating mechanism.

(5) Observe for, withhold drug for, and report early symptoms of *jaundice* and bile tract obstruction, high fever, upper abdominal pain, nausea, diarrhea, rash; monitor liver function.

(6) Relieve excessive *mouth dryness:* mouth rinse, increased fluid intake.

(7) Relieve gastric irritation, *constipation:* take with and increase fluids and roughage in diet.

(8) Observe for and report changes in carbohydrate metabolism (glycosuria, weight gain, polyphagia): change diet.

b. Goal: *health teaching.*

(1) Dangers of drug potentiation with alcohol or sleeping pills.

(2) Advise about driving or occupations where blurred vision may be a problem.

(3) Caution against abrupt cessation at high doses.

(4) Warn regarding dark urine.

(5) Have client with respiratory disorder breathe deeply and cough as drug is a cough depressant.

(6) Need for continuous use of drug and follow-up care.

(7) Prompt reporting of hypersensitivity symptoms: fever, laryngeal edema; abdominal distention (constipation, urinary retention); jaundice; blood dyscrasia.

◆ 4. **Evaluation/outcome criteria:**

a. Behavior is less agitated.

b. Knows side effects to observe for, lessen, and/or prevent.

c. Continues to use drug.

II. Antidepressants

A. Tricyclic (imipramine HCl [Tofranil], desipramine HCl [Norpramin], nortriptyline HCl [Pamelor, Aventyl], trimipramine [Surmontil], amitriptyline HCl [Elavil], amitriptyline HCl/perphenazine [Triavil], protriptyline HCl [Vivactil], doxepin HCl [Sinequan])—effective in 1–3 wk.

1. *Use*—elevate mood in depression, increase physical activity and mental alertness; may bring relief of symptoms of depression so that client can attend individual or group therapy; bipolar disorder, depressed; dysthymic disorder.

◆ 2. **Assessment**—*side effects:*

a. *Behavioral*—activation of latent schizophrenia; hypomania; suicide attempts; mental confusion. Withhold drug if observed.

b. *Central nervous system* (CNS)—tremors, ataxia, jitteriness.

c. *Autonomic nervous system* (ANS)—dry mouth, nasal congestion, aggravation of glaucoma, constipation, urinary retention, edema, paralysis, ECG changes (flattened T waves; arrhythmia severe in overdose).

◆ 3. **Nursing care plan/implementation:**

a. Goal: *assess risk of suicide during initial improvement:* careful, close observation.

b. Goal: *prevent risk of cardiac arrhythmias and hypotension:* use caution with client with hyperthyroidism, having ECT or surgery (gradually discontinue 2–3 d *prior* to surgery). Monitor BP, pulse ×2/d; ECGs, 2–3/wk until dose adjusted.

c. Goal: *observe for signs of urinary retention, constipation:* monitor I&O and weight gain.

d. Goal: *cautious drug use with glaucoma or history of seizures.* Observe seizure precautions due to lowered seizure threshold.

e. Goal: *health teaching:*

(1) Advise against driving car or participating in activities requiring mental alertness, due to *sedative* effects.

(2) Encourage increased fluid intake and frequent mouth rinsing to combat dry mouth.

(3) *Avoid* smoking, which decreases drug effects.

(4) *Avoid* use of alcohol and other drugs, due to adverse interactions, especially OTC (e.g., antihistamines).

(5) Advise of delay in desired effect (2–4 wk).

(6) Instruct gradual discontinuance to avoid withdrawal symptoms.

◆ 4. **Evaluation/outcome criteria:** diminished symptoms of agitated depression and anxiety.

B. Monoamine oxidase inhibitors (MAOIs) (phenelzine sulfate [Nardil], isocarboxazid [Marplan], tranylcypromine sulfate [Parnate], iproniazid [Marsilid], pargiline HCl [Eutonyl], nialamide [Niamid]).

◆ 1. **Assessment**—*side effects:*

a. *Behavioral*—may activate latent schizophrenia, mania, excitement.

b. *CNS*—tremors; *hypertensive crisis* (avoid cheese, colas, caffeine, wine, beer, yeast, chocolate, chicken liver, or other substances high in tyramine or pressor amine, e.g., amphetamines and cold and hay fever medication); *intracerebral hemorrhage; hyperpyrexia.*

c. *ANS*—dry mouth, aggravation of glaucoma, bowel and bladder control problems; edema, paralysis, ECG changes (arrhythmia severe in overdose).

d. *Allergic* hepatocellular jaundice.

◆ 2. **Nursing care plan/implementation:**

a. Goal: *reduce risk of hypertensive crisis:* diet restrictions of foods high in *tyramine* content.

b. Goal: *observe for urinary retention:* measure I&O.

c. Goal: *health teaching.*

(1) Therapeutic response takes 2–3 wk.

(2) *Food and alcohol restrictions:* avocado, bananas, raisins, licorice, chocolate, cheese, yogurt, sour cream, liver, herring, soy sauce, meat tenderizers, wine, beer, caffeine.

(3) Change position gradually to prevent postural hypotension.

(4) Report any stiff neck, palpitations, chest pain, headaches because of possible hypertensive crises (can be fatal).

(5) Take *no nonprescribed* drugs.

◆ 3. **Evaluation/outcome criteria:**

a. Improvement in sleep, appetite, activity, interest in self and surroundings.

b. Lessening of anxiety and complaints.

III. Antianxiety

A. Chlordiazepoxide (Librium)

1. *Use*—alcoholism, tension, and irrational fears; has muscle relaxant and anticonvulsant properties.

◆ 2. **Assessment**—*side effects:* hypotension, drowsiness, motor uncoordination, confusion, skin eruptions, edema, menstrual irregularities, constipation, extrapyramidal symptoms, blurred vision, lethargy; ↑ or ↓ libido.

◆ 3. **Nursing care plan/implementation:**

a. Goal: *administer cautiously, as drug may:*

(1) Be habituating (causing withdrawal convulsions; therefore gradual withdrawal necessary).

(2) Potentiate CNS depressants.

(3) Have adverse effect on pregnancy.

(4) Be dangerous for those with suicidal tendencies or severe psychoses.

(5) Reduce GI effects: crush tablet or take with meals or milk; give antacids 1 h before.

(6) Alter liver function; check chart for results of periodic liver function tests and blood counts, especially with upper respiratory infection.

b. Goal: *health teaching.*

(1) Advise against suddenly stopping drug (withdrawal symptoms begin in 5–7 d).

(2) Talk with physician if plans to be or is pregnant.

(3) Urge to drink fluids.

(4) Avoid alcohol, OTC drugs, and heavy smoking.

◆ 4. **Evaluation/outcome criteria:** decreased alcohol withdrawal symptoms or preoperative anxiety.

B. Diazepam (Valium)

1. *Use*—muscle relaxant; *not* used for psychotics.

◆ 2. **Assessment**—*side effects:* same as for chlordiazepoxide, plus double or blurred vision, difficult speech, headache, hypotension, incontinence, tremor, urinary retention, liver damage.

◆ 3. **Nursing care plan/implementation:**

a. Goal: *anticipate, observe for, and check for side effects,* especially depression, suicidal risk, and constipation.

b. Goal: *reduce risk of hypotension, respiratory depression, phlebitis, venous thrombosis.* Give IM, in large muscles, slowly, and rotate sites, have client lie down; IV: over 1-min period.

c. Goal: *observe for psychological and physical dependence:* avoid abrupt discontinuation.

d. Goal: *health teaching:* sedative effects, potentiation of other CNS depressant drugs and alcohol, and problem of habituation.

◆ 4. **Evaluation/outcome criteria:** relief of tension, anxiety, skeletal muscle spasm.

IV. Antimanic

A. Lithium—effect occurs 1–3 wk after first dose.

1. *Use*—acute manic attack and prevention of recurrence of cyclic manic-depressive episodes of bipolar disorders.

◆ 2. **Assessment**—*side effects:* levels from 1.6–2.0 mEq/L may cause tremors, nausea and vomiting, diarrhea, polvuria, polydipsia; levels >2 mEq/L may cause motor weakness, headache, edema, and lethargy; *signs of severe toxicity:* neurologic, for example, twitching, marked drowsiness, slurred speech, dysarthria, athetotic movements, convulsions, delirium, stupor, coma.

a. *Precautions*—cautious use with clients on *diuretics;* with disturbed *electrolytes* (sweating, dehydrated, and postoperative clients); with *thyroid* problems, on *low-salt diets;* with congestive *heart failure;* and with impaired *renal function.* Risk of suicide.

b. *Dosage*—*therapeutic* level 0.8–1.6 mEq/L; dose for maintenance 300–1500 mEq/d; *toxic* level >2.0 mEq/L; blood sample drawn in acute phase 10–14 h after last dose, taken tid.

◆ 3. **Nursing care plan/implementation:**

a. Goal: *anticipate, observe for, and check for signs and symptoms of toxicity.*

(1) Reduce GI symptoms: take with meals.

(2) Check for edema: daily weight.

⚗ (3) Monitor blood levels (1.6–2.0 mEq/L) for signs of *toxicity:* nausea, vomiting, diarrhea, anorexia, ataxia, weakness, drowsiness, fine tremor or muscle twitching, slurred speech.

⚗ (4) Monitor results from repeat thyroid and kidney function tests.

b. Goal: *report fever right away.*

⚗ c. Goal: *monitor effect* (therapeutic and toxic): through blood samples taken:

(1) 10–14 h after last dose.

(2) Every 2–3 d until 1.6 mEq/L is reached.

(3) Once a week while in hospital.

(4) Every 2–3 mo to maintain blood levels <1 mEq/L.

d. Goal: *health teaching.*

(1) Advise client of 7–10 d lag time for effect.

(2) Urge to drink adequate liquids (2–3 L/d).

(3) Report polyuria and polydipsia.

(4) *Diet:* avoid caffeine, crash diets, diet pills, self-prescribed low-salt diet, antacids, high-sodium foods (which increase lithium excretion and reduce drug effect); take with meals.

(5) Caution against driving, operating machinery that requires mental alertness until drug is effective.

(6) Warn *not* to change or omit dose.

◆ 4. **Evaluation/outcome criteria:**

a. Changed facial affect.

b. Improved posture, ability to concentrate, sleep patterns.

c. Assumption of self-care.

V. Antiparkinson agents

A. Trihexyphenidyl HCl (Artane).

B. Benztropine mesylate (Cogentin).

1. *Use*—counteract extrapyramidal reactions.

◆ 2. **Assessment:**

a. Trihexyphenidyl HCl

(1) *Side effects*—dry mouth, blurred vision, dizziness, nausea, constipation, drowsiness, urinary hesitancy or retention, pupil dilation, headache, and weakness.

(2) *Precautions*—cautious use with cardiac, liver, or kidney disease or obstructive gastrointestinal-genitourinary disease. Do not give if glaucoma present.

b. Benztropine mesylate—*side effects:* same as for trihexyphenidyl HCl plus:

(1) Effect on *body temperature* may result in life-threatening state.

(2) *Gastrointestinal (GI) distress.*

(3) *Inability to concentrate,* memory difficulties, and mild confusion (often mistaken for senility).

(4) May lead to toxic psychotic reactions.

(5) *Subjective sensations*—light or heavy feelings in legs, numbness and tingling of extremities, light-headedness or tightness of head, and giddiness.

◆ 3. **Nursing care plan/implementation:**

a. Goal: *relieve GI distress* by giving after or with meals or at bedtime.

b. Goal: *monitor adverse effects:*

(1) Hypotension, tachycardia: check pulse, blood pressure.

(2) Constipation and fecal impaction: add roughage to *diet.*

(3) Dry mouth: increase *fluid* intake; encourage frequent mouth rinsing.

(4) Blurred vision, dizziness: assist with ambulation; use siderail.

c. *Health teaching:*

(1) *Avoid* driving, and limit activities requiring alertness.

(2) Delayed drug effect (2–3 d).

(3) Potential abuse due to hallucinogenic effects.

(4) *Avoid* alcohol and other CNS depressants.

◆ 4. **Evaluation/outcome criteria:**

a. Less rigidity, drooling, and oculogyric crisis.

b. Improved gait, balance, posture.

❏ Absorption Rates

Table 4.1.

■ TABLE 4.1   Rates of Absorption by Different Routes

Route of Administration	Time Until Drug Takes Effect*
Topical	Hours to days
Oral	30–90 min
Rectal	5–30 min (unpredictable)
Subcutaneous injection	15–30 min
Intramuscular injection	10–20 min
Sublingual tablet	3–5 min
Sublingual injection	3 min
Inhalation	3 min
Endotracheal	3 min
Intravenous	30–60 sec
Intracardiac	15 sec

*In a healthy person with normal perfusion.
Source: Caroline NL. *Emergency Care in the Streets* (5th ed). Boston: Little, Brown, 1995.

❏ Regional Analgesia-Anesthesia in Labor and Delivery

Table 4.2.

❏ Mind-Altering Substances

Major substances used by the public to alter mental states are compared in Table 4.3.

❏ Common Drugs

Table 4.4.

❏ Food and Drug Considerations

Table 4.5.

❏ Classification of Anticancer Drugs

Table 4.6.

❏ Properties of Selected Anti-inflammatory Agents

Table 4.7.

■ **TABLE 4.2   Regional Analgesia-Anesthesia for Labor and Birth**

Types	Characteristics	Nursing Implications
Common Agents in 0.5–1.0% Solution Lidocaine (Xylocaine) Bupivacaine (Marcaine) HCl Tetracaine (Pontocaine) HCl Mepivacaine HCl (Carbocaine) Chloroprocaine HCl (Nesacaine)	Used with epinephrine (or other vasoconstrictor drug) to delay absorption, prolong anesthetic effect, and decrease chance of hypotension	*Note any history of allergy;* note response: allergic reaction, hypotension, and lack of wearing off of anesthetic effect; observe for hypertensive crisis if agent combined with epinephrine and oxytocin is also being given
Peripheral Nerve Block Pudendal (5–10 mL each side) anesthetizes lower two-thirds of vagina and perineum	Perineal anesthesia of short duration (30 min); local anesthesia; simple and safe; does not depress neonate; may inhibit bearing-down reflex	To get cooperation, give explanation during procedure
Paracervical (uterosacral) block (5–10 mL given into each side) anesthetizes cervix and upper two-thirds of vagina; *note:* used more for gynecologic surgery than for labor	May be given between 3 and 8 cm by physician when woman is having at least three contractions in 10 min; lasts 45–90 min; can be repeated; can be followed by local, epidural, or other; may cause temporary fetal bradycardia	Explain: especially length and type of needle; take maternal vital signs and FHR; have her void; help position; monitor FHR continuously; monitor contractions; and watch for return of pain
Local infiltration	Useful for perineal repairs	No special nursing care
Epidural lumbar block	Useful during first and second stages; can be given "one shot" or continuously; T-10 to S-5 for vaginal birth; T-8 to S-1 for abdominal birth; complete anesthesia for labor and birth	*Hypotension* (with resultant fetal bradycardia): (a) turn from supine to lateral, or elevate legs, (b) administer humidified oxygen by mask at 8–10 L/min, (c) increase rate of IV fluids (use infusate *without* oxytocin); will need coaching to push and low forceps may be required
Subarachnoid spinal Continuous	Useful during first or second stage of labor, or for abdominal surgery	Instruct when to bear down
Low spinal ("saddle," "one shot") block	Same as continuous	Same as continuous
Intrathecal (spinal) morphine	0.5 mg produces marked analgesia for 12–24 h; onset in 20–30 min	*Side effects:* respiratory depression, pruritus, nausea, vomiting, sleepiness, urinary retention; keep naloxone 0.4 mg at bedside and respiratory support equipment readily available

Pharmacology

■ TABLE 4.3   Major Substances Used for Mind Alteration

Official Name	Slang Name	Usual Single Adult Dose/Duration	Legitimate Medical Uses (Present and Projected)	Short-Term Effects	Long-Term Effects
Alcohol—whisky, gin, beer, wine	Booze, hooch, suds	1½ oz gin or whisky, 12 oz beer/2–4 h	Rare: sometimes used as a sedative (for tension)	CNS depressant; relaxation (sedation); euphoria; drowsiness; impaired judgment, reaction time, coordination, and emotional control; frequent aggressive behavior and driving accidents	Diversion of energy and money from more creative and productive pursuits; habituation; possible obesity with chronic excessive use; irreversible damage to brain and liver; addiction with severe withdrawal illness (DTs) with heavy use; many deaths
Caffeine—coffee, tea, Coca-Cola, No-Doz, APC	Java	1–2 cups, 1 bottle, 5 mg/2–4 h	Mild stimulant; treatment of some forms of coma	CNS stimulant; increased alertness; reduction of fatigue	Sometimes insomnia, restlessness, or gastric irritation; habituation
Nicotine (and coal tar)—cigarettes, cigars	Fags, nails	1–2 cigarettes/1–2 h	None (used as an insecticide)	CNS stimulant; relaxation or distraction	Lung (and other) cancer, heart and blood vessel disease, cough, etc.; higher infant mortality; many deaths; habituation; diversion of energy and money; air pollution; fire
Sedatives					
Alcohol—see above	Downers				
Barbiturates—amobarbital (Amytal), pentobarbital (Nembutal), secobarbital (Seconal), phenobarbital	Barbs, blue devils, yellow jackets, dolls, red devils, phennies, goofers	50–100 mg	Treatment of insomnia and tension Induction of anesthesia	CNS depressants; sleep induction; relaxation (sedation); sometimes euphoria; drowsiness; impaired judgment, reaction time, coordination, and emotional control; relief of anxiety/tension; muscle relaxation	Irritability, weight loss, addiction with severe withdrawal illness (like DTs); diversion of energy and money; habituation, addiction
Glutethimide (Doriden)		500 mg			
Chloral hydrate		500 mg			
Meprobamate (Miltown, Equanil)		400 mg/4 h[a]			
Stimulants	Uppers				
Caffeine—see above					
Nicotine—see above					
Amphetamines Amphetamine (Benzedrine) Methamphetamine (Methedrine) Dextroamphetamine (Dexedrine)	Pep pills, wake-ups, Bennies, cartwheels, Crystal, speed, meth, Dexies or Xmas trees (spansules)	2.5–15.0 mg	Treatment of obesity, narcolepsy, fatigue, depression	CNS stimulants; increased alertness; reduction of fatigue; loss of appetite; insomnia; often euphoria	Restlessness, weight loss, toxic psychosis (mainly paranoid); diversion of energy and money; habituation; extreme irritability, toxic psychosis

continued

Pharmacology

■ **TABLE 4.3** *(Continued)*

Official Name	Slang Name	Usual Single Adult Dose/Duration	Legitimate Medical Uses (Present and Projected)	Short-Term Effects	Long-Term Effects
Stimulants *(continued)*					
Phenmetrazine HCl (Preludin)		25 mg			
Cocaine	Coke, snow	Variable/4 h[a]	Anesthesia of the eye and throat		
Tranquilizers					
Chlordiazepoxide (Librium)		5–25 mg	Treatment of anxiety, tension, alcoholism, neurosis, psychosis, psychosomatic disorders, and vomiting	Selective CNS depressants; relaxation, relief of anxiety/tension; suppression of hallucinations or delusions, improved functioning	Sometimes drowsiness, dryness of mouth, blurring of vision, skin rash, tremor; occasionally jaundice, agranulocytosis, or death
Phenothiazines Chlorpromazine HCl (Thorazine)		10–50 mg			
Perchlorperazine (Compazine)		5–10 mg			
Trifluoperazine HCl (Stelazine)		2–5 mg			
Reserpine (rauwolfia)		0.10–0.25 mg/4–6 h[a]			
Marijuana or cannabis[b]	Pot, grass, tea, weed, stuff, hash, joint, reefers	Variable—1 cigarette or pipe, or 1 drink or cake (India)/4 h[a]	Treatment of depression, tension, loss of appetite, and high blood pressure	Relaxation, euphoria, increased appetite, some alteration of time perception, possible impairment of judgment and coordination; mixed CNS depressant-stimulant	Usually none; possible diversion of energy and money; habituation; occasional acute panic reactions
Antidepressants					
Ritalin		5–10 mg	Treatment of moderate to severe depression	Relief of depression (elevation of mood), stimulation	Basically the same as tranquilizers above
Dibenzazepine (imipramine [Tofranil], amitriptyline HCl [Elavil])		25 mg, 10 mg			
MAO inhibitors (phenelzine sulfate [Nardil], tranylcypromine sulfate [Parnate])		10 mg, 15 mg/4–6 h[a]			

Pharmacology

Name	Slang names	Dose/Duration	Medical use	Short-term effects	Long-term effects
Narcotics (Opiates, Analgesics)					
Opium	Op	10–12 "pipes" (Asia)/4 h[a]	Treatment of severe pain, diarrhea, and cough	CNS depressants; sedation, euphoria, relief of pain, impaired intellectual functioning and coordination	Constipation, loss of appetite and weight, temporary impotency or sterility; habituation, addiction with unpleasant and painful withdrawal illness
Heroin	Horse, H, smack, shit, junk	Variable—bag or paper with 5–10% heroin			
Morphine		10–15 mg			
Codeine		15–30 mg			
Aspirin/oxycodone HCl (Percodan)		1 tablet			
Meperidine HCl (Demerol)		50–100 mg			
Methadone					
Cough syrups (Cheracol, Hycodan, Romilar, etc.)		2.5–40.0 mg 2–4 oz (for euphoria)/4–6 h[a]			
Hallucinogens					
LSD	Acid, sugar cubes, trip	150 μg/10–12 h	Experimental study of mind and brain function; enhancement of creativity and problem solving; treatment of alcoholism, mental illness, and the dying person; chemical warfare	Production of visual imagery, increased sensory awareness, anxiety, nausea, impaired coordination; sometimes consciousness expansion	Usually none; sometimes precipitates or intensifies an already existing psychosis; more commonly can produce a panic reaction
Psilocybin	Mushrooms	25 mg			
STP		6 mg			
DMT					
Mescaline (peyote)	Cactus	350 mg/12–14 h			
Miscellaneous					
Glue, gasoline, and solvents		Variable	None except for antihistamines used for allergy and amyl nitrite for fainting	When used for mind alteration generally produces a "high" (euphoria) with impaired coordination and judgment	Variable—some of the substances can seriously damage the liver or kidney, and some produce hallucinations
Amyl nitrite		1–2 ampules			
Antihistamines		25–50 mg			
Nutmeg		Variable/2 h			
Nonprescription "sedatives" (Compoze)					
Catnip					
Nitrous oxide					

[a] Time given pertains to all drugs listed.

[b] Hashish or charas is a more concentrated form of the active ingredient THC (tetrahydrocannabinol) and is consumed in smaller doses, analogous to vodka-beer ratios.

■ **TABLE 4.4 Common Drugs**

Drug and Dosage	Use	Action	Assessment: Side Effects
Adrenergics			
Alpha and beta agonists			
Epinephrine (Adrenalin)—SC or IM 0.2–1 mg in 1:1000 solution; IV—intracardiac 1:10,000 solution; ophthalmic 1:1000–1:50,000 solution	Asystole, bronchospasm, anaphylaxis, glaucoma	Stimulates pacemaker cells; inhibits histamine and mediates bronchial relaxation; ↓ intraocular pressure	Ventricular arrhythmias, fear, anxiety, anginal pain, decreased renal blood flow, burning of eyes, headache

NURSING IMPLICATIONS: Use TB syringe for greater accuracy; massaging injection site hastens action; repeated injections may cause tissue necrosis; *avoid* injection in buttocks because bacteria in area may lead to gas gangrene; may make mucous plugs in lungs more difficult to dislodge

Norepinephrine (Levophed)— IV 2–4 µg/min titrated to desired response	Acute hypertension, cardiogenic shock	Increases rate and strength of heartbeat; increases vasoconstriction	Palpitations, pallor, headache, hypertension, anxiety, insomnia, dilated pupils, nausea, vomiting, glycosuria, tissue sloughing

NURSING IMPLICATIONS: Observe vital signs, mentation, skin temperature, and color (earlobes, lips, nailbeds); tissue necrosis occurs with infiltration; antidote is phentolamine 5–10 mg in 10–15 mL normal saline

Beta agonists			
Dobutamine (Dobutrex)—IV 2.5–10 µg/kg/min	Acute heart failure	Stimulates cardiac contractile force (positive inotropy); fewer changes in heart rate than dopamine or isoproterenol	Tachycardia, arrhythmias

NURSING IMPLICATIONS: Mix with 5% dextrose; do not dilute until ready to use; protect from light; administer with infusion pump; check vital signs constantly; extravasation can produce tissue necrosis; see Norepinephrine

Dopamine (Intropin)—IV 2–5 µg/kg/min titrated to desired response	Acute heart failure	↑ Cardiac contractility; ↑ renal blood flow	Ectopic beats, nausea, vomiting, tachycardia, anginal pain, dyspnea, hypotension

NURSING IMPLICATIONS: Monitor vital signs, urine output, and signs of peripheral ischemia; will cause tissue sloughing if infiltration occurs

Isoproterenol (Isuprel)—10–15 mg sublingually; IV 0.5–4.0 µg/min in solution	Cardiogenic shock, heart block, bronchospasm—asthma, emphysema	↑ Cardiac contractility: facilitates AV conduction and pacemaker automaticity	Tachyarrhythmias, hypotension, headache, flushing of skin, nausea, tremor, dizziness

NURSING IMPLICATIONS: Monitor vital signs, ECG: oral inhalation solutions must *not* be injected

Adrenocortical Steroids			
Cortisone acetate—PO or IM 20–100 mg qd in single or divided doses	ACTH insufficiency; rheumatoid arthritis; allergies; ulcerative colitis; nephrosis	Anti-inflammatory effect of unknown action	Moon facies, hirsutism, thinning of skin, striae, hypertension, menstrual irregularities, delayed healing, psychoses

NURSING IMPLICATIONS: Give oral form pc, with snack at bedtime; give deep IM (*never* deltoid); monitor vital signs; observe for behavior changes; skin care and activity to tolerance; *diet*—salt restricted, high protein, KCl supplement; protect from injury

Desoxycorticosterone acetate (hydrocortisone)—IM 1–5 mg	Addison's disease; burns; surgical shock; adrenal surgery	Promotes reabsorption of sodium, and restores plasma volume, BP, and electrolyte balance	Edema, hypertension, pulmonary congestion, hypokalemia

NURSING IMPLICATIONS: Salt restriction according to BP readings; monitor vital signs; weigh daily

Dexamethasone (Decadron)— PO 0.5–5.0 mg qd; IM or IV 4–20 mg qd	Addison's disease; allergic reactions; leukemia; Hodgkin's disease; iritis; dermatitis; rheumatoid arthritis	Anti-inflammatory effect	See Cortisone acetate

NURSING IMPLICATIONS: *Contraindicated* in tuberculosis; see Cortisone acetate for nursing care

Methylprednisolone sodium (Solu-Medrol)—IV, IM 10–40 mg, slowly	Glucocorticoid, corticosteroid	See Dexamethasone	See Dexamethasone

NURSING IMPLICATIONS: See Dexamethasone

continued

■ TABLE 4.4 *(Continued)*

Drug and Dosage	Use	Action	Assessment: Side Effects
Adrenocortical Steroids *(continued)*			
Prednisone—PO 2.5–15.0 mg qd	Rheumatoid arthritis; cancer therapy	Anti-inflammatory effect of unknown action	Insomnia and gastric distress
NURSING IMPLICATIONS: See Cortisone acetate			
Analgesics			
Acetaminophen (Tylenol, Datril, Panadol)—PO 325–650 mg q4h	Simple fever or pain	Analgesic and antipyretic actions; no anti-inflammatory or anticoagulant effects	No remarkable side effects when taken for a short period
NURSING IMPLICATIONS: Consult with physician if no relief after 4 d of therapy			
Alphaprodine HCl (Nisentil)—SC 40–60 mg	**Obstetric use:** control pain, especially during labor	Synthetic narcotic similar to meperidine HCl; subcutaneous peak action 1–2 h; IV peak action first hour	Addictive; may depress fetus, especially if used with barbiturate; respiratory depression; dizziness; sweating, nausea, vomiting, and restlessness
NURSING IMPLICATIONS: See Meperidine HCl			
Aspirin (acetylsalicylic acid)—PO or rectal 0.3–0.6 g	Minor aches and pains; fever of colds and influenza; rheumatoid arthritis; anticoagulant therapy	Selectively depresses subcortical levels of CNS	Erosive gastritis with bleeding, coryza, urticaria, nausea, vomiting, tinnitus, impaired hearing, and respiratory alkalosis
NURSING IMPLICATIONS: Administer *with food or after meals;* observe for nasal, oral, or subcutaneous bleeding; push fluids; check *Hct, Hgb, prothrombin times* frequently; *avoid* use in children with flu			
Codeine—PO, IM, or SC 15–60 mg (gr ¼ to 1)	Control pain; may be used during the puerperium	Nonsynthetic narcotic analgesic	Of little use during labor; allergic response; constipation; GI upset
NURSING IMPLICATIONS: Note response to the medication; less respiratory depression; preferred for head injury patient			
Ecotrin (enteric coated aspirin)	See Aspirin	See Aspirin	See Aspirin
NURSING IMPLICATIONS: See Aspirin			
Etodolac (Lodine)—PO 400–1200 mg/d, 300–400 mg q6–8h	Management of osteoarthritis; mild to moderate pain	Inhibits prostaglandin synthesis; suppression of inflammation and pain (NSAID)	Dyspepsia, asthma, drowsiness, dizziness, rash, tinnitus, anaphylaxis
NURSING IMPLICATIONS: Give 30 min *before or 2 h after* meals for rapid effect; may be taken with food to decrease GI irritation			
Fentanyl transdermal (Duragesic)—25–100 µg/h	Chronic pain; not recommended for postoperative pain	Binds to opiate receptors in the CNS to alter response and perception of pain	Drowsiness, confusion, weakness, constipation, dry mouth, nausea, vomiting, anorexia, sweating
NURSING IMPLICATIONS: Apply to upper torso, flat, nonirritated surface; when applying, hold firmly with palm of hand 10–20 sec			
Hydromorphone (Dilaudid)—PO 2–4 mg q3–6h; IM 1–2 mg q3–6h up to 2–4 mg q4–6h; IV 0.5–1.0 mg q3h	Moderate to severe pain; antitussive	Binds to opiate receptors in the CNS; alters perception and response to pain	Sedation, confusion, hypotension, constipation
NURSING IMPLICATIONS: Give PO with *food or milk;* give IV 2 mg over 3–5 min; *fluids, bulk,* and laxatives to minimize constipation			
Ibuprofen (Motrin)—300–800 mg oral 3–4/d not to exceed 3200 mg/d	Nonsteroid anti-inflammatory, antirheumatic used in chronic arthritis pain	Inhibition of prostaglandin synthesis or release	GI upset; leukopenia; sodium/water retention
NURSING IMPLICATIONS: Give on *empty stomach* for best result; may mix with food if GI upset severe; teach caution when using other medications			
Indomethacin (Indocin)—25 mg 3–4/d; increase to max 200 mg daily in divided doses	Rheumatoid arthritis; bursitis; gouty arthritis	Antipyretic/anti-inflammatory action; inhibits prostaglandin biosynthesis	GI distress; GI bleeding; rash; headache; blood dyscrasias; corneal changes
NURSING IMPLICATIONS: Monitor GI side effects; administer *after* meals for best effect or *with* food, milk, or antacids if GI symptoms severe			

continued

■ **TABLE 4.4** *(Continued)*

Drug and Dosage	Use	Action	Assessment: Side Effects
Analgesics *(continued)*			
Ketorolac (Toradol)—PO 10 mg q4–6h; IM 30–60 mg initially, then 15–30 mg q6h; ophthalmic 1 gtt qid for 1 wk	Short-term management of pain; ocular itching due to allergies (NSAID)	Inhibits prostaglandin synthesis producing peripherally mediated analgesia; antipyretic/anti-inflammatory	Drowsiness, dizziness, dyspnea, prolonged bleeding time, dyspepsia
NURSING IMPLICATIONS: May be given routinely or prn; *advise* dentist or MD before any procedure			
Meperidine HCl (Demerol)—PO or IM 50–100 mg q3–4h	Pain due to trauma or surgery; allay apprehension prior to surgery	Acts on CNS to produce analgesia, sedation, euphoria, and respiratory depression	Palpitations, bradycardia, hypotension nausea, vomiting, syncope, sweating, tremors, and convulsions
NURSING IMPLICATIONS: Check *respiratory rate* and depth before giving drug; give IM, as subcutaneous administration is painful and can cause local irritation			
	Obstetric use: maternal relaxation may either slow labor or speed up labor	Depresses CNS, maternal and fetal; allays apprehension; PO peak action—1–2 h; IM peak action first hour	As above; also can depress fetus
NURSING IMPLICATIONS: Monitor maternal vital signs, contractions, progress of labor, and response to drug; fetal heart rate; if delivery occurs during peak action, prepare to give narcotic antagonist to mother and/or neonate			
Morphine SO₄—PO 10–30 mg (Roxanol, MS Contin); SC 8–15 mg; IV 4–10 mg; rectal 10–20 mg	Control pain and relieve fear, apprehension, restlessness, as in pulmonary edema	Depresses CNS reception of pain and ability to interpret stimuli; depresses respiratory center in medulla	Nausea, vomiting, flushing, confusion, urticaria, depressed rate and depth of respirations, and decreased blood pressure
NURSING IMPLICATIONS: Check rate and depth of *respirations* before administering drug; observe for gas pains and *abdominal distention;* smaller doses for aged; monitor vital signs; observe for postural hypotension			
	Obstetric use: preeclampsia-eclampsia; uterine dysfunction; pain relief	Increases cerebral blood flow; provides antihypertensive action; CNS depressant	Respiratory and circulatory depression in mother and neonate; may depress contractions
NURSING IMPLICATIONS: Observe for level of sedation, respirations, arousability, and deep-tendon reflex; give narcotic antagonist as necessary; check I&O (*urinary retention* possible).			
Naproxen (Naprosyn)—PO 250–500 mg bid	Mild to moderate pain; dysmenorrhea; rheumatoid arthritis; osteoarthritis (NSAID)	Inhibits prostaglandin synthesis; suppression of inflammation	Headache, drowsiness, dizziness, nausea, dyspepsia, constipation, bleeding
NURSING IMPLICATIONS: Take with a full glass of *water; avoid* exposure to sun			
Oxycodone HCl (Percodan, Tylox)—PO 3–20 mg; SC 5 mg	**Postpartum use:** control pain; may be used during puerperium; 5–6 times more potent than codeine	Less potent and addicting than morphine; for moderate pain—episiotomy and "after pains"; peak action 1 h	See Morphine SO₄
NURSING IMPLICATIONS: Administer per order and observe for effect			
Pentazocine (Talwin)—PO 50–100 mg; IM 30–60 mg q3–4h	Relief of moderate to severe pain	Narcotic agonist, opioid antagonist properties, equivalent to codeine	Respiratory depression, nausea, vomiting, dizziness, light-headedness, seizures
NURSING IMPLICATIONS: Monitor *respirations,* BP; *caution* with patients with MI, head injuries, COPD			
Antacids (see Antiulcer)			
Antianemics			
Ferrous sulfate (Feosol, Fer-in-Sol)—adults, PO 300 mg–1.2 g qd; children under 6 yr, PO 75–225 mg qd; 6–12 yr, PO 120–600 mg qd	Iron deficiency anemia; prophylactically during infancy, childhood, pregnancy	Corrects nutritional Fe deficiency anemia	Nausea, vomiting, anorexia, constipation, diarrhea, yellow-brown discoloration of eyes, teeth
NURSING IMPLICATIONS: To minimize GI distress, give *with* meals; do *not* give with antacids or tea; liquid form should be taken through straw to prevent *staining* of teeth; causes dark-green/black stool			

continued

■ TABLE 4.4 *(Continued)*

Drug and Dosage	Use	Action	Assessment: Side Effects
Antianginals			
Atenolol (Tenormin)—PO 50–150 mg daily; IV 5 mg initially, wait 10 min, then another 5 mg	Hypertension; angina; arrhythmias	Blocks beta$_1$ (cardiac) adrenergic receptors	Fatigue, weakness, bradycardia, congestive heart failure, pulmonary edema
NURSING IMPLICATIONS: Give 1 mg/min IV; check vital signs; assess for signs of fluid *overload*			
Isosorbide dinitrate (Isordil, Isorbid)—sublingual 2.5–10.0 mg q5–10min for 3 doses; PO 5–20 mg initially, 10–40 mg q6h	Acute angina; long-term prophylaxis for angina; heart failure	Produces vasodilation, decreases preload	Headache, dizziness, hypotension, tachycardia
NURSING IMPLICATIONS: *Avoid* eating, drinking, or smoking until sublingual tablets are dissolved; change positions *slowly;* aspirin or acetaminophen for headache			
Nitroglycerin—sublingual 0.15–0.3 mg prn; transdermal (patch) 2.5–15.0 mg/d; topical 2–3 in. q8h; IV 10–20 µg/min	Angina pectoris; adjunctive treatment in MI, heart failure, hypertension (IV form)	Directly relaxes smooth muscle, dilating blood vessels; lowers peripheral vascular resistance; increases blood flow	Faintness, throbbing headache, vomiting, flushing, hypotension, visual disturbances
NURSING IMPLICATIONS: Instruct patient to sit or lie down when taking drug, to reduce *hypotensive* effect; onset 1–3 min; may take 1–3 doses at 5-min intervals to relieve pain; up to *10/d* may be allowed; if headache occurs, tell patient to expel tab as soon as pain relief occurs; keep drug at bedside or on person; watch *expiration* dates—tabs lose potency with exposure to air and humidity; *alcohol* ingestion soon after taking may produce shocklike syndrome from drop in BP; *smoking* causes vasoconstricting effect; causes burning under tongue; may crush between teeth to ↑ absorption.			
Antiarrhythmics			
Bretylium (Bretylol)—IV 0.5–10 mg/kg q6h; IM 5–10 mg/kg (max 250 mg in one site)	Ventricular fibrillation; ventricular tachycardia	Inhibits norepinephrine release from sympathetic nerve endings; increased fibrillation threshold	Worsening of arrhythmia; tachycardia, and increased BP initially; nausea, vomiting; hypotension later
NURSING IMPLICATIONS: Monitor BP and cardiac status closely; *rotate* IM injection sites; no more than 5 mL/site			
Diphenylhydantoin (Dilantin)—PO 100–200 mg 3–4 times daily; IV loading dose 10–15 mg/kg (not to exceed 50 mg/min), 50–100 mg over 5–10 min	Digitalis toxicity; ventricular ectopy	Depresses pacemaker activity in SA node and Purkinje tissue without slowing conduction velocity	Severe pain if administered in small vein; ataxia, vertigo, nystagmus, seizures, confusion, skin eruptions, hypotension if administered too fast
NURSING IMPLICATIONS: With IV use monitor vital signs; observe for CNS side effects; have O$_2$ on hand; seizure precautions (padded siderails, nonmetal airway, suction, mouth gag); also see Anticonvulsants			
Lidocaine HCl—IV 50–100 mg; bolus; 1–4 mg/min IV drip	Ventricular tachycardia; PVCs	Depresses myocardial response to abnormally generated impulses	Drowsiness, dizziness, nervousness, confusion, and paresthesias
NURSING IMPLICATIONS: Monitor vital signs; observe for signs of CNS toxicity; monitor ECG for *prolonged PR* interval			
Procainamide HCl (Pronestyl)—PO, IM 500–1000 mg 4–6 times qd; IV 1 g	Atrial and ventricular arrhythmias; PVCs; overdose of digitalis; general anesthesia	Depresses myocardium, and lengthens conduction time between atria and ventricles	Polyarthralgia, fever, chills, urticaria, nausea, vomiting, psychoses, and rapid decrease in BP
NURSING IMPLICATIONS: Check pulse rate *before* giving; monitor heart action during IV administration			
Propranolol HCl (Inderal)—0.5–1.0 mg IV push (up to 3 mg); 20–60 mg orally 3–4 times daily	Ventricular ectopy; angina unresponsive to nitrites, paroxysmal atrial tachycardia; hypertension	Beta adrenergic blocker, ↓ cardiac contractility, ↓ heart rate, ↓ myocardial oxygen requirements	Bradycardia, hypotension, vertigo, paresthesia of hands
NURSING IMPLICATIONS: Instruct patient to take pulse *before* each dose; do *not* give to patients with history of asthma or obstructive pulmonary disease; no smoking, as hypertension may occur			

continued

■ **TABLE 4.4** *(Continued)*

Drug and Dosage	Use	Action	Assessment: Side Effects
Antiarrhythmics *(continued)*			
Quinidine SO_4—PO 0.2–0.6 g q2h loading dose; maintenance: 400–1000 mg tid, qid; IV 5–10 mg/kg over 30–60 min	Atrial fibrillation; PAT; ventricular tachycardia; PVCs	Lengthens conduction time in atria and ventricles; blocks vagal stimulation of heart	Nausea, vomiting, diarrhea, vertigo, tremor, headache, abdominal cramps, AV block, and cardiac arrest
NURSING IMPLICATIONS: *Count pulse before* giving; report changes in rate, quality, or rhythm; give drug *with food;* monitor BP daily; supine during IV administration			
Antiasthmatics			
Cromolyn sodium—inhale, 1 cap 4 times qd	Perennial bronchial asthma (not acute asthma or status asthmaticus)	Inhibits release of bronchoconstrictors—histamine and SRS-A; suppresses allergic response	Cough, hoarseness, wheezing, dry mouth, bitter aftertaste, urticaria, urinary frequency
NURSING IMPLICATIONS: Instruct on use of inhaler—exhale; tilt head back; inhale rapidly, deeply, steadily; remove inhaler; exhale—repeat until dose is taken; gargle or drink water after treatment			
Anticholinergics (antimus-carinics)			
Atropine SO_4—0.3–1.2 mg PO, SC, IM, or IV; ophthalmic 0.5–1.0% up to 6 times qd	Peptic ulcer; spasms of GI tract; Stokes-Adams syndrome; control excessive secretions during surgery	Blocks parasympathomimetic effects of acetylcholine on effector organs	Dry mouth, dysphasia, skin rash, face and upper trunk, skin flushing, urinary retention; *contraindications:* glaucoma and paralytic ileus
NURSING IMPLICATIONS: Observe for postural *hypotension* in ambulating patients; administer cautiously in aged; and monitor vital signs for pulse and respiratory rate changes			
Propantheline bromide (Pro-Banthine)—PO 15 mg qid; IM or IV 30 mg	Decreases hypertonicity and hypersecretion of GI tract; ulcerative colitis; peptic ulcer	Blocks neural transmission at ganglia of autonomic nervous system and at parasympathetic effector organs	Nausea, gastric fullness, constipation, and mydriasis
NURSING IMPLICATIONS: Give *before* meals; observe urinary output to *avoid retention,* particularly in elderly; mouth care pc will relieve dryness; contraindicated with glaucoma			
Tincture of belladonna—0.3–0.6 mL tid	Hypermotility of stomach; bowel, biliary, and renal colic; prostatitis	Blocks parasympathomimetic effects of acetylcholine	Dry mouth, thirst, dilated pupils, skin flushing, elevated temperature, and delirium
NURSING IMPLICATIONS: Administer 30–60 min *before* meals; observe for side effects; *physostigmine salicylate* is antidote			
Anticoagulants			
Heparin—initial dose: SC 10,000–20,000 U; IV 20,000–40,000 U	Acute thromboembolic emergencies	Prevents thrombin formation	Hematuria, bleeding gums, and ecchymosis
NURSING IMPLICATIONS: Observe clotting times—should be 20–30 min; antagonist is *protamine sulfate*			
Warfarin sodium (Coumadin)—initial dose: PO 10–15 mg; maintenance dose—PO 2–10 mg qd	Venous thrombosis; atrial fibrillation with embolization; pulmonary emboli; myocardial infarction	Depresses liver synthesis of prothrombin and factors VII, IX, and X	Minor or major hemorrhage, alopecia, fever, nausea, diarrhea, and dermatitis
NURSING IMPLICATIONS: Drug effects last 3–4 d; antagonist is vitamin K; *avoid* foods high in vitamin K; *no* aspirin			
Anticoagulant Antidotes			
Protamine sulfate 1%—IV 10 mg/mL slowly; 1 mg/100 U heparin	Overdose of heparin	Positive electrostatic charge inactivates negatively charged heparin molecules	Excessive coagulation; hypotension; bradycardia; dyspnea
NURSING IMPLICATIONS: Slow IV; no more than 50 mg in 10-min period; monitor VS continuously; Check APTT for effectiveness			
Vitamin K_1 (Aquamephyton, Konakion)—PO, IM, SC 2.5–25.0 mg; 0.5–1.0 mg in newborns	Warfarin (Coumadin) hypoprothrombinemia; hemorrhagic disease in newborns	Counteracts the inhibitory effects of oral anticoagulants on hepatic synthesis of vitamin K–dependent clotting factors	Flushing; hypotension; allergic reactions; reappearance of clotting problems (high doses)
NURSING IMPLICATIONS: Give IV only if absolutely necessary; dilute with preservative-free 0.9% NaCl, D5W, or D_5NaCl; protect solution *from light;* repeated injection may cause redness and pain; check PT for drug effect			

continued

■ **TABLE 4.4** *(Continued)*

Drug and Dosage	Use	Action	Assessment: Side Effects
Anticonvulsants			
Clonazepam (Klonopin)—PO 1.5 mg in 3 doses initially, 0.5–1.0 mg q third d	Absence (petit mal) seizures, myoclonic seizures	Produces anticonvulsant and sedative effects in the CNS, mechanism unknown	Drowsiness, ataxia, behavioral changes
NURSING IMPLICATIONS: Give *with* food; evaluate *liver, CBC,* and *platelets; avoid* abrupt withdrawal—may cause status epilepticus			
Diazepam (Valium)—PO 2–10 mg bid–qid; IM or IV 5–10 mg	All types of seizures	Induces calming effect on limbic system, thalamus, and hypothalamus	Drowsiness, ataxia, and paradoxical increase in excitability of CNS
NURSING IMPLICATIONS: IV may cause phlebitis; give IV injection slowly, as respiratory arrest can occur; inject IM deeply into tissue			
Ethosuximide (Zarontin)—PO 500 mg/d, increase by 250 mg/d until effective	Absence seizures	Depresses motor cortex and reduces CNS sensitivity to convulsive nerve stimuli	GI distress: nausea, vomiting, cramps; diarrhea; anorexia; blood dyscrasias
NURSING IMPLICATIONS: Administer *with* meals; regular *CBC;* precautions to avoid injury from drowsiness			
Magnesium sulfate—PO 1–5 g/IM or IV 1–4 g at rate of 1.5 mL/min	Control seizures in pregnancy, epilepsy; relief of acute constipation; reduces edema, inflammation, and itching of skin; may inhibit preterm contractions	Depresses CNS as well as smooth, cardiac, and skeletal muscle; promotes osmotic retention of fluid	Flushing, sweating, extreme thirst, complete heart block, dehydration, depressed or absent reflexes, ↓ respirations
NURSING IMPLICATIONS: If given IV, monitor vital signs continuously; I&O; do *not* give during the 2 h preceding birth; observe mother and newborn for signs of toxicity if given near birth. Antidote: Calcium gluconate.			
Phenytoin or diphenylhydantoin (Dilantin) SO₄—PO 30–100 mg 3–4 times qd; IM 100–200 mg 3–4 times qd; IV 150–250 mg	Psychomotor epilepsy; convulsive seizures; ventricular arrhythmias	Depresses motor cortex by preventing spread of abnormal electrical impulses	Nervousness, ataxia, gastric distress, nystagmus, slurred speech, hallucinations, and gingival hyperplasia
NURSING IMPLICATIONS: Give *with* meals *or* pc; frequent and diligent mouth care; advise patient that urine may turn *pink to red-brown;* teach patient signs of adverse reactions; mix IV with normal saline (precipitates with D5W)			
Primidone (Mysoline)—PO 100–250 mg, increase over 10 d	Tonic-clonic, focal, or local seizures	Inhibits abnormal brain electrical activity; dose-dependent CNS depression	Excessive sedation or ataxia; vertigo
NURSING IMPLICATIONS: Careful neurologic, cardiovascular, and respiratory assessment; have resuscitation equipment available			
Valporic acid (Depakene)—PO 15 mg/kg/d, increase up to 60 mg/kg/d	Absence, tonic-clonic, myoclonic, focal, or local seizures	Inhibits spread of abnormal discharges through brain	Nausea, vomiting, diarrhea (disappear over time); drowsiness or sedation if taken in combination with other anticonvulsants
NURSING IMPLICATIONS: Assess responses; monitor blood levels; precautions against excessive sedation; *discourage alcohol* use			
Antidiarrheals			
Diphenoxylate HCl with atropine sulfate (Lomotil)—PO 5–10 mg tid–qid	Diarrhea	Increases intestinal tone and decreases propulsive peristalsis	Rash, drowsiness, dizziness, depression, abdominal distention, headache, blurred vision, and nausea
NURSING IMPLICATIONS: May *potentiate* action of barbiturates, opiates, and other depressants; closely observe patients receiving these drugs, and administer narcotic antagonists such as levallorphan (Lorfan) tartrate, naloxone HCl (Narcan), and nalorphine HCl (Nalline) as ordered; administer cautiously to patients with hepatic dysfunction—may precipitate *hepatic coma*			
Kaolin with pectin (Kaopectate)—adults, PO 60–120 mL after each bowel movement (BM); children over 12, PO 60 mL; 6–12 yr, PO 30–60 mL; 3–6 yr, PO 15–30 mL after each BM	Diarrhea	Reported to absorb irritants and soothe	Granuloma of the stomach
NURSING IMPLICATIONS: Do *not* administer for more than 2 d, in presence of fever, or to children younger than 3 yr			

continued

Pharmacology

■ **TABLE 4.4** *(Continued)*

Drug and Dosage	Use	Action	Assessment: Side Effects
Antidiarrheals *(continued)*			
Paregoric or camphorated opium tincture—5–10 mL q2h, not more than qid	Diarrhea	Acts directly on intestinal smooth muscle to increase tone and decrease propulsive peristalsis	Occasional nausea; prolonged use may produce dependence

NURSING IMPLICATIONS: Contains approximately 1.6 mg morphine or 16 mg opium and is subject to federal narcotic regulations; administer with partial glass of water to facilitate passage into stomach; observe number and consistency of stools—discontinue drug as soon as diarrhea is controlled; keep in tight *light-resistant* bottles

Drug and Dosage	Use	Action	Assessment: Side Effects
Antiemetics			
Chlorpromazine (Thorazine)—preop IM 12.5–25.0 g 1–2 h before; N/V PO 10–25 mg q4–6h; IM 25–50 mg q3–4h; suppository 50–100 mg q6–8h	Nausea, vomiting, hiccups, preoperative sedation, psychoses	Alters the effects of dopamine in the CNS; anticholinergic, alpha adrenergic blocking	Sedation, extrapyramidal reactions, dry eyes, blurred vision, hypotension, constipation, dry mouth, photosensitivity

NURSING IMPLICATIONS: Keep *flat* 30 min after IM; change positions slowly; frequent mouth care; may turn urine *pink* to *red-brown*

Drug and Dosage	Use	Action	Assessment: Side Effects
Prochlorperazine dimaleate (Compazine)—5–30 mg qid PO, IM, rectal	Nausea, vomiting, and retching	See Trimethobenzamide HCl	Drowsiness, orthostatic hypotension, palpitations, blurred vision, diplopia, and headache

NURSING IMPLICATIONS: Use *cautiously* in children, pregnant women, and patients with liver disease

Drug and Dosage	Use	Action	Assessment: Side Effects
Trimethobenzamide HCl (Tigan)—250 mg qid, PO, IM, rectal	Nausea; vomiting	Suppresses chemoreceptors in the trigger zone located in the medulla oblongata	Drowsiness, vertigo, diarrhea, headache, hypotension, jaundice, blurred vision, and rigid muscles

NURSING IMPLICATIONS: Give deep IM to prevent escape of solution; can cause edema, pain, and burning

Drug and Dosage	Use	Action	Assessment: Side Effects
Antifungal			
Amphotericin B (Fungizone)—IV 5 mg/250 mL dextrose over 4–6h (to 1 mg/kg body weight)	Severe fungal infections; histoplasmosis	Fungistatic or fungicidal; binds to sterols in cell membrane, altering cell permeability	Febrile reactions; chills, N/V, muscle/joint pain; renal damage; hypotension, tachycardia arrhythmias; hypokalemia

NURSING IMPLICATIONS: Monitor for side effects; thrombophlebitis at IV site; BUN >40; creatinine 3 or >; stop drug because of *nephrotoxicity*

Drug and Dosage	Use	Action	Assessment: Side Effects
Ketoconazole (Nizoral)—oral 200–400 mg daily	Histoplasmosis, systemic fungal infections	Antifungal	Headache, fatigue, dizziness; N/V; decreased libido, impotence; gynecomastia, esp. in males

NURSING IMPLICATIONS: Administer *with* food; *avoid* concomitant use of antacids, H₂ blockers; advise to report side-effect symptoms

Drug and Dosage	Use	Action	Assessment: Side Effects
Nystatin (Nilstat)—PO, rectal, vaginal 100,000–1,000,000 U 3–4 times qd	Skin, mucous membrane infections (*Candida albicans*); oral thrush, vaginitis; intestinal candidiasis	Fungistatic and fungicidal; binds to sterols in fungal cell membrane	Nausea, vomiting, GI distress, diarrhea

NURSING IMPLICATIONS: *Oral* use—clear mouth of food; keep medication in mouth several minutes before swallowing; *vaginal*—usually requires 2-wk therapy; continue use during menses; consult physician before using anti-infective douches; determine predisposing factors to infection (diabetes, pregnancy, antibiotics, tight-fitting nylon pantyhose)

Drug and Dosage	Use	Action	Assessment: Side Effects
Antigout			
Allopurinol (Lopurin, Zyloprim)—PO 100 mg initially, 300 mg daily with meals or pc	Primary hyperuricemia, secondary hyperuricemia with cancer therapy	Lowers plasma and urinary uric acid levels; no analgesic, anti-inflammatory, or uricosuric actions	Rash, itching, nausea, vomiting, anemia, drowsiness

NURSING IMPLICATIONS: Report side effects, particularly *rash,* as drug must be stopped; avoid driving or other complex tasks until drug effects known; give at least *3000 mL* fluid daily; minimum urine output of *2000 mL/d;* keep urine neutral or *alkaline* with sodium bicarbonate or potassium citrate; use *cautiously* with liver disease, impaired renal function, history of peptic ulcers, lower GI disease, or bone marrow depression

continued

■ **TABLE 4.4** *(Continued)*

Drug and Dosage	Use	Action	Assessment: Side Effects
Antigout *(continued)*			
Colchicine—PO 1.0–1.2 mg acute phase; 0.5–2.0 mg nightly with milk or food; IV 1–2 mg initially	Gouty arthritis, acute gout	Inhibits leukocyte migration and phagocytosis in gouty joints; nonanalgesic, nonuricosuric	Nausea, vomiting, diarrhea, abdominal pain, peripheral neuritis, bone marrow depression (sore throat, bleeding gums, sore mouth), tissue and nerve necrosis with IV use

NURSING IMPLICATIONS: Do *not* dilute IV form with normal saline or 5% dextrose—use sterile water to prevent precipitation; infuse over 3–5 min IV; potentiate drug action with *alkaline ash foods* (milk, most fruits and vegetables)

Probenecid (Benemid)—PO 0.25–0.50 g twice daily pc	Chronic gouty arthritis, no value in acute; adjuvant therapy with penicillin to increase plasma levels	Inhibits renal tubular reabsorption of uric acid; no analgesic or anti-inflammatory activity; competitively inhibits renal tubular secretion of penicillin and many weak organic acids	Headache, nausea, vomiting, anorexia, sore gums, urinary frequency, flushing

NURSING IMPLICATIONS: Give *with* food, milk, or prescribed antacid; 3000 mL/d fluids; *avoid* alcohol, which increases serum urates; do *not* take with aspirin—inhibits action of drug; renal function and hematology should be evaluated frequently; during acute gout, give with colchicine (Colbenemid)

Antihistamines			
Astemizole (Hismanyl)—PO 10 mg/d	Relief of allergic symptoms (rhinitis, urticaria); less sedating	Blocks the effects of histamine	Drowsiness, headache, fatigue, stimulation, dry mouth, rash, increased appetite (none of these are frequent)

NURSING IMPLICATIONS: Take *1 h before* or *2 h after* eating; good oral hygiene; may need to reduce calories

Chlorpheniramine maleate (Chlor-Trimeton)—PO 2–4 mg tid–qid; SC, IM, or IV 10–20 mg	Asthma; hay fever; serum reactions; anaphylaxis	Inhibits action of histamine	Nausea, gastritis, diarrhea, headache, dryness of mouth and nose, nervousness and irritability

NURSING IMPLICATIONS: IV may drop BP; give slowly; caution patient about drowsiness

Diphenhydramine HCl (Benadryl)—PO 25–50 mg tid–qid; IM or IV 10–20 mg	Allergic and pyrogenic reactions; motion sickness; radiation sickness; hay fever; Parkinson's disease	Inhibits action of histamine on receptor cells, and decreases action of acetylcholine	Sedation, dizziness, inability to concentrate, headache, anorexia, dermatitis, nausea, diplopia, and insomnia

NURSING IMPLICATIONS: *Avoid* use in newborn or preterm infants and patients with glaucoma; supervise ambulation; caution against driving or operating mechanical devices; excitation or hallucinations may occur in children

Terfenadine (Seldane)—PO 60 mg 2 times daily	Relief of allergic symptoms, nasal and dermatoses	Blocks the effects of histamine	Drowsiness, sedation, headache, nausea, abdominal pain, dry mouth

NURSING IMPLICATIONS: Risk of *arrhythmias* if taking certain antibiotics; false-negative skin test reactions; take *with* food or milk

Antihyperglycemics			
Sulfonylureas Acetohexamide (Dymelor)— 200–1500 mg qd; 1–2/d; duration 12–24 h	Oral hypoglycemic; antidiabetic	Lowers blood glucose by stimulating insulin release from beta cells; effective only if pancreas has ability to produce insulin	Hypoglycemia (profuse sweating, hunger, headache, nausea, confusion, ataxia, coma), skin rashes, bone marrow depression, liver toxicity

NURSING IMPLICATIONS: Drug therapy must be combined with diet therapy, weight control, and planned, graded exercise; alcohol intolerance may occur (disulfiram reaction—flushing, pounding headache, sweating, nausea, vomiting); should *not* be taken at bedtime unless specifically ordered (nocturnal hypoglycemia more likely); take at *same time* each day; *contraindicated* in liver disease, renal disease, pregnancy

Chlorpropamide (Diabinese)— 100–500 mg; 1/d; duration 30–60 h	See Acetohexamide	See Acetohexamide	See Acetohexamide

NURSING IMPLICATIONS: See Acetohexamide

continued

■ **TABLE 4.4**   *(Continued)*

Drug and Dosage	Use	Action	Assessment: Side Effects
Antihyperglycemics *(continued)*			
Glyburide (Micronase)— 2.5–5 mg initially; 1.25–20 mg/d.	See Acetohexamide	See Acetohexamide	See Acetohexamide
NURSING IMPLICATIONS: See Acetohexamide			
Tolazamide (Tolinase)—100– 500 mg; 1/d; duration 10– 14 h	See Acetohexamide	See Acetohexamide	See Acetohexamide
NURSING IMPLICATIONS: See Acetohexamide			
Tolbutamide (Orinase)—500– 2000 mg; 2–3/d; duration 6– 12 h	See Acetohexamide	See Acetohexamide	See Acetohexamide
NURSING IMPLICATIONS: See Acetohexamide			
Insulin—rapid acting Crystal-line zinc (Regular) (Humulin R) (clear)—onset 0.5–1.0 h; peak 2–4 h; duration 6–8 h	Poorly controlled diabetes; trauma; surgery, coma	Enhances transmembrane passage of glucose into cells; promotes CHO, fat, and protein metabolism	Hypoglycemia (profuse sweating, nausea, hunger, headache, confusion, ataxia, coma), allergic reaction at injection site
NURSING IMPLICATIONS: Monitor blood and urine for glucose and acetone levels; insulin currently being used can be kept at *room temperature for 1 mo;* refrigerate stock insulin only; rotate injection sites; cold insulin leads to lipodystrophy, reduced absorption, and local reaction; only form of insulin that is given IV			
Prompt insulin zinc suspension (Semilente) purified pork (cloudy)—onset 1–2 h; peak 4–10 h; duration 12–16 h	Patients allergic to Regular; used in combination with longer-lasting insulin	See Crystalline zinc (Regular)	See Crystalline zinc (Regular)
NURSING IMPLICATIONS: See Crystalline zinc (Regular); compatible with all Lente preparations			
Insulin—intermediate acting NPH insulin (isophane insulin suspension) purified pork (Humulin N+) (cloudy)—onset 1–2 h; peak 5–12 h; duration 18–24 h	Patients who can be controlled by one dose per day	See Crystalline zinc (Regular)	See Crystalline zinc (Regular)
NURSING IMPLICATIONS: Gently rotate vial between palms, invert several times to mix; do *not* shake; see Crystalline zinc (Regular)			
Insulin zinc suspension (Lente insulin) (cloudy)—onset 1–3 h; peak 6–12 h; duration 18–24 h	Patients allergic to NPH	See Crystalline zinc (Regular)	See Crystalline zinc (Regular)
NURSING IMPLICATIONS: See Crystalline zinc (Regular)			
Insulin—slow acting Extended insulin zinc suspension (Ultralente, Humulin U) purified beef (cloudy)—onset 4–8 h; peak 12–24 h; duration 36 h	Often mixed with Semilente for 24-h curve	See Crystalline zinc (Regular)	See Crystalline zinc (Regular)
NURSING IMPLICATIONS: See Crystalline zinc (Regular)			
Antihypertensives			
Captopril (Capoten)—PO 50 mg tid	Hypertension, heart failure	Prevents production of angiotensin II; vasodilation	Hypotension, loss of taste perception, proteinuria, rashes
NURSING IMPLICATIONS: Monitor VS and weight; take 1 h *before* and 2 h *after* meals; change positions slowly; *avoid* salt and salt substitutes			
Guanfacine hydrochloride (Tenex)—PO 1 mg daily to maximum dose of 3 mg/d	Hypertension, in combination with thiazidelike diuretics	Centrally-acting alpha$_2$ adrenergic receptor agonist	Drowsiness; weakness; dizziness; dry mouth; constipation; impotence
NURSING IMPLICATIONS: Warn patient *not* to drive or perform activities requiring alertness; take at *bedtime* to minimize sedation; monitor BP and pulse			

continued

Pharmacology

■ **TABLE 4.4** *(Continued)*

Drug and Dosage	Use	Action	Assessment: Side Effects
Antihypertensives *(continued)*			
Guanethidine SO₄ (Ismelin)—PO 10–50 mg qd in divided doses	Severe to moderately severe hypertension	Blocks norepinephrine at post-ganglionic synapses	Orthostatic hypotension, diarrhea, and inhibition of ejaculation
NURSING IMPLICATIONS: *Postural hypotension* is marked in the morning and *accentuated* by hot weather, alcohol, and exercise; teach to rise slowly, with assistance			
Hydralazine HCl (Apresoline)—PO 10–50 mg qid	Moderate hypertension	Dilates peripheral blood vessels, increases renal blood flow	Palpitations, tachycardia, angina pectoris, tremors, and depression
NURSING IMPLICATIONS: Encourage moderation in exercise and identification of stressful stimuli			
	Obstetric use: preeclampsia-eclampsia	Relaxes peripheral blood vessels (opens vascular bed—physiologic dehydration)	Headache, heart palpitation, gastric irritation, coronary insufficiency, edema, chills, fever, and severe depression
NURSING IMPLICATIONS: Siderails up; must *not* stand without assistance; may be given with diuretics; observe carefully; IM route only; monitor BP			
Methyldopa (Aldomet)—PO 500 mg–2 g in divided doses	Severe to moderately severe hypertension	Inhibits formation of dopamine, a precursor of norepinephrine	Initial drowsiness, depression with feelings of unreality, edema, jaundice, and dry mouth
NURSING IMPLICATIONS: *Contraindicated* in acute and chronic liver disease; encourage not to drive car if drowsy			
Phentolamine hydrochloride (Regitine)—PO 50 mg 4–6 doses daily; IV, IM, or local 5–10 mg, diluted in minimum 10 mL normal saline	Prevents dermal necrosis; hypertensive crisis; diagnosis pheochromocytoma	Blocks alpha adrenergic receptors	Weakness, dizziness, orthostatic hypotension, nausea, vomiting, abdominal pain
NURSING IMPLICATIONS: When giving parenterally, patient should be *supine;* monitor for overdosage (precipitous drop in BP); do *not* give with epinephrine			
Reserpine (Serpasil)—PO 0.25 mg qd	Mild and moderate hypertension	Depletes catecholamines and decreases peripheral vasoconstriction, heart rate, and BP	Depression, nasal stuffiness, increased gastric secretions, rash, and pruritus
NURSING IMPLICATIONS: Watch for signs of *mental depression;* closely monitor pulse rates of patients also receiving digitalis; *avoid* alcohol			
	Obstetric use: preeclampsia-eclampsia	CNS depressant, tranquilizer; sedation is major effect; decreases neural transmission to nerves; decreases tone in in blood vessels	Low level of toxicity; nasal stuffiness; weight gain; diarrhea; allergic reactions—dry mouth, itching, skin eruptions
NURSING IMPLICATIONS: Siderails up; must not stand up without assistance; observe carefully; monitor *BP*			
Timolol (Timoptic)—PO 20–40 mg/d; ophthalmic 1 gtt 1–2 times/d	Hypertension, migraine, glaucoma	Blocks stimulation of myocardial (beta₁) and pulmonary/vascular (beta₂) receptors	Fatigue, weakness, depression, insomnia, peripheral vasoconstriction, diarrhea, nausea, vomiting
NURSING IMPLICATIONS: Check VS and evidence of congestive heart failure; do not take if pulse <50; *avoid* OTC cold remedies, coffee, tea, and cola			
Anti-infectives			
Cefazolin (Ancef, Kefzol)—IM or IV 250 mg–1.5 g q6–12h	*Staphylococcus aureus; Escherichia coli; Klebsiella;* group A and B *Streptococcus; Pneumococcus*	Bactericidal	Allergic reaction: urticaria, rash; abnormal bleeding
NURSING IMPLICATIONS: See Penicillin; may cause *false-positive* lab tests (Coombs, urine glucose); oral probenecid may be taken concurrently to prolong effects of drug			

continued

■ **TABLE 4.4** *(Continued)*

Drug and Dosage	Use	Action	Assessment: Side Effects
Anti-infectives *(continued)*			
Cephalexin (Keflex)—PO 1–4 g daily in 2–4 equally divided doses	Infections caused by gram-positive cocci; infections; respiratory, biliary, urinary, bone, septicemia, abdominal; surgical prophylaxis	Bactericidal effects on susceptible organisms; inhibition of bacterial cell wall synthesis	Nausea, vomiting; urticaria; toxic paranoid reactions; dizziness; increased alkaline phosphatase; nephrotoxicity; bone marrow suppression
NURSING IMPLICATIONS: Peak blood levels delayed when given with food; *report* nausea, flushing, tachycardia, headache; monitor for *nephrotoxicity* and for bleeding			
Cephalothin (Keflin, Seffin)—IM, IV 2–12 g/d in 4–6 equally divided doses	Same as Cephalexin except not recommended for biliary tract infections	Same as Cephalexin	Same as Cephalexin
NURSING IMPLICATIONS: Same as Cephalexin; pain at site of IM; given in large muscle; rotate sites			
Ciprofloxacin (Cipro)—PO 250–750 mg q12h; IV 200–400 mg q12h; ophthalmic 1–2 gtt q15–30min, then 4–6 times daily	Lower respiratory tract infections; skin, bone, and joint infections; UTI	Inhibits bacterial DNA synthesis	Restlessness, nausea, diarrhea, vomiting, abdominal pain
NURSING IMPLICATIONS: Give PO on an *empty* stomach unless GI irritation occurs, then take with food; *do not* take with milk or yogurt; IV over 60 min			
Cloxacillin (Tegopen)—PO 250–500 mg q6h	Penicillinase-producing staphylococci infections: respiratory, sinus, and skin	Binds to bacterial cell wall, leading to cell death	Nausea, vomiting, diarrhea, rashes, allergic reactions, seizures (high doses)
NURSING IMPLICATIONS: *Give around the clock* on an *empty* stomach; observe for signs of *superinfection* (black, furry tongue, vaginal itching, loose stools)			
Co-trimoxazole (Bactrim, Septra)—PO 160 mg twice daily or 20 mg/kg/d for *P. carinii* pneumonia	Acute otitis media; urinary tract infection; shigellosis; *P. carinii* pneumonia; prostatitis	Bacteriostatic; anti-infective; antagonizes folic acid production; combination of sulfamethoxazole and trimethoprim	Hypersensitivity; see Sulfisoxazole
NURSING IMPLICATIONS: IV administration can cause phlebitis and *tissue damage* with extravasation			
Erythromycin—adults, PO 250 mg q6h; children, PO 30–50 mg/kg qd	Pneumonia; pelvic inflammatory disease; intestinal amebiasis; ocular infections; used if allergic to penicillin	Inhibits protein synthesis of microorganism; more effective against gram positive	Abdominal cramping, distention, diarrhea
NURSING IMPLICATIONS: Be sure culture and sensitivity done *before* treatment; give on *empty* stomach 1 h before or 3 h after meals; do *not* crush or chew tabs; do *not* give with fruit juice			
Gentamicin (Garamycin, Jenamicin)—IM, IV 3–5 mg/kg/d in 3–4 divided doses; topical; skin, eye	Serious gram-negative bacillary infections; possible *S. aureus,* uncomplicated urinary infections	Bactericidal effects on susceptible gram-positive and gram-negative organisms and mycobacteria	Serious toxic effects: kidneys, ear; causes muscle weakness/paralysis
NURSING IMPLICATIONS: Monitor *plasma* levels (peak is 4–10 µg/mL); patients with burns, cystic fibrosis may need higher doses			
Penicillin—penicillin G, penicillin G potassium, penicillin G procaine, ampicillin	*Streptococcus; Staphylococcus; Pneumococcus; Gonococcus; Treponema pallidum*	Primarily bactericidal	Dermatitis and delayed or immediate anaphylaxis
NURSING IMPLICATIONS: Outpatients should be observed for *20 min postinjection;* hospitalized patients should be observed at frequent intervals for 20 min postinjection			
Pentamidine (Pentam)—IV 4 mg/kg once daily; inhale 300 mg via nebulizer	Prevention or treatment of *P. carinii* pneumonia	Appears to disrupt DNA or RNA synthesis to protozoa	Anxiety, headache, bronchospasm, cough, hypotension, arrhythmias, nephrotoxicity, hypoglycemia, leukopenia, thrombocytopenia, anemia, chills
NURSING IMPLICATIONS: Assess for infection and respiratory status; unpleasant metallic taste may occur, not significant			

continued

■ **TABLE 4.4** *(Continued)*

Drug and Dosage	Use	Action	Assessment: Side Effects
Anti-infectives *(continued)* Sulfisoxazole (Gantrisin), sulfa-methizole (Thiosulfil), and sulfisomidine (Elkosin)	Acute, chronic, and recurrent urinary tract infections	Bacteriostatic and bactericidal	Nausea, vomiting, oliguria, anuria, anemia, leukopenia, dizziness, jaundice, skin rashes, and photosensitivity

NURSING IMPLICATIONS: Maintenance of blood levels very important; encourage *fluids* to prevent crystal formation in kidney tubules—push up to 3000 mL/d

Drug and Dosage	Use	Action	Assessment: Side Effects
Tetracyclines—chlortetracy-cline (Aureomycin), doxycy-cline (Vibramycin hyclate), oxytetracycline (Terramycin), and tetracycline HCl (Sumycin)	Wide-spectrum antibiotic	Primarily bacteriostatic	GI upsets such as diarrhea, nausea, and vomiting; sore throat; black, hairy tongue; glossitis; and inflammatory lesions in anogenital region

NURSING IMPLICATIONS: *Phototoxic* reactions have been reported; patients should be advised to stay out of direct sunlight, and medication should *not* be given with milk or snacks, as food interferes with absorption of tetracyclines; do *not* give to pregnant women and children under 8 yr

Drug and Dosage	Use	Action	Assessment: Side Effects
Trimethoprim (TMP)/sulfa-methoxazole (SMZ) (Bac-trim)—PO 160 mg TMP or 800 mg SMZ q12h for 14–21 d; IV 8–10 mg/kg TMP/40–50 mg/kg SMZ q6–12h	Bronchitis, *Shigella* enteritis, otitis media, *P. carinii* pneumonia, UTI, traveler's diarrhea	Combination inhibits the metabolism of folic acid in bacteria; bactericidal	Nausea, vomiting, rashes, phlebitis at IV site, aplastic anemia, hepatic necrosis

NURSING IMPLICATIONS: Check IV site frequently; do *not* give IM; give PO on *empty* stomach; take *around the clock; avoid* exposure to sun

Drug and Dosage	Use	Action	Assessment: Side Effects
Antilactogenics Deladumone (estradiol valer-ate)—IM 200 mg once	**Postpartum use:** suppresses lactation; prevents breast engorgement when given immediately prior to third stage labor	Depresses production of lactogenic hormone by anterior pituitary	Rare, following one dose; masculinization and electrolyte imbalance with long-term therapy

NURSING IMPLICATIONS: Observe for *hypercalcemia,* edema; *contraindicated* in pregnant women

Drug and Dosage	Use	Action	Assessment: Side Effects
Testosterone cypionate—IM 100 mg	**Postpartum use:** suppresses lactation; controls breast engorgement; palliative therapy for breast cancer and menopausal symptoms	See Deladumone	See Deladumone

NURSING IMPLICATIONS: See Deladumone

Drug and Dosage	Use	Action	Assessment: Side Effects
Bromocriptine mesylate (Parlo-del)—PO 2.5 mg bid for 14 d	Prevents lactation; also used for Parkinson's	Inhibits prolactin secretion	Fatigue; ovulation returns; hypertension; postural hypotension; nausea/vomiting; dizziness

NURSING IMPLICATIONS: Contraceptive counseling; monitor VS; take *with* meals to ↓ GI upset. Caution: Withdrawn from obstetric use—no longer used as an antilactogenic.

Drug and Dosage	Use	Action	Assessment: Side Effects
Antilipemics Cholestyramine (Questran)—PO 4 g 1–6 times/d	Hypercholesterolemia; pruritus from increased bile	Binds bile acids in GI tract, increased clearance of cholesterol	Nausea, constipation, abdominal discomfort

NURSING IMPLICATIONS: Take *before* meals; *do not* take with other medications; give others 1 h before or 4–6 h after

Drug and Dosage	Use	Action	Assessment: Side Effects
Gemfibrozil (Lopid)—1200 mg/d	Hypercholesterolemia	May inhibit peripheral lipolysis and reduce triglyceride synthesis in liver	GI upset (abdominal pain, epigastric pain, diarrhea, nausea, vomiting), rash, headache, dizziness, blurred vision

NURSING IMPLICATIONS: Use *caution* when driving or doing tasks requiring alertness; take *before* meals

continued

Pharmacology

■ **TABLE 4.4**   *(Continued)*

Drug and Dosage	Use	Action	Assessment: Side Effects
Antilipemics *(continued)*			
Lovastatin (Mevacor)—PO 20–80 mg daily with evening meal	Primary hypercholesterolemia	Inhibits enzyme that catalyzes synthesis of cholesterol; decreases synthesis of LDL	Headache, constipation, diarrhea, altered taste, blurred vision, muscle cramps
NURSING IMPLICATIONS: Give *with* food; *restrict* fat, cholesterol, CHO, and alcohol in diet			
Niacin (vitamin B$_3$, nicotinic acid)—PO 1.5–6.0 g	Hypercholesterolemia	Decreases liver's production of low-density lipoproteins (LDLs) and synthesis of triglycerides	GI upset, flushing, pruritus, hyperuricemia, hyperglycemia
NURSING IMPLICATIONS: Take the drug *with* meals; prevent flushing by taking an *aspirin 30 min before;* monitor closely during first year of therapy			
Antiplatelet			
Dipyridamole (Persantine)—PO 70–100 mg 4 times/d; IV 570 µg/kg	Prevent thromboembolism; surgical graft patency; *diagnostic* agent in myocardial perfusion studies	Decreases platelet aggregation; coronary vasodilator	Headache, dizziness, hypotension, nausea; MI, arrhythmias with IV
NURSING IMPLICATIONS: Take at *evenly* spaced intervals; *avoid* use of alcohol; if no GI irritation, take 1 h before or 2 h after meals			
Antituberculous*			
First-line drugs			
Isoniazid—5–10 mg/kg up to 300 mg PO or IM	Tuberculosis	Suppresses or interferes with biosynthesis; bacteriostatic	Peripheral neuritis, hepatitis, hypersensitivity
NURSING IMPLICATIONS: Give pyridoxine (B$_6$) 10 mg as prophylaxis for neuritis; 50–100 mg as treatment			
Ethambutol—15–25 mg/kg PO			Optic neuritis (reversible with discontinuation of drug; very rare at 15 mg/kg), skin rash
NURSING IMPLICATIONS: Use with caution with renal disease or when eye testing is not feasible; used in combination *with* other drug			
Rifampin—10–20 mg/kg up to 600 mg PO			Hepatitis, febrile reaction, purpura (rare)
NURSING IMPLICATIONS: *Orange* urine color; *negates* effect of birth control pills			
Streptomycin—15–20 mg/kg up to 1 g IM			*Eighth cranial* nerve damage, *nephrotoxicity*
NURSING IMPLICATIONS: Use with caution in *older* patients or those with *renal* disease			
Pyrazinamide—15–30 mg/kg up to 3 g PO			Hyperuricemia, hepatotoxicity
NURSING IMPLICATIONS: Combination with an aminoglycoside is bactericidal			
Antiulcer			
Aluminum hydroxide gel (Amphojel)—PO 5–10 mL q2–4h or 1 h pc	Gastric acidity; peptic ulcer; phosphatic urinary calculi; ↓ phosphorus level in chronic renal failure	Buffers HCl in gastric juices without interfering with electrolyte balance	Constipation and fecal impaction
NURSING IMPLICATIONS: *Shake well* before administering; encourage *fluids* to prevent impaction and milk-alkali syndrome			
Calcium carbonate (Titralac, Ducon)—PO 1–2 g taken with H$_2$O after meals and at bedtime	Peptic ulcer and chronic gastritis	Reduces hyperacidity	Constipation or laxative effect
NURSING IMPLICATIONS: See Aluminum hydroxide gel			
Cimetidine (Tagamet)—PO 300–600 mg q6h (qid); IM, IV 300 mg q6h	Duodenal ulcers, GERD, gastric hypersecretion	Inhibits action of histamine at H$_2$ receptor site, inhibits gastric secretion	Confusion, dizziness, nausea, rash, diarrhea, constipation
NURSING IMPLICATIONS: Give *with* meals or immediately *after; avoid* smoking			

Note: To minimize resistant strains, combination therapy is used long term.

continued

■ **TABLE 4.4** *(Continued)*

Drug and Dosage	Use	Action	Assessment: Side Effects
Antiulcer *(continued)*			
Magnesium and aluminum hydroxides (Maalox suspension)—PO 5–30 mL 1–3h pc and hs	Gastric hyperacidity; peptic ulcer; heartburn; reflux esophagitis	Neutralizes gastric acids, heals ulcers	Constipation from aluminum hydroxide; diarrhea from magnesium hydroxide
NURSING IMPLICATIONS: Encourage fluid intake; *contraindicated* for debilitated patients or those with renal insufficiency			
Rantidine (Zantac)—PO 150 mg bid; IM 50 mg q6–8h; IV 50 mg q6–8h	Duodenal ulcer, gastric ulcer, GERD, gastric hypersecretion	Inhibits action of histamine at H_2 receptor site, inhibits gastric acid secretion	Headache, malaise, nausea, constipation, diarrhea
NURSING IMPLICATIONS: Food does *not* affect absorption; give 1 h *apart* from antacids; *smoking* interferes with action			
Sucralfate (Carafate)—PO 1 g qid	Prevention and treatment of duodenal ulcer	Reacts with gastric acid to form a thick paste that adheres to the ulcer surface	Constipation
NURSING IMPLICATIONS: Give 1 h *before* meals and at *bedtime; do not* crush or chew tablets; take *antacids* 30 min before or 1 h after sucralfate; increase *fluids and dietary* bulk			
Antiviral			
Acyclovir (Zovirax)—PO 200 mg, 3–5 times/d; IV 5 mg/kg q8h over 1 h; topical 6 times daily for 1 wk	Herpes simplex 1, 2; genital herpes	Converts to an active cytotoxic metabolite that inhibits viral DNA replication	Headache; nausea and vomiting; diarrhea; increased serum BUN and creatinine
NURSING IMPLICATIONS: Measure I&O q8h; ensure adequate *hydration;* assess for common side effects; apply topical with *finger cot* or rubber glove; refer for counseling			
Zidovudine (AZT, Retrovir)—PO 200 mg q4h	AIDS and related disorders	Inhibits replication of human immunodeficiency virus (HIV)	Blood disorders, especially anemia and granulocytopenia; headache; nausea; insomnia; myalgia
NURSING IMPLICATIONS: Monitor for signs of opportunistic infection and adverse drug effects; drug must be taken *around* the clock; regular blood tests (q2wk)			
Bronchodilators			
Albuterol (Ventolin)—PO 2–6 mg 3–4 times/d; inhale q4–6h or 2 puffs 15 min before exercise	Bronchodilator	Results in accumulation of cAMP at beta adrenergic receptors	Nervousness, restlessness, tremor, hypertension, nausea
NURSING IMPLICATIONS: Give *with* meals; allow 1 min *between* inhalations; rinse mouth with water *after* inhalation			
Aminophylline—PO 250 mg bid–qid; rectal 250–500 mg; IV 250–500 mg over 10–20 min	Rapid relief of bronchospasm; asthma; pulmonary edema	Relaxes smooth muscles and increases cardiac contractility; interferes with reabsorption of Na^+ and Cl^- in proximal tubules	Nausea, vomiting, cardiac arrhythmias, intestinal bleeding, insomnia, restlessness, and rectal irritation from suppository
NURSING IMPLICATIONS: Give oral *with* or *after meals;* monitor *vital signs* for changes in BP and pulse; weigh daily; IM injections are painful			
Ephedrine SO_4—PO, SC, or IM 25 mg tid–qid	Asthma; allergies; bradycardia; nasal decongestant	Relaxes hypertonic muscles in bronchioles and GI tract	Wakefulness, nervousness, dizziness, palpitations, and hypertension
NURSING IMPLICATIONS: Monitor vital signs; *avoid* giving dose near bedtime; *check urine* output in older adults			
Isoproterenol HCl (Isuprel)—inhalation of 1:100 or 1:200 solution	Mild to moderately severe asthma attack; bronchitis; pulmonary emphysema	Relaxes hypertonic bronchioles	Nervousness, tachycardia, hypertension, and insomnia
NURSING IMPLICATIONS: Monitor vital signs *before and after* treatment; teach patient how to use nebulizer			

continued

■ **TABLE 4.4** *(Continued)*

Drug and Dosage	Use	Action	Assessment: Side Effects
Bronchodilators *(continued)*			
Theophylline—PO 400 mg/d in divided doses; max adult dose: 900 mg divided dose	Treatment/prevention of emphysema, asthma (broncho-constriction); chronic bronchitis	Bronchodilation	Restlessness; increased respiration/heart rate; palpitations, arrhythmias; N/V; increased urine output → dehydration

NURSING IMPLICATIONS: Monitor theophylline levels: $\boxed{10\text{–}20 \ \mu g/mL;}$ monitor signs of toxicity; take with 8 oz water or *with* meals to decrease GI symptoms

| Terbutaline (Brethine)—PO 2.5–5.0 mg q6h (not to exceed 20 mg/24 h); SC 0.25 mg, repeat 15–30 min (not to exceed 0.5 mg/h); inhalation—2 puffs (0.2 mg each) q4–6h | Bronchospasm | See Isoproterenol | See Isoproterenol |

NURSING IMPLICATIONS: See Isoproterenol

| **Calcium Channel Blocker** | | | |
| Diltiazem (Cardizem)—PO 30–120 mg 3–4 times/d; IV 5–15 mg/h | Angina, hypertension, atrial arrhythmias | Calcium channel blocker, inhibits excitation-contraction; decreased SA, AV node conduction | Headache, fatigue, arrhythmias, edema, hypotension, constipation, rash |

NURSING IMPLICATIONS: May take *with* meals; take pulse; do *not* give drug if pulse < *50* bpm; change positions slowly; may take nitroglycerin sublingually concurrently

| Nicardipine (Cardene)—PO 20–40 mg tid | Angina, hypertension | Calcium channel blocker, inhibits excitation-contraction | Dizziness, light-headedness, headache, peripheral edema, flushing |

NURSING IMPLICATIONS: Give on an *empty* stomach; chest pain may occur 30 min after dose, temporary from *reflex tachy*

| Nifedipine (Procardia)—PO 10–30 mg tid not to exceed 180 mg/d; sublingual 10 mg repeated in 15 min | Angina, hypertension | Calcium channel blocker, vasodilation | Dizziness, light-headedness, giddiness, headache, nervousness, nasal congestion, sore throat, dyspnea, cough, wheezing, nausea, flushing, warmth |

NURSING IMPLICATIONS: May take *with* meals; make position changes slowly; angina may occur 30 min after dose, temporary

| Verapamil (Calan, Isopten)—PO 240–480 mg, 3–4 times/d; IV 75–150 μg/kg over 2 min | Angina; supraventricular arrhythmias; essential hypertension | Inhibits calcium movement into smooth-muscle cells; lowers pressure by reducing cardiac contractility | Constipation; AV block; hepatotoxicity |

NURSING IMPLICATIONS: Monitor VS and ECG for *bradycardia* and *arrhythmias;* observe for *jaundice, abdominal pain;* encourage *fluids* and *bulk-forming* foods

| **Cardiac Glycosides** | | | |
| Digitoxin—digitalizing dose: PO 200 μg twice/d; IM or IV 200–400 μg; maintenance dose: PO 50–300 μg qd | Heart failure; atrial fibrillation and flutter; supraventricular tachycardia | Increases force of cardiac contractility, slows heart rate, decreases right atrial pressures, promotes diuresis | Arrhythmias; nausea; vomiting; anorexia, malaise, color vision, yellow or blue |

NURSING IMPLICATIONS: Hold medication if pulse rate less than *50* or over *120;* encourage foods high in *potassium* (e.g., bananas, orange juice); observe for signs of electrolyte depletion, apathy, disorientation, and anorexia

| Digoxin (Lanoxin)—digitalizing dose: PO up to 750 μg; IM or IV up to 600 μg; maintenance dose: PO 200 μg qd | See Digitoxin | See Digitoxin | See Digitoxin |

NURSING IMPLICATIONS: See Digitoxin

continued

■ **TABLE 4.4** *(Continued)*

Drug and Dosage	Use	Action	Assessment: Side Effects
Chemotherapy (see Tables 2.37 and 4.6)			
Cholinergic Drugs			
Bethanechol Cl (Urecholine)— PO, 5–30 mg; SC, 2.5—5.0 mg; neostigmine bromide (Prostigmin)—PO, 10–30 mg; IM or SC 0.25–1.00 mg	Postoperative abdominal atony and distention; bladder atony with retention; postsurgical or postpartum urinary retention; myasthenia gravis	Increases GI and bladder tone; decreases sphincter tone	Belching, abdominal cramps, diarrhea, nausea, vomiting, incontinence, profuse sweating, salivation, and respiratory depression
NURSING IMPLICATIONS: Check *respirations;* have urinal or bedpan close at hand and answer calls quickly; atropine SO₄ is the *antidote* for cholinergic drugs			

NURSING IMPLICATIONS: Check *respirations;* have urinal or bedpan close at hand and answer calls quickly; atropine SO$_4$ is the *antidote* for cholinergic drugs

Drug and Dosage	Use	Action	Assessment: Side Effects
Edrophonium (Tensilon)—IV 2 mg; IM 10 mg	Diagnosis of myasthenia gravis; reversal of neuromuscular blockers	Inhibits breakdown of acetylcholine; anticholinesterase, cholinergic	Excess secretions, bronchospasm, bradycardia, abdominal cramps, vomiting, diarrhea, excess salivation, sweating

NURSING IMPLICATIONS: Effects last up to 30 min; give IV *undiluted* with *TB* syringe

Drug and Dosage	Use	Action	Assessment: Side Effects
Neostigmine (Prostigmin)—PO 15 mg q3–4h; SC, IM 0.5 mg	Myasthenia, postoperative bladder distention, urinary retention, reversal of neuromuscular blockers	Inhibits breakdown of acetylcholine; cholinergic	Excess secretions, bronchospasm, bradycardia, abdominal cramps, nausea, vomiting, diarrhea, excess salivation, sweating

NURSING IMPLICATIONS: Take oral form *with* food or milk; with chewing difficulty, take 30 min before eating

Cholinergic Miotics

Drug and Dosage	Use	Action	Assessment: Side Effects
Pilocarpine HCl—1–2 gtts 1–2% solution up to 6 times/d. Physostigmine salicylate (Eserine)—0.1 mL of 0.25–10.00% solution; not more than qid	Chronic open-angle and acute angle-closure glaucoma	Contraction of the sphincter muscle of iris, resulting in miosis	Brow ache, headache, ocular pain, blurring and dimness of vision, allergic conjunctivitis, nausea, vomiting, and profuse sweating; bronchoconstriction in patients with bronchial asthma

NURSING IMPLICATIONS: Initially the medication may be irritating; teach proper sterile technique for instilling drops—wipe excess solution to prevent systemic symptoms; discard cloudy solutions

Drug and Dosage	Use	Action	Assessment: Side Effects
Pyridostigmine (Mestinon)— PO 600 mg/d; IM, IV 2 mg q2–3h	Myasthenia gravis, reversal of neuromuscular blockers	Inhibits breakdown of acetylcholine and prolongs its effects	See Neostigmine

NURSING IMPLICATIONS: See Neostigmine

CNS Stimulants

Drug and Dosage	Use	Action	Assessment: Side Effects
Amphetamine SO₄—PO 5–60 mg qd in divided doses	Mild depressive states; narcolepsy; postencephalitic parkinsonism; obesity control; minimal brain dysfunction in children (attention deficit disorder)	Raises BP, decreases sense of fatigue, elevates mood	Restlessness, dizziness, tremors, insomnia; increases libido; suicidal and homicidal tendencies; palpitations; angina pain

NURSING IMPLICATIONS: Give *before* 4 P.M. to avoid sleep disturbance; dependence on drug may develop; *contraindicated* with MAO inhibitors, hyperthyroidism, and psychotic states

Drug and Dosage	Use	Action	Assessment: Side Effects
Methylphenidate hydrochloride (Ritalin)—PO 0.3 mg/kg/d or adults 20–60 mg in divided doses	Childhood hyperactivity; narcolepsy; MBD (attention deficit disorder) in children	Mild CNS and respiratory stimulation	Anorexia, dizziness, drowsiness, insomnia, nervousness, BP and pulse changes

NURSING IMPLICATIONS: To avoid insomnia take last dose 4–5 h before bedtime; monitor vital signs; check weight 2–3 times weekly and report losses

continued

■ **TABLE 4.4**   *(Continued)*

Drug and Dosage	Use	Action	Assessment: Side Effects
Decongestants			
Phenylephrine (Neo-Synephrine, Sinex)—SC, IM 2–5 mg q10–15 min not to exceed 5 mg; IV 40–60 µg/min; nasal 2–3 gtts or 1–2 sprays q3–4h; ophthalmic 3 gtt/d	Shock, hypotension, decongestant, adjunct to spinal anesthesia, mydriatic	Constricts blood vessels by stimulating alpha adrenergic receptors	Dizziness, restlessness, dyspnea, tachycardia, arrhythmias; ophth-burning, photophobia, tearing
NURSING IMPLICATIONS: Check for correct concentration; protect eyes from *light sensitivity;* blow nose before using; *rebound congestion* will occur with prolonged use			
Pseudoephedrine (Sudafed)—PO 60 mg q4–6h	Nasal congestion, allergies, chronic ear infections	Produces vasoconstriction in respiratory tract and possibly bronchodilation	Nervousness, anxiety, palpitations, anorexia
NURSING IMPLICATIONS: Give at least 2 h before bedtime to minimize *insomnia*			
Diuretics			
Acetazolamide (Diamox)—PO 250–1000 mg/d; IV 500 mg	Glaucoma; congestive heart failure; convulsive disorders	Weak diuretic; produces acidosis; self-limiting effect; increases bicarbonate excretion	Electrolyte depletion symptomatology—lassitude, apathy, decreased urinary output, and mental confusion
NURSING IMPLICATIONS: Weigh daily; I&O; assess edema; give *early* in day to allow sleep at night; observe for side effects; replace electrolytes as ordered			
Ethacrynic acid (Edecrin)—PO 50–200 mg qd in divided doses	Pulmonary edema; ascites; edema of congestive heart failure	Inhibits the reabsorption of Na^+ in the ascending loop of Henle	Nausea, vomiting, diarrhea, hypokalemia, hypotension, gout, dehydration, deafness, and metabolic acidosis
NURSING IMPLICATIONS: Assess for dehydration—skin turgor, neck veins; hypotension; *KCl* supplement			
Furosemide (Lasix)—PO 40–80 mg qd in divided doses	Edema and associated heart failure; cirrhosis; renal disease; nephrotic syndrome; hypertension	Inhibits Na^+ and Cl^- reabsorption in the loop of Henle	Dermatitis pruritis, paresthesia, blurring of vision, postural hypotension, nausea, vomiting, diarrhea, dehydration, electrolyte depletion, and hearing loss (usually reversible)
NURSING IMPLICATIONS: Assess for weakness, lethargy, leg cramps, anorexia; peak action in 1–2 h; duration 6–8 h; do *not* give at bedtime; supplementary *KCl* indicated; may induce *digitalis toxicity*			
Hydrochlorothiazide (HydroDIURIL and Esidrix 25–100 mg tid)—PO Diuril 0.5–1.0 g qd	Edema; congestive heart failure; Na^+ retention in steroid therapy; hypertension	Inhibits sodium chloride and water reabsorption in the distal ascending loop and the distal convoluted tubule of the kidneys	Hypokalemia, nausea, vomiting, diarrhea, dizziness, and paresthesias; may accentuate diabetes
NURSING IMPLICATIONS: Watch for muscle weakness; give well-diluted potassium chloride supplement; *monitor* urine for changes in sugar and acetone			
Osmotic diuretic 30% urea, 10% invert sugar, 20% mannitol	Cerebral edema	Hypertonic solution that kidney tubules cannot reabsorb, thereby causing obligatory water loss	↑ Extracellular fluid volume
NURSING IMPLICATIONS: Usually Foley catheter required; monitor *cardiac and respiratory* status			
Spironolactone (Aldactone)—PO 25 mg bid–qid	Cirrhosis of liver; when other diuretics are ineffective	Inhibits effects of aldosterone in distal tubules of kidney	Headache, lethargy, diarrhea, ataxia, skin rash, gynecomastia
NURSING IMPLICATIONS: Potassium-sparing drug; do *not* give supplemental KCl; monitor for signs of electrolyte imbalance			

continued

Pharmacology

■ **TABLE 4.4** *(Continued)*

Drug and Dosage	Use	Action	Assessment: Side Effects
Emetics			
Ipecac syrup—PO 15–30 mL for emesis, followed by 1–2 glasses H_2O (adults and children >1 yr); 5–10 mL followed by ½–1 glass H_2O (children <1 yr)	Emergency emetic for poison ingestion	NH_4 ions cause gastric irritation	Violent emesis, tachycardia, decreased BP, and dyspnea

NURSING IMPLICATIONS: *Contraindicated* in liver and renal disease; if given for emesis, follow dose with as much *water* as patient will drink

Enzymes			
Pancrelipase (Viokase)— adults, PO 325 mg–1 g qd, during meals; children, PO 300–600 mg tid	Chronic pancreatitis; cystic fibrosis; gastrectomy; pancreatectomy; sprue	Assists in digestion of starch, protein, and fats; decreases nitrogen and fat content of stool	Anorexia, nausea, vomiting, diarrhea, buccal/anal soreness (infants), sneezing, skin rashes, diabetes

NURSING IMPLICATIONS: May be taken with antacid or cimetidine; do *not* crush or chew tabs; *monitor* I&O, weight; be alert for signs of diabetes; children may use sprinkles

Expectorants			
Guaifenesin (Robitussin) 100–400 mg q4h	Respiratory congestion	Increases expectoration by causing irritation of gastric mucosa; reduces adhesiveness/surface tension of respiratory tract fluid	Low incidence of GI upset; drowsiness

NURSING IMPLICATIONS: Encourage to stop smoking; increase fluid intake; respiratory hygiene

Terpin hydrate—PO 5–10 mL q3–4h	Bronchitis; emphysema	Liquefies bronchial secretions	Nausea, vomiting, and gastric irritation

NURSING IMPLICATIONS: Give undiluted; *push* fluids

Fibrinolytic Agents			
Alteplase, recombinant (Activase, tPA)—IV bolus, 6–10 mg over 1–2 min; IV infusion, 60 mg first h, 20 mg second h, 20 mg third h	Acute MI; under investigation for pulmonary emboli, deep-vein thrombosis, and peripheral artery thrombosis	Promotes conversion of plasminogen to plasmin, which is fibrinolytic	Internal or local bleeding; urticaria; dysrhythmias related to reperfusion; hypotension, nausea, and vomiting

NURSING IMPLICATIONS: Assess for signs of reperfusion (relief of chest pain, no ST segment elevation); observe for *bleeding;* avoid IM injection; *do not* mix other meds in line

Streptokinase IV—250,000 IU over 30 min; 100,000 IU/h	Lysis of pulmonary or systemic emboli or thrombi; acute MI	Reacts with plasminogen, dissolves fibrin clots	Prolonged coagulation; allergic reactions; mild fever

NURSING IMPLICATIONS: Monitor for signs of excessive *bleeding,* particularly at injection sites; avoid nonessential handling of patient

Urokinase—IV 4400 IU/kg over 10 min; 1.0–1.8 mL of 5000 IU/mL into catheter	Massive pulmonary emboli, coronary artery thrombi, occluded IV catheter	Directly activates plasminogen	Bleeding, anaphylaxis, rash

NURSING IMPLICATIONS: Vital signs; check *q15min* for bleeding during first h; q15–30min for 8 h; have *epinephrine* ready

Fibrinolytic Antidote			
Aminocaproic acid (Amicar)— PO, IV 5 g loading dose; 1 g/h to 30 g in 24 h	Management of streptokinase or urokinase overdose	Inhibits plasminogen activator and antagonizes plasmin	Hypotension; bradycardia; cardiac arrhythmias

NURSING IMPLICATIONS: Give slowly IV to prevent side effects; not recommended for DIC

Hormones			
Chlorotrianisene (TACE), estrogen—PO 12–50 mg	Suppresses lactation; prostatic cancer; menopause	Nonsteroidal synthetic estrogen	Rare after one course of treatment; thromboembolism; impotence and gynecomastia in males

NURSING IMPLICATIONS: *Rebound engorgement* may occur; supply patient with package insert; *contraindicated* in blood coagulation disorders

continued

Pharmacology

■ **TABLE 4.4**   *(Continued)*

Drug and Dosage	Use	Action	Assessment: Side Effects
Hormones *(continued)*			
Diethylstilbestrol (DES)—PO or IM 0.2–5.0 mg qd; vaginal suppository 0.1–0.5 mg at bedtime	Prostate carcinoma; menopausal symptoms; osteoporosis; pain; mammary carcinoma; atrophic vaginitis	Synthetic nonsteroidal compound with estrogenic effects on pituitary, ovaries, myometrium, endometrium, and other tissues	Anorexia, nausea, vomiting, headache, diarrhea, dizziness, and fainting—many side effects with long-term use
NURSING IMPLICATIONS: *Never* give if woman is pregnant—predisposes to vaginal cancer in female offspring at puberty			
Estradiol—PO 1–2 mg up to 10 mg for CA qd–tid; cyclic (on 3 wk, off 1 wk)	Menopausal symptoms; osteoporosis; hypogenitalism; sexual infantilism; postpartum breast engorgement; breast and prostatic carcinoma	Inhibits release of pituitary gonadotropins; promotes growth of female genital tissues	Anorexia, nausea, vomiting, diarrhea, fluid retention, mental depression, headache, thromboembolism and feminization in males
NURSING IMPLICATIONS: Baseline VS; weigh daily; encourage frequent physical checkups to check serum lipids; teach BSE			
Hydroxyprogesterone caproate (Delalutin)—IM 250 mg/2 mL q4wk	Menstrual disorders; ovarian and uterine dysfunction	Synthetic derivative of progesterone; long-acting	GI symptoms, headache, and allergy
NURSING IMPLICATIONS: Requires test for endogenous estrogen production; tell patient onset of menstrual cycle may take 2–3 mo after treatment; BSE			
Medroxyprogesterone (Provera)—PO 2.5–10.0 mg; IM 400–1000 mg weekly	Amenorrhea; functional uterine bleeding; threatened abortion; dysmenorrhea; adjunctive and palliative with renal cancer and endometriosis; PMS	Similar to progesterone, but can be taken orally; thickens uterine decidua	Drowsiness: cyclic menstrual withdrawal bleeding; GI upset; headache; edema; breast congestion
NURSING IMPLICATIONS: Teach patient regarding self-administration; breast self-exam for possible breast changes			
Menotropins (Pergonal)—IM 1 amp (FSH + LH)/d for 9–12 d (followed by 5000–10,000 U HCG, if ovulation does not occur, repeat with 2 ampules)	**Infertility use:** treatment of secondary anovulation; stimulation of spermatogenesis	Human gonadotropic responses; induces ovulation; sperm stimulation	Abortions occur in 25%; failure rate 55–80% of patients; possible multiple births; ovarian enlargement; gynecomastia in males
NURSING IMPLICATIONS: Assist in collection of urine to assess estrogen levels; counsel regarding couple's need to have daily intercourse from day of HCG injection until ovulation			
Progesterone—SC or IM 5–10 mg qd; sublingual 5–10 mg	Amenorrhea; dysmenorrhea; endometriosis; habitual abortion	Converts endometrium into secreting structure; prevents ovulation; stimulates growth of mammary tissue	Nausea, vomiting, dizziness, edema, headache, protein metabolism
NURSING IMPLICATIONS: Give deep IM and rotate sites; weigh daily to ascertain fluid retention			
Testosterone—PO 5–10 mg qd; IM 25–50 mg 2–3 times/wk; 200–400 mg IM q2–4wk for breast cancer	Hypogonadism; eunuchism; impotence; advanced cancer of breast	Growth of sex organs and appearance of secondary male sex characteristics; counteracts excessive amounts of estrogen	Nausea, dyspepsia, masculinization, hypercalcemia, menstrual irregularities, renal calculi, and Na$^+$, K$^+$, and H$_2$O retention
NURSING IMPLICATIONS: Observe for edema; weigh daily; I&O; *push fluids* for bedridden patients, to prevent renal calculi			
Mucolytic Agents			
Acetylcysteine (Mucomyst)—1–10 mL of 20% solution per nebulizer tid	Emphysema; pneumonia; tracheostomy care; atelectasis; cystic fibrosis	Lowers viscosity of respiratory secretions by opening disulfide linkages in mucus	Stomatitis, nausea, rhinorrhea, bronchospasm
NURSING IMPLICATIONS: Observe *respiratory rate;* maintain open airway with suctioning as necessary; observe asthmatics carefully for *increased bronchospasm;* discontinue treatment immediately if this occurs; odor disagreeable initially			
Muscle Relaxants			
Baclofen (Lioresal)—5 mg tid up to 10–20 mg 4/d maintenance dose	Relief of spasticity of multiple sclerosis, spinal cord injury	Centrally acting skeletal-muscle relaxant; depresses polysynaptic afferent reflex activity at spinal cord level	Pruritis, tinnitus; N/V, diarrhea or constipation; drowsiness
NURSING IMPLICATIONS: Administer *with* food if GI symptoms; monitor for safety when ambulating; do not discontinue abruptly			

continued

Pharmacology

■ **TABLE 4.4** *(Continued)*

Drug and Dosage	Use	Action	Assessment: Side Effects
Muscle Relaxants *(continued)*			
Dantrolene sodium (Dantrium)—25 mg/day to 25 mg bid–qid to 100 mg qid max	See Baclofen	See Baclofen	See Baclofen
NURSING IMPLICATIONS: See Baclofen			
Narcotic Antagonists			
Naloxone (Narcan) HCl—IV 0.1–0.2 mg repeated	Reverses respiratory depression due to narcotics	Reverses respiratory depression of morphine SO_4, meperidine HCl, and methadone HCl; does not itself cause respiratory depression, sedation, or analgesia	No known side effects
NURSING IMPLICATIONS: Note time, type of narcotic, dosage received; not useful with CNS depression from other drugs; respiratory depression *may return;* monitor closely			
Sedatives and Hypnotics			
Chlordiazepoxide (Librium) HCl—PO 5–10 mg; IM or IV 50–100 mg	Psychoneuroses; preoperative apprehension; chronic alcoholism; anxiety	CNS depressant resulting in mild sedation; appetite stimulant; and anticonvulsant	Ataxia, fatigue, blurred vision, diplopia, lethargy, nightmares, and confusion
NURSING IMPLICATIONS: Ensure anxiety relief by allowing patient to verbalize feelings; advise patient to avoid driving and alcoholic beverages			
Chloral hydrate—PO 250 mg tid; hypnotic: PO 0.5–1.0 g; rectal supplement 0.3–0.9 g	Sedation for elderly; delirium tremens; pruritus; mania; barbiturate and alcohol withdrawal	Depresses sensorimotor areas of cerebral cortex	Nausea, vomiting, gastritis; pinpoint pupils; delirium; rash; decreased BP, pulse, respirations, and temperature; hepatic damage
NURSING IMPLICATIONS: *Caution*—should not be taken in combination with alcohol; dependency is possible			
Diazepam (Valium)—PO 2–10 mg tid–qid; IM or IV 2–10 mg q3–4h	Anxiety disorders; alcohol withdrawal; adjunctive therapy in seizure disorders; status epilepticus; tetanus; preoperative or preprocedural sedation (also see Midazolam)	Induces calming effect on limbic system, thalamus, and hypothalamus	CNS depression—sedation or ataxia (dose related); dry mouth; blurred vision; mydriasis; constipation; urinary retention
NURSING IMPLICATIONS: *Do not* mix with other drugs; IM injection painful; observe for *phlebitis;* monitor response; measures to ensure patient safety (e.g., falls); high potential for abuse; *contraindicated* in acute angle-closure glaucoma and porphyria			
Flurazepam (Dalmane)—PO>15 yr, 30 mg hs; elderly or debilitated, 15 mg hs	Hypnotic	Fastest acting; see Diazepam	See Diazepam
NURSING IMPLICATIONS: See Diazepam			
Hydroxyzine pamoate (Vistaril)—PO 25–100 mg qid	See Chlordiazepoxide (Librium); antiemetic in postoperative conditions; adjunctive therapy	CNS relaxant with sedative effect on limbic system and thalamus	Drowsiness, headache, itching, dry mouth, and tremor
NURSING IMPLICATIONS: Give deep IM only; *potentiates* action of warfarin (Coumadin), narcotics, and barbiturates			
Lorazepam (Ativan)—PO 1–2 mg bid–tid (up to 10 mg); 2–4 mg hs; IM 4 mg max; IV 2 mg max	Anxiety disorders; insomnia; alternative to diazepam for status epilepticus; preanesthesia	See Diazepam	See Diazepam
NURSING IMPLICATIONS: See Diazepam			
Meprobamate (Equanil, Miltown)—PO 400 mg tid–qid	Anxiety; stress; absence seizures	See Hydroxyzine pamoate (Vistaril)	Voracious appetite, dryness of mouth, and ataxia
NURSING IMPLICATIONS: Older patients prone to drowsiness and hypotension; observe for *jaundice*			

continued

■ **TABLE 4.4**   *(Continued)*

Drug and Dosage	Use	Action	Assessment: Side Effects
Sedatives and Hypnotics *(continued)*			
Midazolam (Versed)—IM 0.05– 0.08 mg/kg; IV 0.1–0.15 mg/ kg	Preanesthesia; prediagnostic procedures; induction of general anesthesia	Penetrates blood-brain barrier to produce sedation and amnesia	Respiratory depression; apnea; disorientation and behavioral excitement
NURSING IMPLICATIONS: Monitor ventilatory status and oxygenation; prevent injuries from CNS depression; nonirritating to vein			
Phenobarbital Na—sedative, PO 20–30 mg tid; hypnotic, PO 50–100 mg; IV or IM 100–300 mg. Butabarbital Na (Butisol), pentobarbital Na (Nembutal), secobarbital Na (Seconal)	Preoperative sedation; emergency control of convulsions; absence seizures	Depresses CNS, promoting drowsiness	Cough, hiccups, restlessness, pain, hangover, and CNS and circulatory depression
NURSING IMPLICATIONS: Observe for hypotension during IV administration; put up siderails on bed of older patients; observe for increased tolerance			
Promethazine (Phenergan) 25– 50 mg IV, IM, PO	Preoperative sedation; postoperative sedation	Antihistaminic; sedative, antiemetic, antimotion sickness	Drowsiness, coma, hypo/hypertension; leukopenia; photosensitivity; irregular respirations; blurred vision; urinary retention; dry mouth, nose, throat
NURSING IMPLICATIONS: Administer oral med *with* food, milk; IM deep into large muscles, rotate sites; verify compatibility with other drugs; safety concerns due to sedative effect			
Thyroid Hormone Inhibitor			
Lugol's solution—PO 2–6 drops tid 10 d prior to thyroidectomy	To reduce size, vascularity of thyroid before thyroid surgery; emergency treatment of thyroid storm; or control of hyperthyroid symptoms after radioiodine (^{131}I) therapy	Inhibits thyroid hormone secretion, synthesis	GI distress; stains teeth; increased respiratory secretions; rashes, acne
NURSING IMPLICATIONS: *Dilute in juice,* give through *straw;* bloody diarrhea/vomiting indicates acute poisoning			
Propylthiouracil—PO 300–400 mg/d, divided initial dose; 100–150 mg/d maintenance dose; methimazole (Tapazole) 15–60 mg/d initial dose; 5– 15 mg/d maintenance dose	Hyperthyroidism; return patient to euthyroid state; also used preoperatively	Inhibits functional thyroid hormone synthesis by blocking reactions; responsible for iodide conversion to iodine; inhibition of T_4 conversion to T_3	Blood dyscrasias; hepatotoxicity; hypothyroidism
NURSING IMPLICATIONS: Teach importance of compliance with med protocol; *avoid* iodine-rich foods (seafood, iodized salt); caution when using other drugs			
Saturated potassium iodide (SSKI)—300 mg tid–qid	Same as Lugol's solution	Same as Lugol's solution	Same as Lugol's solution
NURSING IMPLICATIONS: Same as Lugol's solution			
Thyroid Hormone Replacement			
Levothyroxine (Levothroid, Synthroid)—PO 0.05–0.10 mg/d oral	Hypothyroidism	Replacement therapy to alleviate symptoms	Symptoms of hyperthyroidism
200–500 µg IV	Myxedema coma	Emergency replacement therapy	
NURSING IMPLICATIONS: Teach signs and symptoms of hyper/hypothyroidism; monitor bowel activity; teach diet to combat constipation; keep meds in tight light-proof containers; *avoid foods* that inhibit thyroid secretion (turnips, cabbage, carrots, peaches, peas, strawberries, spinach, radishes)			
Liothyronine (Cytomel)—25 µg/d to maintenance dose 25–75 µg	Mild hypothyroidism in adults	Replacement therapy	See Levothyroxine
NURSING IMPLICATIONS: See Levothyroxine			

continued

■ **TABLE 4.4** *(Continued)*

Drug and Dosage	Use	Action	Assessment: Side Effects
Uterine Contractants			
Ergonovine maleate (Ergotrate)—PO, IM, IV 0.2 mg (gr 1/320)	Postabortal or postpartum hemorrhage; promotes involution after delivery of placenta	Stimulates uterine contractions for 3 h or more	Nausea, vomiting, occasional transient hypertension, especially if given IV; cramping
NURSING IMPLICATIONS: Store in *cool* place; monitor maternal BP and pulse; *do not use in labor*			
Methylergonovine maleate (Methergine)—PO 0.2 mg; IM, IV 0.2 mg (gr 1/320)	Postpartum hemorrhage, after delivery of placenta	Stimulates stronger and longer contractions than ergonovine maleate (Ergotrate)	Nausea, vomiting, transient hypertension, dizziness, tachycardia; cramping
NURSING IMPLICATIONS: Do *not* give if mother is hypertensive; do *not* use if solution is discolored; *do not use in labor*			
Oxytocin (Pitocin, Syntocinon)—IM 0.3–1.0 mL; IV 1 mL (10 U) in 1000 mL solution	Stimulates rhythmic contractions of uterus	Induces labor; augments contractions; prevents or controls postpartum atony; antidiuretic effect	Tetanic contractions, uterine rupture, cardiac arrhythmias, FHR deceleration
NURSING IMPLICATIONS: *Contraindicated* if cervix is unripe, in CPD, abruptio placentae, and cardiovascular disease; *monitor* FHR, contractions, maternal BP, pulse, I&O; watch for signs of water intoxication with prolonged IV use; drug of choice in presence of hypertension; *never* use undiluted; DC if tetanic contractions occur. Antidote: Propanolol.			

❏ Questions

Select the one best answer for each question.

1. A patient has meperidine, 75 mg every 3–4 hours prn, ordered for postoperative pain. Prior to administering this narcotic, the nurse should:
   1. Position in a semi-Fowler's position to minimize respiratory effects.
   2. Assess the type, location, and intensity of discomfort.
   3. Evaluate whether the pain is real.
   4. Try other measures to relieve discomfort, such as position change.

2. Neostigmine bromide (Prostigmin), 0.5 mg subcutaneously stat, is ordered by a patient's physician to relieve urinary retention. The nurse knows that this drug is classified as:
   1. A cholinergic.
   2. An anticholinesterase.
   3. An anticholinergic.
   4. A beta blocker.

3. The nurse explains to a patient that although salicylates are given to relieve pain in rheumatoid arthritis, they also function as an:
   1. Analgesic.
   2. Anti-inflammatory.
   3. Anticholinergic.
   4. Antiadrenergic.

4. Drug therapy goals for a patient included strengthening cardiac contraction and increasing glomerular filtration rate. Which medication would the nurse prepare to accomplish both goals?
   1. Epinephrine.
   2. Digoxin.
   3. Furosemide (Lasix).
   4. Hydralazine.

5. Which outcome is the best indicator that digoxin has been effective?
   1. Increased systolic and diastolic pressures.
   2. Unlabored respirations and increased urinary output.
   3. Decreased pulse rate and increased urinary output.
   4. Increased blood pressure and decreased pulse rate.

6. Patient teaching includes the side effects of theophylline administration, which are:
   1. Tachycardia and palpitations.
   2. Anorexia, nausea, and gastritis.
   3. Restlessness and tremors.
   4. Headache and nausea.

7. Based on the peak action of furosemide (Lasix) PO, the nurse will evaluate the drug's effects in:
   1. 30–60 minutes.
   2. 1–2 hours.
   3. 3–4 hours.
   4. 6–8 hours.

8. The nurse administers sodium polystyrene sulfonate (Kayexalate) knowing that the drug reduces hyperkalemia by:
   1. Exchanging sodium ions for potassium ions in the GI tract, thereby increasing potassium excretion in the feces.
   2. Inhibiting potassium absorption sites in the GI tract.
   3. Promoting diarrhea, thereby decreasing potassium absorption from the gut.
   4. Altering the effects of aldosterone in the kidney tubules.

9. The nurse knows that the best time to give oral iron preparations is:
   1. With meals, to decrease gastric upset.
   2. 1 hour before eating, to enhance absorption.
   3. 1 hour after eating, to slow absorption.
   4. At bedtime.

10. A patient is instructed to report the following side effect of neomycin administration:
    1. Deafness.
    2. Nausea.
    3. Diarrhea.
    4. Anaphylaxis.

11. Before administering morphine sulfate, the nurse should check:
    1. Apical and radial pulse.
    2. Respiratory rate.
    3. Urinary output.
    4. Skin color and turgor.

■ **TABLE 4.5   Guide to Important Food and Drug Considerations**

Key to Nursing Implications (with codes for medication administration records):

1. Take with food or milk (F-M).
2. Take on empty stomach (1 hour ac or 2 to 3 hours pc).
3. Don't drink milk or eat other dairy products (M-D).
4. Take with full glass of water ($+ H_2O$).
5. Take before meals (½ hour ac).
6. May take without regard to meals (OK c̄ meals).

A

acebutolol   6
Achromycin V   2, 3
allopurinol   1
Amcill   2
aminophylline   1
amiodarone   1
amoxicillin   6
amoxicillin/clavulanate   6
Amoxil   6
ampicillin   2
aspirin   1
Augmentin   6
Azo Gantrisin   4, 6
Azolid   1

B

Bactrim   4, 6
Benemid   4
bisacodyl   3
Butazolidin   1

C

Capoten   2
captopril   2
Carafate   2
Carprofen   1
Ceclor   6
cefaclor   6
Ceftin   6
cefuroxime axetil   6
cephalexin   6
chlorothiazide   1
cimetidine   1
Cipro   6
ciprofloxacin   6
Cleocin   4, 6
clindamycin   4, 6
cloxacillin sodium   2
Cloxapen   2
ColBENEMID   1, 4
Cordarone   1

co-trimoxazole   4, 6
Cuprimine   2

D

Declomycin   2, 3
Deltasone   1
demeclocycline   2, 3
Depen   2
Desyrel   1
dicloxacillin sodium   2
diflunisal   1
Diuril   1
Dolobid   1
Donnatal   5
Dopar   1
doxycycline hyclate   3, 6
Dulcolax   3
Dynapen   2

E

Ecotrin   3
E.E.S.   2
E-Mycin   6
enalapril   6
ERYC   2
Ery-Tab   6
Erythrocin   2
erythromycin estolate   6
erythromycin ethylsuccinate   6
erythromycin stearate   2
etretinate   1

F

famotidine   6
Feldene   1
ferrous sulfate   3
Flagyl   1
flecainide   6
fluoxetine   6
Fulvicin   1
Furadantin   1

G

Gantrisin   4, 6
glycopyrrolate   5
Grifulvin V   1
Grisactin   1
griseofulvin   1

H

Hydropres   1
Hytrin   6

I

Ilosone   6
Indocin   1
indomethacin   1
INH   2
isoniazid   2

K

Kaon   1
Kay Ciel   1
Keflex   6
ketoconazole   1
ketoprofen   1
K-Lor   1
K-Lyte   1

L

Larodopa   1
Larotid   6
levodopa   1
Lincocin   2
lincomycin   2
lisinopril   6
Lorelco   1
lovastatin   1

M

Macrodantin   1
Marax   1
methysergide maleate   1
metronidazole   1
Mevacor   1
mexiletine   1
Mexitil   1
Minocin   3, 6
Minocyline   3, 6

N

nafcillin   2
nitrofurantoin   1
nitrofurantoin macrocrystals   1
Nizoral   1
norfloxacin   2, 4
Noroxin   2, 4

O

Omnipen   2
Orazinc   3
Orudis   1
oxacillin sodium   2
oxytetracycline   2, 3

P

penicillamine   2
penicillin G (oral)   2
penicillin V   6
Pen-Vee K   6
Pepcid   6
phenylbutazone   1
pindolol   6
piroxicam   1
Polycillin   2
potassium chloride   1
prednisone   1
Prinivil   6

K

Pro-Banthine   5
probenecid   4
probucol   1
procainamide   6
Pronestyl   6
propantheline bromide   5
Prostaphlin   2
Prozac   6

R

ranitidine   6
Raudixin   1
rauwolfia serpentina   1
Regroton   1
reserpine   1
Rifadin   2
rifampin   2
Rimactane   2
rimadyl   1
Robinul   5

S

Sansert   1
Sectral   6
Septra   4, 6
Ser-Ap-Es   1
Serpasil   1
Sinemet   1
Slow-K   1
Somophyllin   1
sucralfate   2
sulfisoxazole   4, 6
Sumycin   2, 3

T

Tagamet   1
Tambocor   6
Tedral   1
Tegison   1
terazosin   6
Terramycin   2, 3
tetracycline HCl   2, 3
Theobid   6
Theo-Dur   6

U

Unipen   2

V

Vasotec   6
V-Cillin K   6
Vibramycin   3, 6
Visken   6

Z

Zantac   6
Zestril   6
zinc sulfate   3
Zyloprim   1

Source: McGavin K. 10 Golden Rules for Administering Drugs Safely. *Nursing 88,* 18(8): 40, 1988.

■ **TABLE 4.6 Classification of the Anticancer Drugs**

I. Alkylating agents
  A. Nitrogen mustards
    1. Mechlorethamine hydrochloride (*Mustargen*, HN₂, nitrogen mustard)
    2. Cyclophosphamide (*Cytoxan*)
    3. Chlorambucil (*Leukeran*)
    4. Melphalan (*Alkeran, L-PAM*, L-phenylalanine mustard)
    5. Ifosfamide (*Ifex*)
  B. Alkyl sulfonates
    1. Busulfan (*Myleran*)
  C. Nitrosoureas
    1. Carmustine (BCNU, *BiCNU*)
    2. Lomustine (CCNU, *CeeNU*)
    3. Semustine (methyl-CCNU)
    4. Streptozocin (*Zanosar*, streptozotocin)
  D. Ethylenimines
    1. Thiotepa
  E. Triazenes
    1. Dacarbazine (*DTIC-Dome*)
II. Antimetabolites
  A. Folate antagonist
    1. Methotrexate (*Folex, Mexate*)
  B. Purine analogues
    1. Thioguanine (6-TG, 6-thioguanine)
    2. Mercaptopurine (6-MP, *Purinethol*)
    3. Fludarabine (*Fludara*)
    4. Pentostatin (deoxycoformycin, *Nipent*)
    5. Cladribine (2-chloro-deoxyadenosine, *Leustatin*)
  C. Pyrimidine analogues
    1. Cytarabine (cytosine arabinoside, *Cytosar-U*, ara-C)
    2. Fluorouracil (5-FU, 5-fluorouracil)
III. Antibiotics
  A. Anthracyclines
    1. Doxorubicin hydrochloride (*Adriamycin*)
    2. Daunorubicin (daunomycin, *Cerubidine*)
    3. Idarubicin (*Idamycin*)
  B. Bleomycins
    1. Bleomycin sulfate (*Blenoxane*)
  C. Mitomycin (mitomycin C, *Mutamycin*)
  D. Dactinomycin (actinomycin D, *Cosmegen*)
  E. Plicamycin (*Mithracin*)

IV. Plant-derived products
  A. Vinca alkaloids
    1. Vincristine (*Oncovin*)
    2. Vinblastine (*Velban*)
  B. Epipodophyllotoxins
    1. Etoposide (VP-16, *Vepesid*)
    2. Teniposide (VM-26, *Vumon*)
  C. Taxanes: paclitaxel (*Taxol*)
V. Enzymes
  A. L-Asparaginase (*Elspar*)
VI. Hormonal agents
  A. Glucocorticoids
  B. Estrogens/antiestrogens
    1. Tamoxifen citrate (*Nolvadex*)
    2. Estramustine phosphate sodium (*Emcyt*)
  C. Androgens/antiandrogens
    1. Flutamide (*Eulexin*)
  D. Progestins
  E. Luteinizing hormone–releasing hormone (LH-RH) antagonists
    1. Buserelin (*Suprefact*)
    2. Leuprolide (*Lupron*)
  F. Octreotide acetate (*Sandostatin*)
VII. Miscellaneous agents
  A. Hydroxyurea (*Hydrea*)
  B. Procarbazine (*N*-methylhydrazine, *Matulane, Natulan*)
  C. Mitotane (o,p′-DDD, *Lysodren*)
  D. Hexamethylmelamine (HMM)
  E. Cisplatin (*cis*-platinum II, *Platinol*)
  F. Carboplatin (*Paraplatin*)
  G. Mitoxantrone (*Novantrone*)
VIII. Monoclonal antibodies
IX. Immunomodulating agents
  A. Levamisole (*Ergamisol*)
  B. Interferons
    1. Interferon alfa-2a (*Roferon-A*)
    2. Interferon alfa-2b (*Intron A*)
  C. Interleukins: aldesleukin (interleukin-2, IL-2, *Proleukin*)
X. Cellular growth factors
  A. Filgrastim (G-CSF, *Neupogen*)
  B. Sargramostim (GM-CSF, *Leukine, Prokine*)

Source: Craig C, Stitzel R. *Modern Pharmacology*. Boston: Little, Brown, 1994.

Pharmacology

12. The nurse administers spironolactone (Aldactone) knowing that it is classified as:
  1. An aldosterone antagonist.
  2. A carbonic anhydrase inhibitor.
  3. A thiazide.
  4. An osmotic diuretic.

13. Which supplement would the nurse not ordinarily administer to the patient receiving spironolactone?
  1. Vitamin B₆.
  2. Potassium chloride.
  3. Ascorbic acid.
  4. Calcium carbonate.

14. The primary objective in giving prednisone along with aspirin for acute rheumatoid arthritis is:
  1. To inhibit the autoimmune factors associated with rheumatoid arthritis.
  2. To prevent further joint destruction.
  3. To decrease inflammation and suppress symptomatology.
  4. To increase glucose levels for tissue repair.

15. The nurse would recognize prednisone toxicity if which of the following occurred?
  1. Tinnitus.
  2. Exfoliative dermatitis.
  3. Glucosuria.
  4. Nausea and vomiting.

16. Propantheline bromide (Pro-Banthine) is given to patients with cholelithiasis and cholecystitis because it:
  1. Reduces gastric secretions and intestinal hypermobility.
  2. Decreases bile secretion by the liver and gallbladder.
  3. Slows the emptying of the stomach, thereby reducing chyme in the duodenum.
  4. Inhibits contraction of the gallbladder and the bile duct.

17. The nurse would most likely give papaverine HCl for relief of gallbladder pain rather than morphine SO₄ because:
  1. Morphine depresses gallbladder contractions, thereby decreasing bile secretions.

■ **TABLE 4.7 Properties of Selected Anti-inflammatory Agents**

Specific Group	Analgesic	Antipyretic	Anti-inflammatory	Uricosuric
Salicylate derivatives				
Acetylsalicylic acid (aspirin)	*	*	*	*
Pyrazolone derivatives				
Phenylbutazone	*	*	*	*
Oxyphenbutazone	*	*	*	*
Sulfinpyrazone	0	0	0	*
Paraaminophenol derivatives				
Acetaminophen	*	*	0	0
Phenacetin	*	*	0	0
Propionic acid derivatives				
Ibuprofen	*	*	*	0
Naproxen	*	*	*	0
Fenoprofen	*	*	*	0
Flurbiprofen	*	*	*	0
Ketoprofen	*	*	*	0
Newer drugs				
Indomethacin	*	*	*	0
Sulindac	*	0	*	0
Mefenamic acid	*	0	*	0
Tolmetin	*	*	*	0
Diflunisal	*	0	*	0
Piroxicam	*	*	*	0
Diclofenac	*	*	*	0
Etodolac	*	0	*	0
Nabumetone	*	*	*	0

* = possesses the property assigned; 0 = lacks the property assigned.
Source: Ebadi M. *Pharmacology* (2nd ed). Boston: Little, Brown, 1993.

2. Opiates tend to mask symptoms in patients with acute abdomens.
3. Morphine tends to increase contractions of the sphincter of Oddi, thereby increasing intraductal pressures.
4. Morphine relaxes smooth muscles, thereby increasing bile production.

18. The nurse can anticipate side effects of hydrochlorothiazide because it is classified as:
    1. An aldosterone inhibitor.
    2. A carbonic anhydrase inhibitor.
    3. A potassium-sparing drug.
    4. A potassium-wasting drug.

19. The nurse knows that hydrochlorothiazide exerts its primary effect on:
    1. The proximal and distal tubules of the kidney.
    2. The distal convoluted tubule of the kidney only.
    3. The ascending loop of Henle and the distal tubule of the kidney.
    4. The descending loop of Henle and the proximal tubule of the kidney.

20. Assessment for the side effects of hydrochlorothiazide includes signs of:
    1. Hypernatremia.
    2. Hyperkalemia.
    3. Hypochloremia.
    4. Hypouricemia.

21. A 2-year-old patient (diagnosis: meningitis) is to be sedated with phenobarbital, 18 mg PO q6h. The label reads "20 mg per 5 mL." How much phenobarbital should the nurse administer to this patient?
    1. 4 mL.
    2. 4.3 mL.

3. 4.5 mL.
4. 4.8 mL.

22. A patient's CSF culture is positive for *Hemophilus influenzae* meningitis. To protect other members of the patient's family who have been exposed to meningitis, the nurse should explain that they may be given:
    1. Amoxicillin/clavulanate potassium (Augmentin).
    2. Sulfisoxazole.
    3. Rifampin.
    4. Immune serum globulin.

23. The nurse is to administer pancreatin to a 5-year-old patient with cystic fibrosis. To evaluate the effect of this medication, the nurse should know that the primary purpose of this medication is to increase the absorption of:
    1. Glucose.
    2. Vitamin C.
    3. Sodium chloride.
    4. Fats.

24. The nurse about to administer medication to a 5-year-old patient notes that the child has no ID bracelet. The best way for the nurse to identify this patient would be to ask:
    1. The child, "Is your name _____?"
    2. The adult visiting, "The child's name is _____?"
    3. The other children in the room what the child's name is.
    4. Another staff nurse to identify this child.

25. Elixir of digoxin (Lanoxin) is available with 0.05 mg of the drug in 1 mL of solution. How much of this elixir should the nurse administer if the physician's order reads "0.125 mg PO bid"?
    1. 2 mL.

2. 2.25 mL.

3. 2.5 mL.

4. 2.75 mL.

26. In teaching a parent how to administer Cortisporin eye drops to an infant, the nurse would be most correct in advising the parent to place the drops:
    1. Directly onto the infant's sclera.
    2. In the inner canthus of the infant's eye.
    3. In the outer canthus of the infant's eye.
    4. In the middle of the lower conjunctival sac of the infant's eye.

27. The doctor orders ferrous sulfate (Fer-in-Sol), 0.6 cc PO tid. For maximum absorption, the nurse plans to administer this medication:
    1. Between meals.
    2. Before meals.
    3. During meals.
    4. After meals.

28. Two weeks after starting an oral iron supplement, the patient's mother tells the nurse that the child's stools are black in color. The nurse should tell her:
    1. "This is a normal side effect and means the medication is working."
    2. "I will notify the doctor, who will probably decrease the dosage slightly."
    3. "I will need a specimen to check the stool for possible bleeding."
    4. "You sound quite concerned. Would you like to talk about this further?"

29. A pregnant woman's history reveals 12 weeks' gestation, severe pruritus, dysuria, and thick creamy vaginal discharge for the past 3 days. Which assessment factor is considered predisposing to the development of monilial vaginitis?
    1. Pregnancy.
    2. Late adolescence.
    3. High-carbohydrate diet.
    4. Sickle cell anemia.

30. Health teaching for a patient with vaginal infection with *Candida albicans* should be planned and implemented to ensure her consistent and appropriate use of the prescribed medication. Which medication is effective in the treatment of monilial (yeast) vaginitis?
    1. Metronidazole (Flagyl) oral tablets.
    2. Nystatin (Mycostatin) vaginal suppositories.
    3. Local applications of podophyllin.
    4. Antibiotic (bacitracin) ointment.

31. Reviewing the results of a patient's routine prenatal lab work, the nurse notes that her VDRL is positive. To protect the fetus from congenital syphilis, the patient must receive treatment before weeks 18–20. History suggests possible allergy to penicillin. Which drug would be ordered to treat venereal disease in the penicillin-allergic patient?
    1. Streptomycin.
    2. Sulfisoxazole (Gantrisin).
    3. Chloramphenicol (Chloromycetin).
    4. Erythromycin.

32. Health teaching regarding uncomfortable signs and symptoms of side effects of oral antibiotic therapy includes:
    1. Tinnitus (ringing in the ears).
    2. Nausea, vomiting, and abdominal pain.
    3. Nausea and glossitis.
    4. Nausea, diarrhea, and vaginal yeast infections.

33. Which medication is ordered most commonly to attempt to inhibit premature labor?
    1. Magnesium sulfate.

2. Betamethasone.

3. Ritodrine (Yutopar).

4. Bromocryptine mesylate (Parlodel).

34. In evaluating a patient's response to beta-mimetic therapy used to inhibit premature labor, to which sign of side effects must the nurse be alert?
    1. Maternal hypertension.
    2. Fetal bradycardia.
    3. Maternal and fetal tachycardia.
    4. Uterine hypertonia.

35. When a parturient is given a paracervical block, the nurse can expect:
    1. Low forceps birth.
    2. Depression of contractions, maternal hypotension, fetal bradycardia, postnatal uterine atony.
    3. Depression of contractions and fetal bradycardia.
    4. Loss of bearing-down reflex, low forceps birth.

36. When a parturient is given an epidural (or caudal) anesthesia, the nurse could expect:
    1. Maternal hypotension, low forceps birth, need to remain flat in bed for some hours after birth.
    2. Loss of bearing-down reflex, depression of contractions, maternal hypotension, fetal bradycardia, low forceps birth.
    3. Loss of bearing-down reflex, depression of contractions, maternal hypotension, fetal bradycardia, low forceps birth, postnatal bladder atony, postnatal uterine atony.
    4. Depression of contractions, maternal hypotension.

37. When a parturient is given a saddle block (low spinal) anesthesia, the nurse can expect:
    1. Loss of bearing-down reflex, maternal hypotension, low forceps birth, need to remain flat in bed for some hours after birth.
    2. Fetal bradycardia, low forceps birth, postnatal uterine atony, need to remain flat in bed for some hours after birth.
    3. Loss of bearing-down reflex, low forceps birth, postnatal bladder atony, postnatal uterine atony.
    4. Loss of bearing-down reflex, maternal hypotension, low forceps birth, need to remain flat in bed for some hours after birth, fetal bradycardia, postnatal uterine atony, postnatal bladder atony.

38. A patient is receiving tetracycline preoperatively in preparation for bowel surgery. Which common side effect should the nurse instruct the patient to expect with tetracycline?
    1. Urticaria.
    2. Urinary retention.
    3. Jaundice.
    4. Deafness.

39. The following activities have been planned for a patient who is mute and autistic. In which activity will it be important for the nursing staff to take precautionary measures for a common side effect of Thorazine (chlorpromazine), which has been prescribed for this patient?
    1. Shopping in an enclosed mall after lunch.
    2. Attending the symphony on Wednesday evening.
    3. A day at the beach, if the weather permits.
    4. A morning at the art museum.

40. Some patients who are on phenothiazines are also given benztropine mesylate (Cogentin). The nurse administers this medication in order to:
    1. Prevent skin reactions.
    2. Increase the effectiveness of the phenothiazines.
    3. Decrease motor restlessness.
    4. Reduce extrapyramidal side effects.

41. A patient has been on IM fluphenazine (Prolixin) for 3 years now. This patient has recently complained of frequent sore throats and malaise. What potentially serious side effect might these symptoms indicate to the nurse?
    1. Agranulocytosis.
    2. Akathisia.
    3. Dystonia.
    4. Dyskinesia.

42. When nialamide (Niamid) or isocarboxazid (Marplan) is administered, what must the nurse know about the effects of these drugs?
    1. They lower the threshold for seizures.
    2. They potentiate the effects of many other drugs and common foods.
    3. They decrease muscular contractions.
    4. They commonly cause obstructive jaundice.

43. Lithium salts are frequently used to treat manic disorders. What side effect is the nurse *least* likely to observe?
    1. Slurred speech.
    2. Twitching and athetotic movements.
    3. Motor weakness.
    4. Tardive dyskinesia.

44. A 9-month-old patient has been diagnosed with Hirschsprung's disease. At this time, the child is admitted to the hospital for a temporary colostomy; preoperatively, the doctor orders kanamycin. The nurse caring for this child should know that kanamycin is being given to:
    1. Increase peristalsis.
    2. Decrease amount of GI secretions.
    3. Promote passage of stool and flatus.
    4. Decrease number of intestinal flora.

45. A 22-month-old patient is admitted to the pediatrics unit for observation following accidental ingestion of 17 children's acetaminophen (Tylenol) caplets. In the first 2–3 days following this child's admission, it is essential that the nurse plan to observe the child closely for signs of:
    1. Hepatic failure.
    2. Renal failure.
    3. Hyperthermia.
    4. Hemorrhage.

46. In an acetaminophen (Tylenol) overdose situation, the nurse should have on hand the antidote to acetaminophen, which is:
    1. Acetylcysteine (Mucomyst).
    2. Potassium chloride.
    3. Aspirin.
    4. Heparin.

47. The doctor orders aminophylline, 100 mg via IV, for a child who is having an acute asthmatic attack. The nurse should know that the main reason the doctor ordered aminophylline is because it is a(n):
    1. Bronchodilator.
    2. Anticholinergic.
    3. Expectorant.
    4. Mucolytic agent.

48. The nurse is to administer 100 mg of aminophylline IV. The ampule contains 500 mg (gr 7½) of aminophylline in 10 mL of solution. How much solution should the nurse withdraw from the ampule?
    1. 2 mL.
    2. 4 mL.
    3. 6 mL.
    4. 8 mL.

49. While aminophylline is infusing, the nurse should plan to closely monitor the patient's:

    1. Level of consciousness.
    2. Blood pressure.
    3. Cardiac rhythm.
    4. Temperature.

50. The nurse should know that, to prevent future asthmatic attacks, a patient will most likely receive:
    1. Theophylline.
    2. Cromolyn sodium.
    3. Prednisone.
    4. Diphenhydramine.

51. A 15-year-old patient is admitted to the hospital with a diagnosis of infectious hepatitis (type A). To protect other members of this patient's family who have been exposed to infectious hepatitis, the nurse should explain that they may be given:
    1. Amoxicillin/clavulanate potassium (Augmentin).
    2. Sulfisoxazole.
    3. Rifampin.
    4. Immune serum globulin.

52. A 17-month-old child has retropharyngeal abscess and is to receive ampicillin four times a day. The child weighs 15 kg (33 lb). The nurses' reference indicates that the correct dosage is 75 mg/kg/day. Which dose should the nurse give to this patient at 10 A.M.?
    1. 11 mg.
    2. 28 mg.
    3. 280 mg.
    4. 1125 mg.

53. A 4-year-old patient is scheduled for repair of left undescended testicle. To administer a pentobarbital sodium (Nembutal) suppository preoperatively to this patient, in which position should the nurse place him?
    1. Prone with legs abducted.
    2. Sitting on a potty seat.
    3. Supine with foot of bed elevated.
    4. Side-lying with upper leg flexed.

54. A 4-year-old boy appears very anxious and frightened prior to receiving a rectal suppository as a preoperative medication. Which statement by the nurse would be most appropriate in helping the child take this medication?
    1. "Be a big kid! Everyone's waiting for you."
    2. "You look so scared. Want to know a secret? This won't hurt a bit!"
    3. "Lie still now and I'll let you have one of your presents before you even have your operation."
    4. "Take a nice, big, deep breath and then let me hear you count to five."

55. A 10-year-old patient is scheduled for an appendectomy. In preparing this child's preop injections, which size needle should the nurse select to administer this child's IM injection?
    1. 25 G, ⅝ in.
    2. 22 G, 1 in.
    3. 20 G, 1½ in.
    4. 18 G, 1½ in.

❏ Answers/Rationale

1. **(2)** Prior to administering any narcotic, the nurse should assess the type, location, and intensity of pain, as well as factors that seem to precipitate or relieve it. Meperidine, like morphine, has hypotensive and respiratory depressant effects. Positioning in anticipation of respiratory changes is not indicated **(No. 1)**. Pain and discomfort are subjective symptoms that are always real to the patient **(No. 3)**. Based on the information gained

in No. 2, it is then possible to decide whether the patient needs supportive measures (such as back rub or position change as in **No. 4**), the bedpan, and/or the administration of a narcotic. **AS,3,PhI**

2. **(2)** Neostigmine bromide (Prostigmin) is an anticholinesterase. It enhances bladder tone and contraction, enabling complete emptying of the bladder. It is also used in the treatment of myasthenia gravis. Bethanecol chloride (Urecholine) is an example of a cholinergic drug **(No. 1)**, also used to treat postoperative urinary retention. Atropine is an example of an anticholinergic drug **(No. 3)**, which would act to inhibit initiation of urination. Beta blockers **(No. 4)** such as propranolol do not affect the bladder. **PL,8,PhI**

3. **(2)** Salicylates, particularly acetylsalicylic acid (aspirin), are given in divided doses after each meal and at bedtime for their analgesic (reduced pain), anti-inflammatory (reduced swelling), and antipyretic (reduced fever) effects. **No. 1** is incorrect because relief of pain was already described in the question. **Nos. 3 and 4** are incorrect because salicylates neither inhibit nor stimulate the autonomic nervous system synapses. **IMP,3,PhI**

4. **(2)** Digoxin increases the force and velocity of cardiac contraction and slows the heart rate by delaying conduction through the atrioventricular node. The hemodynamic effects of its action include increased cardiac output, decreased right atrial and venous pressures, decreased left ventricular filling pressure, and increased excretion of sodium and water. Epinephrine **(No. 1)** increases the force of cardiac contractions but also increases heart rate, which in this case would increase cardiac embarrassment. Furosemide (Lasix) **(No. 3)** is a rapidly acting diuretic that enhances excretion of sodium and water. However, although its use is indicated to reduce fluid volume during the acute phase of pulmonary edema, it has no known direct effects on the cardiac musculature. Hydralazine **(No. 4)** is a peripheral vasodilator used in hypertensive therapy. It is not indicated in this situation. **PL,6,PhI**

5. **(3)** The best indicator that digoxin has been effective in strengthening cardiac contraction and increasing glomerular filtration is a decrease in heart rate (vagal effect) and increased urinary output. As a result of these drug effects, cardiac output is improved, raising blood pressure and decreasing pulmonary congestion. **Nos. 1, 2, and 4** are only partially correct. **EV,6,PhI**

6. **(2)** Theophylline relaxes bronchial smooth muscles, which helps to relieve the wheezing and coughing associated with bronchospasm. Side effects are rare, but the earliest signs of overdose are usually anorexia, nausea, and vomiting. Tachycardia **(No. 1)**, restlessness and tremors **(No. 3)**, headache **(No. 4)**, and insomnia are side effects associated with catecholamine bronchodilators, such as ephedrine and isoproterenol. **IMP,6,PhI**

7. **(2)** Furosemide is a rapidly acting diuretic with a peak action in 1–2 hours and a duration of 6–8 hours. The

peak time is too rapid for **No. 1** and too long for **Nos. 3 and 4**. **EV,8,PhI**

8. **(1)** Sodium polystyrene sulfonate (Kayexalate) is a cation-exchange resin. As it passes along the intestine or is retained in the colon after enema administration, sodium ions are partially released and replaced by potassium ions, allowing for fecal excretion of potassium ions. This drug is extremely unpalatable and may be administered in syrup, chilled, or mixed in the diet, and if necessary, administered directly into the stomach per nasogastric tube. Side effects of administration include anorexia, nausea, vomiting, constipation, hypokalemia, hypocalcemia, and sodium retention. **Nos. 2, 3, and 4** are not actions of sodium polystyrene sulfonate. **IMP,8,PhI**

9. **(1)** Ideally, oral iron preparations should be taken on an empty stomach **(No. 2)**. However, they tend to irritate the gastric mucosa, so they should be administered with or immediately after meals to ensure patient compliance. Thus **Nos. 2, 3, and 4** are not the best answers. Patients may complain of constipation or loose stools. Stools will change color (dark green to black). Ferrous sulfate is apt to deposit on teeth and gums, so frequent oral hygiene is necessary, and therapy will need to continue even after hemoglobin levels return to normal, to ensure adequate iron stores in the body. **PL,4,PhI**

10. **(1)** Toxic doses of neomycin may result in eighth cranial nerve damage much like that produced by streptomycin. Kidney damage may also occur, extending from milk albuminuria to elevation in blood urea nitrogen. Nausea **(No. 2)** is common with ingestion of antibiotics, though not specific to neomycin. Erythromycin most commonly causes nausea, vomiting, and diarrhea **(No. 3)**. Anaphylactic reactions **(No. 4)** are associated most commonly with penicillin administration. **EV,2,PhI**

11. **(2)** Morphine strongly depresses the medullary respiratory centers. Therefore, before administering the narcotic, the nurse should assess the patient's respiratory rate and depth to prevent severe respiratory depression. **Nos. 1, 3, and 4** are not affected by morphine. **AS,6,PhI**

12. **(1)** Spironolactone (Aldactone) is an aldosterone inhibitor, inhibiting the effects of hyperaldosteronemia, which is common in cirrhosis. This drug safely increases sodium and water excretion but does not cause concomitant losses of potassium as do other diuretics. For this reason, potassium supplements are not generally given to the patient. An example of a carbonic anhydrase inhibitor **(No. 2)** is acetazolamide (Diamox); of a thiazide **(No. 3)** is chlorothiazide (Diuril) or hydrochlorothiazide (HydroDIURIL); and of an osmotic diuretic **(No. 4)** is mannitol. **IMP,6,PhI**

13. **(2)** Potassium chloride. Spironolactone (Aldactone) is an aldosterone inhibitor, inhibiting the effects of hyperaldosteronemia, which is common in cirrhosis. This drug safely increases sodium and water excretion but does not cause concomitant losses of potassium as do other diuretics. For this reason, potassium supplements are not generally given to the patient. Spironolactone would not contraindicate the administration of vitamin B_6 **(No. 1)**, ascorbic acid **(No. 3)**, or calcium gluconate **(No. 4)**. **PL,4,PhI**

14. **(3)** The primary objective in giving corticosteroids is to lessen the symptoms of the disease process. Most patients initially respond well to these drugs; however, as the disease progresses, higher and higher doses are required to relieve symptoms. **Nos. 1 and 2** are incorrect because corticosteroids have no curative effects, only palliative. Many of the side effects of corticosteroid administration are due to the effects of these drugs on glu-

---

Key to codes following rationales Nursing process: **AS,** Assessment; **AN,** Analysis; **PL,** Plan; **IMP,** Implementation; **EV,** Evaluation. Category of human function: **1,** Protective; **2,** Sensory-perceptual; **3,** Comfort, Rest, Activity, and Mobility; **4,** Nutrition; **5,** Growth and Development; **6,** Fluid-Gas Transport; **7,** Psychosocial-Cultural; **8,** Elimination. Client need: **SECE,** Safe, Effective Care Environment; **PhI,** Physiologic Integrity; **PsI,** Psychosocial Integrity; **HPM,** Health Promotion/Maintenance. See appendices for full explanation.

Pharmacology

cose metabolism (**No. 4**), such as Cushing-like syndrome. **AN,3,PhI**

15. **(3)** Side effects of prednisone therapy mimic the manifestations of Cushing's syndrome (moon facies, abnormal fat deposits, purple striae, hyperglycemia with glucosuria, hypertension, obesity, and emotional disturbances). Side effects of other drugs utilized in the management of rheumatoid arthritis include tinnitus (**No. 1**), nausea, vomiting (**No. 4**), headaches, and vertigo with indomethacin (Indocin) administration, and dermatitis ranging from erythema to exfoliative dermatitis (**No. 2**) with gold salts therapy. **EV,8,PhI**

16. **(4)** Although the primary use of propantheline bromide in many clinical situations involving the gastrointestinal tract is to reduce gastric secretions and intestinal hypermobility, it is used in gallbladder disease because of its antispasmodic effects on the gallbladder and bile duct. **No. 1** is therefore correct, but *not the best* choice. **Nos. 2 and 3** are incorrect because propantheline bromide does not reduce bile secretions; its calming effect on gastric motility does not reduce the amount of chyme entering the duodenum. **IMP,4,PhI**

17. **(3)** Morphine sulfate causes spasms of the sphincter of Oddi, thereby increasing intraductal pressures and abdominal pain. Papaverine and meperidine, both synthetic opiates, as well as nitroglycerin may be administered to relieve pain associated with gallbladder disease. **No. 1** is incorrect because the effect of morphine is to increase spasms in the gallbladder. **No. 2**, though correct, is not the *best* answer. Opiates are withheld when a patient has an acute abdomen and the diagnosis is unknown or tentative. In this case, the patient has an established history of gallbladder disease and rather specific symptomatology. **No. 4** is incorrect, in that although morphine does relax vascular smooth muscle, this effect does not increase bile synthesis in the liver. **EV,3,PhI**

18. **(4)** Hydrochlorothiazide is a thiazide diuretic that promotes the excretion of water, sodium, and chloride by inhibiting the reabsorption of sodium ions in the distal ascending limb of the loop of Henle and in the distal convoluted tubule of the nephron. Natriuresis promotes the secondary loss of potassium, so this drug is classified as potassium wasting. Spironolactone is an example of an aldosterone inhibitor and is a potassium-sparing diuretic (**Nos. 1 and 3**). Acetazolemide (Diamox) is the most frequently employed carbonic anhydrase inhibitor (**No. 2**). **EV,8,PhI**

19. **(3)** Hydrochlorothiazide is a thiazide diuretic that promotes the excretion of water, sodium, and chloride by inhibiting the reabsorption of sodium ions in the distal ascending limb of the loop of Henle and in the distal convoluted tubule of the nephron. Natriuresis promotes the secondary loss of potassium, so this drug is classified as potassium wasting. **No. 1** describes the effect of the carbonic anhydrase inhibitors, e.g., acetazolemide (Diamox). **No. 2** would be the effect of the potassium-sparing diuretics such as spironolactone (Aldactone). Finally, **No. 4** is the site for the osmotic diuretics, e.g., mannitol, urea. **AN,8,PhI**

20. **(3)** Thiazide diuretics promote the excretion of sodium, chloride, bicarbonate, and potassium. However, chloride excretion tends to be proportionately greater than bicarbonate excretion, so therapy may result in hypochloremic alkalosis. Hyponatremia, not hypernatremia (**No. 1**) occurs. Hypokalemia, not hyperkalemia (**No. 2**), may develop, especially with brisk diuresis. Supplemental KCl therapy and/or increased dietary intake of potas-

sium is indicated with thiazide therapy. **No. 4** is incorrect because it says hypouricemia and hyperuricemia results, which may precipitate frank gout. **AS,8,PhI**

21. **(3)** The formula for finding the correct answer is: dose desired/dose on hand = x/amount on hand.
$$18/20 = x/5$$
$$20x = 18(5)$$
$$x = \frac{18(5)}{20}$$
$$x = 4.5 \text{ mL}$$
IMP,2,SECE

22. **(3)** Rifampin is the drug of choice for the prophylactic treatment of *Hemophilus influenzae* meningitis. The usual dose is 20 mg/kg/d in a single dose for 4 days. Amoxicillin/clavulanate potassium (Augmentin) (**No. 1**), sulfisoxazole (**No. 2**), and immune serum globulin (**No. 4**) are not the drugs of choice to prevent *H. influenzae* meningitis. **IMP,1,HPM**

23. **(4)** Pancreatin (Viokase) is an exocrine pancreatic supplement used as a digestive aid in cystic fibrosis; its primary use is to promote the absorption of fats. Pancreatin has no effect on the absorption of glucose (**No. 1**), vitamin C (**No. 2**), or sodium chloride (**No. 3**). **AN,4,SECE**

24. **(4)** The only acceptable way to identify a 5-year-old patient is to have a parent or another staff member identify the patient. **No. 1** is incorrect because most 5-year-old children, under the age of reason, cannot legally be held accountable for self-identification. **No. 2** is incorrect unless the nurse is sure this adult is this patient's parent. Also, it would be better to ask, "What is the child's name?" **No. 3** is also incorrect; children cannot legally be held accountable for identifying other children. **IMP,1,SECE**

25. **(3)** The correct answer is found using the following formula:
dose desired/dose on hand = x/amount on hand.
$$0.125/0.05 = x/1$$
$$0.05x = 0.125(1)$$
$$x = \frac{0.125(1)}{0.05}$$
$$x = 2.5 \text{ mL}$$
IMP,6,SECE

26. **(4)** The recommended procedure for administering eye drops to any patient calls for the drops to be placed in the middle of the lower conjunctival sac. Placing drops directly onto the sclera (**No. 1**) is irritating and less effective. Placing drops in the inner canthus of the eye (**No. 2**) may lead to systemic effects from absorption via tear ducts. Placing drops in the outer canthus of the eye (**No. 3**) results in loss of medication and may also cause infection. **IMP,2,HPM**

27. **(1)** Maximum absorption of Fer-in-Sol occurs between meals, when hydrochloric acid is freely available in the stomach. When given before meals (**No. 2**), it may cause GI upset, which will interfere with eating. When given during meals (**No. 3**) or after meals (**No. 4**), there is slowed absorption of the drug; however, GI upset is minimized. **PL,4,SECE**

28. **(1)** When oral iron preparations are given correctly, the stools normally turn dark green/black in color. Parents of children receiving this medication should be advised that this side effect indicates the medication is being absorbed and is working well. **Nos. 2, 3, and 4** would only increase the parent's anxiety and lead them to believe that the stool color was abnormal. **EV,8,SECE**

29. **(1)** Normal pregnancy alters vaginal pH and favors the growth of yeast organisms (*Candida*). **No. 2** is wrong be-

cause age is not a factor in the development of yeast vaginitis. **No. 3** is wrong because ingestion of large amounts of carbohydrates does not alter vaginal pH. **No. 4** is wrong because sickle cell anemia is not a predisposing factor in yeast vaginitis. **AS,5,PhI**

30. **(2)** Nystatin is the drug of choice for treatment of vaginal infections caused by *Candida albicans*. **No. 1** is wrong because metronidazole is used in treatment of trichomonal vaginitis. **No. 3** is wrong because podophyllin is used in treating venereal warts. **No. 4** is wrong because bacitracin ointment is used in treating skin infections. **IMP,1,PhI**

31. **(4)** Erythromycin or tetracycline is commonly used in treating penicillin-allergic patients with venereal disease. **No. 1** is wrong because streptomycin is used in treating tuberculosis. **No. 2** is wrong because sulfisoxazole is most commonly used to treat urinary tract infections. Further, its use is contraindicated in pregnancy. **No. 3** is wrong because chloramphenicol is used in treating *Salmonella* infections and is also contraindicated during pregnancy. **PL,1,PhI**

32. **(4)** Prolonged, heavy doses of oral antibiotics are irritating to the GI tract and result in nausea and diarrhea; yeast infections are common sequelae of antibiotic therapy. **No. 1** is wrong; tinnitus is a symptom of streptomycin toxicity. **No. 2** is wrong because abdominal pain is more commonly associated with sulfisoxazole therapy. **No. 3** is wrong because glossitis and stomatitis are associated with chloramphenicol therapy. **IMP,1,PhI**

33. **(3)** Ritodrine is the drug of choice when attempting to inhibit labor. **No. 1** is wrong because magnesium sulfate is used most commonly in treating preeclampsia/eclampsia. **No. 2** is wrong because betamethasone is used to stimulate production of fetal pulmonary surfactant. **No. 4** is wrong because bromocryptine mesylate is used to inhibit lactation in nonbreastfeeding mothers. **PL,5,PhI**

34. **(3)** Persistent maternal tachycardia (over 140 bpm) is a sign of impending pulmonary edema in patients receiving beta-mimetic drugs; fetal tachycardia is a common result of ritodrine therapy. **No. 1** is wrong because ritodrine commonly results in maternal hypotension. **No. 2** is wrong because the common fetal reaction to beta-mimetics is tachycardia. **No. 4** is wrong because ritodrine is given to reduce uterine hyperirritability and threatened premature labor. **EV,5,PhI**

35. **(3)** Depression of contractions and fetal bradycardia are expected effects of paracervical block. **No. 1** is incorrect because the bearing-down reflex is not affected by this anesthesia and therefore low forceps birth is usually not needed. **No. 2** is incorrect because maternal blood pressure and postnatal uterine contractility are not affected by paracervical block. **No. 4** is incorrect because the bearing-down reflex is not affected, and therefore forceps birth is usually not needed. **AN,5,PhI**

36. **(3)** The medication never mixes with cerebral spinal fluid, and therefore there is no need for the woman to lie flat for several hours after receiving this form of anesthesia **(No. 1)**. **Nos. 2 and 4** are incorrect because their lists are incomplete. **AN,5,PhI**

37. **(4)** All of the listed effects are to be expected following spinal anesthesia: loss of bearing-down reflex, depression of contractions, maternal hypotension, fetal bradycardia, low forceps birth, postnatal bladder atony, need to remain flat in bed for some hours after birth, and postnatal uterine atony. **Nos. 1, 2, and 3** are incorrect because their lists are incomplete. **AN,1,PhI**

38. **(1)** Hypersensitivity reactions (urticaria and hives) are common drug reactions. Photosensitization (exaggerated sunburn) in certain hypersensitive persons may also occur with exposure to direct or artificial sunlight during tetracycline use. Urinary retention **(No. 2)** is a side effect of anticholinergic and antihistamine drugs. Jaundice **(No. 3)** from drug toxicity is more common with isoniazid (INH), acetaminophen, phenothiazines (chlorpromazine [Thorazine]), sulfonamides, and antidiabetic drugs (e.g., tolbutamide [Orinase]). Hepatotoxicity may occur with tetracycline, but it is less common. **No. 4**, deafness (ototoxicity), is a major side effect of the aminoglycoside antibiotics (e.g., gentamicin, neomycin, streptomycin, tobramycin) and diuretics, such as furosemide and ethacrynic acid. **IMP,1,PhI**

39. **(3)** The patient needs to be protected against photosensitivity and dermatitis when exposed to the sun; a sunscreen preparation should be applied to exposed parts of the skin, and the patient should wear long sleeves and cover-up clothing. **Nos. 1, 2, and 4** refer to *indoor* activities, where there is no danger of sunburn. **PL,3,PhI**

40. **(4)** This is the best choice as it *encompasses* **No. 3**. **Nos. 1 and 2** are definitely incorrect. **PL,7,PhI**

41. **(1)** Blood dyscrasias often are overlooked when first symptoms of possible adverse drug effects appear in the form of a minor cold. **Nos. 2, 3, and 4** refer to extrapyramidal tract symptoms that are *not* life-threatening. **AN,7,PhI**

42. **(2)** Hypertensive crisis can be precipitated by combining this drug with common cold medications and foods high in tyramine or pressor amines (yogurt, Chianti wine, cheese, Coca-Cola, and coffee, for example). All other options are incorrect. **EV,7,PhI**

43. **(4)** This effect is seen in patients taking a *major tranquilizer*. All of the other options *are likely* side effects of lithium salts. **EV,7,PhI**

44. **(4)** Kanamycin is an antibiotic that, although poorly absorbed in the GI tract, is often used as part of bowel prep prior to abdominal surgery. It acts as a bactericidal agent, thus significantly decreasing the number of intestinal flora and reducing risk of peritonitis in the postop period. Kanamycin does not increase peristalsis **(No. 1)**, promote passage of stool or flatus **(No. 3)**, or decrease amount of GI secretions **(No. 2)**. **AN,1,SECE**

45. **(1)** The major toxic effect of an overdose of acetaminophen (Tylenol) is liver failure; liver function should be closely monitored during the first 2–3 days following the ingestion of acetaminophen. Renal failure **(No. 2)** may occur as a **late** complication of acetaminophen toxicity, as may bleeding and hemorrhage **(No. 4)**. Hyperthermia **(No. 3)** is not a major symptom of this type of ingestion; it is more common in salicylate ingestions. **PL,1,PhI**

46. **(1)** Acetylcysteine (Mucomyst) is the antidote for acetaminophen poisoning; it serves to protect the liver. It is usually given orally in a carbonated beverage (e.g., cola), but it can also be given via nasogastric tube. A loading dose is followed by q4h doses until a total of 18 doses have been given. KCl **(No. 2)**, aspirin **(No. 3)**, and heparin **(No. 4)** are not antidotes for acetaminophen and do not serve to protect the child's liver. **IMP,1,SECE/PhI**

47. **(1)** Aminophylline, a bronchodilator that acts as a smooth-muscle relaxant, is used to prevent and relieve symptoms of bronchial asthma. Anticholinergics **(No. 2)** are used to treat muscle spasms along the GI tract. Aminophylline is neither an expectorant **(No. 3)**, which would assist in the removal of mucus from the respiratory tract, nor a mucolytic agent **(No. 4)**, which would help thin out viscid secretions. **AN,6,SECE/PhI**

48. **(1)** The formula for finding the correct answer is:
dose desired/dose on hand = x/amount on hand.

$$100/500 = x/10$$
$$500x = 100(10)$$
$$x = \frac{100(10)}{500}$$
$$x = 2 \text{ mL}$$

IMP,6,SECE

49. **(3)** A transient side effect of IV aminophylline is an increase in heart rate; toxic effects include a prolonged increase in heart rate and abnormalities in cardiac rhythm. While receiving IV aminophylline, the patient should be on a cardiac monitor, and both rate and rhythm should be closely monitored and documented by the nurse. Aminophylline may also cause a transient change in the blood pressure **(No. 2)**, but this is not as much a concern as the patient's cardiac rhythm. Aminophylline should not affect level of consciousness **(No. 1)** or temperature **(No. 4)**; thus, there is no particular need for the nurse to monitor these specifically at this time. **PL,6,SECE**

50. **(2)** Cromolyn sodium, an uncategorized drug used as an adjunct in the treatment of asthma, is used only after the acute attack is relieved; its primary intent is prophylaxis, i.e., to prevent future attacks. Cromolyn is used in an inhaler. It is absorbed into the systemic circulation after its inhalation into the lungs. It acts on the mast cells and also inhibits the release of histamine. Theophylline **(No. 1)**, prednisone **(No. 3)**, and diphenhydramine **(No. 4)** do not prevent future asthmatic attacks and have no prophylactic value. **AN,6,SECE**

51. **(4)** Immune serum globulin (ISG) offers the family members some protection against type A infectious hepatitis. It contains antibodies against the organism and will aid the family members in resisting this infectious disease. Amoxicillin/clavulanate potassium (Augmentin) **(No. 1)** and sulfisoxazole **(No. 2)** are antibiotics used for a variety of infections, but they would not prevent hepatitis. Rifampin **(No. 3)** is used prophylactically for *Hemophilus influenzae* meningitis and to treat TB but, again, would not prevent hepatitis. **IMP,1,HPM**

52. **(3)** The nurse should give 280 mg at 10 A.M. Using the formula of 75 mg/kg/d, 75 mg × 15 kg = 1125 mg per day, to be divided into 4 doses. 1125 mg divided by 4 doses = 280 mg per dose. **IMP,1,SECE**

53. **(4)** The recommended position to administer rectal medications to children is side-lying with the upper leg flexed. This position allows the nurse to safely and effectively administer the medication while promoting comfort for the child. If the child were to lie prone **(No. 1)**, the nurse could not administer the medication as safely or effectively, even if the legs were abducted; further, this position would most likely cause the child some discomfort. If the child were sitting on a potty seat **(No. 2)**, the nurse could not reach the rectum to insert the suppository, and it is very likely the suppository would be immediately expelled. If the child were to lie supine **(No. 3)**, again the nurse could not administer the medication comfortably for the child. **IMP,1,SECE**

54. **(4)** Preschool children commonly experience fears and fantasies regarding invasive procedures. The nurse should attempt to momentarily distract the child with a simple task that can be easily accomplished while the child remains in the side-lying position. The suppository can be slipped into place while the child is counting, and then the nurse can praise the child for cooperating, while holding the buttocks together to prevent expulsion of the suppository. The nurse should not pressure the child into acting like a "big kid" **(No. 1)** in such a frightening situation (use of the word "kid" is also not appropriate). The nurse should not lie, breaking a trust by saying something "won't hurt a bit" **(No. 2)**. Finally, the nurse should never "bribe" **(No. 3)** a child with gifts to ensure cooperation. **IMP,5,PsI**

55. **(2)** In selecting the correct needle to administer an IM injection to a school-age child, the nurse should always look at the child and use judgment in evaluating muscle mass and amount of subcutaneous fat. In this case, in the absence of further data, the nurse would be most correct in selecting a needle gauge and length appropriate for the "average" school-age child. A medium-gauge needle (22 G) that is 1 in. long would be most appropriate. A ⅝ in. needle **(No. 1)** would be too small, and a 1½ in. (18–20 G) needle would be too long and unnecessarily large **(Nos. 3 and 4)**. A 23 or 25 G needle would be too thin to use on most school-age children **(No. 1)** and would be better suited for use with a newborn or an infant. **IMP,1,SECE**

Unit 5

Common Diagnostic Procedures, Treatments, and Nursing Care

❑ Common Diagnostic Procedures

I. Noninvasive diagnostic procedures are those procedures that provide an indirect assessment of organ size, shape, and/or function; these procedures are considered safe, are easily reproducible, need less complex equipment for recording, and generally do not require the written consent of patient and/or guardian.

◆ **A. General nursing responsibilities:**
1. Reduce patient's anxieties and provide emotional support by:
   a. Explaining purpose and procedure of test.
   b. Answering questions regarding safety of the procedure, as indicated.
   c. Remaining with patient during procedure when possible.
2. Utilize procedures in the collection of specimens that avoid contamination and facilitate diagnosis—clean-catch urine and sputum specimens after deep breathing and coughing, for example.

B. Graphic studies of heart and brain
1. *Electrocardiogram (ECG)*—graphic record of electrical activity generated by the heart during depolarization and repolarization; *used to* diagnose abnormal cardiac rhythms and coronary heart disease.
2. *Echocardiography* (ultrasound cardiography)—graphic record of motions produced by cardiac structures as high-frequency sound vibrations are echoed through chest wall into the heart; transesophageal echo-

cardiography produces a clearer image, particularly in obese, barrel chested, or COPD patients; *used to* demonstrate valvular or other structural deformities, detect pericardial effusion, diagnose tumors and cardiomegaly, or evaluate prosthetic valve function.
3. *Phonocardiogram*—graphic record of heart sounds; *used to* keep a permanent record of patient's heart sounds before and after cardiac surgery.
4. *Electroencephalogram (EEG)*—graphic record of the electrical potentials generated by the physiologic activity of the brain; *used to* detect surface lesions or tumors of the brain and presence of epilepsy.
5. *Echoencephalogram*—beam of pulsed ultrasound is passed through the head, and returning echoes are graphically recorded; *used to* detect shifts in cerebral midline structures caused by subdural hematomas, intracerebral hemorrhage, or tumors.

C. Roentgenologic studies (X ray)
1. *Chest—used to* determine size, contour, and position of the heart; size, location, and nature of pulmonary lesions; disorders of thoracic bones or soft tissue; diaphragmatic contour and excursion; pleural thickening or effusions; and gross changes in the caliber or distribution of pulmonary vasculature.
2. *Kidney, ureter, and bladder (KUB)—used to* determine size, shape, and position of kidneys, ureters, and bladder.
3. *Mammography*—examination of the breast with or without the injection of radiopaque

dye into the ducts of the mammary gland; *used to* determine the presence of tumors or cysts. *Patient preparation:* no deodorant, perfume, powders, or ointment in underarm area on day of X ray. May be uncomfortable.

4. *Skull*—outline configuration and density of brain tissues and vascular markings; *used to* determine the size and location of intracranial calcifications, tumors, abscesses, or vascular lesions.

D. **Roentgenologic studies (fluoroscopy)**—require the ingestion or injection of a radiopaque substance to visualize the target organ.

◆ 1. *Additional nursing responsibilities* may include:

a. Administration of *enemas or cathartics* prior to the procedure and a laxative after.

b. Keeping the patient *NPO* 6–12 h prior to examination; check with MD regarding oral medications.

c. Ascertaining patient's *history of allergies* or allergic reactions (e.g., iodine, seafood).

d. Observing for *allergic* reactions to contrast medium following procedure.

e. Providing fluid and food following procedure, to counteract dehydration.

f. Observing stool for color and consistency until barium passes.

2. Common fluoroscopic examinations:

a. *Upper GI*—ingestion of barium sulfate or meglumine diatrizoate (Gastrografin, a white, chalky, radiopaque substance), followed by fluoroscopic and X-ray examination; *used to* determine:

(1) Patency and caliber of *esophagus;* may also detect esophageal varices.

(2) Mobility and thickness of *gastric* walls, presence of ulcer craters, filling defects due to tumors, pressures from outside the stomach, and patency of pyloric valve.

(3) Rate of passage in small bowel and presence of structural abnormalities.

b. *Lower GI*—rectal instillation of barium sulfate followed by fluoroscopic and X-ray examination; *used to* determine contour and mobility of colon and presence of any space-occupying tumors; perform

◆ before upper GI. *Patient preparation:* explain purpose; *no food after evening meal* the evening before test; *stool softeners, laxatives, enemas, and suppositories* to cleanse the bowel before the test; *NPO after midnight* prior to test; oral medications *not* permitted day of test. *After completion of exam:* food, *increased liquid* intake, and rest; *laxatives for at least 2 d* or until stools are normal in color and consistency.

c. *Cholecystogram* (done if gallbladder not seen with ultrasound)—ingestion of organic iodine contrast substance Telepaque (iopanoic acid), or Oragrafin (preparation of calcium or sodium salt of ipodate) followed in 12 h by X-ray visualization; gallbladder disease is indicated with *poor* or no visualization of the bladder; accurate only if GI and liver function is intact; perform before barium

◆ enema or upper GI. *Patient preparation:* explain purpose; administer large amount of *water* with contrast capsules; *low-fat meal* evening *before* X ray; *oral laxative or stool softener after meal; no food* allowed after contrast capsules; water, tea, or coffee, with no cream or sugar, usually allowed. *After completion of exam:* fluids, food, and rest; observe for any signs of allergy to contrast capsules.

d. *Cholangiogram*—intravenous injection of a radiopaque contrast substance, followed by fluoroscopic and X-ray examination of the bile ducts; failure of the contrast substance to pass certain points in the bile duct pinpoints *obstruction.*

e. *Intravenous urography (IVU) or pyelography (IVP)*—injection of a radiopaque contrast substance, followed by fluoroscopic and X-ray films of kidneys and urinary tract; *used to* identify lesions in kidneys and ureters and provide a rough estimate of kidney function.

f. *Cystogram*—installation of radiopaque medium through a catheter into the bladder; *used to* visualize bladder wall and evaluate ureterovesical valves for reflux.

g. *Phlebography* (lower limb venography)—determines patency of the tibial-popliteal, superficial femoral–common femoral, and saphenous veins. A contrast medium is injected into the superficial and/or deep veins of the involved extremity, followed by X rays, while the leg is placed in a variety of positions; *used to* detect deep-vein thrombosis and to select a vein for use in arterial bypass grafting; localized clotting may result.

E. **Computerized axial tomography (CAT or CT scan)**—an X-ray beam sweeps around the body, allowing measurement of various tissue densities; provides clear radiographic definition of structures that are not visible by other techniques, permitting earlier diagnosis and treatment and more effective and efficient follow-up. Initial scan may be followed by "contrast enhancement" using an injection of an intravenous contrast agent (iodine), followed

◆ by a repeat scan. *Patient preparation:* instructions for eating before test vary. Clear liquids up to 2 h before are usually permitted.

F. Magnetic resonance imaging (MRI)—non-invasive, nonionic technique produces cross-sectional images by exposure to magnetic energy sources. Provides superior contrast of soft tissue, including healthy, benign, and malignant tissue, along with veins and arteries; utilizes no contrast medium; takes 30–90 min to complete; patient must *stay still* for periods
◆ of 5–20 min at a time. *Patient preparation:* patient can take food and medications except for low abdominal and pelvic studies (food/fluids withheld 4–6 h to decrease peristalsis). *Restrictions:* patients who have metal implants, permanent pacemakers, or implanted medication pumps such as insulin, or who are pregnant or on life support systems. Obese patients may not be able to have full body MRI because they may not fit in the scanner tunnel.

G. Multiple-gated acquisition scan (MUGA)—also known as blood pool imaging. Red blood cells are tagged with a radioactive isotope. A computer-operated camera takes sequential pictures of actual heart wall motion; *complement* to cardiac catheterization; *used to* determine valvular effectiveness, follow progress of heart disease, diagnose cardiac aneurysms, detect coronary artery disease, determine effects of cardiovascular drug therapy. No special preparation. Painless, except for
◆ injections. Wear *gloves* if contact with patient urine occurs within 24 h after scan.

H. Ultrasound (sonogram)—scanning by ultrasound is used to diagnose disorders of the thyroid, kidney, liver, uterus, gallbladder, fetus, and the intracranial structures in the neonate. It is not useful when visualization through air or bone is required (lung studies). In some hospitals the sonogram has taken the place of the oral cholecystogram in diagnosing gallbladder distention, bile duct distention, and
◆ calculi. *Patient preparation* is minimal, i.e., NPO for at least 8 h for gallbladder studies. No X radiation. Thirty-two ounces of water PO 30 min prior to studies of lower abdomen or uterus.

I. Pulmonary function studies
1. Ventilatory studies—utilization of a spirometer to determine how well the lung is ventilating.
   a. *Vital capacity (VC)*—largest amount of air that can be expelled after maximal inspiration.
      (1) *Normally* 4000–5000 mL.
      (2) Decreased in restrictive lung disease.
      (3) May be normal, slightly increased, or decreased in chronic obstructive lung disease.

   b. *Forced expiratory volume (FEV$_T$)*—percentage of vital capacity that can be forcibly expired in 1, 2, or 3 sec.
      (1) *Normally* 81–83% in 1 sec, 90–94% in 2 sec, and 95–97% in 3 sec.
      (2) *Decreased* values indicate expiratory airway obstruction.
   c. *Maximum breathing capacity (MBC)*—maximum amount of air that can be breathed in and out in 1 min with maximal rates and depths of respiration.
      (1) Best overall measurement of ventilatory ability.
      (2) *Reduced* in restrictive and chronic obstructive lung disease.
2. Diffusion studies—measure the rate of exchange of gases across alveolar membrane. Carbon monoxide single-breath, re-breathing, and steady-state techniques—utilized because of special affinity of hemoglobin for carbon monoxide; *decreased* when fluid is present in alveoli or when alveolar membranes are thick or fibrosed.

J. Sputum studies
1. Gross sputum evaluations—collection of sputum samples to ascertain quantity, consistency, color, and odor.
2. *Sputum smear*—sputum is smeared thinly on a slide so that it can be studied microscopically; *used to* determine cytologic changes (malignant cell) or presence of pathogenic bacteria, e.g., tubercle bacilli.
3. *Sputum culture*—sputum samples are implanted or inoculated into special media; *used to* diagnose pulmonary infections.
4. *Gastric lavage or analysis*—insertion of a nasogastric tube into the stomach to siphon out swallowed pulmonary secretions; *used to* detect organisms causing pulmonary infections; especially useful for detecting tubercle bacilli in children.

K. Examination of gastric contents
1. *Gastric analysis*—aspiration of the contents of the fasting stomach for analysis of free and total acid.
   a. Gastric acidity is generally *increased* in presence of duodenal ulcer.
   b. Gastric acidity is usually *decreased* in pernicious anemia, cancer of the stomach.
2. Stool specimens—*examined for* amount, consistency, color, character, and melena; *used to* determine presence of urobilinogen, fat, nitrogen, parasites, and other substances.

L. Thermography—a picture of the surface temperature of the skin using infrared photography (not ionizing radiation) detects the circulation pattern of areas in the breasts. Tumors produce more heat than normal breast tissue. Useful with large tumors, but may not detect small or deep lesions. Requires expensive equipment and is difficult to interpret accurately.

🔬 **M. Doppler ultrasonography**—*used to* measure blood flow in the major veins and arteries. The transducer of the test instrument is placed on the skin, sending out bursts of ultra-high-frequency sound. The ratio of ankle to brachial systolic pressure (API ≥1) provides information about vascular insufficiency. Sound varies with respiration and the Valsalva maneuver. No discomfort to the patient.

🔬 **N. Caloric stimulation test**—*used to* evaluate the vestibular portion of the eighth cranial nerve, identify the impairment or loss of thermally induced nystagmus. Reflex eye movements (nystagmus) result in response to cold or warm irrigations of the external auditory canal if the nerve is intact. A *diminished or absent* response occurs with Meniere's or acoustic neuroma. Nausea, vomiting, or dizziness can be precipitated by the test.

🔬 **O. 24-h urine collection:** a true and accurate evaluation of kidney function, primarily glomerular filtration. Substances excreted by the kidney are excreted at different rates, amounts, and times of day or night. Timed urine collection is done for protein, creatinine, electrolytes, urinary steroids, etc. A large container is used with or without preservative. Label with patient name, type of test, and exact time test starts and ends. Not usually necessary to measure urine. Have patient void, discard urine; test starts at this time. Have patient void as close to the end of the 24-h period as possible. If refrigeration is required, urine may be stored in iced container.

🔬 **P. Glucose testing:** to detect disorder of glucose metabolism, such as diabetes.
1. *Fasting (FBS):* Blood sample is drawn after a 12-h fast (usually overnight). H_2O is allowed. If diabetes is present, value will be >140 mg/dL.
2. *2-h postprandial (PPBS):* blood is taken after a meal. For best results, patient should be on a high CHO diet for 2–4 d before testing. Patient fasts overnight, eats a high CHO breakfast; blood sample is drawn 2 h after eating. Patient should rest during 2-h interval. Smoking and coffee may increase glucose level.
3. *Glucose tolerance test (GTT):* done when sugar in urine, or FBS or 2-h PPBS is not conclusive. A timed test, usually 2 h. High CHO diet is eaten 3 d before test. Blood is drawn after overnight fast. Patient drinks a very sweet glucose liquid. All of the solution must be taken. Blood and urine sample usually taken at 30 min, 1 h, 2 h, and sometimes 3 h after drinking solution. Blood glucose peaks in 30–60 min, and returns to normal, usually within 3 h.

II. Invasive diagnostic procedures—procedures that directly record the size, shape, or function of an organ and that are often complex or expensive or require utilization of highly trained personnel; these procedures may result in morbidity and occasionally mortality of the patient and therefore require the written consent of the patient or guardian.

◆ **A. General nursing responsibilities:**
1. *Prior to procedure:* institute measures to provide for patient's safety and emotional comfort.
   a. Have patient sign permit for procedure.
   b. Ascertain and report any patient history of allergy or allergic reactions.
   c. Explain procedure briefly, and accurately advise patient of any possible sensations, such as flushing or a warm feeling, as when a contrast medium is injected.
   d. Keep patient NPO 6–12 h before procedure if anesthesia is to be used.
   e. Allow patient to verbalize concerns, and note attitude toward procedure.
   f. Administer preprocedure sedative, as ordered.
   g. If procedure done at bedside:
      (1) Remain with patient, offering frequent reassurance.
      (2) Assist with optional positioning of patient.
      (3) Observe for indications of complications—shock, pain, or dyspnea.
2. *Following procedure:* institute measures to avoid complications and promote physical and emotional comfort.
   a. Observe and record vital signs.
   b. Check injection cut-down or biopsy sites for bleeding, infection, tenderness, or thrombosis.
      (1) Report untoward reactions to physician.
      (2) Apply warm compresses to ease discomfort, as ordered.
   c. If topical anesthetic is used during procedure (e.g., gastroscopy, bronchoscopy), do *not* give food or fluid until gag reflex returns.
   d. Encourage relaxation by allowing patient to discuss experience and verbalize feelings.

🔬 **B. Procedures to evaluate the cardiovascular system:**
1. *Angiocardiography*—intravenous injection of a radiopaque solution or dye for the purpose of studying its circulation through the patient's heart, lungs, and great vessels; *used to* check the competency of heart valves, diagnose congenital septal defects, detect occlusions or coronary arteries, confirm suspected diagnoses, and study heart

function and structure prior to cardiac surgery.

2. *Cardiac catheterization*—insertion of a radiopaque catheter into a vein to study the heart and great vessels.

   a. *Right-heart catheterization*—catheter is inserted through a cut-down in the antecubital vein into the superior vena cava and through the right atrium, ventricle, and into the pulmonary artery.

   b. *Left-heart catheterization*—catheter may be passed retrograde to the left ventricle through the brachial or femoral artery; it can be passed into the left atrium after right-heart catheterization by means of a special needle that punctures the septa; or it may be passed directly into the left ventricle by means of a posterior or anterior chest puncture.

   c. Cardiac catheterizations are *used to:*

     (1) Confirm diagnosis of heart disease and determine the extent of disease.

     (2) Determine existence and extent of congenital abnormalities.

     (3) Measure pressures in the heart chambers and great vessels.

     (4) Obtain estimate of cardiac output.

     (5) Obtain blood samples to measure oxygen content and determine presence of cardiac shunts.

 ◆ d. *Specific nursing interventions*

     (1) *Preprocedure patient teaching:*

       (a) Fatigue due to lying still for 3 h or more is a common complaint.

       (b) Some fluttery sensations may be felt—occur as catheter is passed backward into the left ventricle.

       (c) Flushed, warm feeling may occur when contrast medium is injected.

     (2) *Postprocedure observations:*

       (a) Monitor ECG pattern for arrhythmias.

       (b) Check extremities for color and temperature, peripheral pulses (femoral and dorsalis pedis) for quality.

3. *Angiography (arteriography)*—injection of a contrast medium into the arteries to study the vascular tree; *used to* determine obstructions or narrowing of peripheral arteries.

4. *Pericardiocentesis (pericardial aspiration)*—puncture of the pericardial sac is performed to remove fluid accumulating with pericardial effusion. The goal is to prevent cardiac tamponade (compression of the

 ◆ heart). *Nursing responsibilities:* monitor ECG and CVP during the procedure, have resuscitative equipment ready. HOB elevated to *45–60 degrees.* Maintain peripheral IV with saline or glucose. Following the procedure, monitor BP, CVP, and heart sounds for recurrence of tamponade (pulsus paradoxus).

🧪 **C. Procedures to evaluate the respiratory system:**

1. *Pulmonary circulation studies—used to* determine regional distribution of pulmonary blood flow.

   a. *Lung scan*—injection of radioactive isotope into the body, followed by lung scintiscan, which produces a graphic record of gamma rays emitted by the isotope in lung tissues; *used to* determine lung perfusion when space-occupying lesions or pulmonary emboli and infarction are suspected.

   b. *Pulmonary angiography*—X-ray visualization of the pulmonary vasculature after the injection of a radiopaque contrast medium; *used to* evaluate pulmonary disorders, e.g., pulmonary embolism, lung tumors, aneurysms, and changes in the pulmonary vasculature due to such conditions as emphysema or congenital defects.

2. *Bronchoscopy*—introduction of a special lighted instrument (bronchoscope) into the trachea and bronchi; *used to* inspect tracheobronchial tree for pathologic changes, remove tissue for cytologic and bacteriologic studies, remove foreign bodies or mucus plugs causing airway obstruction, assess functional residual capacity of diseased lung, and apply chemotherapeutic agents.

 ◆ a. *Prebronchoscopy nursing actions*

     (1) Oral hygiene.

     (2) Postural drainage is indicated.

   b. *Postbronchoscopy nursing actions*

     (1) Instruct patient not to swallow oral secretions but to let saliva run from side of mouth.

     (2) Save expectorated sputum for laboratory analysis, and observe for frank bleeding.

     (3) NPO until gag reflex returns.

     (4) Observe for subcutaneous emphysema and dyspnea.

     (5) Apply ice collar to reduce throat discomfort.

3. *Thoracentesis*—needle puncture through the chest wall and into the pleura; *used to* remove fluid and, occasionally, air from the

 ◆ pleural space. *Nursing responsibilities prior* to thoracentesis:

   a. *Position:* high Fowler's position or sitting up on edge of bed, with feet supported on chair to facilitate accumulation of fluid in the base of the chest.

   b. If patient is unable to sit up—turn on unaffected side.

c. Evaluate continually for signs of: shock, pain, cyanosis, increased respiratory rate, and pallor.

▲ D. Procedures to evaluate the renal system:

1. *Renal angiogram*—small catheter is inserted into the femoral artery and passed into the aorta or renal artery, radiopaque fluid is instilled, and serial films are taken.
   a. *Used to* diagnose renal hypertension and pheochromocytoma and differentiate renal cysts from renal tumors.
   ◆ b. *Postangiogram nursing actions:* check pedal pulse for signs of decreased circulation.
2. *Cystoscopy*—visualization of bladder, urethra, and prostatic urethra by insertion of a tubular, lighted, telescopic lens (cystoscope) through the urinary meatus.
   a. *Used to* directly inspect the bladder, collect urine from the renal pelvis, obtain biopsy specimens from bladder and urethra, remove calculi, and treat lesions in the bladder, urethra, and prostate.
   ◆ b. *Nursing actions following* procedure
      (1) Observe for urinary retention.
      (2) Warm sitz baths to relieve discomfort.
3. *Renal biopsy*—needle aspiration of tissue from the kidney for the purpose of microscopic examination.

▲ E. Procedures to evaluate the digestive system:

1. *Celiac angiography, hepatoportography, splenoportography, and umbilical venography*—injection of a contrast medium into the portal vein or related vessel; *used to* determine patency of vessels supplying target organ or detect lesions in the organs that distort the vasculature.
2. *Esophagoscopy and gastroscopy*—visualization of the esophagus, the stomach, and sometimes the duodenum by means of a lighted tube inserted through the mouth.
3. *Proctoscopy*—visualization of rectum and colon by means of a lighted tube inserted through the anus.
4. *Peritoneoscopy*—direct visualization of the liver and peritoneum by means of a peritoneoscope inserted through an abdominal stab wound.
5. *Liver biopsy*—needle aspiration of tissue for the purpose of microscopic examination; *used to* determine tissue changes, facilitate diagnosis, and provide information regarding a disease course. *Nursing action:* place patient on *right side* and position pillow for pressure, to prevent bleeding.
6. *Paracentesis*—needle aspiration of fluid from the peritoneal cavity; *used to* relieve excess fluid accumulation or for diagnostic studies.
   ◆ a. *Specific nursing actions prior to paracentesis*
      (1) Have patient void—to prevent possible injury to bladder during procedure.
      (2) *Position*—sitting up on side of bed, with feet supported by chair.
      (3) Check vital signs and peripheral circulation frequently throughout procedure.
      (4) Observe for signs of hypovolemic shock—may occur due to fluid shift from vascular compartment following removal of protein-rich ascitic fluid.
   ◆ b. *Specific nursing actions following paracentesis*
      (1) Apply pressure to injection site and cover with sterile dressing.
      (2) Measure and record amount and color of ascitic fluid; send specimens to lab for diagnostic studies.
7. *Small-bowel biopsy*—a specimen is obtained by passing a tube through the oral cavity and is microscopically examined for changes in cellular morphology. *Nursing responsibilities: no* food or fluids 8 h prior to procedure. Obtain written consent. Remove dentures if present. Monitor vital signs prior to, during, and after procedure for indications of hemorrhage. Procedure takes about an hour.

▲ F. Procedures to evaluate the reproductive system in women:

1. *Culdoscopy*—operative procedure in which a culdoscope is inserted into the posterior vaginal cul-de-sac; *used to* visualize uterus, fallopian tubes, broad ligaments, and peritoneal contents.
2. *Hysterosalpingography*—X-ray examination of uterus and fallopian tubes following insertion of a radiopaque dye into the uterine cavity; *used to* determine patency of fallopian tubes and detect pathology in uterine cavity.
3. *Breast biopsy*—needle aspiration or incisional removal of breast tissue for microscopic examination; *used to* differentiate among benign tumors, cysts, and malignant tumors in the breast tissue.
4. *Cervical biopsy and cauterization*—removal of cervical tissue for microscopic examination and cautery; *used to* control bleeding or obtain additional tissue samples.
5. *Uterotubal insufflation (Rubin's test)*—injection of carbon dioxide into the cervical canal; *used to* determine fallopian tube patency.

▲ G. Procedures to evaluate the neuroendocrine system:

1. *Radioactive iodine uptake test (iodine 131 uptake)*—ingestion of a tracer dose of ^{131}I,

followed in 24 h by a scan of the thyroid for amount of radioactivity emitted.

  a. *High* uptake indicates hyperthyroidism.

  b. *Low* uptake indicates hypothyroidism.

2. *Eight-hour intravenous ACTH test*—administration of 25 units of ACTH in 500 mL of saline over an 8-h period.

  a. *Used to* determine function of adrenal cortex.

  b. 24-h urine specimens are collected, before and after administration, for measurement of 17-ketosteroids and 17-hydroxycorticosteroids.

  c. In *Addison's* disease, urinary output of steroids does *not increase* following administration of ACTH; *normally* steroid excretion *increases three- to fivefold* following ACTH stimulation.

  d. In *Cushing's* syndrome, hyperactivity of the adrenal cortex *increases* the urine output of steroids in the second urine specimen tenfold.

3. *Cerebral angiography*—fluoroscopic visualization of the brain vasculature after injection of a contrast medium into the carotid or vertebral arteries; *used to* localize lesions (tumors, abscesses, intracranial hemorrhages, and occlusions) that are large enough to distort cerebral vascular blood flow.

4. *Myelogram*—through a lumbar-puncture needle, a contrast medium is injected into the subarachnoid space of the spinal column to visualize the spinal cord; *used to* detect herniated or ruptured intervertebral disks, tumors, or cysts that compress or

◆ distort spinal cord. *Nursing responsibilities: elevate HOB* with water-soluble contrast; *flat* with oil contrast; check for bladder distention with metrizamide (water soluble); vital signs every 4 h for 24 h.

5. *Brain scan*—intravenous injection of a radioactive substance, followed by a scan for emission of radioactivity.

  a. *Increased* radioactivity at site of pathology.

  b. *Used to* detect brain tumors, abscesses, hematomas, and arteriovenous malformations.

6. *Lumbar puncture*—puncture of the lumbar subarachnoid space of the spinal cord with a needle to withdraw samples of cerebral spinal fluid (CSF); *used to* evaluate CSF for infections and determine presence of hemorrhage. Not done if ↑ ICP suspected.

♣ **H. Procedures to evaluate the skeletal system:** *Arthroscopy*—examination of a joint through a fiberoptic endoscope called an arthroscope. Usually done in the OR (same day surgery) under aseptic conditions using a local anesthetic, although a general anesthetic may be used. A tourniquet is used to reduce blood

flow to the area while the scope is introduced through a cannula. Saline is used as the viewing medium. Biopsy or removal of loose bodies from the joint may be done. A compression dressing (e.g., Ace bandage) is applied. Restrictions vary according to surgeon preference

◆ and nature of procedure. Weight bearing may be immediate or restricted for 24 h. Teach patient to observe for signs of infection.

❏ Intravenous Therapy

I. Infusion systems

  A. Plastic bag

    1. Contains no vacuum—needs no air to replace fluid as it flows from container.

    2. Medication can be added with syringe and needle through a resealable latex port.

      a. During infusion, administration set should be completely clamped before medications are added.

      b. Prevents undiluted, and perhaps toxic, dose from entering administration set.

  B. Closed system

    1. Requires partial vacuum—however, only filtered air enters container.

    2. Medication may be added during infusion through air vent in administration set.

  C. Administration sets

    1. *Standard*—deliver 10–15 drops/mL.

    2. *Pediatric or minidrop sets*—deliver 60 drops/mL.

    3. *Controlled-volume sets*—permit accurate infusion of measured volumes of fluids.

      a. Particularly valuable when piggybacked into primary infusion.

      b. Solutions containing drugs can then be administered intermittently.

    4. *Y-type administration sets*—allow for simultaneous or alternate infusion of two fluids.

      a. May contain filter and pressure unit for blood transfusions.

      b. *Air embolism* significant hazard with this type of administration set.

    5. *Positive-pressure sets*—designed for rapid infusion of replacement fluids.

      a. In emergency, built-in pressure chamber increases rate of blood administration.

      b. Pump chamber *must* be filled at all times to avoid air embolism.

      c. Application of positive pressure to infusion fluids is responsibility of *physician*.

    6. *Infusion pumps*—utilized to deliver small volumes of fluid or doses of high-potency drugs.

      a. Used primarily in neonatal, pediatric, and adult intensive-care units.

      b. Have increased the safety of parenteral therapy and reduced nursing time.

II. Fluid administration

  A. Factors influencing rate:

Treatments

1. Patient's size.
2. Patient's physical condition.
3. Age of patient.
4. Type of fluid.
5. Patient's tolerance to fluid.

B. Flow rates for parenteral infusions can be computed using the following formula:

$$\frac{gtt/mL\ of\ given\ set}{60\ min/h} \times total\ volume/h = gtt/min$$

If 1000 mL is to be infused in an 8-h (125 mL/h) period and the administration set delivers 15 gtt/mL, the rate is 31.2 gtt/min:

$$\frac{15}{60} \times 125 = \frac{1}{4} \times 125 = 31.2\ gtt/min$$

C. Generally the type of fluid administration set determines its rate of flow.
1. *Fluid* administration sets—approximately 15 gtt/min.
2. *Blood* administration sets—approximately 10 gtt/min.
3. *Pediatric* administration sets—approximately 60 gtt/min.
4. Always check information on the administration set box to determine the number of gtt/mL before calculating; varies with manufacturer.

D. Factors influencing flow rates:
1. *Gravity*—a change in the height of the infusion bottle will increase or decrease the rate of flow; for example, raising the bottle higher will increase the rate of flow, and vice versa.
2. *Blood clot* in needle—stopping the infusion for any reason or an increase in venous pressure may result in partial or total obstruction of needle by clot due to:
   a. *Delay* in changing infusion bottle.
   b. Blood pressure cuff on, or restraints *on* or *above* infusion needle.
   c. Patient *lying on arm* in which infusion is being made.
3. Change in *needle position*—against or away from vein wall.
4. *Venous spasm*—due to cold blood or irritating solution.
5. *Plugged vent*—causes infusion to stop.

III. Fluid and electrolyte therapy
   A. Types of therapy
   1. Maintenance therapy—provides water, electrolytes, glucose, vitamins, and in some instances, protein to meet daily requirements.
   2. Restoration of deficits—in addition to maintenance therapy, fluid and electrolytes are added to replace *previous* losses.
   3. Replacement therapy—infusions to replace *current* losses in fluid and electrolytes.

B. Types of intravenous fluids (Table 5.1)
   1. *Isotonic solutions*—fluids that approximate the osmolarity (290 mOsm/L) of normal blood plasma.
      a. Sodium chloride (0.9%)—normal saline.
         (1) *Indications*
            (a) Extracellular fluid replacement when Cl^- loss is equal to or greater than Na^+ loss.
            (b) Treatment of metabolic alkalosis.
            (c) Na^+ depletion.
            (d) Initiating and terminating blood transfusions.
         (2) Possible *side effects*
            (a) Hypernatremia.
            (b) Acidosis.
            (c) Hypokalemia.
            (d) Circulatory overload.
      b. 5% dextrose in water (D5/W).
         (1) *Provides calories* for energy, *sparing body protein* and development of ketosis from fat breakdown.
            (a) 3.75 calories are provided per gram of glucose.
            (b) USP standards require use of monohydrated glucose, so only 91% is actually glucose.
            (c) 5% D/W yields 170.6 calories; 5% D/W means 5 g glucose/L.

            $$50 \times 3.75 = 187.5\ calories$$
            $$0.91 \times 187.5 = 170.6\ calories$$

         (2) *Indications*
            (a) Dehydration.
            (b) Hypernatremia.
            (c) Drug administration.
         (3) Possible *side effects*
            (a) Hypokalemia.
            (b) Osmotic diuresis—dehydration.
            (c) Transient hyperinsulinism.
            (d) Water intoxication.
      c. 5% dextrose in normal saline.

■ **TABLE 5.1   Commonly Used Intravenous Fluids**

Solution	Glucose (dL)	Cations (mEq/L)			Anions (mEq/L)	
		Na$^+$	K$^+$	Ca^{2+}	Cl$^-$	Lactate
D5/W	5					
D50	50					
0.45% NaCl		77			77	
0.9% NaCl*		154			154	
Ringer's		147.5	4	4.5	156	
Ringer's lactate		130	4	3	109	28
D5/LR	5	130	4	3	109	28

*Also known as normal saline
Source: Caroline NL. *Emergency Care in the Streets* (5th ed). Boston: Little, Brown, 1995.

(1) *Prevents* ketone formation and *loss* of potassium and intracellular water.
(2) *Indications*
  (a) Hypovolemic shock—temporary measure.
  (b) Burns.
  (c) Acute adrenocortical insufficiency.
(3) Same *side effects* as normal saline.

d. Isotonic multiple-electrolyte fluids—utilized for replacement therapy; ionic composition approximates blood plasma.
(1) Types—Plasmanate, Polysol, and lactated Ringer's.
(2) *Indicated in* vomiting, diarrhea, excessive diuresis, and burns.
(3) Possible *side effect*—circulatory overload.
(4) Lactated Ringer's is *contraindicated* in severe metabolic acidosis and/or alkalosis and liver disease.
(5) Same *side effects* as normal saline.

2. *Hypertonic solutions*—fluids with an osmolarity much higher than 290 mOsm (+50 mOsm); increase osmotic pressure of blood plasma, thereby drawing fluid from the cells.
a. 10% dextrose in normal saline.
(1) Administered in large vein to dilute and prevent venous trauma.
(2) *Used for* nutrition and to replenish Na^+ and Cl^-.
(3) Possible *side effects*
  (a) Hypernatremia (excess Na^+).
  (b) Acidosis (excess Cl^-).
  (c) Circulatory overload.
b. 3% and 5% sodium chloride solutions.
(1) Slow administration essential to prevent overload (100 mL/h).
(2) *Indicated in* water intoxication and severe sodium depletion.

3. *Hypotonic solutions*—fluids whose osmolarity is significantly less than that of blood plasma (−50 mOsm); these fluids lower plasma osmotic pressures, causing fluid to enter cells.
a. 0.45% sodium chloride—utilized for replacement when requirement for Na^+ use is questionable.
b. 2.5% dextrose in 0.45% saline, 5% dextrose in 0.45% saline, and 5% dextrose in 0.2% saline—these are all hydrating fluids.
(1) *Indications*
  (a) Fluid replacement when some Na^+ replacement is also necessary.

(b) Encourage diuresis in patients who are dehydrated.
(c) Evaluate kidney status before instituting electrolyte infusions.
(2) Possible *side effects*
  (a) Hypernatremia.
  (b) Circulatory overload.
  (c) Use with *caution* in edematous patients with cardiac, renal, or hepatic disease.
  (d) After adequate renal function is established, appropriate electrolytes should be given to avoid hypokalemia.

4. *Alkalizing agents*—fluids used in the treatment of *metabolic acidosis:*
a. Sodium bicarbonate
(1) *Indications*
  (a) Replace excessive loss of bicarbonate ion.
  (b) Emergency treatment of life-threatening acidosis.
(2) Administration
  (a) Depends on patient's weight, condition, and carbon dioxide level.
  (b) Usual dose is 500 mL of a 1.5% solution (89 mEq).
(3) *Side effects*
  (a) Alkalosis.
  (b) Hypocalcemic tetany.
  (c) Rapid infusion may induce cellular acidity and death.

5. *Acidifying solutions*—fluids used in treatment of *metabolic alkalosis.*
a. Types
(1) Normal saline (see B.1. *Isotonic solutions,* p. 298).
(2) Ammonium chloride.
b. Administration—dosage depends on patient's condition and serum lab values.
c. *Side effects*
(1) Hepatic encephalopathy in presence of decreased liver function since ammonia is metabolized by liver.
(2) Toxic effects of irregular respirations, twitching, and bradycardia.
(3) *Contraindicated* with renal failure.

6. *Blood and blood products* (Table 5.2).
a. *Indications*
(1) Maintenance of blood volume.
(2) Supply red blood cells to maintain oxygen-carrying capacity.
(3) Supply clotting factors to maintain coagulation properties.
(4) Exchange transfusion.

IV. Intravenous cancer chemotherapy

■ **TABLE 5.2   Transfusion with Blood or Blood Products**

Blood or Blood Product	Indications	Assessment: Side Effects	Nursing Care Plan/ Implementation
Whole blood	1. Acute hemorrhage 2. Hypovolemic shock	1. Hemolytic reaction 2. Fluid overload 3. Febrile reaction 4. Pyogenic reaction 5. Allergic reaction	1. See Table 2.19, Postoperative Complications, pp. 108–111, for complete discussion of nursing responsibilities 2. Protocol for checking blood before transfusion is begun varies with each institution; however, at least *two* people must verify that the unit of blood has been cross-matched for a specific patient
Red blood cells, packed	1. Acute anemia with hypoxia 2. Aplastic anemia 3. Bone marrow failure due to malignancy 4. Patients who need red blood cells but not volume	See Whole blood	See Whole blood
Red blood cells, frozen	1. See Red blood cells, packed 2. Patients sensitized by previous transfusions	1. Less likely to cause antigen reaction 2. Decreased possibility of transmitting hepatitis	See Whole blood
White blood cells (leukocytes)	Currently being used in severe leukopenia with infection (research still being done)	1. Elevated temperature 2. Graft-versus-host disease	1. Careful monitoring of temperature 2. *Must* be given as soon as collected
Platelet concentrate	1. Severe deficiency 2. Bleeding thrombocytopenic patients with platelet counts *below* 10,000	1. Fever, chills 2. Hives 3. Development of antibodies that will destroy platelets in future transfusions *Contraindications:* 1. Idiopathic thrombocytopenic purpura 2. Disseminated intravascular coagulopathy	Monitor temperature
Single-donor fresh plasma	1. Clotting deficiency or concentrates not available or deficiency not fully diagnosed 2. Shock	1. Side effects rare 2. Heart failure 3. Possible hepatitis	Use sterile, pyrogen-free filters
Plasma removed from whole blood (up to 5 d after expiration date, which is 21 d)	1. Shock due to loss of plasma 2. Burns 3. Peritoneal injury 4. Hemorrhage 5. While awaiting blood cross-match	See Single-donor fresh plasma	See Single-donor fresh plasma
Freeze-dried plasma	See Plasma removed from whole blood	See Single-donor fresh plasma	Must be reconstituted with sterile water before use
Single-donor fresh-frozen plasma	1. See Single-donor fresh plasma 2. Inherited or acquired disorders of coagulation 3. Presurgical hemophiliac	See Single-donor fresh plasma	1. Notify blood bank to thaw about 30 min before administration 2. Give *immediately*
Cryoprecipitate concentrate (factor VIII—antihemophilic factor)	For hemophilia: 1. Prevention 2. Preoperatively 3. During bleeding episodes	Rare	0.55 mL of cryoprecipitate concentrate has same effect on serum level as 1600 mL of fresh frozen plasma
Factors II, VII, IX, and X compiled	Specific deficiencies	Hepatitis	Commercially prepared

continued

■ **TABLE 5.2** *(Continued)*

Blood or Blood Product	Indications	Assessment: Side Effects	Nursing Care Plan/ Implementation
Fibrinogen (factor I)	Fibrinogen deficiency	Increased risk of hepatitis since the hepatitis virus combines with fibrinogen during fractionation	1. Reconstitute with sterile water 2. Do *not* warm fibrinogen or use hot water to reconstitute 3. Do *not* shake 4. Must be given with a filter
Albumin or salt-poor albumin	1. Shock due to hemorrhage, trauma, infection, surgery, or burns 2. Treatment of cerebral edema 3. Low serum-protein levels	None; these are heat-treated products	Commercially prepared
Dextran	Hypovolemic shock	1. Rare allergic reaction 2. Patients with heart or kidney disease susceptible to heart failure or pulmonary edema	Commercially prepared

A. Usual sites: forearm, dorsum of hand, wrist, antecubital fossa.

B. Procedure:

1. Normal saline infusion usually started first, to verify vein patency, position of needle. Chemotherapy "piggybacked" into IV line that is running.
2. Rate: usually 1 mL/min. Running slowly decreases nausea, vomiting, and the degree of vein damage.
3. Check vein patency every 3–5 min.
4. If more than one drug is to be infused, normal saline should be infused between drugs.
5. Never infuse against resistance.
6. Stop treatment if patient reports pain at needle site. Extravasation (infiltration of toxic drugs into tissue surrounding vessel) may be present.
7. If extravasation present, begin protocol appropriate to drug administered (e.g., flushing of line with saline, applying ice or heat, local injection of site with antidote drugs, topical application of steroid creams).
8. Once treatment is completed, remove needle, apply Band-Aid, exert pressure to prevent hematoma formation.

V. Complications of IV therapy: Table 5.3.

❏ Oxygen Therapy

I. Purpose—to relieve hypoxia and provide adequate tissue oxygenation.

II. Clinical indications

A. Any patient who is likely to have significant *shunt* from:

1. Fluid in the alveoli.
   a. Pulmonary edema.
   b. Pneumonia.
   c. Near drowning.
   d. Chest trauma.
2. Collapsed alveoli (atelectasis).
   a. Airway obstruction.
   (1) Any unconscious patient.
   (2) Choking.
   b. Failure to take deep breaths.
   (1) Pain (rib fracture).
   (2) Paralysis of the respiratory muscles (spine injury).
   (3) Depression of the respiratory center (head injury, drug overdose).
   c. Collapse of an entire lung (pneumothorax).
3. Other gases in the alveoli.
   a. Smoke inhalation.
   b. Toxic inhalations.
   c. Carbon monoxide poisoning.
4. Respiratory arrest.

B. Cardiac arrest.

C. Shock.

D. Shortness of breath.

E. Signs of respiratory insufficiency.

F. Breathing fewer than 10 times per minute.

G. Chest pain.

H. Stroke.

I. Anemia.

J. Fetal decelerations during labor.

III. Precautions

A. Patients with chronic obstructive pulmonary disease should receive oxygen at *low* flow rates, to prevent inhibition of hypoxic respiratory drive.

B. *Excessive* amounts of oxygen for prolonged periods of time will cause retrolental fibroplasia and blindness in premature infants.

C. Oxygen delivered *without* humidification will result in drying and irritation of respiratory mucosa, decreased ciliary action, and thickening of respiratory secretions.

Treatments

■ **TABLE 5.3   Complications of IV Therapy**

| Complication | Assessment | | Nursing Care Plan/ Implementation |
	Subjective Data	Objective Data	
Infiltration—fluid infusing into surrounding tissue rather than into vessel	Pain around needle insertion	1. Infusion rate slow 2. Swelling, hardness, coolness, blanching of tissue at site of needle 3. Blood does not return into tubing when bag/bottle lowered 4. Puffiness under surface of arm	1. Stop IV 2. Apply warm towel to area 3. Restart at another site 4. Record
Thrombophlebitis—inflammatory changes in vessel; *Thromboemboli*—the development of venous clots within the inflamed vessel	Pain along the vein	Redness, swelling around affected area (red line)	1. Stop IV 2. Notify physician 3. Cold compresses or warm towel, as ordered 4. Restart in another site 5. *Rest affected limb; do not rub* 6. See nursing care of Thrombophlebitis, Unit 2
Pyrogenic reaction—contaminated equipment/solution	1. Headache 2. Backache 3. Nausea 4. Anxiety	1. ↑ Temperature 2. Chills 3. Face flushed 4. Vomiting 5. ↓ BP 6. Cyanosis	1. Discontinue IV 2. Vital signs 3. Send equipment for culture/analysis 4. Antibiotic ointment, as ordered, at injection site 5. *Prevention:* change tubing q24–48h; meticulous sterile technique; check for precipitation, expiration dates, damage to containers, tubings etc.; refrigerate hyperalimentation fluids; discard hyperalimentation fluids that have been at room temperature from 8–12 h and use new bag regardless of amount left in first bag (change, to prevent infection—excellent medium for bacterial growth)
Fluid overload—excessive amount of fluid infused; infants/elderly at risk	1. Headache 2. Shortness of breath 3. Syncope 4. Dyspnea	1. ↑ pulse, venous pressure 2. Venous distention 3. Flushed skin 4. Coughing 5. ↑ respirations 6. Cyanosis, pulmonary edema 7. Shock	1. Stop IV 2. Semi-Fowler's *position* 3. Notify physician 4. Be prepared for diuretic therapy 5. *Preventive measures:* monitor flow rate and patient's response to IV therapy (see Fluid volume excess, p. 75, for subjective and objective data)
Air emboli—air in circulatory system	Loss of consciousness	1. Hypotension, cyanosis 2. Tachycardia 3. ↑ venous pressure 4. Tachypnea	1. Turn on *left* side, with head *down* 2. Administer oxygen therapy 3. **Medical emergency—call physician**
Nerve damage—improper position of limb during infusion or *tying* limb down too tight during infusion → damage to nerve	Numbness: fingers, hands	Unusual position for limb	1. Untie 2. Passive ROM exercises 3. Monitor closely for return of function 4. Record limb status
Pulmonary embolism—blood clot enters pulmonary circulation and obstructs pulmonary artery	Dyspnea	1. Orthopnea 2. Signs of circulatory and cardiac collapse	1. Slow IV to keep vein open (rate: 5–6 drops/min) 2. Notify physician 3. **Medical emergency** 4. Be prepared for lifesaving measures and anticoagulation therapy

D. Oxygen supports combustion, and *fire* is a potential hazard during its administration.
   1. Ground electrical administration.
   2. Prohibit smoking.
   3. Institute measures to decrease static electricity.

E. *High* flow rates of oxygen per ventilator or cuffed tracheostomy and endotracheal tubes can produce signs of oxygen toxicity in 24–48 h.
   1. Cough, sore throat, decreased vital capacity, and substernal discomfort.
   2. Pulmonary manifestations due to:
      a. Atelectasis.
      b. Exudation of protein fluids into alveoli.
      c. Damage to pulmonary capillaries.
      d. Interstitial hemorrhage.

IV. Oxygen administration
   A. Oxygen is dispensed from cylinder or piped-in system.
   B. Methods of delivering oxygen:
   1. Nasal catheter
      a. Effective and comfortable.
      b. Delivers 30–50% oxygen at flow rates of 6–8 L/min.
      c. Can produce excoriation of nares.
      d. Do not use in comatose patient.
   2. Nasal prongs/cannula
      a. Comfortable and simple, and allows patient to move about in bed.
      b. Delivers 25–40% oxygen at flow rates of 4–6 L/min.
      c. Difficult to keep in position unless patient is alert and cooperative.
   3. Venturi mask
      a. Allows for accurate delivery of prescribed concentration of oxygen.
      b. Delivers 24–40% oxygen at flow rates of 4–8 L/min.
      c. Useful in long-term treatment of chronic obstructive pulmonary disease.
   4. Face mask
      a. Poorly tolerated—utilized for short periods of time; feeling of "suffocation."
      b. Delivers 50–60% oxygen at flow rates of 8–12 L/min.
      c. Significant rebreathing of carbon dioxide at low oxygen flow rates.
      d. Hot—may produce pressure sores around nose and mouth.
   5. Partial rebreathing mask
      a. About one-third of exhaled air is rebreathed.
      b. Reservoir contains mostly oxygen inspired during previous inhalation.
      c. Delivers 35–60% oxygen at flow rates of 6–10 L/min.
   6. Nonrebreathing mask
      a. Reservoir bag has one-way valve preventing the patient from exhaling back into the bag.
      b. Oxygen flow rate prevents collapse of bag during inhalation.
      c. Delivers 100% oxygen at flow rates of 10–12 L/min.
      d. Ideal for severe hypoxia, but patient may complain of feelings of suffocation.
   7. T-tube
      a. Provides humidification and enriched oxygen mixtures to tracheostomy or ET tube.
      b. Delivers 40–60% oxygen at flow rates of 4–12 L/min.

V. Ventilators
   A. *Indications*
   1. Hypoventilation.
   2. Hypoxia.
   3. Counteract pulmonary edema by changing pressure gradient.
   4. Decrease work of breathing.
   B. *Contraindications*
   1. Tuberculosis—may rupture tubercular bleb.
   2. Hypovolemia—increased intrathoracic pressures decrease venous return.
   3. Air trapping—increased because adequate exhalation is not allowed.
   C. *Complications*
   1. Decreased blood pressure; impaired venous return.
   2. Atelectasis.
   3. Infection.
   4. Oxygen toxicity.
   5. Difficulties weaning.
   6. Gastric dilatation.
   7. Pneumothorax.
   8. Hyper- or hypoventilation.
   9. Tracheal injury.
   D. *Types of ventilators*
   1. Oscillating or rocking bed.
      a. Indirectly aids respirations by using weight and gravity of abdominal contents to change position of diaphragm.
      b. *Used with* paralytic disease, as an aid in weaning.
   2. Iron lung and chest respirators.
      a. Driven by motors that create negative pressure within tank or shell and thus allow air to enter patient's lungs.
      b. *Used for* neuromuscular disease.
   3. Intermittent positive-pressure breathing (*IPPB*).
      a. Produces greater-than-atmospheric pressures, intermittently.
      b. Improves tidal volume and minute volume and aids in overcoming respiratory insufficiency.
      c. Produces more uniform distribution of alveolar aeration and reduces work of breathing.
      d. *Used to* deliver both oxygen and medications during treatment and rehabili-

Treatments

tative pulmonary therapy, particularly if patient has decreased tidal volume.

   e. *Contraindicated in* pneumothorax, active tuberculosis, and history of recent hemoptysis.

4. Pressure-constant ventilators.
   a. *Bird*—Mark VII.
     (1) Pressure cycled, pneumatic powered.
     (2) When preset pressure is reached, valve closes, terminating inspiration.
     (3) Flow rate, sensitivity, and pressure limit are all adjustable.
     (4) Adjustable flow rate allows for increasing tidal volume.
     (5) Disadvantage—changes in compliance or airway resistance can affect oxygen concentration and tidal volume.
   b. *Bennett*—PR II.
     (1) Positive-pressure cycled, time cycled, flow sensitive.
     (2) May be triggered by patient's inspiration or controlled by pressure or time setting.
     (3) Oxygen delivery variable, so frequent monitoring is *essential*.

5. Volume-constant ventilators.
   a. *Bennett*—MA 1.
     (1) Delivers preset tidal volume.
     (2) Oxygen concentration adjusted by lighter flow being fed into machine.
     (3) Sophisticated alarms.
     (4) Has a sigh mechanism and positive end-expiration pressure *(PEEP)*, which maintains lung inflation.
     (5) *Used for* decreased compliance (stiff lungs).
     (6) Excellent humidification system.

6. Minute volume ventilators—Servo 990 C.
   a. Delivers preset inspiratory minute volume.
   b. Has PEEP, continuous positive airway pressure *(CPAP)*, spontaneous intermittent mandatory ventilation *(SIMV)*, and inverse ratio ventilation *(IRV)* capabilities.
   c. *Used for* patients with ARDS who have not responded to conventional treatment (PEEP, IMV) and need the advantage of IRV and prolonged inspiratory ventilation.

❏ Positioning the Patient

Table 5.4.

❏ Commonly Used Tubes

Table 5.5.

❏ Colostomy Care

Tables 5.6 and 5.7.

❏ Basic Prosthetic Care

Tables 5.8 and 5.9.

❏ Universal Precautions

Table 5.10.

❏ Questions

Select the one best answer for each question.

1. A patient's laboratory values indicate hemoconcentration secondary to fluid loss. Which of the following intravenous solutions should the nurse anticipate will be ordered as the most appropriate during initial fluid replacement therapy?
   1. 10% dextrose and saline.
   2. 5% dextrose and water with 60 mEq KCl.
   3. 5% dextrose and water only.
   4. Distilled water.

2. Prior to surgery, a patient was instructed in the use of an incentive spirometer. The *primary* purpose of this activity is:
   1. To encourage coughing.
   2. To arouse and stimulate the patient.
   3. To encourage deep breathing.
   4. To measure tidal volume and expiratory reserve volume.

3. The nurse explains to a patient's family that humidification is given with oxygen administration because:
   1. Oxygen is highly permeable in water, thereby increasing gaseous diffusion.
   2. Oxygen is very drying to the mucous membranes.
   3. The partial pressures of oxygen are increased by water dilution, allowing more oxygen to reach the alveoli.
   4. Water acts as a carrier substance facilitating movement of oxygen across the respiratory membrane.

4. To correctly administer 1000 mL of 5% dextrose/water in 10 hours using a standard 15-drop administration set, the nurse would adjust the infusion rate to:
   1. 32 drops per minute.
   2. 25 drops per minute.
   3. 20 drops per minute.
   4. 15 drops per minute.

5. The nurse would conclude that a patient's fasting serum-glucose levels are normal if the results are:
   1. 30–60 mg/dL of blood.
   2. 80–120 mg/dL of blood.
   3. 120–140 mg/dL of blood.
   4. 140–200 mg/dL of blood.

6. A laboratory test to measure serum- and urine-glucose levels before and after ingestion of a glucose load has been ordered. The nurse knows that the test to be done is called:
   1. Fasting blood sugar.
   2. Glucose tolerance test.
   3. Postprandial blood glucose.
   4. Tolbutamide response test.

■ **TABLE 5.4 Positioning the Patient for Specific Surgical Conditions**

Surgical Condition	Key Points	Rationale
Amputation: lower extremity	*No* pillows under stump after first 24 h. Turn patient prone several times a day	Prevents flexion deformity of the limb
Appendicitis: ruptured	Keep in Fowler's position—not flat in bed	Keeps infection from spreading upward in the peritoneal cavity
Burns (extensive)	Usually *flat* for first 24 h	Potential problem is hypovolemia, which will be more symptomatic in a sitting position
Cast, extremity	Keep extremity elevated	Prevents edema
Coronary surgery	May be ordered flat on back for 24 h	Important to prevent possible hypotension, which may occur if head of bed raised
Craniotomy	Head *elevated* with supratentorial incision; flat with cerebellar or brainstem incision	Prevents collection of fluid in surgical area, which might contribute to increased intracranial pressure
Flail chest	Position on *affected* side	Reduces the instability of the chest wall that is causing the paradoxical respiratory movements
Gastric resection	Lie down after meals	May be useful in preventing dumping syndrome
Hiatal hernia (*before repaired*)	Head of bed elevated on shock blocks	Prevents esophageal irritation from gastric regurgitation
Hip prosthesis	1. Keep affected leg in *abduction* (splint or pillow between legs) 2. Avoid adduction and flexion of the hip 3. Use trochanter roll along outside of femur anterior joint capsule incision to keep affected leg turned slightly *inward;* no trochanter roll with posterior joint capsule incision as leg is turned slightly *outward*	If affected leg is flexed and allowed to adduct and internally rotate, the head of the femur may be displaced from the socket
Laminectomy; fusion	Avoid twisting motion when getting out of bed, ambulating	Prevents any bending of the spine
Liver biopsy	Place on right side, and position pillow for pressure	Prevents bleeding
Lobectomy	Do *not* put in Trendelenburg position. Position of comfort—sides, back	Pushes abdominal contents against diaphragm; may cause respiratory embarrassment
Mastectomy	1. Do *not* abduct arm first few days 2. Elevate hand and arm *higher* than shoulder if lymph glands removed	Puts tension on suture line Prevents lymphedema
Pneumonectomy	Turn only toward operative side for short periods; no extreme lateral positioning	1. Gives unaffected lung room for full expansion 2. Prevents mediastinal shift 3. In case of bleeding there will be no drainage into the unaffected bronchi
Radium implantation in cervix	Bedrest—usually may elevate head to 30 degrees	Must keep radium insert positioned correctly
Respiratory distress	Orthopnea position usually desirable	Allows for maximum expansion of lungs
Retinal detachment	1. Affected area toward bed—complete bedrest 2. No *sudden* movements of head—may use sand bags to prevent turning	1. Gravity may help retina fall in place 2. Any sudden increase in intraocular pressure may further dislodge retina 3. Necessary to cover both eyes to reduce ocular movements
Traction Straight traction	Check specific orders about how much head may be elevated	Body is used as the countertraction—this must not be less than the pull of the traction
Balanced suspension	May give patient more freedom to move about than in straight traction	In balanced suspension additional weights supply countertraction
Unconscious patient	Turn on side with head slightly *lowered*—"coma" position	1. Important to let secretions drain out by gravity 2. Must prevent aspiration
Vascular Ileofemoral bypass; arterial insufficiency	1. Do *not* elevate legs 2. *Avoid* hip flexion—walk or stand, but do *not* sit	1. Arterial flow is helped by gravity 2. Flexion of the hip compresses the vessels of the extremity
Vein strippings; vein ligations	1. Keep legs elevated 2. Do *not* stand or sit for long periods	1. Prevents venous stasis 2. Prevents venous pooling

Source: Jane Vincent Corbett, RN, MS, EdD, Professor, School of Nursing, University of San Francisco. Used with permission.

Treatments

■ **TABLE 5.5   Review of the Use of Common Tubes**

Tube or Apparatus	Purpose	Examples of Use	Key Points
Chest tubes	1. *Anterior tube* drains mostly air from pleural space 2. *Posterior tube* drains mostly fluid from pleural space 3. Removal of fluid and air from pleural space is necessary to reestablish negative intrapleural pressure	1. *Thoracotomy* 2. *Open heart surgery* 3. *Spontaneous pneumothorax* 4. *Traumatic pneumothorax*	1. See Key Points for each of the three entries under Drainage system, below 2. Sterile technique is used when changing dressings around the tube insertions 3. Fowler's *position* to facilitate air and fluid removal 4. Cough, deep breathe q1h; splint chest; medicate for pain 5. Manage pain carefully in order *not* to depress respirations 6. Prepare for removal when there is little or no drainage, air leak disappears, or fluctuations stop in water seal; have suture set, petrolatum gauze (or other ointment), 4×4s, and sturdy elastic tape ready; medicate for pain before removal; monitor breathing after removal (breath sounds, rate, chest pain)
Drainage system (see Figure 5.1, p. 309)			
#1: drainage compartment	Collects drainage		1. Mark level in bottle each shift to keep accurate record—*not* routinely emptied; replaced when full 2. *Never* raise container above the level of the chest; otherwise back flow will occur
#2: water-seal chamber	Water seal prevents flow of atmospheric air into pleural space; essential to prevent recollapse of the lung		1. Air bubbles from postoperative residual air *will* continue for 24–48 h 2. *Persistent* large amounts of air bubbles in this compartment indicate an *air leak* between the alveoli and the pleural space 3. Clamp tube(s) only to verify a leak, replace a broken, cracked, or full drainage unit, or verify readiness of patient for tube removal; not necessary to clamp when ambulating if water seal intact 4. If tube becomes disconnected, clean off tubing ends and reconnect; if dislodged from chest, seal insertion site *immediately* on expiration if possible; use sterile petrolatum gauze and adhesive tape to form *air-occlusive* dressing 5. If air leak is present, clamping the tube for very long may cause a tension pneumothorax 6. Fluctuation of the fluid level in this bottle is *expected* (when the suction is turned off) because respiration changes the pleural pressure: if there is *no fluctuation* of the fluid in the tube of this bottle (when the suction is turned off), then either the lung is fully expanded or the tube is blocked by kinking or by a clot 7. Although not routinely used, milking (gently squeezing) the tubes, if ordered, will prevent blockage from clots or debris; otherwise gravity drainage is sufficient to maintain patency 8. Drainage of >1 dL in 1 h should be *reported* to physician

continued

Treatments

■ **TABLE 5.5** *(Continued)*

Tube or Apparatus	Purpose	Examples of Use	Key Points
#3: suction control—connected to wall suction	Level of the column of water (i.e., 15–20 cm) is used to control the amount of suction applied to the chest tube—if the water evaporates to only *10-cm* depth, then this will be the *maximum* suction generated by the wall suction		1. Air *should continuously bubble* through this compartment when the suction is on; the bubbles are from the atmosphere—not the patient; when the wall suction is turned higher, the bubbling will increase, but the increased pulling of air is from the atmosphere and *not* from the pleural space 2. Since the level of H_2O determines the maximum negative pressure that can be obtained, make sure the water does *not* evaporate—keep filling the bottle to keep the ordered level; if there is *no* bubbling of air through this container, the wall suction is *too low*
Heimlich flutter valve	1. Has a one-way valve so fluids and air can drain out of the pleural space but cannot flow back 2. Eliminates the need for a water seal—no danger when tube is unclamped below the valve	Same as for other chest tubes	1. Can be connected to suction if ordered 2. Sometimes can just drain into portable bag so patient is more mobile
Tracheostomy tube	1. Maintains patent airway and promotes better O_2-CO_2 exchange 2. Makes removal of secretions by suctioning easier 3. Cuff on trach is necessary if need airtight fit for an assisted ventilation	1. *Acute respiratory distress* due to poor ventilation 2. *Severe burns of head and neck* 3. *Laryngectomy* (trach is permanent)	1. Use oxygen *before* and *after* each suctioning 2. Humidify oxygen 3. Sterile technique in suctioning; clean technique at home 4. Cleanse inner cannula as needed—only leave out 5–10 min 5. Hemostat handy if outer cannula is expelled—have obturator taped to bed and another trach set handy 6. Cuff must be deflated periodically to prevent necrosis of mucosa, unless low-pressure cuff used
Penrose drain	Soft collapsible latex rubber drain inserted to drain serosanguineous fluid from a surgical site; usually brought out to the skin via a stab wound	Bowel resection	1. Expect drainage to progress from serosanguineous to more serous 2. Sterile technique when changing dressing—do often 3. Physician will advance tube a little each day
Nasogastric (NG) tubes Levin tube and small-bore feeding tubes	1. Inserted into stomach to decompress by removing gastric contents and air—prevents any buildup of gastric secretions, which are continuous 2. Used when stomach needs to be washed out (lavage) 3. Used for feedings when patient is unable to swallow (gavage)	1. Any abdominal or other *surgery where peristalsis is absent* for a few days 2. *Overdoses* 3. *Gastrointestinal hemorrhage* 4. *Cancer of the esophagus* 5. *Early postoperative laryngectomy patient or radical neck dissection*	1. Connect to *low* intermittent suction 2. Irrigate prn with normal saline or puffs of air. 3. Clean, but *not* sterile, procedure 4. Mouth care needed 5. Report "*coffee ground*" material (digested blood) 6. For overdose, stomach is pumped out as *rapidly* as possible 7. For hemorrhage, iced normal saline may be used to lavage 8. Critical to make sure tube still in stomach *before* beginning feeding; listen for air passing into stomach, and if possible aspirate gastric contents; small-bore tubes need placement check by X ray 9. Follow feeding with some water to rinse out the tube 10. Clamp tube when ambulating 11. With larger-bore tubes, determine residuals and withhold feeding if large residuals obtained

continued

Treatments

■ **TABLE 5.5** *(Continued)*

Tube or Apparatus	Purpose	Examples of Use	Key Points
Nasogastric tubes (cont.)			
Miller-Abbott tube Cantor tube	Longer than Levin tube—has mercury or air in bags so tube can be used to *decompress the lower intestinal tract*	1. *Small-bowel obstructions* 2. *Intussusception* 3. *Volvulus*	1. Care similar to that for Levin NG tube—irrigated 2. Connected to suction, not sterile technique 3. Orders will be written on how to advance the tube, gently pushing tube a few inches each hour; patient position may affect advancement of tube 4. X rays determine the desired location of tube
Salem sump	Double-lumen tube with vent to *protect gastric mucosa* from trauma of suctioning	Same as Levin tube	1. Irrigate vent (blue tubing) with air only 2. See Levin tube
Gastrostomy tube	1. Inserted into stomach via abdominal wall 2. May be used for decompression 3. Used *long term for feedings*	Conditions affecting *esophagus* where it is impossible to insert a nasogastric tube	1. Principles of tube feedings same as with Levin nasogastric tube, *except* no danger that tube is in trachea 2. If permanent, tube may be replaceable
T-tube	To *drain bile* from the common bile duct *until* edema has subsided	*Cholecystectomy* when a CDE (common duct exploration) or choledochostomy was also done	1. Bile drainage is influenced by *position* of the drainage bag 2. Clamp tube as ordered to see if bile will flow into duodenum normally
Hemovac	A type of closed-wound drainage connected to suction—used to *drain a large amount* of serosanguineous drainage from under an incision	1. *Mastectomy* 2. *Total hip procedures* 3. *Total knee procedures*	1. May compress unit, and have portable vacuum or connect to wall suction 2. Small drainage tubes may get clogged—physician may irrigate these at times
Jackson-Pratt	1. A method of closed-wound suction drainage—indicated when tissue displacement and tissue trauma may occur with rigid drain tubes (i.e., Hemovac) 2. See Hemovac	1. *Neurosurgery* 2. *Neck surgery* 3. *Mastectomy* 4. *Total knee and hip replacement* 5. *Abdominal surgery* 6. *Urologic procedures*	1. Empty reservoir when full, to prevent loss of wound drainage and back-contamination 2. See Hemovac
Three-way Foley	To provide avenues for *constant irrigation and constant drainage* of the urinary bladder	1. Transurethral resection (TUR) 2. *Bladder* infections	1. Watch for blocking by clots—causes bladder spasms 2. Irrigant solution often has antibiotic added to normal saline or sterile water 3. Sterile water rather than normal saline may be used for lysis of clots
Suprapubic catheter	To *drain bladder* via an opening through the abdominal wall above the pubic bone	*Suprapubic* prostatectomy	May have orders to irrigate prn or continuously
Ureteral catheter	To *drain urine* from the pelvis of one kidney, or for *splinting* ureter	1. *Cystoscopy* for diagnostic workups 2. *Ureteral surgery* 3. *Pyelotomy*	1. *Never* clamp the tube—pelvis of kidney only holds 4–8 mL 2. Use *only* 5 mL sterile normal saline if ordered to irrigate

Note: This review focuses on care of the tubes, not on total patient care.
Source: Jane Vincent Corbett, RN, MS, EdD, Professor, School of Nursing, University of San Francisco. Used with permission.

■ **FIGURE 5.1   Chest drainage system.**

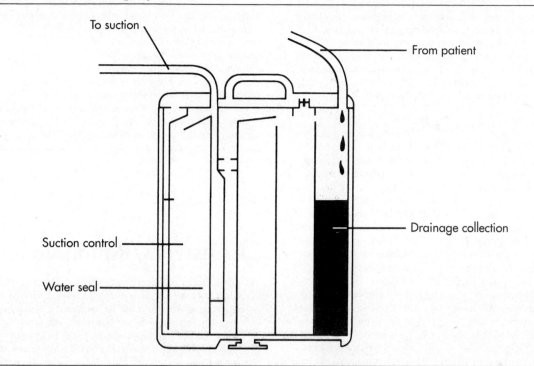

■ **TABLE 5.6   Emptying Colostomy Appliance**

Check for drainage in appliance at least twice during each shift.
If drainage present (diarrhea-type stool):

Do	**Do Not**
1. Unclip the bottom of bag	1. Remove appliance each time it needs emptying
2. Drain into bedpan	2. Use any materials that could irritate bowel
3. Use a squeeze-type bottle filled with warm water to rinse inside of appliance	3. Ignore patient's needs
4. Clean off clamp if soiled	
5. Put a few drops of deodorant in appliance if not odorproof	
6. Fasten bottom of appliance securely (fold bag over clamp 2–3 times before closing)	
7. Check for leakage under appliance every 2–4 h	
8. Communicate with patient while attending to appliance	

7. After a glucose tolerance test, the nurse would look for the blood-glucose levels to return to normal in about how many hours?
   1. One.
   2. Two.
   3. Three.
   4. Four.
8. Following a gastroscopy, the nurse will plan to offer the patient food or fluid:
   1. As soon as he or she returns to the room.
   2. One hour later, or after he or she is fully alert.
   3. Three to 4 hours later, or when the gag reflex returns.
   4. Six to 8 hours later to prevent the electrolyte imbalance that may occur with this procedure.
9. The nurse knows that a 24-hour urine-for-creatinine clear-

ance measures which of the following kidney functions?
   1. Filtration fraction.
   2. Glomerular filtration rate.
   3. Renal blood flow.
   4. Quantity and specific gravity of urinary output.
10. A patient asks why an intravenous pyelogram (IVP) is being done. The nurse tells the patient the purpose is to:
   1. Determine the size, shape, and placement of the kidneys.
   2. Test renal tubular function and the patency of the urinary tract.
   3. Measure renal blood flow.
   4. Outline the kidney vasculature.
11. The nursing care of a patient before an IVP includes:
   1. Warning the patient that the contrast medium may produce a warm, flushed feeling in the face and a salty taste in the mouth.
   2. Administering radiopaque capsules 6 hours before the test.
   3. Ascertaining whether or not the patient has any allergies to mercury.
   4. Pushing fluids until 2 hours before the test, to prevent dehydration.
12. The nurse's preparation of the patient undergoing IV cholangiogram includes:
   1. Administering radiopaque tablets the evening before the examination.
   2. A fatty meal the evening before examination.
   3. Forcing fluids for 6–8 hours before examination.
   4. Informing the patient he or she may experience a feeling of warmth, flushing of face, and/or a salty taste when the contrast medium is injected.
13. The nurse knows that the most important effect of intermittent positive-pressure breathing (IPPB) is:
   1. Mobilization of bronchial secretions.
   2. Increased alveolar ventilation.
   3. Prevention of atelectasis.
   4. Decreased airway resistance.

■ TABLE 5.7   Changing Colostomy Appliance

Gather equipment: gloves, skin prep packet, colostomy appliance measured to fit stoma properly (if new surgical stoma, it will continue to shrink with the healing process; use stoma measuring guide), skin barrier, warm water and soap, face cloth/towel, plastic bag for disposal of old equipment. Remember that bowel is very fragile; also, working near bowel increases peristalsis, and feces and flatulence may be expelled.

Do	**Do Not**
1. Remove old appliance carefully, pulling from area with least drainage to area with most drainage	1. Tear appliance quickly from skin
2. Wash skin area with soap and water	2. Wash stoma with soap; put anything dry onto stoma
3. Observe skin area for potential breakdown	3. Irritate skin or stoma
4. Use packet of skin prep on the skin around the stoma; allow skin prep solution to dry on skin before applying colostomy appliance	4. Put skin prep solution onto stoma; it will cause irritation
5. Apply skin barrier you have measured and cut to size	5. Make opening too large (increases risk of leakage)
6. Put appliance on so that the bottom of the appliance is easily accessible for emptying (e.g., if patient is out of bed most of the time, put the bottom facing the feet; if patient is in bed most of the time, have bottom face the side); picture-frame the adhesive portion of the appliance with 1-in. tape	6. Have appliance attached so patient can't be involved in own care
7. Put a few drops of deodorant in appliance if not odorproof	7. Use any materials that would irritate bowel
8. Use clamp to fasten bottom of appliance	8. Avoid conversation/eye contact
9. Talk to patient (or communicate in best way possible for patient) during and after procedure	9. Contaminate other incisions
10. Use good handwashing technique	

■ TABLE 5.8   Care of Dentures

Wear gloves
If patient cannot remove own dentures, grasp upper plate at the front teeth and move up and down gently to release suction
Lift the upper plate up one side at a time
Use extreme care not to damage dentures while cleaning
Use tepid, not hot, water to clean
Avoid soaking for long periods of time
Inspect for sharp edges
Do oral cavity assessment
Replace moistened dentures in patient's mouth
Use appropriately labeled container for storage when dentures are to remain out of patient's mouth

■ TABLE 5.9   Caring for an Artificial Eye

With gloved hand pull lower eyelid down over the infraorbital bone and exert pressure below the eyelid
Pressure will make the eye pop out
Handle eye prosthesis carefully
Using aseptic techniques, cleanse socket with saline-moistened gauze, stroking from the inner to outer canthus
Wash the prosthesis in warm normal saline
To reinsert, gently pull the patient's lower lid down, raise the upper lid if necessary, slip the saline-moistened eye prosthesis gently into the socket, and release the lids

❑ Answers/Rationale

1. **(3)** Initial fluid therapy is directed toward increasing fluid volume and urine output. **No. 1**, being a hypertonic solution that would act to increase intracellular dehydration, is therefore contraindicated. Once adequate urinary output has been established, potassium salts are added **(No. 2)** to relieve hypokalemia. The amount of added potassium chloride depends on the extent of hypokalemia. **No. 4**, distilled water, is a hypotonic solution; that is, it does not contain any additional electrolytes. Hypotonic solutions, such as 0.45% sodium chloride, are frequently given to relieve hypertonic syndromes. However, distilled water is never given in fluid replacement therapy. **AN,8,PhI**

2. **(3)** The purpose of the incentive spirometer is to encourage deep breathing. The patient is able to directly visualize progress by the number and height of balls he or she is able to raise. *After-effects* of this activity may indeed be coughing up of sputum **(No. 1)** and arousal **(No. 2)** as the patient competes with himself or herself. Incentive spirometry can be used as a rough measure of tidal volume and expiratory reserve volume **(No. 4)** since the patient breathes in deeply and exhales completely into the incentive spirometer. **AN,6,PhI**

3. **(2)** Humidification of oxygen is extremely important in reducing its drying effects on the mucous membranes of the bronchial tree. Humidification of oxygen is generally provided by a water nebulizer. **Nos. 1, 3, and 4** are incorrect because oxygen is not highly permeable in water; thus, water tends to inhibit rather than facilitate oxygen diffusion across the respiratory membrane. Humidification expands the volume of the inhaled gas, but by doing so it decreases the partial pressure of the gas in the alveoli. Normal alveolar partial pressures of oxygen are approximately 100 mm Hg, whereas the partial pressures of oxygen in the atmosphere are approximately 135 mm Hg. **AN,6,PhI**

Key to codes following rationales   Nursing process: **AS,** Assessment; **AN,** Analysis; **PL,** Plan; **IMP,** Implementation; **EV,** Evaluation. Category of human function: **1,** Protective; **2,** Sensory-perceptual; **3,** Comfort, Rest, Activity, and Mobility; **4,** Nutrition; **5,** Growth and Development; **6,** Fluid-Gas Transport; **7,** Psychosocial-Cultural; **8,** Elimination. Client need: **SECE,** Safe, Effective Care Environment; **PhI,** Physiologic Integrity; **PsI,** Psychosocial Integrity; **HPM,** Health Promotion/Maintenance. See appendices for full explanation.

Treatments

■ TABLE 5.10 Universal Blood and Body Fluid Precautions

The Centers for Disease Control recommends universal blood and body fluid precautions (also referred to as *universal precautions*) in the care of *all* patients, especially those in emergency care settings, in which the risk of blood exposure is increased and the infection status of the patient is unknown. In other words, the nurse should treat all body substances or fluids of all patients as if they are potentially infectious.

The CDC recommends that these precautions apply to blood and to body fluids containing visible **blood,** as well as to **semen** and **vaginal** secretions; to tissues, and to the following fluids: **cerebrospinal fluid, synovial fluid, pleural fluid, peritoneal fluid, pericardial fluid,** and **amniotic fluid.** Universal precautions do *not* apply to *nasal secretions, sputum, saliva, sweat, tears, urine, feces,* and *vomitus unless* they contain visible blood. Blood is the single most important source of HIV, HBV, and other bloodborne pathogens in the health care setting.

Protective barriers—gloves, gowns, masks, and protective eyewear—reduce the risk of exposure to potentially infective materials. The following specific precautions are recommended.

- Wash your hands thoroughly and immediately after accidental contact with body substances containing blood, between patients, and immediately after gloves are removed.
- Wear gloves when touching blood and body fluids containing blood as well as when handling items or surfaces soiled with blood or body fluids.
- Change gloves between patient contacts.
- Use sterile gloves for procedures involving contact with normally sterile areas of the body.
- Use examination gloves for procedures involving contact with mucous membranes, unless otherwise indicated, and for other patient care or diagnostic procedures that do not require the use of sterile gloves.
- Do *not* wash or disinfect surgical or examination gloves for reuse. Washing with surfactants may cause *wicking,* i.e., the enhanced penetration of liquids through undetected holes in the glove. Disinfecting agents may cause deterioration.
- Use general-purpose utility gloves (e.g., rubber household gloves) for housekeeping chores involving potential blood contact and for instrument cleaning and decontamination procedures. Utility gloves may be decontaminated and reused but should be discarded if they are peeling, cracked, or discolored or if they have punctures, tears, or other evidence of deterioration.
- Wear gloves when performing phlebotomy (venipuncture):
  - If the nurse has cuts, scratches, or other breaks in the skin.

- In situations where hand contamination with blood may occur, e.g., with an uncooperative patient.
  - When the nurse is learning phlebotomy techniques.
- Wear gloves when performing finger and/or heel sticks on infants and children.
- Wear masks and protective eyewear (glasses, goggles) or face shields to protect the mucous membranes or your mouth, nose, and eyes during procedures that are likely to generate droplets of blood or other body fluids to which universal precautions apply.
- Wear a disposable plastic apron or gown during procedures that are likely to generate splatters of blood or other body fluid (e.g., peritoneal fluid) and soil your clothing.
- To prevent injuries, place used disposable needle-syringe units, scalpel blades, and other sharp items in puncture-resistant containers for disposal. Discard used needle-syringe units *uncapped* and *unbroken.* Puncture-resistant containers should be located as close as practicable to use areas.
- Place mouthpieces, resuscitation bags, or other ventilation devices in areas where the need for emergency mouth-to-mouth resuscitation is predictable—even though saliva has *not* been implicated in HIV transmission.
- If a nurse has exudative lesions or weeping dermatitis, it is necessary to refrain from all direct patient care and from handling patient-care equipment until the condition is resolved.
- Handle soiled linen as little as possible and with minimum agitation to prevent gross microbial contamination of the air and of persons handling the linen. Place and transport linen soiled with blood or body fluids in leakage-resistant bags.
- Put all specimens of blood and listed body fluids in well-constructed containers with secure lids to prevent leakage during transport. When collecting specimens, take care to avoid contaminating the outside of the container.
- Use a chemical germicide that is approved for use as a hospital disinfectant to decontaminate work surfaces after there is a spill of blood or other body fluids. In the absence of a commercial germicide, a solution of sodium hypochlorite (household bleach) in a 1:10 dilution is effective. Before decontaminating areas, first remove visible material. Wear gloves during cleaning and decontaminating procedures.
- Follow agency policies for disposal of infective waste both when disposing of and when decontaminating contaminated materials.
- Carefully pour bulk blood, suctioned fluids, and excretions containing blood and secretions down drains that are connected to a sanitary sewer.

Source: U.S. Department of Health and Human Services. Public Health Service.

4. **(3)** Maintenance of infusion rates as ordered is extremely important. In this example, the nurse can use the following equation:

$$\frac{\text{gtts/mL of given set}}{60 \text{ min/h}} \times \text{total volume/h} = \text{gtts/min}$$

Thus,

$$\frac{15}{60} \times 100 = \frac{1}{4} \times 100 = 25 \text{ gtts/min}$$

IMP,6,PhI

5. **(2)** Normal fasting serum-glucose levels are 80–120 mg/dL of blood. Levels below 60 **(No. 1)** indicate hypoglycemia; levels above 120 mg/dL **(Nos. 3 and 4)** indicate hyperglycemia. **IMP,4,PhI**

6. **(2)** Procedurally, the patient to receive the glucose tolerance test consumes a high-carbohydrate diet for 3 days before the test. All drugs that may influence the test are discontinued during this period (oral contraceptives, aspirin, steroids). On the day of the test, fasting blood **(No. 1)** and urine specimens are collected before the test, to provide control glucose levels. After ingestion of a glucose load, specimens of blood and urine are collected at hourly intervals for 3 hours. In diabetes mellitus, glucose levels are elevated. The postprandial blood glucose **(No. 3)** is determined by giving the patient an oral glucose load only. Blood-glucose levels are then evaluated in 2 hours. Usually glucose levels will return to normal during this period of time. The tolbutamide response test **(No. 4)** may also be utilized to confirm diabetes. After the patient fasts overnight, a baseline fast-

Treatments

ing blood sample is drawn. Intravenous tolbutamide is then given, and blood samples drawn in 20–30 minutes. After this test the patient should be given orange juice and instructed to eat breakfast. **AN,4,PhI**

7. (3) Within 3 hours the patient's serum-glucose levels should not only have returned to normal, but some hypoglycemia should be expected. **Nos. 1, 2, and 4** are incorrect. **EV,4,PhI**

8. (3) Following gastroscopy, food and fluids are withheld until the gag reflex returns (generally 2–3 hours) in order to prevent aspiration. The gag reflex is inactivated by either an anesthetic spray or an oral preparation gargled by the patient prior to insertion of the gastroscopy tube. Inhibition of the gag reflex facilitates insertion. **Nos. 1 and 2** are incorrect because the period of time is too brief. **No. 4** is incorrect not only because it is generally unnecessary to wait 6–8 hours for the gag reflex to return, but because this procedure does not precipitate an electrolyte imbalance. **PL,4,PhI**

9. (2) Decreased amounts of creatinine in the urine are a reflection of the glomerular filtration rate, indicating the ability of the kidney to clear the renal blood of this substance. The filtration fraction is simply the amount of glomerular filtrate entering the tubules **(No. 1)**. Renal blood flow is estimated by measuring renal excretion of PAH (para-aminohippuric acid) **(No. 3)**. Though the amount and specific gravity of urine may be determined, it is not the primary function of this laboratory test **(No. 4)**. **AS,8,PhI**

10. (2) Intravenous pyelogram tests both the function and patency of the kidneys. After the intravenous injection of a radiopaque contrast medium, the size, location, and patency of the kidneys can be observed by roentgenogram, as well as the patency of the urethra and bladder as the kidneys function to excrete the dye. **No. 1** is an example of a KUB, or flat plate of the abdomen, which can reveal gross structural changes in the kidneys and urethra. Renal blood flow (**No. 3**) is determined by the injection of PAH (para-aminohippuric acid) and measurement of its excretion in the urine. **No. 4** is an example of renal angiogram. **IMP,8,SECE**

11. (1) Patient teaching includes telling the patient that a warm, flushed sensation and salty taste may occur from the contrast medium. The contrast medium is given by IV injection during the procedure, not in capsule form (**No. 2**). **No. 3** is incorrect because allergies to iodine, not to mercury, are the concern. Fluids are not pushed prior to this procedure; they are withheld for up to 8 hours prior to testing, to produce a slight dehydration that aids in concentrating the contrast medium in the kidneys and urinary system (**No. 4**). **IMP,8,PhI**

12. (4) The patient is informed of possible reaction to injection of the contrast medium, which is administered by an IV injection at the time of the test, not by tablets the evening before (**No. 1**). **No. 2** is incorrect because patients given anything by mouth are given a low-fat meal the evening before IV cholangiogram or oral cholecystogram. Since the patient is quite ill at this time, he or she may or may not be able to tolerate oral intake. However, in order to have a clear visualization of the gallbladder, the bowel is cleansed, and food and fluids are withheld, not forced (**No. 3**), for 6–8 hours. **PL,4,SECE**

13. (2) The most important effect of intermittent positive-pressure breathing (IPPB) is increased alveolar ventilation. It also helps to mobilize secretions (**No. 1**), decrease the occurrence of atelectasis (**No. 3**), and decrease airway resistance (**No. 4**) through mechanical bronchodilation. **EV,6,PhI**

Nursing Care of Behavioral and Emotional Problems Throughout the Life Span

The chief *objective* of this unit is to highlight the most commonly observed behavioral, emotional problems and disorders in the mental health field. The emphasis is on (a) main points for *assessment,* (b) *analysis* of data based on underlying *basic concepts and general principles* drawn from a psychodynamic and interpersonal theoretical framework, and (c) *nursing interventions* based on the therapeutic use of self as the cornerstone of a helping process. Nursing actions are listed in *priority* whenever possible. Hence the **nursing process framework** is followed throughout. Note that nursing interventions are divided into *planning* and *implementation* (covering long-term and short-term *goals* and stressing *priority* of actions) and *health teaching. Evaluation* of results is listed separately, although this step of the nursing process is circular and relates back to "assessment" and "goals."

I recognize that the categorization of psychiatric-emotional disorders can be complex and controversial. For purposes of clarity and simplicity, an attempt has been made here to capsulize many theoretical principles and component skills of the helping process that these disorders have *in common.* That the term *client* is often used in place of *patient* reflects the interpersonal rather than medical model of psychiatric nursing. The diagnostic categorization of disorders (based on a synthesis of the North American Nursing Diagnosis Association [NANDA] and PND-I classification system for psychiatric nursing diagnoses)* is included here to update the reader in current terminology in the mental health field.

The underlying organizational framework for this unit is based on applicable **categories of human functions** (Growth and Development; Protective Functions; Comfort, Rest, Activity, and Mobility; Sensory-Perceptual Functions; and Psychosocial-Cultural Functions; see Appendices G and H).

These categories have been incorporated into the diagnostic profile sent to the NCLEX-RN examinees as part of a report of their performance on the licensure exam. The categories reflect four **client needs** and are based on clusters of nursing activities designed to meet these needs, for example, protecting the clients, assisting clients with mobility needs.

❏ Growth and Development

Major Theoretical Models

I. **Psychodynamic model (Freud)**
   A. **Assumptions and key ideas**
      1. No human behavior is accidental; each psychic event is determined by preceding ones.
      2. Unconscious mental processes occur with very great frequency and significance.
      3. Psychoanalysis is used to uncover childhood trauma, which may involve conflict and repressed feelings.
      4. Psychoanalytic methods are used: therapeutic alliance, transference, regression, dream association, catharsis.
   B. *Freud*—shifted from classification of behavior to understanding and explaining in psychological terms and changing behavior under structured conditions.
      1. Structure of the mind: id, ego, superego; unconscious, preconscious, conscious.
      2. Stages of psychosexual development.

---

*From ANA Classification of Individual Human Responses of Concern for Psychiatric Mental Health Nursing Practice (PND-I), 1994.

3. Coping mechanisms.

II. Psychosocial development model (Erikson, Maslow, Piaget)

A. *Erik Erikson—Eight Stages of Man* (1963)

1. Psychosocial development—interplay of biology with social factors, encompassing total life span, from birth to death, in progressive developmental tasks.

2. *Stages of life cycle*—life consists of a series of developmental phases. (See Table 6.1 for comparison summary.)

   a. Universal sequence of biologic, social, psychological events.

   b. Each person experiences a series of normative conflicts and crises and thus needs to accomplish specific psychosocial tasks.

   c. Two opposing energies (positive and negative forces) coexist and need to be synthesized.

   d. How each age-specific task is accomplished influences the developmental progress of the next phase and the ability to deal with life.

B. *Abraham Maslow—Hierarchy of Needs* (1962)

1. Beliefs regarding emotional health based on a comprehensive, multidisciplinary approach to human problems, involving all aspects of functioning.

   a. *Premise:* mental illness cannot be understood without prior knowledge of mental health.

   b. *Focus:* positive aspects of human behavior (e.g., contentment, joy, happiness).

2. *Hierarchy of needs*—physiologic, safety, love and belonging, self-esteem and self-recognition, self-actualization, aesthetic. As each stage is mastered, the next stage becomes dominant.

3. *Characteristics of optimal mental health*—keep in mind that wellness is on a continuum with cultural variations.

   a. *Self-esteem:* entails self-confidence and self-acceptance.

   b. *Self-knowledge:* involves accurate self-perception of strengths and limitations.

   c. *Satisfying interpersonal relationships:* able to meet reciprocal emotional needs through collaboration rather than exploitation or power struggles or jealousy; able to make full commitments in close relationships.

   d. *Environmental mastery:* can adapt, change, and solve problems effectively; can make decisions, choose from alternatives, and predict consequences. Actions are conscious, not impulsive.

   e. *Stress-management:* can delay seeking gratification and relief; does not blame or dwell on past; assumes self-responsibility; either modifies own expectations, seeks substitutes, or withdraws from stressful situation when cannot reduce stress.

C. *Jean Piaget—Cognitive and Intellectual Development* (1963)

1. **Assumptions**—child development is steered by interaction of environmental and genetic influences; therefore focus is on environmental and social forces. (See Table 6.1 for comparison with other theories.)

2. **Key concepts**

   a. *Assimilation:* process of acquiring new knowledge, skills, and insights by using what they already know and have.

   b. *Accommodation:* adjusts to change by solving previously unsolvable problems because of newly assimilated knowledge.

   c. *Adaptation:* coping process to handle environmental demands.

3. **Age-specific development levels**—sensorimotor, preconceptual, intuitive, concrete, formal operational thought.

III. Behavioral model (Pavlov, Watson, Wolpe, Skinner)

A. **Assumptions**

1. Roots in neurophysiology.

2. Stimulus-response learning can be *conditioned* through *reinforcement.*

3. Behavior is what one does.

4. Behavior is observable, describable, predictable, and controllable.

5. Classification of mental disease is clinically useless, only provides legal labels.

B. **Aim:** change *observable* behavior. There is *no underlying* cause, *no internal* motive.

IV. Comparison of models—Table 6.1 compares four theories.

Concept of Death Throughout the Life Cycle

I. Ages 1–3

A. No concept per se, but experiences *separation anxiety and abandonment* any time significant other disappears from view over a period of time.

B. *Coping* means: fear, resentment, anger, aggression, regression, withdrawal.

◆ C. **Nursing care plan/implementation**—help the family:

1. Facilitate transfer of affectional ties to another nurturing adult.

2. Decrease separation anxiety of hospitalized child by encouraging family visits and by reassuring child that she or he will not be alone.

3. Provide stable environment through consistent staff assignment.

II. Ages 3–5

A. Least anxious about death.

■ TABLE 6.1 Summary of Theories of Psychosocial Development Throughout the Life Cycle

Freud	Piaget	Sullivan	Erikson
Emphasis on			
Pathology (intrapsychic)	*Normal* children	Pathology (interpersonal)	Both health and illness
Anxiety	*No* emphasis on ego, anxiety, identity, libido	Anxiety	
Unconscious, uncontrollable drives	Cognitive development	Unconscious, uncontrollable drives	Problems are manageable and can be solved
Ego needing defense	Tasks can be accomplished through learning process	Self-system needing defense	Need to integrate individual and society
Pathologic Development Influenced by			
Early feelings; repressed experiences in unconscious mind	Individual differences and social influences on the mind	Unconscious mind *and* interpersonal relationships (IPR)	Ego, anxiety, identity, libido concepts *combined* with social forces
Change Possible with			
Understanding content and meaning of unconscious	Socialization process to facilitate cognitive development	Improved IPR and understanding basic good-bad transformations	Integration of attitudes, libido, and social roles for strong ego identity
Age Group			
First 5 yr of life	Middle childhood years	Adolescence	Middle age, old age
Focus on			
Emotional development	Cognitive skills	Emotional and interpersonal development	Emotional, interpersonal, spiritual
Psychosexual aspects	Cognitive, interactive aspects	Psychosocial aspects	Psychosocial aspects
Cause of Conflicts and Problems			
Oral, anal, genital stage problems (especially unresolved oedipal/castration conflicts)	Faulty adaptation between individual and environment for intellectual development	Threats to self-system; disturbed communication process; 7 stages not complete	Unresolved conflicts, crises in 8 successive life cycle stages
Prognosis			
Few changes possible after age 5	Little change in adult cognitive structure after middle adolescence	Change usually possible with improved IPR	Change not only possible but *expected* throughout life
Sexual problems part of disturbed behavior	Sex as a variable in learning (age, IQ)	Sexual problems are only one type of faulty IPR affecting behavior	Sexual identity as one of many problems solved by interaction of desire and social process

B. Denial of death as inevitable and final process.

C. Death is separation, being alone.

D. Death is *sleep* and sleep is death.

E. "Death" is part of vocabulary; seen as real, gradual, *temporary,* not permanent.

F. Dead person is seen as alive, but in altered form, that is, lacks movement.

G. There are *degrees* of death.

H. Death means not being here anymore.

I. "Living" and "lifeless" are not yet distinguished.

J. Illness and death seen as *punishment* for "badness"; fear and guilt about sexual and aggressive impulses.

K. Death happens, but only to others.

◆ L. **Nursing care plan/implementation** (in addition to above):

1. Encourage play for expression of feelings; use clay, dolls, etc.

2. Encourage verbal expression of feelings using children's books.

3. Model appropriate grieving behavior.

4. Protect child from the overstimulation of hysterical adult reactions by limiting contact.

5. Clearly state what death is—death is final, no breathing, eating, awakening—and that death is *not* sleep.

6. Check child at night and provide support through holding and staying with child.

7. Allow a choice of attending the funeral and, if child decides to attend, describe what will take place.

8. If parents are grieving, have other family or friends attend to child's needs.

III. **Ages 5–10**

A. Death is cessation of life; question of what happens after death.

Mental Health

   B. Death seen as definitive, *universal,* inevitable, *irreversible.*

   C. Death occurs to all living things, including self; may express, "It isn't fair."

   D. Death is distant from self (an eventuality).

   E. Believe death occurs by accident, happens only to the very *old* or very sick.

   F. Death is personified (as a separate person) in fantasies and magical thinking.

   G. Death anxiety handled by *nightmares, rituals,* and *superstitions* (related to fear of darkness and sleeping alone because death is an external person, like a skeleton, who comes and takes people away at night).

   H. Dissolution of bodily life seen as a perceptible result.

   I. Fear of body mutilation.

  ◆ **J.** **Nursing care plan/implementation** (in addition to above):
     1. Allow child to experience the loss of pets, friends, and family members.
     2. Help child talk it out and experience the appropriate emotional reactions.
     3. Understand need for increase in play, especially competitive play.
     4. Involve child in funeral preparation and rituals.
     5. Understand and accept regressive or protest behaviors.
     6. Rechannel protest behaviors into constructive outlets.

IV. Adolescence

   A. Death seen as inevitable, *personal,* universal, and *permanent;* corporal life stops; body decomposes.

   B. Does not fear death, but concerned with how to *live now,* what death feels like, *body changes.*

   C. Experiences *anger, frustration, and despair* over lack of future, lack of fulfillment of adult roles.

   D. Openly asks *difficult,* honest, *direct* questions.

   E. Anger at healthy peers.

   F. Conflict between *developing* body versus *deteriorating* body, *independent* identity versus *dependency.*

  ◆ **G.** **Nursing care plan/implementation** (in addition to above):
     1. Facilitate full expression of grief by answering direct questions.
     2. Help let out feelings, especially through creative and aesthetic pursuits.
     3. Encourage participation in funeral ritual.
     4. Encourage full use of peer group support system, by providing opportunities for group talks.

V. Young adulthood

   A. Death seen as *unwelcome* intrusion, *interruption* of what might have been.

   B. Reaction: *rage, frustration, disappointment.*

◆ **C.** **Nursing care plan/implementation:** all of above, especially peer group support.

VI. Middle age

   A. Concerned with *consequences* of own death and that of significant others.

   B. Death seen as disruption of involvement, responsibility, and *obligations.*

   C. End of plans, projects, experiences.

   D. Death is *pain.*

◆ **E.** **Nursing care plan/implementation** (in addition to above): assess need for counseling when also in midlife crisis.

VII. Old age

   A. *Philosophical* rationalizations: death as inevitable, final process of life, when "time runs out."

   B. *Religious* view: death represents only the dissolution of life and is a doorway to a new life (a preparatory stage for another life).

   C. Time of rest and peace, supreme refuge from turmoil of life.

◆ **D.** **Nursing care plan/implementation** (in addition to above):
     1. Help person prepare for own death by helping with funeral prearrangements, wills, and sharing of mementos.
     2. Facilitate life review and reinforce positive aspects.
     3. Provide care and comfort.
     4. Be present at death.

Death and Dying

Too often the process of death has had such frightening aspects that people have suffered alone. Today there has been a vast change in attitudes; death and dying are no longer taboo topics. There is a growing realization that we need to accept death as a natural process. Elisabeth Kübler-Ross has written extensively on the process of dying, describing the stages of *denial* ("not me!"), *anger* ("why me?"), *bargaining* ("yes me—but"), *depression* ("yes, me"), and *acceptance* ("my time is close now, it's all right"), with implications for the helping person.

   I. Concepts and principles related to death and dying:

   A. Persons may know or *suspect* they are dying and may want to talk about it; often they look for someone to share their fears and the process of dying.

   B. Fear of death can be reduced by helping clients feel that they are *not alone.*

   C. The dying need the opportunity to live their final experiences to the fullest, in their *own* way.

   D. People who are dying remain more or less the *same* as they were during life; their approaches to death are consistent with their approaches to life.

   E. Dying persons' need to review their lives may be a purposeful attempt to reconcile themselves to what "was" and "what could have been."

F. *Three ways* of facing death are (a) quiet acceptance with inner strength and peace of mind; (b) restlessness, impatience, anger, and hostility; and (c) depression, withdrawal, and fearfulness.

G. *Four tasks* facing a dying person are (a) reviewing life, (b) coping with physical symptoms in the end stage of life, (c) making a transition from known to unknown state, and (d) reaction to separation from loved ones.

H. Crying and tears are an important aspect of the grief process.

I. There are many *blocks* to providing a helping relationship with the dying and bereaved:

1. Nurses' unwillingness to share the process of dying—minimizing their contacts and blocking out their own feelings.
2. Forgetting that a dying person may be feeling lonely, abandoned, and afraid of dying.
3. Reacting with irritation and hostility to the person's frequent calls.
4. Nurses' failure to seek help and support from team members when feeling afraid, uneasy, and frustrated in caring for a dying person.
5. Not allowing client to talk about death and dying.
6. Nurses' use of technical language or social chit-chat as a defense against their own anxieties.

◆ **II. Assessment** of death and dying:

A. *Physical*

1. Observable deterioration of physical and mental capacities—person is unable to fulfill physiologic needs, such as eating and elimination.
2. Circulatory collapse (blood pressure and pulse).
3. Renal or hepatic failure.
4. Respiratory decline.

B. *Psychosocial*

1. Fear of death is signaled by agitation, restlessness, and sleep disturbances at night.
2. Anger, agitation, blaming.
3. Morbid self-pity with feelings of defeat and failure.
4. Depression and withdrawal.
5. Introspectiveness and calm acceptance of the inevitable.

◆ **III. Analysis/nursing diagnosis:**

A. *Terminal illness response.*

B. *Altered feeling states* related to fear of being alone.

C. *Altered comfort patterns* related to pain.

D. *Altered meaningfulness* related to depression, hopelessness, helplessness, powerlessness.

E. *Altered social interaction* related to withdrawal.

◆ **IV. Nursing care plan/implementation:**

A. *Long-term goal:* foster environment where person and family can experience dying with dignity.

B. *Short-term goals:*

1. Express feelings (person and family).
2. Support person and family.
3. Minimize physical discomfort.

C. Explore your own feelings about death and dying with team members; form support groups.

D. Be aware of the *normal grief* process.

1. *Allow* person and family to do the work of grieving and mourning.
2. Allow crying and mood swings, anger, demands.
3. Permit yourself to cry.

E. Allow person to *express* feelings, fears, and concerns.

1. Avoid pat answers to questions about "why."
2. Pick up symbolic communication.

F. Provide care and comfort with *relief from pain;* do not isolate person.

G. Stay *physically close.*

1. Use touch.
2. Be available to form a consistent relationship.

H. *Reduce isolation and abandonment* by assigning person to room in which it is less likely to occur and by allowing flexible visiting hours.

I. Keep activities in room as *near normal* and *constant* as possible.

J. Speak in *audible* tones, not whispers.

K. Be alert to cues when person needs to be alone (*disengagement process*).

L. Leave room for *hope.*

M. Help person die with peace of mind by lending support and providing opportunities to express anger, pain, and fears to someone who will accept her or him and not censor verbalization.

N. *Health teaching:* teach grief process to family and friends; teach methods to relieve pain.

◆ **V. Evaluation/outcome criteria:**

A. Remains comfortable and free of pain as long as possible.

B. Dies with dignity.

Grief/Bereavement

Grief is a typical reaction to the loss of a source of psychological gratification. It is a syndrome with somatic and psychological symptoms that diminish when grief is resolved. Grief processes have been extensively described by Erich Lindemann and George Engle.*

I. Concepts and principles related to grief:

---

*Adapted from Engle G. Grief and grieving. *Am J Nurs* 1964;9(64): 93–98. Copyright 1964 American Journal of Nursing Co.

A. Cause of grief: reaction to loss (real or imaginary, actual or pending).

B. Healing process can be interrupted.

C. Grief is universal.

D. Uncomplicated grief is a self-limiting process.

E. Grief responses may vary in degree and kind (e.g., absence of grief, delayed grief, and unresolved grief).

F. People go through stages similar to stages of death described by Elisabeth Kübler-Ross.

G. Many factors influence successful outcome of grieving process:

1. The more *dependent* the person on the lost relationship, the greater the difficulty in resolving the loss.
2. A *child* has greater difficulty resolving loss.
3. A person with *few meaningful relationships* also has greater difficulty.
4. The *more losses* the person has had in the past, the more affected that person will be, as losses tend to be cumulative.
5. The more *sudden* the loss, the greater the difficulty in resolving it.
6. The more *ambivalence* (love-hate feelings, with guilt) there was toward the dead, the more difficult the resolution.
7. *Loss of a child* is harder to resolve than loss of an older person.

◆ **II.** **Assessment**—characteristic stages of grief responses:

A. *Shock and disbelief* (initial and recurrent stage)

1. *Denial* of reality. ("No, it can't be.")
2. Stunned, *numb* feeling.
3. Feelings of loss, *helplessness,* impotence.
4. Intellectual acceptance.

B. *Developing awareness*

1. Anguish about loss.
   a. *Somatic* distress.
   b. Feelings of emptiness.
2. *Anger* and hostility toward person or circumstances held responsible.
3. Guilt feelings—may lead to self-destructive actions.
4. Tears (inwardly, alone; or inability to cry).

C. *Restitution*

1. Funeral *rituals* are an aid to grief resolution by emphasizing the reality of death.
2. Expression and sharing of feelings by gathered family and friends are a source of acknowledgment of grief and support for the bereaved.

D. *Resolving the loss*

1. Increased *dependency* on others as an attempt to deal with painful void.
2. More aware of own *bodily sensations*—may be identical with symptoms of the deceased.
3. Complete *preoccupation* with thoughts and memories of the dead person.

E. *Idealization*

1. All hostile and negative feelings about the dead are *repressed*.

2. Mourner may *assume* qualities and attributes of the dead.
3. Gradual lessening of preoccupation with the dead; *reinvesting* in others.

◆ **III.** **Analysis**—see Table 6.2.

◆ **IV.** **Nursing care plan/implementation** in grief states:

A. *Apply crisis theory and interventions.*

B. *Demonstrate unconditional respect* for cultural, religious, and social mourning customs.

C. *Utilize knowledge of the stages of grief* to anticipate reactions and facilitate the grief process.

1. Anticipate and permit expression of different manifestations of shock, disbelief, and denial.
   a. News of impending death is best communicated to a family group (rather than an individual) in a private setting.
   b. *Let mourners see the dead or dying,* to help them accept reality.
   c. Encourage description of circumstances and nature of loss.
2. *Accept guilt, anger, and rage* as common responses to coping with guilt and helplessness.
   a. Be aware of potential suicide by the bereaved.
   b. Permit crying; stay with the bereaved.
3. Mobilize social support system; promote hospital policy that allows gathering of friends and family in a private setting.
4. Allow dependency on staff for initial decision making while person is attempting to resolve loss.
5. Respond to somatic complaints.
6. Permit reminiscence.
7. Encourage mourner to relate accounts connected with the lost relationship that reflect positive and negative feelings and remembrances; *place loss in perspective.*
8. Begin to encourage and reinforce new interests and social relations with others by the end of the idealization stage, loosen bonds of attachment.
9. Identify high-risk persons for maladaptive responses. (See I.G. Many factors influence successful outcome of grieving process, above.)
10. *Health teaching:*
    a. Explain that emotional response is appropriate and common.
    b. Explain and offer hope that emotional pain will diminish with time.
    c. Describe normal grief stages.

◆ **V.** **Evaluation/outcome criteria:** outcome may take 1 yr or more—can remember comfortably and realistically both pleasurable and disappointing aspects of the lost relationship.

A. Can express feelings of sorrow caused by loss.

■ **TABLE 6.2** Analysis/Nursing Diagnosis: *Altered Feeling States* Related to Grief

Problem Classification	Characteristics
1. Somatic distress	Occurs in waves lasting from 20 min to 1 h
	Deep, sighing respirations most common when discussing grief
	Lack of strength
	Loss of appetite and sense of taste
	Tightness in throat
	Choking sensation accompanied by shortness of breath
2. Preoccupation with image of deceased	Similar to daydreaming
	May mistake others for deceased person
	May be oblivious to surroundings
	Slight sense of unreality
	Fear that he or she is becoming "insane"
3. Feelings of guilt	Accuses self of negligence
	Exaggerates existence and importance of negative thoughts, feelings, and actions toward deceased
	Views self as having failed deceased—"If I had only . . ."
4. Feelings of hostility	Irritability, anger, and loss of warmth toward others
	May attempt to handle feelings of hostility in formalized and stiff manner of social interaction
5. Loss of patterns of conduct	Inability to initiate or maintain organized patterns of activity
	Restlessness, with aimless movements
	Loss of zest—tasks and activities are carried on as though with great effort
	Activities formerly carried on in company of deceased have lost their significance
	May become strongly dependent on whomever stimulates him or her to activity

Source: Wilson HS, Kneisl CR. *Psychiatric Nursing* (3rd ed). Redwood City, CA: Addison-Wesley, 1988.

B. Can describe ambivalence (love, anger) toward lost person, relationship.

C. Able to review relationship, including pleasures, regrets, etc.

D. Bonds of attachment are loosened and new object relationships are established.

Mental and Emotional Disorders in Children and Adolescents

Children have certain developmental tasks to master in the various stages of development (e.g., learning to trust, control primary instincts, and resolve basic social roles; see Unit 8, Nursing Care of Children and Families).

I. Concepts and principles related to mental and emotional disorders in children and adolescents

A. Most emotional disorders of children are related to family dynamics and the place the child occupies in the family group.

B. Children must be understood and treated within the context of their *families.*

C. Many disorders are related to the phases of development through which the children are passing. (Erik Erikson's developmental tasks for children are trust, autonomy, initiative, industry, identity, and intimacy.)

D. Children are not miniature adults; they have special needs.

E. Play and food are important media to make contact with children and help them release emotions in socially acceptable forms, prepare them for traumatic events, and develop skills.

F. Children who are physically or emotionally ill regress, giving up previously useful habits.

G. Adolescents have special problems relating to need for *control* versus need to *rebel, dependency* versus *interdependency,* and search for *identity* and *self-realization.*

H. Adolescents often *act out* their underlying feelings of insecurity, rejection, deprivation, and low self-esteem.

I. Strong feelings may be evoked in nurses working with children; these feelings should be expressed, and each nurse should be supported by team members.

◆ **II. Assessment** of selected disorders:

A. *Autistic disorders* (previously called childhood schizophrenia):

1. Disturbance in how perceptual information is processed; normal abilities present.

a. Behave *as though they cannot* hear, see, etc.

b. Do *not react to external* stimulus.

c. Mute or echolalic.
2. Lack of self-awareness as a unified whole—may not relate bodily needs or parts as extension of themselves.
3. Severe difficulty in communicating with others—may be mute and isolated.
4. Bizarre postures and gestures (banging head, rocking back and forth).
5. Disturbances in learning.
6. Etiology is unknown.
7. Prognosis depends on severity of symptoms and age of onset.

B. *Developmental disorders* (brain injury) characteristics:
1. Hyperactivity.
2. Explosive outbursts.
3. Distractibility.
4. Impulsiveness.
5. Perceptual difficulties (visual distortions, such as figure-ground distortion and mirror reading; body-image problems; difficulty in telling left from right).
6. Receptive or expressive language problems.

C. *Elimination disorders* (functional enuresis)—related to feelings of insecurity due to unmet needs of attention and affection; important to preserve their self-esteem.

D. *Separation anxiety disorders of childhood* (school phobias)—anxiety about school is accompanied by physical distress. Usually observed with fear of leaving home, rejection by mother, fear of loss of mother, or history of separation from mother in early years.

E. *Conduct disorders*—include lying, stealing, running away, truancy, substance abuse, sexual delinquency, vandalism, and fire setting; chief motivating force is either overt or covert hostility; history of disturbed parent-child relations.

◆ III. **Analysis/nursing diagnosis:**
A. *Altered feeling states:* anxiety, fear, hostility related to personal vulnerability and poorly developed or inappropriate use of defense mechanisms.
B. *Altered interpersonal processes:*
1. *Impaired verbal communication* related to cerebral deficits and psychological barriers.
2. *Altered conduct/impulse processes:* aggressive, violent behaviors toward self, others, environment related to feelings of distrust and altered judgment.
3. *Dysfunctional behaviors:* age-inappropriate behaviors, bizarre behaviors; disorganized and unpredictable behaviors related to inability to discharge emotions verbally.
4. *Impaired social interaction:* social isolation/withdrawal related to feelings of suspicion and mistrust.
5. *Altered values:* inability to internalize values associated with refusing limits, related

to unresolved emotions and altered judgment.
6. *Altered parenting* related to ambivalent family relationships and failure of child to meet role expectations.

C. *Sensory/perceptual alterations:* altered attention related to disturbed mental activities.

D. *Altered cognition process:* altered decision making, judgment, knowledge, and learning processes; altered thought content and processes related to perceptual or cognitive impairment and emotional dysfunctioning.

◆ IV. **Nursing care plan/implementation** in mental and emotional disorders in children and adolescents:
A. *General goals:* corrective behavior—*behavior modification.*
B. Help children gain self-awareness.
C. Provide *structured* environment to orient children to reality.
D. Impose *limits* on destructive behavior toward themselves or others without rejecting the children.
1. *Prevent* destructive behavior.
2. *Stop* destructive behavior.
3. *Redirect* nongrowth behavior into constructive channels.
E. Be *consistent.*
F. Meet *developmental and dependency* needs.
G. Recognize and encourage each child's strengths, growth behavior, and reverse regression.
H. Help these children reach the next step in social growth and development scale.
I. Use play and projective media to aid working out feelings and conflicts and in making contact.
J. Offer support to parents and strengthen the parent-child relationship.
K. *Health teaching:* teach parents methods of behavior modification.

◆ V. **Evaluation/outcome criteria:**
A. Destructive behavior is inhibited.
B. Demonstrates age-appropriate behavior on developmental scale.

Midlife Crisis: Phase of Life Problems

Midlife crisis is a time period that marks the passage between early maturity and middle age.

◆ I. **Assessment:**
A. Commonly occurs between ages 35 and 45.
B. Preoccupied with *visible* signs of aging, own mortality.
C. *Feelings: urgency* that time is running out ("last chance") for career achievement and unmet goals; *boredom* with present, *ambivalence, frustration, uncertainty* about the future.

D. Time of *reevaluation:*
  1. Reassess: meaning of time and parental role (omnipotence as a parent is challenged).
  2. Reexamine and contemplate change in career, marriage, family life.
E. *Personality changes* may occur. *Women:* traditional definitions of femininity may be challenged as become more assertive. *Males:* may be more introspective, sensitive to emotions, make external changes (younger mate, improve looks, new sports activity), mood swings.
F. Presence of *helpful elements* necessary to turn life's obstacles into opportunities.
  1. Willingness to take risks.
  2. Strong support system.
  3. Sense of purpose.
  4. Accumulated wisdom.

◆ **II. Analysis/nursing diagnosis:**
  A. *Self-esteem disturbance (low self-esteem)* related to loss of youth, faltering physical powers, and facing discrepancy between youthful ambitions and actual achievement (no longer a promising person with potential).
  B. *Altered role performance (role reversal):* related to parents who previously provided security and comfort but now need care.
  C. *Altered feeling processes (depression):* related to disappointments and diminished optimism as life is reconsidered in light of the reality of aging and death.

◆ **III. Nursing care plan/implementation**—*long-term goal:* help individual to rebuild life structure.
  A. Help client reappraise meaning of his or her life in terms of past, present, and future, and integrate aspects of time. Encourage introspection and reflection with questions.
  1. What have I done with my life?
  2. What do I really get from and give to my spouse, children, friends, work, community, and self?
  3. What are my strengths and liabilities?
  4. What have I done with my early dream, and do I want it now?
  B. Assist client to complete *four major tasks:*
  1. Terminate era of early adulthood by *reappraising* life goals identified and achieved during this era.
  2. Initiate movement into middle adulthood by beginning to make *necessary changes* in *unsuccessful* aspects of the current life while trying out new choices.
  3. Cope with *polarities* that divide life.
  4. Directly confront *death of own parents.*
  C. *Health teaching:* stress-management techniques; how to do self-assessment of aptitudes, interests; how to plan for retirement,

aloneness, and use of increased leisure time; dietary modification and exercise program.

◆ **IV. Evaluation/outcome criteria:**
  A. Gives up *idealized* self of early 20s for more *realistically* attainable self.
  1. Talks *less* of early *hopes of eminence* and *more* on modest goal of *competence.*
  2. Shifts values from sexuality to platonic relationships: replaces romantic dreams with *satisfying* friendships and companionships.
  3. Modifies early illusions about own capacities.
  4. Shifts values away from physical attractiveness and strength to *intellectual* abilities.
  B. Comes to accept that life is finite and reconciles what *is* with what *might have been;* appreciates everyday human experience rather than glamor or power.
  C. Through self-confrontation, self-discovery, and change, experiences time of restabilization; is reinvigorated, adventuresome.
  D. Develops *alternative* abilities that release new energies.
  E. Tries *less* to please everyone; others' opinions less important.
  F. Makes more efficient and well-seasoned decisions from well-developed sense of judgment.

Mental Health Problems of the Aged

In general, problems affecting the elderly are *similar* to those affecting persons of *any* age. This section highlights the *differences* from the viewpoint of etiology, frequency, and prognosis.

I. Concepts and principles related to mental health problems of the aged:
  A. The elderly *do* have capacity for growth and change.
  B. Human beings, regardless of age, need sense of future and *hope* for things to come.
  C. An inalienable right of all individuals should be to make or participate in all decisions concerning themselves and their possessions as long as they can.
  D. Physical disability due to the aging process may enforce dependency, which may be unacceptable to elderly patients and may evoke feelings of anger and ambivalence.
  E. In an attempt to *reduce feelings of loss,* elderly patients may *cling to concrete things* that most represent, in a *symbolic* sense, all that has been significant to them.
  F. As memory diminishes, *familiar objects* in environment and *familiar routines* are important in helping *to keep clients oriented* and in contact with reality.
  G. *Familiarity of environment brings security;* routines bring a sense of security about what is to happen.

H. If individuals feel unwanted, they may tell *stories* about their *earlier* achievements.

I. Many of the traits in the elderly result from *cumulative* effect of *past* experiences of frustrations and *present* awareness of limitations rather than from any primary consequences of physiologic deficit.

◆ **II. Assessment:**

A. *Psychological characteristics of the aged:*

1. Increasingly *dependent* on others, not only for physical needs but also for emotional security.

2. Concerns focus more and more *inward,* with narrowed outside interests.

   a. Decreased emotional energy for concern with social problems unless these issues affect them.

   b. Tendency to *reminisce.*

   c. May appear selfish and unsympathetic.

3. Sources of pleasure and gratification are more childlike: *food, warmth, and affection,* for example.

   a. Tangible and frequent evidence of affection is important (letters, cards, and visits, e.g.).

   b. May hoard articles.

4. *Attention span and memory are short;* may be forgetful and *accuse others of stealing.*

5. Deprivation of any kind is *not* tolerated:

   a. Easily frustrated.

   b. Change is poorly tolerated; need to have favorite chairs and established daily routine, for example.

6. Main *fears* in the aged include fear of *dependency,* chronic *illness, loneliness, boredom,* fear of being unloved, forgotten, *deserted* by those close to them, fear of *death;* fear of *loss of control* of one's own life; a failing *cognition;* loss of *purpose* and *productivity.*

7. *Nocturnal delirium* may be due to problems with night vision and inability to perceive *spatial* location.

B. *Psychiatric problems in aging*

1. *Loneliness*—related to *loss* of mate, diminishing circle of friends and family through death and geographic separation, *decline* in physical energy, loss of work (*retirement*), sharp loss of income, and loss of a lifelong life-style.

2. *Insomnia*—pattern of sleep changes in significant ways: disappearance of *deep* sleep, frequent *awakening, daytime* sleeping.

3. *Hypochondriasis*—anxiety may shift from concern with finances, job, or social prestige to concern about own bodily function.

4. *Depression*—common problem in the aging, with a *high suicide rate;* partly because of bodily changes that influence the *self-concept,* the older person may direct *hostility toward self* and therefore may be subject to feelings of depression and loneliness.

5. *Senility—four early symptoms:*

   a. Change in attention span.

   b. Memory loss for *recent* events and *names.*

   c. Altered intellectual capacity.

   d. Diminished ability to respond to others.

C. *Successful aging*

1. Being able to *perceive* signs of aging and limitations resulting from the aging process.

2. *Redefining* life in terms of effects on social and physical aspects of living.

3. Seeking *alternatives* for meeting needs and finding sources of pleasure.

4. Adopting a *different outlook* about self-worth.

5. *Reintegrating* values with goals of life.

D. *Causative factors* of mental disorder in the aged related to:

1. *Nutritional* problems and *physical ill health* related to *acute and chronic illness:*

   a. Cardiovascular diseases (heart failure, stroke, hypertension).

   b. Respiratory infection.

   c. Cancer.

   d. Alcohol dependence and abuse.

   e. Dentition problems.

2. Faulty adaptation related to *physical* changes of aging, e.g., depression, hypochondriases.

3. Problems related to *loss, grief, and bereavement.*

4. *Retirement* shock related to loss of status and financial security.

5. Social isolation and loneliness related to *inadequate sensory stimulation.*

6. *Environmental change* (relocation within a community or from home to institution): loss of family, privacy.

7. *Hopelessness, helplessness* related to condition and circumstances.

8. *Altered body image* (negative) related to aging process.

9. Depression related to *helplessness, inability to express anger.*

◆ **III. Analysis/nursing diagnosis:**

A. *Self-esteem disturbance* related to body-image disturbance and altered family role.

B. *Impaired social interaction* related to social isolation and environmental changes.

C. *Dysfunctional grieving* related to loss and bereavement.

D. *Altered feeling states and spiritual distress* related to hopelessness, anxiety, fear, powerlessness.

E. *Altered physical regulation processes* related to physical ill health.

F. *Sleep pattern disturbance* related to insomnia and altered sleep/arousal patterns.

◆ **IV. Nursing care plan/implementation:**
  A. *Long-term goal:* to help reduce hopelessness and helplessness.
  B. *Short-term goal:* to focus on ego assets.
  C. Help elderly *preserve* what facet of life they can and *regain* that which has already been lost.
    1. Help *minimize regression* as much as possible.
    2. Help retain their *adult* status.
    3. Help preserve their *self-image* as useful individuals.
    4. Identify and *preserve their abilities* to perform, emphasizing what they *can* do.
  D. Attempt to *prevent* loss of dignity and loss of worth—address them by titles, not "Gramps."
  E. *Reduce* feelings of *alienation* and loneliness. Provide *sensory* experiences for those with visual problems:
    1. Let them *touch* objects of various textures and consistencies.
    2. Encourage heightened *use of remaining senses* to make up for those that are diminished or lost.
  F. *Reduce* depression and feelings of isolation.
    1. Allow time to *reminisce.*
    2. *Avoid changes* in surroundings or routine.
  G. *Protect* from rush and excitement.
    1. Use simple, unhurried conversation.
    2. Allow *extra* time to organize thoughts.
  H. Be sensitive to *concrete* things they may want to *keep.*
  I. *Health teaching:*
    1. How to keep track of time (e.g., by marking off days on a calendar), to promote orientation.
    2. How to keep track of medications.
    3. Exercises to promote blood flow.
    4. *Retirement counseling:*
      a. Obtaining satisfaction from leisure time.
      b. Nurturing relationships with younger generations.
      c. Adjusting to changes: physical health, retirement, loss of loved ones.
      d. Developing connections with own age group.
      e. Taking on new social roles.
      f. Maintaining a satisfactory and appropriate living situation.
      g. Coping with dependence on others, especially one's children.

◆ **V. Evaluation/outcome criteria:**
  A. Less confusion and fewer mood swings.
  B. Increased interest in activities of daily living and interaction with others.
  C. Lessened preoccupation with death, dying, physical symptoms, feelings of sadness.
  D. Reduced insomnia and anorexia.
  E. Expresses feelings of belonging and being needed.

❑ Protective Functions

Common Behavioral Problems

I. Anger
  A. Definition: feelings of resentment in response to anxiety when threat is perceived; need to discharge tension of anger.
◆ **B. Assessment:**
    1. *Degree of anger and frequency:* scope of anger ranges on a continuum from *everyday mild annoyance → frustration* from interference with goal accomplishment → *assertiveness* (behavior used to deal with anger effectively) → *anger* related to helplessness and powerlessness that may interfere with functioning → *rage and fury,* when coping means are depleted or not developed.
    2. *Mode of expression of anger*
      a. *Covert, passive* expression of anger: being overly nice; body language with little or no eye contact, arms close to body, soft voice, little gesturing; sarcasm through humor; *sublimation* through art and music; projection onto others; *denying* and pushing anger out of awareness; *psychosomatic* illness in response to internalized anger, e.g., headache.
      b. *Overt,* active expression of anger: physical activity to work off excess physical energy associated with biologic response (e.g., hitting punching bag, taking a walk); *aggression,* assertiveness.
    3. *Physiologic behaviors*—result of secretion of epinephrine and sympathetic nervous system stimulation preparing for fight-flight.
      a. *Cardiovascular* response: increased blood pressure and pulse, increased free fatty acid in blood.
      b. *Gastrointestinal* response: increased nausea, salivation, decreased peristalsis.
      c. *Genitourinary* response: urinary frequency.
      d. *Neuromuscular* response: increased alertness, increased muscle tension and deep-tendon reflexes, ECG changes.
    4. *Positive functions of anger*
      a. Energizes behavior.
      b. Protects positive image.
      c. Provides ego defense during high anxiety.
      d. Gives greater control over situation.
      e. Alerts to need for coping.
      f. A sign of a healthy relationship.
◆ **C. Analysis/nursing diagnosis:** *defensive coping* related to source of stress (stressors):
    1. *Biologic stressors*—instinctual drives (Lorenz, on aggressive instincts, and Freud), *endocrine imbalances,* seizures, tumors, *hunger, fatigue.*

Mental Health

2. *Psychological stressors*—inability to resolve frustration that leads to aggression; real or imagined threatened loss of self-esteem; conflict, lack of control; anger as a learned expression and a reinforced response. Prolonged stress; an attempt to protect self; a desire for retaliation; a normal part of grief process.

3. *Sociocultural stressors*—lack of early training in self-discipline and social skills; crowding, personal space intrusion; *role modeling of abusive behavior* by significant others and by media personalities.

◆ **D. Nursing care plan/implementation**—*long-term goals:* constructive use of angry energy to accomplish tasks and motivate growth.

1. *Prevent* and *control* violence.
   a. Approach unhurriedly.
   b. Provide atmosphere of acceptance; listen attentively, refrain from arguing and criticizing.
   c. Encourage expression of feelings.
   d. Offer feedback of client's expressed feelings.
   e. Encourage mutual problem solving.
   f. Encourage realistic perception of others and situation and respect for the rights of others.

2. *Limit setting:*
   a. Clearly state *expectations* and *consequences* of acts.
   b. Enforce consequences.
   c. Encourage client to assume responsibility for behavior.
   d. Explore reasons and meaning of negative behavior.

3. Promote *self-awareness* and *problem-solving* abilities. Encourage and assist client to:
   a. Accept self as a person with a right to experience angry feelings.
   b. Explore reasons for anger.
   c. Describe situations where anger was experienced.
   d. Discuss appropriate alternatives for expressing anger (including assertiveness training).
   e. Decide on one feasible solution.
   f. Act on solution.
   g. Evaluate effectiveness.

4. *Health teaching:*
   a. Explore other ways to express feelings, and provide activities that allow appropriate expression of anger.
   b. Recommend that behavioral limits be set (by the family).
   c. Explain how to set behavioral limits.
   d. Advise against causing defensive patterns in others.

◆ **E. Evaluation/outcome criteria:**
1. Demonstrates insight (awareness of factors that precipitate anger; identifies disturbing topics, events, and inappropriate use of coping mechanisms).
2. Uses appropriate coping mechanisms.
3. Reaches out for emotional support before stress level becomes excessive.
4. Evidence of increased reality perception and problem-solving ability.

II. Combative-aggressive behavior
   A. Definition: *acting out* feelings of frustration, anger, anxiety, etc. through *physical or verbal* behavior.

◆ **B. Assessment:** recognize *precombative* behavior:
1. Demanding, fist clenching.
2. Boisterous, loud.
3. Vulgar, profane.
4. Limited attention span.
5. Sarcastic, taunting, verbal threats.
6. Restless, agitated, elated.
7. Frowning.

◆ **C. Analysis/nursing diagnosis:** *risk for violence* related to:
1. Frustration as response to *breakdown of self-control* coping mechanisms.
2. Acting out as customary response to anger (*defensive coping*).
3. Confusion (*sensory/perceptual alterations*).
4. Physical restraints, such as when postoperative patient discovers wrist restraints.
5. Fear of intimacy, intrusion on emotional and physical space (*altered thought processes*).
6. Feelings of helplessness, inadequacy (*situational or chronic low self-esteem*).

◆ **D. Nursing care plan/implementation:**
1. *Long-term goal:* channel aggression—help person express feelings rather than act them out.
2. *Immediate goal: prevent injury to self and others.*
   a. Calmly call for assistance; do *not* try to handle *alone.*
   b. Approach cautiously. Keep client within *eye contact,* observing client's personal space.
   c. *Protect* against self-injury and injury to others; be aware of your position in relation to the weapon, door, escape route.
   d. *Minimize* stimuli, to control the environment—clear the area, close doors, turn off TV so person can hear you.
   e. *Divert* attention from the act; engage in talk and lead away from others.
   f. Assess *triggering* cause.
   g. Identify immediate problem.
   h. Focus on *remedy for immediate* problem.
   i. Choose one calm, quieting individual to interact with person; nonauthoritarian, nonthreatening.
   j. Maintain *verbal contact* to keep communication open; offer empathetic ear, but be firm and consistent in setting *limits* on dangerous behavior.

    k. Negotiate, but don't make false promises or argue.
    l. Restraints may be necessary as a *last* resort.
    m. Place person in quiet room so he or she can calm down.
  3. *Health teaching:*
    a. Explain how to obtain release from stress and how to rechannel emotional energy into acceptable activity.
    b. Advise against causing defensive responses in others.
    c. Explain what is justifiable aggression.
    d. Emphasize importance of how to recognize tension in self.
    e. Explain why self-control is important.
    f. Explain to family, staff, how to set behavioral limits.
    g. Explain causes of maladaptive coping related to anger.
    h. Teach how to use problem-solving method.
◆ E. **Evaluation/outcome criteria:**
  1. Is aware of causes of anger; can recognize the feeling of anger and utilize alternative methods of expressing anger.
  2. Expression of anger is appropriate, congruent with the situation.
  3. Replaces aggression and acting out with assertiveness.

III. **Confusion/disorientation**
  A. **Definition:** loss of reality orientation as to person, time, place, events, ideas.
◆ B. **Assessment:** note unusual behavior:
  1. Picking, stroking movements in the air or on clothing and linens.
  2. Frequent crying or laughing.
  3. Alternating periods of confusion and lucidity (e.g., confused at night, when alone in the dark).
  4. Fluctuating mood, actions, rationality (argumentative, combative, withdrawn).
  5. Increasingly restless, fearful, leading to insomnia, nightmares.
  6. Acts bewildered; has trouble identifying familiar people.
  7. Preoccupied; irritable when interrupted.
  8. Unresponsive to questions; problem with concentration and setting realistic priorities.
  9. Sensitive to noise and light.
  10. Has unrealistic perception of time, place, and situation.
  11. Nurse no longer seen as supportive but as threatening.
◆ C. **Analysis/nursing diagnosis:** *Altered thought processes and sensory/perceptual alterations* related to:
  1. *Physical and physiologic disturbances—* metabolic (uremia, diabetes, hepatic dysfunction), fluid and electrolyte imbalances, cardiac arrhythmias, congestive heart failure; anemia, massive blood loss with low hemoglobin; organic brain disease; nutritional deficiency; pain; sleep disturbance; drugs (antidepressants, tranquilizers, sedatives, antihypertensives, diuretics, alcohol, PCP, street drugs).
  2. *Unfamiliar environment—*unfamiliar routine and people; procedures that threaten body image; *noisy* equipment.
  3. *Loss of sensory acuity* from partial or incomplete reception of orienting stimuli or information.
  4. *Disability in screening out* irrelevant and excessive sensory input.
  5. *Memory impairment.*
◆ D. **Nursing care plan/implementation:**
  1. Check *physical signs,* e.g., vital signs, neurologic status, fluid and electrolyte balance, and blood urea nitrogen.
  2. Be calm; make contact to *reorient to reality:*
    a. Avoid startling if person is alone, in the dark, sedated.
    b. Make sure person can *see, hear, and talk* to you—turn off TV; turn on light, put on client's glasses, hearing aids, dentures.
    c. Call by name, clearly and distinctly.
    d. Approach cautiously, close to *eye* level.
    e. Keep your *hands visible;* for example, on bed.
  3. *Take care of immediate problem,* e.g., disconnected IV tube or catheter.
    a. Give instructions slowly and distinctly; avoid threatening tone and comments.
    b. *Stay* with person until reoriented.
    c. Put *siderails* up.
  4. Use conversation to *reduce* confusion:
    a. Use *simple, concrete phrases;* language the person can understand; *repeat* as needed.
    b. Avoid shouting, arguing, false promises, use of medical abbreviations (e.g., NPO).
    c. Give *more time to concentrate* on what you said.
    d. Focus on *reality-oriented* topics or objects in the environment.
  5. *Prevent confusion by establishing a reality-oriented relationship.*
    a. Introduce self by name.
    b. Jointly establish routines to prevent confusion from unpredictable changes and variations. Determine client's usual routine; attempt to incorporate this to lessen disruption in life-style.
    c. Explain what to expect in understandable words—where client is and why, what will happen, noises and activities client will hear and see, people client will meet, tests and procedures client will have.

Mental Health

d. Find out what meaning hospitalization has to client; reduce anxiety related to feelings of apprehension and helplessness.

e. Spend as much time as possible with client.

6. *Maintain orientation by providing nonthreatening environment.*

a. Assign to room *near nurse's station.*

b. Surround with *familiar* objects from home (e.g., photos).

c. Provide *clock, calendar, and radio.*

d. Have flexible visiting hours.

e. Open curtain for *natural light.*

f. Keep glasses, dentures, hearing aids nearby.

g. Check client often, especially at night.

h. Avoid using intercom to answer calls.

i. *Avoid* low-pitched conversation.

7. *Take care of other needs.*

a. Promote sleep according to usual habits and patterns to *prevent sleep deprivation.*

b. *Avoid sedatives,* which may lead to or increase confusion.

c. Promote independent functions, self-help activities, to *maintain dignity.*

d. Encourage *nutritional* adequacy; incorporate familiar foods, ethnic preferences.

e. Maintain *routine; avoid* being late with meals, medication, or procedures.

f. Have *realistic expectations.*

g. *Discover hidden fears.*

(1) Do not assume confused behavior is unrelated to reality.

(2) Look for clues to meaning from client's background, occupation.

h. *Provide support to family.*

(1) Encourage expression of feelings; avoid being judgmental.

(2) Check what worked in previous situations.

8. *Health teaching:* explain possible causes of confusion. Reassure that it is common. Teach family, friends how to react to confused behavior.

◆ E. **Evaluation/outcome criteria:**

1. Less restlessness, fearfulness, mood lability.

2. More frequent periods of lucidity; oriented to time, place, and person; responds to questions.

IV. **Demanding behavior**

A. **Definition:** a strong and persistent struggle to obtain satisfaction of self-oriented needs (such as control, self-esteem) or relief from anxiety.

◆ B. **Assessment:**

1. Attention-seeking behavior.

2. Multiple requests.

3. Frequency of questions.

4. Lack of reasonableness; irrationality of request.

◆ C. **Analysis/nursing diagnosis:** *defensive coping and impaired social interaction* related to:

1. Feelings of *helplessness* and *hopelessness.*

2. Feelings of *powerlessness* and *fear.*

3. A way of coping with anxiety.

◆ D. **Nursing care plan/implementation:**

1. *Control* own irritation; assess reasons for own annoyance.

2. *Confront* with behavior; discuss reasons for behavior.

3. *Anticipate* and meet client's needs; set time to discuss requests.

4. *Ignore* negative attention seeking and *reinforce appropriate* requests for attention.

5. Make plans with *entire staff* to set *limits.*

6. Set up *contractual* arrangement for brief, frequent, regular, uninterrupted attention.

7. *Health teaching:* teach appropriate methods for gaining attention.

◆ E. **Evaluation/outcome criteria:** fewer requests for attention; assumes more responsibility for self-care.

V. **Denial of illness**

A. **Definition:** an attempt or refusal to acknowledge some anxiety-provoking aspect of oneself or external reality. Denial may be an acceptable first phase of coping as an attempt to allow time for adaptation.

◆ B. **Assessment:**

1. Observe for *coping mechanisms* such as dissociation, repression, selective inattention, suppression, displacement of concern to another person.

2. Note behaviors that may indicate *denial* of diagnosis:

a. Failure to follow treatment plan.

b. Missed appointment.

c. Refusal of medication.

d. Inappropriate cheerfulness.

e. Ignoring symptoms.

f. Use of flippant humor.

g. Use of second or third person in reference to illness.

h. Flight into wellness, overactivity.

3. Use of earliest and most primitive defense by closing eyes, turning head away to separate from what is unpleasant and anxiety provoking.

4. Note *range* of denial: *explicit* verbal denial of obvious facts, disowning or *ignoring* aspects or *minimizing* by understatement.

5. Be aware of situations such as long-term physical disability that make people more prone to denial of anger. *Denial of illness protects the ego from overwhelming anxiety.*

◆ C. **Analysis/nursing diagnosis:** *ineffective denial* related to:

1. Untenable wishes, needs, ideas, deeds, or reality factors.

2. Inability to adapt to full realization of painful experience or to accept changes in body image or role perception.

3. Intense stress and anxiety.

◆ **D. Nursing care plan/implementation:**

1. *Long-term goal:* understand needs met by denial.

2. *Short-term goal:* avoid reinforcing denial patterns.

   a. Recognize behavioral cues of denial of some reality aspect; be aware of level of awareness and degree to which reality is excluded.

   b. Determine if denial interferes with treatment.

   c. Support moves toward greater reality orientation.

   d. Determine person's stress tolerance.

   e. Supportively help person discuss events leading to, and feelings about, hospitalization.

3. *Health teaching:*

   a. Explain that emotional response is appropriate and common.

   b. Explain to family and staff that emotional adjustment to painful reality is done at own pace.

◆ **E. Evaluation/outcome criteria:** indicates desire to discuss painful experience.

VI. Dependence

A. Definition: reliance on other people to meet basic needs, usually for love and affection, security and protection, and support and guidance; *acceptable in early phases* of coping.

◆ **B. Assessment:**

1. Excessive need for advice and answers to problems.

2. Lack of confidence in own decision-making ability and lack of confidence in self-sufficiency.

3. Clinging, too-trusting behavior.

4. Gestures, facial expressions, body posture, recurrent themes conveying "I'm helpless."

◆ **C. Analysis/nursing diagnosis:**

1. *Chronic low self-esteem* related to inability to meet basic needs or role expectations.

2. *Helplessness* and *hopelessness* related to inadvertent reinforcement by staff's expectations.

3. *Powerlessness* related to holding a belief that one's own actions cannot affect life situations.

◆ **D. Nursing care plan/implementation:**

1. *Long-term goal:* increase self-esteem, confidence in own abilities.

2. *Short-term goals:* provide activities that promote independence.

   a. *Limit setting*—clear, firm, consistent; acknowledge when demands are made; accept client but refuse to respond to demands.

   b. *Break cycle* of nurse avoids client when he or she is clinging and demanding → client's anxiety increases → demands for attention increase → frustration and avoidance on nurse's part increase.

   c. *Give attention before* demand exists.

   d. Use *behavior-modification* approaches:

     (1) *Reward* appropriate behavior (such as making decisions, helping others, caring for own needs) with attention and praise.

     (2) Give *no response* to attention-seeking, dependent, infantile behavior; goal is to increase incidence of mature behavior as client realizes little gratification from dependent behavior.

   e. *Avoid secondary gains* of being cared for, which impede progress toward above goals.

   f. Assist in developing *ability to control* panic by responding less to client's high anxiety level.

   g. Help client develop ways to seek gratification other than excessive turning to others.

   h. *Resist* urge to act like a parent when client becomes helpless, demanding, and attention seeking.

   i. *Promote decision making* by not giving advice.

   j. *Encourage accountability* for own feelings, thoughts, and behaviors.

     (1) Help identify feelings through nonverbal cues, thoughts, recurrent themes.

     (2) Convey expectations that client does have opinions and feelings to share.

     (3) Role model how to express feelings.

   k. *Reinforce self-esteem* and ability to work out problems independently. (Consistently ask: "How do you feel about . . ." "What do you think?")

3. *Health teaching:*

   a. Teach family ways of interacting to enforce less dependency.

   b. Teach problem-solving skills, assertiveness.

◆ **E. Evaluation/outcome criteria:**

1. Performs self-care.

2. Asks less for approval and praise.

3. Seeks less attention, proximity, physical contact.

VII. Hostility

A. Definition: a feeling of *intense* anger or an attitude of antagonism or animosity, with the *destructive* component of intent to inflict harm and pain to another or to self; may involve *hate, anger, rage, aggression, regression.*

Mental Health

B. **Operational definition:**
1. Past experience of frustration, loss of self-esteem, unmet needs for status, prestige, or love.
2. Present expectations of self and others not met.
3. Feelings of humiliation, inadequacy, emotional pain, and conflict.
4. Anxiety experienced and converted into hostility, which can be:
   a. Repressed, with result of becoming withdrawn.
   b. Disowned to the point of overreaction and extreme compliance.
   c. Overtly exhibited: verbal, nonverbal.

C. **Concepts and principles:**
1. Aggression and violence are two *outward* expressions of hostility.
2. Hostility is often unconscious, automatic response.
3. Hostile wishes and impulses may be underlying motives for many actions.
4. Perceptions may be *distorted* by hostile outlook.
5. Continuum: from extreme politeness to *externalization* as murderous rage or homicide or *internalization* as depression or suicide.
6. Hostility seen as a defense *against* depression as well as a *cause* of it.
7. Hostility may be repressed, dissociated, or expressed covertly or overtly.
8. *Normal* hostility may come from justifiable fear of *real* danger; *irrational* hostility stems from *anxiety.*
9. Developmental roots of hostility:
   a. *Infants* look away, push away, physically move away from threat; give defiant look. Role modeling by parents.
   b. *Three-year-olds* replace overt hostility with protective shyness, retreat, and withdrawal. Feel weak, inadequate in face of powerful person against whom cannot openly ventilate hostility.
   c. Frustrated or unmet needs for status, prestige, or power serve as a basis for *adult* hostility.

◆ D. **Assessment:**
1. Fault finding, scapegoating, sarcasm, derision.
2. Arguing, swearing, abusiveness, verbal threatening.
3. Deceptive sweetness, joking at others' expense, gossiping.
4. Physical abusiveness, violence, murder, vindictiveness.

◆ E. **Analysis/nursing diagnosis:**
1. *Causes*
   a. *Anxiety* related to a learned means of dealing with an interpersonal threat.
   b. *Risk for violence* related to a reaction to *loss of self-esteem* and *powerlessness.*
   c. *Defensive coping* related to intense frustration, insecurity, and/or apprehension.
   d. *Impaired social interaction* related to low anxiety tolerance.
2. *Situations with high potential for hostility:*
   a. *Enforced illness and hospitalization* cause anxiety, which may be expressed as hostility.
   b. Dependency feelings related to acceptance of illness may result in hostility as a coping mechanism.
   c. Certain illnesses or physical disabilities may be conducive to hostility:
      (1) *Preoperative cancer* client may displace hostility onto staff and family.
      (2) Postoperatively, if diagnosis is *terminal,* the family may displace hostility onto nurse.
      (3) Anger, hostility is a *stage of dying* the person may experience.
      (4) *Amputee* may focus frustration on others due to dependency and jealousy.
      (5) Patients on *hemodialysis* are prone to helplessness, which may be displaced as hostility.

◆ F. **Nursing care plan/implementation:**
1. *Long-term goal:* help alter response to fear, inadequacy, frustration, threat.
2. *Short-term goal:* express and explore feelings of hostility without injury to self or others.
   a. Remain calm, nonthreatening; endure verbal abuse in impartial manner, within limits; speak quietly.
   b. *Protect from self-harm,* acting out.
   c. Discourage hostile behavior while showing acceptance of client.
   d. Offer support to *express* feelings of frustration, anger, and fear *constructively, safely,* and *appropriately.*
   e. Explore hostile feelings *without* fear of retaliation, disapproval.
   f. *Avoid* arguing, giving advice, reacting with hostility, punitiveness, finding fault.
   g. *Avoid* joking, teasing, which can be misinterpreted.
   h. *Avoid* words like *anger, hostility;* use client's words *(upset, irritated).*
   i. Do not minimize problem or give client reassurance or hasty, general conclusions.
   j. *Do not stop verbal* expression of anger unless detrimental.
   k. Respond *matter-of-factly* to attention-seeking behavior, not defensively.
   l. *Avoid* physical contact; allow client to set pace in "closeness."

m. Look for clues to antecedent events and focus *directly* on those areas; *do not evade* or ignore.

n. Constantly focus on *here and now* and affective component of message rather than on content.

o. Reconstruct what happened and why, discuss client's reactions; seek observations, *not* inferences.

p. Learn how client would like to be treated.

q. Look for ways to help client relate better without defensiveness, *when ready.*

r. Plan to channel feelings into *motor* outlets (occupational and recreational therapy, physical activity, games, debates).

s. Explain procedures beforehand; approach frequently.

t. Withdraw attention, *set limits,* when acting out.

3. *Health teaching:* teach acceptable motor outlets for tension.

◆ **G. Evaluation/outcome criteria:** identifies sources of threat and experiences success in dealing with threat.

VIII. Manipulation

A. Definition: process of playing upon and using others by unfair, insidious means to serve own purpose without regard for others' needs; may take many forms; occurs consciously, unconsciously to some extent, in all interpersonal relations.

B. Operational definition (Figure 6.1):

1. Conflicting needs, goals exist between client and other person (e.g., nurse).

2. Other person perceives need as unacceptable, unreasonable.

3. Other person refuses to accept client's need.

4. Client's tension increases, and he or she begins to relate to others as objects.

5. Client increases attempts to influence others to fulfill his or her need.

   a. Appears unaware of others' needs.

   b. Exhibits excessive dependency, helplessness, demands.

   c. Sets others at odds (especially staff).

   d. *Rationalizes,* gives logical reasons.

   e. Uses deception, false promises, insincerity.

   f. Questions and *defies nurse's authority* and competence.

6. Nurse feels powerless and angry at having been used.

◆ **C. Assessment:**

1. Acts out sexually, physically.

2. Dawdles, always last minute.

3. Uses insincere flattery; expects special favors, privileges.

4. Exploits generosity and fears of others.

5. Feels no guilt.

6. Plays one staff member against another.

7. *Tests limits.*

8. Finds weaknesses in others.

9. Makes excessive, unreasonable, unnecessary *demands* for staff time.

10. *Pretends* to be helpless, lonely, distraught, tearful.

11. Can't distinguish between truth and falsehood.

12. *Plays on sympathy* or *guilt.*

13. Offers many excuses, lacks insight.

14. Pursues unpleasant issues without genuine regard for or feelings of individuals involved.

15. *Intimidates,* derogates, threatens, bargains, cajoles, violates rules to obtain reactions or privileges.

16. Betrays information.

17. Uses communication as a medium for manipulation, as verbal, nonverbal means to get others to cooperate, to behave in certain way, to get something from another for own use.

18. May be coercive, illogical, or skillfully deceptive.

19. *Unable to learn from experience,* i.e., repeats unacceptable behaviors despite negative consequences.

◆ **D. Analysis/nursing diagnosis:** *impaired adjustment* related to:

1. Mistrust and contemptuous view of others' motivations.

2. Life experience of rejection, deception.

3. Low anxiety tolerance.

4. Inability to cope with tension.

5. Unmet dependency needs.

6. Need to avoid anxiety when cannot obtain gratification.

7. Need to obtain something that is forbidden, or need for *instant gratification.*

8. Attempt to put something over on another when no real advantage exists.

9. *Intolerance of intimacy,* maneuvering effectively to keep others at a safe distance to dilute the relationship by withdrawing and frustrating others or distracting attention away from self.

10. Attempt to demand attention, approval, disapproval.

◆ **E. Nursing care plan/implementation:**

1. *Long-term goal:* define relationship as a mutual experience in *learning and trust* rather than a struggle for *power and control.*

2. *Short-term goals:* increase awareness of self and others; increase self-control; learn to accept limitations.

3. Promote use of "three Cs"—*cooperation, compromise, collaboration*—rather than exploitation or deception.

4. *Decrease level and extent of manipulation.*

■ **FIGURE 6.1   Operationalization of the behavioral concept of manipulation.**

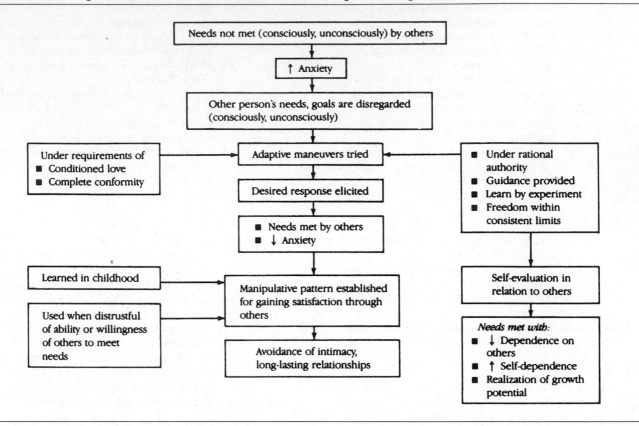

a. Set *firm, realistic goals,* with clear, consistent expectations and limits.
b. *Confront* client regarding exploitation attempts; examine, discuss behavior.
c. Give *positive reinforcement* with concrete reinforcers for nonmanipulation, to lessen need for exploitative, deceptive, and self-destructive behaviors.
d. *Ignore* "wooden-leg" behavior (feigning illness to evoke sympathy).
e. *Allow verbal* anger; don't be intimidated; avoid giving desired response to obvious attempts to irritate.
f. Set *consistent, firm, enforceable limits* on *destructive,* aggressive behavior that impinges on others' health, rights, and interests, and on excessive dependency; *give reasons* when you can't meet requests.
g. Keep staff informed of rules and reasons; obtain staff *consensus.*
h. Enforce *direct* communication; encourage openness about *real* needs, feelings.
i. Do *not* accept gifts, favors, flattery, or other guises of manipulation.

5. Increase responsibility for *self-control* of actions.
   a. Decide who (client, nurse) is responsible for what.

b. Provide opportunities for *success* to increase self-esteem, experiencing acceptance by others.
c. Evaluate actions, *not* verbal behavior; point out the difference between talk and action.
d. Support efforts to be responsible.
e. Assist client to increase emotional repertoire; explore *alternative* ways of relating interpersonally.
f. *Avoid submission* to control based on fear of punishment, retaliation, loss of affection.

6. Facilitate awareness of, and *responsibility* for, manipulative behavior and its *effects on others.*
   a. Reflect back client's behavior.
   b. Discourage distortion and misuse of information.
   c. *Increase tolerance* for differences and *delayed gratification* through behavior modification.
   d. Insist on clear, consistent staff communication.

7. *Avoid:*
   a. Labeling client as a "problem."
   b. Hostile, negative attitude.
   c. Making a public issue of client's behavior.

d. Being excessively rigid or permissive, inconsistent or ambiguous, argumentative or accusatory.

8. *Health teaching:* act as a role model; demonstrate how to deal with mistakes, human imperfections, by admitting mistakes in nonshameful, nonvirtuous ways.

◆ **F. Evaluation/outcome criteria:** accepts limits; able to compromise, cooperate rather than deceive and exploit; acts responsibly, self-dependent.

IX. **Noncompliance and uncooperative behavior**
  A. **Definition:** consistently failing to meet the requirements of the prescribed treatment regimen, e.g., refusing to adhere to dietary restrictions or take required medications.

◆ **B. Assessment:**
  1. Refuses to participate in routine or planned activities.
  2. Refuses medication.
  3. Violates rules, ignores limits, and abuses privileges; acts out anger and frustration.

◆ **C. Analysis/nursing diagnosis:** *noncompliance* related to:
  1. *Psychological factors:* lack of knowledge; attitudes, beliefs, and values; denial of illness; rigid, defensive personality type; anxiety level (very high or very low); can't accept limits or dependency (rebellious counterdependency).
  2. *Environmental factors:* finances, transportation, lack of support system.
  3. *Health care agent–client relationship:* client feels discounted and like an "object"; sees staff as uncaring, authoritative, controlling.
  4. *Health care regimen:* too complicated; not enough benefit from following regimen; results in social stigma or social isolation; unpleasant side effects.

◆ **D. Nursing care plan/implementation:**
  1. *General goal:* reduce need to act out by nonadherence.
     a. Take *preventive* action—be alert to signs of noncompliance, such as intent to leave against medical advice.
     b. *Explore* feelings and reasons for lack of cooperation.
     c. Assess and *allay fears* in client in reassuring manner.
     d. Provide *adequate* information about, and reasons for, rules and procedures.
     e. *Avoid* threats or physical restraints; maintain calm composure.
     f. Demonstrate *tact and firmness* when confronting violations.
     g. Offer *alternatives.*
     h. Firmly insist on cooperation in selected important activities but not all activities.

2. *Health teaching:* increase knowledge base regarding health-related problem, procedures, or treatments and consequences.

◆ **E. Evaluation/outcome criteria:** follows prescribed regimen.

Psychiatric Emergencies*

I. **Definition:** sudden onset (days or weeks, not years) of unusual (for that individual), disordered (without pattern or purpose), or socially inappropriate behavior caused by emotional or physiologic situation. For example: suicidal feelings or attempts, overdose, acute psychotic reaction, acute alcohol withdrawal, acute anxiety.

II. **General characteristics:**
◆ **A. Assessment:** the presence of great distress without reasonable explanation; *extreme* behavior in comparison with antecedent event.
  1. *Fear*—related to a particular person, activity, or place.
  2. *Anxiety*—fearful feeling without any obvious reason, not specifically related to a particular person, activity, or place (e.g., adolescent turmoil).
  3. *Depression*—continual pessimism, easily moved to tears, hopelessness, and isolation (e.g., student despondency around exam time, middle-aged crisis, elderly hopelessness).
  4. *Mania*—unrealistic optimism.
  5. *Anger*—many events seen as deliberate insults.
  6. *Confusion*—diminished awareness of who and where one is; memory loss.
  7. *Loss of reality contact*—hallucinations or delusion (as in acute psychosis).
  8. *Withdrawal*—neglect or giving away of belongings and neglect of appearance; loss of interest in activities; apathy.

◆ **B. Analysis/nursing diagnosis:** *ineffective individual coping* related to degree of seriousness:
  1. *Life-threatening emergencies*—violence toward self or others (e.g., suicide, homicide).
  2. *Serious emergencies*—confused and unable to care for or protect self from dangerous situations (as in substance abuse).
  3. *Potentially serious emergencies*—anxious and in pain; disorganized behavior; can become worse or better (as in grief reaction).

◆ **C. General nursing care plan/implementation:**
  1. *Remove* from stressful situation and persons.
  2. Engage in *dialogue* at a nonthreatening distance, to offer help.
  3. Use *calm, slow, deliberate* approach to relieve stress and disorganization.
  4. *Explain* what will be done about the problem and the likely outcome.

---

*Adapted from Aguilera D, Messick J. *Crisis Intervention,* 5th ed. St. Louis: Mosby, 1986.

Mental Health

5. *Avoid* using force, threat, or counterthreat.
6. Use *confident, firm, reasonable* approach.
7. Encourage client to relate.
8. Elicit *details.*
9. Encourage *ventilation* of feelings without interruption.
10. Accept distortions of reality *without arguing.*
11. Give form and *structure* to the conversation.
12. Contact significant others to gain information and to be with client, including previous therapist.
13. Treat emergency as *temporary* and *readily resolved.*
14. Check every half hour if cannot remain with client.

III. **Categories of psychiatric emergencies:**
   A. *Acute nonpsychotic reactions,* such as acute anxiety attack or panic reaction (for symptoms, see Anxiety and Anxiety Disorders, pp. 352, 353).
   ◆ 1. **Assessment** includes differentiating hyperventilation that is anxiety connected from asthma, angina, and heart disease.
   ◆ 2. **Nursing care plan/implementation** in hyperventilation syndrome—*goal:* prevent paresthesia, tetanic contractions, disturbance in awareness; reassure client that vital organs are not impaired.
      a. Increase CO_2 in lungs by rebreathing from paper bag.
      b. Minimize secondary gains; avoid reinforcing behavior.
      c. *Health teaching:* demonstrate how to slow down breathing rate.
   ◆ 3. **Evaluation/outcome criteria:** respirations slowed down; no evidence of effect of hyperventilation.
   B. *Delirium*—conditions produced by changes in the cerebral chemistry or tissue by metabolic toxins, direct trauma to the brain, drug effects, and/or withdrawal.
      1. *Acute alcohol intoxication* (see also Alcohol Abuse and Dependence, pp. 344–346).
      ◆ a. **Assessment:** signs of head or other injury (past and recent), emotional lability, memory defects, loss of judgment, disorientation.
      ◆ b. **Nursing care plan/implementation:**
         (1) Observe, monitor *vital signs.*
         (2) *Prevent aspiration* of vomitus by positioning.
         (3) *Decrease* environmental stimuli:
            (a) Place in quiet area of emergency room.
            (b) Speak and handle calmly.
         (4) Give medication (diazepam [Valium]) to control agitation.
      ◆ c. **Evaluation/outcome criteria:** oriented to time, place, person; appears calmer.

2. *Hallucinogenic drug intoxication*—LSD, mescaline, amphetamines, cocaine, scopolamine, and belladonna.
   ◆ a. **Assessment:**
      (1) Perceptual and cognitive distortions (e.g., feels heart stopped beating).
      (2) Anxiety (apprehension → panic).
      (3) Subjective feelings (omnipotence → worthlessness).
      (4) Interrelationship of dose, potency, setting, expectations and experiences of user.
      (5) Eyes: *red*—marijuana; *dilated*—LSD, mescaline, belladonna; *constricted*—heroin and derivatives.
   ◆ b. **Nursing care plan/implementation:**
      (1) "Talk down."
         (a) Establish *verbal* contact, attempt to have client verbally express what is being experienced.
         (b) *Environment*—few people, normal lights, calm, supportive.
         (c) Allay fears.
         (d) Encourage to keep eyes *open.*
         (e) Have client focus on *inanimate* objects in room as a bridge to reality contact.
         (f) Use simple, *concrete, repetitive* statements.
         (g) *Repetitively* orient to time, place, and temporary nature.
         (h) Do *not* moralize, challenge beliefs, or probe into life-style.
         (i) Emphasize confidentiality.
      (2) *Medication (minor tranquilizer—diazepam [Valium], chlordiazepoxide HCl [Librium]:*
         (a) Allay anxiety.
         (b) Reduce aggressive behavior.
         (c) Reduce suicidal potential; check client every 5–15 min.
         (d) Avoid anticholinergic crisis (precipitated by use of phenothiazines, belladonna, and scopolamine ingestion) with 2–4 mg IM or PO of physostigmine salicylate.
      (3) *Hospitalization:* if hallucinations, delusions last more than 12–18 h; if client has been injecting amphetamines for extended time; if client is paranoid and depressed.
   ◆ c. **Evaluation/outcome criteria:** less frightened; oriented to time, place, person.
3. *Acute delirium*—seen in postoperative electrolyte imbalance, systemic infections, renal and hepatic failure, oversedation, metastatic cancer.
   ◆ a. **Assessment:**
      (1) Disorientation regarding time, at night.

(2) Hallucinations, delusions, illusions.

(3) Alterations in mood.

(4) Increased emotional lability.

(5) Agitation.

(6) Lack of cooperation.

(7) Withdrawal.

(8) Sleep pattern reversal.

(9) Alterations in food intake.

◆ b. **Nursing care plan/implementation:**

(1) Identify and remove *toxic* substance.

(2) Reality orientation—well-lit room; constant attendance to inform *repetitively* of place and time and to *protect* from injury to self and others.

(3) Simplify environment.

(4) *Avoid* excessive medication and restraints; use low-dose phenothiazines; do not give barbiturates or sedatives (these increase agitation, confusion, disorientation).

◆ c. **Evaluation/outcome criteria:** oriented to time, place, person; cooperative; less agitated.

C. *Acute psychotic reactions*—disorders of mood or thinking characterized by hallucinations, delusions, excessive euphoria (mania), or depression.

1. *Acute schizophrenic reaction* (see also Schizophrenic and other Psychotic Disorders, pp. 359–362).

◆ a. **Assessment:**

(1) History of previous hospitalization, no illicit drug ingestion; use of major tranquilizers and recent withdrawal from them or alcohol.

(2) Auditory hallucinations and delusions.

(3) Violent, assaultive, suicidal behavior directed by auditory hallucinations.

(4) Assault, withdrawal, and panic related to paranoid delusions of persecution; fear of harm.

(5) Disturbance in mental status (associative thought disorder).

◆ b. **Nursing care plan/implementation** (see also II.C. Hallucinations, pp. 359–360).

(1) Hospitalization.

(2) Medication: phenothiazines.

(3) *Avoid* physical restraints or touch when fears and delusions of sexual attack exist.

(4) Allow client to *diffuse* anger and intensity of panic through talk.

(5) Use simple, *concrete* terms, avoid figures of speech or content subject to multiple interpretations.

(6) Do *not* agree with reality distortions; point out that client's thoughts are difficult to understand but you are willing to listen.

◆ c. **Evaluation/outcome criteria:** doesn't hear frightening voices; less fearful and combative behavior.

2. *Manic reaction* (see also Bipolar Disorders, pp. 366–367).

◆ a. **Assessment:**

(1) History of depression requiring antidepressants.

(2) *Thought disorder* (flight of ideas, delusions of grandeur).

(3) *Affect* (elated, irritable, irrational anger).

(4) *Speech* (loud, pressured).

(5) *Behavior* (rapid, erratic, chaotic).

◆ b. **Nursing care plan/implementation:**

(1) Hospitalization to protect from injury to self and others.

(2) Medication: *lithium carbonate.*

(3) Same as for acute schizophrenic reaction, *except do not encourage talk,* as need to decrease stimulation.

(4) Provide food and fluids that can be consumed while on-the-go.

◆ c. **Evaluation/outcome criteria:** speech and activity slowed down; thoughts less disordered.

D. *Homicidal or assaultive reaction*—seen in acutely drug-intoxicated, delirious, paranoid, acutely excited manic, or acute anxiety-panic conditions.

◆ 1. **Assessment**—history of obvious antisocial behavior, paranoid psychosis, previous violence, sexual conflict, rivalry, substance abuse, recent moodiness, and withdrawal.

◆ 2. **Nursing care plan/implementation:**

a. Physically restrain if client has a weapon; use group of trained people to help.

b. Allow person to "save face" in giving up weapon.

c. *Separate* from intended victims.

d. Approach: calm, unhurried; *one person* to offer support and reassurance; use clear, unambiguous statements.

e. Immediate and rapid admission procedures.

f. Observe for *suicidal* behavior that may follow homicidal attempt.

◆ 3. **Evaluation/outcome criteria:** client regains impulse control.

E. *Suicidal ideation*—seen in anxiety attacks, substance intoxication, toxic delirium, schizophrenic auditory hallucinations, and depressive reactions.

1. **Concepts and principles related to suicide:**

a. *Based on social theory:* suicidal tendency is a result of collective social forces rather than isolated individual motives (Durkheim's *Le Suicide*).

(1) Common factor: increased *alienation* between person and social

group; psychological isolation, called "anomie," when links between groups are weakened.

(2) "Egoistic" suicide: results from lack of integration of individual with others.

(3) "Altruistic" suicide: results from insufficient individualization.

(4) *Implication:* increase group cohesiveness and mutual interdependence, making group more coherent and consistent in fulfilling needs of each member.

b. *Based on symbolic interaction theory:*

(1) Person evaluates self according to *others' assessment.*

(2) Thus, suicide stems from *social rejection* and disrupted social relations.

(3) Perceived failure in relationships with others may be inaccurate but seen as real by the individual.

(4) *Implication:* need to recognize difference in perception of alienation between own viewpoint and others'.

c. *Based on psychoanalytic theory:*

(1) Suicide stems mainly from the individual, with external events only as precipitants.

(2) There is a strong life urge in people.

(3) *Universal death instinct* is always present (Freud).

(4) Person may be balancing life wishes and death wishes. When self-preservation instincts are diminished, death instincts may find direct outlet via suicide.

(5) When *love instinct* is frustrated, *hate* impulse takes over (Menninger).

(a) Desire to kill → desire to be killed → desire to kill oneself.

(b) Suicide may be an act of extreme hostility, manipulation, and revenge to elicit guilt and remorse in significant others.

(c) Suicide may also be act of self-punishment to handle own guilt or to control fate.

d. *Based on synthesis of social and psychoanalytic theories:*

(1) Suicide is seen as *running away* from an intolerable situation to interrupt it rather than *running* to something more desirable.

(2) Process *defined in operational terms* involves:

(a) Despair over inability to cope.

(b) Inability to feel hope or adequacy.

(c) Frustration with others when others cannot fill needs.

(d) Rage and aggression experienced toward significant other is turned inward.

(e) Psychic blow acts as precipitant.

(f) Life seen as harder to cope with, with no chance of improvement in life situation.

(g) *Implication:* persons who experience suicidal impulses can gain a certain amount of control over these impulses through the support they gain from meaningful relationships with others.

e. *Based on crisis theory (Dublin):* concept of emotional disequilibrium:

(1) Everyone at some point in life is in a crisis, with temporary inability to solve problems or to master the crisis.

(2) Usual coping mechanisms do not function.

(3) Person unable to relate to others.

(4) Person searches consciously and unconsciously for useful coping techniques, with suicide as one of various solutions.

(5) With inadequate communication of needs and isolation, suicide is possible.

f. *Based on the view that suicide is an individual's personal reaction and decision, a final response to own situation:*

(1) *Process* of anger turned inward → self-inflicted, destructive action.

(2) *Definition* of concept in operational steps:

(a) Frustration of individual needs → anger.

(b) Anger turned inward → feelings of guilt, despair, depression, incompetence, hopelessness, and exhaustion.

(c) Stress felt and perceived as unbearable and overwhelming.

(d) Attempt to communicate hopelessness and defeat to others.

(e) Others do not provide hope.

(f) Sudden change in behavior, as noted when depression appears to lift, may indicate *danger,* as person has more energy to act on suicidal thoughts and feelings.

(g) Decision to end life → plan of action → self-induced, self-destructive behavior.

(3) May be *pseudo-suicide* attempts, where there is no actual or realistic desire to achieve finality of death. Intentions or causes may be:

(a) "Cry for help," where nonlethal attempt notifies others of deeper intentions.

(b) Desire to *manipulate* others.

(c) Need for *attention and pity*.

(d) Self-punishment.

(e) Symbol of *utter frustration*.

(f) Wish to *punish* others.

(g) *Misuse* of alcohol and other drugs.

(4) Other reasons for self-destruction, where the individual *gives his or her life* rather than takes it, include:

(a) Strong parental love that can overcome fear and instinct of self-preservation to save child's life.

(b) "Sacrificial death" during war, such as kamikaze pilots in WWII.

(c) Submission to death for religious beliefs (martyrdom).

◆ 2. **Assessment of suicide:**

a. *Assessment of risk regarding statistical probability of suicide—composite picture:* over-45-yr-old man, unemployed, divorced, living alone, depressed (weight loss, somatic delusions, sleep disturbance, preoccupied with suicide), history of substance abuse and suicide within family.

b. *Ten factors* to predict potential suicide and assess risk:

(1) *Age, sex, and race*—teenage, older age; more women make attempts; more men complete suicide act. Highest risk: older women rather than young boys; older men rather than young girls. Suicide occurs in all races and socioeconomic groups.

(2) *Recent stress*—family problems: death, divorce, separation, alienation; financial pressures; loss of job; loss of status; failing grades.

(3) *Clues to suicide:* suicidal thoughts are usually time limited and do not last forever. Early assessment of behavioral and verbal clues is important.*

(a) *Verbal clues—direct:* "I am going to shoot myself." *Indirect:* "It's more than I can bear." *Coded:* "This is the last time you'll ever see me." "I want you to have my coin collection."

(b) *Behavioral clues—direct:* trial run with pills or razor, for ex-

ample. *Indirect:* sudden lifting of depression, buying a casket, giving away cherished belongings, putting affairs in order, writing a will.

(c) *Syndromes—dependent-dissatisfied:* emotionally dependent but dislikes dependent state, irritable, helpless. *Depressed:* detachment from life; feels life is a burden; hopelessness, futility. *Disoriented:* delusions or hallucinations, confusion, delirium tremens, organic brain syndromes. *Willful-defiant:* active need to direct and control environment and life situation, with low frustration tolerance and rigid set, rage, shame.

(4) *Suicidal plan*—the more details about method, timing, and place, the higher the risk.

(5) *Previous suicidal behavior*—history of prior attempt increases risk. Eight out of ten suicide attempts give verbal and behavioral warnings as listed above.

(6) *Medical status*—chronic ailments, terminal illness, and pain increase suicidal risk.

(7) *Communication*—the more withdrawn and apathetic, the greater potential for suicide, unless extreme psychomotor retardation is present.

(8) *Style of life*—high risks include substance abusers, those with sexual-identity conflicts, unstable relationships (personal and job related). Suicidal tendencies are not inherited but learned from family and other interpersonal relationships.

(9) *Alcohol*—can reinforce helpless and hopeless feelings; may be lethal if used with barbiturates; can decrease inhibitions, result in impulsive behavior.

(10) *Resources*—the fewer the resources, the higher the suicide potential. Examples of resources: family, friends, colleagues, religion, pets, meaningful recreational outlets, satisfying employment.

c. Assess *needs* commonly communicated by individuals who are suicidal:

(1) To trust.

(2) To be accepted.

(3) To bolster self-esteem.

(4) To "fit in" with groups.

(5) To experience success and interrupt the failure syndrome.

*Adapted from the *American Journal of Nursing*, Vol 65, No 5. Copyright May 1965, the American Journal of Nursing Company.

Mental Health

(6) To expand capacity for pleasure.

(7) To increase autonomy and sense of self-mastery.

(8) To work out an acceptable sexual identity.

◆ 3. **Analysis/nursing diagnosis:** *risk for self-directed violence* related to:

a. Feelings of alienation.

b. Feelings of rejection.

c. Feelings of hopelessness, despair.

d. Feelings of frustration and rage.

◆ 4. **Nursing care plan/implementation:**

a. *Long-term goals*

(1) Increase client's self-reliance.

(2) Help client achieve more realistic and positive feelings of self-esteem, self-respect, acceptance by others, and sense of belonging.

(3) Help client experience success, interrupt failure pattern, and expand views about pleasure.

b. *Short-term goals*

(1) Medical: assist as necessary with gastric lavage; provide respiratory and vascular support; assist in repair of inflicted wounds.

(2) Provide protection from self-destruction until client is able to assume this responsibility.

(3) *Allow outward* and *constructive* expression of hostile and aggressive feelings.

(4) Provide for physical needs.

c. *Suicide precautions* to institute under emergency conditions:

(1) One-to-one supervision at *all* times for maximum precautions; check whereabouts every 15 min, if on basic suicide precautions.

(2) Prior to instituting these measures, explain to client what you will be doing and why; MD must also explain; document this explanation.

(3) Do not allow client to leave the unit for tests, procedures.

(4) Look through client's belongings *with* the client and remove any potentially harmful objects, e.g., pills, matches, belts, razors, glass, tweezers.

(5) Allow visitors and phone calls, but maintain one-to-one supervision during visits.

(6) Check that visitors do not leave potentially harmful objects in the client's room.

(7) Serve meals in an isolation meal tray that contains no glass or metal silverware.

(8) Do not discontinue these measures without an order.

d. *General approaches*

(1) *Observe* closely at all times to assess suicide potential.

(2) *Be available.*

(a) Demonstrate concern for client as a person.

(b) Be sensitive, warm, and consistent.

(c) Listen with empathy.

(d) Avoid imposing your own feelings of reality on client.

(e) Avoid extremes in your own mood when with client (especially exaggerated cheerfulness).

(3) *Focus directly* on client's self-destructive ideas.

(a) Reduce alienation and immobilization by discussing this "taboo" topic.

(b) Acknowledge suicidal threats with calmness and without reproach—do not ignore or minimize threat.

(c) *Find out details* about suicide plan and reduce environmental hazards.

(d) Help client verbalize aggressive, hostile, and hopeless feelings.

(e) *Explore death fantasies*—try to take "romance" out of death.

(4) Acknowledge that suicide is one of several options.

(5) *Make a contract* with the client, and structure a plan of alternatives for coping when next confronted with the need to commit suicide (e.g., the client could call someone, express feeling of anger outwardly, or ask for help).

(6) Point out client's *self-responsibility* for suicidal act.

(a) Avoid manipulation by client who says, "You are responsible for stopping me from killing myself."

(b) Emphasize protection against self-destruction *rather than* punishment.

(7) *Support* the part of the client that wants to live.

(a) Focus on *ambivalence.*

(b) Emphasize meaningful past relationships and events.

(c) Look for reasons left for wanting to live. Elicit what is meaningful to the client at the moment.

(d) Point out effect of client's death on others.

(8) *Remove sources of stress.*
  (a) Decrease uncomfortable feelings of *alienation* by initiating one-to-one interactions.
  (b) Make all *decisions* when client is in severe depression.
  (c) Progressively let client make simple decisions: what to eat, what to watch on TV, etc.
(9) *Provide hope.*
  (a) Let client know that problems can be solved with help.
  (b) Bring in new resources for help.
  (c) Talk about likely changes in client's life.
  (d) Review past effective coping behaviors.
(10) *Provide with opportunity to be useful.* Reduce self-centeredness and brooding by planning diversional activities within the client's capabilities.
(11) *Involve as many people as possible.*
  (a) Gradually bring in others, for instance, other therapists, friends, staff, clergy, family, co-workers.
  (b) Prevent staff "burnout," found when only one nurse is working with suicidal client.
(12) *Health teaching:* teach client and staff principles of crisis intervention and resolution. Teach new coping skills.

◆ 5. **Evaluation/outcome criteria:** physical condition is stabilized; client able to verbalize feelings rather than acting them out.

Crisis Intervention

Crisis intervention is a type of brief psychiatric treatment in which individuals and/or their families are helped in their efforts to forestall the process of mental decompensation in reaction to severe emotional stress by direct and immediate supportive approaches.

I. **Definition of crisis:** sudden event in one's life that disturbs homeostasis, during which usual coping mechanisms cannot resolve the problem. Types of crisis:
  A. *Maturational* (internal): see Erik Erikson's eight stages of developmental crises anticipated in the development of the infant, child, adolescent, and adult (Unit 8).
  B. *Situational* (external): occurs at any time, e.g., loss of job, loss of income, death of significant person, illness, hospitalization.

II. **Concepts and principles** related to crisis intervention:
  A. Crises are turning points where changes in behavior patterns and life-styles can occur; individuals in crisis are most amenable to altering old and unsuccessful coping mechanisms and are most likely to learn new and more functional behaviors.
  B. Social milieu and its structure are contributing factors in both the development of psychiatric symptoms and eventual recovery from them.
  C. If crisis is handled effectively, the person's mental stability will be maintained; individual may return to a precrisis state or better.
  D. If crisis is not handled effectively, individual may progress to a worse state with exacerbations of earlier conflicts; future crises may not be handled well.
  E. There are a number of universal developmental crisis periods (maturational crises) in every individual's life.
  F. Each person tries to maintain equilibrium through use of adaptive behaviors.
  G. When individuals face a problem they cannot solve, tension, anxiety, narrowed perception, and disorganized functioning occur.
  H. *Immediate relief* of symptoms produced by crisis is more urgent than *exploring* their cause.

III. **Characteristics** of crisis intervention:
  A. Acute, sudden onset related to a stressful precipitating event of which individual is aware but which immobilizes previous coping abilities.
  B. Responsive to brief therapy with focus on immediate problem.
  C. Focus shifted from the psyche in the individual to the *individual in the environment;* deemphasis on intrapsychic aspects.
  D. Crisis period is *time limited* (usually up to 6 wk).

◆ IV. **Nursing care plan/implementation** in crises:
  A. General goals:
    1. Avoid hospitalization if possible.
    2. Return to precrisis level and preserve ability to function.
    3. Assist in problem solving, with *here-and-now* focus.
  B. *Assess* the crisis:
    1. Identify stressful *precipitating* events: duration, problems created, and degree of significance.
    2. Assess *suicidal and homicidal risk.*
    3. Assess amount of *disruption* in individual's life and effect on significant others.
    4. Assess *current coping skills,* strengths, and general level of functioning.
  C. *Plan* the intervention:
    1. Consider *past coping* mechanisms.
    2. Propose *alternatives* and untried coping methods.
  D. *Implementation:*
    1. Help client relate the crisis event to current feelings.
    2. Encourage expression of all feelings related to disruption.

3. Explore past coping skills and *reinforce adaptive* ones.
4. Use all means available in *social network* to take care of client's *immediate needs* (significant others, law enforcement agencies, housing, welfare, employment, medical, and school, e.g.).
5. Set limits.
6. *Health teaching:* teach additional problem-solving approaches.

◆ **V. Evaluation/outcome criteria:**
   A. Client returns to precrisis level of functioning.
   B. Client learns new, more effective coping skills.
   C. Client can describe realistic plans for future in terms of own perception of progress, support system, and coping mechanisms.

Selected Specific Crisis Situations: Problems Related to Abuse

I. Rape-trauma syndrome
   A. Definition: forcible perpetration of an act of sexual intercourse on the body of an unwilling person.

◆ **B. Assessment:**
   1. *Signs of physical trauma*—physical findings of entry.
   2. *Symptoms of physical trauma*—verbatim statements regarding type of sexual attack.
   3. *Signs of emotional trauma*—tears, hyperventilation, extreme anxiety, withdrawal, self-blame, anger, embarrassment, fears, sleeping and eating disturbances, desire for revenge.
   4. *Symptoms of emotional trauma*—statements regarding method of force used and threats made.

◆ **C. Analysis/nursing diagnosis:** *rape-trauma syndrome* related to phases of response to rape:
   1. *Acute response:* volatility, disorganization, disbelief, shock, incoherence, agitated motor activity, nightmares, guilt (should have been able to protect self), phobias (crowds, being alone, sex).
   2. *Outward coping:* denial and suppression of anxiety and fear (silent rape syndrome), feelings appear controlled.
   3. *Integration and resolution:* confronts anger with attacker; realistic perspective.

◆ **D. Nursing care plan/implementation** in counseling rape victims. Figure 6.2 is a summary of self-care decisions a victim faces the first night following a sexual assault.
   1. Overall goals:
      a. Acknowledge feelings.
      b. Face feelings.
      c. Resolve feelings.
      d. Maintain and restore *self-respect, dignity, integrity,* and *self-determination.*

2. Work through issues:
   a. Handle *legal* matters and police contacts.
   b. Clarify facts.
   c. Get *medical* attention if needed.
   d. Notify *family and friends.*
   e. Understand emotional reaction.
   f. Attend to *practical* concerns.
   g. Evaluate need for psychiatric consultations.
3. *Acute phase:*
   a. Decrease victim's stress, anxiety, fear.
   b. Seek medical care.
   c. Increase self-confidence and self-esteem.
   d. Identify and accept feelings and needs (to be in control, cared about, to achieve).
   e. Reorient perceptions, feelings, and statements about self.
   f. Help resume normal life-style.
4. *Outward coping phase:*
   a. Remain available and supportive.
   b. Reflect words, feelings, and thoughts.
   c. Explore real problems.
   d. Explore alternatives regarding contraception, legal issues.
   e. Evaluate response of family and friends to victim and rape.
5. Integration and resolution phase:
   a. Assist exploration of feelings (anger) regarding attacker.
   b. Explore feelings (guilt and shame) regarding self.
   c. Assist in making own decisions regarding health care.
6. Maintain confidentiality and neutrality—facilitate person's own decision.
7. Search for alternatives to giving advice.
8. *Health teaching:*
   a. Explain procedures and services to victim.
   b. Counsel to avoid isolated areas and being helpful to strangers.
   c. Counsel where and how to resist attack (scream, run unless assailant has weapon).
   d. Teach what to do if pregnancy or STD is outcome.

◆ **E. Evaluation/outcome criteria:** little or no evidence of possible long-term effects of rape (guilt, shame, phobias, denial).

II. Sexual abuse of children
◆ **A. Assessment**—characteristic behaviors:
   1. *Relationship* of offender to victim: many filling paternal role (uncle, grandfather, cousin) with repeated, unquestioned access to the child.
   2. Methods of *pressuring* victim into sexual activity: offering material goods, misrepresenting moral standards ("it's OK"), exploiting need for human contact and warmth.

■ **FIGURE 6.2** Victim decisions following a sexual assault. (From the Rape Crisis Services of the YWCA, Greater Harrisburg, PA.)

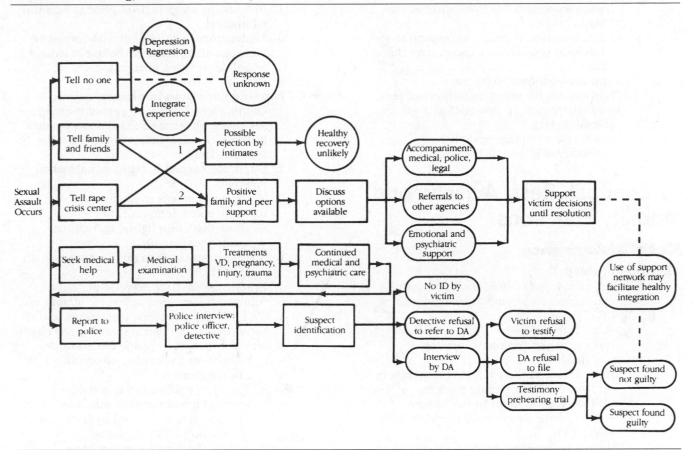

3. Method of pressuring victim to *secrecy* (to conceal the act) is inducing fear of punishment, not being believed, rejection, being blamed for the activity, abandonment.
4. Disclosure of sexual activity via:
   a. Direct visual or verbal confrontation and *observation* by others.
   b. *Verbalization* of act by victim.
   c. *Visible clues:* excess money and candy, new clothes, pictures, notes.
   d. *Signs and symptoms:* bed-wetting, excessive bathing, tears, avoiding school, somatic distress (*GI and urinary* tract pains).

◆ **B. Analysis/nursing diagnosis:**
   1. *Altered protection* related to inflicted pain.
   2. *Risk for injury* related to neglect, abuse.
   3. *Personal identity disturbance* related to abuse as child and feeling guilty and responsible for being a victim.
   4. *Ineffective individual coping* related to high stress level.
   5. *Sleep pattern disturbance* related to traumatic sexual experiences.
   6. *Ineffective family coping.*
   7. *Altered family processes* related to use of violence.

8. *Altered parenting* related to violence.
9. *Powerlessness* related to feelings of being dependent on abuser.
10. *Social isolation/withdrawal* related to shame about family violence.
11. *Risk for altered abuse response patterns.*

◆ **C. Nursing care plan/implementation:**
   1. Establish safe environment and the termination of trauma.
   2. Encourage child to verbalize feelings about incident to dispel tension built up by secrecy.
   3. Ask child to draw a picture or use dolls and toys to show what happened.
   4. Observe for symptoms over a period of time.
      a. *Phobic* reactions when seeing or hearing offender's name.
      b. *Sleep pattern* changes, recurrent dreams, nightmares.
   5. Look for *silent reaction* to being an accessory to sex (i.e., child keeping burden of the secret activity within self); help deal with unresolved issues.
   6. Establish therapeutic alliance with abusive parent.
   7. *Health teaching:*

Mental Health

a. Teach child that his (her) body is private and to inform a responsible adult when someone violates privacy without consent.

b. Teach adults in family to respond to victim with sensitivity, support, and concern.

◆ **D. Evaluation/outcome criteria:**
1. Child's needs for affection, attention, personal recognition, or love met without sexual exploitation.
2. Perpetrator accepts therapy.
3. Conspiracy of silence is broken.

❏ Comfort, Rest, Activity, and Mobility Functions

Sleep Disturbance

I. **Types of sleep:**
   A. *Rapid eye movement (REM) sleep:* colorful, dramatic, emotional, implausible dreams.
   B. *Non-REM sleep—stages:*
   1. Stage 1: lasts 30 sec–7 min—falls asleep, drowsy; easily awakened; fleeting thoughts.
   2. Stage 2: more relaxed; no eye movements, clearly asleep but readily awakens; 45% of total sleep time spent in this stage.
   3. Stage 3 (delta sleep): deep muscle relaxation; ↓ TPR.
   4. Stage 4 (delta sleep): very relaxed; rarely moves.
   C. *Sleep cycle*—common progression of sleep stages:
   1. Stages 1, 2, 3, 4, 3, 2, REM, 2, 3, 4, etc.
   2. *Delta* sleep most common during first third of night, with *REM* sleep periods increasing in duration during night from 1–2 min at start to 20–30 min by early morning.
   3. REM sleep varies.
      a. Adolescents spend 30% of total sleep time in REM sleep.
      b. Adults spend 15% of total sleep time in REM sleep.

II. **Sleep deprivation (dyssomnias):**
   ◆ **A. Assessment:**
   1. *Non-REM sleep loss:* physical fatigue due to less time spent in normal deep sleep.
   2. *REM sleep loss:* psychological effects—irritability, confusion, anxiety, short-term memory loss, paranoia, hallucinations.
   3. *Desynchronized sleep:* occurs when sleep shifts more than 2 h from normal sleep period. Irritability, anoxia, decreased stress tolerance.
   ◆ **B. Analysis/nursing diagnosis:** *sleep pattern disturbance* may be related to:
   1. Interrupted sleep cycles before 90-min sleep cycle is completed.
   2. Unfamiliar sleeping environment.

3. Alterations in normal sleep/activity cycles (e.g., jet lag).
4. Preexisting sleep deficits prior to hospital admission.
5. Medications, e.g., alcohol withdrawal or abruptly discontinuing the use of hypnotic or antidepressant medications.
6. Pain.

◆ **C. Nursing care plan/implementation:**
1. Obtain sleep history as part of nursing assessment. Determine normal sleep hours, bedtime rituals, factors that promote or interrupt sleep.
2. Duplicate normal bedtime rituals when possible.
3. Make *environment* conducive to sleep: lighting, noise, temperature.
   a. Close door, dim lights, turn off unneeded machinery.
   b. Encourage staff to muffle conversation at night.
4. Encourage *daytime* exercise periods.
5. Allow *uninterrupted periods of 90 min of sleep.* Group nighttime treatments and observations that require touching the client.
6. *Minimize* use of hypnotic medications.
   a. Substitute back rubs, warm milk, relaxation exercises.
   b. Encourage physician to consider prescribing hypnotics that minimize sleep disruption (e.g., chloral hydrate and flurazepam HCl [Dalmane]).
   c. *Taper* off hypnotics rather than abruptly discontinuing.
7. Observe client while asleep.
   a. Evaluate quality of sleep.
   b. It may be sleep apnea if client is extremely restless and snoring heavily.
8. *Health teaching:* avoid caffeine and hyperstimulation at bedtime; teach how to promote sleep-inducing environment, relaxation techniques.

◆ **D. Evaluation/outcome criteria:** verbalizes satisfaction with amount, quality of sleep.

❏ Eating Disorders

Anorexia Nervosa/Bulimia Nervosa

Anorexia nervosa is an eating disorder, usually seen in adolescence, when a person is underweight and emaciated and refuses to eat. It can result in death due to irreversible metabolic processes.

Bulimia nervosa is another type of eating disorder, also encountered among older women and younger men. It is characterized by at least two binge-eating episodes of large quantities of high-calorie food over a couple of hours followed by disparaging self-criticism and depression. Self-induced vomiting is commonly associated since it decreases physical pain of abdominal distention, may reduce postbinge anguish, and may provide a method of self-control. Bulimic episodes may occur as part of anorexia nervosa, but these clients rarely become emaciated, and not all have a body-image disturbance.

 I. Concepts and principles related to anorexia nervosa:

 A. *Not* due to lack of appetite or problem with appetite center in hypothalamus.

 B. Normal stomach hunger is *repressed, denied, depersonalized;* no conscious awareness of hunger sensation.

◆ **II. Assessment of** anorexia nervosa:

 A. *Body-image disturbance*—delusional, obsessive (e.g., doesn't see self as thin and is bewildered by others' concern).

 B. Usually *preoccupied* with food, yet dreads gaining too much weight. *Ambivalence:* avoids food, hoards food.

 C. Feels ineffectual, with low sex drive. *Repudiation of sexuality.*

 D. *Pregnancy* fears, including misconceptions of oral impregnation through food.

 E. *Self-punitive* behavior leading to starvation.

 F. *Physical signs and symptoms*

 1. Weight loss (20% of previous "normal" body weight).

 2. Amenorrhea and secondary sex organ atrophy.

 3. *Hyperactivity;* compulsiveness.

 4. Constipation.

 5. *Hypotension, bradycardia,* hypothermia.

 6. *Hyperkeratosis* of skin.

 7. Blood: leukopenia, anemia, hypoglycemia, hypoproteinemia, hypercholesterolemia, hypokalemia.

◆ **III. Analysis/nursing diagnosis:**

 A. *Risk for self-inflicted injury* related to starvation from refusal to eat or ambivalence about food.

 B. *Risk for altered physical regulation processes:* amenorrhea related to starvation; hypotension, bradycardia.

 C. *Altered nutrition, less than body requirements,* related to attempts to vomit food after eating and refusal to eat, related to need to demonstrate control.

 D. *Altered eating:* binge-purge syndrome.

 E. *Compulsive behaviors* related to need to maintain control of self, represented by losing weight.

 F. *Body-image disturbance* related to anxiety over assuming an adult role and concern with sexual identity.

◆ **IV. Nursing care plan/implementation:**

 A. Help reestablish connections between body sensations (hunger) and responses (eating). Use *stimulus-response conditioning* methods to set up eating regimen.

 B. *Monitor* physiologic signs and symptoms (amenorrhea, constipation, hypoproteinemia,

hypoglycemia, anemia, secondary sexual organ atrophy, hypothermia, hypotension, leg cramps and other signs of hypokalemia).

 1. *Weigh* regularly, at same time and with same amount of clothing.

 2. Make sure water drinking is *avoided* before weighing.

 3. Give one-to-one supervision during and 30 min after mealtimes to *prevent* attempts to vomit food.

 C. *Health teaching:*

 1. Explain normal sexual growth and development to improve knowledge deficit.

 2. Use behavior modification to reestablish awareness of hunger sensation and to relate it to the clock and regular meal times.

 3. Teach parents skills in communication related to dependence/independence needs of adolescent.

◆ **V. Evaluation/outcome criteria:**

 A. Attains and maintains minimal normal weight for age and height.

 B. Eats regular meal (standard nutritional diet).

 C. No incidence of self-induced vomiting, bulimia, or compulsive physical activity.

 D. Acts on increased internal emotional awareness and recognition of body sensation of hunger (i.e., talks about being hungry and feeling hunger pangs).

 E. Relates increased sense of effectiveness with less need to control food intake.

❏ Sensory-Perceptual Functions

Sensory Disturbance

 I. Types of sensory disturbance:

 A. *Sensory deprivation*—amount of stimuli *less* than required, such as isolation in bed or room, deafness, stroke victim.

 B. *Sensory overload*—receives *more* stimuli than can be tolerated, e.g., bright lights, noise, strange machinery, barrage of visitors.

 C. *Sensory deficit*—impairment in functioning of sensory or perceptual processes, e.g., blindness, changes in tactile perceptions.

◆ **II. Assessment**—based on awareness of behavioral changes:

 A. *Sensory deprivation*—boredom, daydreaming, increasing sleep, thought slowness, inactivity, thought disorganization, hallucinations.

 B. *Sensory overload*—same as above, plus restlessness and agitation, confusion.

 C. *Sensory deficit*—may not be able to distinguish sounds, odors, and tastes or differentiate tactile sensations.

◆ **III. Analysis/nursing diagnosis:** problems related to sensory disturbance:

 A. *Altered thought processes.*

 B. *Confusion.*

C. *Anger, aggression.*
D. *Body-image disturbance.*
E. *Sleep pattern disturbance.*

◆ IV. **Nursing care plan/implementation:**

A. *Management of existing* sensory disturbances in:
1. *Acute sensory deprivation*
   a. Increase interaction with staff.
   b. Use TV.
   c. Provide touch.
   d. Help clients choose menus that have aromas, varied tastes, temperatures, colors, textures.
   e. Use light cologne or after-shave lotion, bath powder.
2. *Sensory overload*
   a. Restrict number of visitors and length of stay.
   b. Reduce noise and lights.
   c. Reduce newness by establishing and following routine.
   d. Organize care to provide for extended rest periods with minimal input.
3. *Sensory deficits*
   a. Report observations about hearing, vision.
   b. May imply need for new glasses, medical diagnosis, or therapy.

B. *Health teaching: prevention* of sensory disturbance involves *education* of parents during child's growth and development regarding tactile, auditory, and visual stimulation.
1. Hold, talk, and play with infant when awake.
2. Provide bright toys with different designs for children to hold.
3. Change environment.
4. Provide music and auditory stimuli.
5. Give foods with variety of textures, tastes, colors.

◆ V. **Evaluation/outcome criteria:**

A. Client is oriented to time, place, person.
B. Little or no evidence of mood or sleep disturbance.

Delirium, Dementia, and Amnestic and Other Cognitive Disorders

These disorders include etiology associated with (1) the *aging process* (dementias arising in the senium or presenium, including primary degenerative dementia of the Alzheimer type and multi-infarct dementia), (2) *substance-related disorders* (e.g., alcohol, barbiturates, opioids, cocaine, amphetamines, PCP, hallucinogens, *cannabis,* nicotine, and caffeine), and (3) general medical conditions.

I. **Concepts, principles, and subtypes:**

A. Course may be progressive, with steady deterioration.

B. Alternative pathways and compensatory mechanisms may develop to show a clinical picture of remissions and exacerbations.

C. *Delirium* is characterized by a *disturbance of consciousness* with reduced ability to focus, sustain, or shift attention; and a *change in cognition* (e.g., memory deficit, disorientation [time and place], language disturbance); or *development of perceptual disturbance* (e.g., illusions, hallucinations) that develop over a *short* time (hours or days) and *fluctuate* during the course of the day. *Etiology:* a direct physiologic consequence of a general medical condition, substance intoxication or withdrawal, use of a medication, or toxin exposure. *Diagnostic feature:* cannot repeat sequential string of information (e.g., digit span).

D. *Dementia* is characterized by persistent *multiple cognitive deficits* (e.g., aphasia, apraxia, agnosia, disturbance in executive functioning) accompanied by memory impairment and mood and sleep disturbances. *Diagnostic features:* cannot learn (register) new information (e.g., a list of words), or retain, recall, or recognize information.
1. *Possible etiology:* vascular dementia, HIV infection, head trauma, Parkinson's disease, Pick's disease, Alzheimer's disease, Huntington's disease, substance induced, toxin exposure, medication, infections, nutritional deficiencies, endocrine conditions, brain tumors, seizure disorders.
2. *Alzheimer's disease:* progressive, irreversible loss of cerebral function due to cortical atrophy; exists in 2–4% of people over 65 yr old; may have a genetic component; may begin at ages 40–65; may lead to death within 2 yr. Average duration from onset of symptoms to death: 8–10 yr.
   a. Progressive decline in intellectual capacity (recent and remote memory, judgment), affect and motor coordination (apraxia); loss of social sense; apathy or restlessness.
   b. *Problems with* speech (aphasia), recognition of familiar objects (agnosia), disorientation to self (even parts of *own* body).

E. *Amnestic disorder* is characterized by *severe* memory impairment *without* other significant impairments of cognitive functioning (i.e., without aphasia, apraxia, or agnosia). *Diagnostic features:* memory impairment is always manifested by impairment in the ability to learn *new* information and sometimes problems remembering previously learned information or past events. May result in *disorientation* to place and time, but *rarely* to self. Appears bewildered or befuddled.
1. *Etiology:* due to direct physiologic effects of a general medical condition (e.g., physical

trauma or vitamin deficiency) or due to persisting effects of a substance (e.g., drug of abuse, a medication, or toxin exposure).

2. Memory disturbance: sufficiently severe to cause marked impairment in social or occupational functioning and represents a significant decline from a previous level of functioning. May require supervised living situation to ensure appropriate feeding and care.

3. Lacks insight into own memory deficit and may explicitly deny the presence of severe memory impairment despite evidence to the contrary.

4. Altered personality function: apathy, lack of initiative, emotional blandness, shallow range of expression.

◆ **II. Assessment:**

A. *Most common areas of difficulty* can be grouped under the mnemonic term *JOCAM*: J—judgment, O—orientation, C—confabulation, A—affect, and M—memory.

1. *Judgment:* impaired, resulting in socially inappropriate behavior (such as hypersexuality toward inappropriate objects) and inability to carry out activities of daily living.

2. *Orientation:* confused, disoriented; perceptual disturbances (e.g., illusions, misidentification of other persons and objects; misperception to make unfamiliar more familiar; *visual, tactile, and auditory* hallucinations may appear as images and voices or disorganized light and sound patterns). *Paranoid delusions* of persecution.

3. *Confabulation:* common use of this defense mechanism to fill in memory gaps with invented stories.

4. *Affect:* mood changes and unstable emotions; quarrelsome, with outbursts of morbid anger (as in cerebral arteriosclerosis); tearful; withdrawn from social contact; *depression* is a frequent reaction to loss of physical and social function.

5. *Memory:* impaired, especially for names and *recent* events; may compensate by confabulating and by using *circumstantiality and tangential* speaking patterns.

B. *Other areas of difficulty*

1. *Seizures* (in Alzheimer's disease and cerebral arteriosclerosis, e.g.).

2. *Intellectual capacities diminished.*
   a. Difficulty with *abstract* thought.
   b. Compensatory mechanism is to stay with familiar topics; repetition.
   c. Short concentration periods.

3. *Personality changes.*
   a. Loss of ego flexibility; adoption of more rigid attitudes.
   b. *Ritualism* in daily activities.
   c. Hoarding.

   d. Somatic preoccupations (hypochondriases).
   e. *Restlessness.*

◆ **III. Analysis/nursing diagnosis:**

A. *Risk for injury* related to cognitive deficits and altered motor behavior (restlessness, hyperactivity).

B. *Altered conduct/impulse processes* (irritability and aggressiveness) related to neurologic impairment.

C. *Sensory/perceptual alterations:* visual, auditory, kinesthetic, gustatory, tactile, olfactory.

D. *Altered attention and memory* related to progressive neurologic losses.

E. *Total incontinence* related to sensory/perceptual alterations.

F. *Altered nutrition, more or less than body requirements,* related to confusion.

G. *Self-care deficit* (feeding, bathing/hygiene, dressing, toileting) related to physical impairments (poor vision, uncoordination, forgetfulness).

H. *Sleep pattern disturbance* resulting in disorientation at night, related to confusion.

I. *Altered abstract thinking and altered knowledge processes (agnosia)* related to destruction of cerebral tissue and inability to utilize information to make judgments and transmit messages.

J. *Impaired communication* related to poverty of speech and withdrawal behavior, progressive neurologic losses, and cerebral impairment.

K. *Altered role performance* related to decreases in intellectual competence.

◆ **IV. Nursing care plan/implementation:** Also see interventions in III. Confusion/disorientation, p. 325.

A. *Long-term goal:* minimize regression related to memory impairment.

B. *Short-term goal:* provide structure and consistency to increase security.

C. Make *brief, frequent* contacts, as attention span is short.

D. Allow clients *time* to talk and to complete projects.

E. Stimulate *associative* patterns to improve recall (by repeating, summarizing, and focusing).

F. Allow clients to *review* their lives and focus on the past.

G. Utilize *concrete* questions in interviewing.

H. *Reinforce* reality-oriented comments.

I. Keep environment the *same* as much as possible (same room and placement of furniture, e.g.); *routine* is important to diminish stress.

J. Recognize the importance of *compensatory* mechanisms (confabulation, e.g.) to increase self-esteem; build psychological reserve.

K. Give recognition for each accomplishment.

L. Use *recreational* and physical therapy.

M. *Health teaching:* give *specific* instructions for diet, medication, and treatment; how to use

Mental Health

many sensory approaches to learn new information; how to use existing knowledge, old learning, and habitual approaches to deal with new situations.

◆ **V. Evaluation/outcome criteria:**
   A. Symptoms occur *less* frequently and are less severe in areas of emotional lability and appropriateness; false perceptions; self-care ability; disorientation, memory, and judgment; and decision making.
   B. Client is able to preserve optimum level of functioning and independence while allowing basic needs to be met.
   C. Stays relatively calm and noncombative when upset or fearful.
   D. Accepts own irritability and frustrations as part of illness.
   E. Asks for assistance with self-care activities.
   F. Knows and adheres to daily routine; knows own nurse, location of room, bathroom, clocks, calendars.
   G. Uses supportive community services.

Substance-Related Disorders

I. **Definition:** ingesting in any manner a chemical that has an effect on the body.
◆ **II. General assessment:**
   A. *Behavioral* changes exist while under the influence of substance.
   B. Engages in regular *use* of substance.
      1. *Substance abuse:*
         a. Pattern of *pathologic* use (i.e., day-long intoxication; inability to stop use, even when contraindicated by serious physical disorder; overpowering need or desire to take the drug despite legal, social, or medical problems); daily need of substance for functioning; repeated medical complications from use.
         b. *Interference* with social, occupational functioning.
         c. Willingness to obtain substance by any means, including illegal.
         d. Pathologic use for more than 1 mo.
      2. *Substance dependence:*
         a. More severe than substance abuse; body *requires* substance to continue functioning.
         b. Physiologic dependence (i.e., either develops a *tolerance*—must increase dose to obtain desired effect—or has *physical withdrawal symptoms* when substance intake is reduced or stopped).
         c. Person feels it's impossible to get along without drug.
   C. Effects of substance on *central nervous system (CNS)*.
◆ **III. General analysis:** only in recent years has substance abuse been viewed as an illness rather than moral delinquency or criminal behavior. The disorders are very complex and little understood.

There are physiologic, psychological, and social aspects to their causality, dynamics, symptoms, and treatment, where personality disorder has a major part.
   A. *Physiologic aspects*—current unproven theories include "allergic" reaction to alcohol, disturbance in metabolism, genetic susceptibility to dependency, and hypofunction of adrenal cortex. There are *organic effects* of chronic excessive use.
   B. *Psychological aspects*—disrupted parent-child relationship and family dynamics; deleterious effect on ego function.
   C. *Social and cultural aspects*—local customs and attitudes vary about what is excessive.
   D. *Maladaptive behavior related to:*
      1. Low self-esteem.
      2. Anger.
      3. Denial.
      4. Rationalization.
      5. Social isolation.
      6. A rigid pattern of coping.
      7. Poorly defined philosophy of life, values, mores.
◆ **E.** *Nursing diagnosis* in acute phase of abuse, intoxication:
      1. *Risk for injury* related to impaired coordination, disorientation, and altered judgment (worse at night).
      2. *Risk for violence:* self-directed or directed at others, related to misinterpretation of stimuli and feelings of suspicion or distrust of others.
      3. *Sensory/perceptual alterations:* visual, kinesthetic, tactile, related to intake of mind-altering substances.
      4. *Altered thought processes* (delusions, incoherence) related to misinterpretation of stimuli.
      5. *Sleep pattern disturbance* related to mind-altering substance.
      6. *Ineffective individual coping* related to inability to tolerate frustration and to meet basic needs or role expectations, resulting in unpredictable behaviors.
      7. *Noncompliance* with abstinence and supportive therapy, related to inability to stop using substance because of dependence and refusal to alter life-style.
      8. *Impaired communication* related to mental confusion or CNS depression related to substance use.
      9. *Impaired health maintenance management* related to failure to recognize that a problem exists and inability to take responsibility for health needs.

Alcohol Use Disorders: Alcohol Abuse and Dependence

Alcohol dependence is a chronic disorder in which the individual is unable, for physical or psychological reasons or both, to refrain from frequent consumption of alcohol in quantities that produce intoxication and disrupt health and ability to perform daily functions.

◆ **I. Concepts and principles** related to alcohol abuse and dependence:

A. Alcohol affects cerebral cortical functions:
   1. Memory.
   2. Judgment.
   3. Reasoning.

B. Alcohol as a *depressant:*
   1. Relaxes the individual.
   2. Lessens use of repression of unconscious conflict.
   3. Releases inhibitions, hostility, and primitive drives.

C. Drinking represents a tension-reducing device and a relief from feelings of insecurity. Strength of drinking habit equals degree of anxiety and frustration intolerance.

D. Alcohol abuse and dependence is a *symptom* rather than a disease.

E. Underlying fear and anxiety, associated with inner conflict, motivate the alcoholic to drink.

F. Alcoholics can never be cured to drink normally; cure is to be a "sober alcoholic," with total abstinence.

G. The spouse of the alcoholic often unconsciously contributes to the drinking behavior because of own emotional needs (*co-alcoholic* or *co-dependent*).

H. Intoxication occurs with a blood-alcohol level of 0.08% or above. *Signs of intoxication* are:
   1. Incoordination.
   2. Slurred speech.
   3. Dulled perception.

I. Tolerance occurs with alcohol dependence. Increasing amounts of alcohol must be consumed to obtain the desired effect.

◆ **II. Assessment:**

A. *Vicious cycle*—(a) low tolerance for coping with frustration, tension, guilt, resentment; (b) uses alcohol for relief; (c) new problems created by drinking; (d) new anxieties; and (e) more drinking.

B. Coping mechanisms used: *denial, rationalization, projection.*

C. *Complications of abuse and dependence.*
   1. *Alcohol withdrawal delirium (delirium tremens—DTs)* (Figure 6.3)—result of nutritional deficiencies and toxins; requires sedation and constant watchfulness against unintentional suicide and convulsions.
      a. *Impending* signs relate to *CNS*—marked nervousness and restlessness, increased irritability; gross tremors of hands, face, lips; weakness; also *cardiovascular*—increased blood pressure, tachycardia, diaphoresis; *depression; gastrointestinal*—nausea, vomiting, anorexia.
      b. *Actual*—*serious* symptoms of mental confusion, convulsions, hallucinations

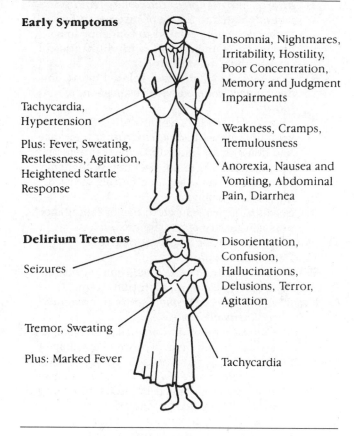

■ **FIGURE 6.3 Symptoms associated with alcohol withdrawal. (From Wilson HS, Kneisl CR. *Psychiatric Nursing* [2nd ed]. Menlo Park, CA: Addison-Wesley, 1983. P 388.)**

Early Symptoms

Tachycardia, Hypertension

Plus: Fever, Sweating, Restlessness, Agitation, Heightened Startle Response

Insomnia, Nightmares, Irritability, Hostility, Poor Concentration, Memory and Judgment Impairments

Weakness, Cramps, Tremulousness

Anorexia, Nausea and Vomiting, Abdominal Pain, Diarrhea

Delirium Tremens

Seizures

Tremor, Sweating

Plus: Marked Fever

Disorientation, Confusion, Hallucinations, Delusions, Terror, Agitation

Tachycardia

(visual, auditory, tactile). Without cure, *15–20%* may die.

   2. *Wernicke's syndrome*—a neurologic disturbance manifested by confusion, ataxia, eye movement abnormalities, and memory impairment. Other problems include:
      a. Disturbed vision.
      b. Wandering mind.
      c. Stupor and coma.
   3. *Alcohol amnestic syndrome (Korsakoff's syndrome)*—degenerative neuritis due to *thiamine* deficiency.
      a. Impaired thoughts.
      b. Confusion, loss of sense of time and place.
      c. Use of confabulation to fill in severe memory loss.
      d. Follows episode of *Wernicke's encephalopathy.*
   4. *Polyneuropathy*—sensory and motor nerve endings are involved, causing pain, itching, and loss of limb control.
   5. *Others*—*gastritis, esophageal varices, cirrhosis, pancreatitis, diabetes,* pneumonia, REM sleep deprivation, *malnutrition.*

Mental Health

◆ **III. Analysis/nursing diagnosis:**

A. *Risk for self-directed violence:* tendency for *self-destructive* acts related to intake of mind-altering substances.

B. *Altered nutrition, less than body requirements,* related to a lack of interest in food.

C. *Defensive coping* related to tendency to be domineering and critical, with difficulties in *interpersonal* relationships.

D. *Conflict with social order* related to extreme dependence coupled with resentment *of authority.*

E. *Spiritual distress* or general dissatisfaction with life related to *low frustration* tolerance and demand for immediate need satisfaction.

F. *Dysfunctional behaviors* related to tendency for *excess* in work, sex, recreation, marked *narcissistic* behavior.

G. *Social isolation* related to use of coping mechanisms that are primarily *escapist.*

◆ **IV. Nursing care plan/implementation:**

A. *Detoxification phase*

   1. *Administer adequate sedation* to control anxiety, insomnia, agitation, tremors.

   2. *Administer anticonvulsants* to prevent *withdrawal seizures.*

   3. *Control nausea and vomiting* to avoid massive GI bleeding or rupture of esophageal varices.

   4. *Assess fluid and electrolyte balance* for dehydration (may need IV fluids) or overhydration (may need a diuretic).

   5. *Reestablish proper nutrition: high protein* (as long as no severe liver damage), carbohydrate, *vitamins C and B complex.*

   6. *Provide calm, safe environment:* bedrest *with rails,* well-lit room to reduce illusions; constant supervision and reassurance about fears and hallucinations, assess depression for suicide potential.

B. *Recovery-rehabilitation phase:* encourage participation in *group* activities; *avoid sympathy* when client tends to rationalize behavior and seeks special privileges—use acceptance and a *nonjudgmental,* consistent, firm, but kind approach; *avoid* scorn, contempt, and moralizing or punitive and rejecting behaviors; do *not* reinforce feelings of worthlessness, self-contempt, hopelessness, or low self-esteem.

C. *Problem behaviors*

   1. *Manipulative*—be firm and consistent; avoid "bid for sympathy."

   2. *Demanding*—set limits.

   3. *Acting out*—set limits, enforce rules and regulations, strengthen impulse control and ability to delay gratification.

   4. *Dependency*—place responsibility on client; avoid giving advice.

   5. *Superficiality*—help client make realistic self-appraisals and expectations in lieu of grandiose promises and trite verbaliza-

tions; encourage formation of lasting interpersonal relationships.

D. *Common reactions among staff*

   1. Disappointment—instead, set realistic goals, take one step at a time.

   2. Moral judgment—instead, support each other.

   3. Hostility—instead, offer support to each other when feeling frustrated from lack of results.

E. Refer client from hospital to *community resources* for follow-up treatment with social, economic, and psychological problems, as well as to self-help groups, to reduce "revolving door" situation in which client comes in, is treated, goes out, and comes in again the next night.

   1. *Alcoholics Anonymous (AA)*—a self-help group of addicted drinkers who confront, instruct, and support fellow drinkers in their efforts to stay sober 1 d at a time through fellowship and acceptance.

   2. *Alanon*—support group for *families* of alcoholics. *Alateen*—support group for *teenagers* when parent is alcoholic.

   3. *Aversion therapy*—client is subjected to revulsion-producing or pain-inducing stimuli at the same time he or she takes a drink, to establish alcohol rejection behavior. Most common is disulfiram (Antabuse), a drug that produces intense headache, severe flushing, extreme nausea, vomiting, palpitations, hypotension, dyspnea, and blurred vision when alcohol is consumed while person is taking this drug.

   4. *Group psychotherapy*—the goals of group psychotherapy are for the client to give up alcohol as a tension reliever, identify cause of stress, build different means for coping with stress, and accept drinking as a serious symptom.

F. *Health teaching:* teach improved coping patterns to tolerate increased stress; teach substitute tension-reducing strategies; prepare in advance for difficult, painful events; teach how to reduce irritating or frustrating environmental stress.

◆ **V. Evaluation/outcome criteria:** everyday living patterns are restructured for a satisfactory life without alcohol; demonstrates feelings of increased self-worth, confidence, and reliance.

Other Substance-Related Disorders

I. Concepts and principles:

A. *Three* interacting key factors give rise to dependence—*psychopathology* of the individual; frustrating *environment;* and *availability* of powerful, addicting, and temporarily satisfying drug.

B. According to conditioning principles, substance abuse and dependence proceed in *several phases:*

1. *Use* of sedatives-hypnotics, CNS stimulants, hallucinogens and narcotics, for relief from daily tensions and discomforts or anticipated withdrawal symptoms.
2. Habit is *reinforced* with each relief by drug use.
3. Development of *dependency*—drug has less and less efficiency in reducing tensions.
4. Dependency is further reinforced as addict *fails* to maintain adequate drug intake—increase in frequency and duration of periods of tension and discomfort.

◆ **II. Assessment:**
  A. Abuse
    1. *Hallucinogens* (LSD, marijuana, STP, PCP, peyote): euphoria and rapid mood swings, flight of ideas; perceptual impairment, feelings of omnipotence, "bad trip" (panic, loss of control, paranoia), flashbacks, suicide.
    2. *CNS stimulants* (*amphetamines* and *cocaine* abuse): euphoria, hyperactivity, hyperalertness, irritability, persecutory delusions; insomnia, anorexia → weight loss; tachycardia; tremulousness; hypertension; hyperthermia → convulsions.
    3. *Narcotics* (*opium* and its derivatives, e.g., morphine, heroin, codeine, meperidine HCl [Demerol]): used by "snorting," "skin popping," and "mainlining." May lead to abscesses and hepatitis. Decreased pain response, respiratory depression; apathy, detachment from reality; impaired judgment; loss of sexual activity; pinpoint pupils.
    4. *Sedatives-hypnotics (barbiturate abuse):* like alcohol-induced behavior, e.g., euphoria followed by depression, hostility; decreased inhibitions; impaired judgment; staggering gait; slurred speech; drowsiness; poor concentration; progressive respiratory depression.
  B. *Withdrawal symptoms*
    1. *Narcotics* (e.g., heroin): begins within 12 h of last dose, peaks in 24–36 h, subsides in 72 h, and disappears in 5–6 d.
      a. Pupil *dilation*.
      b. Muscle: twitches, tremors, aches, pains.
      c. Goose flesh (piloerection).
      d. *Lacrimation, rhinorrhea, sneezing, yawning.*
      e. *Diaphoresis*, chills.
      f. Potential for fever.
      g. *Vomiting*, abdominal distress.
      h. Dehydration.
      i. Rapid weight loss.
      j. Sleep disturbance.
    2. *Barbiturates:* may be gradual or abrupt ("cold turkey"); latter is dangerous or *life-threatening;* should be hospitalized.
      a. *Gradual* withdrawal reaction from barbiturates:

(1) Postural hypotension.
(2) Tachycardia.
(3) Elevated temperature.
(4) Insomnia.
(5) Tremors.
(6) Agitation, restlessness.
      b. *Abrupt* withdrawal from barbiturates:
(1) Apprehension.
(2) Muscular weakness.
(3) Tremors.
(4) Postural hypotension.
(5) Twitching.
(6) Anorexia.
(7) *Grand mal seizures.*
(8) *Psychosis-delirium.*
    3. *Amphetamines:* depression, lack of energy, somnolence.
  C. *Difference* between alcohol and other abused substances (e.g., opioid).
    1. Above drugs may need to be obtained by illegal means, making it a legal and criminal problem as well as a medical and social problem; *not* so with alcohol abuse and dependency.
    2. Opium and its derivatives *inhibit* aggression, whereas alcohol *releases* aggression.
    3. As long as she or he is on large enough doses to avoid withdrawal symptoms, abuser of narcotics, sedatives, or hypnotics is comfortable and functions well, whereas chronically intoxicated alcoholic *cannot* function normally.
    4. Direct physiologic effects of long-term opioid abuse and dependence on above drugs are much *less critical* than those with chronic alcohol dependence.

◆ **III. Analysis/nursing diagnosis:**
  A. *Risk for altered physical regulation processes* (cardiac, circulatory, gastrointestinal, sleep pattern disturbance) related to use of mind-altering drugs.
  B. *Altered conduct/impulse processes* related to rebellious attitudes toward authority.
  C. *Altered social interaction* (manipulation, dependency) related to hostility and personal insecurity.
  D. *Altered judgment* related to misinterpretation of sensory stimuli and low frustration tolerance.
  E. *Altered feeling states* (denial) related to underlying self-doubt and personal insecurity.

◆ **IV. Nursing care plan/implementation:** generally the same as in treating antisocial personality and alcohol abuse and dependence.
  A. Maintain *safety* and optimum level of *physical* comfort. Supportive physical care: vital signs, nutrition, hydration, seizure precautions.
  B. *Assist with medical treatment* and offer support and *reality orientation* to reduce feelings of panic.

Mental Health

1. *Detoxification (or dechemicalization)*—give medications according to detoxification schedule.
   2. *Withdrawal*—may be gradual (barbiturates, hypnotics, tranquilizers) or abrupt ("cold turkey" for heroin). Observe for symptoms and report immediately.
   3. *Methadone*—person must have been dependent on narcotics at least 2 yr and have failed at other methods of withdrawal before admission to program of readdiction by methadone.
       a. *Characteristics*
           (1) Synthetic.
           (2) Appeases desire for narcotics without producing euphoria of narcotics.
           (3) Given by mouth.
           (4) Distributed under federal control (*Narcotic Addict Rehabilitation Act*).
           (5) Given with urinary surveillance.
       b. *Advantages*
           (1) Prevents narcotic withdrawal reaction.
           (2) Tolerance not built up.
           (3) Person remains out of prison.
           (4) Lessens perceived need for heroin or morphine.

C. *Participation in group therapy—goals:* peer pressure, support, and identification.

D. *Rehabilitation phase:*
   1. Refer to halfway house and group living (e.g., Day-top).
   2. Support *employment* as therapy (work training).
   3. Expand client's *range of interests* to relieve characteristic boredom and stimulus hunger.
       a. Provide *structured* environment and planned routine.
       b. Provide educational therapy (academic and vocational).
       c. Arrange activities to include current events discussion groups, lectures, drama, music, and art appreciation.

E. Achieve role of *stabilizer and supportive* authoritative figure; this can be achieved through frequent, regular contacts with the same client.

F. *Health teaching:* how to cope with pain, fatigue, and anxiety without drugs.

V. Evaluation/outcome criteria: replaces addictive life-style with self-reliant behavior.

❑ Psychosocial-Cultural Functions

The Therapeutic Nursing Process

A *therapeutic nursing process* involves an interaction between the nurse and client in which the nurse offers a series of planned, goal-directed activities that are use-

ful to a particular client in relieving discomfort, promoting growth, and satisfying interpersonal relationships.

I. Characteristics of therapeutic nursing:
A. Movement from first contact through final outcome:
   1. *Eight general phases* occur in a typical unfolding of a natural process of problem solving.
   2. Stages are not always in the same sequence.
   3. Not all stages are present in a relationship.

B. Phases*
   1. *Beginning* the relationship. *Goal:* build trust.
   2. *Formulating* and clarifying a problem and concern. *Goal:* clarify client's statements.
   3. *Setting a contract* or working agreement. *Goal:* decide on terms of the relationship.
   4. *Building* the relationship. *Goal:* increase depth of relationship and degree of commitment.
   5. *Exploring goals* and solutions, gathering data, expressing feelings. *Goals:* (a) maintain and enhance relationship (trust and safety), (b) explore blocks to goal, (c) expand self-awareness, and (d) learn skills necessary to reach goal.
   6. *Developing action plan. Goals:* (a) clarify feelings, (b) focus on and choose between alternate courses of action, and (c) practice new skills.
   7. *Working through* conflicts or disturbing feelings. *Goals:* (a) channel earlier discussions into specific course of action and (b) work through unresolved feelings.
   8. *Ending* the relationship. *Goals:* (a) evaluation of goal attainment and (b) leave taking.

II. Therapeutic nurse-client interactions
◆ A. Plans/goals:
   1. Demonstrate unconditional *acceptance,* interest, concern, and respect.
   2. Develop trust—be *consistent and congruent.*
   3. Make *frequent* contacts with the client.
   4. Be *honest* and *direct, authentic* and spontaneous.
   5. Offer support, security, and empathy, *not* sympathy.
   6. Focus comments on concerns of client (*client centered*), not self (social responses). *Refocus* when client changes subject.
   7. Encourage expression of *feelings;* focus on feelings and *here-and-now* behavior.
   8. Give attention to a client who complains.
   9. Give information at client's level of understanding, at appropriate time and place.

*From Brammer, LM. *The Helping Relationship: Process and Skills.* P 55. Copyright © 1973, Prentice-Hall, Inc, Englewood Cliffs, NJ.

Mental Health

10. Use open-ended questions; ask *how, what, where, who,* and *when* questions; avoid *why* questions; avoid questions that can be answered by *yes* or *no.*
11. Use feedback or reflective listening.
12. Maintain hope, but *avoid* false reassurances, clichés, and pat responses.
13. *Avoid* verbalizing value judgments, giving personal opinions, or moralizing.
14. Do not change the subject *unless* the client is redundant or focusing on physical illness.
15. Point out *reality;* help the client leave "inner world."
16. Set *limits* on behavior when client is acting out unacceptable behavior that is self-destructive or harmful to others.
17. Assist clients in arriving at their own decisions by demonstrating problem solving or involving them in the process.
18. Do not talk if it is not indicated.
19. Approach, sit, or walk with agitated clients; stay with the person who is upset, if he or she can tolerate it.
20. Focus on nonverbal communication.
21. Remember the *psyche has a soma!* Do not neglect appropriate physical symptoms.

B. Examples of **therapeutic** responses as interventions:
1. Being *silent*—being able to sit in silence with a person can connote acceptance and acknowledgment that the person has the right to silence. (*Dangers:* The nurse may wrongly give the client the impression that there is a lack of interest, or the nurse may discourage verbalization if acceptance of this behavior is prolonged; it is not necessarily helpful with acutely psychotic behavior.)
2. Using *nonverbal communication*—nodding head, moving closer to the client, and leaning forward, for example; use as a way to encourage client to speak.
3. Give encouragement to continue with *open-ended leads*—nurse's responses: "Then what?" "Go on," "For instance," "Tell me more," "Talk about that."
4. *Accepting, acknowledging*—nurse's responses: "I hear your anger," or "I see that you are sitting in the corner."
5. *Commenting on nonverbal behavior* of client—nurse's responses: "I notice that you are swinging your leg," "I see that you are tapping your foot," or "I notice that you are wetting your lips." Client may respond with, "So what?" If she or he does, the nurse needs to reply why the comment was made—for example, "It is distracting," "I am giving the nonverbal behavior meaning," "Swinging your leg makes it difficult for me to concentrate on what you

are saying," or "I think when people tap their feet it means they are impatient. Are you impatient?"
6. Encouraging clients to *notice with their senses* what is going on—nurse's response: "What did you see (or hear)?" or "What did you notice?"
7. Encouraging *recall and description* of details of a particular experience—nurse's response: "Give me an example," "Please describe the experience further," "Tell me more," or "What did you say then?"
8. *Giving feedback by reflecting, restating, and paraphrasing* feelings and content:
   Client: I cried when he didn't come to see me.
   Nurse: You cried. You were expecting him to come and he didn't?
9. *Picking up on latent content* (what is implied)—nurse's response: "You were disappointed. I think it may have hurt when he didn't come."
10. *Focusing, pinpointing,* asking "what" questions:
    Client: They didn't come.
    Nurse: Who are 'they'?
    Client: [Rambling.]
    Nurse: Tell it to me in a sentence or two. What is your main point? What would you say is your main concern?
11. *Clarifying*—nurse's response: "What do you mean by 'they'?" "What caused this?" or "I didn't understand. Please say it again."
12. *Focusing on reality* by expressing doubt on "unreal" perceptions:
    Client: Run! There are giant ants flying around after us.
    Nurse: That is unusual. I don't see giant ants flying.
13. *Focusing on feelings,* encouraging client to be aware of and describe personal feelings:
    Client: Worms are in my head.
    Nurse: That must be a frightening feeling. What did you feel at that time? Tell me about that feeling.
14. Helping client to *sort and classify impressions, make speculations, abstract* and *generalize* by making connections, seeing common elements and similarities, making comparisons, and placing events in logical sequence—nurse's responses: "What are the common elements in what you just told me?" "How is this similar to . . .?" "What happened just before?" or "What is the connection between this and . . .?"
15. *Pointing out discrepancies* between thoughts, feelings, and actions—nurse's response: "You say you were feeling sad when she yelled at you; yet you laughed.

Mental Health

Your feelings and actions do not seem to fit together."

16. *Checking perceptions* and *seeking agreement* on how the issue is seen, *checking* with the client to see if the message sent is the same one that was received—nurse's response: "Let me restate what I heard you say," "Are you saying that . . .?" "Did I hear you correctly?" "Is this what you mean?" or "It seems that you were saying . . .?"

17. *Encouraging client to consider alternatives*—nurse's response: "What else could you say?" or "Instead of hitting him, what else might you do?"

18. *Planning a course of action*—nurse's response: "Now that we have talked about your on-the-job activities and you have thought of several choices, which are you going to try out?" or "What would you do next time?"

19. *Imparting information*—give additional data as new input to help client; e.g., state facts and reality-based data that client may lack.

20. *Summing up*—nurse's response: "Today we have talked about your feelings toward your boss, how you express your anger, and about your fear of being rejected by your family."

21. *Encouraging client to appraise and evaluate* the experience or outcome—nurse's response: "How did it turn out?" "What was it like?" "What was your part in it?" "What difference did it make?" or "How will this help you later?"

C. Examples of **nontherapeutic** responses:

1. *Changing the subject, tangential response,* moves away from problem and/or focuses on incidental, superficial content:

Client: I hate you.
Nurse: Would you like to take your shower now?

Suggested responses reflect, "You hate me; tell me about this," or "You hate me; what does hate mean to you?"

Client: I want to kill myself today.
Nurse: Isn't today the day your mother is supposed to come?

Suggested responses: (a) give open-ended lead, (b) give feedback: "I hear you saying today that you want to kill yourself," or (c) clarifying: "Tell me more about this feeling of wanting to kill yourself."

2. *Moralizing:* saying with approval or disapproval that the person's behavior is good or bad, right or wrong; *arguing* with stated belief of person; directly opposing the person:

Nurse: That's good. It's wrong to shoot yourself.
Client: I have nothing to live for.
Nurse: You certainly do have a lot!

Suggested responses: similar to those in 1. (See C.1., p. 350.)

3. *Agreeing with client's autistic inventions:*

Client: The eggs are flying saucers.
Nurse: Yes, I see. Go on.

Suggested response: use clarifying response first: "I don't understand," and then, depending on client's response, use either *accepting and acknowledging, focusing on reality,* or *focusing on feelings.*

4. *Agreeing with client's negative view of self:*

Client: I have made a mess of my life.
Nurse: Yes, you have.

Suggested response: use clarifying response about "mess of my life"—"Give me an example of one time where you feel you messed up in your life."

5. *Complimenting, flattering:*

Client: I have made a mess of my life.
Nurse: How could you? You are such an attractive, intelligent, generous person.

Suggested response: same as in 4. (See above.)

6. *Giving opinions and advice* concerning client's life situation—examples of poor responses include: "In my opinion . . ." "I think you should . . ." or "Why not?"

Suggested responses: (a) encourage the client to consider alternatives ("What else do you think you could try?"); (b) encourage the client to appraise and evaluate for himself or herself ("What is it like for you?").

7. *Seeking agreement* from client with nurse's personal opinion—examples of poor responses include: "I think . . . Don't you?" and "Isn't that right?"

Suggested responses: (a) it is best to keep personal opinion to oneself and only to give information that would aid the client's orientation to reality; (b) if you give an opinion as a *model* of orienting to reality, ask client to *state his or her* opinion ("My opinion is . . . What is your opinion?").

8. *Probing* and/or *offering premature solutions and interpretations;* jumping to conclusions:

Client: I can't find a job.
Nurse: You could go to an employment agency.
Client: I'd rather not talk about it.

Nurse: What are you unconsciously doing when you say that? What you really mean is . . .

Client: I don't want to live alone.

Nurse: Are you afraid of starting to drink again?

Suggested responses: use responses that seek clarification and elicit more data.

9. *Changing client's words* without prior validation:

Client: I am *not feeling well* today.

Nurse: What makes you feel so *depressed?*

Suggested response: "In what way are you not feeling well?" Use the same language as the client.

10. *Following vague content* as if understood or *using vague global* pronouns, adverbs, and adjectives:

Client: People are so *unfair.*

Nurse: I know what you mean.

Suggested response: clarify vague referents such as "people" and "unfair."

Client: I feel sad.

Nurse: Everyone feels that way at one time or another.

Suggested response: "What are you sad about?"

11. *Questioning on different topics without waiting for a reply:*

Client: [Remains silent.]

Nurse: What makes you so silent? Are you angry? Would you like to be alone?

Suggested response: choose one of the above and wait for a response before asking the next question.

12. *Ignoring client's questions or comments:*

Client: Am I crazy, nurse?

Nurse: [Walking away as if he or she did not hear the client.]

Suggested responses: "I can't understand what makes you bring this up at this time," or "Tell me what makes you bring this up at this time." Ignoring questions or comments usually implies that the nurse is feeling uncomfortable. It is important not to "run away" from the client.

13. *Closing off exploration* with questions that can be answered by *yes* or *no:*

Client: I'll never get better.

Nurse: Is something making you feel that way?

Suggested response: "What makes you feel that way?" Use open-ended questions that start with *what, who, when, where,* etc.

14. *Using clichés* or stereotyped expressions:

Client: The doctor took away my weekend pass.

Nurse: The doctor is only doing what's best for you. Doctor knows best. [Comment: also an example of moralizing.]

Suggested response: "Tell me what happened when the doctor took away your weekend pass."

15. *Overloading:* giving too much information at one time:

Nurse: Hello, I'm Mr. Brown. I'm a nurse here. I'll be here today, but I'm off tomorrow. Ms. Anderson will assign you another nurse tomorrow. This unit has five RNs, three LVNs, and students from three nursing schools who will all be taking care of you at some time.

Suggested response: "Hello, I'm Mr. Brown, your nurse today." Keep your initial orienting information simple and brief.

16. *Underloading:* not giving enough information, so that meaning is not clear; withholding information:

Client: What are visiting hours like here?

Nurse: They are flexible and liberal.

Suggested response: "They are flexible and liberal, from 10 A.M. to 12 noon and from 6 to 8 P.M." Use specific terms and give specific information.

17. *Saying no without saying no:*

Client: Can we go for a walk soon?

Nurse: We'll see. Perhaps. Maybe. Later.

Suggested response: "I will check the schedule in the nursing office and let you know within an hour." Vague, ambiguous responses can be seen as "putting the client off." It is best to be clear, specific, and direct.

18. *Using double-bind communication:* sending conflicting messages that do not have "mutual fit," or are incongruent:

Nurse: [Continuing to stay and talk with the client.] It's time for you to rest.

Suggested response: "It's time for you to rest and for me to leave [proceeding to leave]."

19. *Protecting:* defending someone else while talking with client; implying client has no right to personal opinions and feelings:

Client: This hospital is no good. No one cares here.

Nurse: This is an excellent hospital. All the staff were chosen for their warmth and concern for people.

Suggested response: focus on feeling tone or on clarifying information.

20. *Asking "why" questions* implies that the person has immediate conscious aware-

ness of the reasons for his or her feelings and behaviors. Examples of this include: "Why don't you?" "Why did you do that?" or "Why do you feel this way?"

Suggested response: ask clarifying questions using *how, what,* etc.

21. *Coercion:* using the interaction between people to force someone to do *your* will, with the implication that if he or she doesn't "do it for your sake," you won't love or stay with him or her:

Client: I refuse to talk with him.
Nurse: Do it for my sake, before it's too late.

Suggested response: "Something keeps you from wanting to talk with him?"

22. Focusing on *negative* feelings, thoughts, actions:

Client: I can't sleep; I can't eat; I can't think; I can't do anything.
Nurse: How long have you not been sleeping, eating, or thinking well?

Suggested response: "What *do* you do?"

23. *Rejecting* client's behavior or ideas:

Client: Let's talk about incest.
Nurse: Incest is a bad thing to talk about; I don't want to.

Suggested response: "What do you want to say about incest?"

24. *Accusing, belittling:*

Client: I've had to wait five minutes for you to change my dressing.
Nurse: Don't be so demanding. Don't you see that I have several people who need me?

Suggested response: "It must have been hard to wait for me to come when you wanted it to be right away."

25. *Evading a response* by asking a question in return:

Client: I want to know your opinion, nurse. Am I crazy?
Nurse: Do you think you are crazy?

Suggested response: "I don't know. What do you mean by 'crazy'?"

26. *Circumstantiality:* communicating in such a way that the main point is reached only after many side comments, details, and additions:

Client: Will you go out on a date with me?
Nurse: I work every evening. On my day off I usually go out of town. I have a steady boyfriend. Besides that, I am a nurse and you are a client. Thank you for asking me, but no, I will not date you.

Suggested response: abbreviate your response to: "Thank you for asking me, but no, I will not date you."

27. *Making assumptions* without checking them:

Client: [Standing in the kitchen by the sink, peeling onions, with tears in her eyes.]
Nurse: What's making you so sad?
Client: I'm not sad. Peeling onions always makes my eyes water.

Suggested response: use simple acknowledgment and acceptance initially, such as "I notice you have tears in your eyes."

28. *Giving false, premature reassurance:*

Client: I'm scared.
Nurse: Don't worry; everything will be all right. There's nothing to be afraid of.

Suggested response: "I'd like to hear about what you're afraid of, so that together we can see what could be done to help you." Open the way for clarification and exploration, and offer yourself as a helping person—not someone with magic answers.

Anxiety

Anxiety is a subjective warning of danger in which the specific nature of the danger is usually not known. It occurs when a person faces a new, unknown, or untried situation. Anxiety is also felt when a person perceives threat in terms of past experiences. It is a general concept underlying most disease states. In its milder form, anxiety can contribute to learning and is necessary for problem solving. In its severe form, anxiety can impede a client's treatment and recovery. The general feelings elicited on all levels of anxiety are nervousness, tension, and apprehension.

It is essential that nurses recognize their own sources of anxiety and behavior in response to anxiety as well as help clients recognize the manifestations of anxiety in themselves.

◆ **I. Assessment:**

  A. *Physiologic* manifestations:

    1. Increased heart rate and palpitations.
    2. Increased rate and depth of respiration.
    3. Increased urinary frequency and diarrhea.
    4. Dry mouth.
    5. Decreased appetite.
    6. Cold sweat and pale appearance.
    7. Increased menstrual flow.
    8. Increased or decreased body temperature.
    9. Increased or decreased blood pressure.
    10. Dilated pupils.

  B. *Behavioral* manifestations—stages of anxiety:

    1. *Mild anxiety:*
      a. Increased perception (visual and auditory).

Mental Health

b. Increased awareness of meanings and relationships.

c. Increased alertness (notice more).

d. Ability to utilize problem-solving process.

2. *Moderate anxiety:*

a. Selective inattention (e.g., may not hear someone talking).

b. Decreased perceptual field.

c. Concentration on relevant data; "tunnel vision."

d. Muscular tension, perspiration, GI discomfort.

3. *Severe anxiety:*

a. Focus on many fragmented details.

b. Physical and emotional discomfort (headache, nausea, dizziness, dread, horror, trembling).

c. Not aware of total environment.

d. Automatic behavior aimed at getting immediate relief instead of problem solving.

e. Poor recall.

f. Inability to see connections between details.

g. Drastically reduced awareness.

4. *Panic state of anxiety:*

a. Increased speed of scatter; does not notice what goes on.

b. Increased distortion and exaggeration of details.

c. Feeling of terror.

d. Dissociation (hallucinations, loss of reality, and little memory).

e. Inability to cope with any problems; no self-control.

C. *Reactions in response to anxiety:*

1. *Fight:*

a. Aggression.

b. Hostility, derogation, belittling.

c. Anger.

2. *Flight:*

a. Withdrawal.

b. Depression.

3. *Somatization* (psychosomatic disorder).

4. *Impaired cognition:* blocking, forgetfulness, poor concentration, errors in judgment.

5. *Learning* about or searching for causes of anxiety, and identifying behavior.

◆ **II. Analysis/nursing diagnosis:** *Anxiety* related to:

A. *Physical causes:* threats to biologic well-being (e.g., sleep disturbances, interference with sexual functioning, food, drink, pain, fever).

B. *Psychological causes:* disturbance in self-esteem related to:

1. Unmet wishes or expectations.

2. Unmet needs for prestige and status.

3. *Impaired adjustment:* inability to cope with environment.

4. *Altered role performance:* not utilizing own full potential.

5. *Altered meaningfulness:* alienation.

6. *Conflict with social order:* value conflicts.

7. Anticipated disapproval from a significant other.

8. *Altered feeling states: guilt.*

◆ **III. Nursing care plan/implementation:**

A. *Moderate to severe anxiety*

1. Provide *motor outlet* for tension energy, such as working at a simple, concrete task, walking, crying, or talking.

2. Help clients *recognize* their anxieties by talking about how they are behaving and by exploring their underlying feelings.

3. Help the clients *gain insight* into their anxieties by helping them to understand how their behavior has been an expression of anxiety and to recognize the threat that lies behind this anxiety.

4. Help the clients *cope* with the threat behind their anxieties by reevaluating the threats and learning new ways to deal with them.

5. *Health teaching:*

a. Explain and offer hope that emotional pain will decrease with time.

b. Explain that some tension is normal.

c. Explain how to channel emotional energy into activity.

d. Explain need to recognize highly stressful situations and to recognize tension within oneself.

B. *Panic state*

1. Give simple, clear, *concise* directions.

2. *Avoid* decision making by client. Do not try to reason with client, for he or she is irrational and cannot cooperate.

3. *Stay* with client.

a. Do not isolate.

b. *Avoid* touching.

4. Allow client to seek *motor* outlets (walking, pacing).

5. *Health teaching:* advise activity that requires no thought.

◆ **IV. Evaluation/outcome criteria:**

A. Uses more positive thinking and problem-solving activities and is less preoccupied with worrying.

B. Uses values clarification to resolve conflicts and establish realistic goals.

C. Demonstrates regained perspective, self-esteem, and morale; expresses feeling more in control, more hopeful.

D. Fewer or absent physical symptoms of anxiety.

Anxiety Disorders (Anxiety and Phobic Neuroses)

I. Definition: emotional illnesses characterized by *fear* and *autonomic nervous system symptoms* (palpitations, tachycardia, dizziness, tremor); related to *intrapsychic conflict* and psychogenic origin where instinctual impulse (related to sexual-

Mental Health

ity, aggression, or dependence) may be in conflict with the ego, superego, or sociocultural environment; related to sudden object loss.

An *anxiety disorder* is a mild to moderately severe functional disorder of personality in which *repressed* inner conflicts between drives and fears are manifested in behavior patterns, including *generalized anxiety* and *phobic, obsessive-compulsive disorders.* (Other related disorders are *dissociative, conversion,* and *hypochondriasis.*)

II. General concepts and principles related to anxiety disorders:

  A. Behavior may be an attempt to "bind" anxiety: to *fix* it in some particular area (hypochondriasis) or to *displace* it from the rest of personality (phobic, conversion, and dissociative disorders—amnesia, fugue, multiple personalities; obsessive-compulsive disorders).

  B. *Purpose of symptoms:*

    1. To intensify *repression* as a defense.

    2. To exhibit some repressed content in *symbolic* form.

◆ **III. General assessment** of anxiety disorders:

  A. Uses behavior to *avoid* tense situations.

  B. Frightened, suggestible.

  C. Prone to *minor* physical complaints (e.g., fatigue, headaches, and indigestion) and reluctance to admit recovery from physical illnesses.

  D. Attitude of martyrdom.

  E. Often feels helpless, insecure, inferior, inadequate.

  F. Uses *repression, displacement, and symbolism* as key coping mechanisms.

Anxiety Disorders

  I. *Generalized anxiety disorder:*

◆ **A. Assessment:**

    1. Persistent, diffuse, free floating, painful anxiety for at least 1 mo.

    2. Motor tension, autonomic hyperactivity.

    3. Hyperattentiveness expressed through vigilance and scanning.

◆ **B. Analysis/nursing diagnosis:**

    1. *Anxiety: excessive worry* related to threat to security.

    2. *Altered attention* related to overwhelming anxiety.

    3. *Fear* related to sudden object loss.

    4. *Guilt* related to inability to meet role expectations.

    5. *Risk for alteration in self-concept* related to feelings of inadequacy.

    6. *Altered role performance* related to inadequate support system.

    7. *Impaired social interaction* related to use of avoidance in tense situations.

    8. *Distractibility* related to pervasive anxiety.

    9. *Hopelessness* related to feelings of inadequacy.

◆ **C. Nursing care plan/implementation:**

    1. Fulfill needs as promptly as possible.

    2. Listen attentively.

    3. Stay with client.

    4. Avoid decision making and competitive situations.

    5. Promote rest; decrease environmental stimuli.

    6. *Health teaching:* teach steps of anxiety reduction.

◆ **D. Evaluation/outcome criteria:** symptoms are diminished.

  II. *Panic disorder:*

◆ **A. Assessment:**

    1. Three acute, terrifying panic attacks within 3-wk period, *unrelated* to marked physical exertion, life-threatening situation, presence of organic illness, or exposure to specific phobic stimulus.

    2. Discrete periods of apprehension, fearfulness (lasting from few moments to an hour).

    3. *Mimics cardiac* disease: dyspnea, chest pain, smothering or choking sensations, palpitations, tachycardia, dizziness, fainting, sweating.

    4. Feelings of unreality, paresthesias.

    5. Hot, cold flashes and dilated pupils.

    6. Trembling, sense of impending death, fear of becoming insane.

◆ **B. Analysis/nursing diagnosis:**

    1. *Ineffective individual coping* related to undeveloped interpersonal processes.

    2. *Altered comfort pattern:* distress, anxiety, fear related to threat to security.

    3. *Decisional conflict* related to apprehension.

    4. *Altered thought processes* related to impaired concentration.

◆ **C. Nursing care plan/implementation:**

    1. *Reduce immediate anxiety* to more moderate and manageable levels.

     a. Stay *physically close* to reduce feelings of alienation and terror.

     b. *Communication approach:* calm, serene manner; short, simple sentences; firm voice to convey that nurse will provide external controls.

     c. *Physical environment:* remove to smaller room to minimize stimuli.

    2. Provide *motor outlet* for diffuse energy generated at high anxiety levels, e.g., moving furniture, scrubbing floors.

    3. Administer *antianxiety medications* as ordered.

    4. *Health teaching:* recommend more effective methods of coping.

◆ **D. Evaluation/outcome criteria:** can endure anxiety while searching out its causes.

  III. *Obsessive-compulsive disorder:*

◆ **A. Assessment**—chief characteristic: fear that client can harm someone or something.

    1. *Obsessions*—recurrent, persistent, involuntary, senseless *thoughts, images, ideas,*

or desires that may be trivial or morbid, e.g., fear of germs, doubts as to performance of an act, thoughts of hurting family member, death, suicide.

2. *Compulsions*—uncontrollable, persistent urge to perform repetitive, stereotyped *behaviors* that provide relief from unbearable anxiety, e.g., handwashing, counting, touching, checking and rechecking doors to see if locked, elaborate dressing and undressing rituals.

◆ **B. Analysis/nursing diagnosis:**
1. *Ineffective individual coping* related to:
   a. *Intellectualization and avoidance* of awareness of feelings.
   b. Limited ability to express emotions (may be disguised or delayed).
   c. Exaggerated feelings of *dependence and helplessness.*
   d. High need to *control* self, others, and environment.
   e. Rigidity in thinking and behavior.
   f. Poor ability to tolerate anxiety and depression.
2. *Social isolation* related to:
   a. Resentment.
   b. Self-doubt.
   c. Exclusion of pleasure.

◆ **C. Nursing care plan/implementation:**
1. *Accept* rituals permissively (excessive handwashing, e.g.); stopping ritual will increase anxiety.
2. *Avoid* criticism or "punishment," making demands, or showing impatience with client.
3. *Allow* extra time for slowness and client's need for precision.
4. *Protect* from rejection by *others.*
5. *Protect* from *self-inflicted* harmful acts.
6. Engage in nursing therapy *after* the ritual is over, when client is most comfortable.
7. *Redirect* client's actions into substitute outlets.
8. *Health teaching:* teach how to prevent health problems related to rituals, e.g., use rubber gloves, hand lotion.

◆ **D. Evaluation/outcome criteria:** avoids situations that increase tension and thus reduces need for ritualistic behavior as outlet for tension.

IV. *Phobic disorders*—intense, *irrational, persistent* fear in response to *external* object, activity, or situation; e.g., *agoraphobia*—fear of being alone or in public places; *claustrophobia*—fear of closed places; *acrophobia*—fear of heights; *simple phobias* such as *mysophobia*—fear of germs. *Social phobias:* fear of situations that may be humiliating or embarrassing. *Dynamics: displacement* of anxiety from original source onto avoidable, *symbolic,* external, and specific object (or activity or situation); i.e., phobias help person control inten-

sity of anxiety by providing specific object to attach it to, which he or she can then avoid.

◆ **A. Assessment:** same as for anxiety symptoms; fear that someone or something will harm them.

◆ **B. Analysis/nursing diagnosis:** *social isolation;* avoidance; irrational *fear* out of proportion to actual danger; *defensive coping* with high need to control self, others, environment.

◆ **C. Nursing care plan/implementation:** promote psychological and physical calm:
1. *Use systematic desensitization:* never force contact with feared object or situation.
2. *Health teaching:* progressive relaxation, meditation, biofeedback training, or other behavioral conditioning techniques.

◆ **D. Evaluation/outcome criteria:** phobia is eliminated (i.e., able to come into contact with feared object with lessened degree of anxiety).

V. *Acute stress disorder and posttraumatic stress disorder:*

◆ **A. Assessment:**
1. *Acute stress disorder:* symptoms occur *within 1 mo* of extreme stressor.
2. *Posttraumatic stress disorder:* symptoms occur *after* 1 mo.
3. Precipitant: severe traumatic event (natural or man-made disaster) that is not an ordinary occurrence, e.g., rape, fire, flood, earthquake, tornado, bombing, torture, kidnapping.
4. Self-report of reexperiencing incident; intrusive memories.
5. Numb, unresponsive, detached, estranged reaction to external world (unable to feel tenderness, intimacy).
6. Change in sleep pattern (insomnia, recurrent dreams, nightmares), memory loss, hyperalertness (startle response).
7. Guilt rumination about survival.
8. Avoids activities reminiscent of trauma; phobic responses.
9. Difficulty with task completion and concentration.
10. Depression.
11. Increased irritability may result in unpredictable, explosive outbursts.
12. Impulsive behavior, sudden life-style changes.

◆ **B. Analysis/nursing diagnosis:**
1. *Posttrauma response* related to overwhelming traumatic event.
2. *Fear* related to environmental stressor.
3. *Sleep pattern disturbance* related to fear and rumination.
4. *Decisional conflict (impaired decision making)* related to perceived threat to personal values and beliefs.
5. *Guilt* related to lack of social support system.

Mental Health

6. *Altered feeling states:* emotional lability related to diminished sense of control over self and environment.

◆ **C. Nursing care plan/implementation:**
1. Crisis counseling (listen with concern and sympathy).
   a. Ease way for client to *talk out* the experience and express fear.
   b. Help client to become aware and accepting of what happened.
2. *Health teaching:* suggest how to resume concrete activity and reconstruct life with available social, physical, and emotional resources. Help make contact with friends, relatives, and other resources.

◆ **D. Evaluation/outcome criteria:** can cry and express anger, loss, frustration, and despair; begins process of social and physical reconstruction.

Dissociative Disorders (Hysterical Neuroses, Dissociative Type)

◆ **I. Assessment:**
A. *Dissociative amnesia:* partial or total inability to recall the past; occurs during highly stressful events; client may have conscious desire to escape but be unable to accept escape as a solution; uses *repression.*
B. *Dissociative fugue:* client not only forgets but also *flees* from stress.
C. *Dissociative identity disorder:* client exhibits two or more complete personality systems, each very different from the other; alternates from one personality to the other without awareness of change (*one* personality *may* be aware of others); each personality has well-developed emotions and thought processes that are in conflict; uses *repression.*
D. *Depersonalization disorder:* loss of sense of self; feeling of self-estrangement (as if in a dream); fear of going insane.

◆ **II. Analysis/nursing diagnosis:**
A. Sudden *alteration in:*
1. *Memory (short- and long-term memory loss:* can't recall important personal events) related to repression.
2. *Personal and social identity* (amnesia: forgets own identity; becomes another identity) related to intense anxiety.
B. *Confusion* related to use of repression.
C. *Spiritual despair* related to conversion of conflict into physical or mental flights.
D. *Sensory/perceptual alteration* of external environment related to repression and escapism.
E. *Altered meaningfulness* (hopelessness, helplessness, powerlessness) related to lack of control over situation.

◆ **III. Nursing care plan/implementation:**
A. *Remove* client from immediate environment to reduce pressure.

B. *Alleviate* symptoms using behavior-modification strategies.
C. *Divert* attention to topics other than symptoms (not remembering names, addresses, and events).
D. Encourage *socialization* rather than isolation.
E. *Avoid* sympathy, pity, and oversolicitous approach.
F. *Health teaching:* teach families to avoid reinforcing dissociative behavior; teach client problem solving, with goal of minimizing stressful aspects of environment.

◆ **IV. Evaluation/outcome criteria:** recall returns to conscious awareness; anxiety kept within manageable limits.

Somatoform Disorders

I. Main characteristic: involuntary, physical symptoms *without* demonstrable organic findings or identifiable physiologic bases; involve psychological factors or nonspecific conflicts.

◆ **II. General assessment:**
A. *Precipitant:* major emotional, interpersonal stress.
B. Occurrence of secondary gain from illness.

◆ **III. General analysis/nursing diagnosis:**
A. *Fear* related to loss of dependent relationships.
B. *Powerlessness* related to chronic resentment over frustration of dependency needs.
C. *Altered feeling states:* inhibition of anger, which is discharged physiologically and is related to control of anxiety.
D. *Impaired judgment* related to denial of existence of any conflicts or relationship to physical symptoms.
E. *Altered role performance:* regression related to not having dependency needs met.

Somatization Disorder

Repeated, multiple, vague or exaggerated physical complaints of several years' duration *without* identifiable physical cause; clients constantly seek medical attention, undergo numerous tests; at risk for unnecessary surgery or drug abuse.

◆ **A. Assessment:**
1. Onset and occurrence—teen years, more common in women.
2. Reports illness most of life.
   a. *Neuromuscular* symptoms—fainting, seizures, dysphagia, difficulty walking, back pain, urinary retention.
   b. *Gastrointestinal* symptoms—nausea, vomiting, flatus, food intolerance, constipation or diarrhea.
   c. *Female reproductive* symptoms—dysmenorrhea, hyperemesis gravidarum.
   d. *Psychosexual* symptoms—sexual indifference, dyspareunia.
   e. *Cardiopulmonary* symptoms—palpitations, shortness of breath, chest pain.

f. *Rule out:* multiple sclerosis, systemic lupus erythematosus, porphyria, hyperparathyroidism.
3. Appears anxious and depressed.

◆ **B. Analysis/nursing diagnosis:**
1. *Anxiety* related to threat to security and inability to meet role expectations.
2. *Self-care deficit* related to development of physical symptoms to escape stressful situations.
3. *Impaired social interaction* related to inability to accept that physical symptoms lack a physiologic basis.
4. *Body-image disturbance and altered role performance* related to passive acceptance of disabling symptoms.

Conversion Disorder (Hysterical Neuroses, Conversion Type)

Sudden symptoms of *symbolic* nature developed under *extreme* psychological stress (e.g., war, loss, natural disaster) that *disappear* through hypnosis.

◆ **A. Assessment:**
1. *Neurologic* symptoms—paralysis, aphonia, tunnel vision, seizures, blindness, paresthesias, anesthesias.
2. *Endocrinologic* symptoms—pseudocyesis.
3. Hysterical, dependent *personality profile:* exhibitionistic dress and language; self-indulgent; suggestible; impulsive and global impressions and hunches; little capacity to concentrate, integrate, and organize thoughts or plan action or outcomes; little concern for symptoms, despite severe impairment ("La Belle Indifference").

◆ **B. Analysis/nursing diagnosis:**
1. Prolonged *loss or alteration of physiologic processes* related to severe psychological stress and conflict that results in disuse, atrophy, contractures. *Primary gain*—internal conflict or need is kept out of awareness; there is a close relationship in time between stressor and occurrence of symbolic symptoms.
2. *Impaired social interaction:* chronic sick role related to attention seeking.
3. *Noncompliance* with expected routines related to *secondary gain*—avoidance of upsetting situation, with support obtained from others.
4. *Impaired adjustment* related to *repression* of feelings through somatic symptoms, *regression, denial* and *isolation,* and *externalization.*
5. *Ineffective individual coping,* e.g., daydreaming, fantasizing, superficial warmth and seductiveness related to inability to control symptoms voluntarily or to explain them by known physical disorder.

Hypochondriasis (Hypochondriacal Neurosis)

Exaggerated concern for one's physical health; *unrealistic* interpretation of signs or sensations as abnormal; *preoccupation with fear* of having serious disease, *despite* medical reassurance of no diagnosis of physical disorder.

◆ **A. Assessment:**
1. Preoccupation with symptoms; sweating, peristalsis, heartbeat, coughing, muscular soreness, skin eruptions.
2. Occurs in both men and women in adolescence, 30s, or 40s.
3. History of long, complicated shopping for doctors and refusal of mental health care.
4. *Organ neurosis* may occur (e.g., cardiac neurosis).
5. Personality trait: *compulsive.*
6. Prevalence of anxiety and depression.
7. *Controls* relationships through physical complaints.

◆ **B. Analysis/nursing diagnosis:**
1. *Personal identity disturbance* related to perception of self as ill in order to meet needs for dependency, attention, affection.
2. Displaced *anxiety* related to inability to verbalize feelings.
3. *Fear* related to not being believed.
4. *Powerlessness* related to feelings of insecurity.
5. *Altered role performance:* disruption in work and interpersonal relations related to regression and need gratification through preoccupation with fantasized illness; and related to control over others through physical complaints.

◆ **IV. General nursing care plans/implementation** for somatoform disorders:
A. *Long-term goals:*
1. Develop interests *outside* of self. Introduce to new activities and people.
2. Facilitate experiences of increased feelings of *independence.*
3. Increase *reality perception* and *problem-solving ability.*
4. Emphasize *positive* outlook and promote positive thinking. Reassure that symptoms are anxiety related, not a result of physical disease.
5. Develop mature ways for meeting *affection* needs.
B. *Short-term goals:*
1. *Prevent* anxiety from mounting and becoming uncontrollable by recognizing symptoms, for early intervention.
2. *Environment:* warm, caring, supportive interactions; instill hope that anxiety can be mastered.
3. Encourage client to *express* somatic concerns verbally. Encourage awareness of body processes.
4. Provide *diversional* activities.

Mental Health

5. Develop ability to relax rather than ruminate or worry. Help find palliative relief through anxiety reduction (slower breathing, exercise).
   C. *Health teaching:*
      1. Relaxation training as self-help measures.
      2. Increase knowledge of appropriate and correct information on physiologic responses that accompany anxiety.
◆ V. **General evaluation/outcome criteria:**
   A. Does not isolate self.
   B. Discusses fears, concerns, conflicts that are self-originated and not likely to be serious.
   C. Decides which aspects of situation can be overcome and ways to meet conflicting obligations.
   D. Looks for things of importance and value.
   E. Deliberately engages in new activities other than ruminating or worrying.
   F. Talks self out of fears.
   G. Decrease in physical symptoms; is able to sleep, feels less restless.
   H. Makes fewer statements of feeling helpless.
   I. Can freely express angry feelings in *overt* way and not through symptoms.

Other Conditions in Which Psychological Factors Affect Medical Conditions (Psychophysiologic Disorders)

This group of disorders occurs in various organs and systems, whereby emotions are expressed by affecting body organs.

I. **Concepts and principles** related to psychological factors affecting physical conditions:
   A. Majority of organs involved are usually under control of *autonomic* nervous system.
   B. Coping mechanisms
      1. *Repression or suppression* of unpleasant emotional experiences.
      2. *Introjection*—illness seen as punishment.
      3. *Projection*—others blamed for illness.
      4. *Conversion*—physical symptoms rather than underlying emotional stresses are emphasized.
   C. Clients often exhibit the following underlying *needs in excess:*
      1. Dependency.
      2. Attention.
      3. Love.
      4. Success.
      5. Recognition.
      6. Security.
   D. Need to distinguish between:
      1. Factitious disorders—deliberate, *conscious* exhibit of physical or psychological illness to avoid an uncomfortable situation.
      2. *Conversion disorder*—affecting *sensory* systems that are usually under *voluntary* control; generally *non-life-threatening;*

symptoms are symbolic solution to anxiety; *no* demonstrable *organic* pathology.
   3. *Psychological factors affecting physical condition*—e.g., psychophysiologic disorders; under *autonomic* nervous system control; structural *organic* changes; may be life-threatening.
   E. A *decrease in emotional security* tends to produce an *increase in symptoms.*
   F. When treatment is confined to physical symptoms, emotional problems are *not* usually relieved.
◆ II. **Assessment of physiologic factors:**
   A. Persistent psychological factors may produce structural *organic* changes resulting in *chronic diseases,* which may be *life-threatening* if untreated.
   B. *All* body systems are affected:
      1. Skin (pruritus and dermatitis, e.g.).
      2. Musculoskeletal (*backache,* muscle cramps, and rheumatism, e.g.).
      3. Respiratory (*asthma,* hiccups, and hay fever, e.g.).
      4. Gastrointestinal (*ulcers,* ulcerative colitis, irritable colon, heartburn, constipation, and diarrhea, e.g.).
      5. Cardiovascular (paroxysmal tachycardia, *migraines,* palpitations, and hypertension, e.g.).
      6. Genitourinary (dysuria and *dysmenorrhea,* e.g.).
      7. Endocrine (hyperthyroidism, e.g.).
      8. Nervous system (general fatigue, anorexia, and exhaustion, e.g.).
◆ III. **Analysis/nursing diagnosis:** *ineffective individual coping* related to inappropriate need-gratification through illness (actual illness used as means of meeting needs for attention and affection). Absence of life experiences that gratify needs for attention and affection.
◆ IV. **Nursing care plan/implementation** in disorders in which psychological factors affect physical conditions:
   A. *Long-term goal: release* of feelings through verbalization.
   B. *Short-term goals:*
      1. Take care of *physical* problems during acute phase.
      2. *Remove* client from anxiety-producing stimuli.
   C. Prompt attention in meeting clients' *basic needs,* to gratify appropriate needs for dependency, attention, and security.
   D. Maintain an attitude of *respect and concern;* clients' pains and worries are very real and upsetting to them; do not belittle the symptoms. Do not say, "There is nothing wrong with you" because emotions do in fact cause somatic disabilities.
   E. *Treat organic* problems as necessary, but without undue emphasis (i.e., do not reinforce preoccupation with bodily complaints).

F. Help clients *express their feelings,* especially anger, hostility, guilt, resentment, or humiliation, which may be related to such issues as sexual difficulties, family problems, religious conflicts, and job difficulties. Help clients recognize that when stress and anxiety are not released through some channel such as verbal expression, the body will release the tension through *"organ language."*

G. Provide *outlets* for release of tensions and diversions from preoccupation with physical complaints.
   1. Provide social and recreational activities to decrease time for preoccupation with illness.
   2. Encourage clients to use physical and intellectual capabilities in constructive ways.

H. *Protect* clients from any disturbing stimuli; help the healing process in the acute phase of illnesses (myocardial infarct, e.g.).

I. Help clients feel *in control* of situations and be as independent as possible.

J. Be *supportive;* assist clients to bear painful feelings through a helping relationship.

K. *Health teaching:*
   1. Teach how to express feelings.
   2. Teach more effective ways of responding to stressful life situations.
   3. Teach the family supportive relationships.

◆ **V. Evaluation/outcome criteria:** can verbalize feelings more fully.

Schizophrenia and Other Psychotic Disorders

Schizophrenia is a group of interrelated symptoms with a number of common features involving disorders of *mood, thought content, feelings, perception,* and *behavior.* The term means "splitting of the mind," alluding to the discrepancy between the content of *thought processes* and their emotional expression; this should *not* be confused with "multiple personality" (dissociative reaction).

Half of the clients in mental hospitals are diagnosed as schizophrenic; many more schizophrenics live in the community. The onset of symptoms for this disorder generally occurs between 15 and 27 yr of age. Causes, psychodynamics, and psychopathology are still a matter of controversy.

I. Common subtypes of schizophrenia (without clear-cut differentiation):

disorganized type disordered, thinking ("word salad"), *inappropriate affect* (blunted, silly), regressive behavior, incoherent speech, preoccupied and withdrawn,

catatonic type disorder of muscle tension, with rigidity, *waxy flexibility, posturing, mutism, violent rage* outbursts, negativism, and frenzied activity. Marked decrease in involvement with environment and in spontaneous movement.

paranoid type disturbed perceptions leading to disturbance in thought content of *persecutory, grandiose,* or hostile nature; *projection* is key mechanism, with religion a common preoccupation.

residual continued difficulty in thinking, mood, perception, and behavior after schizophrenic episode.

undifferentiated type unclassifiable schizophreniclike disturbance with mixed symptoms of delusions, hallucinations, incoherence, gross disorganization.

II. Concepts and principles related to schizophrenic disorders:

A. *General:*
   1. *Symbolic* language used expresses schizophrenic's life, pain, and progress toward health; all symbols used have meaning.
   2. *Physical care* provides media for relationship; nurturance may be initial focus.
   3. *Consistency, reliability,* and *empathic* understanding build trust.
   4. *Denial, regression,* and *projection* are key defense mechanisms.
   5. Felt anxiety gives rise to distorted thinking.
   6. Attempts to engage in verbal communication may result in tension, apprehensiveness, and defensiveness.
   7. Person *rejects real world* of painful experiences and *creates fantasy* world through illness.

B. *Withdrawal:*
   1. Withdrawal from and resistance to forming relationships are attempts to reduce anxiety related to:
      a. Loss of ability to experience satisfying human relationships.
      b. Fear of rejection.
      c. Lack of self-confidence.
      d. Need for protection and restraint against potential destructiveness of *hostile* impulses (toward self and others).
   2. *Ambivalence* results from need to *approach* a relationship and need to *avoid* it.
      a. Cannot tolerate swift emotional or physical closeness.
      b. Needs more time than usual to establish a relationship; time to test sincerity and interest of nurse.
   3. Avoidance of client by others, especially staff, will reinforce withdrawal, thereby creating problem of mutual withdrawal and fear.

C. *Hallucinations:*
   1. It is possible to replace hallucinations with satisfying interactions.
   2. Person can relearn to focus attention on real things and people.
   3. Hallucinations originate during *extreme* emotional stress when unable to cope.
   4. Hallucinations are very real to client.

5. Client will react as the situation is perceived, *regardless* of reality or consensus.
6. Concrete experiences, *not* argument or confrontation, will correct sensory distortion.
7. Hallucinations are *substitutes* for human relations.
8. Purposes served by or expressed in falsification of reality:
   a. Reflection of problem in inner life.
   b. Statement of criticism, censure, self-punishment.
   c. Promotion of self-esteem.
   d. Satisfaction of instinctual strivings.
   e. Projection of unacceptable unconscious content in disguised form.
9. Perceptions *not* as *totally* disturbed as they seem.
10. Client attempts to restructure reality through hallucinations to *protect remaining ego integrity.*
11. Hallucinations may result from a variety of psychological and biologic conditions (extreme fatigue, drugs, pyrexia, and organic brain disease, e.g.).
12. Hallucinating person needs to feel free to describe his or her perceptions if he or she is to be understood by the nurse.

◆ **III. Assessment** of schizophrenic disorders:
   A. Eugene Bleuler described four classic and *primary symptoms as the "four As":*
   1. *Associative looseness*—impairment of logical thought progression, resulting in confused, bizarre, and abrupt thinking. *Neologisms*—making up new words or condensing words into one.
   2. *Affect*—exaggerated, apathetic, blunt, flat, inappropriate, inconsistent feeling tone that is communicated through face and body posture.
   3. *Ambivalence*—simultaneous, conflicting feelings or attitudes toward person or object.
      a. Stormy outbursts.
      b. Poor, weak interpersonal relations.
   4. *Autism*—*withdrawal* from external world; preoccupation with fantasies and idiosyncratic thoughts.
      a. *Delusions*—false, fixed beliefs, not corrected by logic; a defense against intolerable feeling. The two most common delusions are:
         (1) *Delusions of grandeur*—conviction in a belief related to being famous, important, or wealthy.
         (2) *Delusions of persecution*—belief that one's thoughts, moods, or actions are controlled or influenced by strange forces or by others.
      b. *Hallucinations*—false sensory impressions without observable external stimuli.

         (1) *Auditory*—affecting hearing (e.g., hears voices).
         (2) *Visual*—affecting vision (e.g., sees snakes).
         (3) *Tactile*—affecting touch (e.g., feels electric charges in body).
         (4) *Olfactory*—affecting smell (e.g., smells rotting flesh).
         (5) *Gustatory*—affecting taste (e.g., food tastes like poison).
      c. *Ideas of reference*—clients interpret cues in the environment as having reference to them. Ideas *symbolize guilt, insecurity, and alienation;* may become delusions, if severe.
      d. *Depersonalization*—feelings of strangeness and unreality about self or environment or both; difficulty in differentiating boundaries between self and environment.
   B. *Regression*—extreme *withdrawal* and social isolation.
   C. *Prodromal or residual symptoms:*
   1. Social isolation, *withdrawal.*
   2. Marked impairment in *role* functioning (e.g., as student, employee).
   3. Markedly *peculiar* behavior (e.g., collecting garbage).
   4. Marked impairment in personal *hygiene.*
   5. *Affect:* blunt, inappropriate.
   6. *Speech:* vague, overelaborate, circumstantial, metaphorical.
   7. *Thinking:* bizarre ideation or magical thinking, e.g., ideas of reference, "others can feel my feelings."
   8. Unusual *perceptual* experiences, e.g., sensing the presence of a force or person not physically there.

◆ **IV. Analysis/nursing diagnosis:**
   A. *Sensory/perceptual alterations* related to inability to define reality and distinguish the real from the unreal (hallucinations, illusions) and misinterpretation of stimuli.
   B. *Altered communication process* with inability to *verbally* express needs and wishes related to difficulty with processing information and unique patterns of speech.
   C. *Altered thought processes* related to intense anxiety and blocking (delusions).
   D. *Altered feeling states* related to anxiety about others (*inappropriate emotions*).
   E. *Self-care deficit* with *inappropriate* dress and poor physical hygiene related to perceptual or cognitive impairment.
   F. *Altered judgment* related to lack of trust, fear of rejection, and doubts regarding competence of others.
   G. *Altered self-concept* related to *feelings of inadequacy* in coping with the real world.
   H. *Body-image disturbance* related to inappropriate use of defense mechanisms.

Mental Health

I. *Disorganized behaviors:* impaired relatedness to others, related to withdrawal, distortions of reality, and lack of trust.

J. *Diversional activity deficit* related to personal ambivalence.

◆ **V. Nursing care plan/implementation** in schizophrenic disorders:

A. *General:*

1. Set *short-range* goals, realistic to client's levels of functioning.
2. Use *nonverbal* level of communication to demonstrate concern, caring, and warmth, as client often distrusts words.
3. Set climate for free expression of *feelings* in whatever mode, without fear of retaliation, ridicule, or rejection.
4. Seek client out in his or her own fantasy world.
5. Try to understand meaning of symbolic language; help him or her communicate less symbolically.
6. Provide *distance,* as client needs to feel safe and to observe nurses for sources of threat or promises of security.
7. Help client tolerate nurses' presence and learn to *trust* nurses enough to move out of isolation and share painful and often unacceptable (to client) feelings and thoughts.
8. Anticipate and accept negativism; do *not* personalize.
9. *Avoid* joking, abstract terms, and figures of speech when client's thinking is literal.
10. Give antipsychotic medications.

B. *Withdrawn behavior:*

1. *Long-term goal:* develop satisfying interpersonal relationships.
2. *Short-term goal:* help client feel safe in *one-to-one* relationship.
3. Seek client out at every chance, and establish some bond.
   a. Stay with client, in silence.
   b. Initiate talk when he or she is ready.
   c. Draw out, but do not demand, response.
   d. Do *not* avoid the client.
4. Use *simple language, specific words.*
5. Use an *object or activity* as medium for relationship; initiate activity.
6. Focus on *everyday* experiences.
7. *Delay* decision making.
8. *Accept one-sided* conversation, with silence from the client; *avoid* pressuring to respond.
9. Accept the client's outward attempts to respond and inappropriate social behavior, without remarks or disdain; teach social skills.
10. Avoid making demands on client or exposing client to failure.
11. *Protect* from aggressive persons and from impulsive attacks on self and others.

12. Attend to *nutrition, elimination, exercise,* hygiene, and signs of physical illness.
13. Add structure to the day; tell him or her, "This is your 9 A.M. medication."
14. *Health teaching:* assist family to understand client's needs, to see small sign of progress; teach client to perform simple tasks of self-care to meet own biologic needs.

C. *Hallucinatory behavior:*

1. *Long-term goal:* establish satisfying relationships with *real* persons.
2. *Short-term goal:* interrupt *pattern* of hallucinations.
3. Provide a *structured* environment with routine activities. Use *real* objects to keep client's interest or to stimulate new interest (in painting or crafts, e.g.).
4. *Protect* against injury to self and others resulting from "voices" client thinks he or she hears.
5. *Short, frequent* contacts initially, increasing social interaction gradually (one person → small groups).
6. Ask person to describe experiences as hallucinations occur.
7. *Respond to anything real* the client says, e.g., with acknowledgment or reflection. Focus more on *feelings,* not on delusional, hallucinatory content.
8. *Distract* client's attention to something real when he or she hallucinates.
9. *Avoid* direct confrontation that voices are coming from client himself or herself; do not argue, but listen.
10. *Clarify* who "they" are:
    a. Use personal pronouns, avoid universal and global pronouns.
    b. Nurse's own language needs to be clear and unambiguous.
11. Use one sentence, ask only one question, at a time.
12. Encourage *consensual validation.* Point out that experience is not shared by you; voice doubt.
13. *Health teaching:*
    a. Recommend more effective ways of coping (e.g., consensual validation).
    b. Advise that highly emotional situations be avoided.
    c. Explain the causes of misperceptions.
    d. Recommend methods for reducing sensory stimulation.

D. *Delusions* (see IV. Nursing care plan/implementation in paranoid disorders, p. 362 in following section).

◆ **VI. Evaluation/outcome criteria:**

A. Small behavioral changes occur (e.g., eye contact, better grooming).

B. Evidence of beginning trust in nurse (keeping appointments).

C. Initiates conversation with others; participates in activities.

Mental Health

D. Decreases amount of time spent alone.
E. Demonstrates appropriate behavior in public places.
F. Articulates relationship between feelings of discomfort and autistic behavior.
G. Makes positive statements.

Delusional (Paranoid) Disorders

Paranoid disorders have a concrete and pervasive delusional system, usually *persecutory. Projection* is a chief coping mechanism of this disorder.

I. Concepts and principles related to paranoid disorders:
  A. Delusions are attempts to cope with stresses and problems.
  B. May be a means of allegorical or symbolic communication and of testing others for their trustworthiness.
  C. Interactions with others and activities interrupt delusional thinking.
  D. To establish a rational therapeutic relationship, gross distortions, misorientation, misinterpretation, and misidentification need to be overcome.
  E. Delusional people have extreme need to maintain self-esteem.
  F. False beliefs cannot be changed without first changing experiences.
  G. A delusion is held because it *performs a function.*
  H. When people who are experiencing delusions become at ease and comfortable with people, delusions will not be needed.
  I. Delusions are misjudgments of reality based on a series of mental mechanisms: (a) *denial,* followed by (b) *projection* and (c) *rationalization.*
  J. There is a *kernel of truth* in delusions.
  K. Behind the anger and suspicion in a paranoid, there is a *lonely, terrified* person who *feels vulnerable* and *inadequate.*

◆ **II. Assessment** of paranoid disorders:
  A. Chronically *suspicious,* distrustful (thinks "people are out to get me").
  B. Distant, but *not* withdrawn.
  C. Poor insight; blames others (*projects*).
  D. Misinterprets and *distorts reality.*
  E. Difficulty in admitting own errors; takes pride in intelligence and in being correct (superiority).
  F. Maintains false persecutory belief despite evidence or proof (may refuse food and medicine, insisting they are poisoned).
  G. Literal thinking (*rigid*).
  H. Dominating and provocative.
  I. Hypercritical and intolerant of others; *hostile,* quarrelsome, and aggressive.
  J. *Very sensitive* in perceiving minor injustices, errors, and contradictions.
  K. Evasive.

◆ **III. Analysis/nursing diagnosis:**
  A. *Severe anxiety* related to projection of threatening, aggressive impulses and misinterpretation of stimuli.
  B. *Ineffective individual coping* related to lack of trust, fear of close human contact.
  C. *Impaired cognitive functioning* related to rigidity of thought.
  D. *Chronic low self-esteem* related to feelings of inadequacy.
  E. *Impaired social interaction* related to lack of tender, kind feelings, feelings of grandiosity and/or persecution.
  F. *Altered thought processes* related to lack of insight.

◆ **IV. Nursing care plan/implementation** in paranoid disorders:
  A. *Long-term goals:* gain clear, correct perceptions and interpretations through corrective experiences.
  B. *Short-term goals:*
    1. Help client recognize distortions, misinterpretations.
    2. Help client feel safe in exploring reality.
  C. Help client learn to *trust self;* help to develop self-confidence and ego assets through positive reinforcement.
  D. Help to *trust others.*
    1. Be consistent and honest at all times.
    2. *Do not whisper, act secretive, or laugh with others* in client's presence when he or she cannot hear what is said.
    3. Do not mix medicines with food.
    4. Keep promises.
    5. Let client know ahead of time what he or she can expect from others.
    6. Give *reasons* and careful, complete, and *repetitive* explanations.
    7. Ask permission to contact others.
    8. Consult client first about all decisions concerning him or her.
  E. Help to *test reality.*
    1. Present and repeat reality of the situation.
    2. Do not confirm or approve distortions.
    3. Help accept responsibility for own behavior rather than project.
    4. *Divert* from delusions to reality-centered focus.
    5. Let client know when behavior does not seem appropriate.
    6. Assume nothing and leave no room for assumptions.
    7. *Structure* time and activities to limit delusional thought, behavior.
    8. Set limit for *not* discussing delusional content.
    9. Look for underlying needs expressed in delusional content.
  F. Provide *outlets* for anger and aggressive drives.
    1. Listen matter-of-factly to angry outbursts.

2. *Accept* rebuffs and abusive talk as symptoms.
3. *Do not* argue, disagree, or debate.
4. *Allow* expression of negative feelings without fear of punishment.
G. Provide *successful group experience.*
   1. *Avoid competitive* sports involving *close physical* contact.
   2. Give recognition to skills and work well done.
   3. Utilize *managerial* talents.
   4. Respect client's intellect and engage him or her in activities with others requiring *intellect* (chess, puzzles, and Scrabble, e.g.).
H. *Limit* physical contact.
I. *Health teaching:* teach a more rational basis for deciding whom to trust by identifying behaviors characteristic of trusting and trustworthy people.

◆ **V. Evaluation/outcome criteria:** able to differentiate trustworthy from untrustworthy people; growing self-awareness, and able to share this awareness with others; accepting of others without need to criticize or change them; is open to new experiences; able to delay gratification.

Personality Disorders

Subtypes of personality disorders include *antisocial, histrionic, narcissistic, avoidant,* and *dependent personalities.* A *personality disorder* is a syndrome in which the person's inner difficulties are revealed through general behaviors and by a pattern of living that seeks *immediate gratification of impulses* and instinctual needs without regard to society's laws, mores, and customs and *without censorship* of personal conscience.

Borderline personality disorder is a subtype in which the client is unstable in many areas: she or he has unstable but intense interpersonal relationships, impulsive and unpredictable behavior, wide mood swings, chronic feelings of boredom or emptiness, intolerance of being alone, and uncertainty about identity, and is physically self-damaging.

I. **Concepts and principles** related to *antisocial personality disorders:*
   A. One defense against severe anxiety is "acting out," or dealing with distressful feelings or issues through action.
   B. Faulty or arrested emotional development in preoedipal period has interfered with development of adequate social control or superego.
   C. Since there is a malfunctioning or *weakened superego,* there is little internal demand and therefore no tension between ego and superego to evoke guilt feelings.
   D. The defect is *not* intellectual; person shows *lack of moral responsibility, inability to control emotions* and impulses, and *deficiency in normal feeling* responses.
   E. "Pleasure principle" is dominant.

F. Initial stage of treatment is most crucial; treatment situation is very threatening because it mobilizes client's anxiety, and client ends treatment abruptly. Key underlying emotion: fear of closeness, with threat of exploitation, control, and abandonment.

◆ **II. Assessment** of antisocial personality disorders:
   A. Onset *before* age 15.
   B. History of behavior that *conflicts with society:* truancy, expulsion, or suspension from school for misconduct; delinquency, thefts, vandalism, running away from home; persistent lying; repeated substance abuse; initiating fights; chronic violation of rules at home or school; school grades below IQ level.
   C. Inability to sustain consistent *work* behavior (e.g., frequent job changes or absenteeism).
   D. Lack of ability to function as *responsible* parent (evidence of child's malnutrition or illness due to lack of minimal hygiene standards; failure to obtain medical care for seriously ill child; failure to arrange for caretaker when parent is away from home).
   E. Failure to accept *social norms* with respect to *lawful* behavior (e.g., thefts, multiple arrests).
   F. Inability to maintain enduring *intimate* relationship (e.g., multiple relations, desertion, multiple divorces); lack of respect or loyalty.
   G. *Irritability* and *aggressiveness* (spouse, child abuse; repeated physical fights).
   H. Failure to honor *financial* obligations.
   I. Failure to *plan ahead.*
   J. *Disregard for truth* (lying, "conning" others for personal gain).
   K. *Recklessness* (driving while intoxicated, recurrent speeding).
   L. *Violating* rights of others.
   M. Does not appear to profit from experience; *repeats* same punishable or antisocial behavior; usually does not feel guilt or depression.
   N. Exhibits *poor judgment;* may have intellectual, but not emotional, insight to guide judgments. Inadequate problem solving and reality testing.
   O. Uses *manipulative* behavior patterns in treatment setting (see VIII. Manipulation, pp. 329–331).
      1. Demands and controls.
      2. Pressures and coerces, threatens.
      3. Violates rules, routines, procedures.
      4. Requests special privileges.
      5. Betrays confidences and lies.
      6. Ingratiates.
      7. Monopolizes conversation.

◆ **III. Analysis/nursing diagnosis:**
   A. *Ineffective individual coping* related to:
      1. Inability to tolerate frustration (altered conduct/impulse processes).
      2. Verbal, nonverbal manipulation (*lying*).
      3. Destructive behavior toward self or others.

4. Overuse of denial, projection, rationalization, intellectualization.
5. Inability to learn from experience.

B. *Personal identity disturbance* related to:
1. *Self-esteem disturbance* as evidenced by grandiosity, depression.
2. Lack of responsibility, accountability, commitment.
3. Distancing relationships.

C. *Social intrusiveness* related to fear of real or potential loss.

D. *Noncompliance* related to excess need for independence.

◆ **IV. Nursing care plan/implementation** in personality disorders:

A. *Long-term goal:* help person accept responsibility and consequences of own actions.

B. *Short-term goal: minimize manipulation* and acting out.

C. Set *fair, firm, consistent limits and follow through on consequences* of behavior; let client know what she or he can expect from staff and what the unit's regulations are, as well as the consequences of violations. Be explicit.

D. *Avoid* letting staff be played against one another by a particular client; staff should present a unified approach.

E. Nurses should *control* their *own* feelings of anger and defensiveness aroused by any person's manipulative behavior.

F. Change focus when client persists in raising inappropriate subjects (such as personal life of a nurse).

G. Encourage expression of *feelings* as an alternative to acting out.

H. Aid client in realizing and accepting responsibility for own actions and *social responsibility* to others.

I. Use group therapy as a means of *peer control* and multiple feedback about behavior.

J. *Health teaching:* teach family how to use behavior-modification techniques to reward client's acceptable behavior (i.e., when he or she accepts responsibility for own behavior, is responsive to rights of others, adheres to social and legal norms).

◆ **V. Evaluation/outcome criteria:** less use of lying, blaming others for own behavior; more evidence of following rules; less impulsive, explosive behavior.

Mood Disorders

Mood disorders include (1) *depressive disorders* and (2) *bipolar disorders.* Bipolar disorders are further divided into (a) *manic,* (b) *depressed,* (c) *mixed,* or (d) *cyclothymia.* The mood disturbance may occur in a number of patterns of severity and duration, alone or in combination, where client feels extreme sadness and guilt, withdraws socially, expresses self-deprecatory thoughts *(major depression),* or experiences an elevated, expansive mood with hyperactivity, pressured speech, inflated self-esteem, and decreased need for sleep *(manic episode or disorder).*

Another specific mood disorder is *dysthymic* disorder (depressive neuroses), in which there is a chronic mood disturbance involving a depressed mood or loss of interest and pleasure in all usual activities, but not of sufficient severity or duration to be classified as a *major depressive episode.* Table 6.3 *summarizes* the main points of *difference between the two types of depression.*

These affective disorders should be *distinguished from grief.* Grief is *realistic* and proportionate to what has been *specifically* lost and involves *no loss of self-esteem.* There is a *constant* feeling of sadness over a period of 3–12 mo or longer, with good reality contact (no delusions).

Major Depressive Disorder

I. Concepts and principles:

A. Self-limiting factors—most depressions are self-limiting disturbances, making it important to look for a change in functioning and behavior.

B. *Theories of cause of depression:*
1. Aggression turned inward—*self-anger.*
2. Response to separation or object *loss.*
3. *Genetic* and/or *neurochemical* basis.
4. *Cognitive*—negative mind-set of hopelessness.
5. *Personality*—negative self-concept, low self-esteem affect belief system and appraisal of stressors.
6. *Learned helplessness*—environment can't be controlled.
7. *Behavioral*—loss of positive reinforcement.
8. *Integrated*—interaction of chemical, experiential, and behavioral variables acting on diencephalon.

◆ **II. General assessment:**

A. *Physical:* early-morning awakening, *insomnia* at night, increased need for sleep during the day, fatigue, constipation, *anorexia* with weight loss, loss of sexual interest, *psychomotor retardation,* physical complaints, amenorrhea.

B. *Psychological:* inability to remember, decreased *concentration,* slowing or blocking of thought, all-or-nothing thinking, *less interest* and involvement with external world and own appearance, feeling worse at certain times of day or after any sleep, difficulty in enjoying activities, monotonous voice, *repetitive* discussions, *inability to make decisions* due to ambivalence, impaired coping with "practical problems."

C. *Emotional:* loss of self-esteem, feelings of *hopelessness* and *worthlessness,* shame and self-derogation due to *guilt, irritability,* despair and *futility* (leading to *suicidal* thoughts), alienation, *helplessness,* passivity, avoidance, *inertia,* powerlessness, denied an-

■ **TABLE 6.3   Comparison of the Two Different Types of Depressive Disorders**

Dimension	Major Depressive Disorder	Dysthymic Disorder
Cause	Primary disturbance in structure and function of brain and nervous system	Severe, prolonged stress, unresolved conflicts; chronic anxiety, fears, anger
Onset	Rapid and without apparent cause	Gradual
Form of depression	Restlessness and agitation, *or* psychomotor retardation; severe; tends to be worse in morning and better in evening	Mixed; mild to severe; unpredictable mood; usually optimistic in morning and depressed in evening
Sleep	Insomnia after being awakened	Easily awakened, but goes back to deep sleep in morning
Appetite	Anorexia leading to weight loss	Varied (anorexia leading to compulsive eating)
Activity	Chronically tired; needs structure at all times	Occasional energy bursts (feels embarrassed at lack of energy)
Self-esteem	Very low	Fluctuates from high to low
Fears	Intense fear of being alone	Multiple fears about present and future
Decision making	Totally indecisive	OK on minor decisions; indecisive on important decisions
Memory	Poor	Unreliable
Contact with reality	Poor; paranoid, self-deprecatory delusions, distorted judgment	Varies

ger; uncooperative, tense, crying, demanding, and *dependent* behavior.

◆ **III. Analysis/nursing diagnosis:**

   A. *Altered nutrition* (anorexia) related to lack of interest in food.

   B. *Risk for violence* toward self (suicide) related to inability to verbalize emotions.

   C. *Sleep pattern disturbance* (insomnia or excessive sleep) related to emotional dysfunctioning.

   D. *Self-care deficit* related to disinterest in activities of daily living.

   E. *Chronic low self-esteem* with self-reproaches and blame related to feelings of inadequacy.

   F. *Altered feeling states and meaning patterns* (sadness, loneliness, apathy) related to overwhelming feeling of unworthiness and dysfunctional grieving.

   G. *Altered social interaction* related to social isolation/withdrawal.

◆ **IV. Nursing care plan/implementation:**

   A. Promote sleep and food intake: take nursing measures to ensure the *physical* well-being of the client.

   B. Provide steady company to assess *suicidal* tendencies and to diminish feelings of loneliness and alienation.

      1. Build trust in a one-to-one relationship.

      2. Interact with client on a nonverbal level if that is his or her immediate mode of communication; this will promote feelings of being recognized, accepted, and understood.

      3. Focus on *today,* not the past or far into the future.

   4. Reassure that present state is temporary and that he or she will be protected and helped.

   C. Make the *environment* nonchallenging and nonthreatening.

      1. Use a kind, firm attitude, with warmth.

      2. See that client has favorite foods; respond to other wishes and likes.

      3. Protect from overstimulation and coercion.

   D. Postpone client's *decision making* and resumption of duties.

      1. Allow *more time* than usual to complete activity (dressing, eating) or thought process and speech.

      2. Structure the environment for client to help reestablish a set schedule and predictable *routine* during ambivalence and problems with decisions.

   E. *Provide nonintellectual activities* (for instance, sanding wood): avoid chess and crossword puzzles, e.g., as thinking capacity at this time tends to be circular.

   F. Encourage expression of emotions, denial, hopelessness, helplessness, guilt, regret; provide *outlets for anger* that may be underlying the depression; as client becomes more verbal with anger and recognizes the origin and results of anger, help client resolve feelings—allow client to complain and be *demanding* in initial phases of depression.

   G. Discourage *redundancy in speech and thought:* redirect focus from a monologue of painful recounts to an appraisal of more neutral or positive attributes and aspects of situations.

H. Encourage client to *assess own* goals, unrealistic expectations, and perfectionist tendencies.
1. May need to change goals or give up some goals that are incompatible with abilities and external situations.
2. Assist client to recapture what was lost through substitution of goals, sublimation, or relinquishment of unrealistic goals—reanchor client's self-respect to other aspects of his or her existence; help him or her free self from *dependency* on one person or single event or idea.

I. Indicate that success is possible and not hopeless.
1. Explore what steps client has taken to achieve goals and suggest new or alternate ones.
2. Set *small, immediate goals* to help attain mastery.
3. Recognize client's efforts to mobilize self.
4. Provide positive reinforcement for client through exposure to activities in which client can experience a sense of *success, achievement, and completion* to build *self-esteem* and self-confidence.
5. Help client experience *pleasure;* help client start good relationships in social setting.

J. *Long-term goal:* to encourage interest in external surroundings, outside of self, to increase and strengthen social relationships.
1. Encourage purposeful activities.
2. Let client advance to activities at own pace (graded task assignments).
3. Gradually encourage activities with others.

K. *Health teaching:* explain need to recognize highly stressful situation and fatigue as stress factor; advise that negative responses from others be regarded with minimum significance; explain need to maintain positive self-attitude; advise occasional respite from responsibilities; emphasize need for realistic expectation of others.

◆ **V. Evaluation/outcome criteria:** performs self-care; expresses increased self-confidence; engages in activities with others; accepts positive statements from others; identifies positive attributes and skills in self.

Bipolar Disorders

Bipolar disorders are major emotional illnesses characterized by mood swings, alternating from depression to elation, with periods of relative normality between episodes. Most persons experience a *single* episode of manic or depressed type; some have *recurrent* depression or recurrent mania or *mixed.* There is increasing evidence that a biochemical disturbance may exist and that most individuals with manic episodes eventually develop depressive episodes.

I. Concepts and principles related to bipolar disorders:
A. The psychodynamics of manic and depressive episodes are related to hostility and guilt.
B. The struggle between unconscious impulses and moral conscience produces feelings of *hostility, guilt,* and *anxiety.*
C. To relieve the internal discomfort of these reactions, the person *projects* long-retained hostile feelings onto others or onto objects in the environment during *manic* phase; during *depressive* phase, hostility and guilt are *introjected* toward self.
D. Demands, irritability, sarcasm, profanity, destructiveness, and threats are signs of the *projection of hostility;* guilt is handled through *persecutory delusions and accusations.*
E. Feelings of inferiority and fear of rejection are handled by being light and amusing.
F. Both phases, though appearing distinctly different, have the *same objective: to gain attention, approval, and emotional support.* These objectives and behaviors are unconsciously determined by the client; this behavior may be either biochemically determined or *both* biochemically and unconsciously determined.

◆ **II. Assessment** of bipolar disorders:
A. Manic and depressed types are *opposite* sides of the *same* disorder.
1. Both are disturbances of mood and self-esteem.
2. Both have underlying aggression and hostility.
3. Both are intense.
4. Both are self-limited in duration.
B. Comparison of behaviors associated with mania and depression: see Table 6.4.

◆ **III. Analysis/nursing diagnosis:**
A. *Risk for injury* related to poor judgment.
B. *Altered nutrition, less than body requirements,* related to inability to sit down long enough to eat.
C. *Sleep pattern disturbance:* lack of sleep and rest related to restlessness, hyperactivity, emotional dysfunctioning.
D. *Self-care deficits* related to altered motor behavior due to anxiety.
E. *Altered feeling state* (anger), *judgment, thought content* (magical thinking), *thought processes* (altered concentration and problem solving) related to disturbance in self-concept.
F. *Altered feeling processes* (mood swings).
G. *Altered attention:* hyperalertness.
H. *Impaired social interaction* related to internal and external stimuli (overload, underload).

◆ **IV. Nursing care plan/implementation:**
A. *Manic:*
1. Prevent *physical* dangers stemming from suicide and exhaustion—promote rest, sleep, and intake of nourishment.
   a. Use *suicide* precautions.

■ **TABLE 6.4   Behaviors Associated with Mania and Depression**

Mania (Periods of Predominantly and Persistently Elevated, Expansive, or Irritable Mood)	Depression (Loss of Interest or Pleasure in Usual Activities)
Affect Lack of shame or guilt; inflated self-esteem; euphoria; intolerance of criticism	Anger, anxiety, apathy, denial, delusions of guilt, helplessness, feelings of doom, hopelessness, loneliness, low self-esteem (self-degradation)
Physiology Insomnia; inadequate nutrition, weight loss	Insomnia; anorexia, constipation, indigestion, nausea, vomiting → weight loss
Cognition Denial of realistic danger *Thoughts:* flight of ideas, loose associations; illusions, delusions of grandeur; lack of judgment; distractibility	Ambivalence, confusion, inability to concentrate, self-blame; loss of interest and motivation; self-destructive (preoccupied with suicide)
Behavior Hyperactivity (social, sexual, work) → irrationality, aggressiveness, sarcasm, exhibitionism, and acting out in behavior and dress Hostile, arrogant, argumentative, demanding, and controlling *Speech:* rapid, rhyming, punning, witty, pressured	Altered activity level, social isolation, substance abuse, overdependency, underachievement, inability to care for self, *psychomotor retardation*

b. Reduce outside stimuli or remove to quieter area.
c. *Diet:* provide *high-calorie beverages, finger* foods within sight and reach.
2. Attend to client's personal care.
3. Absorb with understanding and without reproach behaviors such as talkativeness, provocativeness, criticism, sarcasm, dominance, profanity, and dramatic actions.
    a. Allow, postpone, or partially fulfill demands and freedom of expression *within limits* of ordinary social rules, comfort, and safety of client and others.
    b. *Do not* cut off manic stream of talk, as this increases anxiety and need for release of hostility.
4. Constructively utilize excessive energies with *activities* that do *not* call for concentration or follow-through.
    a. Outdoor walks, gardening, putting, and ball tossing are therapeutic.
    b. Exciting, disturbing, and highly *competitive* activities should be *avoided*.
    c. Creative occupational therapy activities promote release of hostile impulses, as does creative writing.
5. Give tranquilizers as ordered until lithium affects symptoms (*3 wk*); then give lithium carbonate as ordered.
6. Help client to recognize and express *feelings* (denial, hopelessness, anger, guilt, blame, helplessness).
7. Encourage realistic self-concept.
8. *Health teaching:* how to monitor effects of lithium; instructions regarding salt intake.
B. *Depressed:*
1. Take routine *suicide* precautions.

2. Give attention to *physical* needs for food and sleep and to hygiene needs. Prepare warm baths and hot beverages to aid sleep.
3. Initiate *frequent* contacts:
    a. *Do not allow long periods of silence* to develop or client to remain withdrawn.
    b. Use a kind, understanding, but emotionally neutral approach.
4. *Allow dependency* in severe depressive phase. Since dependency is one of the underlying concerns with depressive persons, if nurse allows dependency to occur as an initial response, he or she must plan for resolution of the dependency toward himself or herself as an example for the client's other dependent relationships.
5. Slowly repeat simple, direct information.
6. *Assist in daily decision making* until client regains self-confidence.
7. Select *mild* exercise and diversionary *activities* instead of stimulating exercise and competitive games, as they may overtax physical and emotional endurance and lead to feelings of inadequacy and frustration.
8. Give antidepressive drugs.
9. *Health teaching:* how to make simple decisions related to health care.
◆ **V. Evaluation/outcome criteria:**
    A. *Manic:* speech and activity are slowed down; affect is less hostile; able to sleep; able to eat with others at the table.
    B. *Depressed:* takes prescribed medications regularly. Does not engage in self-destructive activities. Able to express feelings of anger, helplessness, hopelessness.

Mental Health

❏ Questions

Select the one best answer for each question.

1. A patient is in a withdrawn catatonic state and exhibits waxy flexibility. During the initial phase of hospitalization for this patient, the nurse's first priority is to:
   1. Watch for edema and cyanosis of the extremities.
   2. Encourage the patient to discuss concerns that led to the catatonic state.
   3. Provide a warm, nurturing relationship, with therapeutic use of touch.
   4. Identify the predisposing factors in the illness.

2. An elderly client who has dementia related to cerebral arteriosclerosis says to the nurse, "I'm going to the university today to be their guest lecturer on aerodynamics." Which response by the nurse would be most therapeutic?
   1. "Do you know that you are in the hospital now?"
   2. "Are you saying that you would like to be asked to give a lecture at the university?"
   3. "How about watching a movie on television instead?"
   4. "It's more important that you don't tire yourself out."

3. Which nursing approach would be best for a client with symptoms of severe depression?
   1. Allow the client time for quiet thought; remain silent.
   2. Ask the client to join the nurse and the other clients in the TV lounge.
   3. State that the nurse would like to go with the client for a short walk around the outside grounds, and assist the client with his or her coat.
   4. Give the client a choice of recreational activities.

4. When assessing clients who are exhibiting a depressed episode and those who are exhibiting a manic episode of bipolar mood disorders, which characteristic common to both episodes of the disorder is the nurse likely to note?
   1. Suicidal tendency.
   2. Underlying hostility.
   3. Delusions.
   4. Flight of ideas.

5. A patient who is overweight is referred by the physician to the nurse for diet counseling. What action would the nurse take?
   1. Develop a weight control plan, together with the patient, that will allow gradual weight loss.
   2. Ask the patient to describe his or her eating patterns.
   3. Support the patient's interests in other activities.
   4. Put the patient on a diet with very limited number of calories so he or she will have an immediate weight loss.

6. A patient begins having auditory hallucinations. When the nurse approaches, the patient whispers, "Did you hear that terrible man? He is scary!" Which would be the best response for the nurse to make initially?
   1. "What is he saying?"
   2. "I didn't hear anything. What scary things is he saying?"
   3. "Who is he? Do you know him?"
   4. "I didn't hear a man's voice, but you look scared."

7. After seeing a number of doctors for nonspecific complaints of chest pains, with no conclusive findings of organic disease, a client is referred to a local mental health center. The client has read extensively about coronary disease and talks continuously about the symptoms in great detail. Which approach by the nurse would be best when meeting this client for the first time?
   1. Allow the client to describe the physical problems to become familiar with them.
   2. Comment on a neutral topic instead of using the usual conversation opener of "How are you today?"
   3. Give the client a simple but direct explanation of the physiologic basis for the symptoms.
   4. Let the client know that the nurse is familiar with the psychogenic problems and guide the discussion to other areas.

8. A 35-year-old married clerk had surgery for ulcerative colitis 3 days ago. The physical symptoms have abated, but he continues to complain angrily and to be demanding of the nursing staff. He makes numerous requests, such as to open or close the windows and to bring him fresh water. The nurse needs to understand that this behavior might be saying:
   1. "You aren't doing your job."
   2. "I am alone and helpless and need to depend on you to take care of me when I need you."
   3. "Everyone needs attention."
   4. "I'm going to get even with you for thinking I'm a crank by making you work."

9. The nurse is aware that the main function confabulation serves in clients, especially those with dementia, is to:
   1. Impress others.
   2. Protect their self-esteem.
   3. Control others by distance maneuvers.
   4. Maintain a sense of humor.

10. A 19-year-old patient is brought to the emergency room because she slashed her wrists. What is the nurse's first concern?
    1. Stabilization of physical condition.
    2. Determination of antecedent, causal factors relevant to the wrist slashing.
    3. Reduction of anxiety.
    4. Obtaining a detailed nursing history.

11. An agitated patient begins to shout insults and threats at others, and starts demolishing the recreation room. What is the best response or action by the nurse?
    1. Firmly set limits on the behavior.
    2. Allow the patient to continue, since the patient is seeking to express herself or himself.
    3. Tell the patient he or she is trying to intimidate other clients.
    4. Let the patient know that he or she doesn't need to express anger at the nurse by demolishing the recreation room.

12. A second-grade girl starts at a new school, and the child's grades suffer while focusing on adjusting to new peers. The father severely reprimands the child and forces the child to study after school rather than play with other children. These data indicate to the nurse that this child is deprived of forming which normal phase of development?
    1. A love relationship with the father.
    2. Close relationships with peers.
    3. Heterosexual relationships.
    4. A dependency relationship with the father.

13. The nurse is interviewing a teenage patient with acting-out behaviors. The teenager complains that no one will let him "do his own thing," and sits glaring at the nurse. What is the nurse's best response?

1. "I know you are angry, but how does being angry help?"
2. "Stop being angry and tell me what is wrong."
3. "I think you are angry because you feel you don't need any help."
4. "We have to meet because your parents are concerned about you."

14. A patient looks at a mirror and cries out, "I look like a bird. My face is no longer me." Which would be the best response by the nurse?
    1. "Which bird?"
    2. "That must be a distressing experience; your face doesn't look different to me."
    3. "Maybe it was the light at that particular time. Would you like to use another mirror?"
    4. "What makes you think that your face looks like a bird?"

15. A patient with ulcerative colitis and the patient's family are ready to make discharge plans jointly with the staff. Which assessment will have the greatest bearing on the patient's rehabilitation course?
    1. The amount of emotional support the family gives the patient.
    2. The spouse's interest in, and ability to take care of the postoperative dietary needs.
    3. The family expectations of the patient to resume his or her role in the home.
    4. The spouse's understanding that the course of the illness may have exacerbations and remissions.

16. A 10-year-old child diagnosed with acute leukemia, terminal stage, asks the nurse one morning: "I am going to die, aren't I?" What would be the most appropriate response by the nurse?
    1. "No, you're not. You are getting the latest treatment available and you have a very good doctor. Your white count was better yesterday."
    2. "We are all going to die sometime."
    3. "What did the doctor tell you?"
    4. "I don't know. You have a serious illness. Do you have feelings that you want to talk about now?"

17. For a patient with a diagnosis of a somatoform disorder, which would be the appropriate initial nursing goal?
    1. Help the patient learn how to live with the functional organic disturbance without using the symptoms to control others.
    2. Assist the patient in developing new and varied interests outside of himself or herself at which he or she can be successful.
    3. Accept the patient as a person who is sick and needs help.
    4. Help the patient see how he or she uses the illness to avoid looking at or dealing with problems.

18. An acutely ill patient hospitalized with metastatic lung carcinoma begs for a pass to attend her son's high school graduation in a city 100 miles from the hospital. "If only I could do this one thing, then I'll be ready to die," the patient says. The nurse identifies this behavior as an example of:
    1. Being unrealistic and denying the degree of illness.
    2. Using bargaining as a reaction to death and dying.
    3. Being manipulative to get the patient's way.
    4. Being unaware of the diagnosis.

19. A patient who is overweight says to the nurse, "My therapist told me I eat because I didn't get enough love from my mother. What does the therapist mean?" What is the best response for the nurse to offer?
    1. "Tell me what you think the therapist means."

2. "We are here to deal with your diet, not with your psychological problems."
3. "You need to ask your therapist."
4. "What do you think is the connection between your not getting enough love and your overeating?"

20. An elderly patient who is hard of hearing repeats, over and over again, the same story of the patient's family coming "out West" in a covered wagon. Which interpretation by the nurse would not demonstrate understanding of this behavior?
    1. The patient has better recall for past events than for recent ones.
    2. The patient enjoys reliving the pleasurable aspects of life, since the present and future are bleak.
    3. Repeating stories is one way of interacting, to compensate for a two-way conversation that is difficult for the patient to sustain.
    4. The patient wants to impress others.

21. A nursing care plan for a hospitalized hyperactive client in a manic episode needs to include:
    1. Involvement in a group activity and encouragement to talk.
    2. Attention to adequate food and fluid intake.
    3. Protection against suicide.
    4. Permissive acceptance of bizarre behavior.

22. The nurse finds an elderly patient with Alzheimer's in the hallway at 4:00 A.M., trying to open the door to the fire escape. Which response by the nurse would probably indicate the most accurate assessment of the situation?
    1. "You look confused. Would you like to sit down and talk with me?"
    2. "That door leads to the fire escape. Why do you want to go outside now?"
    3. "This is the fire escape door. Are you looking for the bathroom?"
    4. "Something seems to be bothering you. Let's go back to your room and talk about it."

23. Since the death of her baby, a woman has lost weight, will not eat, spends most of her time immobile, and speaks only in monosyllabic responses. She pays little attention to her appearance. One afternoon, this patient comes to lunch with her hair combed and traces of lipstick. What could the nurse say to reinforce this change of behavior?
    1. "What happened? You combed your hair!"
    2. "This is the first time I've seen you look so good."
    3. "You must be feeling better. You look much better."
    4. "I see that your hair is combed and you have lipstick on."

24. While the nurse is interviewing a teenage patient, the patient says, "I suppose you have to tell my parents everything." What would be the best response by the nurse?
    1. "What are you going to tell me that is so secret that I can't tell your parents?"
    2. "If you tell me you are going to do something to hurt yourself I will have to tell your parents, but I will tell you first before I tell them."
    3. "Everything you tell me is confidential. I will not tell your parents anything."
    4. "Everything you tell me I will need to tell your parents. They have a right to know."

25. In paranoid disorder, the part of the personality that is weak is called the:
    1. Id.
    2. Ego.
    3. Superego.
    4. "Not me."

26. A key consideration in planning the general care of clients with dementia is that:
    1. They be protected from suicide attempts.
    2. Their capacity for physical activity is diminished.
    3. Team effort be aimed at increasing their independence.
    4. The staff be sympathetic when clients mention their failing abilities.

27. A college student was doing exceptionally well and was complimented by her chemistry professor, who arranged for her to become his lab assistant and to do advanced research. Although very thorough in her work, when given constructive criticism this student becomes angry and stalks out of the lab for a few hours. The most plausible theoretical explanation is that the student:
    1. Knows she is right.
    2. Thinks the professor is jealous of her.
    3. Needs to feel and know that she is perfect.
    4. Feels anxiety as a result of a threat to her security and self-image.

28. One therapeutic nursing attitude is to be accepting and permissive. To convey this attitude most therapeutically, the nurse might:
    1. Wait for a client to initiate contact.
    2. Let the client make decisions.
    3. Ignore undesirable behavior.
    4. Meet the client at his or her level of functioning.

29. The basic goal of nursing in a mental health setting is to:
    1. Plan activity programs for clients.
    2. Maintain a therapeutic environment.
    3. Understand various types of family therapy and psychological tests and how to interpret them.
    4. Advance the science of psychiatry by initiating research and gathering data for current statistics on emotional illness.

30. Which nursing intervention is inappropriate with a person who is expressing anger?
    1. Stating observations of the expressed anger.
    2. Assisting the person to describe the feelings.
    3. Helping the person find out what preceded the anger.
    4. Helping the person refrain from expressing anger verbally.

31. The client tells the nurse about the client's parents' impending divorce. The client said, "I couldn't believe that he was going to leave us for someone else." Which would be best for the nurse to reply?
    1. "Was your mother expecting this to happen?"
    2. "Yes, go on."
    3. "Did you cry?"
    4. "I can understand how you must feel."

32. A crisis intervention nurse meets with a young patient who was admitted after attempting suicide by slashing the wrists. The nurse's initial goal at this time is to:
    1. Determine the precipitating event, determine how many people are involved in the incident, and determine how angry the patient is.
    2. Determine if the patient has an immediate support system, determine what the people in the support system think of the patient cutting the wrists, and determine how angry the patient is.
    3. Determine the precipitating event, determine if the patient has an immediate support system, and assess the likelihood of immediate recurrence of the suicidal act.

4. Assess the likelihood of immediate recurrence of the suicidal act.

33. A client states, "the nofas are coming." In response to this neologism, it would be best for the nurse to:
    1. Divert the client's attention to an aspect of reality.
    2. State that what the client is saying has not been understood and then divert attention to something that is reality bound.
    3. Acknowledge that the word has some special meaning for the client.
    4. Try to interpret what the client means.

34. Which nursing approach is important in depression?
    1. Providing motor outlets for aggressive, hostile feelings.
    2. Protecting against harm to others.
    3. Reducing interpersonal contacts.
    4. Deemphasizing preoccupation with elimination, nourishment, and sleep.

35. One evening the nurse sees a client in the dayroom without any clothes, shouting vulgarities and dancing wildly about the room while other clients are watching TV. The best initial response by the nurse at this time would be:
    1. "Let's sit down with the others and watch TV; I'll put this blanket over you to keep you warm."
    2. "We do not allow this behavior in the hospital. It is embarrassing the other clients."
    3. "Please put your clothes on."
    4. "Come put your clothes on. I will help you."

36. The nurse discovers a client crouched in a corner, looking pale and frightened, and holding a gushing wrist wound. A razor is nearby on the floor. What should the nurse do first?
    1. Sit down on the floor, next to the client, and in a quiet, reassuring tone, say, "You seem frightened. Can I help?"
    2. Ask the aide to watch the client and run to get the doctor.
    3. Apply pressure on the wrist, saying to the client, "You are hurt. I will help you."
    4. Go back down the hall to get the emergency cart.

37. Which characteristic should the nurse recognize as common in a person engaged in gradual self-destructive behavior (such as in obesity, drug addiction, and smoking)?
    1. Acceptance of the death wish.
    2. Denial of possibility of death.
    3. Ability to control own behavior.
    4. Ignorance of the consequences of own behavior.

38. A divorced woman learns that her ex-husband has died. Her reaction is stunned silence, followed by anger that he left no insurance money for their young children. The nurse should understand that:
    1. The woman is experiencing a normal bereavement reaction.
    2. To explain the woman's reaction, the nurse needs more information about the relationship and breakup.
    3. The children and the injustice done to them by their father's death are the woman's main concern.
    4. The woman is not reacting normally to the news.

39. What will the nurse most commonly note in the clinical picture of dementia?
    1. Memory loss for events in the distant past.
    2. Quarrelsome behavior directly related to the extent of lack of blood supply to the brain.
    3. Increased resistance to change.

4. Insight into one's situation, its probable causes, and its logical consequences.

40. A man is hospitalized following a car accident in which his wife died, and is unable to attend the funeral due to his severe chest injuries. What would the nurse consider in forecasting this surviving spouse's potential for difficulty with grief resolution?
    1. Feelings of anger toward the hospital staff for keeping him hospitalized during the funeral.
    2. Feelings of anger toward himself for having been injured but not killed in the accident.
    3. His inability to participate in the cultural rituals of grief, wherein the reality of his wife's death is emphasized.
    4. His preoccupation with his own physical distress at this time.

41. A patient who is depressed says, "I don't cry because my wife can't bear it." The nurse needs to be aware that this is an example of:
    1. Suppression.
    2. Undoing.
    3. Repression.
    4. Rationalization.

42. When interacting with clients who have autistic thinking and speaking patterns, what is likely to pose the *greatest difficulty* for the nurse?
    1. Showing acceptance for their incomprehensible acts and verbalizations.
    2. Ignoring their bizarre behavior.
    3. Speaking in a way that clients can understand.
    4. Determining which of the clients' needs are being met by their autistic expressions.

43. A patient refuses to eat meals in the hospital, stating that the food is poisoned. The nurse is aware that the patient is expressing an example of:
    1. Hallucination.
    2. Illusion.
    3. Delusion.
    4. Negativism.

44. An adolescent has a history of truancy from school, running away from home, and "borrowing" other people's things without their permission. The adolescent denies stealing, rationalizing instead that as long as no one was using the items, it was all right to borrow them. It is important for the nurse to understand that psychodynamically, this behavior may be largely attributed to a developmental defect related to the:
    1. Id.
    2. Ego.
    3. Superego.
    4. Oedipal complex.

45. What is the nurse likely to note in a patient being admitted for alcohol withdrawal?
    1. Perceptual disorders.
    2. Impending coma.
    3. Recent alcohol intake.
    4. Depression with mutism.

46. A patient says he must wash his hands from 9:00 to 9:45 A.M. each day and therefore cannot attend 9:00 A.M. group therapy sessions. Which concept does the nursing staff need to keep in mind in planning nursing interventions for this patient?
    1. Fears and tensions are often expressed in disguised form through symbolic processes.
    2. Unmet needs are discharged through ritualistic behavior.
    3. Ritualistic behavior makes others uncomfortable.
    4. Depression underlies ritualistic behavior.

47. To formulate an effective care plan for a client with a somatoform disorder, the nurse needs to have an understanding of which related psychodynamic principle?
    1. The major fundamental mechanism is regression.
    2. An extensive, prolonged study of the symptoms will be reassuring to the client, who seeks sympathy, attention, and love.
    3. The symptoms of a somatoform disorder are an attempt to adjust to painful life situations or to cope with conflicting sexual, aggressive, or dependent feelings.
    4. The client's symptoms are imaginary and the suffering is faked.

48. In evaluating a patient who has somatoform symptoms, the nurse is aware that the patient will probably show the most improvement when he or she:
    1. Accepts the fact that the physical symptoms have an emotional component.
    2. Finds more satisfying ways of expressing feelings through verbalization.
    3. Becomes involved in group activities and focuses less on the symptoms.
    4. Understands that the current way of reacting to stress is not healthy.

49. An important part of the nursing care for a client with dementia would be:
    1. Minimizing regression.
    2. Correcting memory loss.
    3. Rehabilitating toward independent functioning.
    4. Preventing further deterioration.

50. In explaining the goal of therapy in crisis intervention to a new colleague, the nurse states that the goal is to:
    1. Restructure the personality.
    2. Remove specific symptoms.
    3. Remove anxiety.
    4. Resolve immediate problems.

51. The steps in therapeutic nursing intervention with an angry client would be to describe the situation, then:
    1. Discuss alternative solutions, decide on several, try them out, and evaluate their effectiveness.
    2. Focus on one solution, try it out, and evaluate its effectiveness.
    3. Outline to the client exactly what to do about the anger.
    4. Discuss alternative solutions, decide on one, use it, evaluate its effectiveness, and continue repeating the process until the client is satisfied.

52. On a routine physical, a woman learns she has a lump in her breast. It is found to be malignant, and a modified mastectomy is performed. Immediately following the surgery, what behaviors could the nurse expect this patient to display?
    1. Signs of grief reaction.
    2. Signs of deep depression.
    3. Relief that the operation is over.
    4. Denial of the possibility of carcinoma.

53. A 19-year-old patient's overcompliance with his parents' expectations for his behavior could result in:
    1. Lack of development of a separate identity.
    2. Confusion of his sex role.
    3. Successful development of a separate identity.
    4. Identification of a weak superego.

54. A doctor asks the nurse to activate a patient who hears voices and is withdrawn and negativistic. What would be the nurse's best approach?
    1. Give the patient a long explanation of the benefits of activity.

2. Tell the patient that the nurse needs a partner for an activity.
3. Demand that the patient join a group activity.
4. Mention that the "voices" would want the patient to participate.

55. When an experiment in the laboratory goes wrong, a researcher complains of a plot against her, and accuses the lab assistants of sending signals about her to each other. The nurse would determine that this behavior is related to:
    1. Delusions of grandeur.
    2. Illusion.
    3. Ideas of reference.
    4. Echolalia.

56. A teenager with acting-out behaviors says to the nurse, "I want you to go tell the teacher I am sick and I am to be allowed to do what I want." The nurse determines that this statement best represents:
    1. Insight.
    2. Manipulation.
    3. Dependency.
    4. Trust.

57. A 52-year-old patient who appears lucid learns that after surgery, he will wake up in the recovery room without his thick glasses and hearing aid. He immediately states that without these he will be confused and upset. The nurse determines that the patient is trying to say that he:
    1. Has periods of confusion and may have a psychiatric problem.
    2. Is psychologically dependent on the hearing aid and glasses.
    3. Needs the hearing aid and/or glasses to correctly perceive what is going on around him, and misperception will cause confusion.
    4. Needs the hearing aid and/or glasses because he wants to be sure people are taking proper care of him.

58. A patient relates angrily to the nurse that his wife says he is selfish. Which would be the most helpful response by the nurse?
    1. "That's just her opinion."
    2. "I don't think you're that selfish."
    3. "Everybody is a little bit selfish."
    4. "You sound angry—tell me more about what went on."

59. When a client has dementia, it is most important that the nurse plan the daily activities to:
    1. Be highly structured.
    2. Be changed each day to meet the client's needs for variety.
    3. Be simplified as much as possible to avoid problems with decision making.
    4. Provide many opportunities for making choices to stimulate the client's involvement and interest.

60. A woman tells the nurse that she refuses to eat her husband's cooking because she thinks he is poisoning her. The nurse is aware that this behavior is related to:
    1. Delusion of persecution.
    2. Ideas of reference.
    3. Illusion.
    4. Hallucination.

61. The crisis nurse explains to a colleague that the focus of treatment in crisis intervention is on the:
    1. Present and on restoration to the usual level of functioning.
    2. Past and on freeing the unconscious.
    3. Past in relation to the present.

4. Present and on the repression of unconscious drives.

62. A patient in the postoperative period following surgery for ulcerative colitis suddenly becomes angry with another patient who is monopolizing the group therapy meeting. Which interpretation of this noted change in behavior would indicate that the nurse understands the dynamics of this patient's somatoform disorder?
    1. The patient is intolerant of others.
    2. The patient has strong competitive drives.
    3. The patient has his or her own ideas of how the group members should act.
    4. The patient is repressing fewer feelings.

63. A client has a somatoform disorder, paralysis of the arm. It would not be helpful for the nurse to use logic and reason to divert this client's attention from this physical state because:
    1. The client is not in contact with reality and thus is unable to "hear" or understand the nurse.
    2. The client may need the symptoms to handle feelings of guilt or aggression.
    3. The nature of the client's particular illness makes the client suspicious of all medical personnel.
    4. Paralysis of the arm has become a habitual response to stress.

64. While communicating with a patient who is withdrawn, what would be important for the nurse to do at first?
    1. Remain silent and not encourage the patient to talk.
    2. Talk with the patient as one would to a normal person.
    3. Allow the patient to do all the talking.
    4. Use simple, concrete language in speaking to the patient.

65. The nurse bases a plan of care on the knowledge that persons engaged in gradual self-destructive behavior:
    1. Believe they can stop this behavior at any time.
    2. Have decreased anxiety when they stop the behavior.
    3. Believe the behavior controls them.
    4. Believe the behavior, in some manner, is "good" for them.

66. When a patient with symptoms of severe depression says to the nurse, "I can't talk; I have nothing to say," and continues being silent, what should the nurse do?
    1. Say, "All right. You don't have to talk. Let's play cards, instead."
    2. Explain that talking is an important sign of getting well and that the patient is expected to do so.
    3. Be silent until the patient speaks again.
    4. Say, "It may be difficult for you to speak at this time; perhaps you can do so at another time."

67. When talking with a client who is exhibiting a manic episode with flight of ideas, the nurse primarily needs to:
    1. Speak loudly and rapidly to keep the client's attention, as the client is easily distracted.
    2. Focus on the feelings conveyed rather than the thoughts expressed.
    3. Encourage the client to complete one thought at a time.
    4. Allow the client to talk freely.

68. A patient relates to the nurse, "I was going to kill myself last night." What is the best initial response by the nurse?
    1. Say nothing. Wait for the patient's next comment.
    2. "What were you going to do this time?"
    3. "Have you felt this way before?"

4. "You seem upset. I am going to be here with you; perhaps you will want to talk about it."

69. Which feeling is the nurse likely to identify as antecedent of self-destructive behavior?
   1. Omnipotence.
   2. Grandiosity.
   3. Low self-esteem.
   4. Self-satisfaction.

70. Resolution of grief related to death is likely to be complicated when:
   1. There are ambivalent feelings for the deceased.
   2. The death was due to a chronic illness.
   3. It is the first loss to be experienced.
   4. There was little emotional dependency on the deceased.

71. Which behavior might the nurse expect from a patient with congestive heart failure who is in the grief stage of developing awareness of the loss of a spouse?
   1. Crying and/or anger.
   2. Appearing dazed and repeatedly saying, "No, it can't be."
   3. Preoccupation with thoughts of how ideal the marriage had been.
   4. Responding with a brief complaint about the patient's own physical pain.

72. What feeling tone is the nurse most likely to see the client demonstrate during major depression with psychotic features?
   1. Suspicion.
   2. Agitation.
   3. Loneliness.
   4. Worthlessness.

73. When a client's behavior is considered abnormal, the nurse first needs to:
   1. Ignore the client.
   2. Serve as a role model.
   3. Point out the client's disturbed behavior.
   4. Focus on the feelings communicated by the client's behavior.

74. A hospitalized patient cannot find his slippers and accuses other patients and staff of stealing them. The most therapeutic approach is to:
   1. Listen without reinforcing the patient's belief.
   2. Logically point out that the patient is jumping to conclusions.
   3. Inject humor to defuse the intensity.
   4. Divert the patient's attention.

75. In interacting with a patient with an antisocial personality disorder, what would be the most therapeutic approach?
   1. Reinforce the patient's self-concept.
   2. Gratify the patient's inner needs.
   3. Give the patient opportunities to test reality.
   4. Provide external controls.

76. To relate therapeutically with a patient who is dependent on alcohol, it is important that the nurse base his or her care on the understanding that alcohol dependence:
   1. Is hereditary.
   2. Is due to lack of willpower and true remorse.
   3. Results in always breaking promises.
   4. Cannot be cured.

77. A patient uses repetitive handwashing. To help the patient use less maladaptive means of handling stress, the nurse could:
   1. Provide varied activities on the unit, as change in routine can break this ritualistic pattern.
   2. Give the patient ward assignments that do not require perfection.
   3. Tell the patient of changes in routine at the last minute to avoid buildup of anxiety.
   4. Provide an activity in which positive accomplishment can occur so the patient can gain recognition.

78. The most common coping mechanisms utilized in somatoform disorders are:
   1. Repression and symbolism.
   2. Sublimation and regression.
   3. Substitution and displacement.
   4. Reaction formation and rationalization.

79. A patient who has been hospitalized with ulcerative colitis asks the doctor about the prognosis. The patient becomes alternately depressed and agitated when hearing of the impending discharge. Which nursing approach would be best at this time?
   1. "You *are* much better than when you first were hospitalized. You have to decide whether you need to be hospitalized longer or whether you are ready to go home."
   2. "You seem to have concerns about going home."
   3. "What is it about going home that bothers you?"
   4. "You seem sad about going home. Would you like to talk about it?"

80. It is important for the nurse to be aware that the mental health of an aged client is most directly influenced by:
   1. The attitude of relatives in providing for the client's needs.
   2. Societal factors such as role change, loss of loved ones, and loss of physical energy.
   3. The client's level of education and economic situation.
   4. The attitudes the client has toward life circumstances.

81. In crisis intervention therapy, the nurse plans her or his goals based on the principle that crises:
   1. May go on indefinitely.
   2. Seldom occur in normal people's lives.
   3. Usually are resolved in 4–6 weeks.
   4. Are related to deep, underlying problems.

82. The nurse can determine that the expression of hostility is appropriate and useful when the:
   1. Energy from anger is utilized to accomplish what needs to be done.
   2. Expression intimidates others.
   3. Degree of hostility is less than the provocation.
   4. Expression of anger dissipates the energy.

83. Two days after a mastectomy, a woman is crying and saying, "My husband won't love me anymore." The nurse is aware that this statement might stem from:
   1. The woman's deep insecurity about her marriage.
   2. Preexisting marital disharmony.
   3. The woman's concerns about her body and a resultant change in her beliefs about her own self-worth.
   4. A momentary fear about her husband's fidelity.

84. The nurse establishes a nurse-client relationship with a patient with a schizophrenic disorder. One of the goals is to help the patient develop a separate self-identity. One way to do this is to:
   1. Call the patient by a "pet" name frequently.
   2. Use "you" and "I" rather than "we."
   3. Correct the patient's opinions.
   4. Encourage "should" responses.

85. A patient is diagnosed as having a paranoid disorder. What implication might this have for the nurse?

Mental Health

   1. Let the patient talk about her or his suspicions without correcting misinformation.
   2. Avoid talking to other nurses when the patient can see them but can't hear what is being said.
   3. Placate the patient by agreeing with what he or she says.
   4. Argue with the patient about his or her ideas.

86. A teenage patient says to the nurse, "I want you to go tell the teacher I am sick and I am to be allowed to do what I want." What is the nurse's best response?
   1. "Certainly. You are sick and need some relaxation of rules in the classroom."
   2. "I am glad you recognize you are sick."
   3. "No, you are expected to follow the rules of the classroom."
   4. "All teachers are too strict. I agree some rules need to be relaxed."

87. A 50-year-old patient says he needs his glasses and hearing aid with him in the recovery room after surgery, or he will be upset and confused. What is the nurse's best response?
   1. "You won't need your glasses or hearing aid. The nurses will take care of you."
   2. "I understand. You will be able to cooperate best if you know what is going on, so I will find out how I can arrange to have your glasses and hearing aid available to you in the recovery room."
   3. "I understand you might be more cooperative if you have your aid and glasses, but that is just not possible. Rules, you know."
   4. "Do you get upset and confused often?"

88. A mother talks about her daughter who is mentally retarded: "She's really an inspiration to me, do you know what I mean?" Which would be the most appropriate initial comment by the nurse?
   1. "What makes her an inspiration?"
   2. "It seems to be important to you to find something positive about her."
   3. "No, explain more about what you mean."
   4. "Tell me more about her."

89. At the first therapy session with a patient who recently attempted suicide, what does the crisis nurse need to do?
   1. Discourage discussion of the suicide attempt.
   2. Encourage the patient to focus on feelings about how badly the patient was treated as a child.
   3. Encourage the patient to discuss the suicide attempt in detail.
   4. Help the patient see how the suicide attempt hurt others.

90. A mother relates to the nurse, "When my baby had asthma 5 years ago, I thought he was going to die." What would be most appropriate for the nurse to say?
   1. "What made you think that he was going to die?"
   2. "What did you do?"
   3. "You thought he was dying?"
   4. "What were some of your feelings at that time?"

91. In preparing the nursing care plan for an elderly man, the *most* common basic need that must be met is:
   1. Sexual outlet and security.
   2. Unconditional acceptance by others of his impairments and deficits.
   3. Preservation of self-esteem.
   4. Socialization.

92. One effective way for a nurse to start an interaction with a client who is silent is to:
   1. Tell the client something about himself or herself and hope that the client does the same.
   2. Remain silent, waiting for the client to bring up a topic.
   3. Bring up a controversial topic to elicit the client's response.
   4. Introduce a neutral topic, giving the client a broad opening.

93. What would be the most realistic statement a nurse could make about a patient's prognosis after a course of necessary treatment for ulcerative colitis?
   1. The symptoms will recur.
   2. The ulcerative lesions will heal, but under stress the same symptoms will reappear.
   3. It is not possible to prognosticate the future course.
   4. Ongoing psychotherapy is essential for the patient to be free of symptoms.

94. What might be the most therapeutic response the nurse could make to a student who begins crying on hearing that he or she failed an exam?
   1. "You'll make it next time."
   2. "Failing an exam is an upsetting thing to happen."
   3. "How close were you to passing?"
   4. "It won't seem so important 5 years from now."

95. Which adaptive behavior by a client with somatoform disorders might indicate to the nurse the greatest improvement in the client's condition?
   1. The client recognizes that the behavior is unreasonable.
   2. The client agrees to go to occupational therapy and recreational therapy every day.
   3. The symptoms are replaced by expressions of hostility.
   4. The client is verbalizing feelings instead of demonstrating them by pathologic body languages.

96. A client tells the nurse that he has something he wants to say but does not want the nurse to tell anyone else. The nurse should:
   1. Agree not to "tell."
   2. Refuse to agree to this.
   3. Say nothing, allowing him to go on.
   4. Let him know that the nurse cannot promise this.

97. Which is an example of *limit setting* as an effective nursing intervention in ritualistic handwashing behavior?
   1. "I don't want you to wash your hands so often anymore."
   2. "If you continue to wash your hands so frequently, the skin on your hands will break down."
   3. "You may wash your hands before the group therapy meeting if you wish, but not during group therapy."
   4. "The doctor wrote an order that you are to stop washing your hands so often."

98. Which nursing intervention is effective when clients are severely anxious?
   1. Encourage group participation.
   2. Give detailed instructions before treatment procedures.
   3. Impart information succinctly and concretely.
   4. Increase opportunities for decision making.

99. A nursing care plan for a patient with a history of alcohol abuse and dependency will need to incorporate which physical consequence?
   1. Cardiac arrhythmia.
   2. Convulsive disorder.
   3. Psychomotor hyperactivity.
   4. Cirrhosis of the liver.

100. When a client tells the nurse that he or she cannot sleep at night because of fear of dying, what would be the best initial response?

1. "Don't worry, you won't die. You're just here for some tests."
2. "Why are you afraid of dying?"
3. "Try to sleep. You need the rest before tomorrow's test."
4. "It must be frightening for you to feel that way. Tell me more about it."

101. A new nurse is assigned to take clients for an outing. A patient with an antisocial disorder approaches the nurse and says, "I like you. I'm glad you'll be the one to take us out. My doctor told me that I can go too." Which initial response by the nurse is best?
1. "Since I am new here and not familiar with unit routine, I will go check with the staff and be back."
2. "It's a beautiful day, and I'm glad that you have ground privileges now."
3. "When did the doctor tell you that?"
4. "You seem pleased."

102. Which common physiologic reaction occurring in response to anxiety is the nurse likely to note?
1. Clammy hands and increased perspiration.
2. Palpitations and pupillary constriction.
3. Diarrhea and vomiting.
4. Pupillary dilation, retention of feces and urine.

103. Clients with paranoid behavior use projection. The nurse is aware that this mechanism is chiefly a way to:
1. Provoke anger in others.
2. Control delusional thought.
3. Handle their own unacceptable feelings.
4. Manipulate others.

104. Which most characteristic behavior of a panic response is the nurse likely to note?
1. Goal-directed behavior aimed at a "flight" from apparent threat.
2. Automatic behavior with poor judgment.
3. A severity of reaction that is not related to the severity of the threat to self-esteem.
4. A delayed reaction in perceiving the danger.

105. At times, a client seems preoccupied with her own thoughts as she grins, giggles, grimaces, and frowns. Although she is 23 years old, her behavior seems childish and regressed. She is unkempt, voids on the floor, disrobes, and openly masturbates. The main nursing care at this time should be directed toward:
1. Improving the client's social conduct to meet hospital standards.
2. Controlling the narcissistic impulses.
3. Finding out why the client is behaving this way.
4. Showing acceptance of the client.

106. The nurse is aware that the two major types of precipitating factors in anxiety are:
1. Fear of disapproval and shame.
2. Conflicts involving avoidance and pain.
3. Threats to one's biologic integrity and threats to one's self-system.
4. A person's poor health and poor financial condition.

107. After a patient with major depression visits with the spouse, the spouse reports that it was a stressful time. In an interview, the patient says, "We had a marvelous visit." The nurse is aware that this is an example of:
1. Compensation.
2. Denial.
3. Symbolism.
4. Identification.

108. Psychomotor manifestations of anxiety that a nurse may observe include:
1. Decreased activity.
2. Increased activity.

3. Increased lability of emotions.
4. Decreased lability of emotions.

109. A patient whose significant other recently died shows signs of grief resolution when he or she:
1. Wants to enter into another relationship soon.
2. Talks of both the positive and negative aspects of their relationship.
3. Makes up for deficiencies in the relationship, saying, "Things would have been better if we had only had more time."
4. Expresses anger toward the deceased.

110. The nurse needs to know that anxiety may increase intellectual functioning because anxiety may:
1. Increase the perceptual field.
2. Increase ability to concentrate.
3. Decrease the perceptual field.
4. Decrease random activity.

111. In planning patient care, a nurse needs to know that self-destructive behavior may be interpreted as the:
1. Directing of hostile feelings toward self.
2. Directing of hostile feelings toward others.
3. Directing of hostile feelings toward an internalized love object.
4. Internalization of the fear of death.

112. Based on knowledge of Erikson's stages of growth and development, the nurse determines that the task of old age is primarily concerned with:
1. Ego integrity versus despair.
2. Autonomy versus shame and doubt.
3. Trust versus mistrust.
4. Industry versus inferiority.

113. The nurse must assess for high risk of suicide when a patient's behavior suggests:
1. Major depression with melancholia features.
2. Schizophrenic disorders.
3. Bipolar mood disorder, manic episode.
4. Psychological factors affecting physical condition.

114. In working with clients who are depressed, the nurse must know that depression may stem from:
1. A sense of loss—actual, imaginary, or impending.
2. Revived memories of a painful childhood.
3. A confused sexual identity.
4. An unresolved oedipal conflict.

115. When working with a person who is anxious, what is the *overall* goal of nursing intervention?
1. Remove anxiety.
2. Develop the person's awareness of anxiety.
3. Protect the person from anxiety.
4. Develop the person's capacity to tolerate mild anxiety and to use it constructively.

116. In discussions between parents and adolescents about their relationship, a desired outcome is that adolescents benefit because they will be able to:
1. See themselves as the victims.
2. View their parents and themselves realistically.
3. Enlist the therapist's aid as an ally against their parents.
4. See their parents as victims.

117. The main nursing goal with clients with schizophrenic disorders is to:
1. Set limits on their bizarre behavior.
2. Establish a trusting, nonthreatening, reality-based relationship.
3. Quickly establish a warm, close relationship to counteract their aloofness.
4. Protect them from self-destructive impulses.

118. A patient is placed in isolation for seclusion due to agitated behavior. The nurse knows it is essential that:

1. Restraints be applied.
2. All the furniture be removed from the isolation room.
3. A staff member have frequent contacts with the patient.
4. The patient be allowed to come out after 4 hours.

119. Which activity would be best for the nurse to suggest to a depressed client?
    1. Folding laundry or stapling paper sheets for charts.
    2. Playing checkers.
    3. Doing a crossword puzzle.
    4. Ice skating.

120. A woman patient says to the nurse, "That patient over there is a lesbian." What is the best response by the nurse?
    1. "Are you afraid she will attack you?"
    2. "That woman is not a lesbian."
    3. "What did the woman do that makes you think she is a lesbian?"
    4. "Then stay away from her."

121. Which activity could a nurse suggest would be best for a client with hyperactive behavior?
    1. Solitary activity, such as reading.
    2. Hammering on metal in a jewelry-making class.
    3. Playing chess.
    4. Competitive games.

122. A patient says to his mother, "You are controlling me." The mother asks the nurse what he may have meant. What is the best response by the nurse?
    1. "He is upset and thinks you are taking charge of him."
    2. "He resents always having to meet your expectations."
    3. "I can't tell you. You will have to ask him."
    4. "I think you can ask your son that. Do you want me to stay with you while you ask him?"

123. When a client exhibits signs of amnesia, the nurse knows that this behavior is probably related to:
    1. Selective forgetting and storing unacceptable thoughts, wishes, and impulses in the unconscious mind.
    2. Conscious, deliberate forgetting.
    3. Transferring to another situation an emotion felt in a previous situation where its expression would not have been acceptable.
    4. Unconscious imitating of the manners, behavior, and feelings of another.

124. In caring for a patient at risk for suicide, the most important nursing action is to:
    1. Maintain constant awareness of the patient's whereabouts.
    2. Ignore the patient as long as he or she is talking about suicide, because a suicide attempt is unlikely.
    3. Relax vigilance when the patient seems to be recovering from depression.
    4. Administer medication.

125. A client who attempted suicide recently remarked to the nurse the next morning, "Let's not think about that now. Maybe I'll feel like thinking about it later." The nurse identifies this as:
    1. Blocking.
    2. Denial.
    3. Suppression.
    4. Repression.

126. After a mastectomy, a woman says, "My husband won't love me anymore." What would be the most therapeutic response by the nurse?
    1. "Of course your husband loves you."

2. "Tell me what has happened that makes you think your husband won't love you anymore."
3. "If you stop crying and fix yourself up, you will look good to your husband."
4. "Do you think your husband won't love you because you have lost a breast?"

127. Repetitive handwashing is often seen when a client is experiencing guilt feelings. This ritualistic behavior can be described as a mechanism whereby the client attaches significance to the act of washing. The nurse would identify this behavior as:
    1. Symbolism.
    2. Fantasy.
    3. Isolation.
    4. Conversion.

128. In conducting an assessment interview, the nurse needs to be aware that self-destructive behavior is determined by:
    1. A variety of factors, with the same factors present in each individual.
    2. Genetic disturbances.
    3. Interpersonal disturbances.
    4. A variety of factors, different for each individual.

129. A client shouts at the nurse one morning, "Why do you waste your time on me? I'm not sick; I don't need you. Go talk to other patients. They are really sick!" The nurse identifies this as:
    1. Reaction formation.
    2. Denial.
    3. Intellectualization.
    4. Rationalization.

130. Which term would the nurse use to describe the experience of an individual who thought he heard a machine gun when his neighbor's lawnmower backfired as she was mowing the lawn?
    1. Delusion.
    2. Hallucination.
    3. Identification.
    4. Illusion.

131. It would be important for the nurse to implement definite suicide precautions for a depressed patient if the patient's mood changed suddenly to one of:
    1. Cheerfulness.
    2. Psychomotor retardation.
    3. Agitation.
    4. Hostility.

132. The nurse knows that the most characteristic task of puberty and adolescence, according to Erikson's stages of psychosexual development, is:
    1. Identity versus role confusion.
    2. Initiative versus guilt.
    3. Ego integrity versus despair.
    4. Intimacy versus isolation.

133. A patient recently attempted suicide by slashing the wrists. The crisis intervention nurse and physician agree that hospitalization is not necessary for this patient; therefore, the nurse needs to:
    1. Wish the patient luck and terminate the session.
    2. Make an appointment for tomorrow and give the patient a telephone number where the nurse can be reached tonight.
    3. Make an appointment for the patient in 2 weeks, when the wrists might be healed.
    4. Tell the patient to make an appointment when she or he wants to, at the local mental health clinic.

134. A 10-year-old boy was admitted to the hospital for a tonsillectomy. In the morning, the nurse notes that the bedding is wet. There are several boys his age in the

room. Which initial approach would best demonstrate a nurse's understanding of enuresis and this patient's stage of growth and development?

1. While proceeding to change the wet linens, ask him what sports he likes best, purposely ignoring the wet bed by staying on impersonal topics.
2. Draw the curtains around his bed while changing the linen, saying, "I know that this must be embarrassing to you."
3. Say nothing while changing the bed; return at another time, when the other boys are not in the room, and explain to him the medical-emotional reasons for enuresis.
4. Sit down on the bed and convey acceptance of him as a person rather than focusing on the wet bed.

135. A patient with an antisocial personality disorder arouses anxiety and frustration in the staff and tends to intimidate by manipulative behaviors. One morning the patient shouts at the nurse, "Since you won't give me a pass, go away, you fat pig, or I'll hit you." What is the most effective response by the nurse to a client who threatens or derogates?

1. "You are rude and I don't like it. It makes me not want to talk with you."
2. "That kind of talk will keep you here longer."
3. "What did I do wrong?"
4. "I don't like to hear insults and threats. What is important about getting the pass today?"

136. In assessing the behavior of an autistic child, the nurse notes that a symptom that characteristically differentiates an autistic child from one with Down syndrome is:

1. Retardation of activity.
2. Short attention span.
3. Difficulty in responding to a nurturing relationship.
4. Poor academic performance.

137. It is important for a nurse to understand that a patient's repetitive handwashing is probably an attempt to:

1. Punish himself or herself for guilt feelings.
2. Control unacceptable impulses or feelings.
3. Do what the voices the patient hears tell him or her to do.
4. Seek attention from the staff.

138. In establishing a therapeutic nursing approach with a client who abuses and is dependent on substances, the nurse primarily needs to:

1. Promote a permissive, accepting environment.
2. Use a straightforward and confronting approach.
3. Meet the client's need for a chemical substitute for the drug.
4. Prevent the client's use of the addictive drug.

139. At 2:30 A.M., a client walks out to the nurse's station complaining that he is choking, suffocating, weakening, and dying. He demands a cigarette. What is the best response by the nurse?

1. Refuse and tell him it is against the rules.
2. Call the doctor and inform the doctor of the client's request and behavior.
3. Refuse and tell him the cigarettes are locked.
4. Give him a cigarette and stay with him while he smokes.

140. What approach can the nurse use to best handle a client's disturbed behavior?

1. Approve the behavior.
2. Maintain consistency of approach.
3. Encourage the client not to express negative opinions.
4. Interpret for the client the reasons for the behavior.

141. The overall client goal in rape counseling is to help the victim:

1. Forget the incident and repress her feelings in order to be able to carry on with her life.
2. Identify the rapist in a court of law.
3. Accept her part in the rape.
4. Acknowledge, face, and resolve the reaction she is experiencing.

142. Which is the most appropriate response to a client who states emphatically, "I hate them"?

1. "I will stay with you as long as you feel this way."
2. "Tell me about your hate."
3. "I understand how you can feel this way."
4. "For whom do you have these feelings?"

143. The nurse observes for signs of heroin withdrawal, which may include:

1. Rhinorrhea, sneezing, and high fever.
2. Pupillary dilation, diaphoresis, and weight loss.
3. Pupillary constriction, vomiting, and pruritus.
4. Choreiform movements and frequent lip wetting.

144. The nurse will look for what likely outcome of methadone treatment for heroin abuse and dependence?

1. Sedation.
2. Euphoria.
3. Neuritis.
4. Blocking of the euphoric effect of heroin and elimination of craving.

145. An acutely agitated client becomes increasingly aggressive. The staff's verbal attempts to stop the aggressive behavior are not effective. The client begins to shout threats at the staff and other clients, throws furniture, breaks windows, hits and kicks and bites other clients and staff. The client has a prn order for medication when agitated. Which action should the nurse take initially?

1. Orient the client to reality and place the client in a well-lit, quiet room.
2. Give the ordered tranquilizer and put the client in bed with the siderails up.
3. Lock the client in his or her room and call the doctor.
4. Have at least two staff members physically restrain the client and take the client to a quiet room.

146. A teenage patient has a history of stealing cars and traffic violations. The home environment has been permissive, and the teenager has been overly familiar and obsequious with the nurses. A new nurse, about to leave the locked unit, is holding the key as the patient approaches and eagerly offers to unlock the door for the nurse, saying, "The other nurses let me." Which first response by the nurse would be most appropriate?

1. Let the patient turn the key in the lock, but stay close while the patient does it.
2. Ask the patient why he or she wants to unlock the door.
3. Tell the patient in a nice way that this is not allowed.
4. Go to the head nurse and ask if it is all right for the patient to unlock the door.

147. Several staff members voice their frustrations about a patient's constant questions, such as "Should I go to the dayroom or should I stay in my room?" and "Should I have a cup of tea or a cup of coffee?" Which interpretation about this behavior will help the nursing staff deal effectively?

1. The patient's inability to make decisions reflects a basic anxiety about making a mistake and being a failure.

2. The patient's indecisiveness is aimed at testing the staff's reaction and acceptance of him or her.
3. The patient's dependence on others (staff) is a symptom that needs to be interrupted by firm limit setting.
4. The patient's need to ask questions is a bid for attention.

❑ Answers/Rationale

1. (1) Circulation may be severely impaired in a patient with waxy flexibility who tends to remain motionless for hours unless moved. **No. 2** is *not the first* priority. "Touch" is *not* used in this stage, as in choice **No. 3**. And **No. 4** is incorrect because the patient is *mute* and also because intellectual discussion of predisposing factors *ignores* the *feelings* of the patient. **PL,3,PhI**

2. (2) The other choices are *not* helpful, for the following reasons: **Nos. 3 and 4** *switch* the focus and *ignore* the client's statement; **No. 1** is too brusque an attempt to bring client back to reality. **IMP,5,PsI**

3. (3) This will reduce the isolation and withdrawal while at the same time not putting the burden of decision making on the client. The client needs a structured routine that is simple. The client may not be able to handle close proximity to more than one person at this point, as in **No. 2**. **No. 1** incorrectly allows the client to *remain* isolated; **No. 4** is incorrect because the client needs a *structured* routine until he or she can make decisions for himself or herself. **IMP,7,PsI**

4. (2) In the depressed episode, anger is turned inward; in the manic, it is noted in sarcasm, demanding behavior, and angry outbursts. **Nos. 3 and 4** occur in the manic episode. **No. 1** is a particular problem in the depressed phase. **AS,2,PsI**

5. (1) The nurse should formulate a weight control plan, in *cooperation* with the patient, that allows for a *gradual* weight loss, *not immediate* loss as in **No. 4**. **Nos. 2 and 3** *are incorporated* into **No. 1**. **IMP,4,PsI**

6. (4) This is a reality-based response, as well as one that acknowledges the patient's nonverbal reaction. The other choices are *not* the best because **Nos. 1 and 3** focus on "voice," which reinforce the hallucination, and no doubt is placed; in **No. 2** doubt is placed but focus is on "voice" and *not* on patient's *feelings*. **IMP,2,PsI**

7. (1) It shows acceptance by listening to the client's initial account of the physical problems. Neither a superficial focus nor a technical explanation of physical problems (**Nos. 2 and 3**) conveys acceptance of the client as a person; **No. 4** is too abrupt for an initial response. **IMP,7,PsI**

8. (2) Characteristic underlying needs in somatoform disorders are dependency, attention, and the need for security through trust. **Nos. 1 and 4** are incorrect because the patient's complaints are not aimed at blaming others or at seeking vengeance but at expressing dependency needs and seeking security. **No. 3** is inappropriate because the patient is expressing his or

her *own* need for attention; the patient is not speaking for everyone. **AN,7,PsI**

9. (2) Since confabulation is a coping mechanism, the best choice is the one that defines one of the main functions of coping mechanisms—to protect self-esteem. **Nos. 1 and 3** are incorrect because they focus on *others,* not on self. **No. 4** is completely *irrelevant.* **AN,2,PsI**

10. (1) Deal first with the *lifesaving* situation. **Nos. 2 and 3** are incorrect because they are done *following* stabilization of physical condition. **No. 4** is incorrect because it is *not* a necessary lifesaving concern. **PL,7,PhI**

11. (1) The nurse needs to set limits to ensure the safety of the patient and others. **No. 2** is incorrect because the patient may hurt herself or himself or others. **Nos. 3 and 4** are incorrect because they are interpretations that may or may not be correct, and they do *not control* the *unsafe* behavior. **IMP,1,SECE**

12. (2) In second grade a person needs to form close relationships with *peers.* **No. 1** needs to occur *earlier* than second grade or *later* in early teen years. **No. 3** occurs *later.* **No. 4** is incorrect because the father's actions *make* the child dependent on him rather than on peers. **AN,5,HPM**

13. (3) This tells the teenager the nurse heard his statement about "not doing his own thing" and *thinks* he is angry. **No. 1** is incorrect because this states the nurse *knows* he is angry. **No. 2** is incorrect because an angry person *can't stop* being angry on command. **No. 4** is incorrect because focusing on the parents puts the nurse on their side. **IMP,7,PsI**

14. (2) This acknowledges the experience and points out reality as the nurse sees it. **Nos. 1, 3, and 4** do not focus on the patient or attempt to explore feelings. **IMP,2,PsI**

15. (1) Emotional support is a key need. **No. 2** does *not* focus on emotional support. **No. 3**, role expectation, in itself has *no* bearing; emotional support of role would. **No. 4** would help the spouse and his or her own emotional reaction but would *not* help the patient. **AS,7,HPM**

16. (4) An honest, direct answer that focuses on feelings is the best approach. **Nos. 1, 2, and 3** stop any further exploration of the client's feelings. **IMP,7,HPM**

17. (3) Showing *acceptance* and gaining trust and confidence are usually the key initial nursing goals. You need to show acceptance before *helping* (**Nos. 1 and 4**) or *assisting* (**No. 2**). Note the lead verb: *accept* before *help* or *assist*. **PL,7,PsI**

18. (2) Refer to Elisabeth Kübler-Ross's emotional stages of death and dying. She is being neither unrealistic (**No. 1**), manipulative (**No. 3**), nor unaware of her diagnosis (**No. 4**). **EV,7,HPM**

19. (1) This reply asks for information that the nurse can use. If the patient understands the statement, the nurse can support the therapist when focusing on connections between food, love, and mother. If the patient does not understand the statement, the nurse can help get clarification from the therapist. **No. 2** alienates the client, and the nurse loses the chance for collaboration with the therapist. **No. 3** shuts the patient off. **No. 4** is incorrect because it is asked before the nurse is sure the patient understands the therapist's statement. **IMP,7,PsI**

20. (4) Redundancy is *not* meant to impress others but is aimed at *pleasure* gained through focus on the *past* and need to *control* the conversation when memory or hearing deficit is present. **Nos. 1, 2, and 3** *would* demonstrate understanding of this behavior. **AN,5,PsI**

Key to codes following rationales Nursing process: **AS,** Assessment; **AN,** Analysis; **PL,** Plan; **IMP,** Implementation; **EV,** Evaluation. Category of human function: **1,** Protective; **2,** Sensory-perceptual; **3,** Comfort, Rest, Activity, and Mobility; **4,** Nutrition; **5,** Growth and Development; **6,** Fluid-Gas Transport; **7,** Psychosocial-Cultural; **8,** Elimination. Client needs: **SECE,** Safe, Effective Care Environment; **PhI,** Physiologic Integrity; **PsI,** Psychosocial Integrity; **HPM,** Health Promotion/Maintenance. See appendices for full explanation.

Mental Health

21. (2) During a manic episode, the client may be too busy to eat and sleep. **Nos. 1 and 3** are more appropriate for a depressive episode; **No. 4** is more appropriate for schizophrenia with bizarre behavior. Clients in manic episode exhibit hyperactive behavior. **PL,2,PsI**

22. (3) Nocturnal urination is a most common need, complicated by disorientation related to the patient's age, disorder, and unfamiliar environment by night. To sit down **(No. 1)** or to go back to the patient's room and talk **(No. 4)** does not take care of the possible problem, the need to urinate. Asking a person "why" questions **(No. 2)** is not helpful and is too literal a response to the behavior. **IMP,7,SECE**

23. (4) A simple acknowledgment of what the nurse sees is the best response. **No. 3** makes an assumption that the patient feels better if she looks better. **Nos. 1 and 2** can be taken as a put-down. **IMP,7,PsI**

24. (2) Confidentiality cannot be guaranteed if there is a danger to the patient or to others. **No. 1** is incorrect because it is a *sarcastic* response and *denies* that the patient has serious problems. **No. 3** *contradicts* No. 2. **No. 4** is incorrect because parents *do not* have the right to know the content of therapy sessions except in the circumstances described in **No. 2**. **IMP,7,SECE**

25. (2) A diagnosis of a paranoid disorder implies weak *ego* development. **Nos. 1, 3, and 4** are incorrect because a client with a paranoid disorder might have *strong* id, superego, and "not me" components. **AN,5,PsI**

26. (2) An important principle to remember here is that a program of care should not increase physiologic losses by overtaxing the client's physical capacities. It is important to remember that suicide is the *main* concern of *depression* and *not* a key concern of dementia, as in **No. 1**. Empathy *rather than* sympathy **(No. 4)** is a helpful behavior. **No. 3**, increasing independence, is *not realistic; maintaining* it *is*. **PL,2,SECE**

27. (4) This is the all-inclusive answer. **Nos. 1, 2, and 3** may be part of No. 4. **AN,7,PsI**

28. (4) If a particular client is nonverbal, for example, the nurse should not expect that client to function at a verbal level until ready. In **No. 1**, if the nurse waits for a withdrawn client, for example, to make contact, it may not be helpful. In **No. 2**, an ambivalent client may need assistance in making decisions. In **No. 3**, the client's undesirable behavior may be adversely affecting others. **IMP,7,PsI**

29. (2) This is the most neutral answer by process of elimination. **No. 1** is *mainly* the function of a *recreational-occupational* therapist, although nurses participate. **No. 3** is *usually* filled by *psychologists* and social workers, and **No. 4** is carried out *primarily by psychologists* or *statisticians,* although nurses are involved. "Maintenance of a therapeutic environment" fits more readily into a nursing role by virtue of the number of hours per day a nurse spends with the clients on a unit, in comparison with the number spent by other professionals. **PL,7,SECE**

30. (4) A person needs to be allowed to express anger appropriately. **Nos. 1, 2, and 3** are *incorrect* choices here because they *are* things the nurse assists a person to do when intervening in anger. **IMP,1,PsI**

31. (2) Offering a broad opening by giving a general lead is most therapeutic to elicit further description of the client's reaction and to clarify feelings, which were vaguely stated. **No. 1** is a *switch of focus* from the client to the mother. **No. 3** is nontherapeutic because a question that can be *answered by a yes or no* often closes off further exploration. **No. 4** could be a helpful intervention but is *premature* acknowledgment before feelings have been elaborated. **IMP,7,HPM**

32. (3) It incorporates all information a crisis intervention nurse needs immediately. **Nos. 1 and 2** are incorrect because the nurse does not need to know about other people's involvement at this time. **No. 4** is incorrect because it is *not as complete* an answer as No. 3. **PL,7,PsI**

33. (3) It is important to acknowledge a statement, even if it is not understood. **No. 1** is not a *direct* response; **No. 2** leaves out the importance of the meaning of the neologism to the client; and **No. 4** is less valid and important than *acknowledgment* of the meaning to the client. **PL,2,PsI**

34. (1) It is important to externalize the anger away from self. **No. 2** is incorrect because usually the client is turning anger *inward,* toward the self. **No. 3** increases the client's sense of isolation. The needs in **No. 4** should be emphasized, not *deemphasized,* as the depressed client often has somatic delusions. **PL,7,PsI**

35. (4) It is a matter-of-fact statement that is direct, while offering assistance and setting limits on inappropriate behavior. The other choices are not useful because **No. 1** reinforces inappropriate social behavior; **No. 2** sets limits but does not state a positive expectation for the client to follow; and **No. 3** neither offers assistance nor sets limits, which the patient needs. **IMP,2,PsI**

36. (3) In **Nos. 1 and 2** the client could suffer extensive blood loss if the nurse focuses on feelings at this point or leaves the client without first attempting to control the bleeding. In **No. 4**, the client is left alone, bleeding, frightened, and with a razor still at the side. **AN,7,PsI**

37. (2) Persons engaged in self-destructive behavior other than active suicide behavior fantasize *they can control* their behavior and deny the likelihood of death as a result. Thus **Nos. 1, 3, and 4** are incorrect. **AN,7,PsI**

38. (1) Shock and anger are commonly the primary initial reactions. **No. 2** is irrelevant. **No. 3** is a literal, concrete interpretation of the patient's reaction, not aimed at the possible latent feelings. **No. 4** is incorrect because it contradicts the correct answer, No. 1. **AN,7,PsI**

39. (3) One of the main needs experienced by most clients with dementia is the need for most things to be the same. The other choices are wrong for the following reasons: there has been no demonstrable evidence of relationship between any behavior symptom and the extent or severity of pathophysiologic condition **(No. 2)**; intellectual *blunting* usually occurs, which interferes with ability to deal with insight and abstract thoughts **(No. 4)**; and memory loss is for *recent* events and names, *not* those in the distant past, as in **No. 1**. **AS,2,PsI**

40. (3) One way to enhance the development of unresolved grief is *not* to participate in activities that demonstrate death. **Nos. 1, 2, and 4** may occur, but they are *not* the best predictors of grief resolution difficulties. **AN,7,PsI**

41. (4) *Rationalization* is the process of constructing plausible reasons for one's responses. **No. 1**, *suppression,* is the intentional exclusion of material from consciousness. **No. 2**, *undoing,* is an act that partially negates a previous one. **No. 3**, *repression,* is the involuntary exclusion of painful or conflicting thoughts or feelings from awareness. **AN,7,PsI**

42. (4) Decoding symbolic, autistic expressions calls for skill and sensitivity in understanding latent messages. **No. 1** is not a good choice, since showing "acceptance" is a basic, initial nursing goal that does not require a complexity of skills. **No. 2** points out a nontherapeutic

nursing action, which is best not to use at all. **No. 3** implies that the nurse use short sentences with clear, concise, unambiguous meaning; this *can* be accomplished with practice. Nos. 1 and 3 need to be accomplished before No. 4 is possible. **IMP,7,PsI**

43. **(3)** This is a false belief developed in response to an emotional need. In **No. 1**, the situation is *not* a perceptual disorder. In **No. 2**, the situation is *not* a misperception. In **No. 4**, although the patient refuses meals, the reason for this is a false belief (delusion). **AN,7,PsI**

44. **(3)** This shows a weak sense of moral consciousness. According to Freudian theory, personality disorders stem from a *weak* superego. **No. 1** is incorrect, as the id is *strong*. These disorders are *not* characterized by a weak ego, as in **No. 2**, whereas schizophrenia is. **No. 4** is of relevance in sexual-identity difficulties rather than in personality disorders. **AN,5,PsI**

45. **(1)** Frightening visual hallucinations are especially common. **No. 2**, coma, is usually *not* an immediate consequence of alcohol withdrawal. **No. 3** is incorrect because the diagnosis is *withdrawal* from alcohol, not alcohol intoxication (intake). **No. 4** is incorrect because the patient will be *agitated* and *rambling* in conversation, not mute and depressed. **AS,7,PsI**

46. **(1)** Anxiety is generated by group therapy at 9 A.M. The ritualistic behavioral defense of handwashing decreases anxiety by avoiding group therapy. **No. 2** is incorrect because *tension,* not unmet needs, is discharged through ritualistic behavior. **No. 3** may be true, but it is not essential to planning care. **No. 4** is incorrect, as depression is *not* characteristic of ritualism. **AN,7,PsI**

47. **(3) No. 1** is incorrect because conversion, *not regression,* is the major coping mechanism. **No. 2** is incorrect because if a possible cause is identified and treatment relieves the discomfort, the client often develops another symptom. Frequently, clients do not want to be cured of their symptoms because they *need* the symptoms to control the behavior of others or because they do not know how else to get attention. In **No. 4**, the converse is true: the symptoms *are* real, not imagined or faked. **AN,7,PsI**

48. **(2)** All the other choices are correct but can be dovetailed into **No. 2**. **EV,7,PsI**

49. **(1)** Use of regression as a coping response *can* be minimized. Memory loss is usually permanent, not correctable; thus, **No. 2** is wrong. However, disorientation attributed to loss of memory can be minimized. Clients usually become *more* dependent in the course of illness *and* deteriorate progressively. Thus, **Nos. 3 and 4** are incorrect. Use of regression as a coping response (No. 1) *can* be minimized. **PL,2,SECE**

50. **(4)** The major goal of crisis intervention is to resolve immediate problems. **No. 1** is incorrect because restructuring personality is the goal of *psychoanalytic* therapy. **Nos. 2 and 3** are incorrect because they are goals of *brief* psychotherapy, and although they may occur in the resolution of immediate problems, they are *not the* goal. **IMP,7,SECE**

51. **(4)** It provides the complete steps. **No. 1** is incorrect because of the phrase "decide on *several*"; it should be *one* solution at a time. **No. 2** is incorrect because it *doesn't include* "discuss alternative solutions." **No. 3** is incorrect because it does not describe a requested *series* of steps and because *giving* a person one answer is untherapeutic. **IMP,7,SECE**

52. **(1)** It is most likely that grief would be expressed because of object loss. **No. 2** is incorrect because deep depression, if it occurs, would be the result of *lack* of res-

olution of grief over object loss. **No. 3** is incorrect because relief is *not part* of the grief process. **No. 4** is incorrect because the question asks for the client's *immediate* response. Denial of carcinoma, if it occurs, would probably occur *later*. **AS,7,PsI**

53. **(1)** Overcompliance leads to lack of development of self-identity, one of the major problems in schizophrenic disorders. **No. 2** is incorrect because there are *no substantiating data*. **No. 3** is incorrect because it *contradicts* the correct statement in No. 1. **No. 4** is incorrect because the patient probably has a *strong* superego due to an implied "should" system (overcompliance with parents' expectations of behavior). **AN,7,HPM**

54. **(2)** The nurse helps do things by doing something *with* the patient. **No. 1** is incorrect because the patient won't hear a long explanation. **No. 3** is incorrect because demanding won't work; the patient can't join in unless you are with the patient (as in No. 2). **No. 4** is incorrect because you should not produce psychosis to motivate a person. **IMP,7,PsI**

55. **(3)** The meaning of "ideas of reference" is that all that goes on is somehow connected to a person. **No. 1** is incorrect because delusions of grandeur mean a person has an *exalted* opinion of self. **No. 2** is incorrect because illusion is a false perceptual experience occurring in response to a stimulus. **No. 4** is incorrect because echolalia is a person's automatic *repetition* of what is said. **AN,7,PsI**

56. **(2)** Manipulation is the attempt to control the behavior of others to achieve one's own goals. **No. 1**, insight, is understanding and using understanding to correct one's behavior. **Nos. 3 and 4** are incorrect because although the client may be trying to con the nurse into believing he or she *needs* the nurse to do something for him or her and the client *trusts* the nurse, the *real* purpose of the request is manipulation. **AN,7,PsI**

57. **(3)** A person with limited hearing and sight becomes confused and disturbed. **Nos. 1 and 4** are *unwarranted* assumptions. **No. 2** is incorrect because the patient's situation is *not psychological* dependency but actual *sensory* need. **AN,2,PhI**

58. **(4)** It is important to pick up on a feeling tone and encourage exploration of the feelings and the situation. **No. 1** *stops* exploration of the patient's feeling. **Nos. 2 and 3** *shift* the focus away from feelings to content of selfishness. **IMP,7,HPM**

59. **(1)** Clients with dementia feel more secure when they can count on their environment being the same, predictable, and consistent in detail from day to day (hence, structured) to compensate for feelings of loss of the familiar in terms of body functions, social environment, and so on. **Nos. 2 and 4** imply change, not routine. **No. 3**, while correct, is not the *most* important. **PL,5,SECE**

60. **(1)** The patient has ideas that someone (her husband) is out to kill her. **No. 2** is incorrect because the problem is *beyond* just an "idea of reference" (she fears bodily harm). **No. 3** is incorrect because illusion is a false perceptual experience occurring in response to a stimulus. **No. 4** is incorrect because a hallucination is a sensory experience triggered by a person's inner needs, functioning independently of stimulation from the environment. **AN,7,PsI**

61. **(1)** To resolve immediate problems, focus on a person's ability to cope and usual level of functioning. **No. 2** is incorrect because it is a *psychoanalytic* focus. **Nos. 3 and 4** are incorrect because they are the focus of *brief* psychotherapy. **IMP,7,SECE**

62. (4) One coping mechanism often seen in somatoform disorders is repression. As the patient is better able to handle the anxiety connected with underlying feelings, the *need for repression lessens*. **Nos. 1, 2, and 3** may be the content of the patient's feelings, but they do not explain the dynamics, the *reason* the patient is expressing more feelings. **AN,7,PsI**

63. (2) This is a better choice than **No. 4**, which may be true but is a tangential and irrelevant reason. **No. 1** is not correct because the client *is* aware of reality but may not understand the *cause* for the somatoform disorder. **No. 3** is more relevant in a *paranoid* reaction. **AN,7,PsI**

64. (4) Patients with withdrawn behavior in schizophrenic disorders tend to think in concrete terms. Therefore, use of simple language enables them to grasp meaning. **No. 1** is incorrect because if the nurse remains silent the patient will remain silent. **No. 2** is incorrect because if the nurse is not concrete the patient might have trouble understanding some terms in normal conversation. **No. 3** is incorrect, as the patient has difficulty talking. **PL,7,PsI**

65. (1) These persons have not faced up to the idea that they are controlled by their behavior, and this relieves their anxiety. Contrary to **No. 2**, persons have *increased* anxiety if they stop the behavior. **No. 3** is also incorrect because they fantasize that they control their behavior. **No. 4** is incorrect because these persons *know* the behavior is bad for them. **AN,7,PsI**

66. (4) Meet the patient at her or his level of functioning, and provide support and encouragement for a higher level in the near future. **No. 1** implies that the nurse agrees that the patient has nothing to say. **No. 2** conveys no empathy or understanding. **No. 3** is incorrect because silence reinforces silence and a sense of isolation. **IMP,7,PsI**

67. (2) Often the verbalized ideas are jumbled, but the underlying feelings are discernible and need to be acknowledged. Flight of ideas should be *curtailed;* thus, **No. 4** is incorrect. The client may not be able to control the internal stimuli to focus on one idea at a time as in **No. 3**. A louder and more rapid tone by the nurse may only increase the external stimuli for the client, making **No. 1** incorrect. **PL,2,PsI**

68. (4) The patient needs to have his or her feelings acknowledged, with encouragement to discuss feelings, and be reassured about the nurse's presence. The patient may interpret the nurse's silence as discomfort in talking about suicidal feelings and thoughts (**No. 1**). **No. 2** focuses on facts too swiftly without providing an opportunity for the patient to express feelings. Also, **No. 2** would be most appropriate in *crisis* intervention when the patient is *first* admitted, *not* the next morning. **No. 3** moves away from focus on here-and-now to focus on the past. **IMP,7,PsI**

69. (3) When feelings of low self-esteem are prevalent, self-destructive behavior reaches its peak. Hence, **Nos. 1, 2, and 4** are incorrect. **AN,7,PsI**

70. (1) Love-hate feelings take longer to resolve. Reactions to loss tend to be cumulative in effect, in that the more loss experienced in the past, the greater the reaction the next time; thus, **No. 3** is wrong. Reactivation of feelings connected with previous losses by the current loss accounts for the increased intensity of the reaction. Sudden, unexpected death, *rather* than death due to a chronic illness, as in **No. 2**, is harder to resolve, and strong, *not little*, emotional dependency (as in **No. 4**) also complicates grief resolution. **AN,7,PsI**

71. (1) Correct according to Lindemann's and Engle's grief stages. Hence, incorrect are **No. 2** ("shock" stage), **No. 3** ("idealization" stage), and **No. 4** ("resolving the loss" stage). **AS,7,PsI**

72. (4) Feelings of worthlessness or low self-esteem are the underlying problem in depression. **Nos. 1, 2, and 3** may occur but are *not most* apt. **AN,7,PsI**

73. (4) Focusing on feelings is usually the best choice. Ignoring the client is rarely an acceptable intervention (**No. 1**). Pointing out disturbed behavior and role modeling by the nurse are valid, but *not* as first interventions (**Nos. 2 and 3**). **PL,7,PsI**

74. (1) Listening is probably the most effective response of the four choices. A key consideration in interacting with patients who are suspicious is to *avoid* the use of logic and argument; thus, **No. 2** is incorrect. Humor usually intensifies the anger and suspicion; thus, **No. 3** is incorrect. Changing the topic, as in **No. 4**, may serve to reinforce the patient's belief in the guilt of others. **PL,7,PsI**

75. (4) Personality disorders stem from a weak superego, implying a lack of adequate controls. **No. 1** is not relevant, as the patient's *self-identity* is *not* a focus here. **No. 2** is incorrect because the patient typically gratifies his or her own inner needs; this is part of the difficulty with a strong id, and requires external controls as in **No. 4**. **No. 3** is incorrect because the patient is *not* psychotic, but has a personality disorder for which reality testing is *not* impaired. The patient *is* aware of reality. **PL,7,PsI**

76. (4) Arrest of the disease is possible through abstinence, not through change in psychophysiologic response to alcohol. **Nos. 1, 2, and 3** are stereotyped statements, not generally or universally accepted. **AN,7,PsI**

77. (4) The *opposite* of what is stated in the first three choices is true. The patient seems to do best when **(1)** *routine* activities are set up and anxiety-provoking changes are avoided; **(2)** *perfection-type* activities bring satisfaction (cleaning and straightening a linen closet, for example); and **(3)** the patient knows *ahead of time* about changes in routine. **IMP,7,PsI**

78. (1) The original source of conflict, pain, and/or guilt is repressed (pushed out of awareness), only to surface in a symbolic way. **Nos. 2, 3, and 4** are only partially correct: in somatoform disorders, regression is common, *not sublimation;* displacement is common, *not substitution;* reaction formation is common, *not rationalization.* **AN,7,PsI**

79. (2) It reflects the patient's underlying concerns in the *most* open-ended manner. **No. 1** is incorrect because the *nurse* cannot say how the patient is feeling; this assumes here that the patient *is* better, which is inappropriate. **No. 4** only focuses on *one* aspect: *sadness*. What about the *agitation* the patient *also* expresses? **No. 3** is not incorrect, but it is also not the *best* choice because it asks a direct question when a simple acknowledgment (as in **No. 2**) would be better *initially.* **IMP,7,PsI**

80. (4) Although all the other choices *are* valid and important, the fourth answer encompasses them all and is therefore the most *comprehensive* answer. **AN,7,PsI**

81. (3) Part of the definition of a crisis is a time span of 4–6 weeks. **No. 1** is incorrect because by definition, crises do *not* continue indefinitely. **No. 2** is incorrect because *all* people have crises, and having crises does not determine normality. **No. 4** is incorrect because although crises may be related to deep, underlying problems, one of the principles of crisis intervention therapy is to deal with the immediate situation, not the underlying problem. **PL,7,SECE**

82. **(1)** This is the proper use of anger. **No. 2** is incorrect because although anger can be used to intimidate others, that use creates interpersonal problems. **No. 3** is incorrect because in order for hostility to be a good communication mechanism, the degree of hostility must be *appropriate* to the provocation. **No. 4** is incorrect because this expression of anger does not produce positive accomplishment. **EV,7,PsI**

83. **(3)** A change in body image has made the patient feel unloved and unworthy of love. **Nos. 1, 2, and 4** are incorrect because there are *no supporting data.* **AN,7,PsI**

84. **(2)** Use of "you" and "I" forces the patient to acknowledge separate identities. **No. 1** is incorrect because "pet" names are usually not a person's choice. The patient needs to be called by his or her real name. **No. 3** is incorrect because the patient has no identity if he or she can't have his or her own opinions. **No. 4** is incorrect because "should" responses imply others' ideas, not the patient's. **IMP,7,PsI**

85. **(2)** A patient with paranoid disorder is suspicious, so a nurse must make every effort not to engage in behavior the patient can misinterpret. **Nos. 1 and 3** are incorrect because a nurse *should* give correct information about what the patient says and *not* placate him or her (the patient will sense the falseness). **No. 4** is incorrect because arguing just solidifies the patient's ideas. In a neutral voice, the nurse should give correct information. **IMP,7,PsI**

86. **(3)** This response *stops* the manipulation and suggests the patient is responsible for his or her own behaviors. **Nos. 1, 2, and 4** are incorrect because they indicate the nurse has been conned and manipulated. **IMP,7,PsI**

87. **(2)** The patient will be easier to care for if he has his hearing aid and glasses. In **No. 1**, the nurse is *denying* the patient his right to the full information of his senses. **No. 3** is incorrect because the nurse has the responsibility to change rules for clearly therapeutic reasons. **No. 4** does *not* respond to the patient's needs. **IMP,2,PsI**

88. **(3)** An appropriate direct response to a "you know what I mean" comment is to say you do *not* automatically know what is meant. **Nos. 1, 2, and 4** are not the best response because they *shift the focus* from the client's experience to the characteristics of the *other* person. **IMP,7,HPM**

89. **(3)** The patient needs to be aware of his or her actions and the possible ramifications of those actions. **No. 1** is incorrect because the patient *needs to discuss* the actions. **No. 2** is incorrect because the purpose of crisis intervention is to deal with the *present* problem and situation, *not* the past. **No. 4** is incorrect because the focus needs to be on the patient, *not* on others. **PL,7,PsI**

90. **(4)** Attempts to focus on encouraging the client to describe feelings are important. **Nos. 1 and 2** ask for facts rather than focusing on feelings, and **No. 3** is an example of reflecting—a therapeutic response, but in this case it only reflects a *thought*, not a feeling. **IMP,7,HPM**

91. **(3)** Self-esteem is *the most basic* psychological need at *any* age, especially so for the elderly. **Nos. 1, 2, and 4**, although also important, are not the most basic needs. **PL,5,PsI**

92. **(4)** This is the least threatening. **No. 2** is not good because the nurse *needs* to intervene into a pattern of silence. It is not therapeutic for the focus to be on the nurse, as in **Nos. 1 and 3**, and bringing up a *controversial* topic (such as religion or politics) usually results in an exchange of opinions and arguments. **PL,7,PsI**

93. **(3)** This answer is the best choice because the other choices seem *too certain* for a disorder that, although it has a pattern, can be altered *if* and *when* the patient adopts different outlets for expressing emotions. **EV,7,PsI**

94. **(2)** **Nos. 1 and 4** focus on *"there-and-then"* rather than "here-and-now" feelings and events, and **No. 3** is *irrelevant* because the focus is on a *fact* rather than a feeling. **IMP,7,PsI**

95. **(4)** This answer also incorporates **No. 3**. Agreement to attend activities (**No. 2**) does not indicate the *greatest* improvement. The client *already* recognizes that the behavior is irrational but cannot understand the cause or banish the behavior by will, as in **No. 1**. **EV,7,PsI**

96. **(4)** Information that is given to the nurse that may interfere with the client's recovery needs to be related to other team members. The other choices are not the best response because **No. 1** is withholding information from other staff who are also responsible for care and may interfere with recovery needs; **No. 2** is a refusal that may stop the interaction—a negotiation is needed; and **No. 3** does not provide a client with the clear feedback needed to work through conflict. **IMP,7,SECE**

97. **(3)** This is the best example of setting limits on the behavior. **Nos. 1 and 4** may be closely linked to nontherapeutic use of power. **No. 2** is more of an example of a punishment approach. **IMP,7,PsI**

98. **(3)** Brief and specific information *can* be processed during severe anxiety. In severe anxiety, the person cannot respond to the social environment (as in **No. 1**); giving detailed information results in overload, as the client cannot retain and recall data (as in **No. 2**). Only directive information that is brief and specific is effective when the client cannot focus on what is happening. Decision making needs to be postponed until the person is less anxious; hence, **No. 4** is wrong. **PL,7,SECE**

99. **(4)** The liver is affected by both the direct effect of alcohol and nutritional deficiencies associated with alcohol abuse and dependence. **Nos. 1, 2, and 3** are areas not usually affected by alcohol abuse and dependence. **AN,7,PhI**

100. **(4)** Acknowledging a feeling tone is the most therapeutic response and provides a broad opening for the client to elaborate feelings. The other choices are not the best response because **No. 1** is false *reassurance* that does not allay feelings; **No. 2** is asking a *"why"* question, which is confrontive and may increase anxiety; and **No. 3** gives *advice,* which stops exploration of underlying feelings. **IMP,3,PsI**

101. **(1)** This response aims to prevent use of manipulative patterns. In **Nos. 2, 3, and 4**, the nurse needs to seek validation, and these responses indicate acceptance without validation. **IMP,7,PsI**

102. **(1)** No. 1 is the best choice. Common reactions: pupillary dilation, *not* constriction (**No. 2**); diarrhea, *not* constipation (**No. 4**). Vomiting is not typical of an anxiety response (**No. 3** is incorrect). **AS,7,PhI**

103. **(3)** This response refers to the definition of *projection* as a coping mechanism (attributing one's own unacceptable thoughts, feelings, and behaviors to another). **Nos. 1, 2, and 4** are incorrect because they have nothing to do with the coping mechanism of projection. Coping mechanisms in general function in the service of "self"—that is, they protect the ego and preserve

self-esteem in an effort to cope with anxiety; the focus is *not* on *others,* as in **Nos. 1 and 4.** Symptoms of projection do in fact *express* delusional thought rather than *control* it, contrary to **No. 2. AN,7,PsI**

104. **(2)** In panic, a person is highly suggestible and follows "herd instinct" rather than exercising independent judgment and problem solving **(No. 1)**. No. 3 is incorrect because the severity of the reaction *is* related to the severity of the threat. The more severe the perceived threat (actual or imaginary), the more intense the reaction to the danger, and *not* delayed as in **No. 4. AN,7,PsI**

105. **(4)** The primary initial focus of the nurse-client relationship is in showing the client, through acceptance, that it is *the client* one is concerned about, *not* the *symptoms.* **Nos. 1 and 2** are incorrect because the focus of *initial* nursing care is on the client, not on meeting hospital standards or controlling impulses. **No. 3** is incorrect because it is an attempt to analyze the *whys* of behavior, which is not an appropriate *basic* nursing intervention and certainly *not* an initial aspect of care. **PL,7,PsI**

106. **(3)** This is the most inclusive answer. **Nos. 1, 2, and 4** are all *incorporated* into **No. 3. AN,7,PsI**

107. **(2)** *Denial* is the act of avoiding disagreeable realities by ignoring them. **No. 1** is incorrect because *compensation* is the process by which a person makes up for a deficiency in self-image by emphasizing an asset. **No. 3,** *symbolism,* is the use of one mental image to represent another. **No. 4,** *identification,* is the process of taking on another person's attribute. **AN,7,PsI**

108. **(2)** Research shows *increased* activity is a psychomotor manifestation of anxiety; **No. 1** is therefore wrong. **Nos. 3 and 4** are incorrect because emotion is *not* a psychomotor manifestation. **AS,7,PhI**

109. **(2)** When the mourner can pass through the idealization stage and be more realistic about the positive and negative aspects of the loss, resolution of grief is beginning. **Nos. 3 and 4** occur in *earlier* stages of grief. **No. 1** could be a sign of denial of grieving, an initial grief reaction. **EV,7,PsI**

110. **(3)** Research shows that anxiety *decreases* the perceptual field—**No. 1** therefore is incorrect. Research also shows that anxiety *decreases* the ability to concentrate and *increases* random activity; therefore, **Nos. 2 and 4** are incorrect. **AN,7,PsI**

111. **(3)** This is correct by Freudian theory. **Nos. 1, 2, and 4** are incorrect because they are incomplete. **AN,7,PsI**

112. **(1) No. 2** relates to toddler; **No. 3,** to infancy; **No. 4,** to latency period in childhood. **AN,5,HPM**

113. **(1)** Another name for major depression is depression with psychotic features. Suicide risk is a part of all depressions. **Nos. 2, 3, and 4** are incorrect because the diagnosis alone does not indicate suicide risk like the diagnosis of depression. **AN,7,PsI**

114. **(1)** "Loss" is *most basic* to the development of depression. **Nos. 2, 3, and 4** are *not essential* to development of depression. **AN,7,PsI**

115. **(4)** Some anxiety is necessary to learn. **No. 2** is incorrect because it is *incomplete.* **Nos. 1 and 3** are incorrect because anxiety *is necessary* for learning and growth. **PL,7,PsI**

116. **(2)** Part of maturing is learning to view one's parents *and* oneself realistically. **Nos. 1, 3, and 4** are incorrect because they represent the *misinformation* that creates problems between individuals. **EV,7,HPM**

117. **(2)** A permissive atmosphere is the key, as well as a *slowly* evolving relationship (not quickly evolving, as in

No. 3) with room for *distance.* Self-destruction is *not a persistent* problem requiring *major* focus for concern, as in **No. 4. No. 1** is not the best response because "acceptance" of *bizarre* behavior is more important than setting limits. **PL,7,PsI**

118. **(3)** Frequent contacts at times of stress are important, especially when a patient is isolated. The other choices are not useful because **No. 1,** isolation does not automatically imply the use of restraints; **No. 2,** *all* furniture need not be removed, depending on the institution and the type of behavior exhibited by the patient; and **No. 4,** there is *no specific* time limit, as time depends on individual behavior and the patient's individual needs. **PL,1,SECE**

119. **(1)** An undemanding task that the client could finish would allow a feeling of successful accomplishment. **Nos. 2 and 3** require intellectual activity that is usually slowed down during a depressive phase. **No. 4** requires a skill that the client may not have and that might frustrate the client to learn; also, the client may not have the psychomotor energy for ice skating. **IMP,3,PsI**

120. **(3)** The nurse should encourage the patient to *explain* her statement in order to understand the experience she is having. **No. 1** is incorrect because it offers an *interpretation* that may or may not be true. **No. 2** is incorrect because it denies the patient's perception without clarification. **No. 4** is incorrect because the nurse agrees with an unsupported statement. **IMP,7,PsI**

121. **(2)** It will provide energy release without the external stimuli and pressure of *competitive games* **(Nos. 3 and 4).** Reading usually requires sitting, which a hyperactive client cannot readily do, as in **No. 1. IMP,3,PsI**

122. **(4)** The mother needs to ask the patient, not the nurse, but the nurse should also support the mother and encourage her to interact with her son. **Nos. 1 and 2** are incorrect because they are *interpretations* that state opinions about the patient without his participation. **No. 3** is incorrect because *no support is given* to the mother. **IMP,7,PsI**

123. **(1)** By definition, **No. 2** is suppression; **No. 3,** displacement; and **No. 4,** identification. **AN,7,PsI**

124. **(1)** The patient needs to be constantly observed. **No. 2** is incorrect because all suicidal talk and gestures are to be taken seriously. If the patient *talks* about suicide, there *may* be an attempt. **No. 3** is incorrect because suicide risk is greater when depression is lifting, requiring greater vigilance. **No. 4** is incorrect because medication for depression may take up 2 weeks to decrease symptoms, and the patient needs vigilant surveillance *now.* **PL,7,PsI**

125. **(3)** By definition, this is the conscious, deliberate effort to avoid talking or thinking about painful, anxiety-producing experiences. **AN,7,PsI**

126. **(2)** This question attempts to get a specific description of what has happened and will allow the client to describe grief and feelings of low self-worth because of loss of breast. **No. 1** is incorrect because it offers *false* reassurance. **No. 3** is incorrect because it is a *stereotyped* response to a female and denies the client's actual loss. **No. 4** is incorrect because it is an *interpretation* that, although possibly true, the client may reject. Resolution of grief, etc., is better achieved if the client can state connection. **IMP,7,PsI**

127. **(1)** Symbolism is the most clearly descriptive mechanism. **No. 2,** fantasy, is a mental activity; **No. 3,** isolation, is the exclusion from awareness of a feeling; and

No. 4, conversion, is a disruption of motor or sensory functioning. **AN,7,PsI**

128. **(4)** A variety of factors can cause self-destructive behavior, and these differ for each individual. Hence, **Nos. 1, 2, and 3** are not the best choices because, although correct, they are *examples* of a *variety* of factors; **No. 4** is more inclusive. **AS,7,PsI**

129. **(2)** Denial is the mind's way of protecting the self-system from a disturbing reality. **No. 1**, reaction formation, is an expression of an attitude opposite to unconscious feelings; **No. 3**, intellectualization, is giving rational reasons without expression of underlying feelings; **No. 4**, rationalization, is the attempt to make one's behavior look like the result of logical thinking. **AN,7,PsI**

130. **(4)** This is correct by definition. **No. 1** is incorrect because delusion is a fixed *idea* arising out of a person's inner needs and contrary to observed facts. **No. 2** is incorrect because a hallucination is a misperception that is *unrelated to an external stimulus*. **No. 3** is incorrect because identification is the process of taking on another person's attribute. **AN,7,PsI**

131. **(1)** A person who has settled on a plan for suicide will become more cheerful. **No. 2** is incorrect because a person who is severely retarded in the psychomotor area cannot carry out a suicide act. **Nos. 3 and 4** are incorrect because the patient is more likely to be hostile and agitated if he or she does not have a suicide plan. Agitated behavior can also represent the need to "repent" for sins thought to be committed. **EV,7,PsI**

132. **(1) No. 2** refers to preschool age, **No. 3** is characteristic of "maturity" in later years of life, and **No. 4** refers to young adulthood. **AN,5,HPM**

133. **(2)** On principle, the crisis intervention nurse needs to be *immediately* available to the patient. **No. 1** is incorrect because it abandons the patient. **No. 3** is incorrect because the patient needs to deal with the situation *immediately*. **No. 4** is incorrect because the patient might decide that the crisis intervention nurse is not interested in helping, and the patient needs *immediate* assistance. **IMP,7,SECE**

134. **(4)** The goal is to preserve ego strength through acceptance and respect of the patient as a person. **No. 1** focuses on the tangential and irrelevant; **No. 2** makes the problem more obvious to others in the room and makes an assumption without validation about how the patient must feel; **No. 3** is incorrect because it is usually not helpful to give a rational explanation for an emotional difficulty related to enuresis. **IMP,5,HPM**

135. **(4)** The nurse must state feelings, without anger, and show no intimidation, then help the patient examine what he or she is doing and why. **No. 1** is incorrect because it points the finger in an angry, accusatory way and labels the patient in turn ("*You* are rude"). **No. 2** patient sounds like "Big Nurse"—authoritarian and punitive. **No. 3** may place the nurse in a position to be intimidated and "kicked" by the patient. **IMP,7,PsI**

136. **(3)** Most children with Down syndrome are affectionate and enjoy being held and cuddled, whereas the *opposite* is usually the case with an autistic child. All other responses may apply to *both* Down syndrome and autism. **AS,5,PsI**

137. **(2)** A ritual, such as compulsive handwashing, is an attempt to allay anxiety caused by unconscious impulses that are frightening. **No. 1** is incorrect because it is the opposite of what the handwashing ritual is intended to do—the ritual is aimed at *absolving* guilt, not *punishing*. **No. 3** is related to *psychotic* symptoms and not at

all relevant to symptoms of ritualism. **No. 4** is incorrect because handwashing is aimed at relief of guilt and self-help to reduce anxiety, *not* at seeking attention from staff. **AN,7,PsI**

138. **(2)** It is important to provide external support in helping develop the superego. **No. 1** may promote manipulative behavior in the client. **No. 3** may foster additional dependence. And preventing the client's use of drugs **(No. 4)** is *not* the primary step in building a nurse-client relationship based on therapeutic communication. **PL,7,PsI**

139. **(4)** The client is anxious and needs someone with him. **No. 1** is incorrect because it *ignores* the client's anxiety and needs. **No. 2** is incorrect because it also *ignores* the client's anxiety and uses the doctor as an excuse to ignore his needs. **No. 3** is incorrect because it also *ignores* the client's anxiety and needs and gives a poor reason for refusal. **IMP,7,PsI**

140. **(2)** Consistency lets clients know consequences of behavior and develops trust. **No. 1** is incorrect because the nurse *cannot approve all* behavior (e.g., destructive behavior). **No. 3** is incorrect because it can be therapeutic *to express* negative opinions. **No. 4** is incorrect because interpretation of behavior is *not* always advisable. Clients may use interpretations of behavior to avoid consequences of behavior or may see them as an excuse not to change behavior. **PL,7,SECE**

141. **(4)** The victim needs to engage in *expression* of the experience, which will assist her to work through her feelings so that the experience may not interfere in future interpersonal relations. To repress the incident, as in **No. 1**, would make it continually interfere in her relationships. **No. 2** is only done *after* **No. 4** has been accomplished. **No. 3** is incorrect because the rape victim has *no* "part" in the rape. **PL,1,HPM**

142. **(2)** The nurse is asking the client to clarify and further discuss feelings. **No. 1** is incorrect because while staying with the client *might* convey acceptance, it does *not* help the client clarify or deal with feelings. **No. 3** is incorrect because it cuts off any further response from the client and because it is *doubtful* that the nurse can understand another person's feelings. **No. 4** is incorrect because it is *more* important to *clarify* the client's *feelings* than it is to understand the *object* of hate. **IMP,2,PsI**

143. **(2)** Note the eyes: when a person is *on* heroin, the pupils are constricted; during *withdrawal,* they are dilated. Withdrawal does *not* usually include high fever, pupil constriction, or choreiform movements, as in **Nos. 1, 3, and 4. AS,7,PhI**

144. **(4)** Methadone is a synthetic narcotic and has no euphoric effect. Methadone does not produce sedation **(No. 1)**, euphoria **(No. 2)**, or neuritis **(No. 3)**. **EV,7,PhI**

145. **(4)** With concern for danger to the other clients, staff, and the environment, it is essential for the client to be restrained at this time. The other choices are incorrect because **No. 1**, orientation and a quiet environment *alone* do *not* provide for safety when the client's agitation is out of control; **No. 2**, the initial *delay* in onset of effectiveness of the tranquilizer does not *immediately* provide for the safety needs of other clients, staff, and the environment; and **No. 3**, locking the client in his or her room eliminates only the danger to others, and additional measures would be needed to provide for the safety of this *client.* **IMP,1,SECE**

146. **(4)** Based on the patient's history of antisocial behavior, he or she is probably attempting to use the nurse for his or her own purpose and is not truthful. There-

fore, it is best that the new nurse on the unit go directly to the head nurse to check on what is permissible and not accept the patient's word that it is permissible. **No. 1** is not helpful because allowing the patient to unlock the door may feed into the manipulative attempt by the patient to get off the unit. **No. 2** is incorrect because asking a "why" question is not a therapeutic communication. **No. 3** is incorrect because this option places the new nurse in an argumentative position with the patient, who is likely to become de-

fensive and say, "Oh, yes. I *am* allowed to open doors." **IMP,7,SECE**

147. **(3)** Limit setting is an important intervention with a patient who exhibits excessive, constant dependence on others for simple, seemingly inconsequential decisions in everyday life. The other choices are wrong because the situation presented provides insufficient data on which to base interpretations related to fear of failure (**No. 1**), a need to test for staff acceptance (**No. 2**), or a bid for attention (**No. 4**). **AN,7,SECE**

Unit 7

Nursing Care of the Childbearing Family

❑ Growth and Development

Biologic Foundations of Reproduction

General overview: This review of the structures, functions, and important assessment characteristics of the reproductive system provides essential components of the database required for accurate nursing judgments. Comparing normal characteristics and established patterns with nursing assessment findings assists in identifying patient needs and in planning, implementing, and evaluating appropriate goal-directed nursing interventions.

Female Reproductive Anatomy and Physiology

  I. **Structure of pelvis** (Figure 7.1)
   A. Two hip bones (right and left innominate: sacrum, coccyx).
   B. False pelvis—upper portion above brim, supportive structure for uterus during last half of pregnancy.
   C. True pelvis—below brim; pelvic inlet, mid-cavity, pelvic outlet comprise this structure. Fetus passes through during birth.
 II. **Pelvic measurements**
   A. Diagonal conjugate—12.5 cm or greater is adequate size; measured by examiner.
   B. Conjugate vera—11 cm is adequate size; measured by X ray.
   C. Obstetric conjugate—measured by X ray.
   D. Tuber-ischial diameter—9 to 11 cm indicates adequate size; measured by examiner.
III. **Female external organs**
   A. Mons veneris—protects symphysis.
   B. Labia majora—covers, protects labia minora.
   C. Labia minora—two located within labia majora.
   D. Clitoris—small erectile tissue.

■ **FIGURE 7.1   The female pelvis.**

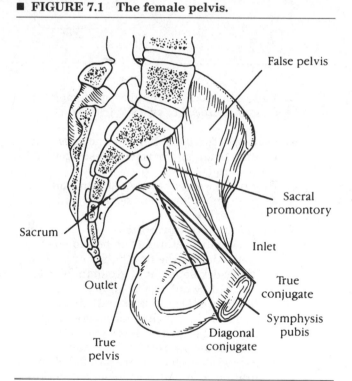

   E. Hymen—thin membrane at opening of vagina.
   F. Urinary meatus—opening of urethra.
   G. Bartholin glands—producer of alkaline secretions that enhance sperm motility, viability.
 IV. **Internal structures** (Figure 7.2)
   A. Vagina—outlet for menstrual flow, depository of semen, lower birth canal.
   B. Cervix—uterine outlet.
   C. Uterus—muscular organ that houses fetus during gestation.

387

Maternal-Infant

■ **FIGURE 7.2   Female internal reproductive organs.**

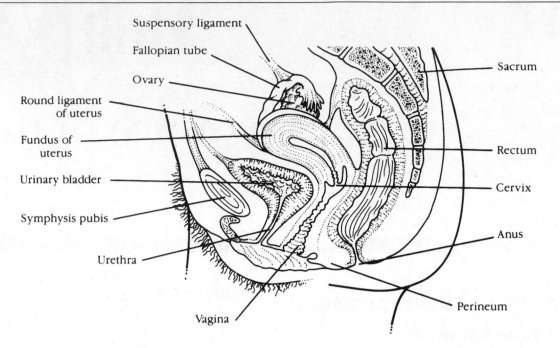

D. Fallopian tubes—two tubes stretching from cornua of uterus to ovaries; transport ovum.

E. Ovaries—two oval-shaped structures that produce ovum and hormones (estrogen and progesterone).

F. Breasts—two mammary glands capable of secreting milk for infant nourishment.

V. Menstrual cycle

  A. Reproductive hormones

  1. *FSH* (follicle stimulating hormone)—secreted during the first half of cycle; stimulates development of graafian follicle; secreted by anterior pituitary.

  2. *ICSH or LH* (interstitial cell stimulating hormone, luteinizing hormone)—stimulates ovulation and development of corpus luteum; secreted by pituitary.

  3. *Estrogen*—assists in ovarian follicle maturation; stimulates endometrial thickening; responsible for development of secondary sex characteristics; maintains endometrium during pregnancy. Secreted by ovaries and adrenal cortex during cycle and by placenta during pregnancy.

  4. *Progesterone*—aids in endometrial thickening; facilitates secretory changes; maintains uterine lining for implantation and early pregnancy; relaxes smooth muscle. Secreted by corpus luteum and placenta.

  5. *Prostaglandins*—substances produced by various body organs that act hormonally on the endometrium to influence the onset and continuation of labor. A medica-

tion that may be used to facilitate onset of second trimester abortion; also used to efface the cervix before induction of labor in term pregnancies.

  B. Ovulation—maturation and release of egg from ovary; generally occurs 14 d *before* beginning of next menses.

  C. Menstruation—vaginal discharge of blood and fragments of the endometrium; cyclic; occurs in response to dropping levels of estrogen and progesterone.

  D. Fertilization—impregnation of ovum by sperm.

  E. Implantation—fertilized ovum attaches to uterine wall for growth.

  F. Menopause—normally occurring cessation of menses with gradual decrease in amount of flow and increase in the time between periods at end of fertility cycle; average age, 53. Early menopause rare but may be influenced by hypothyroidism, surgical ovarian removal, overexposure to radiation. Treatments during menopause for symptom relief: hormonal replacement therapy, vitamins B and E for hot flashes, vaginal creams for dyspareunia (painful intercourse), and calcium for osteoporosis.

  G. Spinnbarkheit—stretchable, thin cervical mucus present at ovulation.

◆ **VI. Assessment of reproductive tract/reproductive health:**

  A. Health history

  1. Menarche: onset and duration.

  2. Menstrual problems.

  3. Contraceptive use.

4. Pregnancy history.
5. Fertility problems.
B. Physical examination
   1. External, internal reproductive organs.
   2. Breast examination
   3. Mammography, if at risk or yearly $\geq$ 40 yr of age.
   4. Periodic Pap smears.
   5. Tests for STDs (sexually transmitted diseases).

◆ **VII. Analysis/nursing diagnosis:**
   A. *Health-seeking behaviors* related to health promotion.
   B. *Health-seeking behaviors* related to menopause.

◆ **VIII. Nursing care plan/implementation:**
   A. Discuss anatomy and physiology of reproductive tract.
   B. Review menstruation, ovulation, fertilization.
   C. Explain need for periodic Pap smears, annual gynecologic exams, including mammography.

◆ **IX. Evaluation/outcome criteria:**
   A. Woman displays basic understanding of anatomy and physiology.
   B. Woman understands cycle and contraception.
   C. Woman regularly seeks preventive care and performs monthly breast self-examination (BSE).

Decision Making Regarding Reproduction

General overview: During the reproductive years, the sexually active woman often faces the decision to postpone, prevent, or terminate a pregnancy. The nursing role focuses on assisting her to make an informed decision consistent with individual needs.

I. Family planning
◆ **A. Assessment:**
   1. Determine interest in and present knowledge of methods of family planning.
   2. Identify factors affecting choice of method: cultural and religious objections, contraindications for individual methods, motivation/ability to follow chosen method successfully, financial considerations.
◆ **B. Analysis/nursing diagnosis:** *knowledge deficit* regarding family planning methods/options.
◆ **C. Nursing care plan/implementation**—Goal: *health teaching*—to facilitate informed decision making, selection of option appropriate to individual needs, desires.
   1. Describe, explain, discuss options available and appropriate to the woman. Include information on advantages and disadvantages of each option (Tables 7.1, 7.2).
   2. Demonstrate, as necessary, method selected.

3. Quick health teaching reminders for missed oral hormone preparations:[a]
   a. Woman should take one pill at the same time every day for 21 (or 28) d.
   b. If woman misses one pill, she should take it as soon as she remembers it; she should then take the next one at the usual time.
   c. If woman misses two or more pills in a row in the first 2 wk of her cycle, she should take 2 pills for 2 d and use a backup method of contraception for the next 7 d.
   d. If woman misses two pills in the third week, or three or more pills anytime:
      (1) A *Sunday starter* should keep taking pills until the next Sunday, then start a new pack that Sunday. She should use a backup method of contraception for the next 7 d.
      (2) A *day 1 starter* should throw out the rest of the pack and start a new pack that day. She should use a backup method of contraception for the next 7 d.
   e. *28-day pill pack:* If woman misses any of the seven pills that do not have any hormones, she should throw out the pills missed and keep taking one pill a day until the pack is empty. She does not need a backup method of contraception.
4. Alert woman to discontinue use of *oral hormone contraceptive* preparations and report any of the following symptoms to the physician stat. Signs of potential problems: **"ACHES"**
   A — **A**bdominal pain: possible problem with the liver or gallbladder.
   C — **C**hest pain or shortness of breath: possible clot within lungs or heart.
   H — **H**eadaches (sudden or persistent): possibly caused by cardiovascular accident or hypertension.
   E — **E**ye problems: possible vascular accident or hypertension.
   S — **S**evere leg pain: possible thromboembolic process.
5. Signs of *potential problems* related to IUD use: **"PAINS"**[b]
   P — **P**eriod (menstrual) late, abnormal spotting or bleeding.
   A — **A**bdominal pain, pain during coitus (dyspareunia).
   I — **I**nfection, abnormal vaginal discharge.
   N — **N**ot feeling well; fever or chills.
   S — **S**tring missing (nonpalpable on vagi-

---

[a]Modified from Family Health International. *An example of OC use instructions for PPIs.* Research Triangle Park, NC: Family Health International, 1990.

[b]Modified from Hatcher RA, et al. *Contraceptive Technology: 1994–1995* (16th ed). New York: Irving Publishers, 1994.

■ **TABLE 7.1 Contraception**

Method	Action/Effectiveness	Advantages	Disadvantages and Side Effects
Hormonal Contraceptives Combination of estrogen and progesterone	Suppresses ovulation by suppressing production of FSH and LH *Most efficient* form of contraception (99.7%) if used consistently	■ Convenient; easy to take ■ Withdrawal bleeding cycles are predictable ■ Not related to sex act ■ Safe for older nonsmoking women until menopause ■ Many noncontraceptive health benefits	■ *Absolute contraindications,* e.g., thromboembolic or coronary artery disease, some cancers or liver disease ■ *Relative contraindications,* e.g., migraines, hypertension, immobility 4 wk or more, abnormal genital bleeding ■ Some decrease in glucose tolerance ■ Effectiveness decreased if taken during use of barbiturates, phenytoin, antibiotics ■ **No protection against STDs**
Estrogen only "Morning-after" pill: estrogen (diethylstilbestrol [DES]) in very high doses (25 mg)	Antifertility; taken within 72 h of unprotected coitus during fertile period	■ Available, prn	■ Because of DES effect on fetus, elective abortion advised if method fails
Progestin only Minipill (0) qd Depo-Provera (IM) q3–6mo Norplant (subdermal) up to 5 yr	Impairs fertility Thickens cervical mucus; decreases sperm penetration Alters endometrial maturation *Effectiveness:* Undetermined; can reach 100% reliability if used exactly as prescribed	■ (0) convenient, easy to take ■ (IM) 2–4 times a yr; lactation OK during this time ■ Subdermal, long term; not related to sex	■ Ovulation may occur ■ Irregular bleeding ■ May change glucose and insulin values ■ **No protection against STDs**
Intrauterine Devices (IUDs) Small T-shaped device inserted into uterine cavity Medicated: ■ Copper ■ Progesterone	Prevents fertility Recommended for women who have had at least one child Damages sperm in transit to fallopian tube Alters cervical mucus and endometrial maturation *Effectiveness* rate: 90–99%	■ Can be used by women who cannot use hormonal contraception; no disruption of ovulation pattern ■ Can be used effectively for 10 yr (Copper) ■ Change every yr (Progesterone) ■ Less blood loss during menses and decreases primary dysmenorrhea	■ *Contraindications:* history of PID, pregnancy, undiagnosed genital bleeding, genital malignancy, abnormal uterine cavity ■ *Risks:* uterine perforation, infection (may be followed by PID) in the first 3 mo of insertion; unnoticed expulsion ■ *Side effects* (especially with copper-T): heavy flow, spotting between periods, and cramping within first few mo of insertion ■ Must check for string after each menses and before intercourse ■ **No protection against STDs**
Mechanical Barriers Diaphragm: shallow rubber device that fits over cervix	Barrier preventing sperm from entering cervix (if it is correct size, undamaged, correctly placed, and is used with spermicide) *Effectiveness:* 83–90%; 99% in highly motivated women	■ Does not interupt sex act, except to add spermicide just before act ■ Insert up to 6 h before intercourse and leave in place for 6 h after last intercourse, but not longer than 24 h[b] ■ Safe: no side effects from well-fitted device if woman is not allergic to diaphragm or spermicide ■ Decreased incidence of vaginitis, cervicitis, PID	■ Requires careful cleansing with warm water and mild soap; powder with cornstarch, and store away from heat. Size/fit must be checked after term birth, second/third trimester abortion, weight gain or loss of 20 lb or more, or every 2 yr ■ Spermicide must be reinserted for additional acts that may follow after initial intercourse

continued

■ **TABLE 7.1**   *(Continued)*

Method	Action/Effectiveness	Advantages	Disadvantages and Side Effects
Mechanical Barriers (*continued*)			
Cervical cap: 1¼″ to 1½″ soft natural rubber dome with a firm but pliable rim	Physical barrier to sperm Spermicide inside cap adds a chemical barrier *Effectiveness* similar to that of diaphragm	■ Worn for 8 h but not longer than 48 h ■ No need to add spermicide for repeated acts of intercourse	■ Need a Pap smear every yr: higher rate of conversion from class I to class III[c] ■ If in place over 48 h, it produces an odor and might be associated with TSS[b] ■ Cannot be worn during menstrual flow (menses) or up to at least 6 wk postpartum ■ *Contraindications:* abnormal Pap smear, hard to fit, history of TSS or genital infection, allergy ■ Change after genital surgery or birth, major change in weight ■ Must be checked each yr ■ **Does not protect against STDs**
Female condom: vaginal sheath of natural latex rubber with flexible rings at both the closed and the open ends	Barrier preventing sperm from entering vagina *Effectiveness* similar to other mechanical methods used with spermicide *Note:* Male and female condoms should not be used at the same time	■ Apply well in advance of intercourse; spermicide added just before intercourse ■ Heightens sensation for man ■ About as satisfying for both woman and man as intercourse without it ■ **Provides protection from STDs**	■ Cost ■ A new one must be used for every act of intercourse
Condom: thin, stretchable latex sheath to cover penis	Barrier preventing sperm from entering vagina, applied over erect penis before loss of preejaculatory drops and is held in place as penis is withdrawn Spermicidal foam, jelly,[a] or cream is also used *Effectiveness* rate: 64–98% when used with spermicide	■ Safety—no side effects ■ **Provides protection from spread of STDs** With spermicide (0.5 g of nonoxynol-9) added to interior or exterior surface, provides protection from STDs, including HIV	■ Check expiration date ■ Requires high motivation to use correctly/constantly ■ Must be properly applied and removed ■ Sheath may tear during intercourse
Chemical Barriers			
Spermicide: aerosol foams, foaming tablets, suppositories, creams, and films (C-Film)	Physical barrier to sperm penetration Chemical action of sperm (kills sperm) Nonoxynol-9 has a bacteriostatic action *Effectiveness* rate: 70–98% when used with diaphragm or condoms	■ Increases effectiveness of mechanical barriers ■ Ease of application. Aids lubrication of vagina ■ Requires no medical examination or prescription ■ May be used during lactation ■ Backup for missed oral contraceptive pills	■ Messy ■ Some people are allergic to preparations ■ Tabs or suppositories take 10–15 min to dissolve ■ If it is only method being used, each intercourse should be preceded (by 30 min) by a fresh application. May be allergenic
Other Methods			
Natural family planning: BBT each morning before any physical activity Symptothermal variation: BBT plus cervical mucus changes Calendar method Predictor test for ovulation	Requires sexual abstinence during woman's fertile period (4 d before ovulation), and for 3 or 4 d after ovulation *Effectiveness:* about 80%	Physically safe to use—no drugs or appliances are used. Meets requirements of most religions	■ Effectiveness depends on high level of motivation and diligence ■ Requires fairly predictable menstrual cycle

[a]Spermicide provides lubrication, but if additional lubrication is needed, use water-based products only, e.g., K-Y jelly.
[b]TSS: toxic shock syndrome. Although there is no direct link between TSS and use of the diaphragm or cervical cap, a possible association remains (see p. 392).
[c]Class I Pap smear: no abnormal cells; Class III Pap smear: suspicious abnormal cells present.

■ **TABLE 7.2 Sterilization**

Action/Effectiveness	Advantages	Disadvantages and Side Effects
Male		
Vas deferens is occluded (ligated and severed; bands; clips) to prevent passage of sperm	■ Relatively simple surgical procedure ■ Does not affect endocrine function, production of testosterone ■ Does not alter volume of ejaculate ■ Tubal reconstruction possible (90%)	■ Sterility is not immediate. Sperm are cleared from vas after about 15 ejaculations ■ Some men become impotent due to psychological response to procedure ■ Fertility after tubal reconstruction (40–60%)
Female ■ Both fallopian tubes are ligated and severed, or occluded with bands or clips to prevent passage of eggs; fulguration of the tubes at the cornu is most effective	■ Abdominal surgery utilizing 1-in incision and laparoscopy ■ Greater than 99.5% effective	■ Major surgery (if done by laparotomy) with possible complications of anesthesia, infection, hemorrhage, and trauma to other organs. Psychological trauma in some ■ Success rate for pregnancy after tubal reanastomosis is about 15%
■ Hysterectomy or oophorectomy or both	■ Abdominal or vaginal surgery ■ Absolute sterility	

nal self-examination, or not seen on speculum examination).

6. *Toxic Shock Syndrome* (TSS)
   a. Signs/symptoms
      (1) Fever of sudden onset—over 102°F (38.9°C).
      (2) Hypotension—systolic pressure <90 mm Hg; orthostatic dizziness; disorientation.
      (3) Rash—diffuse, macular erythroderma (resembling sunburn).
      (4) Sore throat; severe nausea, vomiting.
      (5) Copious vaginal discharge.
   b. Instructions for prevention
      (1) General
         (a) *Avoid* use of tampons, cervical caps, diaphragms, and contraceptive vaginal sponges during the postpartum period (6 wk).
         (b) Do not use any of the above if you have a history of TSS.
         (c) Call physician if you experience sudden onset of a high fever, vomiting, diarrhea, or skin rash.
         (d) Insert clean tampons and contraceptive devices with clean hands.
         (e) Remove within prescribed time limits.
      (2) Tampons
         (a) Change tampons every 3 to 6 h.
         (b) Do not use superabsorbent tampons.
         (c) For overnight protection, substitute other products such as sanitary napkins or minipads.
      (3) Diaphragm or cervical cap
         (a) *Avoid* use during your menstrual period.
         (b) Remove within 8 h after intercourse (diaphragm must be removed no later than 24 h; the cap, no later than 48 h).
      (4) Contraceptive vaginal sponge
         (a) Wet sponge with clean water only.
         (b) *Avoid* using the sponge during your menstrual period.
         (c) Leave in place no longer than 30 h (it is effective up to 24 h).
         (d) *Note:* Production of contraceptive sponge was suspended in 1994 because of increasingly stringent manufacturing requirements from the FDA.

◆ **D. Evaluation/outcome criteria:**
   1. Woman avoids or achieves a pregnancy as desired.
   2. Woman expresses comfort and satisfaction with method selected.

II. Infertility
   A. Definition: inability to conceive after 1 yr of unprotected intercourse.
   B. Pathophysiology: contributing factors—hormonal deficiencies, reproductive system disorders, congenital anomalies, male impotence, sexual knowledge deficit, debilitating disease.
◆ **C. Assessment:**
   1. History—general health, reproduction, social history.
   2. Maternal diagnosis
      a. BBT.
      b. Endocrine studies.
      ▲ c. Sims-Huhner (postcoital).
      ▲ d. Rubins (tubal patency).
      ▲ e. Hysterosalpingogram (tubal patency).

3. Male diagnosis—history, physical examination, laboratory studies, e.g., semen analysis.
◆ **D. Analysis/nursing diagnosis:** *altered sexuality* related to infertility.
◆ **E. Nursing care plan/implementation:**
1. Provide emotional support.
2. Explain testing procedures for diagnosis.
3. Assist with referral process.
◆ **F. Evaluation/outcome criteria:**
1. The couple conceives, or,
2. If the couple does not conceive, they accept referral for help with adoption, other reproductive alternatives, or childlessness.

III. **Interruption of Pregnancy**—also known as elective, voluntary, or therapeutic abortion. Once the diagnosis of pregnancy and the length of gestation are established, the woman faces the decision to interrupt or to maintain the pregnancy (Table 7.3).
A. Decision-making stage:
◆ 1. **Assessment:**
a. Health history:
(1) Determine woman's feelings about the pregnancy, reasons for considering abortion, level of maturity; if decision was already made before she came to clinic, how was decision made? Does she have a support system?
(2) Identify factors influencing/complicating her decisions (religious beliefs, cultural mores, peer and family pressures).
(3) Information needs.
b. Physical examination.
🧪 c. Laboratory tests: blood type, Rh, hemoglobin, hematocrit, urinalysis, pregnancy test, antibody titer, other tests dependent on her health status.
◆ 2. **Analysis/nursing diagnosis:**
a. *Ineffective coping* related to emotional conflicts associated with need for decision to continue/terminate pregnancy.
b. *Altered family process* related to intrafamily conflict associated with need for/decision to continue/terminate pregnancy.
c. *Anticipatory grieving* related to loss of pregnancy/child.
d. *Altered self-concept, self-esteem disturbance* related to possible guilt feelings related to pregnancy/termination.
e. *Knowledge deficit* related to available options.
◆ 3. **Nursing care plan/implementation:**
a. Goal: *emotional support* to minimize impact on self-image and self-esteem.
(1) Maintain accepting, nonjudgmental attitude.

(2) Encourage verbalization of feelings, perceptions, and values.
(3) Support woman's decision.
b. Goal: *health teaching* to facilitate informed decision making.
(1) Explain and discuss available options as applicable (see Table 7.3).
(2) Describe procedure selected and what to expect after procedure.
c. Goal: *minimize impact on intrafamily relations, family process.* Where applicable, encourage open communication between deciding partners.
◆ 4. **Evaluation/outcome criteria:**
a. Woman states she understands all information necessary to give consent.
b. Woman expresses comfort and satisfaction with the decision.
B. Preoperative period
◆ 1. **Assessment:**
a. Reassess woman's emotional and physical status and current feelings regarding decision.
b. Determine woman's current knowledge/understanding of authorization form, anticipated procedure, and consequences (informed consent).
c. Monitor woman's physiologic and (if awake) psychological response to procedure.
◆ 2. **Analysis/nursing diagnosis:**
a. *Anxiety/fear* related to procedure, potential complications
b. *Knowledge deficit* related to ongoing procedure, sights, sounds, and sensations experienced.
◆ 3. **Nursing care plan/implementation:**
a. Goal: *provide opportunity to reconsider decision regarding termination of pregnancy.*
(1) Check to ensure all required permission (informed consent) forms have been signed/filed.
(2) Refer to physician if woman is ambivalent or insecure in decision.
b. Goal: *reduce anxiety/fear related to procedure.*
(1) Explain all anticipated preoperative, operative, and postoperative care.
(2) Assist with procedure;* if woman is awake, explain what is happening and what she may be experiencing.
c. Goal: *emotional support* to facilitate effective coping.
(1) Encourage verbalization of feelings, fears, concerns.
(2) Support woman's decision.

---

*"Conscience" clauses allow nurses to refuse to assist with procedures that go against their moral, religious, or medical judgment.

■ **TABLE 7.3 Interruption of Pregnancy (Elective/Voluntary Abortion)**

Method	Advantages	Disadvantages and Side Effects
First-Trimester Procedures		
Menstrual extraction—aspiration of endometrium through undilated cervix	Performed for women who have not yet missed a menstrual period 100% effective if implantation site is not missed	Cervical trauma may occur and may lead to incompetent cervix Hemorrhage
RU 486 (mifepristone)—a progesterone antagonist; taken up to 5 wk after conception	Prevents implantation of fertilized egg Most effective in early gestation, during luteal phase, within 10 d of first missed period Softens cervix	Slight nausea and fatigue during period of bleeding Uterine aspiration may be needed if RU 486 does not work Controversy of use continues
Uterine aspiration (vacuum or suction curettage)—cannula suction under local anesthesia, following cervical dilatation, usually with laminaria tent	Relatively few complications—minimal bleeding, minimal discomfort Outpatient basis	Performed after one or two missed menstrual periods Cervical or endometrial trauma possible
Surgical D & C—cervix dilated with laminaria tents; endometrium scraped with metal curette or flexible aspiration tip, under local anesthesia (paracervical block)	After cervix is dilated, procedure takes about 15 min Outpatient basis Relatively few complications (≤1%)—bleeding like a heavy period, some cramping	Performed after one or two missed periods Possible but rare: cervical trauma, uterine perforation, infection, hemorrhage
Second-Trimester Procedures		
Intraamniotic infusion between weeks 14 and 16. Transabdominal extraction of 200 mL amniotic fluid and replacement with equal amount of hypertonic NaCl (20%); or 30% urea in D5W	Does not require laparotomy Woman may ambulate until labor starts and during early labor Abortion completed within 36–40 h; ⅔ of fetuses are aborted in 24 h With urea: abortion usually occurs within 12 h; complications less common or serious than with NaCl	Complications increase proportionately with weeks of gestation Risks—*hypernatremia:* tinnitus, tachycardia, and headache *Water intoxication:* edema, oliguria (≤200 mL/8 h), dyspnea, thirst, and restlessness Hemorrhage and possible DIC; fever with sepsis Woman experiences labor May require D & C
Instillation of 40–45 mg prostaglandin F₂, E₂	Labor is usually shorter than with hypertonic NaCl Avoids complications of water intoxication and hypernatremia	May cause vomiting, diarrhea, nausea Fetus may be born alive
D & E (dilation and evacuation)—extends D & C and vacuum curettage up to 20 weeks' gestation	Woman does not experience labor Hospitalization is shortened With a skilled operator, complication rate is lower than with intraamniotic injection methods	Requires 3 d to dilate cervix; procedure done on third day
Second- and Third-Trimester Procedures		
Hysterotomy—cesarean delivery	Available for gestations more than 14–16 wk Preferred method if woman wishes a tubal ligation or hysterectomy to follow	*After:* major surgery complications—hemorrhage and infection possible Fetus may be born alive, causing ethical, moral, religious, and legal problems

◆ 4. **Evaluation/outcome criteria:** woman does not experience physiologic or psychological problems during procedure.

C. **Postoperative period**

◆ 1. **Assessment:**

   a. Monitor *physiologic* response to procedure (vital signs, blood loss, uterine cramping).

   b. Determine *psychological* response (happy, relieved; guilt feelings, lowered self-esteem).

   c. Determine desire for family planning information.

   d. Determine need for Rho (Dᵘ) immune globulin, *Rubella* vaccination

◆ 2. **Analysis/nursing diagnosis:**

   a. *Pain* related to procedure.

   b. *High risk for infection* related to lack of knowledge of postabortal self-care.

◆ 3. **Nursing care plan/implementation:**

   a. Goal: *provide and explain postoperative care.*

(1) Administer IV fluids.

(2) Administer medications prn for discomfort.

 (3) Administer oxytocic meds for uterine atony, prn.

(4) If *Rh-negative* mother, 8 or more weeks' gestation, and laboratory tests indicate no current sensitization (i.e., she is Coombs negative):

(a) Explain rationale for postabortion administration of Rho (D antigen) immune globulin (RhoGAM).

 (b) Administer RhoGAM, as ordered.

(5) Provide and explain perineal care

b. Goal: *health teaching* to facilitate active participation in own health maintenance, informed decision making, provide predischarge anticipatory guidance (also provide in written form with attention to woman's level of reading skill and understanding, and in her native language whenever possible):

(1) Immediately report any cramping, excessive bleeding, signs of infection.

(2) Provide name and telephone number of person to call if she has questions.

(3) Schedule a postabortal check-up.

(4) Discuss contraception, if woman indicates interest; or give her place and name to call for information later.

(5) Discuss resumption of tampon use (3 d to 3 wk as ordered) and sexual intercourse (1 wk to 3 wk as ordered).

(6) Discuss need to avoid douching.

◆ 4. **Evaluation/outcome criteria:**

a. Woman returns for postabortal appointment.

b. Woman suffers no adverse physical sequelae to the procedure.

c. Woman suffers no adverse psychological sequelae to the procedure.

d. Woman is successful in achieving her goal of either contraception or conception at the time she desires.

5. Postabortion psychological impact:

a. Majority—relieved and happy.

b. Small number (5–10%)—negative feelings, such as guilt or low self-esteem.

❏ Childbearing: Pregnancy by Trimester

General overview: This review of the normal physiologic and psychosocial changes occurring during each trimester of pregnancy provides essential components of the database for accurate nursing judgments and anticipatory guidance during the prenatal period. Complications of pregnancy are correlated with the trimester of common occurrence; relationships with other NCLEX categories of human function are described.

I. **General aspects of nursing care**

◆ A. **Assessment**—based on nursing knowledge of:

1. Biophysical and psychosocial aspects of conception and gestation.

2. Parameters of normal pregnancy.

3. Risk factors, signs, symptoms, and implications of deviations from normal patterns of maternal and fetal health.

◆ B. **Analysis/nursing diagnosis:**

1. *Knowledge deficit* related to normal pregnancy-related alterations (physiologic and emotional alterations/trimester).

2. *Pain* related to normal physiologic alterations in pregnancy.

3. *Altered elimination* related to normal physiologic changes during pregnancy (polyuria, constipation).

4. *Altered nutrition* related to increased metabolic needs due to pregnancy.

5. *Impaired adjustment* related to altered self-image; anticipated role change; resurgence of old, unresolved conflicts.

◆ C. **Nursing care plan/implementation:**

1. Goal: *emotional support.*

a. Encourage verbalization of feelings, fears, concerns.

b. Validate normalcy of behavioral response to pregnancy.

2. Goal: *anticipatory guidance.*

a. Facilitate achievement of developmental tasks.

b. Strengthen coping techniques for pregnancy, labor, birth. Suggest appropriate resources (preparation for childbirth classes).

3. Goal: *health teaching.* Describe, explain, discuss:

a. Normal physiologic alterations during pregnancy.

b. Common discomforts of pregnancy, management.

◆ D. **Evaluation/outcome criteria:**

1. Woman takes an active, informed part in her pregnancy-related care.

2. Woman copes effectively with common alterations associated with pregnancy (physiologic, psychological, role change).

3. Woman successfully carries an uneventful pregnancy to term.

II. **Biologic foundations of pregnancy**

A. **Conception**

1. *Egg*—life span, approximately 24 h after ovulation.

2. *Sperm*—life span, approximately 72 h after ejaculation into female reproductive tract.

3. *Conception* (fertilization)—usually occurs 12–24 h after ovulation, within fallopian tube.
4. *Implantation* (nidation)—usually occurs within 7 d of conception, or about day 21 of a 28-day menstrual cycle.
5. *Ovum*—period of conception until primary villi have appeared; usually about 12–14 d.
6. *Embryo*—period from end of ovum stage until measurement reaches approximately 3 cm; 54–56 d.
7. *Fetus*—period from end of embryo stage until birth.

First Trimester
Susceptible to teratogens
Heart functions at 3–4 wk
Eye formation at 4–5 wk
Arm and leg buds at 4–5 wk
Recognizable face at 8 wk
Brain: rapid growth
External genitalia at 8 wk
Placenta formed at 12 wk
Bone ossification at 12 wk
Second Trimester
Less danger from teratogens after 12 wk
Facial features formed at 16 wk
Fetal heartbeat heard by 18 to 20 wk with a stethoscope
Quickening at 18–20 wk
Length: 10 in., weight: 8–10 oz
Vernix: present
Third Trimester
Iron stored
Surfactant production begins in increasing amounts
Size: 15 in., 2–3 lb
Calcium stored at 28–32 wk
Reflexes present at 28–32 wk
Subcutaneous fat deposits at 36 wk
Lanugo shedding at 38–40 wk
Average size: 18–22 in., 7.5–8.5 lb at 38–40 wk

B. **Anatomic and physiologic modifications**
1. *Bases of functional alterations*
   a. *Hormonal*—Table 7.4 discusses the effects of estrogen and progesterone during pregnancy. Nursing implications provide the knowledge base for:
      (1) Anticipatory guidance regarding normal maternal adaptations.
      (2) Early identification of deviations from normal patterns.
   b. *Mechanical*—enlarging uterus → displacement and pressure; increased weight of uterus and breasts → changes in posture and pressure.
2. *Breasts*—enlarged darkened areola; secrete colostrum.
3. *Reproductive organs*
   a. *Uterus*

(1) Amenorrhea. Occasional spotting common, especially at time of first missed menstrual period.
(2) Increased vascularity adds to increase in size and softening of the lower uterine segment (*Hegar's sign*).
(3) Growth is due to hypertrophy and hyperplasia of existing muscle cells and connective tissue.
(4) Fundal height measurement landmarks:

Uterus	Nonpregnant	Pregnant (At Term)
Length	6.5 cm	32 cm
Width	4 cm	24 cm
Depth	2.5 cm	22 cm
Weight	50 g	1000 g

   b. *Cervix*
      (1) Increased vascularity → softening (*Goodell's sign*) and deepened blue-purple coloration (*Chadwick's sign*).
      (2) Edema, hyperplasia, thickening of mucous lining, and increased mucus production; formation of mucus plug by end of second month.
      (3) Becomes shorter, thicker, and more elastic.
   c. *Vagina*
      (1) Hyperemia deepens color (*Chadwick's sign*).
      (2) Hypertrophy and hyperplasia thicken vaginal mucosa.
      (3) Relaxation of connective tissue.
      (4) pH acidic (4.0–6.0).
      (5) Leukorrhea—nonirritating.
   d. *Perineum*
      (1) Increases in size—hypertrophy of muscle cells, edema, and relaxation of elastic tissue.
      (2) Deepened color—increased vascularization/hyperemia.
   e. *Ovaries*
      (1) Ovum production ceases.
      (2) Corpus luteum persists; produces hormones to wk 10–12 until placenta "takes over."
C. **Alterations affecting fluid-gas transport**
1. *Cardiovascular system* (Table 7.5)
   a. **Physiologic changes**
      (1) Heart displaced upward and to the left.
      (2) Circulation:
         (a) Cardiac volume increases by 20–30%.
         (b) Labor—cardiac output increases by 20–30%.
      (3) Hemoglobin and hematocrit values remain between 10–14 g and 35–42%; normal drop is 10% during second trimester.
      (4) Hypercoagulability—increased levels of blood factors VII, IX, and X.

■ **TABLE 7.4 Hormones of Pregnancy**

Primary Effects	Clinical Implications for Nursing Actions
Estrogen	
Level rises in serum and urine	Basis of test for maternal/placental/fetal well-being
Uterine development	Probable sign of pregnancy
Breast development	Probable sign of pregnancy; increased tingling, tenderness
Genital enlargement: increased vascularization, hyperplasia	Vaginal growth facilitates vaginal birth
Softens connective tissue	Results in backache and leg ache; relaxes joints to increase size of birth canal and rib cage
Alters nutrient metabolism:	*GI and metabolic changes:*
Decreases HCl and pepsin	Digestive upsets
Antagonist to insulin—makes glucose available to fetus	Anti-insulin effect challenges maternal pancreas to produce more insulin; failure of β-cells to respond leads to "gestational" diabetes. For the insulin-dependent woman, insulin requirements increase by an average of 67% during the second half of pregnancy
Supports fat deposition	Protect source of energy for fetus
Sodium and water retention; edema of lower extremities (nonpitting)	Meet increased plasma volume needs and maintain fluid reserve
Hematologic changes:	
Increased coagulability	Increased tendency to thrombosis
Increased sedimentation rate (SR)	SR loses diagnostic value for heart disease
Vasodilation: spider nevi; palmar erythema	Resolves spontaneously after birth
Increased production of melanin-stimulating hormone	Resolves spontaneously after birth
Progesterone	
Development of decidua	High levels result in tiredness, listlessness, and sleepiness
Reduces uterine excitability	Protection against abortion/early birth
Development of mammary glands	Prepares breasts for lactation
Alters nutrient metabolism:	*Nutritional significance:*
Antagonist to insulin	Diabetogenic
Favors fat deposition	Energy reserve
Decreases gastric motility and relaxes sphincters	Favors heartburn and constipation
Increased sensitivity of respiratory center to CO_2	Increased depth, some dyspnea, increased sighing
Decreased smooth-muscle tone:	*Decreased tone can lead to:*
Colon	Constipation
Bladder, ureters	Stasis of urine with infection
Veins	Dependent edema; varicosities
Gallbladder	Gallbladder disease
Increased basal body temperature (BBT) by 0.5°C	Discomfort from hot flashes and perspiration
Human Chorionic Gonadotropin	
Maintains corpus luteum during early pregnancy	Placenta must "take over" after a few wk
Stimulates male testes	Increased testosterone in male fetuses
May suppress immune response	May inhibit response to foreign protein, for example, fetal portion of placenta
	Diagnostic value:
	Basis for pregnancy test
	Hydatidiform mole
	Decreased level with threatened abortion
	Increased level with multiple pregnancy

continued

Maternal-Infant

■ **TABLE 7.4**   *(Continued)*

Primary Effects	Clinical Implications for Nursing Actions
Human Placental Lactogen	
Antagonizes insulin	Diabetogenic; may → gestational diabetes or complicate management of existing diabetes
Mobilizes maternal free fatty acids	Increased tendency to ketoacidosis in pregnant diabetic
Prolactin	
Suppressed by estrogen and progesterone	No milk produced before birth
Increased level after placenta is delivered	Milk production 2–3 d after birth
Follicle Stimulating Hormone	
Production suppressed during pregnancy; level returns to prepregnant levels within 3 wk after birth	No ovulation during pregnancy. Ovulation usually returns: within 6 wk for 15%, within 12 wk for 30%
Oxytocin	
Causes uterus to contract when the oxytocin levels exceed those of estrogen and progesterone	Labor induction or augmentation. Treatment for postpartum uterine atony

■ **TABLE 7.5   Blood Values**

Component	Prepregnant	Pregnant	Postpartum*
WBC	4–11,000	9–16,000 (25,000–labor)	20,000–25,000 within 10–12 d of birth, then returns to normal.
RBC volume	1600 mL	1900 mL	Prepregnant level of 1600 mL.
Plasma volume	2400 mL	3700 mL	Prepregnant level of 2400 mL.
Hct (PCV)	37–47%	32–42%	At 72°, returns to prepregnant level of 37–42%.
Hgb (at sea level)	12–16 g/dL	10–14 g/dL	At 72°, returns to prepregnant level of 12–16 g/dL.
Fibrinogen	250 mg/dL	400 mg/dL	At 72°, returns to prepregnant level of 250 mg/dL.

*Postpartum values depend on factors of amount of blood loss, mobilization, and physiologic edema (excretion of extravascular water). Normal blood loss for vaginal birth is 300–400 mL.

(5) Nonpathologic increased sedimentation rate—due to 50% increase in fibrinogen level.
(6) Blood pressure should remain stable with drop in second trimester.
(7) Heart rate often increases 10–15 beats/min at term.
(8) Compression of pelvic veins → stasis of blood in lower extremities.
(9) Compression of inferior vena cava when supine → bradycardia → reduced cardiac output, faintness, sweating, nausea (*supine hypotension*). *Fetal response:* marked bradycardia due to hypoxia secondary to decreased placental perfusion.

◆ b. **Assessment:**
(1) Apical systolic murmur.
(2) Exaggerated splitting of first heart sound.
(3) Physiologic anemia.
(4) Dependent edema in third trimester (Table 7.6).
(5) *Vena cava syndrome* (supine hypotension)—drop in systolic blood pressure may occur due to compression of descending aorta and inferior vena cava when supine.
(6) Varicosities (vulvar, anal, leg).

◆ c. **Nursing care plan/implementation:**
Goal: *health teaching*
(1) Elevate lower extremities frequently.
(2) Apply support hose.
(3) Avoid excess intake of sodium.
(4) Assume side-lying position at rest.
(5) Learn signs and symptoms of pregnancy-induced hypertension.

2. *Respiratory system*
   a. **Physiologic changes:**
   (1) Increased tidal volume, vital capacity, respiratory reserve, oxygen consumption, production of CO_2.
   (2) Diaphragm elevated, increased substernal angle → flaring of rib cage.
   (3) Uterine enlargement prevents maximum lung expansion in third trimester.

◆ b. **Assessment:**
   (1) Shortness of breath or dyspnea on exertion and when lying flat in third trimester.

■ **TABLE 7.6   Common Discomforts During Pregnancy**

Discomfort and Cause	Health Teaching
Morning sickness—first 3 mo; nausea and vomiting; may occur anytime, day or night; *cause:* hormonal, psychological, and empty stomach	Alternate dry carbohydrate and fluids hourly; take dry carbohydrate before rising, stay in bed 15 more minutes; *avoid* empty stomach, offending odors, and food difficult to digest (e.g., food high in fat)
Fatigue (sleep hunger)—first 3 mo; *cause:* possibly hormones. Often returns in late pregnancy when physical load is great	Iron supplement if anemic—foods high in *iron, folic acid,* and *protein.* Adequate rest
Fainting (syncope)—early pregnancy; due to slightly decreased arterial blood pressure; late pregnancy, due to venous stasis in lower extremities	Elevate feet; sit down when necessary. When standing, do not lock knees; *avoid* prolonged standing, fasting
Urinary frequency—enlarging uterus presses on bladder, turgescence of structures from hormone stimulation; relieved somewhat as uterus rises from pelvis; recurs with lightening	*Kegel exercises;* limit fluids just before bedtime to ensure rest. Rule out urinary tract infection
Vaginal discharge—mo 2–9; mucus less acidic, and increases in amount (leukorrhea)	Cleanliness important. Treat only if infection sets in; douche contraindicated in pregnancy
Hot flashes—heat intolerance, due to increased metabolism → diaphoresis	Alter clothing, bathing, and environmental temperature prn
Headache—cause unknown; possibly blood pressure change, nutritional, tension (unless associated with preeclampsia)	If pain relief needed, consult physician (avoid over-the-counter drugs without prescription). Reduce tension
Nasal stuffiness—due to increased vascularization; allergic rhinitis of pregnancy	Antihistamines and nasal sprays by *prescription only*
Heartburn—enlarging uterus and hormones slow digestion; progesterone → reverse peristaltic waves → reflux of stomach contents into esophagus	Physician may prescribe an antacid; *"flying exercise"; avoid* use of antacids containing sodium. Instead of leaning over, bend at the knees, keeping torso straight; sit on firm chairs; *limit fatty and fried* foods; small, frequent meals
Flatulence—altered digestion from enlarging uterus and hormones	Maintain regular bowel habits, *avoid* gas-forming foods. Antiflatulent may be prescribed
Insomnia—fetal movements, fears or concerns, and general body discomfort from heavy uterus	Medication by prescription only. Exercise; side-lying *positions* with pillow supports; change position often; back rubs, ventilate feelings
Shortness of breath—enlarging uterus limits expansion of diaphragm	Good posture; cut down/stop smoking; *position*—supine and upright
Backache—increased elasticity of connective tissue, increased weight of uterus, and increased lumbar curvature	Correct posture, low-heeled, wide-base shoes, and diet; do pelvic rock often; avoid fatigue
Pelvic joint pain—hormones relax connective tissue and joints and allow movement within joints	Rest; good posture; will go away after giving birth, in 6–8 wk
Leg cramps—pressure of enlarging uterus on nerve supplying legs; possible causes: lack of calcium, fatigue, chilling, and tension	Stretch affected muscle and hold until it subsides; *do not rub* (may release a blood clot, if present)
Constipation—decreased motility (hormones, enlarging uterus) and increased reabsorption of water; iron therapy (oral)	*Diet*—prunes, fruits, vegetables, roughage, and fluids; regular habits; exercise; sit on toilet with knees up. *Avoid* enemas, mineral oil, laxatives
Hemorrhoids—varicosities around anus; aggravated by pushing with stool and by uterus pressing on blood vessels supplying lower body	As above, *avoid* constipation. Pure Vaseline or Desitin is mild and sometimes soothing; use any other preparation with prescription only
Ankle edema—normal and nonpitting; gravity	Rest legs often during day with legs and hips raised
Varicose veins—lower legs, vulva, pelvis; pressure of heavy uterus; relaxation of connective tissue in vein walls; hereditary	Progressively worse with subsequent pregnancies and obesity; elevate legs above level of heart; support hose may help
Cramp in side or groin—round ligament pain; stretching of round ligament with cramping	To get out of bed, turn to side, use arm and upper body and push up to sitting position

    (2) Nasal stuffiness due to estrogen-induced edema (see Table 7.6).

    (3) Deeper respiratory excursion.

◆ c. **Nursing care plan/implementation:**
    Goal: *health teaching*

    (1) Sit and stand with good posture.

    (2) When resting assume *semi-Fowler's* position.

    (3) Avoid overdistention of stomach.

D. Alterations affecting elimination

1. *Urinary system*
   a. **Physiologic changes**
      (1) Relaxation of smooth muscle results in conditions that can persist 4–6 wk after birth:
         (a) Dilatation of ureters.
         (b) *Decreased* bladder tone.
         (c) Increased potential for urinary stasis and *infection* (UTI).
      (2) *Increased* glomerular filtration rate (50%) during last two trimesters.
      (3) *Increased* renal plasma flow (25–50%) during first two trimesters; returns to near normal levels by end of last trimester.
      (4) *Increased* renal-tubular reabsorption rate—compensates for increased glomerular activity.
      (5) Glycosuria common—reflects kidney's inability to reabsorb all glucose filtered by glomeruli (urine glucose not reliable index of diabetic status during pregnancy).
      (6) *Increased* renal clearance of urea and creatinine (creatinine clearance used as test of renal function during pregnancy).
      (7) Hormone-induced turgescence of bladder and pressure on bladder from gravid uterus (see Table 7.6).
   b. **Assessment:**
      (1) Urinary frequency, first and third trimesters (see Table 7.6).
      (2) Nocturia.
      (3) Stress incontinence in third trimester.
   c. **Nursing care plan/implementation:**
      Goal: *health teaching*
      (1) Void with urge to prevent bladder distention.
      (2) Learn signs and symptoms of UTI.
      (3) Decrease fluid intake in late evening.
      (4) Perform *Kegel* exercises to reduce incontinence.
2. *Gastrointestinal system* (see Table 7.6)
   a. **Physiologic changes**
      (1) General decrease in smooth-muscle tone and motility due to actions of progesterone.
      (2) *Intestines:* slowed peristalsis, increased water reabsorption in bowel.
      (3) *Stomach*
         (a) Gastric emptying time is delayed (e.g., 3 h vs. 1½ h).
         (b) Gastric secretion of HCl and pepsin decreases.
         (c) Decreased motility delays emptying; increased acidity.
      (4) *Cardiac sphincter* relaxes.
      (5) Increasing size of *uterus* and displacement of *intraabdominal organs*.
      (6) *Gallbladder:* decreased emptying.

   b. **Assessment**
      (1) Nausea and vomiting in first trimester.
      (2) Constipation and flatulence.
      (3) Hemorrhoids.
      (4) Heartburn, reflux esophagitis, indigestion.
      (5) Hiatal hernia.
      (6) Epulis—edema and bleeding of gums.
      (7) Ptyalism—excessive salivation.
      (8) Jaundice.
      (9) Gallstones.
      (10) Pruritus due to increased retention of bile salts.
   c. **Nursing care plan/implementation:**
      Goal: *health teaching*
      (1) Nausea and vomiting
         (a) *Avoid* fatty food; increase carbohydrates.
         (b) Eat small, frequent meals.
         (c) Eat dry crackers in A.M.
         (d) *Decrease* liquids with meals.
         (e) *Avoid* odors that predispose to nausea.
      (2) Constipation and flatulence
         (a) *Increase* fluids (6–8 glasses/d).
         (b) Maintain exercise regimen.
         (c) Add *fiber* to diet.
         (d) *Avoid* mineral oil laxatives.
         (e) *Avoid* gas-producing foods (i.e., beans, cabbage).
      (3) Heartburn and indigestion
         (a) *Eliminate* fatty or spicy foods.
         (b) Eat small, frequent meals (6/d).
         (c) Eat slowly.
         (d) *Avoid* gastric irritants (i.e., alcohol, coffee).
         (e) Perform "flying exercises."
         (f) *Avoid* lying flat.
         (g) Take antacids without sodium or phosphorus.
         (h) Sip milk or eat yogurt if heartburn occurs.
         (i) *Avoid* sodium bicarbonate.
      (4) Hemorrhoids
         (a) Increase *fluid and fiber* intake.
         (b) Maintain exercise regimen.
         (c) *Avoid* constipation and straining to defecate.
         (d) Take warm sitz baths.
         (e) Apply witch hazel pads.
         (f) Elevate hips and legs frequently.
         (g) Use hemorrhoidal ointments only with advice of health care provider.
E. **Alterations affecting nutrition**
   1. **Physiologic changes**
      a. *Gastrointestinal system*
         (1) Gingivae soften and enlarge due to increased vascularity.
         (2) Increased saliva production.

b. *Endocrine system*
(1) *Increased* size and activity of pituitary, parathyroids, adrenals.
(2) *Increased* vascularity and hyperplasia of thyroid.
(3) Pancreas—*increased* insulin production during second half of pregnancy, needed to meet rising maternal needs; placental HPL and insulinase deactivate maternal insulin; may precipitate *gestational diabetes* in susceptible women.

c. *Metabolism*
(1) Basal metabolic rate (BMR)—*increases* 25% as pregnancy progresses, due to increasing oxygen consumption; protein-bound iodine (PBI) *increases* to 7–10 μg/dL; metabolism returns to normal by sixth postpartal week.
(2) Protein—need *increased* for fetal and uterine growth, maternal blood formation.
(3) Water retention—*increased.*
(4) Carbohydrates—need *increases* to spare protein stores.
   (a) *First half of pregnancy*—glucose rapidly and continuously siphoned across placenta to meet fetal growth needs; may lead to hypoglycemia and faintness.
   (b) *Second half of pregnancy*—placental production of antiinsulin hormones; normal maternal hyperglycemia; affects coexisting diabetes.
(5) Fat—*increased* plasma-lipid levels.
(6) Iron—supplements recommended to meet *increased* need for red blood cells (RBCs) by maternal/placental/fetal unit.

◆ 2. **Assessment:**
a. Weight gain: 20–30 lb (average gain, 24 lb).
b. Normal pattern: first trimester, 1 lb/mo; remainder of gestation, 0.9–1 lb/wk.

◆ 3. **Nursing care plan/implementation:**
Goal: *health teaching*
a. Evaluate diet for adequacy of nutrient and caloric intake.
b. Evaluate cultural, religious, and economic influences on diet.
c. Review dietary recommendation for pregnancy with woman.
d. *Avoid* dieting in pregnancy (even if obese).
e. Supplement diet with *vitamins, iron,* or *folic acid* on advice of health provider.
f. *Ptyalism:*
   (1) Suck hard candies.
   (2) Perform frequent oral hygiene.
(3) Maintain adequate oral intake (6–8 glasses/d).
(4) Use lip balm to prevent chapping.
g. *Epulis:*
   (1) Frequent oral hygiene.
   (2) Use soft toothbrush.
   (3) Floss gently.
   (4) See dentist regularly.

F. **Alterations affecting protective functions**—*integumentary system*
1. **Physiologic changes**—estrogen-induced vascular and pigment changes.

◆ 2. **Assessment:**
a. Increased pigmentation.
b. Striae gravidarum (stretch marks).
c. Increased sebaceous and sweat gland activity.
d. Palmar erythema.
e. Angiomas—vascular "spiders."

◆ 3. **Nursing care plan/implementation:**
Goal: *health teaching*
a. Bathe or shower daily.
b. Reassure woman that skin changes decrease after pregnancy.

G. **Alterations affecting comfort, rest, mobility**—*musculoskeletal system*
1. **Physiologic changes**
a. Progesterone, estrogen, and relaxin-induced relaxation of joints, cartilage, and ligaments.
b. Function in childbearing—increases anteroposterior diameter of rib cage and enlarges birth canal.

◆ 2. **Assessment:**
a. Complaint of pelvic "looseness."
b. Duck-waddle walk.
c. Tenderness of symphysis pubis.
d. Lordosis (exaggerated lumbar curve)—*increased* weight of pelvis tilts pelvis forward; to compensate, woman throws head and shoulders backward; complaint of leg and back strain and fatigue (see Table 7.6)

◆ 3. **Nursing care plan/implementation:**
Goal: *health teaching*
a. Good body alignment—tuck pelvis under; tighten abdominal muscles.
b. Pelvic-rock exercises.
c. Squat; bend at knees, *not* at waist.
d. Wear low-heeled, sturdy shoes.
e. *Avoid* tight-fitting clothing that interferes with circulatory return in legs.

III. **Psychosocial-cultural alterations**
A. *Emotional changes*—affected by age, maturity, support system, amount of current stresses, coping abilities, physical and mental health status. *Developmental tasks of pregnancy:*
1. Accept the pregnancy as real: "I am pregnant"; progress from symbiotic relationship with the fetus to perceiving the child as an individual.

2. Seek and ensure acceptance of child by others.
3. Seek protection for self and fetus through pregnancy and labor ("safe passage").
4. Prepare realistically for the coming child and for necessary role change: "I am going to be a parent."

B. *Physical bases of changes*
   1. *Increased* metabolic demands may result in anemia and fatigue.
   2. *Increased* hormone levels (steroids, estrogen, progesterone)—affect mood as well as physiology.

C. *Characteristic behaviors*—Table 7.7 describes behaviors commonly exhibited in each trimester.

D. *Sexuality and sexual expression*—feelings and expressions of sexuality may vary during pregnancy due to maternal adaptations.

E. *Intrafamily relationships*
   1. Pregnancy is a maturational crisis for the family.
   2. Requires changes in life-style and interactions:
      a. Increased financial demands.
      b. Changing family and social relationships.
      c. Adapting communication patterns.
      d. Adapting sexual patterns.

e. Anticipating new responsibilities and needs.
f. Responding to reactions of others.

Prenatal Management

◆ **I. Initial assessment:** Goal: *establish baseline for health supervision, teaching, emotional support, or referral.*

II. Objectives:
   A. Determine woman's present health status and validate pregnancy.
   B. Identify factors affecting or affected by pregnancy.
   C. Describe current gravidity and parity.
   D. Identify present length of gestation.
   E. Establish an estimated date of birth (EDB). Nägele's determination of EDB—subtract 3 mo, add 7 d to LMP.
   F. Determine relevant knowledge deficit.

◆ **III. Assessment:** *history*
   A. *Family*—inheritable diseases, reproductive problems.
   B. *Personal*—medical, surgical, gynecologic, past obstetric, average nonpregnant weight.
      1. *Gravida*—a pregnant woman.
         a. *Nulligravida*—woman who has *never* been pregnant.
         b. *Primigravida*—woman with a *first* pregnancy.

■ **TABLE 7.7   Behavioral Changes in Pregnancy**

Assessment/Characteristics	Nursing Care Plan/Implementation
First Trimester	
Emotional lability (mood swings)	Encourage verbalization of feelings, concerns
Displeasure with subjective symptoms of early pregnancy (nausea, fatigue, etc.)	Validate normalcy of feelings, behaviors
Feelings of ambivalence	*Health teaching:* diet, rest, relaxation, diversion
Second Trimester	
Accepts pregnancy (usually coincides with awareness of fetal movement, i.e., "quickening")	Encourage exploration of feelings of dependency, introspection, mood swings
Becomes introspective: resolves old conflicts (feelings toward mother, sexual intimacy, masturbation)	Discuss childbirth preparation and preparation-for-parenthood classes; refer, as necessary
Reevaluates self, life-style, marriage	
Daydreams, fantasizes self as "mother"	
Seeks out other pregnant women and new mothers	
Third Trimester	
Altered body image	Encourage verbalization of concerns, discomforts of late pregnancy
Fears body mutilation (stretching of body tissues, episiotomy, cesarean birth)	Help meet dependency needs; offer reassurance, as possible
Distress over loss of control over body functions (ptyalism, colostrum leakage, leukorrhea, urinary frequency, constipation, stress incontinence)	*Health teaching:* Kegel exercises; preparation for labor. Anticipatory guidance and planning for needs of self, baby, and family in early postpartum
Anxiety for baby (deformity, death)	
Fears pain, loss of control in labor	
Acceptance of impending labor during last 2 wk (ready to "move on")	

c. *Multigravida*—woman with a *second or later* pregnancy.

2. *Para*—refers to *past pregnancies* (not number of babies) that reached viability (20–22 wk) (whether or not born alive).

   a. *Nullipara*—woman who has *not* carried a pregnancy to viability; e.g., may have had one or more abortions.

   b. *Primipara*—woman who has carried *one* pregnancy to viability.

   c. *Multipara*—woman who had *two or more* pregnancies that reached viability.

   d. *Grandmultipara*—woman who has had *six or more* viable pregnancies.

3. *Examples of gravidity / parity.* Several methods of describing gravidity and parity are in common use. One method (GTPAL) describes number of "*G*ravida" (pregnancies), *T*erm (or full-term infants), *P*reterm infants, *A*bortions, and number of *L*iving children.

   a. A woman who is pregnant for the *first* time and is currently *undelivered* is designated as 1-0-0-0-0. *After* giving birth to a full-term living neonate, she becomes 1-1-0-0-1.

   b. If a woman's second pregnancy ends in abortion and she has a living child from a previous pregnancy, born at term, she is designated as 2-1-0-1-1.

   c. A woman who is pregnant for the fourth time and whose previous pregnancies yielded one full-term neonate, premature twins, and one abortion (spontaneous or induced), and who now has three living children, may be designated as 4-1-1-1-3.

   d. Others record as follows: number gravida/number para. Applying this system to the examples given above, those mothers would be designated as follows: a—G1P1; b—G2P1; c—G4P2.

   e. Others include recording of abortions:
   G1P1 Ab0
   G2P1 Ab1
   G4P2 Ab1

◆ **IV. Assessment:** *initial physical aspects:*

  A. Height and weight.

  B. Vital signs.

  C. Blood work—hematocrit and hemoglobin for anemia; type and Rh factor; tests for sickle cell trait, syphilis, and rubella antibody titer (see also Table 7.5).

  D. Urinalysis—glucose, protein, acetone, signs of infection, and pregnancy test (HCG).

  E. Breast examination.

  F. Pelvic examination.

   1. Signs of pregnancy.

   2. Adequacy of pelvis and pelvic structures.

   3. Size and position of uterus.

   4. Papanicolau smear.

   5. Smears for monilial and trichomonal infections.

6. Signs of pelvic inflammatory disease.

7. Tests for STD: GC, chlamydia.

G. *Validation of pregnancy*—physician or midwife makes differential diagnosis between presumptive/probable signs/symptoms of early pregnancy and other signs.

  1. *Presumptive symptoms*—subjective experiences.

   a. Amenorrhea—more than 10 d past missed menstrual period.

   b. Breast tenderness, enlargement.

   c. Nausea and vomiting.

   d. Quickening (wk 16–18).

   e. Urinary frequency.

   f. Fatigue.

   g. Constipation (50% of women).

  2. *Presumptive signs*

   a. Striae gravidarum, linea nigra, chloasma (after wk 16).

   b. Increased basal body temperature (BBT)

  3. *Probable signs*—examiner's objective findings.

   a. Positive pregnancy test.

   b. Enlargement of abdomen/uterus.

   c. Reproductive organ changes (after sixth week):

    (1) *Goodell's sign*—cervical softening.

    (2) *Hegar's sign*—softening of lower uterine segment.

    (3) Vaginal changes (*Chadwick's sign*): purple hue in vulvar/vaginal area.

   d. Ballottement (after 16–20 wk).

   e. *Braxton-Hicks* contractions.

  4. *Positive signs of pregnancy:*

   ▶ a. Fetal heart tones.

    (1) Doptone: wk 10–12.

    (2) Fetoscope: wk 20.

   b. Examiner visualizes and feels fetal movements (usually after wk 24).

   c. Sonographic examination (after wk 14) when fetal head is sufficiently developed for accurate diagnosis.

◆ **V. Assessment:** *nutritional status:*

  A. Physical findings suggesting poor nutritional status:

   1. Skin: rough, dry, scaly.

   2. Lips: lesions in corners.

   3. Hair: dull, brittle.

   4. Mucous membranes: pale.

   5. Dental caries.

  B. Height, weight, age—average weight gain approximately 24 lb. Range from 24 to 32 lb is best for mother and neonate.

  C. Laboratory values—Hemoglobin: <10.5/100 mg. Hct: <32% indicates anemia.

  D. Nutrition history.

◆ **E. Analysis/nursing diagnosis:**

   1. *Altered nutrition: less than body requirements* related to anemia, vitamin/mineral deficit.

2. *Altered nutrition: more than body re-quirements* related to obesity.

◆ **F. Nursing care plan/implementation:**
Goal: *health teaching.* Nutritional counseling for diet in pregnancy and/or lactation.

◆ **G. Evaluation/outcome criteria:**
1. If *underweight* at conception: should gain more than 24 lb.
2. If *obese* at conception: should gain approximately 24 lb; dieting contraindicated.

◆ **VI. Assessment:** *psychosocial aspects:*
A. Pregnancy: planned or not; desired or not.
B. Present plans:
1. Carry pregnancy, keep baby.
2. Carry pregnancy, adoption.
3. Abortion.
C. Cultural, ethnic influences on decisions: will influence range of activities, types of safeguarding actions, diet, and health-promotion behaviors.
D. Parenting potential: actively seeking medical care and information about pregnancy, childbirth, parenthood.
E. Family readiness for childbearing/childrearing:
1. Physical maintenance.
2. Allocation of resources: identify support system.
3. Division of labor.
4. Socialization of family members.
5. Reproduction, recruitment, launching of family members into society.
6. Maintenance of order (relationships within family).
F. Perceptions of present and projected family relationships.
G. Review life-style for smoking, drugs, alcohol (ETOH), attitudes to pregnancy, and health care practices.

◆ **VII. Analysis/nursing diagnosis:**
A. *Altered role performance* related to stress imposed by developmental tasks.
B. *Ineffective coping: individual, family* related to stress caused by developmental tasks/crises.
C. *Altered family process* related to developmental tasks. First baby may precipitate individual or family developmental crisis.

◆ **VIII. Nursing care plan/implementation:**
A. Goal: *anticipatory guidance/support.*
1. Discuss mood swings, ambivalent feelings, negative feelings.
2. Reinforce "normalcy" of such feelings.
B. Goal: *increase individual/family coping skills, reduce intrafamily stress.*
1. Reinforce family strengths (both partners), sense of family identity.
a. Encourage open communication between partners; share feelings and concerns.

b. Increase understanding of mutual needs, encourage mutuality of support.
c. Increase tendency of mother to turn to partner as most significant person (as opposed to physician).
d. Enhance bond, success of childbirth preparation classes.
2. Promote understanding/acceptance of role change.
a. Facilitate/support achievement of developmental tasks.
b. Reduce probability of postpartal psychological problems.
c. Promote family bonding.
C. Goal: *health teaching.*
1. *Siblings:*
a. Alert parents to sibling needs for security, love.
b. Include sibling in pregnancy experience.
c. Provide clear, simple explanations of happenings.
d. Continue demonstrations of love.
e. Describe increased status ("big sister/brother").
f. Discuss possible misbehavior to gain attention.
2. *Relatives:* alert parents to possible negative feelings of in-laws.
3. Referral to childbirth preparation/parenting classes.
4. Appropriate community referrals for financial relief to decrease stress and provide aid.

◆ **IX. Evaluation/outcome criteria:**
A. Actively participates in pregnancy-related decision making.
B. Expresses satisfaction with decisions made.
C. Demonstrates growth and development in parenting role.
D. Prepared for the birth and for early parenthood.

Antepartum

I. Nursing care and obstetric support
A. **General aspects of prenatal management**
1. *Scheduled visits:*
a. Once monthly—until wk 32.
b. Every 2 wk—wk 32–36.
c. Weekly—wk 36 until labor.
◆ 2. **Assessment:**
a. General well-being, signs of deviations, concerns, questions.
b. Weight gain pattern.
c. Blood pressure (right arm, sitting).
d. Abdominal palpation:
(1) Fundal height; tenderness, masses, hernia.
(2) Fetal heart rate (FHR).

    (3) Leopold's maneuvers for presentation (after wk 32).

e. Laboratory tests:

    (1) Urinalysis—for protein, sugar, signs of asymptomatic infection.

    (2) Venous blood—for Hgb, Hct; done initially: VDRL, anti-Rh titer, sickle cell. HIV recommended for high-risk groups.

    (3) Cultures (vaginal discharge; cervical scrapings, for *Chlamydia trachomatis*) prn.

    (4) Tuberculosis screening in high-risk areas.

    (5) Maternal alpha-fetoprotein screen, 16–18 wk optimum time.

    (6) Serum-glucose screen, 24–28 wk.

f. Follow-up on medications (vitamins, iron) and nutrition.

B. Common minor discomforts during pregnancy (for **Assessment,** see Table 7.6, p. 399.)

1. **Etiology:** normal maternal physiologic/psychological alterations in pregnancy.

◆ 2. **Nursing care plan/implementation:**

a. Goal: *anticipatory guidance.* Discuss the importance of adequate rest, exercise, diet, and hydration in minimizing symptoms.

b. Goal: *health teaching* (see Table 7.6).

◆ 3. **Evaluation/outcome criteria:** woman avoids, minimizes, or copes effectively with minor usual discomforts of pregnancy.

C. Danger signs:

1. **Etiology:** Specific disease processes are discussed under Complications, below.

◆ 2. **Nursing care plan/implementation:**

Goal: *health teaching*—to safeguard status. Signs to report *immediately:*

a. Persistent vomiting beyond first trimester or severe vomiting at any time. *Possible cause:* Hyperemesis gravidarum

b. Fluid discharge from vagina—bleeding or amniotic fluid (anything other than leukorrhea). *Possible causes:* Placental problem, rupture of membranes (ROM)

c. Severe or unusual pain: abdominal. *Possible cause:* Abruptio placentae

d. Chills or fever. *Possible cause:* Infection

e. Burning on urination. *Possible cause:* UTI

f. Absence of fetal movements after quickening. *Possible cause:* Intrauterine fetal death

g. Visual disturbances—blurring, double vision, "spots before eyes." *Possible cause:* Preeclampsia

h. Swelling of fingers or face. *Possible cause:* Preeclampsia

i. Severe, frequent, or continual headache. *Possible cause:* Preeclampsia

j. Muscle irritability or convulsions. *Possible cause:* Preeclampsia

◆ 3. **Evaluation/outcome criteria:**

a. Actively participates in own health maintenance/pregnancy management.

b. Identifies early signs of potentially serious complications during the antepartal period.

c. Promptly reports and seeks medical attention.

II. Complications during the antepartum

A. General aspects:

1. **Etiology:**

a. Normal alterations and increasing physiologic stress of pregnancy affect status of coexisting medical disorders.

b. Conditions affecting mother's general health also affect ability to adapt successfully to normal physiologic stress of pregnancy.

c. Aberrations of normal pregnancy.

2. Goal: *reduce incidence of health problems affecting maternal/fetal health and pregnancy outcome.*

a. Identify presence of risk factors and signs and symptoms of complications early.

b. Treat emerging complications promptly and effectively.

c. Minimize effects of complications on pregnancy outcome.

◆ 3. **Assessment:** risk factors:

a. Age:

    (1) Adolescent.

    (2) Primigravida, age 35 or older.

    (3) Multigravida, age 40 or older.

b. Socioeconomic level: lower.

c. Ethnic group

d. Previous pregnancy history:

    (1) Habitual abortion.

    (2) Multiparity greater than 5.

    (3) Previous stillbirths.

    (4) Previous cesarean birth.

    (5) Preterm labor.

e. Multifetal pregnancy.

f. Prenatal care:

    (1) Enters health care system late in pregnancy.

    (2) Irregular/episodic prenatal care visits.

    (3) Noncompliance with medical/nursing recommendations.

g. Preexisting or coexisting medical disorders:

    (1) Cardiovascular: hypertension, heart disease.

    (2) Diabetes.

    (3) Other: renal, respiratory, infections, acquired immunodeficiency syndrome (AIDS).

h. Substance abuse.

◆ 4. **Nursing care plan/implementation:**

a. Goal: *health teaching* (discussed under specific health problem).

b. Goal: *early identification/treatment of emerging health problems* (if any).

(1) Monitor status and progress of pregnancy.

(2) Refer for medical management, as necessary.

c. Goal: *emotional support.*

◆ 5. **Evaluation/outcome criteria:**

a. Understands present health status, interactions of coexisting disorder and pregnancy.

b. Accepts responsibility for own health maintenance.

c. Makes informed decisions regarding pregnancy.

d. Minimizes potential for complications of coexisting disorder/pregnancy.

(1) Avoids factors predisposing to health problems.

(2) Understands and implements therapeutic management of coexisting disorder/pregnancy.

(3) Increases compliance with medical/nursing recommendations.

e. Carries uneventful pregnancy to successful termination.

B. **Disorders affecting fluid-gas transport: cardiac disease**

1. **Pathophysiology:** cardiac overload → cardiac decompensation → right-sided failure → pulmonary edema.

2. **Etiology:**

a. Congenital heart defects.

b. Valvular damage—due to rheumatic fever (most common lesion is mitral stenosis, which can lead to pulmonary edema and emboli).

c. Increased circulating-blood volume and cardiac output—exceeds cardiac reserve. Greatest risk: *after 28 weeks' gestation*—reaches maximum (30–50%) volume increase; *postpartum*—due to diuresis.

d. Secondary to treatment (tx) (e.g., tocolysis and B methasone)

e. Pregnancy after valve replacement.

3. Normal physiologic alterations during pregnancy that *mimic cardiac disorders:*

a. Systolic murmurs, palpitations, tachycardia, and hyperventilation with some dyspnea on normal moderate exertion.

b. Edema of lower extremities.

c. Cardiac enlargement.

d. Elevated sedimentation rate near term.

◆ 4. **Assessment:**

a. Medical evaluation of cardiac status. Classification of severity of cardiac involvement.

(1) *Class I*—least affected; asymptomatic with ordinary activity.

(2) *Class II*—activities somewhat limited; ordinary activities cause fatigue, dyspnea, angina.

(3) *Class III*—moderate/marked limitation of activity; common activities result in severe symptoms of fatigue, etc.

(4) *Class IV*—most affected; symptomatic (dyspnea, angina) at rest; should avoid pregnancy.

b. **Cardiac decompensation:**

(1) *Subjective symptoms*

Palpitations; feeling that the heart is "racing"

Increasing fatigue or difficulty breathing, or both, with the usual activities

Feeling of smothering and/or frequent cough

Periorbital edema; edema of face, fingers (e.g., rings do not fit anymore), feet, legs

(2) *Objective signs*

Irregular weak, rapid pulse (≥100 beats/min)

Rapid respirations (≥25 breaths/min)

Progressive, generalized edema

Crackles (rales) at base of lungs, after two inspirations and exhalations

Orthopnea; increasing dyspnea on minimal physical activity

Moist, frequent cough

Cyanosis of lips and nailbeds

◆ 5. **Analysis/nursing diagnosis:**

a. *Fluid volume excess* related to inability of compromised heart to handle increased workload (decreased cardiac reserve → congestive heart failure).

b. *Impaired gas exchange* related to pulmonary edema secondary to congestive heart failure.

◆ 6. **Nursing care plan/implementation:**

a. *Medical management:*

(1) Diuretics, electrolyte supplements.

(2) Digitalis (dose may need to be higher because of dilution in the increased blood volume of pregnancy).

(3) Antibiotics—prophylaxis against rheumatic fever; treatment of bacterial infections during pregnancy.

(4) Anticoagulants. Heparin is preferred because its large molecule cannot easily cross placenta. Occasionally, sequelae may include maternal hemorrhage, preterm birth, stillbirth.

(5) Oxygen, as needed.

(6) Mitral valvotomy for mitral stenosis often brings dramatic relief.

b. Goal: *health teaching.*

(1) Need for compliance with therapeutic regimen, medical/nursing recommendations.

(2) Drug actions, dosage, necessary actions (how to take own pulse, reportable signs/symptoms).

(3) Methods for *decreasing work of heart:*

(a) Adequate *rest*—minimum 10 h sleep each night; ½ h nap after each meal.

(b) *Avoid* heavy physical *activity* (including housework), fatigue, excessive weight gain, emotional stress, infection.

(c) *Avoid situations* of reduced ambient O_2, such as smoking, exposure to pollutants, flight in unpressurized small planes.

c. Goal: *nutritional counseling.*

(1) Well-balanced *diet;* adequate protein, fresh fruits and vegetables, water.

(2) *Avoid* "junk food," stimulants (caffeine), excessive salt intake.

d. *Anticipatory planning:* management of **labor.**

(1) Goal: *minimize physiologic and psychological stress.*

(2) Medical management:

(a) Reevaluation of cardiac status before EDB and labor.

(b) Regional anesthesia for labor/birth.

(c) Low-outlet forceps birth; episiotomy.

◆ (3) **Assessment:** continuous.

(a) Physiologic response to labor stimuli—*frequent vital signs* (pulse rate most sensitive and reliable indicator of impending congestive heart failure).

(b) Color, respiratory effort, diaphoresis.

(c) Contractions, etc.—same as for any laboring mother.

◆ (4) **Nursing care plan/implementation:** *labor.*

(a) Goal: *safeguard status.*

(1) Report *promptly:* pulse rate over 100; respirations more than 24 between contractions.

(2) Oxygen at 6 liters, as needed.

(b) Goal: *emotional support*—to reduce anxiety, facilitate cooperation.

(1) Encourage verbalization of feelings, fears, concerns.

(2) Explain all procedures.

(c) Goal: *promote cardiac function. Position*—semirecumbent; support arms and legs.

(d) Goal: *promote relaxation/control over labor discomfort.* Encourage Lamaze (or other) breathing/relaxation techniques.

(e) Goal: *reduce stress on cardiopulmonary system.* Discourage bearing-down efforts.

(f) Goal: *relieve stress of pain, eliminate bearing-down.* Prepare for regional anesthesia.

(g) Goal: *maintain effective cardiac function.* Administer medications, as ordered (e.g., digitalis, diuretics, antibiotics).

e. *Anticipatory planning:* **postpartal** management.

(1) Factors increasing risk of cardiac decompensation:

(a) Delivery → rapid, decreased intraabdominal pressure → vasocongestion and rapid rise in cardiac output.

(b) Loss of placental circulation.

(c) Normal diuresis increases circulating blood volume.

◆ (2) **Assessment:**

(a) Observe for tachycardia or respiratory distress.

(b) Monitor blood loss, I&O—potential hypovolemic shock, cardiac overload due to diuresis.

(c) Pain level—potential neurogenic shock.

(d) Same as for any postpartum mother (fundus, signs of infection, etc.).

◆ (3) **Nursing care plan/implementation:** *postpartum.*

(a) Goal: *minimize stress on cardiopulmonary system.*

(1) Rest, dangle, ambulate with aid.

(2) Gradual increase in activity—as tolerated without symptoms.

(3) *Position,* semi-Fowler's if needed.

(4) Extra help with newborn care.

◆ (4) **Evaluation/outcome criteria:**

(a) Successfully carries uneventful pregnancy to term.

(b) Experiences no cardiopulmonary embarrassment during labor, birth, or postpartum.

C. **Disorders affecting fluid-gas transport in fetus: Rh incompatibility**

1. **Pathophysiology**—in an Rh-negative mother: Rh-positive fetal red blood cells enter the maternal circulation → maternal antibody formation → antibodies cross placenta and enter fetal bloodstream → attack fetal red blood cells → hemolysis → anemia, hypoxia.

a. The pregnant Rh-positive mother carries her infant (Rh negative *or* positive) without incident.

b. The pregnant Rh-negative mother carries an Rh-negative infant without incident.

c. The pregnant Rh-negative mother *usually* carries her first Rh-positive child without problems *unless* she has been sensitized by inadvertent transfusion with Rh-positive blood. *Note:* Fetal cells do not usually enter the maternal bloodstream until placental separation (at abortion, abruptio placentae, amniocentesis, or birth).

2. **Etiology**
   a. The Rh factor is an antigen on the red blood cells of some people (these people are Rh positive); the Rh factor is dominant; a person may be homozygous or heterozygous for Rh factor.
   b. An Rh-negative person is homozygous for this recessive trait—does *not* carry the antigen; develops antibodies when exposed to Rh-positive red blood cells (isoimmunization) through transplacental (or other) transfusion.
   c. Following birth of an Rh-positive infant, if fetal cells enter the mother's bloodstream, maternal antibody formation begins; antibodies remain in the maternal circulation.
   d. At time of next pregnancy with Rh-positive fetus, antibodies cross placenta → hemolysis. *Note: Degree* of hemolysis depends on amount (titer) of maternal antibodies present.

3. Possible serious complication (fetal)—rare today. Hydrops fetalis—most severe hemolytic reaction: severe anemia, cardiac decompensation, hypoxia, edema, ascites, hydrothorax; may be stillborn.

◆ 4. **Assessment:**
   🧪 a. *Prenatal*—diagnostic procedures:
      (1) Maternal blood type and Rh factor.
      (2) Indirect Coombs test—to determine presence of Rh sensitization (titer indicates amount of maternal antibodies).
      (3) Amniocentesis—as early as 26 weeks' gestation—amount of bilirubin by-products indicates severity of hemolytic activity.
      (4) RhoGAM between 28–32 wk to prevent antibody formation.
   🧪 b. *Intrapartal* observation of amniotic fluid (after membrane rupture).
      (1) Straw-colored fluid—mild disease.
      (2) Golden fluid—severe fetal disease.
   🧪 c. *Postnatal*—see III.A. Rh Incompatibility, p. 477.

◆ 5. **Nursing care plan/implementation:**
   a. Goal: *prevent isoimmunization in Coombs-negative women*
      (1) *Postabortion*—if no evidence of Rh sensitization (antibody formation) in the Rh-negative mother, administer RhoGAM.
      (2) *Prenatal*—if no evidence of sensitization, administer RhoGAM at 28

weeks' gestation, as ordered, to all Rh− women.
      (3) *Postpartum*—if no evidence of sensitization, administer RhoGAM within 72 h of birth to Rh− women who gave birth to Rh+ baby.

   > **Give RhoGAM to:**
   > 1. Rh− mother who gives birth to Rh+ neonate.
   > 2. Rh− mother after spontaneous or induced abortion (>8 wk).
   > 3. Rh− mother after amniocentesis or chorionic villus sampling (CVS).
   > 4. Rh− mother between 28 and 32 weeks' gestation.

   b. Goal: *health teaching.*
      (1) Explain, discuss that RhoGAM suppresses antibody formation in susceptible Rh-negative women carrying Rh-positive fetus. *Note:* Cannot reverse sensitization if already present.
      (2) Required during and after each pregnancy with Rh+ fetus.

◆ 6. **Evaluation/outcome criteria:**
   a. Successfully carries pregnancy to term.
   b. No evidence of Rh isoimmunization.
   c. Birth of viable infant.

D. **Disorders affecting nutrition: diabetes mellitus**
   1. **Pathophysiology**—increased demand for insulin exceeds pancreatic reserve → inadequate insulin production; enzyme (insulinase) activity breaks down circulating insulin → further reduction in available insulin; increased tissue resistance to insulin; glycogenolysis/gluconeogenesis → ketosis.
   2. **Etiology**—increased metabolic rate; action of placental hormones (see below), enzyme (insulinase) activity.
   3. *Normal physiologic* alterations during pregnancy that may *affect* management of the *diabetic* woman, or *precipitate gestational diabetes* in susceptible women:
      a. Hormone production:
         (1) Human placental lactogen (HPL)
         (2) Progesterone.
         (3) Estrogen.
         (4) Cortisol.
      b. *Effects of hormones:*
         (1) Decreased glucose tolerance.
         (2) Increased metabolic rate.
         (3) Increased production of adrenocortical and pituitary hormones.
         (4) Decreased effectiveness of insulin (increased resistance to insulin by peripheral tissues).
         (5) Increased gluconeogenesis.
         (6) Increased size and number of islets of Langerhans to meet increased maternal needs.

(7) Increased mobilization of free fatty acids.

(8) Decreased renal threshold, increased glomerular filtration rate; glycosuria common.

(9) Decreased CO_2-combining power of blood; higher metabolic rate increases tendency to acidosis.

c. *Effect of pregnancy on diabetes:*

(1) Nausea and vomiting—predispose to ketoacidosis.

(2) Insulin requirements—relatively stable or may decrease in first trimester; rapid *increase* during second and third trimesters; rapid *decrease* after birth to prepregnant level.

(3) Pathophysiologic progression (nephropathy, retinopathy, and arteriosclerotic changes) may appear; existing pathology may worsen.

4. *Effect of poorly controlled diabetes on pregnancy*—increased incidence of:

a. Infertility.

b. UTI.

c. Vaginal infections (moniliasis).

d. Spontaneous abortion.

e. Congenital anomalies (three times as prevalent).

f. Preeclampsia/eclampsia.

g. Hydramnios.

h. Preterm labor and birth.

i. Fetal macrosomia—cephalopelvic disproportion (CPD).

j. Stillbirth.

◆ 5. **Assessment:** *gestational diabetes (mellitus)*

a. History:

(1) Family history.

(2) Previous infant 4200 g or more.

(3) Unexplained fetal wastage—abortion, stillbirth, or early neonatal death.

(4) Obesity with very rapid weight gain.

(5) Hydramnios (excessive amniotic fluid).

(6) Previous infant with congenital anomalies.

(7) Increased tendency for intense vaginal or urinary tract infections.

b. Symptoms: *3 "Ps"—polydipsia, polyphagia, polyuria*—and weight loss.

c. *Abdominal assessment:*

(1) Fetal heart rate.

(2) Excessive fundal height.

(a) Hydramnios.

(b) Large-for-gestational-age (LGA) fetus. *Note:* With vascular pathology, small-for-gestational-age (SGA) fetus.

d. *Medical diagnosis*—procedures:

▲ (1) Abnormal glucose tolerance test (GTT): two or more of the following

findings are not within normal limits (normal values follow):

(a) Fasting blood sugar (FBS)—60–80 mg/dL (90 mg/dL may be normal during first trimester).

(b) One hour—under 200 mg/dL.

(c) Two hours—under 150 mg/dL (~120).

(d) Three hours—under 150 mg/dL (~120).

(2) *Diabetic classification criteria*

(a) Class A—gestational or chemical diabetes (abnormal GTT).

(b) Class B—overt diabetes, onset after age 20, duration less than 10 yr, no vascular involvement.

(c) Class C—overt diabetes, onset before age 20, duration 10–20 yr, no vascular involvement.

(d) Class D—overt diabetes, onset before age 10, duration longer than 20 yr, vascular involvement, benign retinopathy, leg calcification.

(e) Class F—renal impairment.

e. Woman with known diabetes—all classes.

(1) Knowledge and acceptance of disease and its management:

(a) Signs and symptoms of hyperglycemia/hypoglycemia (pp. 126, 470).

(b) Appropriate behaviors (e.g., skim milk for symptoms of hypoglycemia).

(2) Skill and accuracy in monitoring serum glucose (dextrometer use).

(3) Skill and accuracy in preparing and administering insulin dosage; site rotation; subcutaneous injection.

(4) Close monitoring—prenatal status assessment every 2 wk until 30 wk, then weekly until birth. Alert to signs of emerging problems (need for insulin adjustment, hydramnios, macrosomia).

(5) Other—as for any pregnant woman.

◆ 6. **Analysis/nursing diagnosis:**

a. *Knowledge deficit* related to pathophysiology, interactions with pregnancy, management (e.g., insulin administration).

b. *Altered nutrition, more or less than body requirements,* related to weight gain.

c. High-risk pregnancy: high risk for infection, ketosis, perinatal wastage, fetal macrosomia, cephalopelvic disproportion, hydramnios, preterm labor and birth, congenital anomalies.

◆ 7. **Nursing care plan/implementation:**

a. Goal: *health teaching.*

(1) Pathophysiology of diabetes, as necessary; effect of pregnancy on management.

(2) Signs and symptoms of hyperglycemia, hypoglycemia; appropriate management of symptoms.

(3) Hygiene—to reduce probability of infection.

(4) Exercise—needed to control serum-glucose levels, regulate weight gain, and for feeling of well-being.

(5) Need for close monitoring during pregnancy.

(6) Insulin regulation:

(a) Requirements vary through pregnancy: *first trimester*—may decrease with some periods of hypoglycemia due to fetal drain; *second trimester*—increased need for insulin; *third trimester*—needs may be triple prepregnant dose; acidosis more common in late pregnancy (precipitated by emotional stress, infection).

(b) Serum-glucose testing—dextrometer, Acucheck, or other.

(c) Preparation and self-administration of insulin injection, as necessary.

(d) Prompt reporting of fluctuating serum-glucose levels.

(7) Diagnostic testing/hospitalization:

(a) Nonstress test.

(b) Sonography.

(c) Amniocentesis.

b. Goal: *dietary counseling.*

(1) Optimal weight gain—about 24 lb.

(2) Needs 35 calories/kg of ideal body weight.

(3) Protein—20% (2 g/kg, or about 70 g daily).

(4) Carbohydrates: 30–45% in complex form (milk, bread).

(5) Fats—unsaturated.

(6) Appropriate exchanges.

c. *Medical management:* hospitalize woman for:

(1) Regulation of insulin (oral hypoglycemics **contraindicated** in pregnancy, due to teratogenicity).

(2) Control of infection.

(3) Determination of fetal jeopardy or indications for early termination of pregnancy.

8. **Evaluation/outcome criteria:**

a. Understands and accepts diagnosis of diabetes.

b. Actively participates in effective management of diabetes and pregnancy.

c. Maintains serum-glucose levels within acceptable parameters (e.g., 60–90 mg/dL after fasting; 2 hr postprandial, less than 120 mg/dL).

(1) Monitors serum-glucose levels accurately (dextrometer, Acucheck, urine testing).

(2) Prepares and self-administers insulin appropriately.

(3) Complies with dietary regimen.

9. **Antepartal** *hospitalization*

a. **Assessment:**

(1) *Medical evaluation*—procedures:

(a) Serum-glucose levels (↓ 120 mg).

(b) Sonography for fetal growth: biophysical profile (BPP) evaluates fetal physical well-being and volume of amniotic fluid.

(c) Nonstress testing/contraction stress testing.

(d) Amniocentesis for fetal maturity (*Note:* L/S ratio may be elevated in diabetic women; *phosphatidylglycerol [PG]* more accurate for diabetic women.)

(2) **Nursing assessment:**

(a) Daily weight, vital signs, FHR q4h, I&O.

(b) Fundal height and Leopold's maneuvers on admission.

b. **Nursing care plan/implementation.** Goal: *emotional support*—to reduce anxiety and tension, which contribute to insulin imbalance.

(1) Explain all procedures.

(2) Assist with tests for fetal status.

(3) Prepare for possibility of preterm or caesarean birth.

10. *Anticipatory planning*—management of **labor**

a. **Assessment:** continuous.

(1) Signs and symptoms of hyperglycemia, hypoglycemia (pp. 126, 470).

(2) Electronic fetal monitoring—to identify signs of fetal distress.

(3) Other—as for any laboring woman.

b. **Nursing care plan/implementation:** Goal: *safeguard maternal/fetal status. Position:* lateral Sims'—to reduce compression of inferior vena cava and aorta due to hydramnios or LGA baby. (Supine hypotensive syndrome results from compression; reduced placental perfusion increases incidence of fetal hypoxia/anoxia.)

c. *Medical management*—varies widely.

(1) Timing—amniocentesis to determine PG and phosphatidylinositol levels (estimate fetal pulmonary surfactant).

(2) Insulin added to intravenous infusion of 5–10% D/W, and titrated to maintain serum glucose between 100 and 150 mg/dL. D/W needed to prevent hypoglycemia that may lead to maternal ketoacidosis; hy-

perglycemia may result in newborn hypoglycemia.

(3) Ultrasound or X-ray pelvimetry to identify CPD.

11. *Anticipatory planning*—management of **postpartum**

a. Factors influencing serum-glucose levels:

(1) Loss of placental hormones that degrade insulin.

(2) Lower metabolic rate. Woman requiring large doses of insulin may need to triple caloric intake and decrease insulin by one-half.

◆ b. **Assessment:**

(1) Observe for:

(a) Hypoglycemia.

(b) Infection.

(c) Preeclampsia/eclampsia (higher incidence in diabetic women).

(d) Hemorrhage (associated with hydramnios, macrosomia, induction of labor, forceps birth, or caesarean birth).

(2) Monitor healing of episiotomy/abdominal incision.

◆ c. **Nursing care plan/implementation:**

(1) *Medical management:* insulin calibration—requirement may drop to one-half or two-thirds pregnant dosage on first postpartum day if woman is on full diet (due to loss of human placental lactogen and conversion of serum glucose to lactose).

(2) *Nursing management*

(a) Goal: *euglycemia.* Acucheck, insulin as ordered.

(b) Goal: *avoid trauma, reduce risk of UTI.* Avoid catheterization, where possible.

(c) Goal: *health teaching.* Nipple care—to prevent fissures and possible mastitis.

(d) Goal: *reduce serum-glucose and insulin needs.* Encourage/support breastfeeding → antidiabetogenic effect. *Note:* If *acetonuria* occurs, stop breastfeeding while physician readjusts diet/insulin balance; may pump breasts to maintain lactation. If *hypoglycemic,* adrenaline level rises → decreased milk supply and let-down reflex.

12. *Anticipatory guidance*—**discharge plan implementation**

a. Goal: *counseling.* Reinforce recommendations of physicians/genetic counselors.

(1) Risk of infant inheriting gene for diabetes is greater if mother has early-onset disease.

(2) Increased risk of congenital disorders.

b. Goal: *family planning*

(1) Oral contraceptives **contraindicated** because they decrease carbohydrate tolerance; IUD contraindicated because of impaired response to infection. Barrier contraceptives (diaphragm or condoms with spermicides) recommended.

(2) Tubal ligation: if mother has vascular involvement, i.e., retinopathy or nephropathy, increased risk with later pregnancies (see Table 7.2, p. 392).

c. Goal: *health teaching.*

(1) Self-care measures.

(2) Importance of eating on time, even if infant must wait to breastfeed or bottle feed.

(3) Importance of adequate rest and exercise to maintain insulin/glucose balance.

(4) Organize schedule to care for infant, other children, and her diabetes. Allow time for self.

◆ d. **Evaluation/outcome criteria:**

(1) Successfully completes an uneventful pregnancy, labor, and birth of a normal, healthy newborn.

(2) Makes informed judgments regarding parenting, family planning, management of her diabetes.

E. **Disorders affecting psychosocio-cultural behaviors: substance abuse**

◆ 1. **Assessment:** pregnant substance abuser

a. *Medical history*

(1) Infections: HIV-positive status, AIDS, STDs, hepatitis, cirrhosis, cellulitis, endocarditis, pancreatitis, pneumonia.

(2) Psychiatric illness: depression, paranoia, irritability.

(3) Trauma related to violence.

b. *Obstetric history*

(1) Spontaneous abortions.

(2) History of abruptio placentae.

(3) Preterm labor.

(4) Preterm rupture of membranes.

(5) Fetal death.

(6) Low-birthweight infants.

c. *Current pregnancy*

(1) Preterm labor contractions.

(2) Hypoactivity or hyperactivity in fetus.

(3) Poor or decreased weight gain.

(4) STD.

(5) Undiagnosed vaginal bleeding.

(6) Drugs being used and methods of self-administration.

d. *Psychosocial history*

(1) Attitudes re: pregnancy.

(2) Current support system: lacking.

(3) Current living arrangements; lifestyle.

(4) History of psychiatric illness.

(5) History of physical, sexual abuse.

(6) Involvement with legal system.

e. *Physical examination*

f. *Commonly abused substances*

(1) Nicotine.

(2) Alcohol (FAS [fetal alcohol syndrome] or FAE [fetal alcohol effects]).

(3) Marijuana.

(4) Stimulants—cocaine, crack, ice.

(5) Opiates—heroin, methadone, Darvon, Tylenol.

(6) Sedatives, hypnotics.

(7) Caffeine.

g. *Neonatal outcomes*

(1) LBW, small heads.

(2) Irritable, difficult to console.

(3) Disorganized suck-swallow reflex.

(4) Impaired motor development.

(5) Congenital anomalies: genitourinary, gastrointestinal, limb anomalies.

(6) Cerebral infarctions (CVAs).

(7) Breastfeeding contraindicated unless mother is drug-free for 3 months.

(8) Poor, slow weight gain; failure to thrive.

◆ 2. **Analysis/nursing diagnosis:**

a. *Altered nutrition: more than body requirements*—weight gain related to poor nutrition.

b. *Altered nutrition: less than body requirements*—slow fetal growth related to slow gain in weight.

c. *Altered placental function* related to high risk for abruptio placentae.

d. *Noncompliance* with health care protocols related to persistent drug use.

e. *Altered parenting* related to psychological illness (substance dependence).

◆ 3. **Nursing care plan/implementation:**

a. Early identification of substance abuser.

b. Stabilize physiologic status.

c. Fetal surveillance

d. Urge consistent obstetric care.

e. Refer for social services.

◆ 4. **Evaluation/outcome criteria:**

a. Seeks out and uses social services and drug treatment program.

b. Abstains from illicit substances during pregnancy.

c. Successfully completes an uneventful pregnancy, labor, and birth of normal healthy infant.

III. Other high-risk women

A. The pregnant adolescent

1. *General aspects:*

a. Pregnancy in female between 12 and 17 yr old.

b. Incidence increasing dramatically; approximately one-third of all births are to adolescents.

c. *Predisposing factors:* early menarche, early experimentation with sex, poor family relationships, poverty, late or no prenatal care.

d. *Associated health problems:* pregnancy-induced hypertension (PIH), preterm labor, SGA infants, anemia, bleeding disorders, infections, CPD.

e. *Social problems:* poorly educated mothers, child abuse, single-parent families, mothers who are unemployed or working at minimum wage or who lack support system.

◆ 2. **Assessment:**

a. Present physical/health status.

b. Feelings toward pregnancy.

c. Plans for the future.

d. Factors influencing decisions related to self, pregnancy, baby.

e. Signs and symptoms of complications of pregnancy (see A.1.d. *Associated health problems,* above).

f. Potential for gestational diabetes.

g. Need/desire for health maintenance information (family planning).

◆ 3. **Analysis/nursing diagnosis:**

a. *Ineffective coping, individual/family,* related to need to alter life-style, plans, expectations.

b. *Altered family processes,* related to unexpected/unwanted pregnancy.

c. *Altered parenting* related to intrafamily stress secondary to unexpected pregnancy, developmental tasks.

d. *Self-esteem disturbance* related to altered self-concept, body image, role performance, personal identity.

e. *Knowledge deficit* related to family planning, health maintenance, risk factors, pregnancy options.

f. *Altered nutrition* related to life-style

◆ 4. **Nursing care plan/implementation:**

a. Goal: *emotional support.*

(1) Ensure confidentiality.

(2) Establish acceptant, supportive environment.

(3) Encourage verbalization of feelings, concerns, fears, desires, etc.

(4) Maintain continuity of care—consistency of nursing approach, to establish trust, confidentiality.

b. Goal: *facilitate informed decision making.* Discuss available options; aid in exploring implications of possible decisions.

c. Goal: *nutritional counseling* (anemia).

(1) Needs for own growth and that of fetus.

(2) High-quality diet—value for character of skin, return to prepregnant figure.

(3) Include pizza, hamburgers, milkshakes as acceptable—to minimize anger at being "different."

  d. Goal: *health teaching.*

    (1) Rest, exercise, hygiene—as for other women.

    (2) Prevention of infection—STD, UTI, etc.

    (3) Breast self-exam; Pap smear.

    (4) Future family planning options (see Table 7.1, pp. 390–391).

  e. Goal: *assist in achievement of normal developmental tasks.* Encourage exploration of new role and responsibilities.

  f. Goal: *referral to appropriate resources.*

    (1) Abortion.

    (2) Preparation for childbirth and parenting classes.

    (3) Family counseling.

    (4) Social services.

  g. Goal: *assist in facilitating/continuing/completing basic education.*

    (1) Communicate with school nurse.

    (2) Explore other options available in community.

◆ 5. **Evaluation/outcome criteria:**

  a. Makes informed decisions appropriate to individual and family needs, desires.

  b. Actively participates in own health maintenance.

    (1) Complies with medical/nursing recommendations.

    (2) Minimizes potential for complications of pregnancy.

  c. Copes effectively with normal physiologic and psychosocial alterations of pregnancy.

  d. Both woman and baby's father express satisfaction with decision and management of this pregnancy. If parenthood is chosen and pregnancy is successful, accepts parenting role.

B. Older parents: primigravida over age 35

  1. *General aspects*—higher incidence of congenital anomalies (e.g., Down syndrome), increased possibility of complications of pregnancy. However generally it is a conscious decision to have postponed childbearing. Individuals are usually used to making own decisions regarding career and health care.

◆ 2. **Assessment:**

  a. Same as for other pregnant women.

  b. Reaction to reality of pregnancy.

  c. Family response to pregnancy.

◆ 3. **Analysis/nursing diagnosis:**

  a. *Fear* related to threat to pregnancy.

  b. *Knowledge deficit* related to aspects of pregnancy care.

◆ 4. **Nursing care plan/implementation:**

  a. Goal: *anticipatory guidance.* Preparation for parenthood, altered life-style, potential change of career. Assist with realistic expectations. Refer to "over 30" parents' support group.

  b. Goal: *health teaching.* Explain, discuss special diagnostic procedures. See III.F. Amniocentesis, p. 426.

  c. Other—same as for other pregnant women.

◆ 5. **Evaluation/outcome criteria:**

  a. Experiences normal, uncomplicated pregnancy, labor, and birth of normal, healthy newborn.

  b. Expresses satisfaction with decision and outcome of this pregnancy.

C. Older parents: multipara over age 40

  1. *General aspects*

  a. Increased incidence of preexisting and coexisting medical disorders (hypertension, diabetes, arthritis).

  b. Increased incidence of complications of pregnancy (preeclampsia/eclampsia, hemorrhage).

  c. Smoking is major risk factor.

◆ 2. **Assessment:**

  a. Same as for other pregnant women.

  b. Reaction to pregnancy (varies from pleasure at still being "young enough," to despair, if facing decision to abort).

  c. History, signs and symptoms of coexisting disorders.

  d. Indications of reduced physical ability to cope with normal physiologic alterations of pregnancy.

  e. Family constellation: stage of family developmental cycle, responses to this pregnancy (especially adolescents' reaction to parents' pregnancy).

◆ 3. **Analysis/nursing diagnosis:** same as for over-35 age group.

◆ 4. **Nursing care plan/implementation:**

  a. Goal: *emotional support.* Encourage verbalization of feelings, fears, concerns.

  b. Goal: *referral to appropriate resource.*

    (1) Genetic counseling.

    (2) Abortion/support groups.

    (3) Preparation for childbirth and parenthood classes.

  c. Goal: *facilitate/support effective family process.* Involve family in preparation for birth and integration of newborn into family unit.

  d. Other—same as for other pregnant women.

◆ 5. **Evaluation/outcome criteria:**

  a. Makes informed decisions related to pregnancy.

  b. Expresses satisfaction with decision and outcome of this pregnancy.

c. Experiences uncomplicated pregnancy, labor, and birth of normal, healthy newborn.

D. AIDS

1. *General aspects*—AIDS is a serious condition affecting the immune system. Heterosexual females are considered at risk if they or their sexual partners:
   a. Are HIV positive.
   b. Are IV drug users (50%).
   c. Received blood between 1977 and 1985 (9%).
   d. Are homosexual or bisexual males (39%).
   e. Are hemophiliacs.

◆ 2. **Assessment**—general symptoms:
   a. Malaise.
   b. Chronic cough; possible tuberculosis (Tbc).
   c. Chronic diarrhea.
   d. HIV positive.
   e. Weight loss: 10 lb in 2 mo.
   f. Night sweats; lymphadenopathy.
   g. Skin lesions; thrush.
   h. PID; STDs; vulvovaginitis (usually, yeast [*Candidiasis*]), often refractory and severe.
   i. Cervical cytologic abnormalities; often infected with human papillomavirus (HPV).

◆ 3. **Analysis/nursing diagnosis:**
   a. *Altered nutrition, less than body requirements,* related to general malaise.
   b. *Fatigue,* related to altered health status, weight loss.
   c. *Fear* related to progressively debilitating disease.
   d. *Knowledge deficit* related to disease progression, treatment, life expectancy.
   e. *Ineffective individual coping* related to disease progression.

◆ 4. **Nursing care plan/implementation:**
   a. Identify women at risk.
   b. Protect confidentiality.
   ▶ c. Implement universal precautions.
   d. Use proper gloves, gown, handwashing.
   e. Use protective eyewear and mask in labor, birth.

◆ 5. **Evaluation/outcome criteria:**
   a. No further transmission of virus.
   b. Woman's confidentiality maintained.
   c. Universal precautions implemented.
   d. Emotional support implemented.
   e. Supportive groups contacted.

6. **HIV-positive women**—prenatal care:
   a. *Antepartum*
      (1) Increased incidence of other STD (gonorrhea, syphilis, herpes, HPV).
      (2) Increased incidence of CMV.
      (3) Differential diagnosis for all pregnancy-induced complaints.
      (4) Counsel regarding nutrition.
      (5) Advise about risk to infant.
      (6) Counsel regarding safer sex.
   b. *Intrapartum*
      (1) Focus on prevention of transmission.
      (2) External EFM (electronic fetal monitoring) preferred.
      (3) Mode of birth not based on disease.
      (4) Avoid use of fetal scalp electrodes or sampling.
   c. *Postpartum*
      (1) No remarkable alteration in disease progression.
      (2) Breastfeeding contraindicated.
      (3) Implement universal precautions for mother and infant.
      (4) Refer to specialists in AIDS care and treatment.

7. **Newborn or neonate:**
   a. *General aspects:* Neonatal AIDS—exact mode of transmission unknown, but possibly transplacental, contact with maternal blood at birth, or postnatal exposure to infected parent (i.e., breastfeeding). Classic signs evident in adult often not present. Common signs: lymphadenopathy, hepatosplenomegaly, oral candidiasis, bacterial infections, failure to thrive.
   b. Provide supportive nursing care (thermoregulation, respiratory).
   c. Encourage parent-infant contact.
   d. Provide opportunities for sensory stimuli and touch.
   e. Monitor intake and weight gain.
   f. Observe for signs of infection.
   g. Initiate social service consultation.

Common Complications of Pregnancy

First Trimester Complications

I. Complications affecting fluid-gas transport: hemorrhagic disorders

A. General aspects (review Table 7.8)

◆ 1. **Assessment:**
   a. Vital signs, output, general status.
   b. Evidence of internal/external bleeding (pad count).
   c. Pain.
   d. Emotional response.
   e. Perineal pads saturated and number.
   f. Speculum examination.

◆ 2. **Analysis/nursing diagnosis:**
   a. *Knowledge deficit* related to diagnosis, prognosis, treatment, sequelae.
   b. *Anxiety/fear* related to loss of pregnancy, surgery.
   c. *Fluid volume deficit, potential/actual,* related to excessive blood loss.
   d. *Pain.*

■ **TABLE 7.8 Emergency Conditions**

First Trimester		
Assessment/Observations	**Possible Problem**	**Nursing Care Plan/Implementation**

Fluid-Gas Transport

a. *Cramping*—with or without bleeding or passage of tissue	Abortion (before 24 wk)
	  Threatened
	  Imminent, incomplete, septic
		Bedrest, sedation, *avoid* coitus—if threatened; bedrest, start IV fluids and draw blood for laboratory work; CBC, type/crossmatch, electrolytes, platelets, HCG levels

b. *Passage of tissue* (products of conception; grapelike vesicles) or *brown spotting; fundus* too high for gestational age; *blood pressure* elevated. Often associated with hyperemesis gravidarum and preeclampsia	Hydatidiform mole (trophoblastic disease)	Vital signs q5–15min, prn
c. Severe *pain, shock* out of proportion to amount of overt blood; shoulder-strap pain (*Kehr's sign*), a "referred pain" that indicates intraabdominal bleeding (or rupture of ovarian cyst); amenorrhea of 6–12 wk	Ectopic pregnancy	Save all pads or tissue passed through vagina for physician evaluation No rectal or vaginal examination until physician is present
d. Malodorous *discharge; hyperthermia and chills;* tender abdomen	Septic abortion (self-induced or "criminal")	Take complete history, if possible Convulsion precautions if hypertensive
e. *Ecchymosis or bleeding*—with a history that includes any or all of the following: had symptoms of pregnancy, but they subsided; pregnancy test negative; uterine size diminishing; no FHT	Missed abortion with possible DIC (Retained dead fetus syndrome)	Emotional support for loss of pregnancy (through nurse's manner, tone of voice, touch, use of woman's name, keep her informed of what is happening). Oxygen, prn

Second Trimester		
Assessment/Observations	**Possible Problem**	**Nursing Care Plan/Implementation**

Fluid-Gas Transport

a. Cramping; passage of products of conception	Late abortion	Same as for first trimester
b. Labor—cervical changes, "show"	Incompetent cervical os	See physician immediately for possible cerclage
c. *Prolonged* nausea and vomiting; unexplained *hypertension* or *preeclampsia;* passage of dark blood or grapelike vesicles; *absent FHTs;* excessive fundal height for gestation	Hydatidiform mole	Maintain hydration; assess for dehydration; refer to physician

Sensory-Perceptual

a. *Preeclampsia/eclampsia* *Assessment:* hypertension first noted after 24 wk; followed by increased proteinuria *Symptoms:* blurred or double vision; pain: headache, epigastric (late sign) *Signs:* BP 160/110; 3⁺ proteinuria Edema: facial, digital; pulmonary Oliguria Hyperreflexia	With increased severity: renal failure, circulatory collapse, CVA, coagulation defects (DIC); abruptio placentae	Pharmacologic management of hypertension (see Unit 2) *Convulsion precautions:* 1. Emergency tray at bedside 2. Oxygen/suction 3. Start IV 4. Padded siderails 5. Indwelling urinary catheter 6. Constant observation 7. Deep-tendon reflexes 8. Daily weight 9. I&O 10. Note any complaints and changes 11. Prepare for lab work (type and crossmatch, CBC, platelets, BUN, and creatinine)

b. *Convulsions* in absence of hypertension, proteinuria, or facial edema	CVA, epilepsy, drug toxicity; intracranial injury; diabetic complications; encephalopathy	*Convulsion care:*
		1. Oxygen/mask; drugs (magnesium sulfate IV)
		2. Observe:
		  a. Uterine tone, FHTs, fetal activity
		  b. Signs of labor
		3. Emotional support for woman and family

continued

■ **TABLE 7.8** *(Continued)*

Third Trimester		
Assessment/Observations	**Possible Problem**	**Nursing Care Plan/Implementation**
Fluid-Gas Transport		
a. *Bleeding:* painless, bright red, vaginal Contractions or uterine tone normal	Placenta previa	**No vaginal exam** Apply fetal monitor; assess for labor; *position:* semi- to high Fowler's
b. *Pain:* abdomen rigid and tender to touch Increased uterine tone; signs of shock disproportionate to visible blood loss; may have loss of FHTs; associated with: preeclampsia, multiparity, precipitous labor, oxytocin induction trauma, cocaine use	Abruptio placentae	As for placenta previa; *position:* Sims'

e. *Ineffective coping, individual/family,* related to knowledge deficit and fear.

f. *Anticipatory/dysfunctional grieving,* related to loss of pregnancy.

g. *Disturbance in self-esteem, body image, role performance,* related to threat to self-image as woman and childbearer.

◆ 3. **Nursing care plan/implementation:**

   a. Goal: *minimize blood loss, stabilize physiologic status.*

     (1) Facilitate prompt medical management.

▶   (2) Administer IV fluids, blood, as ordered.

     (3) Administer analgesics, as needed.

   b. Goal: *prevent infection.* Strict aseptic technique.

   c. Goal: *emotional support.*

     (1) Encourage verbalization of anxiety, fears, concerns.

     (2) Supportive care for grief reaction (p. 448).

◆ 4. **Evaluation/outcome criteria:**

   a. Blood loss minimized; physiologic status stable.

   b. Copes effectively with loss of pregnancy.

B. **Spontaneous abortion:** *before viable age of 20–22 wk*

   1. **Etiology:**

     a. Defective products of conception.

     b. Insufficient production of progesterone.

     c. Acute infections.

     d. Reproductive system abnormalities, e.g., incompetent cervical os.

     e. Trauma (physical or emotional).

     f. Rh incompatibility.

◆ 2. **Assessment:** types

     a. *Threatened*—mild bleeding, spotting, cramping; cervix closed.

     b. *Inevitable*—moderate bleeding, painful cramping; cervix dilated, positive Nitrazine test (membranes ruptured).

     c. *Imminent*—profuse bleeding, severe cramping, urge to bear down.

     d. *Incomplete*—fetal parts or fetus expelled; placenta and membranes retained.

e. *Complete*—all products of conception expelled; minimal vaginal bleeding.

f. *Habitual/recurrent*—history of spontaneous loss of three or more successive pregnancies.

g. *Missed*—fetal death with no spontaneous expulsion within four weeks.

     (1) Anorexia, malaise, headache.

     (2) Fundal height—inconsistent with gestational estimate.

     (3) Laboratory—prolonged clotting time, due to resultant concurrent hypofibrinogenemia (disseminated intravascular coagulation [DIC], a major threat to mother).

h. *Induced* abortions (intentionally introduced loss of pregnancy).

◆ 3. **Analysis/nursing diagnosis:**

   a. *Altered family processes* related to pregnancy, circumstances surrounding abortion.

   b. *Sexual dysfunction* related to compromised self-image, altered interpersonal relationship, guilt feelings.

◆ 4. **Nursing care plan/implementation:**

   a. *Threatened*—Goal: *health teaching.* Suggest: avoid coitus and orgasm, especially around normal time for menstrual period.

   b. *Incomplete, inevitable, imminent.*

     (1) Goal: *safeguard status.*

       (a) Save all pads, clots, tissue for expert diagnosis.

       (b) Report immediately any change in status, excessive bleeding, signs of infection, shock.

       (c) Prepare for surgery.

     (2) Goal: *comfort measures.*

       (a) Administer analgesics, as necessary.

       (b) Bedrest, quiet diversional activities.

     (3) Goal: *emotional support.*

       (a) Encourage verbalization of fear, concerns.

       (b) Reduce anxiety, as possible.

(c) If pregnancy terminates, facilitate grieving process; assist in working through guilt feelings (p. 447).

(d) Supportive care for grief reaction (p. 448).

(4) Goal: *prevent isoimmunization.* See III. A. Rh incompatibility, pp. 407, 477.

(5) *Medical management:*

(a) Laboratory—blood type and Rh factor, indirect Coombs, platelets, serum fibrinogen, clotting time.

▶ (b) Replace blood loss; maintain fluid levels with IV.

(c) Dilatation and curettage or dilatation and evacuation.

(d) *Habitual*—determine etiology.

◆ 5. **Evaluation/outcome criteria:**

a. *Threatened*—responds to medical/nursing regimen; abortion avoided, successfully carries pregnancy to term.

b. *Spontaneous abortion*—after uterus emptied.

(1) Her bleeding is controlled.

(2) Her vital signs are stable.

(3) Copes effectively with loss of pregnancy.

(4) Expresses satisfaction with care.

c. *Habitual abortion*—cause identified and corrected; carries subsequent pregnancy to successful termination.

C. **Hydatidiform mole** (complete)

1. **Pathophysiology**—chorionic villi degenerate into grapelike cluster of vesicles; may be antecedent to choriocarcinoma.

2. **Etiology**—genetic base of complete mole (sperm enters empty egg and its chromosomes replicate; 23 pairs of chromosomes are all paternal); rare complication; more common in women over 45 yr of age and Asian women.

◆ 3. **Assessment:**

a. Uterus—rapid enlargement; fundal height inconsistent with gestational estimate.

b. Brownish discharge—beginning about wk 12; may contain vesicles.

c. Signs and symptoms of preeclampsia/eclampsia (before third trimester), increased incidence of hyperemesis gravidarum.

🝪 d. *Medical evaluation*—procedures:

(1) Sonography, X ray, amniography—no fetal parts present; "snow storm."

(2) Laboratory test—for elevated human chorionic gonadotropin (HCG) levels.

(3) Follow-up surveillance of HCG levels for at least 1 yr; persistent HCG level is consistent with choriocarcinoma; X ray.

◆ 4. **Analysis/nursing diagnosis:**

a. *Anxiety/fear* related to treatment, possible sequelae of hydatidiform mole (choriocarcinoma).

b. *Potential for injury* related to hemorrhage, perforation of uterine wall, preeclampsia/eclampsia.

c. *Fluid volume deficit* related to injury.

◆ 5. **Nursing care plan/implementation:**

a. *Medical management*

(1) Monitor for PIH (pregnancy-induced hypertension).

(2) Evacuate the uterus—hysterectomy may be necessary.

(3) Strict contraception for at least 1 yr to enable accurate assessment of status.

◖💊 (4) Choriocarcinoma—chemotherapy (methotrexate plus Dactinomycin) or radiation therapy, or both.

b. *Nursing management*

(1) Goal: *safeguard status.* Observe for hemorrhage, passage of retained vesicles and abdominal pain, or signs of infection (because woman is at risk for perforation of uterine wall).

(2) Goal: *health teaching.*

(a) Explain, discuss diagnostic tests; prepare for tests.

(b) Discuss contraceptive options.

(c) Importance of follow-up.

(3) Goal: *preoperative and postoperative care.*

(4) Goal: *emotional support.* Facilitate grieving (p. 447).

◆ 6. **Evaluation/outcome criteria:**

a. Verbalizes understanding of diagnosis, tests, and treatment.

b. Complies with medical/nursing recommendations.

c. Tolerates surgical procedure well.

(1) Bleeding controlled.

(2) Vital signs stable.

(3) Urinary output adequate.

d. Copes effectively with loss of pregnancy.

e. Returns for follow-up care/surveillance.

f. Selects and effectively implements method of contraception; avoids pregnancy for 1 yr or more.

g. Tests for HCG remain negative for 1 yr; no evidence of malignancy.

h. Achieves a pregnancy when desired.

i. Successfully carries pregnancy to term; normal, uncomplicated birth of viable infant.

D. **Ectopic pregnancy**

1. **Pathology**—implantation outside of uterine cavity.

2. Types:

a. Tubal (most common).

b. Cervical.

c. Abdominal.

d. Ovarian.

3. **Etiology:**

a. PID—pelvic salpingitis and endometritis.

b. 43% caused by STD-related factors: 25%, chlamydial; 20%, previous STD.

c. Tubal or uterine anomalies, tubal spasm.

d. Adhesions from PID or past surgeries.

e. Presence of IUD.

◆ 4. **Assessment:** dependent on implantation site.

a. *Early signs*—abnormal menstrual period (usually following a missed menstrual period), spotting, some symptoms of pregnancy; possible dull pain on affected side.

b. *Impending or posttubal rupture*—sudden, acute, lower abdominal pain; nausea and vomiting; signs of shock; referred shoulder pain (*Kehr's sign*) or neck pain—due to blood in peritoneal cavity; blood in cul-de-sac may → rectal pressure.

c. Sharp, localized pain when cervix is touched during vaginal exam; shock and circulatory collapse in some, usually following vaginal examination.

d. Positive pregnancy test in many women.

◆ 5. **Analysis/nursing diagnosis:**

a. *Fear* related to abdominal pain and pregnancy status.

b. *Grief* related to pregnancy loss.

◆ 6. **Nursing care plan/implementation:**

a. *Medical management:* Surgical removal/repair.

b. *Nursing management:*

(1) Goal: *preoperative and postoperative care, health teaching.*

(2) Goal: *supportive care for grief reaction;* encourage verbalization of anxiety and concerns of further pregnancies.

◆ 7. **Evaluation/outcome criteria:**

a. Woman experiences uncomplicated postoperative course.

b. Woman copes effectively with loss of pregnancy.

II. **Complications affecting nutrition/elimination: hyperemesis gravidarum**

A. **Pathophysiology**—pernicious vomiting during first 14–16 wk (peak incidence around 10 weeks' gestation); excessive vomiting at any time during pregnancy. Potential hazards include:

1. Dehydration with fluid and electrolyte imbalance.

2. Starvation, with loss of 5% or more of body weight; protein and vitamin deficiencies.

3. Metabolic acidosis—due to breakdown of fat stores to meet metabolic needs.

4. Hypovolemia and hemoconcentration; *increased* blood urea nitrogen (BUN); *decreased* urinary output.

B. **Etiology:**

1. Physiologic—secretion of HCG, decrease in free gastric HCl, decreased gastrointestinal motility. Increased incidence in hydatidiform mole and multifetal pregnancy (due to high levels of HCG).

2. Psychological—thought to be related to rejection of pregnancy or sexual relations.

◆ C. **Assessment:**

1. Intractable vomiting.

2. Abdominal pain.

3. Hiccups.

4. Marked weight loss.

5. Dehydration—thirst, tachycardia, skin turgor.

6. Increased respiratory rate (metabolic acidosis).

7. Laboratory—elevated BUN.

8. *Medical evaluation:* rule out other causes (infection, tumors).

◆ D. **Analysis/nursing diagnosis:**

1. *Altered nutrition, less than body requirements,* related to inability to retain oral feedings.

2. *Fluid volume deficit* related to dehydration.

3. *Ineffective individual coping* related to symptoms, insecurity in role, psychological stress of unwanted pregnancy.

4. *Personal identity disturbance* related to symptoms or perception of self as inadequate in role, sick, socially unpresentable.

◆ E. **Nursing care plan/implementation:**

1. Goal: *physiologic stability*

a. Rest GI tract (keep NPO), e.g., maintain IV fluids, parenteral nutrition.

b. Progress diet, as ordered; present small feedings attractively.

c. Weigh daily, assess hydration; note weight gain.

2. Goal: *minimize environmental stimuli.*

a. Limit visitors and phone calls.

b. Bedrest with bathroom privileges.

3. Goal: *emotional support.*

a. Establish accepting, supportive environment.

b. Encourage verbalization of anxiety, fears, concerns.

c. Support positive self-image.

◆ F. **Evaluation/outcome criteria:**

1. Woman's signs and symptoms subside; she takes oral nourishment and gains weight.

2. Woman's pregnancy continues to term without recurrence of hyperemesis.

III. **Complications affecting protective function: STDs.** This NCLEX category measures applications of knowledge about conditions related to patient's capacity to maintain defenses and prevent physical and chemical trauma, injury, *infection,* and threats to health status.

A. **Vaginitis**—inflammation of vagina.

1. **Pathophysiology**—local inflammatory reaction (redness, heat, irritation/tenderness, pain).

2. **Etiology:**

a. Common causative organisms:

(1) Bacteria—streptococci, *Escherichia coli,* gonococci, chlamydia.
(2) *Viruses*—herpes type II, CMV, HPV
(3) Protozoa—*Trichomonas vaginalis.*
(4) Fungi—*Candida albicans.*
b. Atrophic changes—due to declining hormone level (postmenopausal women).
◆ 3. **Assessment:** differentiate among common vaginal infections:
a. Vulvovaginal erythema.
b. Pruritus, dysuria, dyspareunia.
c. Vaginal discharge.
◆ 4. **Analysis/nursing diagnosis:** *pain* related to inflammation, discharge.
◆ 5. **Nursing care plan/implementation:**
a. Goal: *emotional support.*
b. Goal: *health teaching.* Instruct woman in self-care measures to promote comfort and healing:
(1) Perineal care.
(2) Sitz baths.
(3) Douching (as ordered). *Not* recommended during pregnancy.
(4) Exposing vulva to air.
(5) Cotton briefs.
(6) Proper insertion of vaginal suppository.
c. Goal: *prevent reinfection.*
(1) Suggest sexual partner use condom until infection is eliminated—or abstain from intercourse.
(2) Recommend sexual partner seek examination and treatment.
d. Goal: *medical consultation/treatment.* Refer for diagnosis and treatment.
◆ 6. **Evaluation/outcome criteria:**
a. Woman is asymptomatic; unable to recover organism from body fluids or tissue.
b. Woman avoids reinfection.
B. **Gonorrhea**
1. **Pathophysiology:**
a. Male—early infection usually confined to urethra, vestibular glands, anus, or pharynx. Untreated: ascending infection may involve testes, causing sterility.
b. Female—early infection usually confined to vestibular glands, endocervix, urethra, anus (vagina is resistant). May ascend to involve pelvic structures, e.g., PID: fallopian tubes, ovaries; scarring may cause sterility.
c. Pregnant female—may result in preterm rupture of membranes, amnionitis, preterm labor, postpartum salpingitis.
d. Sequelae (untreated):
(1) May develop carrier state (asymptomatic; organism resident in vestibular glands).

(2) Systemic spread may result in gonococcal:
(a) Arthritis.
(b) Endocarditis.
(c) Meningitis.
(d) Septicemia.
e. Newborn—ophthalmia neonatorum (gonococcal conjunctivitis). Untreated sequelae: blindness.
2. **Etiology:** gram-negative diplococcus (*Neisseria gonorrhoeae*).
3. **Epidemiology:**
a. Portal of entry—oral or genitourinary mucous membranes.
b. Mode of transmission—usually sexual contact.
c. Incubation period: 2–5 d; may be asymptomatic.
d. Communicable period—as long as organisms are present; to 4 d after antibiotic therapy begun.
◆ 4. **Assessment:**
a. History of known (or suspected) contact.
b. *Male:*
(1) Complaint of mucoid or mucopurulent discharge.
▲ (2) Medical diagnosis—procedure: urethral discharge gram stain.
c. *Female:*
(1) Often asymptomatic; acute infection: severe vulvovaginal inflammation, venereal warts, greenish-yellow vaginal discharge.
▲ (2) Medical diagnosis—procedure: endocervical culture.
d. Gonococcal urethritis (male and female)—sudden severe dysuria, frequency, burning, edema.
e. Salpingitis/oophoritis—severe, sudden abdominal pain, fever (with or without vaginal discharge).
◆ 5. **Analysis/nursing diagnosis:** *impaired tissue integrity* related to tissue inflammation.
◆ 6. **Nursing care plan/implementation:**
a. Goal: *emotional support.*
b. Goal: *health teaching* to prevent transmission, sequelae, reinfection.
(1) Need for accurate diagnosis and effective treatment, follow-up examination in 7–14 d, and culture.
(2) All sexual partners need examination, treatment.
(3) Possible sequelae/complications (sterility, carrier state).
c. Goal: *medical consultation/treatment.*
(1) Determine allergy to penicillin, erythromycin, probenecid.
(2) Refer for diagnosis and treatment.
(a) Diagnosis.
(b) Treatment—aqueous penicillin G, 2.4 million U in each buttock

(4.8 million U total dose) and probenecid 1 g PO.
- (c) Follow-up culture before birth.
- (d) Notification of sexual partners.

◆ 7. **Evaluation/outcome criteria:**
- a. Verbalizes understanding of mode of transmission, prevention, importance of examination, treatment of sexual contacts.
- b. Informs sexual contacts of need for examination.
- c. Returns for follow-up examinations.
- d. Successfully treated; weekly follow-up cultures: negative on two successive visits.
- e. Avoids reinfection.

C. *Chlamydia trachomatis*
1. **Pathophysiology:**
- a. Most common sexually transmitted disease in U.S.
- b. Initial infection mild in females; inflammation of cervix with discharge.
- c. If untreated, may lead to urethritis, dysuria, PID, tubal occlusion, infertility.

2. **Etiology:**
- a. *Chlamydia trachomatis* has maternal-fetal effects.
- b. Bacteria can exist only within living cells.
- c. Transmission is by direct contact from one person to another.

◆ 3. **Assessment—maternal:**
- a. Inflamed cervix (may be asymptomatic).
- b. Cervical congestion, edema.
- c. Mucopurulent discharge.

◆ 4. **Assessment—fetal-neonatal:**
- a. Increased incidence of stillbirth.
- b. Preterm birth may result.
- c. Contact with infected mucus occurs during birth.
- d. Newborn may be asymptomatic.
- e. Conjunctivitis may lead to scarring.
- f. Respiratory problems—tachypnea, dyspnea, apnea.

◆ 5. **Analysis/nursing diagnosis:**
- a. *Pain* related to inflamed reproductive organs.
- b. *Fatigue* related to inflammation.
- c. *Knowledge deficit* related to mode of treatment, disease transmission.

◆ 6. **Nursing care plan/implementation:**
- a. Treatment with antibiotics, generally erythromycin, tetracycline.
- b. Provide pain relief, analgesics.
- c. Counsel regarding use of condoms, spermicidal agents (containing nonoxynol-9) to prevent reinfection.

◆ 7. **Evaluation/outcome criteria:**
- a. Woman understands treatment and shows compliance.
- b. Woman understands portal of entry and risk for reinfection.

D. *Herpes genitalis*
1. **Pathophysiology**—initial infection: varies in severity of symptoms, may be local or systemic; duration: prolonged; morbidity: severe.
2. **Etiology**—Herpesvirus type II.
3. **Epidemiology:**
- a. Portal of entry—skin, mucous membranes.
- b. Mode of transmission—usually sexual.
- c. Incubation: 3–14 d.
- d. Communicable period—while organisms are present.

◆ 4. **Assessment:**
- a. Lesions—painful, red papules; pustular vesicles that break and form wet ulcers that later crust; self-limiting (three wk).
- b. Severe itching or pain.
- c. Discharge—copious; foul smelling.
- d. Dysuria.
- e. Lymph nodes—enlarged, inflammatory, inguinal.
- f. Pregnant female—vaginal bleeding, spontaneous abortion, fetal death.
- g. May shed virus for 7 wk.
- h. Medical diagnosis: multinucleated giant cells in microscopic examination of lesion exudate; culture for herpes simplex virus (HSV).

◆ 5. **Analysis/nursing diagnosis:**
- a. *Pain* related to inflammation process.
- b. *Fear* related to longevity of disease.
- c. *Fear* related to no cure for disease.
- d. *Knowledge deficit* related to transmission to future partners.

◆ 6. **Nursing care plan/implementation:**
- a. Goal: *emotional support.*
- b. Goal: *health teaching.*
  - (1) Virus remains in body for life (dormant, noninfectious) in 25–30% of population; small percentage have symptoms.
  - (2) Recurrence probable; usually shorter and milder.
  - (3) Annual Pap smear important—associated with later development of cervical cancer.
  - (4) Need for close surveillance during pregnancy; cesarean birth may be indicated if woman has active genital lesions.
- c. Goal: *promote comfort.*
- d. Goal: *accurate definitive treatment.* Refer for diagnosis and treatment.
  - (1) Diagnosis—cervical smears.
  - (2) Treatment—acylovir ointment (Zovirax, but not in pregnancy).

◆ 7. **Evaluation/outcome criteria:**
- a. Woman remains asymptomatic.
- b. Pregnancy continues to term with no newborn effects.

E. **Syphilis**
  1. **Pathophysiology:**
    🧪 a. *Primary stage:* nonreactive VDRL.
      (1) *Male:* 3–4 wk after contact, pain-less, localized penile/anal ulcer (chancre); lymph nodes—enlarged, regional.
      (2) *Female:* often asymptomatic; labial, vaginal, or cervical chancre.
      (3) Medical diagnosis—procedure: dark-field microscopic examination of lesion exudate.
    🧪 b. *Secondary stage:* reactive VDRL.
      (1) 6–8 wk after infection.
      (2) Rash—macular, papular; on trunk, palms, soles.
      (3) Malaise, headache, sore throat, weight loss, low-grade temperature.
    🧪 c. *Latent stage:* reactive serologic test for syphilis (STS). Asymptomatic; noninfectious.
    d. *Tertiary stage:*
      (1) Gumma formation in skin, cardiovascular or central nervous system.
      (2) Psychosis.
  2. **Etiology:** *Treponema pallidum* (spirochete).
  3. **Epidemiology:**
    a. Portal of entry—skin, mucous membranes.
    b. Mode of transmission—usually sexual.
    c. Incubation period—9 d–3 mo.
    d. Communicable period—primary and secondary stages.
  ◆ 4. **Assessment:**
    a. *Primary*—chancre, when detectable.
      🧪 Medical diagnosis—procedure: dark-field examination of lesion exudate.
    b. *Secondary:*
      (1) Malaise, lymphadenopathy, headache, elevated temperature.
      (2) Macular, papular rash on palms and soles; may be disseminated.
      (3) Medical diagnosis—see d., below.
    c. *Tertiary:*
      (1) Subcutaneous nodules (gumma).
      (2) *Note:* Gumma formation may affect any body system; symptoms associated with area of involvement.
    🧪 d. Medical diagnosis—procedures: stages other than primary—STS: VDRL, rapid plasma reagin (RPR), *T. pallidum* immobilization (TPI), fluorescent treponemal antibody absorption (FTA). *False-positive STS* in: collagen diseases, infectious mononucleosis, malaria, systemic tuberculosis.
  ◆ 5. **Analysis/nursing diagnosis:**
    a. *Pain* related to inflammation process.
    b. *Knowledge deficit* related to treatment and transmission of the disease.

◆ 6. **Nursing care plan/implementation:**
    a. Goal: *emotional support*
      (1) Nonjudgmental.
      (2) Caring, supportive manner.
    b. Goal: *health teaching.*
      (1) Need for accurate diagnosis and treatment, follow-up examinations.
      (2) All sexual partners need examination and treatment.
    c. Goal: *medical consultation / treatment.*
      (1) Refer for diagnosis and treatment. *Note:* In pregnancy—treatment by 18th gestational week prevents congenital syphilis in neonate; however, treat at time of diagnosis.
      💊 (2) Treatment:
        (a) Primary, secondary—benzathine penicillin G, 2.4 million U.
        (b) Other stages—7.2 million U over 3-wk period.
        (c) Erythromycin for penicillin-allergic clients.
◆ 7. **Evaluation/outcome criteria:**
    a. If treated by 18th wk of pregnancy, congenital syphilis is prevented.
    b. Appropriate treatment after 18th wk cures both mother and fetus; however, any fetal damage occurring before treatment is irreversible.
    🧪 c. Follow-up VDRL: nonreactive at 1, 3, 6, 9, and 12 mo.
    🧪 d. *Tertiary*—cerebrospinal fluid examination negative at 6 mo and 1 yr following treatment.
    e. Verbalizes understanding of mode of transmission, potential sequelae without treatment, importance of examination/treatment of sexual contacts, preventive techniques.
    f. Informs contacts of need for examination.
    g. Returns for follow-up visit.
    h. Avoids reinfection.

F. **PID**
◆ 1. **Pathophysiology**—ascending pelvic infection; may involve fallopian tubes (salpingitis), ovaries (oophoritis); may develop pelvic abscess (most common complication), pelvic cellulitis, pelvic thrombophlebitis, peritonitis.
  2. **Etiology:**
    a. *C. trachomatis.*
    b. Gonococci.
    c. Streptococci.
    d. Staphylococci.
◆ 3. **Assessment:**
    a. Pain: acute, abdominal.
    b. Vaginal discharge: foul smelling.
    c. Fever, chills, malaise.
    d. Elevated white blood cell (WBC) count.
◆ 4. **Analysis/nursing diagnosis:**
    a. *Pain* related to occluded tubules.

b. Infertility related to permanent block of tubes.

c. *Knowledge deficit* related to transmission of disease.

d. *Altered urinary elimination* related to dysuria.

◆ 5. **Nursing care plan/implementation**—for hospitalized woman:

a. Goal: *emotional support.*

b. Goal: *limit extension of infection.*

(1) Bedrest—*position:* semi-Fowler's, to promote drainage.

(2) *Force fluids* to 3000 mL/d.

(3) Administer antibiotics, as ordered.

c. Goal: *prevent autoinocculation/transmission.*

▶ (1) Strict aseptic technique (handwashing, perineal care).

▶ (2) Contact-item isolation.

(3) *Health teaching:* if untreated: high risk of tubal scarring, sterility, or ectopic pregnancy; pelvic adhesions; transmission of disease.

d. Goal: *promote comfort.*

(1) Analgesics, as ordered.

(2) External heat, as ordered.

◆ 6. **Evaluation/outcome criteria:**

a. Woman responds to therapy; uneventful recovery.

b. Woman avoids reinfection.

Second Trimester Complications

See Table 7.8, pp. 415–416.

I. Complications affecting comfort, rest, mobility: Incompetent cervix

A. **Pathophysiology**—inability of cervix to support growing weight of pregnancy; associated with repeated spontaneous second trimester abortion.

B. **Etiology:**

1. Unknown.

2. Congenital defect in cervical musculature.

3. Cervical trauma during previous birth, abortion; aggressive, deep, or repeated dilatation and curettage.

◆ C. **Assessment:**

1. History of habitual, second trimester abortions.

2. Painless, progressive cervical effacement and dilatation during second trimester.

3. Signs of threatened abortion or (early third trimester) preterm labor.

◆ D. **Analysis/nursing diagnosis:**

1. *Pain* related to early dilatation.

2. *Fear* related to possible pregnancy loss.

◆ E. **Nursing care plan/implementation:**

1. *Medical management*

a. Cerclage surgical procedure (*Shirodkar, McDonald*).

2. *Preoperative nursing management*

a. Goal: *reduce physical stress on incompetent cervix.* Bedrest, supportive care.

b. Goal: *emotional support.* Encourage verbalization of anxiety, fear, concerns.

c. Goal: *health (preoperative) teaching.* Explain procedure—purse-string suture encircles cervix and reinforces musculature.

d. Goal: *preparation for surgery.*

3. *Postoperative nursing management*

a. Goal: *maximize surgical result.* Bedrest, supportive care.

b. Goal: *health teaching.*

(1) *Avoid:* strenuous physical activity; straining.

(2) Report promptly: signs of labor (vaginal bleeding, cramping).

(3) Need for continued, close health surveillance.

◆ 4. **Evaluation/outcome criterion:** woman carries pregnancy to successful termination.

II. Complications affecting sensory/perceptual functions: pregnancy-induced hypertension (PIH); preeclampsia/eclampsia

A. **Pathophysiology**

1. Generalized arteriospasm → increased peripheral resistance, decreased tissue perfusion, and hypertension.

2. *Kidney:*

a. Reduced renal perfusion and vasospasm → glomerular lesions.

b. Damage to membrane → loss of serum protein (albuminuria). *Note:* Reduced serum A/G (albumin/globulin) ratio alters blood osmolarity → edema.

c. Increased tubular reabsorption of sodium → increased water retention (edema).

d. Release of angiotensin contributes to vasospasm and hypertension.

3. *Brain:* decreased oxygenation, cerebral edema, and vasospasm → visual disturbances and hyperirritability, convulsions, and coma.

4. *Uterus:* decreased placental perfusion → increased risk of SGA baby, abruptio placentae.

B. **Etiology:** unknown. *Risk factors:*

1. Pregnancy—occurs only when a functioning trophoblast is present; more common in *first* pregnancies; develops after wk 24 of gestation.

2. Age-related—under 17 and over 35 yr of age.

3. Coexisting conditions—diabetes, multifetal gestation, hydramnios.

4. Diet—low in protein.

◆ C. **Assessment**—types:

1. *Preeclampsia—mild*

a. Hypertension—systolic increase of 30 mm Hg or more over baseline; diastolic rise of 15 mm Hg or more.

b. Proteinuria—1 g/d.

c. Edema—digital and periorbital; weight gain over 0.45 kg (1 lb)/wk.

2. *Preeclampsia—severe*

a. Increasing hypertension—systolic at or above 160 mm Hg or more than 50 mm Hg over baseline; diastolic, 110 mm Hg or more.

b. Urine: proteinuria (5 g or more in 24 h); oliguria (400 mL or less in 24 h).

c. Hemoconcentration, hypoproteinemia, hypernatremia, hypovolemic condition.

d. Persistent vomiting.

e. Epigastric pain—due to edema of liver capsule.

f. Cerebral or visual disturbances (before convulsive state):

(1) Disorientation and somnolence.

(2) Severe frontal headache.

(3) Increased irritability; hyperreflexia.

(4) Blurred vision, halo vision, dimness, blind spots.

3. *Eclampsia*

a. Tonic and clonic convulsions; coma.

b. Renal shutdown—oliguria, anuria.

◆ **D. Assessment—hospitalized** woman:

1. Vital signs (blood pressure, pulse, respirations)—q2–4h, while awake (if mild to moderate preeclampsia) or as necessary. *Note:* Record, report persistent hypertension.

▶ 2. Fetal heart tones at time of vital signs.

▶ 3. Deep-tendon reflexes (DTR) and clonus—to identify/monitor CNS hyperirritability.

4. I&O—to identify diuresis. (*Note:* oliguria indicates pathologic progression.)

5. Urinalysis (clean-catch) for protein, daily or after each voiding, as necessary.

6. Signs of pathologic progression (see C. Assessment—types, p. 422).

7. Signs of labor, abruptio placentae (*Note:* high blood pressure, or a rapid drop, may initiate abruptio), DIC.

8. Emotional status.

9. Daily weight, amount/distribution of edema (pitting; pedal, digital, periorbital)—to identify signs of mobilization of tissue fluid, diuresis.

◆ **E. Analysis/nursing diagnosis:**

1. *Fluid volume excess:* hemoconcentration, edema related to altered blood osmolarity and sodium/water retention.

2. *Altered nutrition, less than body requirements:* protein deficiency related to dietary lack or loss through damaged renal membrane.

3. *Altered tissue perfusion* related to increased peripheral resistance and vasospasm in renal, cardiovascular system.

4. *Altered urinary elimination:* oliguria, anuria related to hypovolemia.

5. *Sensory/perceptual alterations:* visual disturbances, hyperirritability related to cerebral edema, decreased oxygenation to brain.

6. *Anxiety* related to symptoms, implications of pathophysiology.

7. *Diversional activity deficit* related to need for reduced environmental stimuli, bedrest.

8. *Risk for injury* related to seizure.

F. Prognosis:

1. *Good*—symptoms mild, respond to treatment.

2. *Poor*—convulsions (number and duration); persistent coma; hyperthermia, tachycardia (120 beats/min); cyanosis.

3. *Terminal*—pulmonary edema, congestive heart failure, acute renal failure, cerebral hemorrhage. The earlier the symptoms appear, the poorer the outcome for the pregnancy.

◆ **G. Nursing care plan/implementation:** Goal: *health teaching.*

1. *Dietary counseling:* high-protein diet—to increase blood osmolarity, reduce movement of vascular fluid into interstitial space.

2. *Rest*—frequent naps in *lateral Sims' position.*

3. Immediate report of *danger signs.*

a. Digital and periorbital edema.

b. Severe headache, irritability.

c. Visual disturbances.

d. Epigastric pain.

4. *Do roll-over* test (BP while on back and lateral positions).

5. Importance of regular prenatal visits.

6. Monitoring own blood pressure between prenatal visits.

◆ **H. Nursing care plan/implementation—hospitalized** woman:

1. Goal: *reduce environmental stimuli.* To minimize stimulation of hyperirritable CNS. Limit visitors and phone calls.

2. Goal: *emotional support.*

a. Encourage verbalization of anxiety, fears, concerns.

b. Explain all procedures, seizure precautions.

3. Goal: *supportive care.*

a. Encourage bedrest—to increase tissue perfusion, promote diuresis.

b. *Position:* lateral Sims'—to reduce risk of supine hypotensive syndrome.

4. Goal: *health teaching. High protein diet*—to replace protein lost in urine, to retain fluid in the intravascular compartment, to reduce edema; moderate sodium—reduce intake of high-sodium foods, no added salt.

5. Goal: *monitor and administer drugs as ordered.*

a. Anticonvulsants (especially magnesium sulfate).

b. Antihypertensives.

c. Diuretics (used rarely, and only in presence of congestive heart failure [CHF]).
d. Blood volume expanders.

6. Goal: *seizure precautions.* To safeguard maternal/fetal status.
   a. Observe for signs and symptoms of *impending* convulsion:
      (1) Frontal headache.
      (2) Epigastric pain.
      (3) Sharp cry.
      (4) Eyes fixed; unresponsive.
      (5) Facial twitching.
   b. Emergency items (suction equipment, airway, drugs, IV fluids) immediately available.

▶ 7. Goal: *convulsion care* (eclamptic woman).
   a. Maintain patent *airway;* administer oxygen.
   b. *Safety*—padded bed rails.
   c. Reduce environmental stimuli: dim lights, quiet.
   d. Observe, report, and record:
      (1) Onset and progression of convulsion.
      (2) If followed by coma or incontinence.
   e. Observe for labor; check FHR. Close observation for 48 h postpartum, even if no further convulsions (or no convulsions to date).

◆ I. **Evaluation/outcome criteria:**
   1. Woman complies with medical/nursing plan of care.
   2. Woman's symptoms respond to treatment; progression halted.
   3. Woman carries uneventful pregnancy to successful termination.

Third Trimester Complications

See Table 7.8, pp. 415–416.

I. Complications affecting fluid-gas transport
   A. Placenta previa—abnormal implantation; near or over internal os. Increased incidence with smokers.
   ◆ 1. **Assessment:**
      a. Painless vaginal bleeding (may be intermittent); absence of contractions, abdomen soft.
      b. If in labor, contractions usually normal.
      c. Boggy lower uterine segment—palpated on vaginal exam. (*Note:* If placenta previa is suspected, internal examinations are **contraindicated.**)
      ⚗ d. *Medical diagnosis—procedure:* sonography—to determine placental site.
   ◆ 2. **Analysis/nursing diagnosis:**
      a. *Anxiety* related to bleeding, outcome.
      b. *Fluid volume deficit* related to excessive blood loss.
      c. *Altered tissue perfusion* related to blood loss.
      d. *Altered urinary elimination* related to hypovolemia.
      e. *Fear* related to fetal injury or loss.

◆ 3. **Nursing care plan/implementation:**
   a. *Medical management*
      (1) Sterile vaginal examination under double set-up.
      (2) Vaginal birth possible if bleeding minimal, marginal implantation; this is woman's second or later vaginal birth; fetal vertex is presenting so that presenting part acts as tamponade.
      (3) Cesarean birth for complete previa.
   b. *Nursing management.* Goal: *safeguard status.*
◆ 4. **Evaluation/outcome criteria:** see following section on abruptio placentae and Table 7.9.

B. Abruptio placentae—premature separation of normally implanted placenta.
   ◆ 1. **Assessment:**
      a. Sudden onset, severe abdominal pain.
      b. Increased uterine tone—may contract unevenly, fails to relax between contractions; very tender.
      c. Shock usually more profound than expected on basis of external bleeding or internal bleeding.
      ⚗ d. *Medical evaluation—procedures:* DIC screening (bleeding time, platelet count, prothrombin time, activated partial thromboplastin time, fibrinogen).
   ◆ 2. **Analysis/nursing diagnosis:**
      a. *Fluid volume deficit* related to bleeding.
      b. *Potential for fetal injury* related to uteroplacental insufficiency.
      c. *Fear* related to unknown outcome.
      3. *Potential complications:*
         a. Afibrinogenemia and DIC.
         b. Couvelaire uterus—bleeding into uterine muscle.
         c. Amniotic fluid embolus.
         d. Hypovolemic shock.
         e. Renal failure.
         f. Uterine atony, hemorrhage, infection in postpartum.
   ◆ 4. **Nursing care plan/implementation:**
      a. *Medical management*
         (1) Control: hemorrhage, hypovolemic shock, replace blood loss.
         (2) Cesarean birth.
         ▬▶ (3) Fibrinogen, if necessary (avoided if possible, due to chance of hepatitis).
         ▬▶ (4) IV heparin—by infusion pump—to reduce coagulation and fibrinolysis.
      b. *Nursing management.* Goal: *safeguard status.*
   ◆ 5. **Evaluation/outcome criteria:**
      a. Experiences successful termination of pregnancy.
         (1) Woman gives birth to viable newborn (by vaginal or cesarean method).
         (2) Woman has minimal blood loss.
         (3) Woman's assessment findings within normal limits.

■ **TABLE 7.9 Comparison of Placenta Previa and Abruptio Placentae**

Pathology	Etiology	Assessment	Nursing Care Plan/ Implementation
Placenta Previa			
Types:	Unknown	Painless vaginal bleeding	■ *No* vaginal or rectal
Marginal—low-lying	More common with	Usually manifests in 8th mo	examinations or enemas
Partial—partly covers	multiparity, advanced	*Postpartum:* signs of	■ Bedrest (*high Fowler's* if
internal os	maternal age	hemorrhage, infection	marginal previa)
Complete—covers internal os	Fibroid tumors		■ Continuous fetal monitor
	Endometriosis		■ Maternal vital signs q4h, or
	Old scars		prn
	Smoking		■ Note character and amount
			of bleeding
			■ Emotional support
Abruptio Placentae			
Types:	Preeclampsia/eclampsia	Pain: sudden, severe	■ *Position:* supine; elevate (R)
Partial—small part separates	Before birth of second twin	Abdomen: rigid	hip
Complete—total placenta	Traction on cord	Uterus: very tender to touch	■ Monitor: vital signs, blood
separates	Rupture of membranes	Fetal hyperactivity;	loss, fetus
Retroplacental—bleeding	High parity	bradycardia, death	■ I&O (anuria, oliguria;
(concealed)	Chronic renal hypertension	Shock: rapid, profound	hematuria)
Marginal—occurs at edges;	Oxytocin induction/	Port-wine amniotic fluid	■ Prepare for surgery
external bleeding	augmentation of labor	Signs of DIC	■ Emotional support
	Cocaine addiction	*Postpartum:* signs of: atony,	
	Trauma	infection, pulmonary emboli	

(4) Woman retains capacity for further childbearing.

b. No evidence of complications (anemia, hypotonia, DIC) during postpartal period.

II. **Complications affecting comfort, rest, mobility**

A. **Hydramnios**—amniotic fluid over 2000 mL (normal volume: 500–1200 mL).

1. **Etiology:** unknown. Risk factors:
   a. Maternal diabetes.
   b. Multifetal gestation.
   c. Erythroblastosis fetalis.
   d. Preeclampsia/eclampsia.
   e. Congenital anomalies (e.g., anencephaly, upper-GI anomalies, such as esophageal atresia).

◆ 2. **Assessment:**
   a. Fundal height: excessive for gestational estimate.
   b. Fetal parts: difficult to palpate, small in proportion to uterine size.
   c. Increased discomfort—due to large, heavy uterus.
   d. Increased edema in vulva and legs.
   e. Shortness of breath.
   f. GI discomfort—heartburn, constipation.
   g. Susceptibility to supine hypotensive syndrome—due to compression of inferior vena cava and descending aorta while in supine position.

🧪 h. *Medical diagnosis*—procedures:
   (1) Sonography—to diagnose multifetal pregnancy, gross fetal anomaly, locate placental site.

🧪 (2) Amniocentesis—to diagnose anomalies, erythroblastosis.

3. *Potential complications:*
   a. Maternal respiratory embarrassment.
   b. Premature rupture of membranes (PROM) with prolapsed cord or amnionitis.
   c. Preterm labor.
   d. Postpartum hemorrhage—due to overdistention and uterine atony.

◆ 4. **Analysis/nursing diagnosis:**
   a. *Pain* related to excessive size of uterus impinging on diaphragm, stomach, bladder.
   b. *Impaired physical mobility* related to increased lordotic curvative of back, increased weight on legs.
   c. *Altered tissue perfusion* related to decreased venous return from lower extremities, compression of body structures by overdistended uterus.
   d. *Potential fluid volume deficit* related to potential uterine atony in immediate postpartum, secondary to loss of contractility due to overdistention.
   e. *Sleep pattern disturbance* related to respiratory embarrassment and discomfort in side-lying position.
   f. *Anxiety* related to discomfort, potential for complications, associated with congenital anomalies.
   g. *Altered urinary elimination* frequency related to pressure of overdistended uterus on bladder.

◆ 5. **Nursing care plan/implementation:**

a. *Medical management*

▲ (1) Amniocentesis—remove excess fluid very slowly, to prevent abruptio placentae.

(2) Termination of pregnancy—if fetal abnormality present *and* woman desires.

b. *Nursing management*

(1) Goal: *health teaching.*

(a) Need for *lateral Sims' position* during resting; semi-Fowler's may alleviate respiratory embarrassment.

(b) Explain diagnostic or treatment procedures.

(c) Signs and symptoms to be *reported immediately:* bleeding, loss of fluid through vagina, cramping.

(2) Goal: *prepare for diagnostic and/or treatment procedures.*

(a) *Force fluids*—for sonography.

(b) Permit for amniocentesis.

(3) Goal: *emotional support for loss of pregnancy* (if applicable).

(a) Encourage verbalization of feelings.

(b) Facilitate grieving: permit parents to see, hold infant; if desired, take photograph, footprints for them.

◆ 6. **Evaluation/outcome criteria:**

a. Woman complies with medical/nursing management.

b. Woman's symptoms of respiratory embarrassment, etc. reduced; comfort promoted.

c. Woman experiences normal, uncomplicated pregnancy, labor, birth, and postpartum.

III. **Diagnostic tests to evaluate fetal growth and well-being**

▲ A. **Daily fetal movement count (DFMC)**

1. Assesses fetal activity.

2. Noninvasive test done by pregnant woman.

3. Three movements/h normal activity.

4. Two movements or less/h may indicate fetal jeopardy.

5. Assess for fetal sleep patterns; repeat after ingesting glucose.

▲ B. **Nonstress test (NST)**

1. Correlates fetal movement with FHR. Requires electronic monitoring.

2. *Reactive test*—acceleration of FHR 15 beats/min above baseline FHR, lasting for 15 sec or more.

3. *Nonreactive test*—acceleration less than 15 beats/min above baseline FHR. May indicate fetal jeopardy.

▲ C. **Contraction stress test (CST); oxytocin challenge test (OCT)**

1. Correlates fetal heart rate response to induced uterine contractions.

2. Requires electronic monitoring.

3. Indicator of uteroplacental sufficiency.

4. Identifies pregnancies at risk for fetal compromise from uteroplacental insufficiency.

5. Increasing doses of oxytocin are administered to stimulate uterine contractions.

6. Interpretation: *negative* results indicate absence of abnormal deceleration with all contractions.

7. *Positive* results indicate abnormal FHR decelerations with contractions.

8. Nipple stimulation (breast self-stimulation test) may also release enough systemic oxytocin to contract uterus to obtain indicators of fetal well-being or fetal jeopardy.

▲ D. **Biophysical profile (BPP)**

1. Observation by ultrasound of five variables for 30 min:

a. Fetal body movements.

b. Fetal tone.

c. Amniotic fluid volume.

d. Response to nonstress testing.

e. Fetal breathing movements.

2. Variables are scored at 2 if present; score of less than 6 is associated with perinatal mortality.

▲ E. **Ultrasound**

1. Noninvasive procedure involving passage of high-frequency sound waves through uterus to obtain data regarding fetal growth, placental positioning, and the uterine cavity.

2. Purpose may include:

a. Pregnancy confirmation.

b. Fetal viability.

c. Estimation of fetal age.

d. BPD measurement (biparietal diameter).

e. Placenta location.

f. Detect fetal abnormalities.

g. Confirm fetal death.

h. Identify multifetal gestations.

3. No risk to mother with infrequent use. Fetal risk not determined on long-term basis.

▲ F. **Amniocentesis**

1. Invasive procedure for amniotic fluid analysis to assess fetal growth and maturity; done after 14 weeks' gestation.

2. Needle placed through abdominal-uterine wall; designated amount of fluid is withdrawn for examination.

3. Empty bladder if gestation greater than 20 wk.

4. Risk of complications less than 1%. Ultrasound *always* precedes this procedure.

5. *Possible complications:* onset of contractions; infections (probably amnionitis); placental, cord puncture; bladder puncture.

6. Advise women to observe and report to physician: fetal hypoactivity or hyperactiv-

ity, vaginal bleeding, vaginal discharge
(clear or colored), signs of labor.

🔔 **G. Analysis of amniotic fluid**
1. Chromosomal studies to detect genetic aberrations.
2. Biochemical analysis of fetal cells to detect
inborn errors of metabolism.
3. Determination of fetal lung maturity by
assessing *lecithin-sphingomyelin* ratios.
4. Evaluation of *phospholipids* (PG and PI);
aids in determining lung maturity; new
and accurate.
5. Determination of *creatinine* levels, aids in
determining fetal age. (*Greater than 1.8*
mg/dL indicates fetal maturity and the fetal age.)
6. Assesses isoimmune disease.
7. Assesses *alpha-fetoprotein (AFP)* levels for
determination of neural-tube defects.
8. Presence of meconium may indicate fetal
hypoxia.

🔔 **H. Chorionic villus sampling (CVS)**
1. Cervically invasive procedure.
2. Advantage—results can be obtained after
10 weeks' gestation due to fast-growing fetal cells.
3. Procedure—removal of small piece of tissue (chorionic villus) from fetal portion of
placenta. Tissue reflects genetic makeup of
fetus.
4. Determines some genetic aberrations and
allows for earlier decision for induced abortion (if desired) from abnormal results.
Does not diagnose neural tube defects;
CVS patients need further diagnoses with
ultrasound and serum AFP levels.
5. Protects "pregnancy privacy" because results can be obtained before the pregnancy
is apparent and decisions can be made regarding abortion or continuation of gestation.
6. Risks involve spontaneous abortion, infection, hematoma, intrauterine death.

❏ The Intrapartal Experience

General overview: This review of the anatomic and
physiologic determinants of successful labor provides
baseline data against which the nurse compares findings of an ongoing assessment of the woman in labor.
Nursing actions are planned and implemented to meet
the present and emerging needs of the woman in labor.

I. Biologic foundations of labor
  A. Premonitory signs
    1. *Lightening*—process in which the fetus
    "drops" into the pelvic inlet.
      a. *Characteristics*
        (1) Nullipara—usually occurs 2–3 wk
        before onset of labor.
        (2) Multipara—commonly occurs with
        onset of labor.

      b. *Effects*
        (1) Relieves pressure on diaphragm—
        breathing is easier.
        (2) Increases pelvic pressure.
          (a) Urinary frequency returns.
          (b) Increased pressure on thighs.
          (c) Increased tendency to vulvar,
          vaginal, perianal, and leg vari-
          cosities.
    2. *Braxton-Hicks contractions*—may become
    more uncomfortable.

  B. Etiology: unknown. *Theories* include:
    1. Uterine overdistention.
    2. Placental aging—declining estrogen/proges-
    terone levels.
    3. Rising prostaglandin level.
    4. Fetal cortisol secretion.
    5. Maternal/fetal oxytocin secretion.

  C. Overview of labor process—forces of labor
  (uterine contractions) overcome cervical resistance; cervix thins (*effacement*) and opens (0–
  10 cm *dilatation*). (Table 7.10). Voluntary contraction of secondary abdominal muscles (e.g.,
  pushing, bearing-down) forces fetal descent.
  Changing pelvic dimensions force fetal head to
  accommodate to the birth canal by molding
  (cranial bones overlap to decrease head size).
  Stages of labor:
    1. *First*—begins with establishment of regu-
    lar, rhythmic contractions; ends with com-
    plete effacement and dilatation (10 cm); di-
    vided into three phases:
      a. Latent and early active.
      b. Active.
      c. Transitional.
    2. *Second*—begins with complete dilatation
    and ends with birth of infant.
    3. *Third*—begins with birth of infant and ends
    with expulsion of placenta.
    4. *Fourth*—begins with expulsion of placenta;
    ends when maternal status is stable (usu-
    ally 1–2 h postpartum).

  D. Anatomic/physiologic determinants
    1. **Maternal**
      a. *Uterine contractions*—expel products of
      conception, begin process of involution.
        (1) *Characteristics:* rhythmic; increasing
        tone (*increment*), peak (*acme*), relax-
        ation (*decrement*).
        (2) *Effects:*
          (a) Decreases blood flow to uterus
          and placenta.
          (b) Dilates cervix during first stage
          of labor.
          (c) Raises maternal blood pressure
          during contractions.
          (d) With bearing-down efforts, ex-
          pels fetus (second stage) and pla-
          centa (third stage).
          (e) Begins involution.
       ◆ (3) **Assessment:**

■ **TABLE 7.10   First Stage of Labor**

Phases of First Stage	Assessment: Expected Maternal Behaviors	Nursing Care Plan/Implementation
0 to 4 cm: Latent Phase and Early Active Phase		
1. Time: multipara 5–6 h; nullipara 8–10 h, average	1. Usually comfortable, euphoric, excited, talkative, and energetic, but may be fearful and withdrawn	1. Provide encouragement, feedback for relaxation, companionship
2. Contractions: regular, mild, 5–10 min apart, 20–30 seconds' duration	2. Relieved or apprehensive that labor has begun	2. Coach during contractions: signal beginning of contraction, mark the seconds, signal end of contraction; "Follow my breathing," "Watch my lips," etc.
3. Low-back pain and abdominal discomfort with contractions	3. Alert, usually receptive to teaching, coaching, diversion, and anticipatory guidance	3. Comfort measures: position for comfort; praise; keep aware of progress
4. Cervix thins; some bloody show		
5. Station: Multipara ⁻2 to ⁺1; nullipara 0.		
4 to 8 cm: Midactive Phase, Phase of Most Rapid Dilatation		
1. Average time: nullipara 1–2 h; multipara 1½–2 h	1. Tired, less talkative, and less energetic	1. Coach during contractions; husband (coach) may need some relief
2. Contractions: 2–5 min apart, 30–40 seconds' duration, intensity increasing	2. More serious, malar flush between 5 and 6 cm, tendency to hyperventilate, may need analgesia, needs constant coaching	2. Comfort measures (to husband too—as needed): position for comfort while preventing hypotensive syndrome; encourage relaxation, focusing her on areas of tension; provide counterpressure to sacrococcygeal area, prn; praise; keep aware of progress; minimize distractions from surrounding environment (loud talking, other noises); offer analgesics and anesthetics, as appropriate; provide hygiene: mouth care, ice chips, clean perineum; warmth, as needed
3. Membranes may rupture now		3. Monitor progress of labor and maternal/fetal response
4. Increased bloody show		4. If monitors are in use, attention on mother; periodically check accuracy of monitor read-outs
5. Station: ⁻1 to 0		
8 to 10 cm: Transition, Deceleration Period of Active Phase		
1. Average time; nullipara 40 min–1 h; multipara 20 min	1. If not under regional anesthesia, more introverted; may be amnesic between contractions	1. Stay with woman (couple) and provide constant support
2. Contractions: 1½–2 min apart, 60–90 seconds' duration, strong intensity	2. Feeling she cannot make it; increased irritability, crying, nausea, vomiting, and belching; increased perspiration over upper lip and between breasts; leg tremors; and shaking	2. Continue to coach with contractions: may need to remind, reassure, and encourage her to reestablish breathing techniques and concentration with each contraction; coach panting or "he-he" respirations to prevent pushing
3. Increased vaginal show; rectal pressure with beginning urge to bear down	3. May have uncontrollable urge to push at this time	3. Comfort measures: remind her and husband her behavior is normal and "OK"; coach breathing to quell nausea
4. Station: ⁺3 to ⁺4		4. Assist with countertension techniques woman requested: effleurage
		5. Monitor contractions, FHR (after each contraction), vaginal discharge, perineal bulging, maternal vital signs; record every 15 min
		6. Assess for bladder filling
		7. Keep mother (couple) aware of progress
		8. Prepare husband for birth (scrub, gown, etc.)

(a) Frequency—time from beginning of one contraction to beginning of the next.
(b) Duration—time from beginning of contraction to relaxation.
(c) Strength (intensity)—resistance to indentation.
(d) False/true labor—differentiation (Table 7.11).
(e) Signs of dysfunctional labor. See pp. 449–452.
b. *Pelvic structures and configuration:*
(1) *False pelvis*—above linea terminalis (line travels across top of symphysis pubis around to sacral promontory); supports gravid uterus during pregnancy.
(2) *True pelvis*—lies below linea terminalis; divided into:
(a) Inlet—"brim," demarcated by linea terminalis.
    (i) Widest diameter: transverse.
    (ii) Narrowest diameter: anterior-posterior (true conjugate).
(b) Midplane—pelvic cavity.
(c) Outlet.
    (i) Widest diameter: anterior-posterior (requires internal rotation of fetal head for entry).
    (ii) Narrowest diameter: transverse (intertuberous); facilitates birth in occiput anterior (OA) position.
(3) *Classifications*
(a) Gynecoid—normal female pelvis; rounded oval.
(b) Android—normal male pelvis; funnel shaped.
(c) Anthropoid—oval.
(d) Platypelloid—flattened, transverse oval.

2. **Fetal**
a. *Fetal head* (Figure 7.3, p. 430).
(1) Bones—one occipital, one frontal, two parietals, two temporals.
(2) Suture—line of junction or closure between bones; sagittal (longitudinal), coronal (anterior), and lambdoidal (posterior); permit molding.
(3) Fontanels—membranous space between cranial bones during fetal life and infancy.
(a) *Anterior* "soft spot"—diamond shaped; junction of coronal and sagittal sutures; closes (ossifies) in *12–18 mo.*
(b) *Posterior*—triangular; junction of sagittal and lambdoidal sutures; closes by *2 mo of age.*
b. *Fetal lie*—relationship of fetal long axis to maternal long axis (spine).
(1) Transverse—shoulder presents.
(2) Longitudinal—vertex or breech presents.
c. *Presentation*—fetal part entering inlet first (Figure 7.4, p. 430).
(1) *Cephalic*—vertex (most common); face, brow.
(2) *Breech*
(a) *Complete*—feet and legs flexed on thighs; buttocks and feet presenting.
(b) *Frank*—legs extended on torso, feet up by shoulders; buttocks presenting.
(c) *Footling*—single (one foot), double (both feet) presenting.
d. *Attitude*—relationship of fetal parts to one another (e.g., head flexed on chest).
e. *Position*—relationship of presenting fetal part to quadrants of maternal pelvis; vertex most common, occiput anterior on maternal left side (LOA). See Figure 7.4.
3. **Assessment:** determine presentation and position.
a. *Leopold's maneuvers*—abdominal palpation.
(1) *First*—palms over fundus, breech feels softer, not as round as head would be.
(2) *Second*—palms on either side of abdomen, locates fetal back and small parts.
(3) *Third*—fingers just above pubic symphysis, grasp lower abdomen; if unengaged, presenting part is mobile.
(4) *Fourth*—facing mother's feet, run palms down sides of abdomen to symphysis; check for cephalic prominence (usually on right side), and if head is floating or engaged.

■ TABLE 7.11   Assessment: Differentiation of False/True Labor

False Labor	True Labor
Contractions: Braxton-Hicks intensify (more noticeable at night); short, irregular, little change	*Contractions:* begin in lower back, radiate to abdomen ("girdling"), become regular, rhythmic; frequency, duration, intensity increase
Relieved by change of position or activity (e.g., walking)	*Unaffected* by change of position, activity, drinking two glasses of water, or moderate analgesia
Cervical changes—none; *no* effacement or dilatation progress	*Cervical changes*—progressive effacement and dilatation

■ **FIGURE 7.3**   The fetal head. *Bones:* two frontal, two temporal, one occipital. *Sutures:* sagittal, frontal, coronal, lambdoid. *Fontanels:* anterior, posterior. (Reprinted with permission of Ross Laboratories, Columbus, OH, Clinical Education Aid No. 13.)

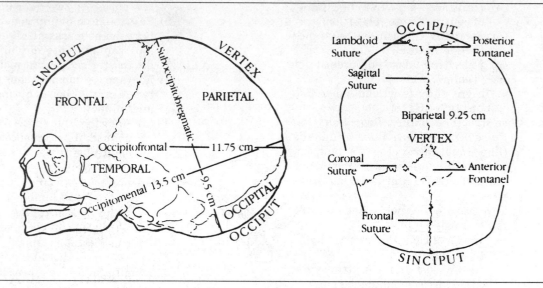

■ **FIGURE 7.4**   Categories of fetal presentation. (a) LOA: fetal occiput is in left anterior quadrant of maternal pelvis. (b) LOP: fetal occiput is in left posterior quadrant of maternal pelvis. (c) ROA: fetal occiput is in right anterior quadrant of maternal pelvis. (d) ROP: fetal occiput is in right posterior quadrant of maternal pelvis. (e) LSP: fetal sacrum is in left posterior quadrant of maternal pelvis. (f) Shoulder presentation with fetus in transverse lie. (g) Prolapse of umbilical cord with fetus in LOA position. (Reprinted with permission of Ross Laboratories, Columbus, OH, Clinical Education Aid No. 18.)

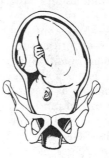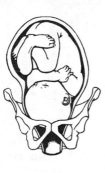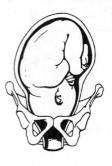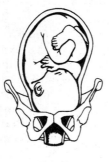

(a) LOA   **(b) LOP**   **(c) ROA**   **(d) ROP**

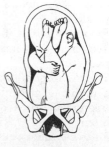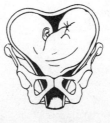

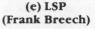

(e) LSP
(Frank Breech)   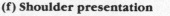**(f) Shoulder presentation**   **(g) Prolapse of cord**

▶ b. *Location of fetal heart tones*—heard best through fetal back or chest.
   (1) *Breech* presentation—usually most audible *above* maternal umbilicus.
   (2) *Vertex* presentation—usually most audible *below* maternal umbilicus.
   (3) Changing location of most audible FHTs (fetal heart tones)—useful indicator of fetal descent.
   (4) Factors affecting audibility:
      (a) Obesity.
      (b) Maternal position.
      (c) Hydramnios.
      (d) Maternal gastrointestinal activity.
      (e) Loud uterine bruit—origin: hissing of blood through umbilical arteries; synchronous with maternal pulse.
      (f) Loud funic souffle—origin: hissing of blood through umbilical arteries; synchronous with fetal heart rate (FHR).
      (g) External noise, faulty equipment.
▲ c. *Vaginal examination:* palpable sutures, fontanels (triangular-shaped superior, diamond-shaped inferior = vertex presentation, OA position).
4. *Cardinal movements of the* **mechanisms of normal labor**—vertex presentation, positional changes of fetal head accommodate to changing diameters of maternal pelvis (Figure 7.5).
   a. *Descent*—head engages and proceeds down birth canal.
   b. *Flexion*—head bent to chest; presents smallest diameter of vertex (suboccipital-bregmatic).
   c. *Internal rotation*—during second stage of labor, transverse diameter of fetal head enters pelvis; occiput rotates 90 degrees to bring back of neck under symphysis (e.g., LOT to LOA to OA); presents smallest diameter (biparietal) to smallest diameter of outlet (intertuberous).
   d. *Extension*—back of neck pivots under symphysis, allows head to be born by extension.
   e. *Restitution*—head returns to normal alignment with shoulders (with LOA, results in head facing right thigh), presents smallest diameter of shoulders to outlet.
   f. *Expulsion*—birth of neonate completed.
◆ g. **Assessment:** relationship of fetal head to ischial spines (**degree of descent**).
   (1) *Engagement*—widest diameter of presenting part has passed through pelvic inlet (e.g., biparietal diameter of fetal head).

   (2) *Station*—relationship of presenting part to ischial spines (IS).
      (a) *Floating*—presenting part above inlet, in false pelvis.
      (b) Station—−5 is at inlet (presenting part well above IS).
      (c) Station 0—presenting part at IS (engaged).
      (d) Station +4—presenting part at the outlet.
E. **Danger signs during labor**
   1. *Contraction*—hypertonic, poor relaxation, or tetanic (greater than 90 sec long and ≤2 min apart).
   2. *Abdominal pain*—sharp, rigid abdomen.
   3. *Vaginal bleeding*—profuse.
   4. *FHR*—late decelerations, prolonged variable decelerations, bradycardia, tachycardia (Figure 7.6, p. 433).
   5. *Maternal hypertension.*
   6. *Meconium-stained amniotic fluid (MSAF).*
   7. *Prolonged ROM.*
II. **Participatory childbirth techniques**
   A. **Psychoprophylaxis—Lamaze method**
      1. Premise—conditioned responses to stimuli occupy nerve pathways, reducing perception of pain. Emphasis is on childbirth as a natural event, with an informed woman as the active participant. The ability to relax effectively reduces the perception of pain, and the involvement of the coach fosters the family concept.
      2. Childbirth partners are taught:
         a. Anatomy and physiology of labor.
         b. Psychology of man and woman.
         c. What to expect in the hospital setting.
         d. Conditioned responses to labor stimuli.
            (1) Concentration on focal point.
            (2) Breathing techniques.
            (3) Need for active coaching to enable woman to:
               (a) Use techniques appropriate to present stage of labor.
               (b) Avoid hyperventilation.
         e. Specific stage—appropriate techniques:
            (1) *First stage of labor*—early: slow, deep chest breathing.
            (2) *Transition* (8–10 cm)—rapid, shallow breathing pattern, to prevent pushing prematurely.
               (a) Panting.
               (b) Pant-blow.
               (c) "He-he" pattern.
            (3) *Second stage of labor*
               (a) Pushing (or bearing-down)—aids fetal descent through birth canal.
               (b) Panting—aids relaxation between contractions; prevents explosive birth of head.
         f. Effects on labor behaviors/coping:
            (1) Help mother cope with and assist contractions.

■ **FIGURE 7.5** Cardial movements in the mechanism of labor with the fetus in vertex presentation. **(a)** Engagement, descent, flexion. **(b)** Internal rotation. **(c)** Extension beginning (rotation complete). **(d)** Extension complete. **(e)** External rotation (restitution). **(f)** External rotation (shoulder rotation). **(g)** Expulsion. (Reprinted with permission of Ross Laboratories, Columbus, OH, Clinical Education Aid No. 13.)

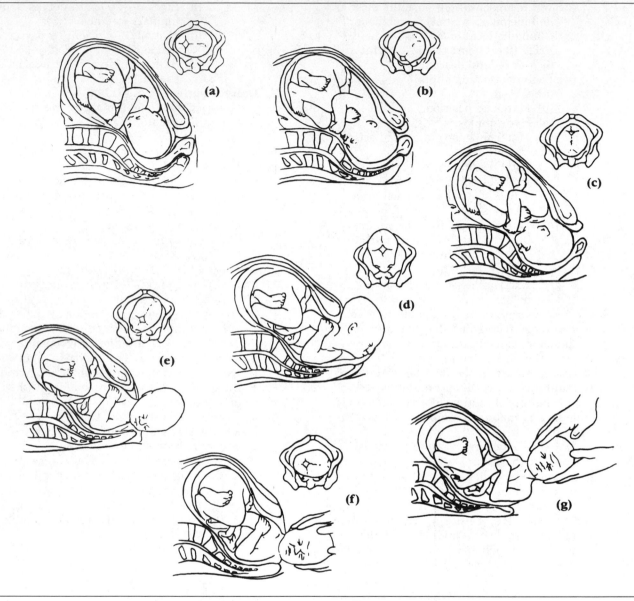

(2) Prevent premature bearing-down; reduce possibility of cervical edema due to pushing on incompletely dilated cervix.

(3) When appropriate, improve efficiency of bearing-down efforts.

B. Other methods—include parent classes, classes for siblings, multiparas, and those who plan cesarean birth.

III. Nursing actions during first stage of labor

◆ **A. Assessment:**—careful evaluation of:

1. *Antepartal history*
   a. EDB
   b. Genetic and familial problems.

c. Preexisting and coexisting medical disorders, allergies.

d. Pregnancy-related health problems (hyperemesis, bleeding, etc.).

e. Infectious diseases (past and present herpes, etc.).

f. Past obstetric history, if any.

g. Pelvic measurements.

h. Height.

i. Weight gain.

j. Laboratory results:
   (1) Blood type and Rh factor.
   (2) Serology.
   (3) Urinalysis.

■ **FIGURE 7.6** Fetal heart rate (FHR) decelerations and nursing interventions.

Pattern	Description	Nursing Intervention

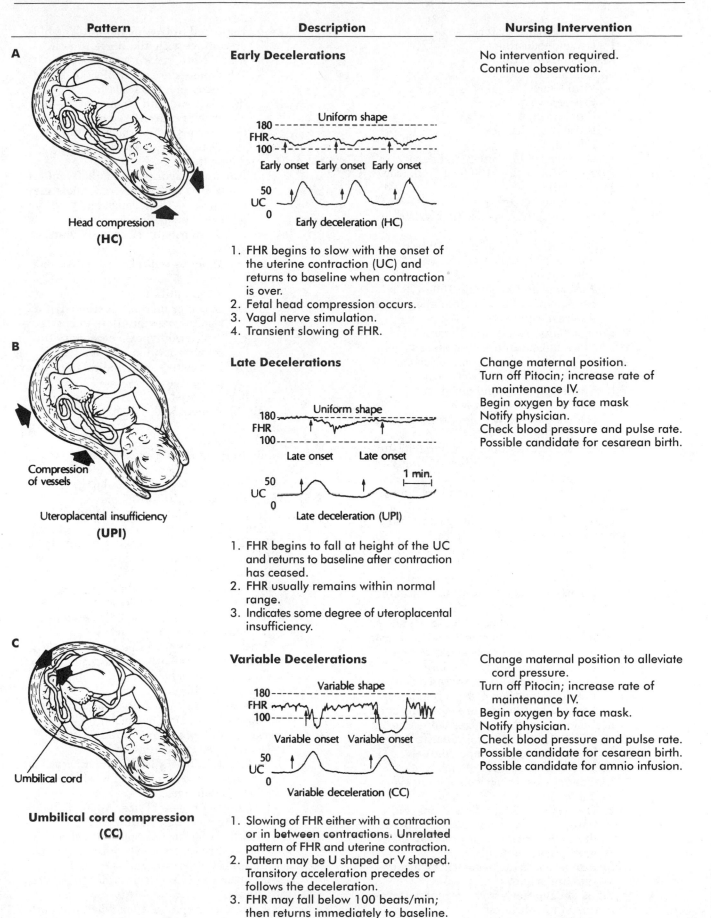

A

Head compression
(HC)

Early Decelerations

Uniform shape

180 -----
FHR
100 -
Early onset Early onset Early onset

50
UC
0
Early deceleration (HC)

1. FHR begins to slow with the onset of the uterine contraction (UC) and returns to baseline when contraction is over.
2. Fetal head compression occurs.
3. Vagal nerve stimulation.
4. Transient slowing of FHR.

No intervention required.
Continue observation.

B

Compression of vessels

Uteroplacental insufficiency
(UPI)

Late Decelerations

Uniform shape

180
FHR
100
Late onset   Late onset

50   1 min.
UC
0
Late deceleration (UPI)

1. FHR begins to fall at height of the UC and returns to baseline after contraction has ceased.
2. FHR usually remains within normal range.
3. Indicates some degree of uteroplacental insufficiency.

Change maternal position.
Turn off Pitocin; increase rate of maintenance IV.
Begin oxygen by face mask
Notify physician.
Check blood pressure and pulse rate.
Possible candidate for cesarean birth.

C

Umbilical cord

**Umbilical cord compression
(CC)**

Variable Decelerations

Variable shape

180 -----
FHR
100 -
Variable onset   Variable onset

50
UC
0
Variable deceleration (CC)

1. Slowing of FHR either with a contraction or in between contractions. Unrelated pattern of FHR and uterine contraction.
2. Pattern may be U shaped or V shaped. Transitory acceleration precedes or follows the deceleration.
3. FHR may fall below 100 beats/min; then returns immediately to baseline.
4. Usually indicates cord compression.

Change maternal position to alleviate cord pressure.
Turn off Pitocin; increase rate of maintenance IV.
Begin oxygen by face mask.
Notify physician.
Check blood pressure and pulse rate.
Possible candidate for cesarean birth.
Possible candidate for amnio infusion.

Maternal-Infant

    k. Prenatal care history.

    l. Use of medications.

  2. *Admission findings*

    a. Emotional status.

    b. Vital signs.

    c. Present weight.

    d. Fundal height.

    e. Present fetal size.

    f. Edema.

    g. Urinalysis (for protein and sugar).

▶ 3. *FHR*—normal, 120–160 beats/min (see Figure 7.6).

    a. Check and record every 30 min—to monitor fetal response to physiologic stress of labor.

    b. *Bradycardia* (mild, 100–119 beats/min, or 30 beats/min lower than baseline reading).

    c. *Tachycardia* (moderate, 160–179 beats/min, or 30 beats/min above baseline reading).

  4. *Contractions*—every 15–30 min.

    a. Place fingertips over fundus, use gentle pressure; contraction felt as hardening or tensing.

    b. Time: frequency and duration.

    c. Intensity/strength at acme:

      (1) Weak—easily indent fundus with fingers.

      (2) Moderate—some tension felt, fundus indents slightly with finger pressure.

      (3) Strong—unable to indent fundus.

  5. *Maternal response to labor*—assess for effective coping, cooperation, and utilizing effective breathing techniques.

  6. *Maternal vital signs*—between contractions.

    a. Response to pain or use of special breathing techniques alters pulse and respirations.

    b. B/P, P, RR—if normotensive: on admission, and then every hour and prn; after regional anesthesia: every 30 min (every 5 min first 20 min).

    c. Temp—if within normal range: on admission, and then every 4 h and prn. Every 2 h after rupture of membranes.

    d. Before and after analgesia/anesthesia.

    e. After rupture of membranes (see Amniotic fluid embolism, p. 450).

  7. Character and amount of bloody show.

  8. Bladder status: encourage voiding every 1–2 h, monitor output.

    a. Determine bladder distention—palpate just above symphysis (full bladder may impede labor progress or result in trauma to bladder).

    b. Admission urinalysis—check for protein and sugar.

  9. Signs of deviations from normal patterns.

 10. Status of membranes:

    a. Intact.

▶   b. Ruptured (nitrazine paper turns blue on contact with alkaline amniotic fluid). Note, record, and report:

      (1) Time—danger of infection if ruptured more than 24 h.

      (2) FHR stat and 10 min later—to check for prolapsed cord.

      (3) Character and color of fluid (see 11.b. and c., below).

⚠ 11. Amniotic fluid.

    a. Amount—hydramnios (>2000 mL)—associated with congenital anomalies.

    b. Character—thick consistency or odor associated with infection.

    c. Color—normally clear with white specks.

      (1) Yellow—indicates fetal distress about 35 h previous; Rh or ABO incompatibility.

      (2) Green or meconium stained; if fetus in vertex position, indicates recent fetal hypoxia secondary to respiratory distress in fetus.

      (3) Port wine—may indicate abruptio placentae.

 12. Labor progress:

    a. Effacement.

    b. Dilatation.

    c. Station.

    d. Bulging membranes.

    e. Molding of fetal head.

 13. Perineum—observe for bulging.

◆ **B. Analysis/nursing diagnosis:**

  1. *Anxiety, fear* related to uncertain outcome, pain.

  2. *Ineffective individual coping* related to lack of preparation for childbirth or poor support from coach.

  3. *Altered nutrition: less than body requirements* related to physiologic stress of labor.

  4. *Altered urinary elimination* related to pressure of presenting part.

  5. *Altered thought processes* related to sleep deprivation, transition, analgesia.

  6. *Fluid volume deficit* related to anemia, excessive blood loss.

  7. *Impaired (fetal) gas exchange* related to impaired placental perfusion.

◆ **C. Nursing care plan/implementation:**

  1. Goal: *comfort measures.*

    a. Maintain hydration of oral mucosa. Encourage sucking on cool washcloth, ice chips, lollipops.

    b. Reduce dryness of lips. Apply lip balm (Chapstick, petrolatum jelly).

    c. Relieve backache. Apply sacral counterpressure (particularly with occiput posterior [OP] presentation).

    d. Encourage significant other to participate.

    e. Encourage ambulation when presenting part engaged.

2. Goal: *management of physical needs.*
   a. Encourage frequent voiding—to prevent full bladder from impeding oncoming head.
   b. Encourage ambulation throughout labor; *lateral Sims' position with head elevated* to:
      (1) Encourage relaxation.
      (2) Allow gravity to assist in anterior rotation of fetal head.
      (3) Prevent compression of inferior vena cava and descending aorta (supine hypotensive syndrome).
      (4) Promote placental perfusion.
   ▶ c. Perineal prep, if ordered—to promote cleanliness.
   ▶ d. Fleet's enema, if ordered—to stimulate peristalsis, evacuate lower bowel. *Note:* **contraindicated** if:
      (1) Cervical dilatation (4 cm or more) with unengaged head—due to possibility of cord prolapse.
      (2) Fetal malpresentation/malposition—due to possible fetal distress.
      (3) Preterm labor—may stimulate contractions.
      (4) Painless vaginal bleeding—due to possible placenta previa.
3. Goal: *management of psychosocial needs. Emotional support:*
   a. Encourage verbalization of feelings, fears, concerns.
   b. Explain all procedures.
   c. Reinforce self-concept ("You're doing well!").
4. Goal: *management of discomfort.*
   a. Analgesia or anesthesia—may be required or desired—to facilitate safe, comfortable birth.
   b. Support/enhance/teach childbirth techniques.
   ▶ (1) Reinforce appropriate *breathing techniques* for current labor status.
      (a) If woman is **hyperventilating,** to increase PaCO$_2$, minimize fetal acidosis, and relieve symptoms of vertigo and syncope, suggest:
         (i) Breathe into paper bag.
         (ii) Breathe into cupped hands.
      (b) Demonstrate appropriate breathing for several contractions—to reestablish rate and rhythm.
   (2) Goal: *sustain motivation.*
      (a) Offer support, encouragement, and praise, as appropriate.
      (b) Keep informed of status and progress.
      (c) Reassure that irritability is normal.

(d) Serve as surrogate coach when necessary (if no partner, before partner arrives, while partner changes clothes, during needed breaks); assist with effleurage, breathing, focusing.
(e) Discourage bearing-down efforts by pant-blow until complete (10 cm) dilatation to avoid cervical edema.
(f) Facilitate informed decision making regarding medication for relaxation or pain relief.
(g) Keep woman and family informed of her progress.
(h) Minimize distractions: quiet, relaxed environment; privacy.

◆ **D. Evaluation/outcome criteria:**
1. Woman manages own labor discomfort effectively.
2. Woman maintains control over own behavior.
3. Woman successfully completes first stage of labor without incident.

IV. **Nursing actions during second stage of labor**
◆ **A. Assessment:**
1. Maternal (or couple's) response to labor.
▶ 2. FHR—continuous electronic monitoring, or after each contraction with fetoscope, Doppler.
3. Vital signs.
4. Time elapsed—average: 2 min to 1 h; prolonged second stage increases risk of fetal distress, maternal exhaustion, psychological stress, intrauterine infection.
5. Contraction pattern—average every 1½– 3 min, lasting 60–90 sec.
6. Vaginal discharge—increases.
7. Nausea, vomiting, disorientation, tremors, amnesia between contractions, panic.
8. Response to regional anesthesia, if administered.
   a. Signs of hypotension—reduces placental perfusion, increases risk of fetal hypoxia.
   b. Effect on contractions—note and report any slowing of labor.
9. Efforts to bear down—increase expulsive effects of uterine contractions.
10. Perineal bulging with contractions—fetal head distends perineum, crowns; head born by extension.

◆ **B. Analysis/nursing diagnosis:**
1. *Pain* related to strong uterine contractions, pressure of fetal descent, stretching of perineum.
2. *High risk for injury:*
   a. Infection related to ruptured membranes, repeated vaginal examinations.
   b. Laceration related to pressure of fetal head exceeding perineal elasticity and

uterine rupture related to fundal pressure.

3. *Impaired skin integrity* related to laceration, episiotomy.

4. *Fluid volume deficit* related to hypotension secondary to regional anesthesia.

5. *Anxiety* related to imminent birth of fetus.

6. *Ineffective individual coping* related to prolonged sensory stimulation (contractions) and anxiety.

7. *Altered urinary elimination* related to anesthesia and contractions.

8. *Sleep pattern disturbance.*

◆ **C. Nursing care plan/implementation:**
1. Goal: *emotional support.*
   a. To sustain motivation/control:
      (1) Never leave mother and significant other alone now.
      (2) Keep informed of progress.
   ▶ (3) Direct bearing-down efforts (pushing) without holding breath* while pushing. Encourage pushing "out through vagina" and encourage mother to touch coming head; position mirror so woman can see perineal bulging with effective efforts; minimize distractions.
   b. To allay significant other's anxiety: reassure regarding mother's behavior if she is not anesthetized.
   c. Support family choices.
2. Goal: *safeguard status.*
   a. Precautions when putting legs in stirrups:
      (1) If varicosities, **do not put legs in stirrups.**
      (2) *Avoid* pressure to popliteal veins; pad stirrups.
      (3) Ensure proper, even alignment by adjusting stirrups.
      (4) Move legs simultaneously into or out of stirrups—to *avoid* nerve, ligament, and muscle strain.
      (5) Provide proper support to woman not using stirrups.
   b. Support woman in whatever position selected for birth, e.g., side-lying.
   ▶ c. Cleanse perineum, thighs, and lower abdomen, maintaining sterile technique.
3. Goal: *maintain a comfortable environment.*
   a. Free of unnecessary noise, light.
   b. Comfortable temperature (warm).
4. *Medical management*

---

*The woman must be discouraged from using the **Valsalva maneuver** (holding one's breath and tightening abdominal muscles) for pushing during the second stage. This activity increases intrathoracic pressure, reduces venous return, and increases venous pressure. Cardiac output and blood pressure increase, and pulse slows temporarily. During the Valsalva maneuver, fetal hypoxia may occur. The process is reversed when the woman takes a breath.

a. Episiotomy may be performed to facilitate birth.

b. Forceps may be applied to exert traction and expedite birth.

c. Vacuum extraction also used.

5. Birthing room birth with alternative positions.

◆ **D. Evaluation/outcome criteria:**
1. Cooperative, actively participates in birth; maintains control over own behavior.
2. Successful, uncomplicated birth of viable infant.
3. All assessment findings within normal limits (vital signs, emotional status, response to birth).
4. Presence of significant other.

V. Nursing actions during third stage of labor

◆ **A. Assessment:**
1. Time elapsed—average: 5 min; prolonged third stage (greater than 25 min) may indicate complications.
2. Signs of *placental separation:*
   a. Increase in bleeding.
   b. Cord lengthens.
   c. Uterus rises in abdomen, assumes globular shape.
3. Assess mother's level of consciousness.
4. Examine placenta for intactness and number of vessels in umbilical cord (normal: three. *Note:* two vessels only—associated with increased incidence of congenital anomalies); condition of placenta for calcification, infarcts, etc.

◆ **B. Analysis/nursing diagnosis:**
1. *Family coping: potential for growth* related to bonding, beginning achievement of developmental tasks.
2. *Fluid volume deficit* related to blood loss during third stage.

◆ **C. Nursing care plan/implementation:**
1. Goal: *prevent uterine atony.* Administer oxytocin, as ordered.
2. Goal: *facilitate parent-child bonding.*
   a. While protecting neonate from cold stress, encourage parents to see, hold, touch neonate.
   b. Comment about neonate's individuality, characteristics, and behaviors.
   c. After neonate assessed for congenital anomalies (cleft palate, esophageal atresia), encourage breastfeeding, if desired.
3. Goal: *health teaching.*
   a. Describe, discuss common neonatal behavior in transitional period (periods of reactivity, sleep, hyperactivity).
   b. Demonstrate removal of mucus by aspiration with bulb syringe.
   c. Demonstrate ways of facilitating breastfeeding.

◆ **D. Evaluation/outcome criteria:**
1. Woman has a successful, uneventful completion of labor.

a. Minimal blood loss.
b. Vital signs within normal limits.
c. Fundus well contracted at level of umbilicus.

2. Parents express satisfaction with outcome, demonstrate infant attachment.

VI. **Nursing actions during the fourth stage of labor**—1–2 h postpartum.

◆ A. **Assessment**—every 15 min four times; then, every 30 min two times—or until stable—to monitor response to physiologic stress of labor/birth.

▶ 1. Vital signs:
a. *Temperature* taken once; if elevated, requires follow-up—may indicate infection, dehydration, excessive blood loss. Note, record, report temperature of 100.4°F (38°C).
b. *Blood pressure*—every 15 min × 4.
(1) Returns to prelabor level—due to loss of placental circulation and increased circulating blood volume.
(2) Elevation may be in response to use of oxytocic drugs or preeclampsia (first 48 h).
(3) Lowered blood pressure—may reflect significant blood loss during labor/birth, or occult bleeding.
c. *Pulse*—every 15 min × 4.
(1) Physiologic bradycardia—due to normal vagal response.
(2) Tachycardia—may indicate excessive blood loss during labor/birth, dehydration, exhaustion, or occult bleeding.

▶ 2. Location and consistency of fundus—every 15 min, to ensure continuing contraction; prevent blood loss due to uterine relaxation.
a. Fundus—firm; at or slightly lower than the umbilicus; in midline.
b. May be displaced by distended bladder—due to normal diuresis; common cause of bleeding in immediate postpartum, uterine atony.

3. Character and amount of vaginal flow.
a. Moderate lochia rubra.
b. If perineal pad saturated in 15 min, or blood pools under buttocks, excessive loss.
c. Bright red bleeding may indicate cervical or vaginal laceration.

4. Perineum.
a. Edema.
b. Bruising—due to trauma.
c. Distention/hematoma, rectal pain.

5. Bladder fullness/voiding—to prevent distention.

6. Rate of IV, if present; response to added medication, if any.

7. Intake and output—to evaluate hydration.

8. Recovery from analgesia/anesthesia.
9. Energy level.
10. Verbal, nonverbal interaction between woman and significant other.
a. Dialogue.
b. Posture.
c. Facial expressions.
d. Touching.
11. Interactions between parent(s) and newborn; signs of bonding.
a. Eye contact with newborn.
b. Calls by name.
c. Explores with fingertips, strokes, cuddles.
12. Signs of postpartal emergencies:
a. Uterine atony, hemorrhage.
b. Vaginal hematoma.

◆ B. **Analysis/nursing diagnosis:**
1. *Fluid volume deficit* related to excessive intrapartal blood loss, dehydration.
2. *Altered urinary elimination* related to intrapartal bladder trauma, dehydration, blood loss.
3. *Impaired skin integrity* related to episiotomy, lacerations, cesarean birth.
4. *Altered family processes* related to role change.
5. *Altered parenting* related to interruption in bonding secondary to:
a. Compromised maternal status.
b. Compromised neonatal status.
6. *Knowledge deficit* related to self-care procedures.
7. *Fatigue* related to sleep disturbances and anxiety.
8. *Anxiety* regarding status of self and infant.
9. *Altered nutrition, less than body requirements,* related to decreased food and fluid intake during labor.

◆ C. **Nursing care plan/implementation:**
1. Goal: *comfort measures.*
a. Position, pad change.
▶ b. Perineal care—to promote healing; to reduce possibility of infection.
c. Ice pack to perineum, as ordered—to reduce edema, discomfort, and pain related to hemorrhoids.
2. Goal: *nutrition/hydration.* Offer fluids, foods as tolerated.
3. Goal: *urinary elimination.*
a. Encourage voiding—to avoid bladder distention.
b. Record: time, amount, character.
c. Anticipatory guidance related to nocturnal diuresis and increased output.
4. Goal: *promote bonding.*
a. Provide privacy, quiet; encourage sustained contact with newborn.
b. Encourage: touching, holding baby; breastfeeding (also promotes involution).

5. Goal: *health teaching.*
   a. Perineal care—front to back, labia closed (after *each* void/bm).
   b. Handwashing—before and after each pad change; after voiding, defecating; before and after baby care.
   c. Signs to report:
      (1) Uterine cramping.
      (2) Increased vaginal bleeding, passage of large clots.
      (3) Nausea, dizziness.

◆ **D. Evaluation/outcome criteria:**
   1. Expresses comfort, satisfaction in fourth stage.
   2. Vital signs stable, fundus contracted, moderate lochia rubra, perineum undistended.
   3. Tolerates food and fluids well.
   4. Voids in adequate amount.
   5. Demonstrates eye contact with infant, cuddles.
   6. Verbalizes abnormal signs to report to physician.
   7. Returns demonstration of appropriate perineal care.
   8. Ambulates without pain, dizziness, numbness of legs.

VII. Nursing management of the newborn immediately after birth
◆ **A. Assessment:**
   1. Mucus in nasophyarynx, oropharynx.
   2. *Apgar score:* note and record—at 1 and 5 min of age (Table 7.12).
      a. Score of 7–10: good condition.
      b. Score of 4–6: fair condition; assess for CNS depression; resuscitate, as necessary.
      c. Score of 0–3: poor condition; requires immediate resuscitative measures. *Asphyxia neonatorum*—fails to breathe spontaneously within 30–60 sec after birth.
   3. Number of vessels in umbilical stump.
   4. Passage of meconium stool, urine.
   5. General physical appearance/status.
      a. Signs of respiratory distress (nasal flaring, grunting, sternal retraction, cyanosis, tachypnea).
      b. Skin condition (meconium-stained, cyanosis, jaundice, lesions).
   c. Cry—presence, pitch, quality.
   d. Signs of birth trauma (lacerations, dislocations, fractures).
   e. Symmetry (absent parts, extra digits, gross malformations, ears, palm creases, sacral dimples).
   f. Molding, caput succedaneum, cephalhematoma.
   g. Assess gestational age.
   6. Identify high-risk infant.

◆ **B. Analysis/nursing diagnosis:**
   1. *Ineffective airway clearance* related to excessive nasopharyngeal mucus.
   2. *Ineffective breathing pattern* related to CNS depression secondary to intrauterine hypoxia narcosis, prematurity, and lack of pulmonary surfactant.
   3. *Impaired gas exchange* related to respiratory distress.
   4. *Fluid volume deficit* related to birth trauma; hemolytic jaundice.
   5. *Impaired skin integrity* related to cord stump.
   6. *High risk for injury* (biochemical, metabolic) related to impaired thermoregulation.
   7. *Ineffective thermoregulation* related to environmental conditions.

◆ **C. Nursing care plan/implementation:**
   1. Goal: *ensure patent airway.*
      a. Suction mouth first, then nose; when stimulated, sensitive receptors around entrance to nares initiate gasp, causing aspiration of mucus present in mouth.
   ▶ b. Suction with bulb syringe.
      (1) If deeper suctioning necessary, use DeLee mucus trap attached to suction. Oral use of DeLee is discouraged due to risk of contact with baby's secretions (new Delee now available that has no such risk).
      (2) *Avoid* prolonged, vigorous suctioning.
         (a) Reduces oxygenation.
         (b) May traumatize tissue, cause edema, bleeding, laryngospasm, and cardiac arrhythmia.
      c. Assist gravity drainage of fluids. *Position:* head dependent (Trendelenburg), and side-lying.

■ **TABLE 7.12   Apgar Score**

Sign	0	1	2
Heart rate	Absent	<100	>100
Respiratory effort	Absent	Slow and irregular	Good and crying
Muscle tone	Flaccid	Some flexion of extremities	Active motions, general flexion
Reflex irritability	No response	Weak cry or grimace	Cry
Color	Blue, pale	Body pink, extremities blue	Completely pink

2. Goal: *maintain body temperature*—to conserve energy, preserve store of brown fat, decrease oxygen needs; prevent acidosis. Prevent chilling:
   a. Minimize exposure; dry quickly.
   b. Warm; apply hat.
   c. Take temperature hourly until stable.
3. Goal: *identify infant:*
   a. Apply Identiband or name beads.
   b. Take infant's footprints and maternal fingerprints.
4. Goal: *prevent eye infection* (gonorrheal and chlamydial ophthalmia neonatorum).
   ▣ Within 2 h of birth apply antibiotic drops (two drops in each eye).
5. Goal: *facilitate prompt identification/vigilance for potential neonatal complications.*
   a. Record significant data from mother's chart:
      (1) History of pregnancy, diabetes, hypertension, current drug abuse, excessive caffeine, medications, alcohol, malnutrition.
      (2) Course of labor, evidence of fetal distress, medications received in labor.
      (3) Birth history of anesthesia.
      (4) Apgar; resuscitative efforts.
   b. Goal: *facilitate prompt identification/intervention in hemolytic problems of the newborn.*
      ⚗ (1) Collect and send cord blood for appropriate tests:
         (a) Blood type and Rh factor.
         (b) Coombs test.
      ▣ (2) Give vitamin K to facilitate clotting.

◆ **D. Evaluation/outcome criteria:** successful transition to extrauterine life.
1. Status satisfactory; all assessment findings within normal limits.
2. Responsive in bonding process with parents.

VIII. Nurse-attended emergency birth (precipitate birth). When woman presents without prenatal care to ER, may represent drug abuse.
IMMINENT BIRTH
◆ **A. Assessment:** identify signs of *imminent birth:*
1. Strong contractions.
2. Bearing-down efforts.
3. Perineal bulging; crowning.
4. Mother states, "It's coming."
◆ **B. Analysis/nursing diagnosis:**
1. *Pain* related to:
   a. Strong, sustained contractions.
   b. Descent of fetal head.
   c. Stretching of perineum.
2. *Anxiety/fear* related to imminent birth.
3. *Ineffective individual coping* related to circumstances surrounding birth; anxiety, fear for self and infant.
4. *Injury* (mother) related to:

a. Lacerations (vaginal, perineal).
b. Infection secondary to unsterile birth.
5. *Fluid volume deficit* related to:
   a. Lacerations.
   b. Uterine atony.
   c. Retained placental fragments.
6. *Impaired gas exchange* (infant) related to intact membranes during birth.
7. *Potential for injury* (infant) related to:
   a. Precipitate birth.
   b. Trauma.
   c. Hypoxia.

◆ **C. Nursing care plan/implementation:**
1. Goal: *reduce anxiety/fear*—reassure mother.
2. Goal: *delay birth,* as possible.
   a. Discourage bearing-down.
   b. Encourage panting.
   c. *Side-lying position* to slow descent and allow for more controlled birth.
▶ 3. Goal: *prevent infection.*
   a. Provide sterile (or clean) field for birth.
   b. Avoid touching birth canal without gloved hands.
   c. Support perineum (and advancing head) with sterile (or clean) towel.
▶ 4. Goal: *prevent, or minimize, infant hypoxia* and perineal lacerations.
   a. If membranes intact as head emerges, tear at neck to facilitate first breath.
   b. Feel for cord around neck (if present, and if possible, slip cord over head; if tight, *and* sterile equipment at hand, clamp cord in two places, cut between clamps, unwrap cord). If unsterile environment, keep fetus and placenta attached—do not cut cord.
▶ 5. Goal: *facilitate/assist birth.*
   a. Hold head in both hands.
   b. After restitution, apply gentle downward pressure to bring anterior shoulder under pubic symphysis.
   c. Gently lift head to ease birth of posterior shoulder.
   d. Support infant as body slips free of mother's body.
▶ 6. Goal: *facilitate drainage of mucus and fluid* → patent airway.
   a. Hold infant in head-dependent position.
   b. Clear mucus with bulb syringe (if available), or use fingertip, wipe with towel.
▶ 7. Goal: *prevent placental transfusion*—hold infant level with placenta until cord stops pulsating.
▶ 8. Goal: *prevent chilling.*
   a. Wrap infant in towel or other clean material.
   b. Place infant on side, head dependent, on mother's abdomen.

   c. Dry head, cover with cap or material.

PLACENTAL SEPARATION

◆ **A. Assessment**—*third stage:* identify signs of *placental separation.*

◆ **B. Nursing care plan/implementation:**
1. Goal: *avoid/minimize potential for complications* (everted uterus, tearing of placenta with fragments remaining, separation of cord from placenta).
   a. *Avoid* traction (pulling) on cord.
   b. *Avoid* vigorous fundal massage.
   c. Discourage maternal bearing-down efforts unless placenta visible at introitus.
   d. With fundus well contracted, and placenta visible at introitus, encourage mother to bear down to expel placenta.
2. Goal: *stimulate respiration.* If neonate *fails to breathe* spontaneously:
   a. Maintain body temperature—dry and cover.
   b. Clear airway.
      (1) *Position:* head down.
      (2) Turn head to side.
   c. Stimulate.
      (1) Rub back gently.
      (2) Flick soles of feet.
   d. If no response to stimulation:
      (1) Slightly extend neck to "sniffing" position (head tilt–chin lift method).
      (2) Place mouth over newborn's nose and mouth and exhale air in cheeks, saying "ho" (prevents excessive pressure).
   ▶ e. Goal: begin *cardiopulmonary resuscitation (CPR)* if no heart rate.
      (1) Place infant on firm, flat surface.
      (2) With 2 fingers on sternum depress ½–1 in. 100 times/min.
      (3) Assist ventilation on upstroke of every fifth compression (5:1 ratio).
      (4) Go immediately to emergency room.
3. Goal: *maintain infant's body temperature.*
   a. Wrap placenta with baby, if cord intact.
   b. Place infant in mother's arms.
4. Goal: *prevent maternal hemorrhage* (uterine atony).
   a. Encourage breastfeeding, or stimulate nipple.
   b. Gently massage fundus, support lower part of uterus, and express clots when uterus is contracted.
   c. Encourage voiding if bladder is full.
   d. Get to a medical facility.
5. Goal: *encourage bonding/stimulate uterine contractions.* Encourage breastfeeding.

6. Goal: *legal accountability* as birth attendant. Record date, time, birth events, maternal and fetal status.

◆ **C. Evaluation/outcome criteria:**
1. Experiences normal spontaneous birth of viable infant over intact perineum.
2. Uncomplicated fourth stage—status satisfactory for both mother and infant.
3. Expresses satisfaction in management and result.

IX. Alterations affecting protective function
  A. Induction of labor—deliberate initiation of uterine contractions.
1. Indications for:
   a. History of rapid or silent labors, precipitate birth.
   b. Woman resides some distance from hospital (controversial).
   c. Coexisting medical disorders:
      (1) Uncontrolled diabetes.
      (2) Progressive preeclampsia.
      (3) Severe renal disease.
   d. PROM—spontaneous rupture of membranes before onset of labor and less than 37 wk from last menstrual period. **Hazards:**
      (1) Maternal—intrauterine infection (amnionitis, endometritis).
      (2) Fetal—sepsis; prolapsed cord.
   e. Rh or ABO incompatibility, fetal hemolytic disease.
   f. Congenital anomaly (e.g., anencephaly).
   g. Postterm pregnancy with nonreactive NST (nonstress test).
   h. Intrauterine fetal demise.
2. *Criteria for induction:*
   a. Absence of CPD, malpresentation, or malposition.
   b. Engaged vertex of single gestation.
   c. Nearing, or at, term.
   d. Fetal lung maturity.
      (1) Survival rate—better at 32 wk or more.
      (2) *Lecithin/sphingomyelin* ratio greater than 2:1.
      (3) Diabetic mother—*PG* is present in amniotic fluid.
   e. "Ripe" cervix—softening, partially effaced, or ready for effacement/dilatation (if not already present). *Note:* Intravaginal or paracervical application of prostaglandin gel, or laminaria, may be used to prepare cervix for labor.
3. *Methods*
   a. Amniotomy—artificial rupture of membranes with fetal head engaged.
   b. Intravenous oxytocin infusion.
4. *Potential complications*
   a. *Amniotomy*—irrevocably committed to birth.
      (1) Prolapsed cord.

(2) Infection.
b. *IV oxytocin infusion:*
   (1) Overstimulation of uterus.
   (2) Decreased placental perfusion/fetal distress.
   (3) Precipitate labor and birth.
   (4) Cervical/perineal lacerations.
   (5) Uterine rupture.
   (6) Water intoxication—if large doses given in D/W over prolonged period (antidiuretic effect increases water reabsorption).
   (7) Hypertensive crisis.

BEFORE INDUCTION:

◆ 5. **Assessment**—*before induction:*
   a. Estimate of gestation (EDB, fundal height, cervical status).
   b. *Bishop score:* evaluation of cervical inducibility
   c. General health status:
      (1) Weight, vital signs, FHR, edema.
      (2) Status of membranes.
      (3) Vaginal bleeding.
      (4) Coexisting disorders.
   d. History of previous labors, if any.
   e. Emotional status.
   f. Knowledge/understanding of anticipated procedures:
      (1) Amniotomy (artificial rupture of membranes).
      (2) IV oxytocin infusion.
      (3) Fetal monitoring.
   g. Preparation for childbirth (Lamaze, etc.); coping strategies. Identify support person.

◆ 6. **Analysis/nursing diagnosis:**
   a. *Knowledge deficit* related to process of induction.
   b. *Anxiety/fear* related to need for induction of labor.
   c. *Ineffective individual coping* related to psychological stress.
   d. *Pain* related to uterine contractions.

◆ 7. **Nursing care plan/implementation:**
   a. Goal: *health teaching.*
      (1) Explain rationale for procedures:
         (a) Amniotomy.
            (i) Induces labor.
            (ii) Relieves uterine overdistention.
            (iii) Increases efficiency of contractions, shortening labor.
         (b) Oxytocin infusion.
            (i) Induces labor.
            (ii) Stimulates uterine contractions.
         (c) Internal fetal monitor.
            (i) Provides continuous assessment of uterine response to oxytocin stimulation.
            (ii) Provides continuous as-

sessment of fetal response to physiologic stress of labor.
      (2) *Describe procedure*—to reduce anxiety and increase cooperation.
      (3) *Explain advantages/disadvantages*—to ensure "informed consent."
   b. Goal: *emotional support*—encourage verbalization of concerns, reassure, as possible.

◆ 8. **Evaluation/outcome criterion:** woman verbalizes understanding of process, rationale, procedures, and alternatives.

DURING INDUCTION AND LABOR:

◆ 9. **Assessment**—*during induction and labor:*
   a. *Amniotomy*—same as for spontaneous rupture of membranes:
      (1) Observe fluid—note color, amount.
      (2) Monitor FHR; assess for fetal distress.
      (3) Observe for signs of prolapsed cord.
      (4) Assess fetal activity.
         (a) Excessive activity may indicate distress.
         (b) Absence of activity may indicate distress or demise.
   b. *IV oxytocin infusion:*
      (1) Continually assess response to oxytocin stimulation/flow rate; always given by controlled infusion.
         (a) Uterine contractions.
         (b) Maternal vital signs, FHR.
      (2) Identify signs of:
         (a) *Deviation* from normal patterns:
            (i) Lack of response to increasing flow rate.
            (ii) Uterine hyperirritability (contractions—less than 2 min apart).
            (iii) Lack of adequate uterine relaxation between contractions.
         (b) *Side effects* of oxytocin: diminished output—potential water intoxication.
         (c) **Hazards** to mother or fetus:
            (i) Sustained (over 90 sec) or tetanic (strong, spasmlike) contractions—potential abruptio placentae, uterine rupture, fetal hypoxia/anoxia/death.
            (ii) *Fetal* arrhythmias, decelerations.
            (iii) *Maternal* hypertension—potential for hypertensive crisis, cerebral hemorrhage.

◆ 10. **Nursing care plan/implementation:**
   a. Same as for other women in labor.

b. If indications of deviations from normal patterns:
  (1) Change maternal position (see Figure 7.6, p. 433).
  (2) Stop oxytocin infusion, maintain IV with 5% D/W or other (Ringer's lactate, etc.).
  ▶ (3) Begin oxygen per mask; up to 8–10 L/min.
  (4) Notify physician promptly.
  (5) Check maternal blood pressure and pulse rate.
c. Anticipatory guidance: may have strong contractions soon after induction starts.

◆ 11. **Evaluation/outcome criteria:**
a. Demonstrates response to oxytocin stimulation.
  (1) Establishes desired contraction pattern, not hyperstimulated.
  (2) Progress through labor—within normal limits:
    (a) Normotensive.
    (b) Voids in adequate amounts.
    (c) No evidence of deviation from normal contraction patterns.
b. No evidence of fetal distress.
c. Experiences normal vaginal birth of viable infant.

B. **Operative obstetrics**—procedures used to prevent trauma/reduce hazard to mother or infant during the birth process.
1. **Episiotomy**—incision of perineum to facilitate infant's birth.
  a. Rationale:
    (1) Surgical incision reduces possibility of laceration.
    (2) Heals more easily than a laceration.
    (3) Protects infant's head from pressure exerted by resistant perineum.
    (4) Shortens second stage of labor.
  b. Types:
    (1) Midline—chance of extension into anal sphincter greater than with mediolateral.
    (2) Mediolateral—healing is more painful than midline.
  ◆ c. **Assessment:**
    (1) *REEDA*:
      (a) *R*edness
      (b) *E*dema
      (c) *E*cchymosis
      (d) *D*ischarge
      (e) *A*pproximation (suture line intact, separated)
    (2) Healing.
    (3) Bruised; hematoma.
    (4) Tenderness; pain. *Note:* Evaluate complaints of pain carefully. If intense, and unrelieved by usual measures, report promptly. May indicate

vulvar, paravaginal, or ischiorectal abscess or hematoma.
◆ d. **Analysis/nursing diagnosis:**
  (1) *Pain* related to labor process.
  (2) *Impaired skin integrity* related to surgical incision.
  (3) *Fluid volume deficit* related to hematoma.
  (4) *Sexual dysfunction* related to discomfort.
◆ e. **Nursing care plan/implementation:**
  (1) Goal: *prevent/reduce edema, promote comfort and healing.*
    (a) Place covered ice pack during immediate postpartum.
    (b) Administer analgesics, topical sprays, ointments, witch hazel pads.
    (c) Encourage use of sitz bath or rubber ring.
    (d) Encourage *Kegel* exercises.
    (e) Do *health teaching:*
      (i) Instruct in tightening gluteal muscles before sitting.
      (ii) Instruct to avoid sitting on one hip.
  (2) Goal: *minimize potential for infection.*
    (a) Teach/provide perineal care during fourth stage of labor.
    (b) *Health teaching:* instruct in self-perineal care after voiding, defecation, and with each pad change.
◆ f. **Evaluation/outcome criteria:**
  (1) Woman's incision heals by primary intention.
  (2) Woman demonstrates appropriate self-perineal care.
  (3) Woman evidences no signs of hematoma, infection, or separation of suture line.
  (4) Woman experiences minimal discomfort.
2. **Forceps-assisted birth**—use of instruments to assist birth of infant.
  a. Indications:
    (1) Fetal distress.
    (2) Maternal need:
      (a) Exhaustion.
      (b) Coexisting disease, such as cardiac disorder.
      (c) Poor progress in second stage.
      (d) Persistent fetal OT or OP position.
  b. *Criteria* for forceps application:
    (1) Engaged fetal head.
    (2) Ruptured membranes.
    (3) Full dilatation.
    (4) Absence of CPD.

(5) Some anesthesia has been given; usually, episiotomy has been performed.

(6) Empty bladder.

c. Types:

(1) Low—outlet forceps.

(2) Mid—applied after head is engaged (rarely used).

(3) Pipers—applied to after-coming head in selected breech births.

d. Potential *complications:*

(1) *Maternal:*

  (a) Lacerations of: birth canal, rectum, bladder.

  (b) Uterine rupture/hemorrhage.

(2) *Neonatal:*

  (a) Cephalohematoma.

  (b) Skull fracture.

  (c) Intracranial hemorrhage, brain damage.

  (d) Facial paralysis.

  (e) Direct tissue trauma (abrasions, ecchymosis).

  (f) Umbilical cord compression.

◆ e. **Assessment:**

▶ (1) FHR immediately before—and after—forceps application (forceps blade may compress umbilical cord); suction.

(2) Observe mother/newborn for injury or signs of complications.

◆ f. **Analysis/nursing diagnosis:**

(1) *Self-esteem disturbance* related to inability to give birth without surgical assistance.

(2) *Anxiety/fear* related to infant's appearance (forceps marks) or awareness of potential complications.

◆ g. **Nursing care plan/implementation:**

(1) Goal: *minimize feelings of failure due to inability to give birth "naturally."*

  (a) Explain, discuss reasons/indications for forceps-assisted birth.

  (b) Emphasize no maternal control over circumstances.

(2) Goal: *reduce parental anxiety, maternal guilt over infant bruising/forceps marks.* Explain condition is temporary and has no lasting effects on child's appearance.

◆ h. **Evaluation/outcome criteria:**

(1) Woman verbalizes understanding of reasons for forceps-assisted birth.

(2) Woman evidences no interruption in bonding with infant.

(3) Woman experiences uncomplicated recovery.

3. Vacuum cap and pump-assisted birth.

4. **Cesarean birth**—incision through abdominal wall and uterus to deliver products of conception.

a. Indications for elective cesarean birth:

(1) Known CPD.

(2) Previous uterine surgery (e.g., myomectomy), repeated cesarean births (depends on type of incision done).

(3) Active maternal genital herpes II infection.

(4) Breech presentation (*Note:* To reduce infant morbidity/mortality, elective cesarean birth is common method of choice).

(5) Neoplasms of cervix, uterus, or birth canal.

(6) Maternal diabetes with placental aging; fetal macrosomia (CPD).

b. *Criteria* for elective cesarean birth: L/S ratio greater than 2:1 —indicates presence of pulmonary surfactant; less risk of respiratory distress syndrome.

c. *Indications for emergency cesarean birth:*

(1) *Fetal:*

  (a) *Fetal distress:* prolapsed cord.

  (b) *Fetal jeopardy:* Rh or ABO incompatibility.

  (c) *Fetal malposition*/malpresentation.

  (d) *Medical evaluation:* fetal blood sampling—low O_2, elevated CO_2, pH below 7.20 (indicates fetal hypoxia, acidosis).

(2) Maternal:

  (a) Uterine dysfunction.

  (b) Placental disorders:

    (i) Placenta previa.

    (ii) Abruptio placentae, with Couvelaire uterus.

  (c) Severe maternal preeclampsia/eclampsia.

  (d) Fetopelvic disproportion.

  (e) Sudden maternal death.

  (f) Carcinoma.

  (g) Failed induction.

d. Types:

(1) Low segment—method of choice:

  (a) Transverse incision through abdominal wall and lower uterine segment.

  (b) Transverse incision through abdominal wall, with vertical incision of lower uterine segment.

  (c) Advantages—fewer complications:

    (i) Less blood loss.

    (ii) More comfortable convalescence.

    (iii) Less adhesion formation.

    (iv) Lower risk of uterine rupture in subsequent pregnancy/labor and birth.

    (v) Cosmetically more acceptable.

(2) Classic—vertical incision through abdominal wall and uterus. Necessary for anterior placenta previa and transverse lie.

(3) Porro's—hysterotomy followed by hysterectomy. Necessary in presence of:

(a) Hemorrhage from uterine atony.

(b) Placenta accreta.

(c) Large uterine myomas.

(d) Ruptured uterus.

(e) Cancer of uterus or ovary.

◆ e. **Assessment:**

(1) Maternal physical status.

(a) Vital signs.

(b) Labor status, if any.

(c) Contractions (if any).

(d) Membranes (intact; ruptured).

(e) Signs of complications.

(2) Fetal status.

(a) FHR pattern.

(b) Color and amount of amniotic fluid.

(c) Biophysical profile (BPP)

(3) Maternal emotional status.

(4) Understanding of procedure, indications for, implications.

(5) Other—as for any abdominal surgery (see Unit 2).

◆ f. **Analysis/nursing diagnosis:**

(1) *Self-esteem disturbance* related to perceived failure to give birth vaginally.

(2) *Anxiety / fear* related to impending surgery and/or reasons for cesarean birth.

(3) *Ineffective individual coping* related to anxiety and fear for self, infant.

(4) *Fluid volume deficit* related to abdominal surgery or reason for cesarean birth.

(5) *Pain* related to abdominal surgery.

(6) *Constipation* related to decreased bowel activity.

(7) *Altered urinary elimination* related to fluid volume deficit.

◆ g. **Nursing care plan/implementation:**

(1) *Preoperative:*

(a) Goal: *safeguard fetal status.*

(i) Monitor fetal heart rate continually.

(ii) Notify neonatology and neonatal intensive care unit (NICU) of scheduled surgical birth.

(b) Goal: *health teaching.*

(i) Describe, discuss anticipated anesthesia.

▪▪ (ii) Explain rationale for preoperative antacids to minimize effects of aspiration: cimetidine, histamine

blocker to decrease production of gastric acid. Reglan (metoclopramide), to hasten gastric emptying.

(iii) Describe, explain anticipated procedures—abdominal shave, indwelling catheter, intravenous fluids—to woman and support person.

(c) Other—as for any abdominal surgery.

(d) Prepare for cesarean birth.

(2) *Postoperative:*

(a) Same as for other abdominal surgical patients (see Unit 2).

(b) Same as for other postpartum women.

◆ h. **Evaluation/outcome criteria:**

(1) Verbalizes understanding of reasons for cesarean birth.

(2) Successful birth of viable infant.

(3) Evidences no surgical/birth complications.

(4) Evidences no interference with bonding.

(5) Expresses satisfaction with procedure and result.

5. **Vaginal birth after cesarean (VBAC)**

a. Candidates for VBAC.

(1) Previous low cervical cesarean birth.

(2) Head well-engaged in pelvis.

(3) Soft anterior cervix.

(4) Preexisting reason for cesarean birth not apparent.

(5) No history of sepsis with previous cesarean birth, which may hinder scar from healing properly.

◆ b. **Assessment:**

(1) Monitor FHR carefully during trial of labor.

(2) Monitor contractions carefully for adequate progress of labor.

(3) Observe mother for signs of complications.

◆ c. **Analysis/nursing diagnosis:**

(1) *Knowledge deficit* related to trial of labor.

(2) *Fear* related to outcome for fetus.

(3) *Ineffective individual coping* related to labor progress and outcome.

Complications During the Intrapartal Period

I. **General aspects**

A. **Pathophysiology**—interference with normal processes and patterns of labor/birth result in maternal or fetal jeopardy (e.g., **preterm** labor, **dysfunctional** labor patterns; **prolonged** [over 24 h] labor; **hemorrhage: uterine rupture**/inversion, **amniotic-fluid embolus**).

B. **Etiology:**

1. **Preterm labor**—unknown.
2. **Dysfunctional labor (dystocia:** see p. 448):
   a. Physiologic response to anxiety/fear/pain—results in release of catecholamines, increasing physical/psychological stress → myometrial dysfunction; painful and ineffectual labor.
   b. Iatrogenic factors: premature or excessive analgesia, particularly during latent phase.
   c. *Maternal factors:*
      (1) Pelvic contractures.
      (2) Uterine tumors (e.g., myomas, carcinoma).
      (3) Congenital uterine anomalies (e.g., bicornate uterus).
      (4) Pathologic contraction ring (*Bandl's* ring).
      (5) Rigid cervix, cervical stenosis/stricture.
      (6) Hypertonic/hypotonic contractions.
      (7) Prolonged rupture of membranes. *Note:* Intrauterine infection may have caused rupture of membranes or may follow rupture.
      (8) Prolonged first or second stage.
      (9) Medical conditions: diabetes, hypertension.
   d. *Fetal factors:*
      (1) Macrosomia (LGA).
      (2) Malposition/malpresentation.
      (3) Congenital anomaly (e.g., hydrocephalus, anencephaly).
      (4) Multifetal gestation (e.g., interlocking twins).
      (5) Prolapsed cord.
      (6) Postterm.
   e. *Placental factors:*
      (1) Placenta previa.
      (2) Inadequate placental function with contractions.
      (3) Abruptio placentae.
      (4) Placenta accreta.
   f. Physical restrictions: when confined to bed, *flat position,* etc.

◆ **C. Assessment:**
   1. Antepartal history.
   2. Emotional status.
   3. Vital signs, FHR.
   4. Contraction pattern (frequency, duration, intensity).
   5. Vaginal discharge.

◆ **D. Analysis/nursing diagnosis:**
   1. *Anxiety/fear* for self and infant related to implications of prolonged or complicated labor/birth.
   2. *Pain* related to hypertonic contractions/dysfunctional labor.
   3. *Ineffective individual coping* related to physical/psychological stress of complicated labor/birth, lowered pain threshold secondary to fatigue.

   4. *High risk for injury* related to prolonged rupture of membranes, infection.
   5. *Fluid volume deficit* related to excessive blood loss secondary to placenta previa, abruptio placentae, Couvelaire uterus, DIC.

◆ **E. Nursing care plan/implementation:**
   1. Goal: *minimize physical/psychological stress during labor/birth.* Assist woman in coping effectively:
      a. Reinforce relaxation techniques.
      b. Support couple's effective coping techniques/mechanisms.
   2. Goal: *emotional support.*
      a. Encourage verbalization of anxiety/fear/concerns.
      b. Explain all procedures—to minimize anxiety/fear, encourage cooperation/participation in care.
      c. Provide quiet environment conducive to rest.
   3. Goal: *continuous monitoring of maternal/fetal status and progress through labor*—to identify early signs of dysfunctional labor, fetal distress; facilitate prompt, effective treatment of emerging complications.
   4. Goal: *minimize effects of complicated labor on mother, fetus.*
      a. *Position* change: lateral Sims'—to reduce compression of inferior vena cava.
      b. Oxygen per mask, as indicated.
      c. Institute interventions appropriate to emerging problems (see specific disorder).

◆ **F. Evaluation/outcome criteria:**
   1. Woman has successful birth of viable infant.
   2. Maternal/infant status stable, satisfactory.

II. Disorders affecting protective functions. Preterm labor—occurs after 20 weeks gestation and before beginning of wk 38.
   A. Pathophysiology—physiologic events of labor (i.e., contractions, spontaneous rupture of membranes, cervical effacement/dilatation) occur before completion of normal, term gestation.
   B. Etiology—unknown. Theory: may be due to fetal factors released when placental function begins to diminish and intrauterine environment is hostile to continuing fetal well-being.
   C. *Coexisting disorders:*
      1. Infections that may cause PROM.
      2. PROM of unknown etiology.
      3. Hypertension (preeclampsia/eclampsia).
      4. Uterine overdistention.
         a. Hydramnios.
         b. Multifetal gestation.
      5. Maternal diabetes, renal or cardiovascular disorder, UTI.
      6. Severe maternal illness (e.g., pneumonia, acute pyelonephritis).
      7. Abnormal placentation.
         a. Placenta previa.

b. Abruptio placentae.

8. Iatrogenic: miscalculated EDB for repeat cesarean birth.

9. Fetal death.

10. Incompetent cervical os (small percentage).

11. Uterine anomalies (rare).
    a. Intrauterine septum.
    b. Bicornate uterus.

12. Uterine fibroids.

D. *Prevention:*
1. *Primary*—close obstetric supervision; education in signs/symptoms of labor.
2. *Secondary*—prompt, effective treatment of associated disorders (see C., p. 445).
3. *Tertiary*—suppression of preterm labor.
   a. Bedrest.
   b. *Position:* side-lying—to promote placental perfusion.
   c. Hydration.
   d. Pharmacologic (may require "informed consent"; follow hospital protocol). Beta-adrenergic agents (take ECG first) to reduce sensitivity of uterine myometrium to oxytocic and prostaglandin stimulation; increase blood flow to uterus.
   e. May be maintained at home with adequate follow-up and health teaching.

E. Contraindications for suppression: Labor is not suppressed in presence of:
1. Placenta previa or abruptio placentae.
2. Chorioamnionitis.
3. Erythroblastosis fetalis.
4. Severe preeclampsia.
5. Severe diabetes (e.g., "brittle").
6. Increasing placental insufficiency.
7. Cervical dilatation of 4 cm or more.
8. Ruptured membranes (depends on cause and if sepsis).

◆ **F. Assessment:**
1. Maternal vital signs. Response to medication:
   a. Hypotension.
   b. Tachycardia, arrhythmia.
   c. Dyspnea, chest pain.
   d. Nausea and vomiting.
2. Signs of infection:
   a. Increased temperature.
   b. Tachycardia.
   c. Diaphoresis.
   d. Malaise.
   e. Increased baseline fetal heart rate.
3. Contractions: frequency, duration, strength.
4. Emotional status—signs of denial, guilt, anxiety, exhaustion.
5. Signs of continuing and progressing labor. *Note:* Vaginal examination *only* if indicated by other signs of continuing labor progress.
   a. Effacement.
   b. Dilatation.
   c. Station.

6. Status of membranes.
7. Fetal heart rate, activity (continuous monitoring).

◆ **G. Analysis/nursing diagnosis:**
1. *Anxiety/fear* related to possible outcome.
2. *Self-esteem disturbance* related to feelings of guilt, failure.
3. *Impaired physical mobility* related to imposed bedrest.
4. *Knowledge deficit* related to medication side effects.
5. *Ineffective individual coping* related to possible outcome.
6. *Impaired gas exchange* related to side effects of medication (circulatory overload; pulmonary edema).
7. *Diversional activity deficit* related to imposed bedrest, decreased environmental stimuli.
8. *Altered urinary elimination* related to bedrest.
9. *Constipation* related to bedrest.

◆ **H. Nursing care plan/implementation:**
1. Goal: *inhibit uterine activity.* Administer medications as ordered—ritodrine (Yutopar), terbutaline, or magnesium sulfate.
2. Goal: *safeguard status.*
   a. Continuous maternal/fetal monitoring.
   b. I&O—to identify early signs of possible circulatory overload.
   c. *Position:* side-lying—to increase placental perfusion, prevent supine hypotension.
   d. Report **promptly** to physician:

(1)	Maternal pulse of 110 or more.
(2)	Diastolic pressure of 60 mm Hg or less.
(3)	Respirations of 24 or more; crackles (rales).
(4)	Complaint of dyspnea.
(5)	Contractions: increasing frequency, strength, duration, or cessation of contractions.
(6)	Intermittent back and thigh pain.
(7)	Rupture of membranes.
(8)	Vaginal bleeding.
(9)	Fetal distress.

3. Goal: *comfort measures.*
   a. Basic hygienic care—bath, mouth care, cold washcloth to face, perineal care.
   b. Back rub, linen change—to promote relaxation.
4. Goal: *emotional support.*
   a. Encourage verbalization of guilt feelings, anxiety, fear, concerns; provide factual information.
   b. Support positive self-concept.
   c. Keep informed of progress.
5. Goal: *provide quiet diversion.* Television, reading materials, handcrafts.
6. Goal: *health teaching.*

a. Explain, discuss proposed management to suppress preterm labor.

b. Describe, discuss side effects of medication.

c. Explain rationale for bedrest, position.

I. If labor continues to progress:

1. Goal: *facilitate infant survival.*

a. Administer betamethasone, as ordered, 24 h before birth—to increase/stimulate production of pulmonary surfactant.

b. Notify perinatal team—to increase chances for fetal survival, ensure prompt, expert management of neonate, and provide information and support to parents.

c. Monitor progress of labor to identify signs of impending birth. *Note:* May give birth before complete (10 cm) dilatation.

d. Consider transfer to high-risk facility.

e. Prepare for birth, or cesarean birth if infant less than 34–36 weeks' gestation.

2. Goal: *emotional support.*

a. Do not leave woman (or couple) alone.

b. Encourage verbalization of anxiety, fear, concern.

c. Explain all procedures.

3. Goal: *comfort measures. Note:* Analgesics contraindicated—to prevent depression of fetus/neonate.

4. Goal: *support effective coping techniques.* Encourage/support Lamaze (or other) techniques—coach, as necessary; discourage hyperventilation.

5. Goal: *health teaching*—for preterm birth.

a. Discuss need for episiotomy, possibility of outlet forceps–assisted birth—to reduce stress on fetal head, *or*

b. Prepare for cesarean birth—to reduce possibility of fetal intraventricular hemorrhage.

c. Rationale for avoiding use of medications to reduce contraction pain.

J. Immediate care of neonate:

1. Goal: *safeguard status.*

a. Stabilize environmental temperature—to prevent chilling (isolette or other controlled-temperature bed).

▶ b. Suction, oxygen, as needed; may need intubation.

c. Parenteral fluids, **as** ordered—to support normal acid-base balance, pH; administer antibiotics, as necessary.

d. Arrange transport to high-risk facility, as necessary.

2. Goal: *continuous monitoring of status.*

a. Electronic monitors—to observe respiratory and cardiac functions.

b. Blood samples—to monitor blood gases, pH, hypoglycemia.

K. Postpartum care: Goal: *emotional support.*

1. Facilitate attachment.

2. If couple, foster sense of mutual experience and closeness.

3. Help her/them maintain a positive self-image.

4. Encourage touching of infant before transport to nursery or high-risk facility; father/partner may accompany infant and report back to mother.

5. Encourage early contact—to facilitate mother's need to ventilate her feelings.

6. Assist parent(s) with grieving process, if necessary.

7. Refer to support group if necessary.

L. *Other*—as for any postpartum woman.

◆ **M. Evaluation/outcome criteria:**

1. Woman verbalizes understanding of medical/nursing recommendations and treatments.

2. Woman complies with medical/nursing regimen.

3. Woman experiences no discomfort from side effects of therapy.

4. Woman experiences successful outcome—labor inhibited.

5. Woman carries pregnancy to successful termination.

6. If preterm birth occurs, woman copes effectively with outcome (physiologically compromised neonate, neonatal death).

III. Grief and childbearing experience. The loss of a pregnancy or a newborn, or the birth of a physiologically compromised child (preterm, congenital disorder), is a crisis situation. The unexpected outcome can cause the parent(s) to suffer a sense of loss of self-esteem, self-concept, positive body image, feelings of worth (see p. 463).

◆ **A. Assessment:**

1. Response to loss of the "fantasy child"/real child.

a. Behavioral—anger, hostility, depression, disinterest in activities of daily living, withdrawal.

b. Biophysical—somatic complaints (stomach pain, malaise, anorexia, nausea).

c. Cognitive—feelings of guilt.

2. Knowledge/understanding/perception of situation.

3. Coping abilities, mechanisms.

4. Support system.

◆ **B. Analysis/nursing diagnosis:**

1. *Ineffective family coping: compromised* related to psychological stress related to fear for infant, guilt feelings, impact on self-image.

2. *Ineffective individual coping* related to anxiety, stress.

3. *Ineffective family coping: disabling* related to disturbance in intrafamily relations secondary to individual coping deficits, recriminations.

4. *Altered parenting* related to lack of effective bonding secondary to emotional separation from infant, feelings of guilt.
5. *Dysfunctional grieving* related to guilt feelings, impact of loss on self-concept.
6. *Disturbance in body image, self-esteem, role performance* related to perceived failure to complete gestational task, produce perfect, healthy infant, sleep deprivation.
7. *Social isolation* related to severe coping deficit, dysfunctional grieving, disturbance in self-esteem.

◆ **C. Nursing care plan/implementation:**
　1. Goal: *emotional support.*
　　a. Provide privacy; encourage open expression/verbalization of feelings, fears, concerns, perceptions.
　　b. Crisis intervention techniques.
　2. Goal: *facilitate bonding, effective coping, or anticipatory grieving processes.*
　　a. Encourage contact and participation in care of premature or compromised infant.
　　b. Keep informed of infant's status.
　　c. Provide realistic data.
　3. Goal: *health teaching.*
　　a. Clarify misperceptions, as appropriate.
　　b. Discuss, demonstrate infant care techniques (e.g., feeding infant who has cleft lip or palate).
　　c. Refer to appropriate community resources.

◆ **D. Evaluation/outcome criteria:**
　1. Woman verbalizes recognition and acceptance of diagnosis.
　2. Woman verbalizes understanding of relevant information regarding treatment, prognosis.
　3. Woman makes informed decision regarding infant care.
　4. Woman demonstrates comfort and increasing participation in care of neonate.
　5. Woman shows evidence of bonding (eye contact, cuddles, calls infant by name).

IV. Disorders affecting comfort, rest, mobility: dystocia
　A. Definition—difficult labor.
　B. *General aspects (MOTHER, "3 Ps": Psych, Placenta, Position):*
　　1. **Pathophysiology**—see specific disorders.
　　2. **Etiology**—due to effects of factors that affect the FETUS (also "3 Ps"):
　　　a. *POWER:* forces of labor (uterine contractions, use of abdominal muscles).
　　　　(1) Premature analgesia/anesthesia.
　　　　(2) Uterine overdistention (multifetal pregnancy, fetal macrosomia).
　　　　(3) Uterine myomas.
　　　b. *PASSAGEWAY:* resistance of cervix, pelvic structures.
　　　　(1) Rigid cervix.
　　　　(2) Distended bladder.

　　　　(3) Distended rectum
　　　　(4) Dimensions of the bony pelvis: pelvic contractures.
　　　c. *PASSENGER:* accommodation of the presenting part to pelvic diameters.
　　　　(1) Fetal malposition/malpresentation.
　　　　　(a) Transverse lie.
　　　　　(b) Face, brow presentation.
　　　　　(c) Breech presentation.
　　　　　(d) CPD.
　　　　(2) Fetal anomalies.
　　　　　(a) Hydrocephalus.
　　　　　(b) Conjoined ("Siamese") twins.
　　　　　(c) Myelomeningocele.
　　　　(3) Fetal size.
　　3. **Hazards:**
　　　a. *Maternal:*
　　　　(1) Fatigue, exhaustion, dehydration—due to prolonged labor.
　　　　(2) Lowered pain threshold, loss of control—due to prolonged labor, continued uterine contractions, anxiety, fatigue, lack of sleep.
　　　　(3) Intrauterine infection—due to prolonged rupture of membranes and frequent vaginal examinations.
　　　　(4) Uterine rupture—due to obstructed labor.
　　　　(5) Cervical, vaginal, perineal lacerations—due to obstetric interventions.
　　　　(6) Postpartum hemorrhage—due to uterine atony or trauma.
　　　b. *Fetal:*
　　　　(1) Hypoxia, anoxia, demise—due to decreased O_2 concentration in cord blood.
　　　　(2) Intracranial hemorrhage—due to changing intracranial pressure.
　C. **Hypertonic dysfunction**
　　1. **Pathophysiology**—increased resting tone of uterine myometrium; diminished refractory period; prolonged latent phase:
　　　a. *Nullipara*—more than 20 h.
　　　b. *Multipara*—more than 14 h.
　　2. **Etiology**—unknown. Theory—ectopic initiation of incoordinate uterine contractions.
◆ 3. **Assessment:**
　　　a. Onset—early labor (latent phase).
　　　b. Contractions:
　　　　(1) Continuous fundal tension, incomplete relaxation.
　　　　(2) Painful.
　　　　(3) Ineffectual—no effacement or dilatation.
　　　c. Signs of fetal distress
　　　　(1) Meconium-stained amniotic fluid.
　　　　(2) FHR irregularities.
　　　d. Maternal vital signs.
　　　e. Emotional status.

🧪 f. Medical evaluation: vaginal examination, X-ray pelvimetry, ultrasonography—to rule out CPD.

◆ 4. **Analysis/nursing diagnosis:**
   a. *Pain* related to hypertonic contractions, incomplete uterine relaxation.
   b. *Anxiety/fear* for self and infant related to strong, painful contractions without evidence of progress.
   c. *Ineffective individual coping* related to fatigue, exhaustion, anxiety, tension, fear.
   d. *Impaired gas exchange (fetal)* related to incomplete relaxation of uterus.
   e. *Sleep pattern disturbance* related to prolonged ineffectual labor.

◆ 5. **Nursing care plan/implementation:**
   a. Medical management:
   💊 (1) Short-acting barbiturates (see Unit 4)—to encourage rest, relaxation.
      (2) Intravenous fluids—to restore/maintain hydration and fluid-electrolyte balance.
      (3) If CPD, cesarean birth.
   b. Nursing management:
      (1) Goal: *emotional support*—assist coping with fear, pain, discouragement.
         (a) Encourage verbalization of anxiety, fear, concerns.
         (b) Explain all procedures.
         (c) Reassure. Keep couple informed of progress.
      (2) Goal: *comfort measures.*
         (a) *Position:* side-lying—to promote relaxation and placental perfusion.
         (b) Bath, back rub, linen change, clean environment.
         (c) Environment: quiet, darkened room—to minimize stimuli and encourage relaxation, warmth.
         (d) Encourage voiding—to relieve bladder distention; to test urine for ketones.
      (3) Goal: *prevent infection.* Strict aseptic technique.
      (4) Goal: *prepare for cesarean birth* if necessary.

◆ 6. **Evaluation/outcome criteria:**
   a. Relaxes, sleeps, establishes normal labor pattern.
   b. Demonstrates no signs of fetal distress.
   c. Successfully completes uneventful labor.

D. Hypotonic dysfunction during labor
1. **Pathophysiology**—after normal labor at onset, contractions diminish in frequency, duration and strength; lowered uterine resting tone; cervical effacement and dilatation slow/cease.
2. **Etiology:**

   a. Premature or excessive analgesia/anesthesia (caudal or epidural block).
   b. CPD.
   c. Overdistention (hydramnios, fetal macrosomia, multifetal pregnancy).
   d. Fetal malposition/malpresentation.
   e. Maternal fear/anxiety.

◆ 3. **Assessment:**
   a. Onset—may occur in latent phase; most common during active phase.
   b. Contractions: normal previously, demonstrate:
      (1) Decreased frequency.
      (2) Shorter duration.
      (3) Diminished intensity (mild to moderate).
      (4) Less uncomfortable.
   c. Cervical changes—slow or cease.
   d. Signs of fetal distress—rare.
      (1) Usually occur late in labor due to infection secondary to prolonged rupture of membranes.
      (2) Tachycardia.
   e. Maternal vital signs may indicate infection (↑ temperature).
   🧪 f. Medical diagnosis—procedures: vaginal examination, X-ray pelvimetry, ultrasonography—to rule out CPD (most common cause).

◆ 4. **Analysis/nursing diagnosis:**
   a. *Knowledge deficit* related to limited exposure to information.
   b. *Anxiety/fear* related to failure to progress as anticipated; fear for fetus.
   c. *High risk for injury* (infection) related to prolonged labor or ruptured membranes.

◆ 5. **Nursing care plan/implementation:**
   a. Medical management:
      (1) Amniotomy—artificial rupture of membranes.
   💊 (2) Oxytocin augmentation of labor—intravenous infusion of oxytocin to increase frequency, duration, strength, and efficiency of uterine contractions (see IX.A. Induction of labor, p. 440).
      (3) If CPD, cesarean birth.
   b. Nursing management:
      (1) Goals: *emotional support, comfort measures, prevent infection*—as for Hypertonic dysfunction, see p. 448.
      (2) Other—see IX.A. Induction of labor, p. 440.

◆ 6. **Evaluation/outcome criteria:**
   a. Reestablishes normal labor pattern.
   b. Experiences successful birth of viable infant.

V. Disorders affecting fluid-gas transport: *maternal*

A. Uterine rupture
1. **Pathophysiology**—stress on uterine muscle exceeds its ability to stretch.
2. **Etiology:**
    a. Overdistention—due to large baby, multifetal gestation.
    b. Old scars—due to previous cesarean births.
    c. Contractions against CPD, fetal malpresentation, pathologic retraction ring (Bandl's).
    d. Injudicious obstetrics—malapplication of forceps (or application without full effacement/dilatation).
    e. Tetanic contraction—due to hypersensitivity to oxytocin (or excessive dosage) during induction/augmentation of labor.
◆ 3. **Assessment:**
    a. Identify predisposing factors early.
    b. *Complete rupture*
        (1) Pain: sudden, sharp, abdominal; followed by cessation of contractions; tender abdomen.
        (2) Signs of shock; vaginal bleeding.
        (3) Fetal heart tones—absent.
        (4) Presenting part—not palpable on vaginal examination.
    c. *Incomplete rupture*
        (1) Contractions: continue, accompanied by abdominal pain and failure to dilate.
        (2) Signs of shock.
        (3) May demonstrate vaginal bleeding.
        (4) Fetal heart tones—absent.
4. *Prognosis*
    a. Maternal—guarded.
    b. Fetal—grave.
◆ 5. **Analysis/nursing diagnosis:**
    a. *Pain* related to rupture of uterine muscle.
    b. *Fluid volume deficit* related to massive blood loss secondary to uterine rupture.
    c. *Anxiety/fear* related to concern for self, fetus.
    d. *Altered tissue perfusion* related to blood loss secondary to uterine rupture.
    e. *Altered urinary elimination* related to necessary conservation of intravascular fluid secondary to blood loss.
    f. *Anticipatory grieving* related to expected loss of fetus; inability to have more children.
◆ 6. **Nursing care plan/implementation:**
    a. Medical management:
        (1) Surgical—laparotomy, hysterectomy.
        (2) Replace blood loss—transfusion, packed cells.
        (3) Reduce possibility of infection—antibiotics.
    b. Nursing management:
        (1) Goal: *safeguard status.*
            (a) Report *immediately;* mobilize staff.
            (b) Prepare for immediate laparotomy.
            ▶ (c) Oxygen per mask—to increase circulating oxygen level.
            (d) Order stat type and crossmatch for blood—to replace blood loss.
            ▶ (e) Establish IV line—to infuse fluids, blood, medications.
            ▶ (f) Insert indwelling catheter—to deflate bladder.
            (g) Abdominal prep—to remove hair, bacteria.
            (h) Surgical permit (informed consent) for hysterectomy.
        (2) Goal: *emotional support*—to allay anxiety (woman and family).
            (a) Encourage verbalization of fears, anxiety, concerns.
            (b) Explain all procedures.
            (c) Keep family informed of progress.
◆ 7. **Evaluation/outcome criteria:**
    a. Experiences successful termination of emergency; minimal blood loss.
    b. Postoperative status stable.

B. Amniotic fluid embolus
1. **Pathophysiology:** acute cor pulmonale—due to embolus blocking vessels in pulmonary circulation; massive hemorrhage—due to DIC resulting from entrance of thromboplastin-like material into bloodstream.
2. **Etiology**—amniotic fluid (with any meconium, lanugo, or vernix) enters maternal circulation through open venous sinuses at placental site; travels to pulmonary arterioles.
    a. Rare.
    b. Associated with: tumultuous labor, abruptio placentae.
3. *Prognosis*—poor; often fatal to mother.
◆ 4. **Assessment:**
    a. May occur during labor, at time of rupture of membranes, or immediately postpartum.
    b. Sudden dyspnea and cyanosis.
    c. Chest pain.
    d. Hypotension, tachycardia.
    e. Frothy sputum.
    f. **Signs of DIC:**
        (1) Purpura—local hemorrhage.
        (2) Increased vaginal bleeding—massive.
        (3) Rapid evolution of shock.
◆ 5. **Analysis/nursing diagnosis:**
    a. *Impaired gas exchange* related to pulmonary edema.

b. *Potential fluid volume deficit* related to DIC.

c. *Anxiety/fear* for self and fetus related to severity of symptoms, perception of jeopardy.

◆ 6. **Nursing care plan/implementation:**

a. Medical management:

(1) IV heparin, whole blood.

(2) Birth: immediate, by forceps, if possible.

(3) Digitalize, as necessary.

b. Nursing management:

(1) Goal: *assist ventilation.*

(a) *Position:* semi-Fowler's.

▶ (b) Oxygen under positive pressure.

▶ (c) Suction prn.

(2) Goal: *facilitate/expedite administration of fluids, medications, blood.*

▶ (a) Establish intravenous line with large-bore needle.

(b) Administer heparin, fluids, as ordered.

(3) Goal: *restore cardiopulmonary functions, if needed.* Cardiopulmonary resuscitation techniques.

(4) Goal: *emotional support* of woman, family.

(a) Allay anxiety, as possible.

(b) Explain all procedures.

(c) Keep informed of status.

◆ 7. **Evaluation/outcome criteria:**

a. Dyspnea relieved.

b. Bleeding controlled.

c. Successful birth of viable infant.

d. Uneventful postpartum course.

VI. **Disorders affecting fluid-gas transport:** *fetal*

A. **Fetus in jeopardy**—general aspects:

1. **Pathophysiology**—maternal hypoxemia, anemia, ketoacidosis, Rh isoimmunization, or decreased uteroplacental perfusion.

2. **Etiology**—maternal:

a. Preeclampsia/eclampsia.

b. Heart disease.

c. Diabetes.

d. Rh or ABO incompatibility.

e. Insufficient uteroplacental/cord circulation due to:

(1) Maternal hypotension/hypertension.

(2) Cord compression:

(a) Prolapsed.

(b) Knotted.

(c) Nuchal.

(3) Hemorrhage; anemia.

(4) Placental problem:

(a) Malformation of the placenta/cord.

(b) Premature "aging" of placenta.

(c) Placental infarcts.

(d) Abruptio placentae.

(e) Placenta previa.

(5) Postterm gestation.

(6) Maternal infection.

(7) Hydramnios.

(8) Hypertonic uterine contractions.

f. PROM (premature rupture of membrane) with chorioamnionitis.

g. Dystocia (e.g., from CPD).

◆ 3. **Assessment**—intrapartal:

🧪 a. Amniotic fluid examination—at or after rupture of membranes. *Signs of fetal distress:* meconium stained, vertex presentation—due to relaxation of fetal anal sphincter secondary to hypoxia/anoxia. *Note:* Fetus "gasps" in utero—may aspirate meconium and amniotic fluid.

b. Fetal activity:

(1) Hyperactivity—due to hypoxemia, elevated CO_2.

(2) Cessation—possible fetal death.

▶ c. Methods of monitoring FHR:

(1) Stethoscope or fetoscope.

(2) Phonocardiography with microphone application.

(3) Internal fetal electrode—attached directly to fetus through dilated cervix after membranes ruptured.

(4) Doppler probe using ultrasound flow.

(5) Cardiotocograph—transducer on maternal abdomen transmits sound.

d. Abnormal FHR patterns (see Figure 7.6).

(1) Persistent irregularity.

(2) Persistent tachycardia of 160 or more beats/min.

(3) Persistent bradycardia of 100 or fewer beats/min.

(4) *Early deceleration*—due to vagal response to head compression.

(5) *Late deceleration*—due to uteroplacental insufficiency.

(6) *Variable deceleration*—due to cord compression.

(7) Decreased or loss of variability in FHR pattern.

e. Medical evaluation—procedures: fetal blood gases, pH.

(1) Purpose—to identify fetal acid-base status.

(2) Requirements for:

(a) Ruptured membranes.

(b) Cervical dilatation.

(c) Engaged head.

🧪 (3) Procedure—under sterile condition, sample of fetal scalp blood obtained for analysis.

(4) Signs of fetal distress:

(a) pH <7.20 (normal range is 7.3–7.4).

(b) Increased CO_2.

(c) Decreased PO_2.

◆ 4. **Analysis/nursing diagnosis:**
   a. *Impaired gas exchange, fetal,* related to decreased placental perfusion/insufficient cord circulation.
   b. *Altered tissue perfusion* related to hemolytic anemia.
   c. *High risk for fetal injury* related to hypoxia.

B. **Prolapsed umbilical cord**
   1. **Pathophysiology**—cord descent in advance of presenting part; compression interrupts blood flow, exchange of fetal/maternal gases → fetal hypoxia, anoxia, death (if unrelieved).
   2. **Etiology:**
      a. Spontaneous or artificial rupture of membranes before presenting part is engaged.
      b. Excessive force of escaping fluid, as in hydramnios.
      c. Malposition—breech, compound presentation, transverse lie.
      d. Preterm or SGA fetus—allows space for cord descent.
   ◆ 3. **Assessment:**
      a. Visualization of cord outside (or inside) vagina.
      b. Palpation of pulsating mass on vaginal examination.
      c. Fetal distress—variable deceleration and persistent bradycardia.
   ◆ 4. **Analysis/nursing diagnosis:**
      a. *Impaired gas exchange, fetal,* related to interruption of blood flow from placenta/fetus.
      b. *Anxiety/fear, maternal,* related to knowledge of fetal jeopardy.
   ◆ 5. **Nursing care plan/implementation:**
      a. Goal: *reduce pressure on cord.*
         (1) *Position:* knee to chest; lateral modified Sims' with hips elevated; modified Trendelenburg.
         (2) With gloved hand, support fetal head off cord.
      ▶ b. Goal: *increase maternal/fetal oxygenation:* oxygen per mask (8–10 L/min).
      ▶ c. Goal: *protect exposed cord:* cover cord with warm sterile wet saline dressing.
      d. Goal: *identify fetal response* to above measures, reduce threat to fetal survival: monitor FHR continuously.
      e. Goal: *expedite termination of threat to fetus:* prepare for immediate vaginal/cesarean birth.
      f. Goal: *support mother and significant other* by staying with them and explaining.
   ◆ 6. **Evaluation/outcome criteria:**
      a. FHR returns to normal rate and pattern.
      b. Uncomplicated birth of viable infant.

VII. Summary of danger signs during labor

A. Contractions—strong, every 2 min or less, lasting 90 secs or more; poor relaxation between contractions.
B. Sudden sharp abdominal pain followed by boardlike abdomen and shock—abruptio placentae or uterine rupture.
C. Marked vaginal bleeding.
D. FHR periodic pattern decelerations—late; variable; absent (see Table 7.6).
E. Baseline.
   1. Bradycardia (<100 beats/min).
   2. Tachycardia (>160 beats/min).
F. Amniotic fluid.
   1. Amount: excessive; diminished.
   2. Odor.
   3. Color: meconium stained; port-wine; yellow.
   4. 24 h or more since rupture of membranes.
G. Maternal hypotension.

❏ The Postpartal Period

General overview: This review of the normal physiologic and psychological changes occurring during the postpartal period (birth to 6 weeks after) provides the database necessary for assessing the woman's progress through involution, planning and implementing care, anticipatory guidance, health teaching, and evaluating the results. Emerging problems are identified by comparing the woman's status against established standards.

I. **Biologic foundations of the postpartal period**
   A. **Uterine involution**—integrated processes by which the uterus returns to normal size, shape, and consistency.
   ◆ 1. **Assessment:**
      a. Contractions ("after pains")—shorten muscles, close venous sinuses, restore normal tone.
         (1) Frequency, intensity, and discomfort decrease after first 24 h.
         (2) More common in: multiparas, and after birth of a large baby; primiparous uterus remains contracted.
         (3) Increased by breastfeeding.
      b. Autolysis—breakdown and excretion of muscle protein (decreasing size of myometrial cells). Lochia—sloughing of decidua and blood.
      c. Formation of *new endometrium*—4–6 wk until placental site healed.
      d. *Cervix*
         (1) *Immediately* following birth—bruised, small tears; admits one hand.
         (2) *Eighteen hours* after birth—becomes shorter, firmer; regains normal shape.
         (3) *One week* postpartum—admits two fingers.

(4) Never returns fully to prepregnant state.
    (1) Parous os is wider and not perfectly round.
    (2) Lacerations heal as scars radiating out from the os.

e. *Fundal height and consistency*
  (1) After birth—at umbilicus; size and consistency of firm grapefruit.
  (2) Day 1 (first 12 h)—one finger above umbilicus.
  (3) Descends by one finger-breadth daily until d 10.
  (4) Day 10—behind symphysis pubis, nonpalpable.

f. *Lochia*
  (1) Character:
    (1) Days 1–3; rubra (red).
    (2) Days 3–7; serosa (pink to brown).
    (3) Day 10; alba (creamy white).
  (2) Amount:
    (1) Moderate: 4–8 pads/d (average 6 pads/d).
    (2) Following cesarean birth: less lochia—due to manipulation during surgery.
  (3) Odor: normal lochia has characteristic "fleshy" odor; foul odor is characteristic of infection.
  (4) Clots: normal: a few small clots, most commonly on arising—due to pooling. *Note:* Clots and *heavy* bleeding are associated with uterine atony, retained placental fragments.

B. Birth canal

1. *Vagina*—never returns fully to prepregnant state.
  a. First few weeks postpartum—thin walled, due to lack of estrogen; few rugae.
  b. Week 3: rugae may reappear.
  c. Hymen—if torn, may heal.

2. *Pelvic floor*
  a. Immediately after birth—infiltrated with blood, stretched, torn.
  b. Month 6: considerable tone regained.

3. *Perineum*
  a. Immediately following birth—edematous; may have episiotomy (or repaired lacerations); hemorrhoids.
  b. Healing, incisional line clean; no separation.
  c. Hematoma—blood in connective tissue beneath skin; complains of pain, unrelieved by mild analgesia or heat; perineal distention; painful, tense, fluctuant mass.

C. Abdominal wall

1. Overdistention during pregnancy may → rupture of elastic fibers, persistent striae, and diastasis of the rectus muscles.

2. Usually takes 6–8 wk to retrogress, depending on previous muscle tone, obesity, and amount of distention during pregnancy.

3. Strenuous exercises discouraged until 8 wk postpartum.

D. Cardiovascular system—characteristic changes:

1. Immediately after birth—*increased* cardiac load, due to:
  a. Return of uterine blood flow to general circulation.
  b. Diuresis of excess interstitial fluid.

2. Volume—returns to prepregnant state (4 L) in about 3 wk. Major reduction—during first week, due to diuresis and diaphoresis.

3. Blood values (see Table 7.5)
  a. High WBC during labor (25,000/mL); drops to normal level in first few days.
  b. Week 1—Hgb, RBC, Hct, elevated fibrinogen return to normal.

4. Blood coagulation
  a. During labor: rapid consumption of clotting factors.
  b. During postpartum: increased consumption of clotting factors. Hypercoagulability maintained during first few days postpartum; predisposes to thrombophlebitis, pulmonary embolism.

◆ 5. **Assessment: potential complications**—vital signs:
  a. *Temperature*—elevated in:
    (1) Excessive blood loss, dehydration, exhaustion, infection.
    (2) Elevation: 100.4°F (38°C) after first day postpartum suggests puerperal infection.
  b. *Pulse*—physiologic bradycardia (50–70) common through second day postpartum; may persist 7–10 days; etiology: unknown. *Tachycardia*—associated with: excessive blood loss, dehydration, exhaustion, infection.
  c. *Blood pressure*—generally unchanged. *Elevation*—associated with: preeclampsia, essential hypertension.

E. Urinary tract—characteristic changes:

1. Output—increased due to: diuresis (12 h to 5 d postpartum); daily output to 3000 mL.

2. Urine constituents:
  a. Sugar—primarily lactose.
  b. Acetonuria—after prolonged labor; dehydration.
  c. Proteinuria—first 3 d in response to the catalytic process of involution.

3. Dilatation of ureters—subsides in first few weeks.

◆ 4. **Assessment: potential complications**—measure first few voidings, palpate bladder to determine emptying.
  a. Edema, trauma, and/or anesthesia may → retention with overflow.

b. Overdistended bladder—common cause of excessive bleeding in immediate post-partum.

F. **Integument (skin)**—characteristic changes:
1. Striae—persist as silvery or brownish lines.
2. Diastasis recti abdominis—some midline separation may persist.
3. Diaphoresis—excessive perspiration for first few (approximately 5) d.
4. Breast changes—see II.A.3. *Breasts,* below.

G. **Legs**
1. Should have no redness, tenderness, local areas of increased skin temperature, or edema.
2. May have some soreness from birth position.
3. *Homans' sign* should be negative (no calf pain when knee is extended and gentle pressure applied to dorsiflex the foot).

H. **Weight**—characteristic changes:
1. Initial weight loss—fetus, placenta, amniotic fluid, excess tissue fluid.
2. Weighs more than in prepregnant state (weight maintained in breasts).
3. Week 6—weight loss is individualized.

I. **Menstruation and ovarian function**—first menstrual cycle may be anovulatory.
1. Nonnursing—ovulation at 4–6 wk; menstruation at 6–8 wk.
2. Nursing—anovulatory period varies (39 d to 6 mo or more); some for duration of lactation; contraceptive value: *very unreliable.*

II. **Nursing management during the postpartal period**
◆ A. **Assessment**—minimum of twice daily.
1. Vital signs.
2. Emotional status, response to baby.
3. *Breasts*
a. Observe: size, symmetry, placement and condition of nipples, leakage of colostrum. Normal: although one breast is usually larger than the other, breasts are essentially symmetrical in shape; nipples: in breast midline, erectile, intact (no signs of fissure); bilateral leakage of colostrum is common.
b. *Note:* reddened areas, elevations, supernumerary nipples, inverted nipples, cracks.
c. Observe for signs of (normal) engorgement (i.e., tenderness, distention, prominent veins). Transient; normally occurs shortly before lactation is established—due to venous and lymphatic stasis.
· d. Palpate for: local heat, edema, tenderness, swelling (signs of localized infection).
4. Fundus, lochia, perineum.
5. Voiding and bowel function.

6. Legs (see G., at left).
7. Signs of complications.
◆ B. **Analysis/nursing diagnosis:** (See VI.B., Nursing actions during the fourth stage of labor, p. 437.)
◆ C. **Nursing care plan/implementation:**
1. Goal: *comfort measures.*
a. Perineal care—to promote healing, prevent infection.
b. Sitz baths—to promote healing.
c. Apply topical anesthetics, witch hazel to episiotomy area, hemorrhoids.
d. Administer mild analgesia, as ordered.
e. Instruct in tensing buttocks on position change—to reduce stress on suture line, discomfort.
f. Breast care: *bottle-feeding mother*
(1) Wash daily with clear water and mild soap.
(2) Support with well-fitting brassiere.
(3) For engorgement:
(a) Prevent with tight binder.
(b) Treat with ice pack and mild analgesic.
(c) Avoid nipple stimulation.
(4) Also see: IV. Breastfeeding and lactation, p. 456.
2. Goal: *encourage normal bowel function.* (Normal to take 1–3 d for function to resume).
a. Administer stool softeners, as ordered.
b. Encourage ambulation.
c. Increase *dietary fiber* (salads, fresh fruit, vegetables, bran cereals).
d. Provide adequate fluid intake.
3. Goal: *health teaching and discharge planning.*
a. Reinforce appropriate perineal self-care.
b. Reinforce handwashing (see VI.B. Nursing actions during the fourth stage of labor, p. 437.).
▶ c. *Infant care*
(1) Bathing, cord care, circumcision care, diapering.
(2) Feeding, burping, scheduling.
(3) Assessment—temperature, skin color, newborn rash, jaundice.
(4) Normal stool cycle and voiding pattern.
(5) Common sleep/activity patterns.
(6) Signs to report **immediately:**
(a) Fever, vomiting, diarrhea.
(b) Signs of inflammation or infection at cord stump.
(c) Bleeding from circumcision site.
d. Self-care
(1) Adequate rest, nutrition, hydration.
(2) Breast self-examination; wear bra to support breasts and promote comfort.
(3) Normal process of involution; lochial patterns.

e. Resumption of intercourse approximately 4 wk postpartum (wait until lochia stops).
   (1) Explain that time interval varies as to first postpartal ovulation.
   (2) Family planning options may resume if desired:
       (a) If not breastfeeding, oral contraceptives after first menstrual period (low dose given to breastfeeding mothers) (see Table 7.1, pp. 390–391).
       (b) Use of IUD or diaphragm decided at postpartal check-up.
       (c) Emphasize need to recheck size and fit of diaphragm.
       (d) Other options: condom plus spermicides.
f. Exercises—to restore muscle tone, relieve tension.
   ▶ (1) Mild exercise during first few weeks.
       (a) Deep abdominal breathing.
       (b) Supine head-raising.
       (c) Stretching from head to toe.
       (d) Pelvic tilt.
       (e) Kegel—to regain perineal muscle tone.
   (2) Strenuous exercises (sit-ups, leg lifts)—deferred until later in postpartum.
g. Maternal signs to report **immediately:**
   (a) Prolonged lochia rubra.
   (b) Cramping.
   (c) Signs of infection.
   (d) Excessive fatigue, depression.
   (e) Dysuria.
4. Goal: *anticipatory guidance*—discharge planning: mothers are discharged earlier in their postpartum recovery today—(6–24 h after birth if asymptomatic).
   a. Discuss, assist in organizing time schedule. Nap, when possible, when infant asleep—to minimize fatigue.
   b. Common maternal emotional/behavior changes, feelings.
      (1) Jealous of infant; guilt feelings.
      (2) "Baby blues"—due to hormonal fluctuations, fatigue, change of life-style.
      (3) Feelings of inadequacy.
   c. Discuss support groups, aid in identifying supportive people.

◆ **D. Evaluation/outcome criteria:**
1. Woman experiences normal, uncomplicated postpartal period. All assessment findings within normal limits.
2. Woman returns demonstrations of appropriate self-care measures/techniques:
   a. Perineal care, pad change, handwashing.
   b. Breast care, breast self-examination.
3. Woman verbalizes understanding of:
   a. Need for adequate rest and diversion.

b. Appropriate time for resumption of intercourse and exercise.
c. Appropriate nutritional intake to meet needs (own and, if breastfeeding, infant's).
d. Signs to be reported immediately.
e. Returns demonstration of appropriate infant care measures.
f. Evidences beginning comfort and increasing confidence in parenting role.

◆ **E. Postpartal assessment**—*6 or less wk after birth:*
1. Weight, vital signs, urine for protein, complete blood count (CBC).
2. Breast examination—lactating or not.
3. Pelvic examination—involution and position of uterus; perineal healing; tone of pelvic floor.
4. Desire for selection of method of contraception.

III. **Psychological/behavioral changes** *Achievement of developmental tasks*—progress in assuming maternal role.

◆ **A. Assessment:**
1. *Taking-in* phase: 1–3 d following birth.
   a. Talkative; verbally relives labor/birth experience.
   b. Passive, dependent, concerned with own needs (eating, sleeping, elimination).
2. *Taking-hold*—d 3 to 2 wk.
   a. Impatient to control own bodily functions, care for self.
   b. Expresses interest/concern in learning how to care for baby (desire to assume "mothering" role).
   c. Responds to positive reinforcement.
3. *Letting-go*—mother "lets go" of former self-concept, role, life-style; begins to integrate new role and self-concept as "mother."
   a. Feelings of insecurity, inadequacy.
   b. Hesitancy in approaching infant care tasks.
4. "Baby blues"—may appear on d 4 or 5. (*Note:* Often, father/partner experiences same feelings.)
   a. Thought to result from fatigue (sleep deprivation), realization of need for role change, recognition of new responsibilities.
   b. Mild depression, cries without provocation.
   c. Frightened—intimidated by own perceptions of responsibilities.
5. Lag in experiencing "maternal feelings"—usually resolved within 6 wk.
   a. May contribute to "baby blues."
   b. Guilt regarding lack of "maternal feelings."
   c. Diminished by prompt bonding experience.

---

*This section is based on a study written by R Rubin.

◆ **B. Analysis/nursing diagnosis:**
1. *Ineffective family coping: compromised,* related to achieving developmental tasks.
2. *Situational low self-esteem* related to perceived inadequacy in acceptance of maternal role.
3. *Ineffective individual coping* related to "baby blues," lag in experiencing maternal feelings.

◆ **C. Nursing care plan/implementation:**
1. *Taking-in.* Goal: *emotional support.*
   a. Encourage verbalization of labor/birth experiences; compliment parents on "how well" they did.
   b. Explore feelings of disappointment, if any.
   c. Meet dependency needs; comment on appearance, hair, personal gowns.
   d. Encourage rooming in.
2. *Taking-hold.* Goal: *health teaching.*
   a. Discuss self-care, postpartal physiologic/psychological changes.
   b. Demonstrate infant care; mother returns demonstration.

◆ **D. Evaluation/outcome criteria:**
1. Woman demonstrates beginning comfort in maternal role.
2. Woman develops confidence and competence in infant care.
3. Woman expresses satisfaction with self, infant; eager to return home.
4. Woman succeeds in breastfeeding. (Tension inhibits let-down reflex; baby nurses poorly.)

IV. Breastfeeding and lactation
   A. Biologic foundations:
   1. *Antepartal* alterations
      a. High estrogen/progesterone levels—stimulate proliferation and development of breast ducts.
      b. High progesterone levels—also → development of mammary lobules and alveoli.
   2. *Postpartum* alterations
      a. Rapid drop in estrogen/progesterone levels.
      b. Increased secretion of prolactin—stimulates alveolar cells → milk.
      c. Suckling—stimulates release of oxytocin → contraction of ducts → milk ejection (let-down reflex).
      d. Engorgement—due to venous and lymphatic stasis.
         (1) Immediately precedes lactation.
         (2) Lasts about 24 h.
         (3) Frequent feeding reduces engorgement.

◆ **B. Assessment:**
1. Colostrum (yellowish fluid)—continues for first 2–3 d; may have some antibiotic, immunologic, and nutritive value.
2. Milk (bluish-white, thin)—secreted on about third day.

◆ **C. Analysis/nursing diagnosis:**
1. *Knowledge deficit* related to breastfeeding techniques.
2. *Pain* related to engorgement.
3. *Personal identity disturbance* related to problems in breastfeeding.
4. *Sleep pattern disturbance* related to discomfort or infant care needs.

◆ **D. Nursing care plan/implementation:**
1. Goal: *promote successful breastfeeding.*
   a. Encourage first feeding right after giving birth.
   b. Encourage emptying both breasts at each feeding and before engorgement to stimulate milk production, prevent mastitis.
   c. Encourage rest, relaxation, fluids.
   d. *Nutritional* counseling (see Unit 3).
      (1) Additional 500 calories daily—may be supplied by one extra pint of milk, one extra egg, and one extra serving of meat, citrus fruit, and vegetable.
      (2) Increase fluid intake to 3000 mL daily.
2. Goal: *prevent or relieve engorgement.*
   ▶ a. Pain: relieved by warm packs, emptying breasts.
   b. Wear good, supportive brassiere.
   ● c. Administer analgesics, as ordered/necessary.
3. Goal: *health teaching.*
   ▶ a. Instruct, demonstrate rooting reflex and putting infant to breast. Infant must grasp nipple and areola over location of milk sinuses.
   b. Demonstrate burping techniques, what to do if infant chokes; removing infant from breast.
   ▶ c. Instruct in *basic nipple care.*
      (1) Teach good handwashing.
      (2) Nurse on each breast, making sure areola is in mouth, alternating position of infant.
      (3) Alternate "beginning" breast.
      (4) Break suction before removing infant from breast.
      (5) Air-dry nipples after each feeding and apply lanolin if abrased. *Note:* Creams, lotions, or ointments block secretion of a natural bacteriostatic oil by Montgomery glands—and infant may refuse breast until it is washed. Instead: expressed milk may be massaged gently around nipple.
      (6) Teach daily hygiene of breasts.
   d. Instruct in care of *cracked or fissured nipples.*
      (1) Encourage and support mothers.
      (2) Air-dry nipples after each feeding.

(3) Use nipple shield if nipples extremely sore.

(4) Discontinue nursing for 48 h; maintain milk supply by expressing milk with pump.

e. Discuss avoiding use of any drugs except under medical supervision—may affect infant or suppress lactation.

f. Discuss possibility of sexual stimulation during breastfeeding.

(1) Validate normalcy and acceptability.

(2) *Note:* During orgasm, milk may squirt from nipples.

g. Explain that contraceptive value of nursing is unpredictable; time ovulation is inhibited varies widely.

▶ h. Explain *contraindications to breastfeeding:*

(1) Active tuberculosis.

(2) Severe chronic maternal disease.

(3) Mastitis (temporary interruption may be necessary).

(4) Narcotic addiction, therapeutic drug dependence.

(5) Severe cleft lip or palate in newborn (may pump and give in special bottles).

(6) HIV-positive status; AIDS.

(7) Drug abusers (must be drug-free 3 mo).

◆ **E. Evaluation/outcome criteria:**

1. Woman verbalizes understanding of breast-feeding techniques, nutritional requirements for successful lactation.

2. Woman successfully demonstrates breast-feeding; infant nurses well.

3. Woman demonstrates appropriate burping techniques; clears excessive mucus from infant's mouth without incident.

4. Woman verbalizes understanding of basic breast care techniques:

a. Self-examination.

b. Clear water bath.

c. Drying nipples after bathing, feeding.

d. Care of cracked or irritated nipples.

Complications During the Postpartal Period

I. Disorders affecting fluid-gas transport

A. Postpartum hemorrhage

1. Definition—loss of 500 mL or more during first 24 postpartal h in vaginal birth; 1000 mL in cesarean birth.

2. **Pathophysiology**—excessive loss of blood secondary to trauma, decreased uterine contractility; results in hypovolemia.

3. **Etiology** (in order of frequency):

a. Uterine atony

(1) Uterine overdistention (multipregnancy, hydramnios, fetal macrosomia).

(2) Multiparity.

(3) Prolonged or precipitous labor.

(4) Anesthesia—deep inhalation or regional (particularly saddle block).

(5) Myomata (fibroids).

(6) Oxytocin induction of labor.

(7) Overmassage of uterus in postpartum.

(8) Distended bladder.

b. Lacerations—cervix, vagina, perineum.

c. Retained placental fragments—usually delayed postpartum hemorrhage.

d. Hematoma—deep pelvic, vaginal, or episiotomy site.

◆ 4. **Assessment:**

a. Uterus—boggy, flaccid; excessive vaginal bleeding (dark; seepage, large clots)—due to uterine atony, retained placental fragments.

b. Signs of shock—air hunger; anxiety/apprehension, tachycardia, tachypnea, hypotension.

c. Blood values (admission and postpartal)—hemoglobin (Hgb), hematocrit (Hct), clotting time.

d. Estimated blood loss: during labor/birth; in early postpartum.

e. Pain: vulvar, vaginal, perineal.

f. Perineum: distended—due to edema; discoloration—due to hematoma. May complain of rectal pressure.

g. Lacerations—bright red vaginal bleeding with firm fundus.

◆ 5. **Analysis/nursing diagnosis:**

a. *Fluid volume deficit* related to excessive blood loss secondary to uterine atony, retained placental fragments.

b. *Anxiety/fear* related to unexpected complication.

c. *Altered tissue perfusion* related to decreased oxygenation secondary to blood loss.

d. *Activity intolerance* related to fatigue.

◆ 6. **Nursing care plan/implementation:**

a. Medical management:

(1) IV oxytocin infusion; IV or oral ergot preparations (ergonovine [Ergotrate maleate]; methylergonovine [Methergine]); carboprost (Prostin/M15), an oxytocic; prostaglandin.

(2) Order blood work: clotting time, fibrinogen level, Hgb, Hct, CBC.

(3) Type and crossmatch for blood replacement.

(4) Surgical:

(a) Repair of lacerations.

(b) Evacuation, ligation of hematoma.

(c) Curettage—retained placental fragments.

b. Nursing management:

(1) Goal: *minimize blood loss.*

(a) Notify physician promptly of abnormal assessment findings.

🝪 (b) Order lab work stat, as directed—to determine blood loss and etiology.

(c) Fundal massage.

💊 (d) Administer medications to stimulate uterine tone. For ergot products and carboplast, monitor blood pressure.

(2) Goal: *stabilize status*.

▶ (a) Establish IV line—to enable administration of medications and rapid absorption/action. Administer whole blood (with larger catheter).

💊 (b) Administer medications, as ordered—to control bleeding, combat shock.

(c) Prepare for surgery, as ordered.

▶ (3) Goal: *prevent infection*. Strict aseptic technique.

(4) Goal: *continual monitoring*. Vital signs, bleeding (do pad count or weigh pads), fundal status.

(5) Goal: *prevent sequelae* (*Sheehan's* syndrome).

(6) Goal: *health teaching*—after episode: Reinforce appropriate perineal care and handwashing techniques.

◆ 7. **Evaluation/outcome criteria:**
   a. Maternal vital signs stable.
   b. Bleeding diminished or absent.
   c. Assessment findings within normal limits.

B. **Subinvolution**—delayed return of uterus to normal size, shape, position.
   1. **Pathophysiology**—inability of inflamed uterus (endometritis) to contract effectively → incomplete uterine involution; failure of contractions to effect closure of vessels in site of placental attachment → bleeding.
   2. **Etiology**
      a. PROM with secondary amnionitis, endometritis.
      b. Retained placental fragments.
      c. Stimulation of overdistended uterine muscle may interfere with involution.
   ◆ 3. **Assessment:**
      a. Uterus: large, flabby; lack of uterine tone; failure to shrink progressively.
      b. Discharge: persistent lochia; painless fresh bleeding, hemorrhagic episodes.
   ◆ 4. **Analysis/nursing diagnosis:**
      a. *Pain* related to tender, inflamed uterus secondary to endometritis.
      b. *Anxiety/fear* related to change in physical status.
      c. *Knowledge deficit* related to diagnosis, treatment, prognosis.
      d. *High risk for injury* related to infection.

e. *Fluid volume deficit* related to excessive bleeding.

◆ 5. **Nursing care plan/implementation:**
   a. Medical management:
      (1) Have woman void or catheterize; massage.
   🝪 (2) Surgical (curettage)—to remove placental fragments.
   💊 (3) Antibiotic therapy—to treat intrauterine infection.
   💊 (4) Oxytocics—to stimulate/enhance uterine contractions.
   b. Nursing management:
      (1) Goal: *health teaching*.
         (a) Explain condition and treatment.
         (b) Describe, demonstrate perineal care, pad change, handwashing.
      (2) Goal: *emotional support*. Encourage verbalization of anxiety regarding return to normal, separation from newborn.
      (3) Goal: *promote healing*.
         (a) Encourage rest, complicance with medical/nursing regimen.
      💊 (b) Administer oxytocics, antibiotics, as ordered.

◆ 6. **Evaluation/outcome criteria:**
   a. Verbalizes understanding of condition and treatment.
   b. Complies with medical/nursing regimen.
   c. Demonstrates normal involutional progress.
   d. All assessment findings (vital signs, fundal height, consistency, lochial discharge) within normal limits.
   e. Expresses satisfaction with care.

C. **Hypofibrinogenemia**
   1. **Pathophysiology**—decreased clotting factors, fibrinogen; may be accompanied by DIC.
   2. **Etiology:**
      a. Missed abortion (retained dead fetus syndrome).
      b. Fetal death, delayed delivery.
      c. Abruptio placentae; Couvelaire uterus.
      d. Amniotic fluid embolism.
      e. Hypertension.
   ◆ 3. **Assessment:**
      a. Observe for bleeding from injection sites, epistaxis, purpura.
      b. See DIC assessment, p. 450, and Unit 2.
      c. Maternal vital signs, color.
      d. I&O.
      e. Medical evaluation—procedures.
         (1) Thrombin clot test—important: size and persistence of clot.
         (2) Prothrombin time—prolonged.
         (3) Bleeding time—prolonged.
         (4) Platelet count—decreased.
         (5) Activated partial thromboplastin time—prolonged.

(6) Fibrinogen (factor I concentration)—decreased.
(7) Fibrin degradation products—present.

◆ 4. **Analysis/nursing diagnosis:**
   a. *Fluid volume deficit* related to uncontrolled bleeding secondary to coagulopathy.
   b. *Anxiety/fear* related to unexpected critical emergency.
   c. *Altered tissue perfusion* related to decreased oxygenation secondary to blood loss.

◆ 5. **Nursing care plan/implementation:**
   a. Medical management:
      (1) Replace platelets
      (2) Replace blood loss
      (3) IV heparin—to inhibit conversion of fibrinogen to fibrin.
   b. Nursing management:
      (1) Goal: *continuous monitoring.*
         (a) Vital signs.
         (b) I&O hourly.
         (c) Skin: color, emergence of petechiae.
         (d) Note, measure (as possible), record, and report blood loss.
      (2) Goal: *control blood loss.*
         (a) Establish IV line, administer fluids or blood products as ordered.
         (b) *Position:* bedrest—to maintain blood supply to vital organs.
      (3) Goal: *emotional support.*
         (a) Encourage verbalization of anxiety, fear, concerns.
         (b) Explain all procedures.
         (c) Remain with woman continuously.
         (d) Keep woman and family informed.

◆ 6. **Evaluation/outcome criteria:**
   a. Bleeding controlled.
   b. Laboratory studies—returning to normal values.
   c. Status stable.

II. **Disorders affecting protective functions:** postpartal infection (Table 7.13).
   A. **General aspects**
      1. Definition—genital tract infection occurring during the postpartal period.
      2. **Pathophysiology**—bacterial invasion of birth canal; most common: localized infection of the lining of the uterus (endometritis).
      3. **Etiology:**
         a. Anaerobic nonhemolytic streptococci.
         b. *E. coli.*
         c. *C. trachomatis* (bacteroides).
         d. Staphylococci.
      4. Predisposing conditions:
         a. Anemia.
         b. PROM.

   c. Prolonged labor.
   d. Repeated vaginal examinations during labor.
   e. Intrauterine manipulation—e.g., manual extraction of placenta.
   f. Retained placental fragments.
   g. Postpartum hemorrhage.

◆ 5. **Assessment:**
   a. Fever 38°C (100.4°F) or more on two or more occasions, after first 24 h postpartum.
   b. Other signs of infection: pain, malaise, dysuria, subinvolution, foul lochial odor.

◆ 6. **Analysis/nursing diagnosis:**
   a. *Fluid volume deficit* related to excessive blood loss, anemia.
   b. *Knowledge deficit* related to danger signs of postpartum period.
   c. *High risk for injury* related to infection.

◆ 7. **Nursing care plan/implementation:** prevention
   a. Goal: *prevent anemia.*
      (1) Minimize blood loss—accurate postpartal assessment and management of bleeding.
      (2) *Diet:* high protein, high vitamin.
      (3) Vitamins, iron—suggest continuing prenatal pattern until postpartum check-up.
   b. Goal: *prevent entrance/transport of microorganisms.*
      (1) Strict aseptic technique during labor, birth, and postpartum (universal precautions).
      (2) Minimize vaginal examinations during labor.
      (3) Perineal care.
   c. Goal: *health teaching.*
      (1) Handwashing—before and after each pad change, after voiding or defecating.
      ▶ (2) Perineal care—from front to back; use clear, warm water or mild antiseptic solution as a cascade; do *not* separate labia.
      (3) Maintain sterility of pads; apply from front to back.
      (4) *Avoid* use of tampons until normal menstrual cycle resumes.

◆ 8. **Evaluation/outcome criteria:**
   a. Woman has assessment findings within normal limits:
      (1) Vital signs.
      (2) Rate of involution (fundal height, consistency).
      (3) Lochia: character, amount, odor.
   b. Woman avoids infection.

   B. **Endometritis**—infection of lining of uterus.
      1. **Pathophysiology**—see A. General aspects, at left.
      2. **Etiology**—most common: invasion by normal body flora (e.g., anaerobic streptococci).

■ **TABLE 7.13   Postpartum Infections**

Condition/Etiology	Assessment: Signs/Symptoms	Nursing Interventions
Postpartum Infection Traumatic labor and birth and postpartum hemorrhage make woman more vulnerable to infection by such bacteria as nonhemolytic streptococci, *Escherichia coli,* and *Staphylococcus* species	Depends on location and severity of infection; usually include fever, pain, swelling, and tenderness Temperature of 100.4°F (38°C) or more after first 24 h after birth on two or more occasions indicates puerperal infection ("childbed fever")	1. Monitor: Signs and symptoms, drainage (e.g., uterine) 2. Obtain culture and sensitivity 3. Administer *antimicrobial* agents and *analgesic* agents 4. Ensure comfort; encourage rest 5. Use *universal* precautions 6. Force *fluids* and provide *high*-calorie diet 7. Keep family informed of mother's and newborn's progress 8. Promote maternal-infant contact as soon as possible 9. Plan and implement discharge and follow-up care
Endometritis Microorganisms invade placental site and may spread to entire endometrium	Temperature, chills, anorexia, malaise, boggy uterus, foul-smelling lochia, and cramps	1. Administer *antimicrobial* agents and *analgesic* agents 2. Encourage *Fowler's position* to promote drainage 3. *Force fluids* 4. Take universal precautions
Pelvic Cellulitis or Parametritis Microorganisms spread through lymphatics and invade tissues surrounding uterus	Fever, chills, lower-abdominal pain, and tenderness	1. Administer *antimicrobial* agents and *analgesic* agents 2. Encourage bedrest 3. *Force fluids*
Perineal Infection Trauma to perineum makes woman more vulnerable to infection	Localized pain, fever, swelling, redness, and seropurulent drainage	1. Administer *antimicrobial* agents and *analgesic* agents 2. Provide sitz baths or other heat/cold applications 3. Take universal precautions
Mastitis Lesions or fissures on nipples allow entry of microorganisms (e.g., *Staphylococcus aureus*) from infant's nose/mouth or mother's unwashed hands (Breast milk is a good medium for growth of organism)	Marked engorgement, pain, chills, fever, tachycardia If untreated, single or multiple breast abscesses may form	1. Order culture and sensitivity studies of mother's milk 2. Administer *antimicrobial* agents and *analgesic* agents 3. Apply heat or cold therapy 4. Assist with incising and draining abscesses 5. Use universal precautions and perform meticulous handwashing
Thrombophlebitis Infected pelvic or femoral thrombi Increased tendency to clot formation during pregnancy; trauma to tissues, and hemorrhage decrease new mother's resistance to infection	Pain, chills and fever *Femoral:* stiffness of affected area or part and positive Homans' sign *Pelvic:* severe chills and wide fluctuations in temperature	*Femoral:* 1. Rest and *elevate* leg 2. Administer antimicrobial agents, analgesic agents, and anticoagulants *Pelvic:* 1. Encourage bedrest 2. *Force fluids* 3. Administer *antimicrobial* agents and *anticoagulants*

3. Characteristics:
   a. Mild, localized—asymptomatic, or low-grade fever.
   b. Severe—may lead to ascending infection, parametritis, pelvic abscess, pelvic thrombophlebitis.

   c. If remains localized, self-limiting; usually resolves within 10 d.
◆ 4. **Assessment:**
   a. Signs of infection: fever, chills, malaise, anorexia, headache, backache.
   b. Uterus: large, boggy, extremely tender.

(1) Subinvolution.

(2) Lochia: dark brown; foul odor.

◆ 5. **Analysis/nursing diagnosis:**

a. *Anxiety/fear* related to effects on self and newborn.

b. *Self-esteem disturbance and altered role performance* related to inability to meet own expectations regarding parenting, secondary to unexpected hospitalization.

c. *Pain* related to inflammation/infection.

d. *Ineffective individual coping* related to physical discomfort and psychological stress associated with self-concept disturbance; worry, guilt, concern regarding newborn at home.

e. *Altered family processes*—interruption of adjustment to altered life pattern related to postpartal infection/hospitalization.

◆ 6. **Nursing care plan/implementation:**

a. Goal: *prevent cross-contamination.* Contact-item isolation.

b. Goal: *facilitate drainage. Position:* semi-Fowler's.

c. Goal: *nutrition/hydration.*

(1) *Diet:* high-calorie, high-protein, high-vitamin.

(2) Push *fluids* to 4000 mL/d (oral or IV, or both, as ordered).

(3) I&O.

d. Goal: *increase uterine tone/facilitate involution.* Administer medications, as ordered (e.g., oxytocics, antibiotics).

e. Goal: *minimize energy expenditure, as possible.*

(1) Bedrest.

(2) Maximize rest, comfort.

f. Goal: *emotional support.*

(1) Encourage verbalization of anxiety, concerns.

(2) Keep informed of progress.

◆ 7. **Evaluation/outcome criteria:**

a. Vital signs stable, within normal limits.

b. All assessment findings within normal limits.

c. Unable to recover organism from discharge.

C. **Urinary tract infections**

1. **Pathophysiology**—normal physiologic changes associated with pregnancy (e.g., ureteral dilatation) and the postpartal period (e.g., diuresis, increased bladder capacity with diminished sensitivity of stretch receptors) → increased susceptibility to bacterial invasion and growth → ascending infections (cystitis, pyelonephritis).

2. **Etiology:** usually bacterial.

3. Predisposing factors:

a. Birth trauma to bladder, urethra, or meatus.

b. Bladder hypotonia with retention (due to intrapartal anesthesia or trauma).

c. Repeated or prolonged catheterization, or poor technique.

d. Weakening of immune response secondary to anemia, hemorrhage.

◆ 4. **Assessment:**

a. Maternal vital signs (fever, tachycardia).

b. Dysuria, frequency (flank pain—with pyelonephritis).

c. Feeling of "not emptying" bladder.

d. Cloudy urine; frank pus.

◆ 5. **Analysis/nursing diagnosis:**

a. *Altered urinary elimination* related to diuresis, dysuria, inflammation/infection.

b. *Pain* related to dysuria secondary to cystitis.

c. *Knowledge deficit* related to self-care (perineal care).

◆ 6. **Nursing care plan/implementation:**

a. Goal: *minimize perineal edema.* Perineal ice pack in fourth stage—to limit swelling secondary to trauma, facilitate voiding.

b. Goal: *prevent overdistention of bladder.*

(1) Monitor level of fundus, lochia, bladder distention. (*Note:* Distended bladder displaces uterus, limits its ability to contract → boggy fundus, increases its vaginal bleeding.)

(2) Encourage *fluids* and voiding; I&O.

▶ (3) Aseptic technique for catheterization.

(4) Slow emptying of bladder on catheterization—to maintain tone.

🧪 c. Goal: *identification of causative organism*—to facilitate appropriate medication (antibiotics). Obtain clean-catch (or catheterized) specimen for culture and sensitivity.

d. Goal: *health teaching.* See previous discussion re: fluids, general hygiene, diet, and medications.

◆ 7. **Evaluation/outcome criteria:**

a. Voiding: quantity sufficient (although small, frequent output may mean overflow with retention).

b. Urine character: clear, amber, or straw-colored.

c. Vital signs: within normal limits.

d. No complaints of frequency, urgency, burning on urination, flank pain.

D. **Mastitis**—inflammation of breast tissue:

1. **Pathophysiology**—local inflammatory response to bacterial invasion; suppuration may occur; organism can be recovered from breast milk.

2. **Etiology**—most common: *Staphylococcus aureus;* source—most common: infant's nose, throat.

◆ 3. **Assessment:**

a. Signs of infection (may occur several weeks postpartum).

(1) Fever.

(2) Chills.

(3) Tachycardia.

(4) Malaise.

(5) Abdominal pain.

b. Breast

(1) Reddened area(s).

(2) Localized/generalized swelling.

(3) Heat, tenderness, palpable mass.

◆ 4. **Analysis/nursing diagnosis:**

a. *Impaired skin integrity* related to nipple fissures, cracks.

b. *Pain* related to tender, inflamed tissue secondary to infection.

c. *Disturbance in body image, self-esteem* related to association of breastfeeding with female identity and role.

d. *Anxiety/fear* related to sexuality; impact on breastfeeding, if any.

◆ 5. **Nursing care plan/implementation:**

a. Goal: *prevent infection.* Health teaching in early postpartum:

(1) Handwashing.

(2) Breast care—wash with warm water only (no soap)—to prevent removing protective body oils.

(3) Let breast milk dry on nipples to prevent drying of tissue.

(4) Clean bra (with no plastic pads or liners) to support breasts, reduce friction, minimize exposure to microorganisms.

(5) Good breastfeeding techniques (see p. 456).

(6) Alternate position of infant for nursing to change pressure areas.

b. Goal: *comfort measures.*

(1) Encourage bra or binder—to support breasts, reduce pain from motion.

▶ (2) Local heat or ice packs as ordered—to reduce engorgement, pain.

💊 (3) Administer analgesics, as necessary.

c. Goal: *emotional support.*

(1) Encourage verbalization of feelings, concerns.

(2) If breastfeeding is discontinued, reassure woman she will be able to resume breastfeeding.

d. Goal: *promote healing.*

(1) Maintain lactation (if desired) by manual expression or breast pump, q4h.

💊 (2) Administer antibiotics as ordered.

◆ 6. **Evaluation/outcome criteria:**

a. Woman promptly responds to medical/nursing regimen.

(1) Symptoms subside.

(2) Assessment findings within normal limits.

b. Woman successfully returns to breastfeeding.

E. Thrombophlebitis

1. **Pathophysiology**—inflammation of a vein secondary to lodging of a clot.

2. **Etiology:**

a. Extension of endometritis with involvement of pelvic and femoral veins.

b. Clot formation in pelvic veins following cesarean birth.

c. Clot formation in femoral (or other) veins secondary to poor circulation, compression, and venous stasis.

◆ 3. **Assessment:**

a. Pelvic—pain: abdominal or pelvic tenderness.

⚗ b. Calf—pain: positive *Homans'* sign (pain elicited by flexion of foot with knee extended).

c. Femoral

(1) Pain.

(2) Malaise, fever, chills.

(3) Swelling—"milk leg."

◆ 4. **Analysis/nursing diagnosis:**

a. *Pain* in affected region related to local inflammatory response.

b. *Anxiety/fear* related to outcome.

c. *Ineffective individual coping* related to unexpected postpartum complications, hospitalization, separation from newborn.

d. *Impaired physical mobility* related to imposed bedrest to prevent emboli formation.

◆ 5. **Nursing care plan/implementation:**

a. Goal: *prevent clot formation.*

(1) Encourage early ambulation.

(2) *Position:* avoid prolonged compression of popliteal space, use of knee gatch.

▶ (3) Apply TED hose, as ordered, preoperatively or postoperatively, or both, for cesarean birth.

b. Goal: *reduce threat of emboli.*

(1) Bedrest, with cradle to support bedding.

(2) Discourage massaging "leg cramps."

💊 c. Goal: *prevent further clot formation.* Administer anticoagulants, as ordered.

d. Goal: *prevent infection.*

💊 (1) Administer antibiotics, as ordered.

(2) Push *fluids.*

e. Goal: *facilitate clot resolution.* Heat therapy, as ordered.

◆ 6. **Evaluation/outcome criteria:**

a. Symptoms subside; all assessment findings within normal limits.

b. No evidence of further clot formation.

III. **Disorders affecting psychosocial-cultural functions**

A. General aspects

1. Can occur in both new parents.

2. Usually occur within 2 wk of birth.

3. Increased incidence among single parents.

4. Most common symptomatology: affective disorders.

5. Psychiatric intervention required in small percentage of cases; if underlying cause unresolved, increased risk in subsequent pregnancies.

B. Etiology—theory: birth of child may emphasize:

1. Unresolved role conflicts.

2. Unachieved normal development tasks.

◆ **C. Assessment:**

1. Withdrawal.

2. Paranoia.

3. Anorexia, sleep disturbance, mood swings.

4. Depression—may alternate with manic behavior.

5. Potential for self-injury or child abuse/neglect.

◆ **D. Analysis/nursing diagnosis:**

1. *Ineffective individual coping* related to perceived inability to meet role expectations ("mother") and ambivalence related to dependence/independence.

2. *Self-esteem disturbance and altered role performance* related to "femaleness" and reaction to responsibility for care of newborn.

3. *High risk for violence,* self-directed or directed at newborn related to anger or depression.

4. *Ineffective family coping* related to lack of support system in early postpartum.

5. *Altered family processes* related to psychological stress, interruption of bonding.

6. *Altered parenting* related to hormonal changes and stress.

◆ **E. Nursing care plan/implementation:**

1. Goal: *emotional support.*

   a. Encourage verbalization of feelings, fears, anxiety, concerns.

   b. Support positive self-image, feelings of adequacy, self-worth.

      (1) Reinforce appropriate comments and behaviors.

      (2) Encourage active participation in self-care, comment on accomplishments.

      (3) Reduce threat to self-image, fear of failure. Maintain support, gradually increase tasks.

2. Goal: *safeguard status of mother/newborn.*

   a. Unobtrusive, protective environment.

   b. Stay with woman when she is with infant.

3. Goal: *nutrition/hydration.*

   a. Encourage selection of favorite foods—to aid security in decision making; counteract anorexia refusal to eat by tempting appetite.

   b. Push *fluids* (juices, soft drinks, milkshakes)—to maintain hydration.

4. Goal: *minimize stress, facilitate effective coping.* Administer therapeutic medications, as ordered.

   a. Schizophrenia—phenothiazines.

   b. Depression—mood elevators.

   c. Manic behaviors—sedatives, tranquilizers.

◆ **F. Evaluation/outcome criteria:**

1. Woman increases interaction with infant.

2. Woman expresses interest in learning how to care for infant.

3. Woman evidences no agitation, depression.

4. Woman actively participates in caring for self and infant.

5. Woman demonstrates increasing comfort in mothering role.

6. Woman has positive family interactions.

❏ The Newborn Infant

General overview: Effective nursing care of the newborn infant is based on: (1) knowledge of the conditions present during fetal life; (2) requirements for independent extrauterine life; and (3) alterations needed for successful transition. The *first 24 hours are the most hazardous.*

I. Biologic foundations of neonatal adaptation—*general aspects:*

A. *Fetal anatomy and physiology*

1. *Fetal circulation*—four intrauterine structures that differ from extrauterine structures:

   a. *Umbilical vein*—carries oxygen and nutrient-enriched blood from placenta to ductus venosus and liver.

   b. *Ductus venosus*—connects to inferior vena cava; allows most blood to bypass liver.

   c. *Foramen ovale*—allows fetal blood to bypass fetal lungs by shunting it from right atrium into left atrium.

   d. *Ductus arteriosus*—allows fetal blood to bypass fetal lungs by shunting it from pulmonary artery into aorta.

   e. *Umbilical arteries* (two)—allow return of deoxygenated blood to the placenta.

2. *Umbilical cord*—extends from fetus to center of placenta; usually 50 cm (18–22 in.) long and 1–2 cm (½–1 in.) in diameter. Contains:

   a. *Wharton's jelly*—protects umbilical vessels from pressure, cord "kinking," and interference with fetal-placental circulation.

   b. Umbilical vein—carries oxygen and nutrients from placenta to fetus.

   c. Two umbilical arteries—carry deoxygenated blood and fetal wastes from fetus to placenta. *Note:* Absence of one artery indicates need to rule out intraabdominal anomalies.

3. *Characteristics of fetal blood*
   a. Fetal hemoglobin (Hb$_f$)
      (1) Higher oxygen-carrying capacity than adult hemoglobin.
      (2) Releases oxygen easily to fetal tissues.
      (3) Ensures high fetal oxygenation.
      (4) Normal range at term: 12–22 g/dL; average: 15–20 g/dL.
   b. Total blood volume at term: 85 mL/kg body weight; Hct: 38–62%, average 53%; RBC 3–7 million, average 4.9 million/U.

B. *Extrauterine adaptation: tasks*
   1. Establish and maintain ventilation, successful gas transfer—requires patent airway and adequate pulmonary surfactant.
   2. Modify circulatory patterns—requires closure of fetal structures.
   3. Absorb and utilize fluids and nutrients.
   4. Excrete body wastes.
   5. Establish and maintain thermal stability.

◆ **C. Nursing care plan/implementation**
   1. Facilitate successful transition to independent life.
   2. Protect infant from physiologic stress and environmental hazards.
   3. Encourage development of a strong family unit.

II. Admission to nursery
   A. Admission assessment of normal, term neonate
      1. Color and reactivity.
      2. General appearance, symmetry.
      3. Length and weight.
      4. Head and chest circumferences.
      5. Vital signs:
         a. Axillary temperature.
         b. Respirations (check rate, character, rhythm).
         c. Apical pulse.
      6. General physical assessment (Table 7.14) and reflexes (Table 7.15).
      7. Estimate of gestational age (Table 7.16).

◆ **B. Analysis/nursing diagnosis:**
   1. *Altered health maintenance* related to separation from maternal support system.
   2. *Impaired skin integrity* related to umbilical stump; incontinence of urine and meconium stool; skin penetration by scalp electrode, injections, heel stick, scalpel during cesarean birth; abrasion from obstetric forceps.
   3. *Ineffective airway clearance* related to excessive mucus.
   4. *Pain* related to environmental stimuli.
   5. *Ineffective thermoregulation* related to immature temperature regulation mechanism.

◆ **C. Nursing care plan/implementation:**
   1. Goal: *promote effective gas transport.*
      a. Maintain patent airway—to promote effective gas exchange and respiratory function.

   b. *Position:* right side-lying, head dependent (gravity drainage of fluid, mucus).
   c. Suction prn with bulb syringe for mucus.
   2. Goal: *establish/maintain thermal stability.*
      a. Avoid chilling—to prevent metabolic acidosis.
      b. Dry, wrap, and apply hat.
      c. Place in heated crib.
      d. Monitor vital signs hourly until stable.
   3. Goal: *reduce possibility of blood loss.*
      a. Check cord clamp for security.
      b. Administer vitamin K injection, as ordered, in anterior or lateral thigh muscle—to stimulate blood coagulability.
   4. Goal: *prevent infection.*
      a. Administer antibiotic treatment to eyes (if not performed in birth room)—to prevent ophthalmia neonatorum.
      b. Treat cord stump (alcohol, Triple Dye antibiotic ointment), as ordered.
      c. Use universal precautions.
   5. Goal: *promote comfort and cleanliness.* Admission bath when temperature stable.
   6. Goal: *promote nutrition, hydration, elimination.*
      a. Encourage breastfeeding immediately after birth.
      b. Check blood sugar (Dextrostix or Chemstrip) at 30 min, 1, 2, and 4 h for infants at risk for hypoglycemia (e.g., SGA, LGA).
      c. First feeding at 1–4 h of age with sterile water if permissible and if not breastfeeding.
      d. Note voiding or meconium stool; report failure to void or defecate within 24 h.
   7. Goal: *promote bonding.*
      a. Encourage parent-infant interaction (holding, touching, eye contact, talking to infant).
      b. Encourage breastfeeding within 1 h of birth, if applicable.
      c. Encourage parent participation in infant care—to develop confidence and competence in caring for newborn.
         (1) Assist with initial efforts at feeding.
         (2) Discuss and demonstrate positioning and burping techniques.
         (3) Demonstrate/assist with basic care procedures, as necessary:
            (a) Bath.
            (b) Cord care.
            (c) Diapering.
            (d) Aid parents in distinguishing normal vs. abnormal newborn characteristics.
   8. Goal: *health teaching*—to provide anticipatory guidance for discharge.
      a. Facilitate sibling bonding.
      b. Describe/discuss normal newborn behavior:

■ **TABLE 7.14**　**Physical Assessment of the Term Neonate**

Criterion	Average Values and Normal Variations	Deviations from Normal
Vital Signs		
Heart rate	120–140/min, irregular, especially when crying, and functional murmur	Faint sound—pneumomediastinum; and heart rate <100 beats/min or >180 beats/min
Respiratory rate	30–60/min with short periods of apnea, irregular; vigorous and loud cry	Distress—flaring of nares, retractions, tachypnea, grunting, excessive mucus, <30 beats/min or >60 beats/min; cyanosis
Temperature	Stabilizes about 8–10 h after birth; 36.5–37°C (97.7–98.6°F) axillary	Unreliable indicator of infection
Blood pressure	80/46; varies with change in activity level	Hypotension: with RDS Hypertension: coarctation of aorta
Measurements		
Weight	3400 g (7½ lb)	Birthweight <2500 g: preterm or SGA infant; >4000 g: LGA infant, evaluate mother for gestational diabetes
Length	50 cm (20 in)	
Chest circumference	2 cm (¾ in) less than head circumference	If relationship varies, check for reason
Head circumference	33–35 cm (13–14 in)	Check for microcephalus and macrocephalus
General Assessment		
Muscle tone	Good tone and generalized flexion; full range of motion; spontaneous movement	Flaccid, and persistent tremor or twitching; movement limited; asymmetrical
Skin color	Mottling, acrocyanosis, and physiologic jaundice; petechia (over presenting part), milia, mongolian spotting, lanugo, and vernix caseosa	Pallor, cyanosis, or jaundice within 24 h of birth Petechiae or ecchymoses elsewhere; all rashes, except erythema toxicum; pigmented nevi; hemangioma; and yellow vernix
Head	Molding of fontanels and suture spaces; comprises ¼ of body length	Cephalhematoma, caput succedaneum, sunken or bulging fontanels, closed sutures; excessively wide sutures
Hair	Silky, single strands; lies flat; grows toward face and neck	Fine, wooly; unusual swirls, patterns, hair line; coarse
Eyes	Edematous eyelids, conjunctival hemorrhage; grayish-blue to grayish-brown; blink reflex; usually no tears; uncoordinated movements may focus for a few seconds; good placement on face; cornea is bright and shiny; pupillary reflex equal and reactive to light; eyebrows distinct	Epicanthal folds (in non-Asians); discharges; agenesis; opaque lenses; lesions; strabismus; "doll's eyes" beyond 10 d; absence of reflexes
Nose	Appears to have no bridge; should have no discharge; preferential nose breathers; sneezes to clear nose	Discharge and choanal atresia; malformed; flaring of nares beyond first few moments of life
Mouth	Epstein's pearls on gum ridges; tongue does not protrude and moves freely, symmetrically; uvula in midline; reflexes present: sucking, rooting, gag, extrusion	*Cleft lip or palate;* teeth, cyanosis, circumoral pallor; asymmetrical lip movement; excessive saliva; thrush; incomplete or absent reflexes
Ears	Well formed, firm; notch of ear should be on straight line with outer canthus	Low placement, clefts; tags; malformed; lack of cartilage
Face	Symmetrical movements and contours	Facial palsy (7th cranial nerve); looks "funny"
Neck	Short, freely movable; some head control	Wry neck, webbed neck; restricted movement; masses; distended veins; absence of head control
Chest	Enlarged breasts, "witch's milk"; barrel shaped; both sides move synchronously; nipples symmetrical	Flattened, funnel-chested, asynchronous movement; lack of breast tissue; fracture of clavicle(s); supernumerary or widely spaced nipples; bowel sounds
Abdomen	Dome shaped, abdominal respirations; soft; may have small umbilical hernia; umbilical cord well formed, containing three vessels; dry around base; bowel sounds within 2 h of birth; voiding; passage of meconium	Scaphoid shaped, omphalocele, diastasis recti, and distention; umbilical cord containing two vessels; redness or drainage around base of cord
Genitalia 　Female	Large labia; may have pseudomenstruation, smegma; vaginal orifice open; increased pigmentation; ecchymosis and edema following breech birth; pink-stained urine (uric acid crystals)	Agenesis and imperforate hymen; ambiguous labia widely separated, fecal discharge per vagina; *epispadias or hypospadias*

continued

■ **TABLE 7.14** *(Continued)*

Criterion	Average Values and Normal Variations	Deviations from Normal
General Assessment *(continued)*		
Genitalia *(continued)*		
Male	Pendulous scrotum covered with rugae, and testes usually descended; voids with adequate stream; increased pigmentation; edema and ecchymosis following breech birth	*Phimosis, epispadias,* or *hypospadias;* ambiguous; scrotum smooth and testes undescended *Hydrocele:* collection of fluid in the sac surrounding the testes
Extremities	Synchronized movements, freely movable through full range of motion; legs appear bowed, and feet appear flat; attitude of general flexion; arms longer than legs; grasp reflex; palmar and sole creases; normal contour	Fractures, brachial nerve palsy, *clubbed foot,* phocomelia or amelia, unusual number or webbing of digits, and abnormal palmar creases; poor muscle tone; asymmetry; hypertonicity; unusual hip contour and click sign (*hip dysplasia*); hypermobility of joints
Back	Spine straight, easily movable, and flexible; may have small pilonidal dimple at base of spine; may raise head when prone	Fusion of vertebrae; pilonidal dimple with tuft of hair; *spina bifida,* agenesis of part of vertebral bodies; limitation of movement; weak or absent reflexes
Anus	Patent, well placed; "wink" reflex	Imperforate, and absence of "wink" (absence of sphincter muscle); fistula
Stools	Meconium within first 24 h; transitional—d 2–5; *breastfed:* loose, golden yellow; *bottlefed:* formed, light yellow (see Table 7.17)	Light-colored meconium (dry, hard), or absent with distended abdomen (*cystic fibrosis* or *Hirschsprung's disease*); diarrhetic
Laboratory Values		
Hemoglobin (cord)	13.6–19.6 g/dL	Evaluate for anemia and persistent polycythemia
Serum bilirubin	2–6 mg/dL	Hyperbilirubinemia (*term:* 12 mg or more; *preterm:* 15 mg or more)
Blood glucose	>30–40 mg/dL for *term;* >20 mg/dL for *preterm*	Identify hypoglycemia before overt or asymptomatic hypoglycemia—do Dextrostix on all suspects (LGA or SGA neonates, or neonates of diabetic mothers)
Neurologic Examination*	Specific to gestational age and state of wakefulness	
1. Behavioral patterns		
a. Feeding	Variations in interest, hunger; usually feeds well within 48 h	Lethargic. Poor suck, poor coordination with swallow, choking, cyanosis
b. Social	Crying is lusty, strong, and soon indicative of hunger, pain, attention seeking. Responds to cuddling, voice by quietness and increased alertness	Absent; no focusing on person holding him/her; unconsolable
c. Sleep–wakefulness	Two periods of reactivity: at birth, and 6–8 h later. Stabilization, with wakeful periods about every 3–4 h	Lethargy, drowsiness Disorganized pattern

d. Elimination	Stooling: see Stools
	Urination:
	  First few days: 3–4 qd
	  End of first week: 5–6 qd
	  Later: 6–10 qd, with adequate hydration
		See Stools
		Diminished number: dehydration

2. Reflex response	Bilateral, symmetric response (see Table 7.15)	Absent, hyperactive, incomplete, asynchronous
3. Sensory capabilities		
a. Vision	Limited accommodation, with clearest vision within 7–8 in. Focuses and follows by 15 min of age. Prefers patterns to plain.	Absence of these responses may be due to absence of or diminished acuity or to sensory deprivation
b. Hearing	By 2 min of age, can move in direction of sound: responds to high pitch by "freezing," followed by agitation; to low pitch (crooning) by relaxing	Absence of response: deafness
c. Touch	Soothed by massaging, warmth, weightlessness (as in water bath)	Unable to be comforted: possible drug dependence Cocaine-addicted newborns avoid eye contact
d. Smell	By fifth d, can distinguish between mother's breasts and those of another woman	
e. Taste	Can distinguish between sweet and sour	
f. Motor	Coordinates body movement to parent's voice and body movement	Absence

*Based on Brazelton's method.

■ **TABLE 7.15 Assessment: Normal Newborn Reflexes***

Reflex	Description	Implications of Deviations from Normal Pattern
Moro (startle)	Symmetric *abduction* and *extension* of arms with fingers extended in response to sudden movement or loud noise	Asymmetrical reflex may indicate brachial (Erb's) palsy or fractured clavicle
Tonic neck (fencing)	When head turned to one side, arm and leg on *that* side *extend,* and *opposite* arm and leg *flex*	Asymmetry may indicate cerebral lesion, if persistent
Rooting and sucking	With stimulus to cheek, turns *toward* stimulus, opens mouth, sucks	Absence of response may indicate prematurity, neurologic problem, or depressed infant (or not hungry)
Palmar grasp	If palm stimulated, fingers *curl;* holds adult finger briefly	Asymmetry may indicate neurologic involvement
Plantar grasp	Pressure on sole will elicit *curling* of toes	Absence/asymmetry associated with defects of lower spinal column
Stepping/dancing	If held in upright position with feet in contact with hard surface, alternately raises feet	Asymmetry may indicate neurologic problem
Babinski	Stroking the sole in a upward fashion elicits *hyperextension* of toes	Same as for plantar grasp
Crawling	When placed in prone position, attempts to crawl	Absence may indicate prematurity or depressed infant

*Reflexes are good indicators of the neurologic system in well infants but not in sick neonates. Infants with infections may not show normal reflexes yet have an intact neurologic system.

(1) *Sleeping*—almost continual (wakes only to feed) or 12–16 h daily.
(2) *Feeding*—from every 2–3 h to longer intervals; establish own pattern; breastfed babies feed more often.
(3) *Weight loss*—5–10% in first few days; regained in 7–14 d.
(4) *Stools*—Table 7.17.
(5) *Cord care*—drops off in 7–10 d.
  (a) Keep clean and dry.
  (b) Alcohol to stump.
  (c) HIV precautions.
(6) *Circumcision care*
  (a) Keep clean and dry; heals rapidly.
  (b) Watch for bleeding.
  (c) Petroleum jelly, gauze prn, if ordered.
  (d) Do not remove yellowish exudate.
(7) *Physiologic jaundice*—occurs 24–72 h after birth.
  (a) Nonpathologic.
  (b) Need for hydration.
(8) Identify need for phenylketonuria (PKU) test after ingestion of milk (done routinely at 24 h of age and later).
(9) Describe suggested sensory *stimulation* modalities (mobiles, color, music).
(10) Discuss *safety* precautions:
  (a) Infant seat for travel and home safety.
  (b) Maintaining contact/control over infant to prevent falls, drowning in bath.
  (c) Instruct parents in infant cardiopulmonary resuscitation (CPR).
(11) Describe signs of *common health problems* to be reported promptly:
  (a) Diarrhea, constipation.
  (b) Colic, vomiting.
  (c) Rash, jaundice.
  (d) Differentiation from normal patterns.

◆ **D. Evaluation/outcome criteria:**
1. Infant demonstrates successful transition to independent life:
  a. Nurses well.
  b. Normal feeding, sleeping, elimination patterns.
  c. No evidence of infection or abnormality.
2. Mother/family evidences bonding.
  a. Eye contact.
  b. Stroking, cuddling.
  c. Crooning, calling baby by name, talking to infant.
3. Mother demonstrates comfort and skill in basic newborn care.
4. Mother verbalizes understanding of subjects discussed:
  a. Safety precautions.
  b. Health maintenance actions.

■ **TABLE 7.16 Estimation of Gestational Age: Common Clinical Parameters**

Characteristic	Preterm	Term
Head	Oval—narrow biparietal (35 cm, 13 in.); large in proportion to body; face looks like "old man"	Square-shaped biparietal prominences; ¼ body length
Ears: form, cartilage	Soft, flat, shapeless	Pinna firm; erect from head
Hair: texture, distribution	Fine, fuzzy, or wooly; clumped; appears at 20 wk	Silky; single strands apparent
Sole creases	Starting at ball of foot: ⅓ covered with creases by 36 wk, ⅔ by 38 wk	Entire sole heavily creased
Breast nodules	0 mm at 36 wk; 4 mm at 37 wk	10 mm or more
Nipples	No areolae	Formed; raised above skin level
Genitalia		
Female	Clitoris large, labia gaping	Labia larger, meet in midline
Male	Small scrotum, rugae on inferior surface only, and testes undescended	Scrotum pendulous, covered with rugae; testes usually descended
Skin: texture, opacity	Visible abdominal veins; thin, shiny	Few indistinct larger veins; thick, dry, cracked, peeling
Vernix	Covers body by 31–33 wk	Small amount or absent at term; postterm: dry, wrinkled
Lanugo	Apparent at 20 wk; by 33–36 wk, covers shoulders	Minimal or no lanugo
Muscle tone	Hypotonia; extension of arms and legs	Hypertonia; well flexed
Posture	Froglike	Attitude of general flexion
Head lag	Head lags; arms have little or no flexion	Head follows trunk; strong arm flexion
Scarf sign	Elbow can extend to opposite axilla	Elbow to midline only; infant resists
Square window	90 degrees	0 degrees
Ankle dorsiflexion	90 degrees	0 degrees
Popliteal angle	180 degrees	<90 degrees
Heel-to-ear maneuver	Touches ear easily	90 degrees
Ventral suspension	Hypotonia; "rag-doll"	Good caudal and cephalic tone
Reflexes		
Moro	Apparent at 28 wk; good, but no adduction	Complete reflex with adduction; disappears 4 mo postterm
Grasp	Fair at 28 wk; arm is involved at 32 wk	Strong enough to sustain weight for a few seconds when pulled up; hand, arm, shoulder involved
Cry	24 wk: weak; 28 wk: high-pitched; 32 wk: good	Lusty; can persist for some time
Length	Under 47 cm (18½ in), usually	50 cm (20 in)
Weight	Under 2500 g (5 lb 5 oz)	3400 g (7½ lb)

■ **TABLE 7.17 Infant Stool Characteristics**

Age (d)	Bottlefed	Breastfed	Implications of Abnormal Patterns
1	Meconium	Meconium	Absence may indicate obstruction, atresia
2–5 (transitional)	Greenish yellow, loose	Greenish yellow, loose, frequent	*Note*—At any time: *Diarrhea*—greenish, mucus or blood tinged, or forceful expulsion, may indicate infection
>5	Yellow to brown, firm, 2–4 daily, foul odor	Bright golden yellow, loose, 6–10 daily	*Constipation*—dry, hard stools or infrequent or absent stools may indicate obstruction

c. Signs of normal infant behavior and health.

Complications During the Neonatal Period: The High-Risk Newborn

I. **General overview**—successful newborn adaptation to the demands of independent extrauterine life may be complicated by environmental insults during the *prenatal* period or those arising in the period immediately surrounding birth. The nursing role focuses on minimizing the effect of present and emerging health problems and on facilitating and supporting a successful transition to extrauterine life.

II. **General aspects**—common neonatal risk factors:
   A. Gestational age profile (see Tables 7.14 and 7.16):
      1. Prematurity.
      2. Dysmaturity.
      3. Postmaturity.
   B. Congenital disorders.
   C. Birth trauma.
   D. Infections.

III. **Disorders affecting protective functions: neonatal infections**
   A. **Assess for intrauterine infections.**
   B. **Oral thrush** (mycotic stomatitis).
      1. **Pathophysiology**—local inflammation of oral mucosa due to fungal infection.
      2. **Etiology:**
         a. Organism—*Candida albicans.*
         b. More common in vulnerable newborn, i.e., sick, debilitated; those receiving antibiotic therapy.
      3. Mode of transmission—direct contact with:
         a. Maternal birth canal, hands, and linens.
         b. Contaminated feeding equipment, staff's hands.
      ◆ 4. **Assessment:**
         a. White patches on oral mucosa, gums, and tongue that bleed when touched.
         b. Occasional difficulty swallowing.
      ◆ 5. **Analysis/nursing diagnosis:**
         a. *Pain* related to irritation of oral mucous membrane secondary to oral moniliasis.
         b. *Altered nutrition, less than body requirements* related to irritability and poor feeding.
      ◆ 6. **Nursing care plan/implementation:**
         Goal: *prevent cross-contamination.*
         a. Aseptic technique; good handwashing.
         b. Chemotherapy, as ordered:
            (1) Aqueous gentian violet, 1–2%: apply to infected area with swab.
            (2) Nystatin (Mycostatin)—instill into mouth with medicine dropper, or apply to lesions with swab, *after*

feedings. *Note:* Before medicating, feed sterile water to rinse out milk.
      ◆ 7. **Evaluation/outcome criteria:**
         a. Oral mucosa intact, lesions healed, no evidence of infection.
         b. Feeds well; maintains weight or regains weight lost, if any.
   C. **Neonatal sepsis**
      1. **Pathophysiology**—generalized infection; may overwhelm infant's immature immune system.
      2. **Etiology:**
         a. Prolonged rupture of membranes.
         b. Long, difficult labor.
         c. Resuscitation procedures.
         d. Maternal infection (i.e., beta-hemolytic streptococcus vaginosis).
         e. Aspiration—amniotic fluid, formula, mucus.
         f. Iatrogenic (nosocomial)—caused by infected health personnel or equipment.
      ◆ 3. **Assessment:**
         a. Respirations—irregular, periods of apnea.
         b. Irritability or lethargy.
      ◆ 4. **Analysis/nursing diagnosis:**
         a. *Fatigue* related to increased oxygen needs.
         b. *High risk for infection* related to septic condition.
      ◆ 5. **Nursing care plan/implementation:**
         a. Cultures (spinal, urine, blood).
         b. Check vitals.
         c. Monitor respirators.
      ◆ 6. **Evaluation/outcome criteria:**
         a. Responds to medical/nursing regimen (all assessment findings within normal limits).
         b. Parent(s) verbalize understanding of diagnosis, treatment; demonstrate appropriate techniques in participating in care (as possible).
         c. Parent(s) demonstrate effective coping with situation; express satisfaction with care.

IV. **Disorders affecting nutrition: infant of the diabetic mother (IDM)**
   A. **Pathophysiology**—hyperplasia of pancreatic beta cells → increased insulin production → excessive deposition of glycogen in muscles, subcutaneous fat, and tissue growth. Results in fetal:
      1. *Macrosomia*—LGA infant.
      2. *Enlarged internal organs*—common.
         a. Cardiomegaly.
         b. Hepatomegaly.
         c. Splenomegaly.
      3. Neonatal—inadequate carbohydrate reserve to meet energy needs.
      4. Associated with *increased incidence of:*

a. Congenital anomalies (five times average incidence)—includes cardiac, pelvic, and spinal anomalies.

b. Preterm birth. Respiratory distress syndrome (RDS). Increased insulin needs prenatally lead to decreased surfactant production.

c. Maternal dystocia—due to CPD.

d. Neonatal metabolic problems:
    (1) Hypoglycemia.
    (2) Hypocalcemic tetany.
    (3) Metabolic acidosis.
    (4) Hyperbilirubinemia.

B. Etiology—high circulating maternal glucose levels during fetal growth and development; loss of maternal glucose supply following birth; decreased hepatic gluconeogenesis.

◆ **C. Assessment:**
1. Characteristics of IDM.
2. Hypoglycemia—apply Dextrostix or Chemstrip to heel stick at:
    a. 30 min.
    b. 1, 2, 4, 6, 9, 12, and 24 h of age.
    c. Hypoglycemia laboratory values for term infant: under 30–40 mg/dL.
    d. Hypoglycemia laboratory values for preterm infant: under 20 mg/dL.
    e. Behavioral signs—tremors, twitching, hypotonia, seizures.
3. Gestational age, since macrosomia may mask prematurity.
4. Hypocalcemia—usually within first 24 h
    a. Irritability.
    b. Coarse tremors, twitching, convulsions.
5. Birth injuries
    a. Fractures: clavicle, humerus, skull.
    b. Brachial palsy.
    c. Intracranial hemorrhage/signs of increased intracranial pressure.
    d. Cephalhematoma.
6. Respiratory distress
    a. Nasal flaring.
    b. Sternal retraction.
    c. Costal breathing.
    d. Cyanosis.
    e. Expiratory grunt.
7. Jaundice.

◆ **D. Analysis/nursing diagnosis:**
1. *High risk for injury* related to CPD, dystocia.
2. *Altered cardiopulmonary tissue perfusion* related to placental insufficiency, RDS.
3. *Impaired gas exchange* related to RDS.
4. *Altered nutrition, less than body requirements,* related to hypoglycemia, hypocalcemia.
5. *Risk for altered endocrine/metabolic processes* related to hyperbilirubinemia and kernicterus.

◆ **E. Nursing care plan/implementation:**

1. Hypoglycemia—administer oral or IV glucose, as ordered (may cause rebound effect).
2. Preterm/immature—institute preterm care prn.
3. Hypocalcemia—administer oral or IV calcium gluconate, as ordered.
4. Inform pediatrician immediately of signs of:
    a. Jaundice.
    b. Hyperirritability.
    c. Birth injury.
    d. Increased intracranial pressure/hemorrhage.

◆ **F. Evaluation/outcome criteria:**
1. Infant makes successful transition to extrauterine life.
2. Infant responds to medical/nursing regimen. Experiences minimal or no metabolic disturbances (hypoglycemia, hypocalcemia, hyperbilirubinemia).
3. Infant exhibits normal respiratory function and gas exchange.

V. Hypoglycemia
A. Pathophysiology—low serum-glucose level → altered cellular metabolism → cerebral irritability, cardiopulmonary problems.

B. Etiology:
1. Loss of maternal glucose supply.
2. Normal physiologic activities of respiration, thermoregulation, muscular activity exceed carbohydrate reserve.
3. Decreased hepatic ability to convert amino acids into glucose.
4. More common in:
    a. Infants of diabetic mothers.
    b. Preterm, postterm infants.
    c. SGA infants.
    d. Smaller twin.
    e. Infant of preeclamptic mother.
    f. Birth asphyxia.

◆ **C. Assessment:**
1. Jitteriness, tremors, convulsions; lethargy and hypotonia.
2. Sweating; unstable temperature.
3. Tachypnea; apneic episodes; cyanosis.
4. High-pitched, shrill cry.
5. Difficulty feeding.

◆ **D. Analysis/nursing diagnosis:**
1. *Altered tissue perfusion (fetal)* related to placental insufficiency associated with maternal diabetes, preeclampsia, renal or cardiac disorders; erythroblastosis.
2. *Risk for altered endocrine/metabolic processes* related to high incidence of morbidity associated with birth asphyxia.
3. *Impaired gas exchange* related to coexisting RDS.
4. *Altered nutrition, less than body requirements,* related to hypoglycemia.
5. *High risk for injury* related to coexisting infection, metabolic acidosis.

◆ **E. Nursing care plan/implementation:** see IV. Infant of the diabetic mother, p. 469.

◆ **F. Evaluation/outcome criteria:** see IV. Infant of the diabetic mother, p. 469.

VI. Disorders affecting psychosocial-cultural functions: drug-dependent (heroin) neonate

  A. General aspects

  1. Maternal drug addiction has been associated with:

     a. Prenatal malnutrition and vitamin deficiencies.

     b. Increased risk of antepartal infections.

     c. Higher incidence of antepartal and intrapartal complications.

  2. Infant at risk for:

     a. Intrauterine growth retardation (IUGR).

     b. Prematurity.

     c. Congenital anomalies.

     d. Fetal distress.

     e. Perinatal death.

     f. Child abuse.

  B. Pathophysiology—withdrawal of accustomed drug levels → physiologic deprivation response.

  C. Etiology—repeated intrauterine absorption of heroin/cocaine/methadone from maternal bloodstream → fetal drug dependency.

◆ **D. Assessment**—degree of withdrawal depends on type and duration of addiction and maternal drug levels at birth.

  1. Irritability, hyperactivity, hypertonicity, exaggerated reflexes, tremors, high-pitched cry, difficult to comfort:

     a. *"Step" reflex* (dancing)—infant places both feet on surface; assumes rigid stance—does not "step" or dance.

     b. *"Head-righting" reflex*—holds head rigid; fails to demonstrate head-lag.

  2. Nasal stuffiness and sneezing; respiratory distress, tachypnea, cyanosis or apnea.

  3. Exaggerated acrocyanosis or mottling in the warm infant.

  4. Sweating.

  5. Hunger—sucks on fists; feeding problems—regurgitation, vomiting, poor feeding, diarrhea, and increased mucus production.

  6. Convulsions with abnormal eye-rolling and chewing motions.

  7. Developmental lags/mental retardation.

◆ **E. Analysis/nursing diagnosis:**

  1. *High risk for injury* related to convulsions secondary to physiologic response to withdrawal, CNS hyperirritability.

  2. *Impaired gas exchange* related to respiratory distress secondary to inhibition of reflex clearing of fluid by the lungs.

  3. *Altered nutrition, less than body requirements,* related to feeding problems secondary to respiratory distress and GI hypermotility.

  4. *High risk for impaired skin integrity* related to scratching secondary to withdrawal symptoms.

◆ **F. Nursing care plan/implementation:**

  1. Goal: *prevent/minimize respiratory distress.*

     a. *Position:* side-lying, head dependent—to facilitate mucus drainage.

     b. Suction prn with bulb syringe for excess mucus—to maintain patent airway.

     c. Monitor respirations and apical pulse.

  2. Goal: *minimize possibility of convulsions.*

     a. Decrease environmental stimuli—quiet, touch only when necessary, offer pacifier.

     b. Keep warm, swaddle for comfort.

  3. Goal: *maintain nutrition/hydration.*

     a. Food/fluids—oral or IV, as ordered.

     b. I&O.

     c. Daily weight.

  4. Goal: *assist in diagnosis of drug and drug level.* Collect all urine during first 24 h for toxicologic studies.

  5. Goal: *maintain/promote skin integrity.*

     a. Mitts over hands—to minimize scratching.

     b. Keep clean and dry.

     c. Medicated ointment/powder, as ordered, q2–4h, to excoriated areas.

     d. Expose excoriated areas to air.

  6. Goal: *minimize withdrawal symptoms.* Administer medications, as ordered.

     a. Paregoric elixir—to wean from drug.

     b. Phenobarbital—to reduce CNS hyperirritability, hyperbilirubinemia.

     c. Chlorpromazine (Thorazine), diazepam (Valium)—to tranquilize, reduce hyperirritability. *Note:* Valium is **contraindicated** for jaundiced neonate because it predisposes to hyperbilirubinemia.

     d. Methadone.

  7. Goal: *emotional support to mother.*

     a. Encourage verbalization of feelings of guilt, anxiety, fear, concerns.

     b. Refer to social service.

◆ **G. Evaluation/outcome criteria:**

  1. Infant responds to medical/nursing regimen.

     a. Maintains adequate respirations.

     b. Feeds well, gains weight.

     c. No evidence of CNS hyperirritability, convulsions; demonstrates normal newborn reflexes.

  2. Infant evidences bonding with parent(s). Responsive to mother's voice.

VII. Disorders affecting psychosocial-cultural function: fetal alcohol syndrome (FAS). *General aspects:*

  A. Maternal alcohol abuse has been associated with:

  1. Malnutrition, vitamin deficiencies.

  2. Bone marrow suppression.

3. Liver disease.
4. Child abuse.
B. **Infant at risk for:**
   1. Congenital anomalies.
   2. Mental deficiency.
   3. IUGR.
C. **Pathophysiology**—permanent damage to developing embryonic/fetal structures; cardiovascular anomalies (ventricular septal defects).
D. **Etiology**—high circulating alcohol levels are lethal to the embryo; lower levels cause permanent cell damage.
◆ E. **Assessment:**
   1. Characteristic craniofacial abnormalities:
      a. Short, palpebral fissure.
      b. Epicanthal folds.
      c. Maxillary hypoplasia.
      d. Micrognathia.
      e. Long, thin upper lip.
   2. Short stature.
   3. Irritable, hyperactive, poor feeding.
   4. High-pitched cry, difficult to comfort.
◆ F. **Nursing care plan/implementation:**
   1. Goal: *reduce irritability.*
      a. Reduce environmental stimuli.
      b. Wrap, cuddle.
      c. Administer sedatives, as ordered.
   2. Goal: *maintain nutrition/hydration.*
   3. Goal: *emotional support to mother.*
◆ G. **Evaluation/outcome criteria:** see VI. Drug-dependent (heroin) neonate, p. 471.
   1. No respiratory distress.
   2. Infant feeding properly.
   3. Maternal bonding apparent.
   4. Social service—home involvement.
VIII. **Classification of infants by weight and gestational age**
   A. Terminology
      1. *Preterm, or premature*—37 wk gestation or less (usually 2500 g [5 lb] or less).
      2. *Term*—38–42 wk gestation.
      3. *Postterm*—over 42 wk.
      4. *Postmature*—gestation greater than 42 wk.
      5. *Appropriate for gestational age (AGA)*—for each week of gestation, there is a normal range of expected weight.
         a. Term infants weighing 2500 g or more are usually mature in physiologic functions.
         b. If respiratory distress occurs, it is usually related to aspiration syndrome.
      6. *SGA or dysmature*—weight falls below normal range for age. *Etiology:*
         a. Preeclampsia.
         b. Malnutrition.
         c. Smoking.
         d. Placental insufficiency.
         e. Alcohol syndrome.
         f. Rubella.

g. Syphilis.
h. Multifetal gestation (twins, etc.).
i. Genetic.
j. Cocaine abuse.
      7. *LGA*—above expected weight for age. *Note:* If **preterm,** at risk for **RDS.** If **postterm,** at risk for **aspiration** and **sudden intrauterine death.**
         a. *Etiology:*
            (1) Maternal diabetes or prediabetes.
            (2) Maternal weight gain over 35 lb.
            (3) Maternal obesity.
            (4) Genetic.
         b. *Associated problems:*
            (1) Hypoglycemia.
            (2) Hypocalcemia.
            (3) Hyperbilirubinemia.
            (4) Birth injury.
   B. *Estimation of gestational age*—planning appropriate care for the newborn requires accurate assessment to differentiate between preterm and term infants.

Preterm Infant

Born at 37 weeks' gestation or less.

A. **Pathophysiology**—anatomic and physiologic immaturity of body systems compromises ability to adapt to extrauterine environment and independent life.
   1. *Interference with* **protective** *functions*
      a. *Heat regulation*—unstable, due to:
         (1) Lack of subcutaneous fat.
         (2) Large body surface area in proportion to body weight.
         (3) Small muscle mass.
         (4) Absent sweat or shiver responses.
         (5) Poor capillary response to changes in environmental temperature.
      b. *Resistance to infection*—low, due to:
         (1) Lack of immune bodies from mother (these cross placenta *late* in pregnancy).
         (2) Inability to produce own immune bodies (immature liver).
         (3) Poor WBC response to infection.
      c. *Immature liver*
         (1) Inability to conjugate bilirubin liberated by normal breakdown of RBCs → increased susceptibility to hyperbilirubinemia and kernicterus.
         (2) Immature production of clotting factors and immune globulins.
         (3) Inadequate glucose stores → increased susceptibility to hypoglycemia.
   2. *Interference with* **elimination:** immature *renal* function—unable to concentrate urine → precarious fluid/electrolyte balance.

3. *Interference with* **sensory-perceptual functions:** CNS—immature → weak or absent reflexes and fluctuating primitive control of vital functions.

B. Etiology: (often unknown); preterm labor.
1. *Iatrogenic*—EDB miscalculated for repeat cesarean birth.
2. *Placental factors*
   a. Placenta previa.
   b. Abruptio placentae.
   c. Placental insufficiency.
3. *Uterine factors*
   a. Incompetent cervix.
   b. Overdistention (multifetal gestation, hydramnios).
   c. Anomalies (e.g., myomas).
4. *Fetal factors*
   a. Malformations.
   b. Infections (rubella, toxoplasmosis, HIV-positive status, AIDS, cytomegalic inclusion disease).
   c. Multifetal gestations (twins, triplets).
5. *Maternal factors*
   a. Severe physical or emotional trauma.
   b. Coexisting disorders (preeclampsia, hypertension, heart disease, diabetes, malnutrition).
   c. Infections (streptococcus, syphilis, pyelonephritis, pneumonia, influenza, leukemia).
6. *Miscellaneous factors*
   a. Close frequency of pregnancies.
   b. Advanced parental age.
   c. Heavy smoking.
   d. High-altitude environment.
   e. Cocaine use.

C. Factors influencing survival:
1. Gestational age.
2. Lung maturity.
3. Anomalies.
4. Size.

D. Causes of mortality (in order of frequency):
1. Abnormal pulmonary ventilation.
2. Infection.
   a. Pneumonia.
   b. Septicemia.
   c. Diarrhea.
   d. Meningitis.
3. Intracranial hemorrhage.
4. Congenital defects.

E. Disorders affecting fluid-gas transport: RDS
1. **Pathophysiology**—insufficient pulmonary surfactant (lecithin) and insufficient number/maturity of alveoli predispose to atelectasis; alveolar ducts and terminal bronchi become lined with fibrous, glossy membrane.
2. **Etiology:**
   a. Primarily associated with prematurity.
   b. Other *predisposing* factors:

(1) Fetal hypoxia—due to decreased placental perfusion secondary to maternal bleeding (e.g., abruptio) or hypotension.
(2) Birth asphyxia.
(3) Postnatal hypothermia, metabolic acidosis, or hypotension.
3. Factors *protecting* neonate from RDS:
   a. Chronic fetal stress—due to maternal hypertension, preeclampsia, or heroin addiction.
   b. PROM.
   c. Maternal steroid ingestion (i.e., betamethasone).
   d. Low-grade chorioamnionitis.

◆ 4. **Assessment:**
   a. Usually appears during first or second day after birth.
   b. Signs of *respiratory distress:*
      (1) Nasal flaring.
      (2) Sternal retractions.
      (3) Tachypnea (60 beats/min or more).
      (4) Cyanosis.
      (5) Expiratory grunt.
      (6) Increasing number and length of apneic episodes.
      (7) Increasing exhaustion.
   c. *Respiratory acidosis*—due to hypercapnea and rising CO_2 level.
   d. *Metabolic acidosis*—due to increased lactic acid levels and falling pH.

◆ 5. **Analysis/nursing diagnosis:**
   a. *Impaired gas exchange* related to lack of pulmonary surfactant secondary to preterm birth, intrapartal stress and hypoxia, infection, postnatal hypothermia, metabolic acidosis, or hypotension.
   b. *Altered nutrition, less than body requirements,* related to poor feeding secondary to respiratory distress.

◆ 6. **Nursing care plan/implementation:**
   a. Goal: *reduce metabolic acidosis, increase oxygenation, support respiratory efforts.*
      (1) Ensure warmth (isolette at 97.6°F).
   ▶ (2) Warmed, humidified O_2 at lowest concentration required to relieve cyanosis, through hood, nasal prongs, or endotracheal tube.
   ▶ (3) Monitor *continuous positive airway pressure (CPAP)*—oxygen–air mixture administered under pressure during inhalation *and* exhalation to maintain alveolar patency.
      (4) *Position:* side-lying or supine with neck slightly extended ("sniffing" position); arms at sides.
   ▶ (5) Suction prn with bulb syringe—for excessive mucus.

▶ b. Goal: *modify care for infant with endotracheal tube.*
   (1) Disconnect tubing at adaptor.
   (2) Inject 0.5 mL sterile normal saline.
   (3) Insert sterile suction tube, start suction, rotate tube, withdraw.
   (4) Suction up to 5 sec.
   (5) Ventilate with bag and mask during procedure.
   (6) Reconnect tubing securely to adaptor.
   (7) Auscultate for breath sounds and pulse.

c. Goal: *maintain nutrition / hydration.*
▶   (1) Administer: fluids, electrolytes, calories, vitamins, minerals PO or IV, as ordered.
   (2) I&O.

d. Goal: *prevent secondary infections.*
   (1) Strict aseptic technique.
   (2) Handwashing.

e. Goal: *emotional support of infant.*
   (1) Gentle touching.
   (2) Soft voices.
   (3) Eye contact.
   (4) Rocking.

f. Goal: *emotional support of parents.*
   (1) Keep informed of status and progress.
   (2) Encourage contact with infant—to promote bonding, understanding of treatment.

g. Goal: *minimize possibility of iatrogenic disorders associated with oxygen therapy* (see F., below).

◆ 7. **Evaluation/outcome criteria:**
a. Respiratory distress treated successfully; infant breathes without assistance.
b. Infant completes successful transition to extrauterine life.

F. **Iatrogenic (oxygen toxicity) disorders: retinopathy of prematurity**
1. **Pathophysiology**—intraretinal hemorrhage → fibrosis → retinal detachment → loss of vision.
2. **Etiology**—prolonged exposure to high concentrations of oxygen.
◆ 3. **Assessment**—only perceptible retinal change is vasoconstriction. *Note:* Arterial blood (PaO_2) gas readings less than 50 or more than 70 mm Hg.
◆ 4. **Nursing care plan/implementation:** Goal: *prevent disorder.* Maintain PaO_2 of 50–70 mm Hg.
◆ 5. **Evaluation/outcome criteria:**
a. Successful recovery from respiratory distress.
b. No evidence of disorder.

G. **Iatrogenic (oxygen toxicity) disorders: bronchopulmonary dysplasia (BPD)**

1. **Pathophysiology**—damage to alveolar cells results in focal emphysema.
2. **Etiology**—positive pressure ventilation (CPAP and PEEP) and prolonged administration of high concentrations of oxygen.
◆ 3. **Assessment**—monitor for signs of:
a. Tachypnea.
b. Increased respiratory effort.
c. Respiratory distress.
◆ 4. **Nursing care plan/implementation:** Goal: *prevent disorder.*
a. Use of *negative* pressure devices.
▶ b. Maintain oxygen concentration *below* 70%.
c. Supportive care.
d. Wean off ventilator, as possible.
◆ 5. **Evaluation/outcome criteria:**
a. Successful recovery from respiratory distress.
b. No evidence of disorder.

H. **Intraventricular hemorrhage**
1. **Pathophysiology**—rupture of thin, fragile capillary walls within ventricles of the brain (more common in preterm).
2. **Etiology:**
a. Hypoxia.
b. Respiratory distress.
c. Birth trauma.
d. Birth asphyxia.
e. Hypercapnia.
◆ 3. **Assessment:**
a. Hypotonia.
b. Lethargy.
c. Hypothermia.
d. Bradycardia.
e. Bulging fontanels.
f. Respiratory distress or apnea.
g. Seizures.
h. Cry: high-pitched whining
◆ 4. **Nursing care plan/implementation:** Goal: *supportive care*—to promote healing.
a. Monitor vital signs.
b. Maintain thermal stability.
▶ c. Ensure adequate oxygenation (may be placed on CPAP).
◆ 5. **Evaluation/outcome criteria:**
a. Condition stable, all assessment findings within normal limits.
b. No evidence of residual damage.

I. **Disorders affecting nutrition**
1. **Pathophysiology**—underdeveloped feeding abilities, small stomach capacity, immature enzyme system, fat intolerance.
2. **Etiology**—immature body systems associated with preterm birth.
◆ 3. **Assessment:**
a. Weak suck, swallow, gag reflexes—tendency to aspiration.

b. Signs of malabsorption and fat intolerance (abdominal distention, diarrhea, weight loss, or failure to gain weight).
c. Signs of vitamin E deficiency (edema, anemia).

◆ 4. **Analysis/nursing diagnosis:**
a. *Altered nutrition, less than body requirements,* related to poor feeding reflexes, reduced stomach capacity, inability to absorb need nutrients.
b. *Impaired gas exchange* related to aspiration.

◆ 5. **Nursing care plan/implementation:**
Goal: *maintain/increase nutrition.*
a. Frequent, small feedings—to avoid exceeding stomach capacity, facilitate digestion.
b. Frequent "burping" during feeding—to avoid regurgitation/aspiration.
c. Supplement vitamin E (alpha-tocopherol) intake, as ordered, in formula-fed infants (*Note:* intake adequate in breastfed babies.)
d. Vitamin E actions:
(1) Antioxidant.
(2) Maintains structure and function of smooth, skeletal, and cardiac muscle.
(3) Maintains structure and function of vascular tissue, liver, and RBC integrity.
(4) Coenzyme in tissue respiration.
(5) Treatment for malnutrition with macrocytic anemia.
e. Encourage parent/family participation.

◆ 6. **Evaluation/outcome criteria:**
a. Feeds well without regurgitation/aspiration.
b. Maintains/gains weight.
c. No evidence of malabsorption, vitamin deficiency.

J. Disorders affecting nutrition/elimination: *necrotizing enterocolitis (NEC)*
1. **Pathophysiology**—intestinal thrombosis, infarction, autodigestion of mucosal lining, and necrotic lesions; incidence increased in preterm.
2. **Etiology**—intestinal ischemia, due to blood shunt to brain and heart in response to:
a. Fetal distress.
b. Fetal/neonatal asphyxia.
c. Neonatal shock.
d. After birth, may result from:
(1) Low cardiac output.
(2) Infusion of hyperosmolar solutions.
e. Complicated by action of enteric bacteria on damaged intestine.

◆ 3. **Assessment**—early identification is **vital.**
a. Abdominal distention or erythema, or both.
b. Poor feeding, vomiting.
c. Blood in stool.
d. Systemic signs associated with sepsis that may need temporary colostomy or iliostomy:
(1) Lethargy or irritability.
(2) Hypothermia.
(3) Labored respirations or apnea.
(4) Cardiovascular collapse.
e. Medical diagnosis:
(1) Increased gastric residual.
(2) X ray shows ileus, air in bowel wall.

◆ 4. **Analysis/nursing diagnosis:**
a. *Altered nutrition, less than body requirements,* related to inability to tolerate oral feedings and gastrointestinal dysfunction secondary to ischemia, thrombosis, or necrosis.
b. *Constipation* related to paralytic ileus with stasis; diarrhea related to water loss.
c. *High risk for injury* related to infection, thrombosis, metabolic alterations (acidosis, osmotic diuresis, dehydration, hyperglycemia) due to parenteral nutrition.
d. *Altered parenting* related to physiologic compromise and prolonged hospitalization.
e. *Impaired skin integrity* when colostomy is necessary.

◆ 5. **Nursing care plan/implementation:**
a. Goal: *supportive care.*
(1) Rest GI tract: *no oral intake*—to achieve gastric decompression.
(2) IV fluids, as ordered—to maintain hydration.
b. Goal: *prevent infection.* Administer antibiotics, as ordered.
c. Goal: *Prevent trauma to skin surrounding stoma.*

◆ 6. **Evaluation/outcome criteria:**
a. Tolerates oral feedings.
b. Demonstrates weight gain.
c. Normal stool pattern.
d. Parents are accepting and knowledgeable about care of infant.

Postterm Infant

Over 42 weeks' gestation.

A. General aspects
1. Labor may be hazardous for mother and fetus because:
a. Large size of infant contributes to maternal dystocia; diagnosis by: ultrasound, X ray.

b. Placental insufficiency → fetal hypoxia; diagnosis by:
  (1) Contraction stress test.
  (2) Nonstress test.
  (3) Maternal urine estriols.

c. Meconium passage (common physiologic response) increases chance of meconium aspiration.

◆ **B. Assessment:**
1. If postmature skin: dry, wrinkled—due to metabolism of fat and glycogen reserves to meet in utero energy needs.
2. Long limbs, fingernails, and toenails—due to continued growth in utero.
3. Lanugo and vernix—absent.
4. Expression: wide-eyed, alert—probably due to chronic hypoxia (oxygen hunger).
5. Placenta—signs of aging.

◆ **C. Analysis/nursing diagnosis:** *High risk for injury* related to high incidence of morbidity and mortality due to dystocia or hypoxia.

◆ **D. Nursing care plan/implementation:**
1. **During labor:**
  a. Goal: *emotional support of mother*—may require cesarean birth due to CPD or fetal distress.
  b. Goal: *Continuous electronic monitoring of FHR.* Report *late* or *variable* decelerations immediately (indicate fetal distress).
2. **After birth:**
  a. Goal: *if born vaginally, prompt identification of birth injuries, respiratory distress.* Continual observation.
  b. Goal: *early identification/treatment of emerging signs of complications.*
    (1) *Hypoglycemia*—Dextrostix readings and behavior.
    (2) Administer oral or intravenous glucose, as ordered.

◆ **E. Evaluation/outcome criterion:** successful transition to extrauterine life (all assessment findings within normal limits).

Congenital Disorders

I. *General overview:* Genetic abnormalities and environmental insults often lead to congenital disorders of the newborn. Successful transition to independent extrauterine life may pose a major challenge to infants compromised by anatomic or physiologic disorders. Knowledge regarding the implications of the neonate's structural or metabolic problems enables the nurse to identify early signs of health problems and to plan, provide, and evaluate appropriate outcome-directed care to safeguard the status of the infant with a congenital disorder.

II. **Disorders affecting fluid-gas transport:** *congenital heart disease*

A. Pathophysiology—altered hemodynamics, due to persistent fetal circulation or structural abnormalities.
1. *Acyanotic defects*—no mixing of blood in the systemic circulation.
  a. *Patent ductus arteriosus.*
  b. *Atrial septal defect.*
  c. *Ventricular septal defect.*
  d. *Coarctation of the aorta.*
2. *Cyanotic defects*—unoxygenated blood enters systemic circulation.
  a. *Tetralogy of Fallot.*
  b. *Transposition of the great vessels.*

B. Etiology—unknown. Associated with maternal:
1. Prenatal viral disease (e.g., rubella, coxsackie).
2. Malnutrition; alcoholism.
3. Diabetes.
4. Ingestion of lithium salts.

◆ **C. Assessment:**
1. *Patent ductus arteriosus* (see Figure 8.3, p. 505)
  a. Characteristic machine murmur, mid to upper left sternal border (cardiomegaly); persists throughout systole and most of diastole; associated with a "thrill."
  b. Widened pulse pressure.
  c. Bounding pulse, tachycardia, "gallop" rhythm.
2. *Atrial septal defect* (see Figure 8.1, p. 504)
  a. Characteristic crescendo/decrescendo systolic ejection murmur.
  b. Fixed S_2 splitting.
  c. Dyspnea, fatigue on normal activity.
  d. Medical diagnosis—cardiac catheterization, X ray.
3. *Ventricular septal defect* (see Figure 8.2, p. 504)
  a. Loud, harsh, pansystolic murmur; heard best at left lower sternal border; radiates throughout precordium. (*Note:* may be absent—due to high pulmonary vascular resistance → equalization of interventricular pressure).
  b. Medical diagnosis—cardiac catheterization, ECG, chest X ray.
4. *Coarctation of the aorta* (see Figure 8.4, p. 505)
  a. Absent femoral pulse.
  b. Late systolic murmur.
  c. Decreased blood pressure in *lower* extremities.
  d. Medical diagnosis: X ray.
5. *Tetralogy of Fallot* ("blue" baby) (see Figure 8.5, p. 506)
  a. Acute hypoxic/cyanotic episodes.
  b. Limp, sleepy, exhausted; hypotonic extended position—postepisode.
  c. Medical diagnosis—cardiac catheterization.

6. *Transposition of the great vessels* (see Figure 8.6, p. 506)
   a. Cyanotic after crying or feeding.
   b. Progressive tachypnea—attempt to compensate for decreased PaO_2, metabolic acidosis.
   c. Heart sounds vary, consistent with defect.
   d. Signs of CHF.
   🧪 e. Medical diagnosis—cardiac catheterization, X ray, ECG.

◆ **D. Analysis/nursing diagnosis:**
  1. *Fluid volume excess* related to persistent fetal circulation, structural abnormalities.
  2. *Impaired gas exchange* related to abnormal circulation, secondary to above pathology.
  3. *Altered nutrition, less than body requirements,* related to exhaustion, dyspnea.

◆ **E. Nursing care plan/implementation:**
  1. Goal: *minimize cardiac workload.*
   a. Minimize crying—snuggle; pacifier—to meet psychological needs.
   b. Keep clean and dry.
  2. Goal: *maintain thermal stability*—to reduce body need for oxygen.
  3. Goal: *prevent infection.*
  ▶ a. Strict aseptic technique; universal precautions.
   b. Handwashing.
  4. Goal: *parental emotional support.*
   a. Encourage verbalization of anxiety, fears, concerns.
   b. Keep informed of status.
  5. Goal: *health teaching*—explain, discuss:
   a. Diagnostic procedures.
   b. Treatment procedures.
   c. Basic care modalities.
  6. Goal: *promote bonding.* Encourage to participate in infant care, as possible.
  7. Medical/surgical management: surgical intervention/repair of congenital cardiac abnormality.

◆ **F. Evaluation/outcome criteria:**
  1. Experiences no respiratory embarrassment in immediate postnatal period.
  2. Completes transfer to high-risk center without incident, if applicable.
  3. Surgical intervention successful, where applicable.

III. **Disorders affecting fluid-gas transport: hemolytic disease of the newborn**
  A. Rh incompatibility
   1. **Pathophysiology**—see p. 407.
   2. **Etiology**—see Rh isoimmunization, p. 408.
  ◆ 3. **Assessment:**
   a. *Prenatal*—maternal Rh titers, amniocentesis.
  🧪 b. *Intrapartal*—amniotic fluid color:
   (1) Straw-colored: mild disease.
   (2) Golden: severe fetal disease.

🧪 c. Direct Coombs test on cord blood; positive test demonstrates Rh antibodies in fetal blood.

◆ 4. **Nursing care plan/implementation—exchange transfusion:**
  a. Goal: *health teaching.*
   (1) Explain purpose and process to parents.
   (2) Removes anti-Rh antibodies and fetal cells that are coated with antibodies.
   (3) Reduces bilirubin levels—indicated when 20 mg/dL in term neonate and 15 mg/dL in preterm.
   (4) Corrects anemia—supplies RBCs that will not be destroyed by maternal antibodies.
   (5) Rh-negative type O blood elicits no reaction; maximum exchange is 500 mL; duration of exchange: 45–60 min.
  ▶ b. Goal: *minimize transfusion hazards.*
   (1) Warm blood to room temperature, since cold blood may precipitate cardiac arrest.
   (2) Use only fresh blood—to reduce possibility of hypocalcemia, tetany, convulsions.
  💊 (3) Give calcium gluconate, as ordered, after each 100 mL of transfusion.
  c. Goal: *prepare for transfusion procedure.* Ready necessary equipment—monitor, resuscitation equipment, radiant heater, light.
  d. Goal: *assist with exchange transfusion.*
   (1) Continuous monitoring of vital signs; record baseline, and every 15 min during procedure.
   (2) Record: time, amount of blood withdrawn; time and amount injected; medications given.
   (3) Observe for: dyspnea, listlessness, bleeding from transfusion site, cyanosis, cardiovascular irregularity or arrest; coolness of lower extremities.
  e. Goal: *posttransfusion care.*
  ◆ (1) **Assessment:**
   (a) Observe for dyspnea, cyanosis, cardiac arrest or irregularities, jaundice, hypoglycemia; frequent vital signs.
   (b) Signs of *sepsis*—fever, tachycardia, dyspnea, chills, tremors.
  ◆ (2) **Nursing care plan/implementation:**
   (a) Maintain thermal stability—to reduce physiologic stress, possibility of metabolic acidosis.
  ▶ (b) Give oxygen—to relieve cyanosis.

(c) Keep cord moist—to facilitate repeat transfusion, if necessary.

(d) Maintain nutrition/hydration—feed per schedule.

◆ 5. **Evaluation/outcome criteria:**

a. Infant's hemolytic process ceases; bilirubin level drops.

b. Infant makes successful transition to extrauterine life.

c. Infant experiences no complications of therapeutic regimen.

d. Infant shows evidence of bonding.

B. **ABO incompatibility**

1. **Pathophysiology**—fetal blood carrying antigens A/B enters maternal type O bloodstream → antibody formation → antibodies cross placenta → hemolyze fetal RBCs. *Note:* less severe than Rh reaction.

2. **Etiology:**

a. Type O mother carries anti-A and anti-B antibodies.

b. Even first pregnancy is jeopardized if fetal blood enters maternal system.

c. Reaction possible if fetus is type A, type B, or type AB and mother is type O.

◆ 3. **Assessment:**

a. Jaundice within first 24 h.

b. Rising bilirubin levels.

c. Enlarged liver and spleen.

◆ 4. **Nursing care plan/implementation:**
Goal: *reduce hazard to newborn.*

▶ a. Prepare for exchange transfusion with O negative blood.

▶ b. Phototherapy may be ordered if bilirubin 10 mg/dL, and anemia is mild or absent.

c. Close monitoring of status.

d. Supportive care.

◆ 5. **Evaluation/outcome criteria:**

a. Infant responds to medical/nursing regimen.

b. Infant's assessment findings within normal limits.

C. **Hyperbilirubinemia**

1. **Pathophysiology**—bilirubin, a breakdown product of hemolyzed RBCs, appears at increased levels; exceeds 13–15 mg/dL. Bilirubin is safe when bound with albumin and conjugated by user for body excretion; danger is when unconjugated and deposits in CNS.

a. WARNING: There is no "safe" serum-bilirubin level; kernicterus is a function of the bilirubin level *and* neonatal age and condition; poor fluid-and-caloric balance subjects the infant (especially the preterm infant) to kernicterus at low serum-bilirubin levels.

b. *Kernicterus*—high bilirubin levels result in deposition of yellow pigment in basal ganglia of brain → irreversible retardation.

2. **Etiology:**

a. Rh or ABO incompatibility, during first 48 h.

b. Resolution of an enclosed hemorrhage (e.g., cephalohematoma).

c. Infection.

d. Drug induced—vitamin K injection, maternal ingestion of sulfisoxazole (Gantrisin).

e. Bile duct blockage.

f. Albumin-binding capacity is exceeded.

g. "Breastfeeding jaundice" (e.g., pregnandiol in milk). Breastfeeding is *not* dangerous and not a cause of physiologic jaundice.

h. Dehydration.

i. Immature liver (interferes with conjugation).

◆ 3. **Assessment:**

a. Jaundice noted after blanching skin to suppress hemoglobin color; noted in sclera or mucosa in dark-skinned neonates; make sure light is adequate; spreads from head down, with increasing severity.

b. Pallor.

c. Concentrated, dark urine.

⚗ d. Blood level determination—hemoglobin or indirect bilirubin (unconjugated, unbound bilirubin deposits in CNS).

e. *Kernicterus*—similar to intracranial hemorrhage.

(1) Poor feeding or sucking.

(2) Regurgitation, vomiting.

(3) High-pitched cry.

(4) Temperature instability.

(5) Hypertonicity/hypotonicity.

(6) Progressive lethargy; diminished Moro reflex.

(7) Respiratory distress.

(8) Cerebral palsy, mental retardation.

(9) Death.

◆ 4. **Analysis/nursing diagnosis:**

a. *Fluid volume (RBC) deficit* related to hemolysis secondary to blood incompatibility.

b. *High risk for injury* (brain damage) related to kernicterus.

c. *Altered thought processes* (mental retardation) related to brain damage secondary to kernicterus.

d. *Knowledge deficit (parental)* related to infant condition.

◆ 5. **Nursing care plan/implementation:**

a. Medical management:

⚗ (1) *Prenatal*—amniocentesis.

(2) *Postnatal*—exchange transfusion, phototherapy.

▶ b. Goal: *assist bilirubin conjugation through phototherapy.*

(1) Cover closed eyelids while under light; remove eyepads when not un-

der light (feeding, cuddling, during parental visits)—to protect eyes.
(2) Expose as much skin as possible—to maximize exposure of circulating blood to light. Remove for only brief periods.
(3) *Change position* q1h—to maximize exposure of circulating blood to light.
(4) *Note:* any loose green stools as bile is cleared through gut; watch for skin breakdown on buttocks.
(5) Monitor temperature—to identify hyperthermia.
(6) *Push fluids* (to 25% more than average) between feedings—to counteract dehydration. Breast milk has natural laxative effects that help clear bile.
c. Goal: *health teaching.* Explain, discuss phototherapy, bilirubin levels, implications.
d. Goal: *emotional support.*
(1) Encourage verbalization of anxiety, fears, concerns.
(2) Encourage contact with infant.
(3) Reassure, as possible.
◆ 6. **Evaluation/outcome criteria:**
a. Infant's hemolytic process ceases; bilirubin level drops.
b. Infant makes successful transition to extrauterine life.
c. Infant experiences no complications of therapeutic regimen.
d. Infant shows evidence of effective bonding.

Emotional Support of the High-Risk Infant

I. General aspects
A. The high-risk infant has the same *developmental needs* as the healthy term infant:
1. Social and tactile stimulation.
2. Comfort and removal of discomfort (hunger, soiling).
3. Continuous contact with a consistent, parenting person.
B. Treatment for serious physiologic compromise may result in:
1. Isolation.
2. Sensory deprivation or noxious stimuli.
3. Emotional stress.
◆ II. **Assessment**—signs of neonatal emotional stress:
A. Does not look at person performing care.
B. Does not cry or protest.
C. Poor weight gain; failure to thrive.
◆ III. **Analysis/nursing diagnosis:** *sensory/perceptual alterations* related to isolation in isolette, oxygen hood.
◆ IV. **Nursing care plan/implementation:**

A. Goal: *provide consistent parenting contact.* Assign same nurses whenever possible.
B. Goal: *emotional support.*
1. Comfort when crying.
2. Provide positive sensory stimulation. Arrange time to:
a. Stroke skin.
b. Hold hand.
c. Hum, sing, talk.
d. Hold in en-face position (nurse looking into infant's eyes).
e. Hold when feeding, if possible.
C. Goal: *encourage parents to participate in care*—to:
1. Reduce their psychological stress, anxiety, fear.
2. Promote bonding.
3. Reduce possibility of later child abuse (higher incidence of child abuse against children who have been high-risk infants).
◆ V. **Evaluation/outcome criteria:**
A. Infant demonstrates successful resolution of physiologic problems.
B. Parents and infant evidence bonding.
C. Parents express satisfaction with care and result.

General Aspects: Nursing Care of the High-Risk Infant and Family

I. *General overview:* The birth of a physiologically compromised neonate is psychologically stressful for both infant and family and physiologically stressful for the neonate. Effective, goal-directed nursing care is directed toward:
A. Minimizing physiologic and psychological stress.
B. Facilitating/supporting successful coping or adaptation.
C. Encouraging parental attachment/separation/grieving, as appropriate.
◆ II. **Assessment**—directed toward determining neonate's present and projected status:
A. Determine neonate's current physical status.
B. Identify specific status and diagnosis-related problems and needs.
C. Describe family psychological status, strengths, and coping mechanisms/skills.
D. Determine medical/surgical/nursing approach to problems—and prognosis.
◆ III. **Analysis/nursing diagnosis:**
A. Parental *anxiety/fear* related to physiologic compromise of neonate.
B. *Self-esteem disturbance* related to feelings of guilt or anger.
C. *Ineffective individual coping* related to severe psychological stress.
D. *Knowledge deficit* related to diagnosis, treatment, prognosis of infant.
E. *High risk for altered parenting* related to concern about infant.
◆ IV. **Nursing care plan/implementation:**

A. Goal: *preoperative and postoperative care.*
   1. Maintain/improve physiologic stability.
      a. Temperature stabilization—keep warm.
      ► b. Oxygenation:
         (1) Position.
         (2) Administer oxygen, as ordered or necessary.
      c. Nutrition/hydration:
         ► (1) Administer/monitor IV fluids.
         (2) Oral fluids, as ordered.
         (3) Feed, as status permits.
   2. Assist with diagnostic testing.
B. Goal: *emotional support of parents.*
   1. Encourage exploring and ventilating feelings.
   2. Involve parents in decision-making process.
C. Goal: *health teaching.*
   1. Determine knowledge/understanding of problem.
   2. Explain/simplify/clarify, as needed, physician's discussions with parents.
   3. Describe/explain/discuss neonate's present status and any auxiliary equipment; teach CPR to family.
   4. Refer, as needed, to hospital/community resources.
D. Goal: *promote bonding.* Encourage parental participation in care of the neonate.
◆ **V. Evaluation/outcome criteria:**
   A. Parents verbalize understanding of relevant information; make informed decisions regarding infant care.
   B. Parents demonstrate comfort and increasing participation in care of neonate.
   C. Infant maintains/increases adequacy of adaptation to extrauterine life.
   D. If relevant, parents demonstrate progress in grieving process.

❏ Questions

Select the one answer that is best for each question.

1. Which contraceptive method is most appropriate for a woman whose history reveals two episodes of thrombophlebitis with her previous pregnancy, repeated *Candida* infections, and gestational diabetes and who wants to postpone pregnancy for at least 1 year?
   1. Oral contraceptive pill.
   2. Tubal ligation.
   3. Diaphragm.
   4. Intrauterine device.
2. Which of the following identifies the basal body temperature (BBT) change characteristic of ovulation?
   1. Falls slightly, then increases by about 0.5°C.
   2. Rises slightly, then falls by about 0.5°C.
   3. Is affected by a surge of FSH.
   4. Is due to an estrogen surge.
3. When calculating the 1-minute Apgar, the nurse adds the following assessment findings: heart rate—over 100; respiratory effort—slow and irregular; muscle tone—flaccid response to slap on soles of feet; weak cry; color—body pink, extremities blue. In view of these as-

sessment findings, which Apgar score should the nurse record?
   1. 5.
   2. 6.
   3. 7.
   4. 8.
4. A woman 36 weeks' pregnant is admitted directly from clinic, with a blood pressure of 146/98, puffy face and hands, and "awful headaches and problems seeing." Admission note states: Admit stat for preeclampsia. Which nursing order should be questioned?
   1. Assess reflexes and amount and distribution of edema every shift.
   2. Up as desired.
   3. Admission and daily weight.
   4. Test urine for protein every 4 hours.
5. Objectives for the initial prenatal visit include determining a woman's present health status, validating pregnancy, and identifying factors that may affect or be affected by a pregnancy. Which assessment finding indicates a need for further evaluation?
   1. Urinary frequency, nausea, fatigue.
   2. Vital signs—T 98.2, P 92, R 20, BP 110/70.
   3. Urine—negative for sugar, trace of protein.
   4. Marked vaginal discharge with itching for the past few days.
6. Health teaching about over-the-counter pregnancy test kits should include which of the following information?
   1. False-negative tests may be due to dilute urine secondary to diuresis and inaccurate technique.
   2. Urine tests are classed as presumptive signs of pregnancy.
   3. Levels of progesterone from the corpus luteum are sufficient to diagnose pregnancy as early as the fourth week.
   4. Urine tests are classed as positive signs of pregnancy.
7. A woman appears excited, euphoric, and eager to learn about her labor status. Her behavior supports the nursing assessment that she is progressing through which phase of labor?
   1. Latent.
   2. Active.
   3. Transitional.
   4. Prodromal.
8. Thirty minutes after the birth of twins, a new mother's fundus is "boggy" and her lochial flow increased. After massage to firm the fundus, and while supporting the uterus with a hand above the symphysis, the nurse expresses several large clots. Which action should the nurse take next?
   1. Notify the physician because the site of her bleeding must be located.
   2. Notify the physician because she needs surgery.
   3. Administer oxytocin according to prn order.
   4. Reapply perineal pad and tell her to keep her thighs together.
9. While performing a newborn assessment, the nurse notes yellowish vernix. The nurse promptly calls this to the physician's attention because this may be a sign of which of the following?
   1. Rh or ABO incompatibility or maternal ingestion of sulfisoxazole (Gantrisin).
   2. An intrauterine gonorrheal infection.
   3. Maternal diabetes mellitus.
   4. Fetal postmaturity.
10. Which plan should the nurse recommend to a pregnant woman for morning nausea?
   1. Try a high-protein snack at bedtime.

2. Eat two dry crackers or toast before arising.

3. Eat a high-protein breakfast.

4. Drink a glass of orange juice immediately on awakening.

11. Which of the following *best* explains indigestion, heartburn, and constipation during pregnancy?
1. Progesterone, produced by the placenta, causes reduced motility of smooth muscle, e.g., intestinal tract.
2. Stress due to developmental tasks of pregnancy results in increased gastric acidity and reflux.
3. Pressure from the growing uterus displaces the stomach and intestines.
4. Increased pancreatic activity results in digestive-tract fat intolerance.

12. When preparing the room for a woman with preeclampsia which of the following equipment items is most important to have ready?
1. Suction and oxygen apparatus.
2. Urinary retention catheter and drainage bag.
3. Electronic blood pressure monitor.
4. Padded tongue blade and airway.

13. A new mother saturates her perineal pad in 15 minutes. Her fundus is firm and smooth, and there is a constant trickle of blood from the vagina. No clots can be expressed when the fundus is massaged. Which of the following should the nurse suspect on the basis of these findings?
1. Atonic bleeding.
2. Traumatic bleeding.
3. Retained placental fragments.
4. Inverted uterus.

14. Which nursing action *increases* a woman's discomfort during a pelvic examination?
1. Explaining why the examination is being done and what she may expect.
2. Offering the nurse's hand for her to squeeze.
3. Suggesting breathing techniques to help her relax.
4. Asking her to empty her bladder before the examination.

15. Which finding is inconsistent with an 8-week gestation?
1. Chadwick's sign.
2. Hegar's sign.
3. Goodell's sign.
4. Ballottement.

16. Four hours after birth, a newborn begins to show signs of respiratory distress. This newborn's history includes: 42 weeks' gestation; two episodes of late FHR decelerations during labor. Which of the following should the nurse suspect?
1. Aspiration syndrome.
2. RDS.
3. Oxygen toxicity.
4. Bronchopulmonary dysplasia.

17. Plans to minimize symptoms of physiologic adaptations to pregnancy include suggesting which of the following?
1. High-carbohydrate diet and decreased fluid intake, to stimulate peristalsis.
2. Pelvic rock-and-tilt exercises, to increase tone of her abdominal muscles.
3. Symptomatic relief by over-the-counter antacids and mild laxatives.
4. Increased fluid intake and small, frequent, high-bulk meals.

18. Which theory provides the basis for the nurse's explanation and teaching regarding gestational diabetes?
1. Anti-insulin effect of human placental lactogen (HPL).
2. Proinsulin effect of HPL.

3. Increased maternal tissue sensitivity to insulin.
4. Diabetes is unrelated to pregnancy; size and production of the islets of Langerhans are unaffected.

19. A new mother wants to breastfeed. She has had no previous experience or instruction. Which of the following should the nurse include in teaching her about good nipple care?
1. Washing nipples and breasts every day with soap and water to prevent infection.
2. Keeping nipples clean with warm water and then air-drying to reduce irritation.
3. Applying dilute alcohol solution to nipples after each feeding, to toughen them.
4. Covering the nipples with a plastic-lined breast shield to protect clothing.

20. A woman in labor is becoming more serious, evidences a malar flush, and tends to hyperventilate with contractions. These signs occur most commonly during which phase?
1. Latent.
2. Active.
3. Transitional.
4. Pushing.

21. A newborn who weighed 7 lb at birth now weighs 6 lb 8 oz. Implementing health teaching, the nurse tells the mother the percentage of birthweight usually lost by normal, healthy babies. Which of the following represents the maximum amount of normal weight loss for this newborn?
1. 6 oz (170 g).
2. 8 oz (227 g).
3. 11 oz (317 g).
4. 16 oz (454 g).

22. For which reason must a preeclamptic woman be carefully assessed for fluid intake and urine output?
1. Oliguria is a grave sign.
2. Daily intake should never exceed 2000 mL.
3. Sudden diuresis can precipitate convulsion.
4. If urine output is less than 100 mL/4 h, repeat dose of magnesium sulfate is needed.

23. A new mother saturates her perineal pad in 15 minutes. Her fundus is firm and smooth, and there is a constant trickle of blood from the vagina. No clots can be expressed when the fundus is massaged. Which action should the nurse take immediately?
1. Notify the physician because she needs surgery.
2. Notify the physician because the site of her bleeding must be located.
3. Administer oxytocin according to prn order.
4. Reapply perineal pad and evaluate bleeding in 15 minutes.

24. If a pregnant woman's vaginal discharge is thick, white, cheeselike, and pruritic, the nurse's therapeutic and educational actions should be based on which of the following?
1. No action needed. This is normal leukorrhea of pregnancy.
2. Metronidazole (Flagyl) is the drug of choice to treat this condition.
3. Even if untreated, this condition presents no hazard to the neonate.
4. This condition is more likely to occur in women who are pregnant or taking oral contraceptives or antibiotics or who are diabetic.

25. If a pregnant woman's last normal menstrual period started August 5, her EDB is:
1. May 12.
2. May 30.

3. June 8.

4. June 12.

26. A pregnant woman complains, "I waddle like a duck, and after even a short walk, my back and legs ache. Why? What can I do about that?" Which of the following provides the basis for appropriate health teaching?
   1. Relaxation of pelvic joint articulations and strain on supporting muscles due to the growing uterus cause these symptoms.
   2. An increased metabolic rate in pregnancy results in excess production of lactic acid in back muscles.
   3. Progesterone causes striated muscle stretching and pain on motion.
   4. Decreased venous return from the legs and the pressure of the heavy uterus cause waddling and discomfort.

27. Which action should the nurse recommend to reduce normal discomforts of pregnancy such as duck-waddle walk and back and leg ache?
   1. Avoid walking whenever possible; get bedrest in side-lying Sims' position several times daily.
   2. Perform pelvic tilt-and-rock exercises; get rest whenever possible, legs elevated.
   3. Wear a maternity girdle to provide support.
   4. Increase calcium intake, perform stretching exercises, and rest frequently during the day.

28. A new mother is distressed because her baby looks a little yellow. She says, "The other nurse said she has 'physical' jaundice. What's that? Is it bad?" The nurse's explanation is based on knowledge of the normal physiologic changes of the newborn. Which of the following is responsible for a newborn's physiologic jaundice?
   1. Liver immaturity and fetal polycythemia.
   2. Oliguria and kidney immaturity.
   3. Infection.
   4. Dehydration.

29. When discussing common complaints arising from normal maternal adaptations to pregnancy, which normal physiologic change has greater implications for the woman with a history of diabetes mellitus and requires more teaching about warning signs and symptoms needing prompt medical evaluation?
   1. Increased venous pressure in lower extremities.
   2. Placental production of HPL (human placental lactogen).
   3. Increased cardiac output.
   4. Relaxation of the cardiac sphincter.

30. Close observation and continuous nursing assessment of a woman with severe preeclampsia are necessary to facilitate prompt identification and management of which of the following?
   1. Abruptio placentae.
   2. Placenta previa.
   3. Hydramnios.
   4. Hyperemesis gravidarum.

31. A pregnant woman is admitted for evaluation of her cardiac status at 24 weeks' gestation. During the evening, she complains of dyspnea and shortness of breath while ambulating. She has a moist cough. Her physician orders complete bedrest. Which nursing intervention is most appropriate to prevent further deterioration of her cardiac condition?
   1. Place her in Trendelenburg position to encourage venous return to the heart.
   2. Assist her with activities of daily living to reduce energy expenditures.
   3. Encourage frequent coughing and deep breathing to prevent pulmonary complications of immobility.

4. Initiate a regimen of lower-limb exercises to prevent venous stasis and leg thrombosis.

32. A new mother tells the nurse she is breastfeeding because she can't stand the thought of the baby's being vaccinated. Which response demonstrates effective health teaching?
   1. "That's great. Vaccinations aren't needed if you breastfeed him."
   2. "Oh, you still need to have him vaccinated against DPT, measles, and polio before he is 6 months old."
   3. "You can only give temporary protection to the infant against the diseases you have had yourself."
   4. "The most protection comes from colostrum just after birth. Unfortunately, you didn't start feeding him right away."

33. A woman says, "My doctor says I'm 5 months (20 weeks) pregnant. What does my baby look like now?" The nurse's response is based on knowledge of normal fetal development. Which of the following describes the average fetus at 20 weeks' gestation?
   1. Viable, able to survive outside of the uterus with minimal assistance.
   2. About 10 inches long, weight about 10 oz, and covered with fine, downy hair and vernix.
   3. Beginning sex differentiation, kidney function, and detectable movements.
   4. Shedding lanugo and vernix, growing rapidly, weighs about 1½ pounds.

34. In discussing "dos and don'ts," which health teaching aspect should be emphasized as important for health maintenance during pregnancy?
   1. Keeping appointments for prenatal visits, remembering to ask questions when necessary, and following the medical/nursing recommendations.
   2. Making preparation for childbirth classes.
   3. Moderate exercise, high-carbohydrate diet, and adequate rest.
   4. Taking multivitamins and iron, drinking six glasses of milk daily, and minimizing physical exertion.

35. Which response is appropriate for a pregnant woman who experiences urinary frequency?
   1. "Placental progesterone causes irritability of the bladder sphincter. Your symptoms will go away after the baby comes."
   2. "Frequency is due to bladder irritation from concentrated urine and is normal in pregnancy. Increase your daily fluid intake to 3000 mL."
   3. "Pregnant women void frequently to get rid of fetal wastes. Limit fluids to 1000 mL daily."
   4. "Try using Kegel (perineal) exercises and limiting fluids before bedtime. If you have frequency associated with fever, pain on voiding, or blood in the urine, call your doctor/nurse-midwife."

36. As a woman progresses through labor, she becomes increasingly irritable with her husband, complaining of lower-back pain and fatigue. Which nursing intervention is most appropriate now?
   1. Have the woman turn on her side and give her a back rub.
   2. Ask her if she would like the nurse to get an order for something for her discomfort.
   3. Reassure the husband that his wife's irritability is normal, and teach him to apply sacral pressure with contractions.
   4. Send the husband for a coffee break, and encourage the woman to try to get some rest.

37. At 37 weeks, a pregnant woman calls the office to say she awakened in a pool of blood and is dizzy and nause-

ated. She denies any abdominal pain or cramping. On the basis of this assessment, the nurse suggests she go to the hospital immediately. The nurse established a nursing diagnosis of *high risk for fluid volume deficit* associated with which of the following?
1. Placenta previa.
2. Abruptio placentae.
3. Preeclampsia.
4. Uterine rupture.

38. An expectant father says, "My wife is a heavy smoker—three packs a day. She won't listen to me. Will you talk to her?" Which approach is appropriate to this problem?
    1. Tell her that, if she continues to smoke that much, the baby will be small and have a greater chance of childhood respiratory infections.
    2. Teach her to substitute snacking on cheese, dried apricots, or raisins to curb her desire to smoke.
    3. Discuss current thoughts about the effects of smoking during pregnancy, and ask her if she can think of ways to cut down.
    4. Ask her how she plans to cut down to 10 cigarettes daily.

39. Which signs and symptoms require immediate medical evaluation during pregnancy?
    1. Excessive saliva, "bumps" around the areolae, and increased vaginal mucus.
    2. Fatigue, nausea, and urinary frequency at any time during pregnancy.
    3. Ankle edema, enlarging varicosities, and heartburn.
    4. Severe abdominal pain or fluid discharge from the vagina.

40. Which signs and symptoms should the nurse teach as possible warning signs of potential problems?
    1. Edema of the lower extremities, vulvar varices, and copious, clear vaginal discharge.
    2. Heartburn, shortness of breath, change in appetite.
    3. Leg cramps, back pain, and increased pigmentation over the bridge of the nose and the cheeks.
    4. Headache, visual disturbances, or feeling of fullness in face and hands.

41. The physician orders a magnesium sulfate infusion. Which nursing assessment is most important when administering this drug to a pregnant woman?
    1. Monitoring the serum magnesium level every 8 hours.
    2. Evaluating the apical heart rate every 4 hours.
    3. Counting the respiratory rate every hour.
    4. Auscultating bowel sounds before meals.

42. A woman with a history of diabetes may require hospitalization during her pregnancy for treatment of any problems associated with her pregnancy or for diagnostic tests. When asked to verbalize her understanding of the discussion, which of this woman's responses indicates a need for further health teaching?
    1. "Pregnancy may change the amount of insulin I need for regulation of my diabetes."
    2. "I may need to be hospitalized to evaluate how well my placenta is functioning."
    3. "If this awful morning sickness keeps up, the doctor may put me in to control it."
    4. "The doctor may need to take a sample of my water (amniocentesis) to see if the baby has the gene for diabetes."

43. Assessment findings at 16 weeks gestation include marked chloasma and secondary pigmented areolae; in addition, the woman's umbilicus is flush with her skin. During which trimester are these physical changes of pregnancy commonly found?

1. First.
2. Second.
3. Third.
4. Fourth.

44. A new mother tells the nurse, "I am afraid the baby will have something wrong with her because I was bad while I was carrying her. Is she really okay?" If observed, which of the following would the nurse note as unusual in a newborn girl?
    1. Enlarged breasts and some pink drainage from the baby's vagina.
    2. A dark line between the baby's umbilicus and symphysis.
    3. Little "blackheads" covering her nose and chin.
    4. A dark discoloration over her sacrum and lower back.

45. An infertility assessment begins with a thorough health history. Which factor is likely to be implicated in female infertility?
    1. Moderate alcohol intake.
    2. Menstrual cycle of 26 to 28 days.
    3. History of PID.
    4. Past use of diaphragm and spermicide for contraception.

46. Which nursing intervention is most likely to be included in the plan of care for a woman with heart disease during the first postpartum day?
    1. Push oral and IV fluid to stimulate diuresis and prevent fluid volume overload.
    2. Encourage early ambulation and exercise to reduce the risk of thrombophlebitis.
    3. Monitor vital signs, skin color, and pulmonary status to identify cardiac decompensation.
    4. Encourage her to defer breastfeeding on the first day to reduce the cardiac workload.

47. The nursing assessment of a newborn reveals a lump on one side of the head that does not cross suture lines. Which of the following should the nurse tell the mother is the cause of the lump?
    1. Bleeding between the periosteum and parietal bone occurred due to pressure against the bony pelvis during birth.
    2. Edema of the scalp occurred due to pressure of the vertex against the cervix during the first stage of labor.
    3. Intracranial hemorrhage occurred due to pressure from the forceps during birth.
    4. Simple swelling of a common hemangioma occurred due to prolonged pushing in the second stage of labor.

48. Assessing for the normal psychological changes in the third trimester, the nurse would expect a pregnant woman to exhibit which normal behavior?
    1. Ambivalence about the pregnancy.
    2. Eagerness to begin Lamaze classes.
    3. Fantasizing about her child.
    4. Withdrawal from other relationships.

49. In reviewing with a pregnant woman those symptoms that require prompt medical evaluation, which of the following would the nurse include?
    1. Increasing pedal edema.
    2. Feelings of dizziness on arising.
    3. Epigastric pain.
    4. Spotting within 24 hours of vaginal examination.

50. A pregnant woman's history reveals a pregnancy at age 15 that was terminated by elective abortion at 10 weeks, birth of twin girls at 37 weeks, and a spontaneous abortion at 12 weeks last year. Analyzing these data, the nurse selects which of the following to describe her present gravidity and parity?

1. Gravida 5 Para 2.
2. Gravida 5 Para 1.
3. Gravida 4 Para 2.
4. Gravida 4 Para 1.

51. The postovulation rise in BBT is due to the high blood level of which hormone?
    1. Follicle stimulating hormone (FSH).
    2. Human placental lactogen (HPL).
    3. Estrogen.
    4. Progesterone.

52. Nursing assessment of a woman in labor notes marked introspection, irritability, and inability to focus. She is diaphoretic, and cries, "I can't take it!" These behaviors are characteristic of which stage or phase of labor?
    1. Active phase.
    2. Transitional phase.
    3. Second stage.
    4. Third stage.

53. During the last month of pregnancy, a pregnant woman comments, "I am sick and tired of this whole thing. I can hardly wait for it to be over." Comparing her statement to the normal psychological responses of other pregnant women during the last trimester, the nurse responds appropriately with which statement?
    1. "I think you should see the psychiatric social worker. You should be feeling more positive about the baby by now."
    2. "I know exactly how you feel. I've seen it a thousand times. It'll pass."
    3. "Well, sounds like you're ready for labor. Do you have any questions about your coming labor?"
    4. "Your pregnancy is getting a bit tiresome and the time is dragging?"

54. A 16-year-old, single woman wants to give her baby up for adoption. Which plan will be of most help to her?
    1. Provide a safe environment, encourage ventilation of her feelings, give no answers or direction so that she makes her own decisions.
    2. Provide the information she needs to understand the situation, place it in perspective in terms of her life goals, and begin to plan for the future.
    3. Support her choice whatever her decision.
    4. Help her see ways of not making the same error again so she can grow in self-esteem and self-respect.

55. The physician determines that a woman's inability to conceive is due to anovulatory cycles. An expected emotional response to this diagnosis indicating that the woman understands the underlying problem would be:
    1. Guilt for past sexual behaviors.
    2. Grief because she will never be able to conceive.
    3. Fears regarding the need for corrective surgery.
    4. Anxiety regarding the side effects of clomiphen citrate (Clomid).

56. A couple has been unable to conceive; the man is being evaluated for possible problems. A semen analysis is ordered. Which instruction regarding collection of a sperm specimen is appropriate?
    1. Collect specimen at night, refrigerate, and bring to clinic the next morning.
    2. Collect specimen in the morning after 24 hours of abstinence and bring to clinic immediately.
    3. Collect specimen after 48 to 72 hours of abstinence and bring to clinic within 2 hours.
    4. Collect a specimen at the clinic, place in iced container, and give to laboratory personnel immediately.

57. In health teaching for women who desire "natural childbirth," which statement should the nurse explain is a myth?

1. Medication may be used to reduce tension and pain during labor.
2. Labor and birth under Lamaze techniques are almost painless.
3. Labor is easier for women who are self-assured, relaxed, and cooperative during the process.
4. Preparation for childbirth may include body-building exercises, breathing techniques, and comfort aids.

58. When admitted to the hospital, a pregnant woman (37 weeks) is having sufficient bleeding for blood to trickle down her leg. Her blood pressure is 102/68, pulse 92. Which nursing action will the admitting nurse perform based on these findings?
    1. Vaginal examination to assess fetal presentation, position, station, effacement, and dilatation.
    2. Position her on her side with a small pillow under her head.
    3. Adjust the bed in semi-Fowler's position.
    4. Prepare her for immediate cesarean birth.

59. Health teaching during the prenatal period should emphasize that expectant primigravida mothers should go to the hospital when which pattern is evident?
    1. Contractions are 2–3 minutes apart, lasting 90 seconds, and membranes have ruptured.
    2. Contractions are 3–5 minutes apart, accompanied by rectal pressure and bloody show.
    3. Contractions are 5 minutes apart, lasting 60 seconds, and increasing in intensity.
    4. Contractions are 5–10 minutes apart, lasting 30 seconds, and are felt as strong menstrual cramps.

60. Assessment findings of Leopold's maneuvers reveal a soft, rounded mass in the fundus, irregular nodules on the right side, and a hard prominence on the right, just above the symphysis. Which of the following accurately describes the fetal presentation and position?
    1. Right sacrum posterior (RSP).
    2. Left sacrum anterior (LSA).
    3. Right occiput posterior (ROP).
    4. Left occiput anterior (LOA).

61. If the fetus is LOA, in which maternal location should the nurse anticipate finding the fetal heart tones (FHTs)?
    1. Below the umbilicus on the left side.
    2. Below the umbilicus on the right side.
    3. Above the umbilicus on the left side.
    4. Above the umbilicus on the right side.

62. Which normal assessment finding can the nurse expect in the 34th week of pregnancy?
    1. Braxton-Hicks contractions, joint hypermobility, and backache.
    2. Dysuria, constipation, hemorrhoids, and lightening.
    3. Feeling of tranquility and heightened introspection.
    4. Morning sickness, breast tenderness.

63. Which suggestion by the nurse may relieve a pregnant woman's heartburn symptoms?
    1. Eat dry bread products before rising.
    2. Bend at the knees when reaching down, not at the waist.
    3. Eat fewer, larger meals and avoid nibbling.
    4. Do pelvic-rock exercise.

64. A new mother complains she is having severe cramping after breastfeeding. Which would be the first action taken by the nurse to reduce her discomfort?
    1. Administer pain medication as per order.
    2. Have her lie on her abdomen with a rolled towel at the level of her fundus.
    3. Ask her to walk around for a few minutes.
    4. Ask her to empty her bladder.

65. In assessing a new mother's response to her son's birth on the first postpartum day, which behavior should the nurse expect to find present?
    1. Talkativeness, dependency, passivity.
    2. Autonomy and independence.
    3. Disinterest in her own body functions.
    4. Interest in learning to bathe the baby.

66. Which technique should the nurse use to assess the frequency, duration, and intensity of uterine contractions?
    1. Spread fingers of one hand lightly over the fundus.
    2. Move the fingers of one hand over the uterus, pressing into the muscle.
    3. Hold fingers and palm of one hand over the area just below the umbilicus.
    4. Indent the uterus in several places, during and between contractions.

67. Ongoing evaluation of a woman with severe preeclampsia reveals 4 plus deep-tendon patellar reflexes with two beats of clonus. The most appropriate nursing diagnosis related to her current status would be:
    1. Pain related to hyperreflexia and clonus.
    2. Potential for injury related to possible eclamptic seizures.
    3. Impaired physical mobility related to alterations in lower limbs.
    4. Sensory/perceptual alterations related to sensory overload.

68. Following a birth, after the physician or midwife has cut the cord, and before the baby is given to the mother, which should the nurse do *first*?
    1. Confirm identification of the infant and apply bracelets to mother and infant.
    2. Examine the infant for any observable abnormalities.
    3. Wrap the infant in a prewarmed blanket and cover the head.
    4. Instill prophylactic medication in the infant's eyes.

69. Which of the following should elicit the Moro reflex in healthy newborns?
    1. Sudden or loud noises.
    2. Stroking the soles of the feet.
    3. Turning a newborn's head to one side.
    4. Stroking a newborn's cheek.

70. Which assessment of a woman in labor can be determined by vaginal examination?
    1. Fetal weight.
    2. Cervical dilatation.
    3. Strength of contractions.
    4. Fetal head circumference.

71. The decision is made to encourage a woman in early labor to walk around the unit for a while, and to then reassess her status. Which assessment distinguishes between true and false labor?
    1. Confirmation of spontaneous rupture of membranes.
    2. Signs and symptoms of increasing discomfort.
    3. Evidence of cervical dilatation.
    4. Presence of copious bloody vaginal discharge.

72. Which of the following should be emphasized as the most important factor in safeguarding cardiac function during pregnancy, for a woman with rheumatic heart disease (RHD)?
    1. Adequate exercise.
    2. Adequate rest.
    3. Low-salt diet.
    4. Ferrous sulfate.

73. Late in pregnancy, which of the following is the *most* likely cause of groin pain that seems worse on the right side?
    1. Bladder infection.

2. Constipation.
3. Tension on the round ligament.
4. Beginning of labor.

74. A pregnant woman's history reveals one pregnancy, terminated by elective abortion at 10 weeks; birth of twins at 37 weeks; and a spontaneous abortion at 12 weeks. According to the TPAL system, which of the following describes her present parity?
    1. 0-2-2-2.
    2. 2-0-2-2.
    3. 0-1-2-2.
    4. 1-0-2-2.

75. Which of the following influences the planning and implementation of postpartum care for a woman who has been diagnosed as severely preeclamptic?
    1. Even if she has had no convulsions during the antepartal and intrapartal periods, she remains at risk for convulsions for the first 48 hours postpartum.
    2. Preeclampsia is associated only with pregnancy. Once the baby has been born, she is cured.
    3. The woman should be advised she may be left with chronic renal damage.
    4. Since subsequent pregnancy is extremely hazardous, family planning should be implemented as soon as possible.

76. For which complication of pregnancy is an Rh-negative woman at risk?
    1. Spontaneous abortion.
    2. Preeclampsia.
    3. Maternal anemia.
    4. Erythroblastosis fetalis.

77. Which assessment findings indicate a 20 weeks gestation?
    1. Lightening, FHR audible by fetoscope, fundus palpable at the umbilicus.
    2. Braxton-Hicks contractions, ballottement, and fundus at umbilicus.
    3. Quickening noted, FHR audible by fetoscope, fundus just below the umbilicus.
    4. Goodell's, Hegar's, and Chadwick's signs present, fundus halfway between symphysis and umbilicus.

78. A new mother tells the nurse she is planning to breast-feed her son until he is 2 years old so she won't have to worry about getting pregnant. Which response demonstrates appropriate health teaching?
    1. "Lactation does suppress ovulation, so you'll be pretty safe."
    2. "You are safe only as long as you don't menstruate."
    3. "It's best to use some other form of birth control. You may not menstruate, but you may ovulate and could get pregnant."
    4. "You'll find you won't be interested in intercourse until you wean your baby."

79. Nursing assessments during the fourth stage of labor following placenta previa will include close monitoring for signs of hemorrhage. This nursing decision is based on which rationale?
    1. Placenta was implanted in lower uterine segment, where there are fewer muscle fibers to contract the placental site.
    2. The area under an abrupted placenta never contracts as strongly as when there is no premature separation.
    3. Since the placenta was surgically removed, the uterine muscle does not contract as efficiently.
    4. The woman lost 250 mL of blood during the third stage of labor.

80. A woman in labor using the Lamaze technique is examined and found to be in transition. Which breathing pattern used at this time would indicate a need for nursing intervention?
1. Rapid, shallow chest breathing.
2. Slow, deep, abdominal breathing.
3. Use of intercostal muscles with diaphragm relaxed.
4. Beginning and ending each contraction with two cleansing breaths.

81. Which of these normal physiologic changes has greater implications for the woman with a history of rheumatic fever at age 8, and requires more teaching about warning signs and symptoms needing prompt medical evaluation?
1. Increased venous pressure in lower extremities.
2. Placental production of HPL.
3. Increased cardiac output.
4. Relaxation of the cardiac sphincter.

82. Following an amniotomy, the nurse remains alert for any signs of complications. In addition to the FHR, which of the following may indicate fetal distress?
1. Crowning and increased fetal activity.
2. Crowning and hypotonic contractions.
3. Increased fetal activity and meconium-stained amniotic fluid.
4. Baseline variability on the monitor strip.

83. A woman in labor insists on remaining in a supine position in bed. Which response should the nurse make regarding this behavior?
1. "It's best for the baby if you lie on your side."
2. "These two pillows under your knees will be good for the baby and more comfortable for you."
3. "You will get nauseated and light-headed if you stay in that position."
4. "This rolled-up towel under your hip will do the job just as well."

84. Which of the following would the nurse note as a deviation from the normal characteristics of the term neonate?
1. Head circumference larger than chest circumference.
2. Diaphragmatic breathing.
3. Passage of meconium stool.
4. Epicanthal folds and simian line.

❑ Answers/Rationale

1. **(3)** Of the family planning options presented, a diaphragm and jelly is the optimum choice for this woman. **(1)** is incorrect because oral contraceptives are contraindicated with a history of thrombophlebitis. **(2)** is incorrect because she is interested only in postponing pregnancy. **(4)** is incorrect because of a strong relative contraindication to use of intrauterine devices by women with impaired responses to infection, such as diabetics. **IMP,5,HPM**

2. **(1)** Basal body temperature falls slightly immediately before ovulation, then rises approximately 0.5°C. This characteristic finding aids women in identifying the fer-

Key to codes following rationales Nursing process: **AS,** assessment; **AN,** analysis; **PL,** plan; **IMP,** implementation; **EV,** evaluation. Category of human function: **1,** protective; **2,** sensory-perceptual; **3,** comfort, rest, activity, and mobility; **4,** nutrition; **5,** growth and development; **6,** fluid-gas transport; **7,** psychosocial-cultural; **8,** elimination. Client need: **SECE,** safe, effective care environment; **PhI,** physiological integrity; **PsI,** psychosocial integrity; **HPM,** health promotion/maintenance. See appendices for full explanation.

tile period of their cycle. **(2)** is incorrect because the pattern described is reversed. **(3)** and **(4)** are wrong because ovulation is related to an LH surge. **IMP,5,HPM**

3. **(1)** Heart rate—2; respiratory effort—1; muscle tone—0; reflex response—1; color—1. Total Apgar score is 5. **(2)**, **(3)**, and **(4)** are incorrect because of inaccurate allocation of points for behaviors described. **AS,5,SECE**

4. **(2)** If avoidable, women hospitalized for treatment of preeclampsia should be on bedrest in a quiet environment to minimize stimuli. **(1)** is incorrect because the nurse should assess the amount and distribution of edema. **(3)** is wrong because weight is an indicator of edema and diuresis and should be assessed in the preeclamptic woman. **(4)** is wrong because I & O relationships and the presence and amount of protein in the urine are important indicators of her status. **IMP,2,HPM**

5. **(4)** Marked vaginal discharge with itching for the past few days indicates a need for further assessment. Itching is most commonly associated with vaginal infections, and the cause should be identified and treated. Altered vaginal pH in pregnancy contributes to increased susceptibility to infection. **(1)** is incorrect because urinary frequency, nausea, and fatigue are common complaints in early pregnancy. **(2)** is wrong because vital signs are within normal limits. **(3)** is wrong because normally increased vaginal discharge in pregnancy may contaminate voided urine and result in a nonpathologic trace of protein. **AS,1,HPM**

6. **(1)** The most common cause of false-negative findings in urine testing for signs of pregnancy (presence of HCG) is faulty technique; further, dilute urine secondary to diuresis may contain too little hormone to register in the routine over-the-counter (or office) pregnancy tests. *Note:* HCG levels peak approximately 50–60 days after conception. **(2)** is incorrect because urine tests are classed as "probable" signs of pregnancy. **(3)** is incorrect because pregnancy tests identify presence/levels of HCG (the biologic marker for pregnancy). **(4)** is wrong because urine tests are classed as "probable" signs of pregnancy. **IMP,5,HPM**

7. **(1)** These behaviors are typical of a woman during the latent phase of labor. **(2)** is incorrect because, as labor progresses, internal stimuli demand more focus. **(3)** is wrong because women in transitional phase are irritable and increasingly aware of their labor as contractions increase in strength, length, and discomfort. **(4)** is wrong because, in the prodromal period of labor, contractions are mild and irregular and her major question may be "Am I really in labor?" **AS,5,HPM**

8. **(3)** The most common cause of bleeding immediately postpartum is uterine atony, and bleeding may be controlled with fundal massage and oxytocic stimulation. **(1)** is incorrect because she has responded to the nursing measures. **(2)** is wrong because her bleeding does not appear associated with lacerations that might require surgery. **(4)** is wrong because perineal pressure is effective only in treating superficial tears. **IMP,6,HPM**

9. **(1)** Yellow vernix results from the breakdown of hemoglobin or bile pigments in meconium. Both maternal anti-Rh-antigen antibodies and ingestion of sulfisoxazole (Gantrisin) are implicated in hemolysis of fetal RBCs. **(2)** is incorrect because gonorrheal infection renders amniotic fluid opaque, thick, and odorous without discoloring vernix. **(3)** is wrong because diabetes does not have any effect on the color of vernix. **(4)** is wrong because the postmature fetus does not have vernix. **AN,6,PhI**

10. **(2)** Carbohydrates taken before arising seem to reduce symptoms of morning nausea; dry crackers may absorb stomach acid and raise blood sugar. **(1)** is incorrect because high-protein snacks at bedtime appear to have no effect on nausea in the morning. **(3)** is wrong because nausea is present before eating and may be severe enough to prevent eating. **(4)** is wrong because orange juice on an empty stomach may precipitate emesis in a woman with "morning sickness." **IMP,4,HPM**

11. **(1)** The effects of progesterone on the GI tract include relaxation of the cardiac sphincter and delayed gastric emptying, which contribute to indigestion and heartburn, and slowed intestinal peristalsis, which increases water reabsorption and predisposes to constipation. **(2)** is incorrect because the major cause of symptoms is described in **(1)**. **(3)** is wrong because displacement due to pressure from the uterus is secondary to the effects of reduced smooth muscle tone. **(4)** is wrong because increased pancreatic activity does not cause fat intolerance. **AS,4,HPM**

12. **(1)** is correct because the nurse's primary responsibility is to prepare for respiratory and cardiac support in case the woman experiences an eclamptic seizure. **(2)** is incorrect because not all preeclamptic women require bladder catheterization. **(3)** is incorrect because the nurse may monitor blood pressures using the standard sphygmomanometer and arm cuff. **(4)** is incorrect because tongue blades are never used to manage seizures today. **IMP,5,SECE**

13. **(2)** Traumatic bleeding is characterized by a firm, smooth uterus and a continuous trickle. **(1)** is incorrect because the uterus remains well contracted. **(3)** is wrong because bleeding from retained placental fragments occurs most commonly later in the postpartum period. **(4)** is wrong because an inverted uterus is characterized by profuse vaginal bleeding and maternal collapse. **AN,6,PhI**

14. **(2)** Offering your hand to squeeze encourages her to tense her muscles, including the pubococcygeus muscle of the pelvic floor, increasing the discomfort of a pelvic examination. **(1)** is incorrect because explaining what she may expect and the reasons for examination procedures is an appropriate nursing action designed to *reduce* her anxiety and tension. **(3)** is wrong because suggesting and demonstrating breathing techniques is an appropriate nursing action designed to assist her to *relax* during the procedures. **(4)** is wrong because asking her to empty her bladder is appropriate anticipatory guidance designed to *reduce* the stress of the pelvic examination. **IMP,5,HPM**

15. **(4)** The finding of ballottement is more consistent with a pregnancy of 19 or more weeks. **(1)** is incorrect because Chadwick's sign (bluish discoloration of the vagina) is usually present at 8 weeks' gestation. **(2)** is wrong because Hegar's sign (softening of the lower uterine segment) is present by 8 weeks. **(3)** is wrong because Goodell's sign (softening of the cervix) is usually present at this point in gestation. **AS,5,HPM**

16. **(1)** Aspiration syndrome occurs commonly among post-term newborns, especially if they are postmature. Hypoxia accompanies progressive placental insufficiency (evidenced by late FHR decelerations) with advancing gestational age. Physiologic response to hypoxia is relaxation of the anal sphincter, with release of meconium into amniotic fluid, and the fetal gasp reflex. **(2)** is incorrect because RDS is associated most commonly with prematurity and insufficient pulmonary surfactant. **(3)** is wrong because oxygen toxicity occurs after a period of oxygen therapy. **(4)** is wrong because bronchopulmonary dysplasia (BPD) is associated with prolonged administration of oxygen at high concentrations; the time since birth is too short for the baby to develop BPD. **AN,6,PhI**

17. **(4)** Increasing fluid and roughage intake will help reduce symptoms of constipation. **(1)** is incorrect because a high-carbohydrate diet and reduced fluid intake may make constipation worse. **(2)** is wrong because exercise does not counteract the effects of progesterone. **(3)** is wrong because many over-the-counter antacids contain sodium and frequent use of laxatives may result in further loss of tone, leading to constipation. **IMP,4,HPM**

18. **(1)** The anti-insulin effects of the placental hormone HPL (a growth hormone) and reduced maternal tissue sensitivity to insulin often may result in development of gestational diabetes in women who previously had no symptoms of diabetes. **(2)** is wrong because the effect of HPL is antagonistic to insulin, not proinsulin. **(3)** is wrong because there is decreased maternal tissue sensitivity to insulin. **(4)** is wrong because the size and production of the islets of Langerhans increase during pregnancy. **AS,4,HPM**

19. **(2)** Nipples cleansed with plain water and air-dried carefully are less likely to develop fissures. **(1)** is incorrect because soap is drying and removes natural oils. **(3)** is incorrect because alcohol would be too drying and promotes fissure development. **(4)** is wrong because a plastic shield would retain body heat and moisture, irritating nipples. **IMP,5,HPM**

20. **(2)** These behaviors are characteristic of the active phase of the first stage of labor, at about 5 cm dilatation. **(1)** is wrong because women are more excited and relaxed during the latent phase when labor is less uncomfortable. **(3)** is wrong because behaviors during transition reveal the woman's focus on completing the process rapidly; irritability is common. **(4)** is wrong because the woman uses sustained inhalations to increase the force of her pushing. **AS,5,HPM**

21. **(3)** Term infants may lose 5–10% of their birthweight. Arithmetic: 7 × 16 oz = 112 oz; 10% of 112 = 11.2 oz (317.5 g). **(1)**, **(2)**, and **(4)** are wrong because of inaccurate computation. **AN,5,PsI**

22. **(1)** Oliguria is an ominous sign in preeclampsia. **(2)** is incorrect because daily intake is individualized for the preeclamptic woman. **(3)** is wrong because sudden diuresis is a good prognostic sign. **(4)** is wrong because urinary output must equal or exceed 120 mL/4 h before magnesium sulfate, if needed, can be given again. **AS,2,HPM**

23. **(2)** The laceration must be located and treated before bleeding will stop. **(1)** is incorrect because, if the laceration is accessible, bleeding may be controlled by insertion of vaginal packing. **(3)** is wrong because bleeding is not related to uterine atony. **(4)** is wrong because perineal pressure would be ineffective with a vaginal laceration. **IMP,6,PhI**

24. **(4)** Her discharge is characteristic of a monilial (yeast) infection. This infection is more common in women whose vaginal pH has changed because of pregnancy or diabetes or who are taking oral contraceptives. Antibiotic therapy is also associated with increased risk for developing an infection by *Candida albicans*. **(1)** is incorrect because normal leukorrhea associated with pregnancy is thin, colorless, and nonpruritic. **(2)** is wrong because mycostatin (Nystatin) is the drug of choice for treating vaginal yeast infections; metronidazole (Flagyl) is used in treating trichomonal infections. **(3)** is wrong because, if present during the baby's

Maternal-Infant

birth, this organism causes neonatal thrush.
IMP,1,HPM

25. (1) Using Nägele's rule to calculate the EDB, the correct date is arrived at by taking the date of the first day of the last menstrual period (LMP) and subtracting 3 months and adding 7 days. (2) is wrong because 7 days have been *subtracted* from her LMP. (3) is wrong because calculations have erroneously included August as one of the 3 months, and only 3 days have been added to the date of LMP. (4) is wrong because, although calculations added 7 days, August was again erroneously included as one of the 3 months subtracted. **AS,5,HPM**

26. (1) Shifting the center of gravity to compensate for the weight of the growing uterus places strain on supporting musculature and contributes to low-back ache during pregnancy; relaxation of joint articulations is responsible for the waddling gait. (2) is wrong because vigorous exercise contributes to the production of lactic acid; the increased metabolic rate during pregnancy has no effect. (3) is wrong because progesterone affects smooth muscle. (4) is wrong because decreased venous return and pressure from the growing uterus contribute to development of varicosities. **AS,3,HPM**

27. (2) Exercises like the pelvic tilt and rock strengthen the abdominal and back muscles, which support the mother in an erect position—and the growing uterus; rest while elevating the legs reduces stress on these muscles and the legs and decreases symptoms. (1) is incorrect because walking is an excellent mild exercise recommended for the pregnant woman. (3) is wrong because a girdle may contribute to decreased venous return from the extremities. (4) is wrong because symptoms are due to strain on supporting muscles and are unrelated to the level of circulating calcium. **IMP,3,HPM**

28. (1) *Physiologic* jaundice is related to inability of the liver to conjugate bilirubin liberated by normal hemolysis of fetal RBCs and polycythemia. (2) is incorrect because jaundice associated with kidney immaturity is *pathologic*. (3) is wrong because jaundice occurring secondary to infection is also *pathologic*. (4) is wrong because, although dehydration may be associated with the jaundice, it also is *pathologic*. **AN,6,PsI**

29. (2) Human placental lactogen (HPL) is an insulin antagonist and may complicate management of diabetes during pregnancy. (1) is incorrect because fatigue and varicosities are common complaints associated with decreased venous return from the lower extremities. (3) is wrong because increased cardiac output places additional work on the heart. (4) is wrong because relaxation of the cardiac sphincter is associated with heartburn and gastric reflux. **IMP,4,PhI**

30. (1) Abruptio placentae may be a complication of severe preeclampsia and places both mother and fetus in jeopardy. (2) is incorrect because placenta previa is due to low implantation, not pathophysiologic changes in preeclampsia. (3) is wrong because hydramnios is most commonly associated with maternal diabetes, and although it may coexist with preeclampsia, it is not a contributing factor. (4) is wrong because hyperemesis gravidarum occurs earlier in pregnancy and is not associated with development or progression of preeclampsia. **AS,6,HPM**

31. (2) Activities of daily living will increase energy expenditures and may contribute to further cardiac decompensation. (1) is incorrect because dyspnea and shortness of breath will be exacerbated in Trendelenburg position. (3) is incorrect because any activity that causes her to perform a Valsalva maneuver (coughing) will cause a sudden increase in blood return to the heart, which is con-

traindicated in cardiac disease. (4) is incorrect because the major goal of care is to reduce all energy expenditures. **IMP,3,PhI**

32. (3) Only disease-specific antibodies produced by the mother in response to that infection can be passed through breast milk to the baby. (1) is incorrect because vaccinations would be needed to develop active immunity. (2) is wrong because measles vaccination is not effective if given before 1 year of age. (4) is wrong because maternal antibodies confer only short-lived passive immunity. **IMP,5,HPM**

33. (2) These are the characteristics of the fetus at 20 weeks gestation (22 menstrual weeks). (1) is incorrect because, although 20 weeks has been identified as viability, most such fetuses are too immature to survive independent extrauterine existence successfully. (3) is wrong because sex differentiation begins at conception and is discernible at 12 weeks, and kidneys begin secreting urine at 11 weeks. (4) is wrong because the fetus begins to exhibit these characteristics at 31 weeks. **AS,5,HPM**

34. (1) The most important factor in reducing morbidity and mortality associated with pregnancy is close health supervision and prompt management of emerging problems and complications. (2) is incorrect because the primary goal of prenatal classes is to prepare the couple for labor and birth. (3) is wrong because high-protein diets are recommended during pregnancy to reduce the possibility of preeclampsia. (4) is wrong because the pregnant woman should drink 1 quart of milk and increase her intake during lactation. **IMP,5,HPM**

35. (4) Progesterone also reduces smooth muscle motility in the urinary tract and predisposes the pregnant woman to urinary tract infections. Women should contact their doctors if they exhibit signs of infection. Kegel exercises will help strengthen the perineal muscles; limiting fluids at bedtime reduces the possibility of being awakened by the necessity of voiding. (1) is incorrect because progesterone does not cause irritability of the bladder sphincter. (2) is wrong because frequency in early and late pregnancy is due to pressure on the bladder from the growing uterus. (3) is wrong because hydration is important in maintaining normal digestion and nutrient transport to body cells, removing wastes, and regulating body temperature. During pregnancy, eight 8-oz glasses of fluid daily are recommended. **IMP,8,HPM**

36. (3) Reassurance that her behavior is normal for this point in labor helps reduce the mate's feelings of guilt and helplessness and fosters the sense of a mutual, shared experience; sacral pressure reduces her discomfort. (1) is wrong because it does not address the partner's feelings. (2) is wrong because it does not facilitate the shared experience and may result in feelings of failure in some women. (4) is wrong because she is progressing well and needs/wants her mate's support. **IMP,5,HPM**

37. (1) Painless vaginal bleeding is associated with placenta previa. (2) is wrong because abdominal pain and a tense abdomen are signs of possible abruptio placentae. (3) is wrong because painless vaginal bleeding is not indicative of preeclampsia. (4) is wrong because the uterine rupture is characterized by sudden sharp abdominal pain, signs of internal bleeding, and shock. **AN,6,PhI**

38. (3) Encouraging her to consider ways to reduce her smoking implies your respect for her ability to deal with the problem and encourages her active participation in her own pregnancy-related care. (1) is incorrect because such comments generate guilt and may threaten her

self-image. **(2)** is wrong because telling her to substitute even "good foods" implies lack of respect for her judgment and assumes that she will comply with your choices for her behavior. **(4)** is wrong because it implies she has no choice in the matter; patient goals are best established mutually. **IMP,6,HPM**

39. **(4)** Severe abdominal pain may indicate complications of pregnancy such as abortion, ectopic pregnancy, or abruptio placentae; fluid discharge from the vagina may indicate premature rupture of the membranes. **(1)** is incorrect because ptyalism, elevated Montgomery tubercles, and leukorrhea are normal physiologic responses during pregnancy. **(2)** is wrong because fatigue, nausea, and frequency are normal in early pregnancy. **(3)** is wrong because ankle edema, varicosities, and heartburn are normal during pregnancy. **IMP,6,HPM**

40. **(4)** Headache and feeling of fullness in face and hands may indicate preeclampsia. **(1)** is wrong because pedal edema, varicosities, and vaginal discharge are related to decreased venous return and increased vascularity in pregnancy. **(2)** is wrong because heartburn, shortness of breath, and change in appetite are normal responses in pregnancy. **(3)** is wrong because leg cramps, low-back ache, and chloasma are associated with normal physiologic changes of pregnancy. **IMP,2,HPM**

41. **(3)** is correct because respiratory depression is a cardinal sign of magnesium toxicity. **(1)** is incorrect because individual variations in respiratory depression are observed at the same serum-magnesium level. **(2)** is incorrect because respiratory compromise normally precedes depressed cardiac function and is a late sign of magnesium toxicity. **(4)** is incorrect because, although decreased peristalsis can occur with a magnesium infusion, it is not the most important assessment to make. **IMP,1,PhI**

42. **(4)** Amniocentesis does not show whether the fetus is a potential diabetic, but it may be performed on diabetic women to test for fetal lung maturity. **(1)** is incorrect because her statement indicates understanding of the interrelationship between her pregnancy and her diabetes. **(2)** is wrong because pregnant diabetics may be hospitalized for testing for placental function. **(3)** is wrong because nausea and vomiting in the pregnant diabetic may lead to acidosis. **EV,4,PhI**

43. **(2)** Chloasma, secondary pigmented areolae, and umbilicus flush with the skin are characteristic changes in the second trimester. **(1)** is wrong because these signs are not present during the normal first trimester. **(3)** is wrong because, although present during the third trimester, these changes begin during the second. **(4)** is wrong because these signs diminish during the fourth trimester. **AS,5,HPM**

44. **(3)** is unusual because milia (unopened sebaceous glands) look like *white*heads. **(1)** is *typical* because enlarged breasts and pink spotting (pseudomenstruation) are effects of high circulating levels of maternal hormones. **(2)** is *typical* because the linea nigra *is evident* due to maternal hormones. **(4)** is *typical* because "mongolian spots" *are found* on the lower back and sacrum of darker-skinned people. **AS,5,PSI**

45. **(3)** PID is associated with adhesions and blockage of the fallopian tubes, preventing transport and joining of the ovum and sperm. **(1)** is incorrect because moderate alcohol intake is not implicated in female infertility. **(2)** is incorrect because a normal menstrual cycle is not associated with infertility. **(4)** is incorrect because use of a diaphragm and spermicidal jelly is not implicated in infertility. **AS,5,PhI**

46. **(3)** is correct because major cardiovascular changes that occur with the termination of pregnancy can result in sudden cardiac decompensation in the first postpartum day. **(1)** is incorrect because pushing fluids can result in fluid volume overload and cardiac decompensation. **(2)** is incorrect because the postpartum woman with heart disease is encouraged to rest in the first day to minimize cardiac stressors while major cardiovascular changes occur. **(4)** is incorrect because breastfeeding is not contraindicated. **IMP,1,PhI**

47. **(1)** Cephalhematoma is caused by subperiosteal bleeding, and the "lump" is limited by the suture lines. **(2)** is incorrect because edema of the scalp is caput succedaneum. **(3)** is wrong because a cephalhematoma is outside the skull. **(4)** is wrong because hemangiomas are benign blood vessel tumors. **IMP,5,HPM**

48. **(2)** During the third trimester, the mother becomes ready to begin learning techniques for her use during labor. **(1)** is wrong because ambivalence about the pregnancy is usually seen in early pregnancy. **(3)** is wrong because fantasizing is most typical during the second trimester. **(4)** is wrong because the period of introspection and introversion occurs in the second trimester. **AS,4,HPM**

49. **(3)** Epigastric pain is associated with edema of the liver capsule in preeclampsia. **(1)** is incorrect because dependent edema is common in late pregnancy, due to reduced venous return from the lower extremities. **(2)** is wrong because orthostatic hypotension may be a common occurrence during the third trimester. **(4)** is wrong because brown spotting is a normal finding within 24 hours of vaginal examination, due to the increased friability of the cervix during pregnancy. **AS,2,HPM**

50. **(4)** Gravidity is defined as the number of pregnancies; she has been pregnant three previous times and is now pregnant for the fourth time. Parity is defined as the number of *pregnancies* carried to viability (20 weeks since conception; 22 menstrual weeks). The woman has had two pregnancies terminated before viability (abortions) and has carried *one* pregnancy, which resulted in viable twin girls. **(1)** is incorrect because this counts the twins as two pregnancies carried to viability. **(2)** is wrong because, although it correctly identifies the twins as one parity, it counts them as two pregnancies. **(3)** is wrong because, although it correctly identifies the woman as gravida 4, it counts the twins twice. **AS,5,HPM**

51. **(4)** High circulating levels of progesterone released by the corpus luteum are thought to be responsible for the immediate postovulation rise in body temperature. **(1)** is incorrect because FSH is responsible for maturation of the follicle before ovulation. **(2)** is wrong because HPL is produced by the placenta and is not present at this time. **(3)** is wrong because estrogen is not implicated in the rise in body temperature postovulation. **IMP,5,HPM**

52. **(2)** These behaviors are characteristic of the transitional phase of labor, approaching 10 cm dilatation. **(1)** is incorrect because the woman shows a more intense, serious demeanor and may hyperventilate with contractions in the active phase. **(3)** is incorrect because the second stage of labor is characterized by expulsive efforts. **(4)** is incorrect because in the third stage of labor, the placenta is expelled and the woman is often euphoric and focuses on the infant. **AS,5,HPM**

53. **(4)** She does need support for her feelings at this point in pregnancy, and validation that they are normal. **(1)** is incorrect because she is evidencing only normal responses to late pregnancy. **(2)** is wrong because such statements tend to inhibit further exploration of her

feelings and convey that such feelings are unimportant to the nurse. **(3)** is wrong because it neither validates the normalcy of her feelings nor encourages any further ventilation. **IMP,7,HPM**

54. **(2)** is correct because the nurse can best fulfill the role of advocate by providing all essential information the adolescent needs to make informed decisions; this allows opportunity for introspection and growth. **(1)** is incorrect because adolescents require and desire some guidance or assistance with major life decisions from supportive adults. **(3)** is incorrect because it may not be appropriate or ethical to support some decisions the adolescent makes. **(4)** is incorrect because such actions are judgmental, tend to destroy rapport, and nullify possible growth. **IMP,7,HPM**

55. **(4)** is correct because clomiphen citrate (Clomid) is used in infertility caused by anovulatory cycles. It increases the secretion of FSH and LH and stimulates ovulation. Side effects include vasomotor flushes, bloating, nausea, vomiting, headache, hair loss, and visual disturbances. **(1)** is incorrect because anovulatory cycles are not caused by past patterns of sexual behavior. **(2)** is incorrect because many women who experience anovulatory cycles may successfully conceive after treatment. **(3)** is incorrect because anovulatory cycles are not treated with surgical intervention. **AS,7,HPM**

56. **(3)** is correct because semen analysis requires that a freshly masturbated specimen be obtained after a rest (abstinence) period of 48 to 72 hours. **(1)** is incorrect because an accurate sperm count and evaluation of motility require that the specimen be examined within 2 hours. Refrigeration will kill sperm. **(2)** is incorrect because 24 hours of abstinence is insufficient for adequate production of sperm. **(4)** is incorrect because ice will reduce motility and kill sperm. **IMP,1,HPM**

57. **(2)** Lamaze techniques, although helpful, do not guarantee freedom from discomfort throughout the labor process. **(1)** is incorrect because medication may be used to assist the woman in controlling her response to the childbearing process and to facilitate a successful experience. **(3)** is wrong because labor is easier for the woman who understands what is happening and is able to relax and cooperate. **(4)** is wrong because many preparation-for-childbirth courses use these aids. **IMP,5,HPM**

58. **(3)** Semi-Fowler's position allows the presenting part to apply pressure to the placenta. **(1)** is incorrect because a vaginal examination is likely to increase the separation and hemorrhage. **(2)** is wrong because this position does not use the presenting part as a tamponade. **(4)** is wrong because some women with placenta previa are able to give birth vaginally. **IMP,6,PhI**

59. **(3)** Although instructions vary among birth centers, primigravidas should seek care when regular contractions are felt about 5 minutes apart, becoming longer and stronger. **(1)** is incorrect because she should have sought care earlier. **(2)** is incorrect because she should have sought care earlier. Rectal pressure may be a sign of impending birth. **(4)** is incorrect because this pattern may reflect "false labor" or very early latent phase labor. **IMP,5,HPM**

60. **(4)** Of the choices given, if the breech is in the fundus, the occiput must be the presenting part; if the irregular nodules (elbows, knee, feet) are on the right side, the fetal back is to the maternal left. **(1)** is incorrect because the "S" refers to the fetal sacrum and describes a breech presentation. **(2)** is wrong because this also describes a breech presentation. **(3)** is wrong because the fetal back is on the maternal left side, as is the occiput. **AS,5,HPM**

61. **(1)** FHR is heard best through the fetal back, which, in LOA presentations, is below the umbilicus on the maternal left side. **(2)** is incorrect because the fetal back is on the maternal left. **(3)** is wrong because, in a vertex presentation, the heart tones are more audible below the umbilicus. **(4)** is wrong because it describes the placement of FHTs in breech presentations. **AS,5,HPM**

62. **(1)** Braxton-Hicks contractions, hypermobility of joints, and backache are all normal findings at this point in pregnancy. **(2)** is incorrect because complaints of dysuria should be explored due to the tendency to urinary tract infection in pregnancy. **(3)** is wrong because a feeling of tranquility and heightened introspection are common in the second trimester. **(4)** is wrong because these symptoms are most common in the first trimester. **AS,3,HPM**

63. **(2)** Bending at the waist facilitates movement of food out of the stomach through a relaxed cardiac sphincter. **(1)** is incorrect because this is the treatment for morning sickness. **(3)** is wrong because this tends to aggravate heartburn. **(4)** is wrong because the pelvic rock relieves backache, not heartburn. **IMP,4,HPM**

64. **(4)** A full bladder may be the major source of her discomfort. **(1)** is incorrect because medication should be given for minor discomforts only after trying other comfort measures. **(2)** is wrong because this measure would be used only after she has voided. **(3)** is wrong because walking does not relieve afterpains. **IMP,3,HPM**

65. **(1)** Talkativeness, dependency, and passivity are all signs of the "taking-in" phase of the postpartum. **(2)** is incorrect because the mother needs to have her needs for nurturing and positive reinforcement met at this time. **(3)** is wrong because she is most interested in her own body functions, her return to normal, and her ability to void and defecate. **(4)** is wrong because she is not ready to "take hold." **AS,7,HPM**

66. **(1)** The frequency, duration, and intensity of uterine contractions are assessed by light palpation of the contractile part, i.e., the fundus. **(2)** is incorrect because moving the hand over the uterus may reduce the accuracy of perceiving contractions; pressure into the muscle may contribute to uterine dysfunction due to manipulation. **(3)** is wrong because the most contractile part of the uterus is the fundus, not the corpus. **(4)** is wrong because uterine manipulation between contractions may contribute to uterine dysfunction. **AS,4,HPM**

67. **(2)** is correct because deep-tendon reflexes indicate the degree of CNS irritability and the potential for seizure activity. **(1)** is incorrect because hyperreflexia and clonus are not associated with pain or discomfort. **(3)** is incorrect because hyperreflexia and clonus do not interfere with motor activity in the lower extremities. **(4)** is incorrect because women with preeclampsia are placed in environments with reduced stimuli to decrease the risk of seizure activity. **AS,1,SECE**

68. **(3)** The first priority (beside maintaining a newborn's patent airway) is body temperature. **(1)** is incorrect because, although important, identification of the newborn may be delayed until the infant's status is stable. **(2)** is wrong because the second priority is to note any abnormalities. **(4)** is wrong because eye prophylaxis may be delayed for 2 hours. **IMP,5,HPM**

69. **(1)** The Moro reflex occurs in response to sudden stimulation of the newborn's CNS by noise, falling, or jolting.

(2) is incorrect because this action elicits the Babinski reflex. (3) is wrong because this action elicits the tonic neck reflex. (4) is wrong because this elicits rooting. **IMP,5,HPM**

70. (2) Cervical dilatation is determined by vaginal examination. (1) is incorrect because fetal weight can only be indirectly estimated by fundal height measurement and sonography. (3) is incorrect because strength of contractions is evaluated by palpation of the uterine fundus. (4) is incorrect because head circumference cannot be determined until after birth. **AS,5,HPM**

71. (3) The criterion used to distinguish true from false labor is evidence of cervical change. (1) is incorrect because spontaneous rupture of membranes can occur before initiation of labor. (2) is incorrect because women who are not in true labor may experience increasing pain due to obstetric complications. (4) is incorrect because copious bloody vaginal discharge can occur without labor (placental problems). **AS,5,HPM**

72. (2) The most important single factor in maintaining good health for the pregnant woman with heart disease is adequate rest. The woman should have approximately 8–10 hours rest each night and should lie down for 30 minutes after each meal. (1) is incorrect because *reduced* activity reduces fatigue and supports preservation of cardiac reserve. (3) is wrong because moderate sodium intake (2000 mg) is allowable for the average class I cardiac; nutritional counseling focuses on increasing dietary intake of iron, protein, and essential nutrients to meet the increased demands of pregnancy. (4) is wrong because ferrous sulfate is prescribed to meet the increased demands for hemoglobin synthesis and to combat nutritional anemia. **IMP,5,PhI**

73. (3) Tension on the round ligaments occurs because of the erect human posture and pressure exerted by the growing uterus. (1) is incorrect because bladder infection is accompanied by frequency and dysuria. (2) is wrong because discomfort from constipation is accompanied by other symptoms, and the location of the discomfort differs. (4) is wrong because groin pain is not characteristic of beginning labor. **AS,3,HPM**

74. (3) 0-1-2-2 describes her present status. She has not carried a pregnancy to term (T); one pregnancy terminated in the preterm (P) birth of twins, two pregnancies ended in abortion (A), and she has two living children (L). (1) is incorrect because only one was a preterm pregnancy. (2) is incorrect because it describes her as having delivered two term infants and no preterm infants. (4) is wrong because it describes her as having carried one pregnancy to term and having *no* preterm infants. **AS,5,HPM**

75. (1) The possibility of postpartum eclampsia, while high, is often overlooked. Nursing care is planned to maintain ongoing status assessments and minimize environmental stimuli. (2) is wrong because, although the risk decreases subsequent to birth, eclamptic convulsions have been known to occur in the postpartum. (3) is wrong because chronic renal disease is not a sequel to preeclampsia. (4) is wrong because preeclampsia does not necessarily occur in subsequent pregnancies. **AN,6,HPM**

76. (4) Even Rh-negative women during their first pregnancy are at some risk for Rh incompatibility; erythroblastosis fetalis results from hemolysis of fetal cells by maternal antibodies. (1) and (2) are wrong because the Rh-negative woman is not more prone to spontaneous abortion or preeclampsia. (3) is wrong because fetal, not maternal, anemia results from Rh incompatibility. **AN,6,PhI**

77. (3) Quickening, audible FHR with fetoscope, and fundal height just below the umbilicus are present in most women by the 20th week of pregnancy. (1) is wrong because lightening usually occurs at 36–38 weeks gestation. (2) is wrong because Braxton-Hicks contractions are palpable around the 30th week and the fundus is at the umbilicus at approximately the 22nd week. (4) is wrong because Goodell's, Hegar's, and Chadwick's signs are first noted at 6–8 weeks of pregnancy, and this fundal height is consistent with the 16th week of gestation. **AS,5,HPM**

78. (3) Although lactation does suppress ovulation, time of ovulation varies widely, making this an unreliable birth-control method (bottle-feeding mothers have ovulated as early as 36 days postpartum; breastfeeding mothers, as early as 39 days postpartum). (1) is incorrect because of the unpredictability of the time of inhibition of ovulation. (2) is wrong because the mother may have anovulatory or ovulatory menses or may ovulate in the absence of menstruation. (4) is wrong because the woman may desire to resume intercourse when lochia stops. **IMP,5,HPM**

79. (1) The lower uterine segment does not contract as effectively as the fundus. Postpartum bleeding is more common in women with placenta previa. (2) is incorrect because the woman did not have abruptio placentae. (3) is wrong because surgical removal of the placenta does not inhibit uterine contraction. (4) is wrong because a loss of 250 mL during the third stage is within normal limits. **AN,6,PhI**

80. (2) is the best choice because *intervention* is needed, since the breathing technique recommended for transition is rapid, shallow chest breathing. (1) is not the best choice because slow, deep abdominal breathing *is advised* in the latent and early active phases of labor. (3) is not the best choice because the use of intercostal muscles with a relaxed diaphragm *is recommended*. (4) is not the best choice because each contraction *should* begin and end with two cleansing breaths in the Lamaze method. **EV,3,HPM**

81. (3) Increased cardiac output has greater implications because her heart has been compromised by rheumatic fever. She should understand and be able to recognize signs of complications associated with her heart function. (1) is wrong because increased venous pressure in the lower extremities presents little more than an annoyance. (2) is wrong because placental production of HPL presents a greater problem for a woman with diabetes. (4) is wrong because relaxation of the cardiac sphincter results in minor complaints. **IMP,6,PhI**

82. (3) Significantly increased fetal activity and meconium-stained amniotic fluid are signs of fetal distress. (1) is incorrect because crowning is followed rapidly by birth and because any fetal distress can be treated promptly. (2) is wrong because crowning is shortly followed by birth. (4) is wrong because baseline variability is a normal fetal pattern. **AS,5,HPM**

83. (4) Tilting the hip moves the heavy uterus off the major blood vessels (the vena cava and aorta), preventing supine hypotension, reduced placental perfusion, and fetal bradycardia. (1) is incorrect because the statement denies the need for comfort at this time. (2) is wrong because the pillows may increase her comfort but will not prevent supine hypotension. (3) is wrong because the statement may be perceived as a threat and does not

recognize the woman's need for comfort and emotional support. **IMP,5,HPM**

84. **(4)** Epicanthal folds and simian lines are associated with a diagnosis of Down syndrome. **(1)** is incorrect because the head is the largest part of the newborn's body and is larger than the chest. **(2)** is wrong because diaphragmatic breathing is the normal newborn pattern of respiration. **(3)** is wrong because passage of meconium stool immediately following birth is within the normal pattern for newborns. **AN,5,HPM**

Unit 8

Nursing Care of Children and Families

❑ Growth and Development

I. Infant (28 d–1 yr)

A. Erikson's theory of personality development

1. *Central task:* basic trust vs. mistrust; central person: primary caretaker.
2. *Behavioral indicators*
   a. Crying is only means of communicating needs.
   b. Quieting usually means needs are met.
   c. Fear of strangers at 6–8 mo.
3. **Parental guidance/teaching**
   a. Must meet infant's needs consistently—cannot "spoil" infant by holding, comforting.
   b. Neonatal *reflexes* fade between 4 and 6 mo, replaced with increase in purposeful behavior, e.g., babbling, reaching.
   c. *Fear of strangers* is normal—indicates attachment between infant and primary caretaker.
   d. Child may repeat over and over newly learned behaviors, e.g., sitting or standing.
   e. *Weaning* can begin around the time child begins walking.
4. For additional information about behavioral concerns for each age group, see Tables 8.3 and 8.4.

B. Physical growth

1. *Height* (length): 50% increase by first birthday.
2. *Weight*
   a. Doubles by 4–7 mo, triples by 1 yr.
   b. Gains 5–7 oz/week in first 6 mo of life.
   c. Gains 3–5 oz/week in second 6 mo of life.
3. *Vital signs:* Table 8.1.
4. *Fontanels*
   a. *Posterior*—closed by 6–8 wk.
   b. *Anterior*—remains open through first 12 mo.
5. *Teething*
   a. Generally begins around 6 mo.
   b. First two teeth: lower central incisors.
   c. By 1 yr: six to eight teeth.

C. Denver Developmental Screening Test (DDST): Table 8.2.

1. *Birth–3 mo*
   a. Personal-social: smiles responsively, then spontaneously.
   b. Fine motor-adaptive:
      (1) Follows 180 degrees, past midline.
      (2) Grasps rattle.
      (3) Holds hands together.
   c. Language: laughs/squeals; vocalizes without crying.
   d. Gross motor: while on stomach, lifts head 45–90 degrees, able to hold head steady and erect; rolls over, from stomach to back.

■ **TABLE 8.1 Normal Vital Signs: Measurements and Variations with Age**

Age (yr)	Heart Rate (beats/min)	Respiratory Rate (breaths/min)	Blood Pressure (mm Hg)
Newborn	120–160	30–40	70/55
1	100–140	25–35	90/55
2	80–120	20–30	90/56
5	70–100	18–24	95/56
10	60–90	18–22	102/62
14	55–90	16–20	110/65
18	55–90	16–18	116/68

Source: Adapted from Wong D. *Whaley and Wong's Nursing Care of Infants and Children* (5th ed). St. Louis: Mosby, 1995.

493

■ **TABLE 8.2 Facts About the Denver Developmental Screening Test (DDST)**

Parents' Questions	Nurse's Best Response
"Will this be used as a measure of my child's IQ?"	"No, it is a screening test for your child's development."
"What ages can be tested?"	"Infants through preschoolers, *or* from birth to 6 years."
"What will they test?"	"There are four areas: personal-social, fine motor-adaptive, language, gross motor."
"Can I stay with my child?"	"Yes, in fact it is preferred you be there."
"If my child fails, does it mean he is retarded?"	"No, this is not a diagnostic tool but rather a screening test."
"If he fails, what do we do?"	"Repeat the test in a week or two to rule out temporary factors."
"Why didn't my child accomplish everything?"	"He is not expected to."
"Why did my child score so poorly?"	"Perhaps it's a bad day for the child, he isn't feeling up to par, etc."

2. *4–6 mo*
   a. Personal-social: works for toy; feeds self (bottle).
   b. Fine motor-adaptive: palmar grasp, reaches for objects.
   c. Language: turns toward voice, imitates speech.
   d. Gross motor: some weight bearing on legs; no head lag when pulled to sitting; sits with support.
3. *7–9 mo*
   a. Personal-social
      (1) Indicates wants
      (2) Plays Pat-a-cake, waves bye-bye.
   b. Fine motor-adaptive: takes two cubes in hands and bangs them together; passes cube hand to hand; crude pincer grasp.
   c. Language: "dada," "mama," nonspecific, jabbers.
   d. Gross motor: gets self up to sitting; pulls self to standing; stands holding on.
4. *10–12 mo*
   a. Personal-social
      (1) Plays ball.
      (2) Imitates activities.
      (3) Drinks from cup.
   b. Fine motor-adaptive: neat pincer grasp.
   c. Language: "dada," "mama," specific.
   d. Gross motor: stands alone well; walks holding on; stoops and recovers.
◆ **D. Nursing interventions/parental guidance, teaching:**
   1. *Play*
      a. First year—generally solitary.
      b. Visual stimulation
         (1) Best color: red.
         (2) Toys: mirrors, brightly colored pictures.
      c. Auditory stimulation
         (1) Talk and sing to infant.
         (2) Toys: musical mobiles, rattles, bells.
      d. Tactile stimulation
         (1) Hold, pat, touch, cuddle, swaddle/keep warm; rub body with lotion, powder.

      (2) Toys: various textures; nesting and stacking; plastic milk bottle with blocks to dump in, out.
      e. Kinetic stimulation
         (1) Cradle, stroller, carriage, infant seat, car rides, wind-up infant swing, jumper seat, walker, furniture strategically placed for walking.
         (2) Toys: cradle gym, push-pull.
   2. *Safety*
      a. *Note:* Most common accident during first 12 mo is the aspiration of foreign bodies.
         (1) Keep small objects out of reach.
         (2) Use one-piece pacifier only.
         (3) *No* nuts, raisins, hot dogs, popcorn.
         (4) *No* toys with small, removable parts.
         (5) *No* balloons or plastic bags.
      b. *Falls*
         (1) Raise crib rails.
         (2) *Never* place child on high surface unsupervised.
         (3) Use restraining straps in seats, swings, high-chairs, etc.
      c. *Poisoning*
         (1) Check that paint on toys/furniture is *lead-free.*
         (2) Treat all medications as drugs, never as "candy."
         (3) Store all poisonous substances in locked cabinet, closet.
         (4) Have telephone number of poison control center on hand.
         (5) Instruct in use of syrup of ipecac (see p. 534).
      d. *Burns*
         (1) Use microwave oven to heat refrigerated formula only; heat only 4 oz or more for about 30 sec. Test formula on top of your hand, not inside wrist.
         (2) Check temperature of bath water; *never* leave infant alone in bath.
         (3) Special care with cigarettes, hot liquids.
         (4) Do *not* leave infant in sun.
         (5) Cover all electrical sockets.

(6) Keep electrical wires out of sight/reach.

(7) Avoid tablecloths with overhang.

(8) Put guards around heating devices.

e. *Motor vehicles*

(1) Use only federally approved car seat for all car rides.

(2) *Never* leave stroller behind parked car.

(3) Do *not* allow infant to crawl near parked cars or in driveway.

II. Toddler (1–3 yr)

A. Erikson's theory of personality development

1. *Central task:* autonomy vs. shame and doubt; central person(s): parent(s)

2. *Behavioral indicators*

a. Does not separate easily from parents.

b. Negativistic.

c. Prefers rituals and routine activities.

d. Active physical explorer of environment.

e. Begins attempts at self-assertion.

f. Easily frustrated by limits.

g. Temper tantrums.

h. May have favorite "security object."

i. Uses "mine" for everything—does not understand concept of sharing.

3. **Parental guidance/teaching**

a. Avoid periods of prolonged separation if possible.

b. Avoid constantly saying "no" to toddler.

c. Avoid "yes"/"no" questions.

d. Stress that child may use "no" even when he or she means "yes."

e. Establish and maintain rituals, e.g., toilet training, going to sleep.

f. Offer opportunities for play, *with* supervision.

g. Allow child to feed self.

h. Offer only allowable choices.

i. Best method to handle temper tantrums: ignore them.

j. Keep security object with child, if so desired.

k. Do not force toddler "to share."

4. Additional information about behavioral concerns for each age group may be found in Tables 8.3 and 8.4.

B. Physical growth

1. *Height*

a. Slow, steady growth at 2–4 in./yr, mainly in *legs* rather than trunk.

b. Adult height is roughly twice child's height at 2 yr of age.

2. *Weight*

a. Slow, steady growth at 4–6 lb/yr.

b. Birth weight *quadruples* by 2½ yr of age.

3. *Vital signs:* refer to Table 8.1.

4. *Anterior fontanel*—closes between 12–18 mo.

5. *Teething*

a. Introduce tooth brushing as a "ritual."

b. By 30 mo: all 20 primary teeth present.

c. First dental check-up should be between 12–18 mo of age.

6. *Vision*

a. Full binocular vision well developed.

b. Visual acuity of toddler: 20/40.

7. *Posture and gait*

a. Lordosis: abdomen protrudes.

b. Walks like a duck: wide-based gait, side-to-side.

C. DDST (see Table 8.2)

1. *12–18 mo*

a. Personal-social

(1) Imitates housework.

(2) Uses spoon, spilling little.

(3) Removes own clothes.

(4) Drinks from cup.

(5) Feeds doll.

b. Fine motor-adaptive

(1) Scribbles spontaneously.

(2) Builds tower with two to four cubes.

c. Language

(1) Three to six words other than "mama," "dada."

(2) Points to at least one named body part.

d. Gross motor

(1) Kicks ball forward.

(2) Walks up steps.

2. *19–24 mo*

a. Personal-social

(1) Puts on clothing.

(2) Washes and dries hands.

(3) Brushes teeth with help.

b. Fine motor-adaptive

(1) Builds tower with four to six cubes.

(2) Imitates vertical line.

c. Language

(1) Combines two or three words.

(2) Speech half-understandable.

(3) Names picture.

d. Gross motor

(1) Throws ball overhand.

(2) Jumps in place.

3. *2–3 yr*

a. Personal-social

(1) Puts on T-shirt.

(2) Can name a friend.

b. Fine motor-adaptive

(1) Thumb wiggles.

(2) Builds tower of eight cubes.

c. Language

(1) Knows two actions and two adjectives.

(2) Names one color.

d. Gross motor

(1) Balances on one foot briefly.

(2) Pedals tricycle.

◆ D. Nursing interventions/parental guidance:

1. *Play:* toddler years—generally parallel.

2. Toys—stimulate multiple senses simultaneously:

a. Push-pull.

■ TABLE 8.3   Pediatric Behavioral Concerns: Nursing Implications and Parental Guidance

Behavioral Concern	Nursing Implications/ Parental Guidance	Behavioral Concern	Nursing Implications/ Parental Guidance
Teething	Begins around age 4 mo—infant may seem unusually fussy and irritable but should *not* run a fever	Sibling rivalry	Fairly common, normal
			Allow older child to "help"
	Provide relief with teething rings, acetaminophen, topical preparations		Give each child "special" time, with individual attention
Thumb sucking	Need to "suck" varies: may be due to hunger, frustration, loneliness	Masturbation	Normal, common in *preschooler*
			Set firm limits
	Do *not* stop *infant* from doing this— usually stops by preschool years		Avoid overreacting
	If behavior persists, evaluate need for attention, peer play	Lying	*In preschooler:* not deliberate; child is often unable to differentiate between "real" and "lie," and by speaking something he often feels it makes a thing real
Temper tantrums	Normal in the *toddler*—occurs in response to frustration		
	Avoid abrupt end to play or making excessive demands		*In older child:* may indicate problems and need for professional attention if persists
	Offer only allowable choices		
	Once a decision is verbalized, *avoid* sudden changes of mind		Serve as role model—no "white lies"
	Provide diversion to achieve cooperation	Cursing	Avoid overreacting
	If it occurs, best means to handle is to *ignore* the outburst		Defuse use of "the word" by simply stating "not here, not now"
Toilet training	Assess child for readiness: awareness of body functions, form of mutual communication, physical control over sphincters		Distract, change subject, substitute activity
			Serve as role model by own language
		"Accidents" (enuresis)	*Occasional*—common and normal through preschool
	Use child-size seat		*If frequent*—need complete physical exam to rule out pathology
	No distractions (food, toys, books)		
	Offer praise for success *or* efforts (never shame accidents)		"Training": after dinner—avoid fluids; before bed—toilet (perhaps awaken once during night)
Discipline	*Not* for infant		
	Can begin with *toddler,* within limits		*Never* put back into diapers or attempt to shame
	Be consistent and clear	Smoking/drinking	May begin in *older school-age* child or adolescent
	Avoid excessively strict measures		
			Serve as role model with own habits

b. Riding toys, e.g., straddle horse or car.
c. Small, low slide or gym.
d. Balls, in various sizes.
e. Blocks—multiple shapes, sizes, colors.
f. Dolls, trucks, dress-up clothes.
g. Drums, horns, cymbals, xylophones, toy piano.
h. Pounding board and hammer, clay.
i. Finger paints, chalk and board, thick crayons.
j. Wooden puzzles with large pieces.
k. Toy record player with kiddie records.
l. Talking toys: dolls, see 'n say, phones.
m. Sand, water, soap bubbles.
n. Picture books, photo albums.
o. Nursery rhymes, songs, music.

3. *Safety*
   a. Accidents are the primary cause of death among toddlers.
   b. *Motor vehicles:* most accidental deaths in children under age 3 are related to motor vehicles.
      (1) Use only federally approved car seat for all car rides, through age 4 or 40 lb or 40 in tall (*"Rule of Fours"*).
      (2) Follow manufacturer directions carefully.
      (3) Make car seat part of routine for toddler.
   c. Drowning
      (1) Always supervise child near water: tub, pool, Jacuzzi, lake, ocean.

■ TABLE 8.4   Pediatric Sleep and Rest Norms: Nursing Implications and Parental Guidance

Pediatric Sleep and Rest Norms	Nursing Implications/Parental Guidance
Infant: 16–20 h/d	No set schedule can be predetermined
3 mo: nocturnal pattern	If waking at night after age 3 mo, investigate hunger as a probable cause
6 mo: 1–2 naps, with 12 h at night	Monitor behavior to determine sleep needs: alert and active? growing, developing?
12 mo: 1 nap, with 12 h at night	Routine fairly well established
Toddler: 12–14 h/night	
"Dawdles" at bedtime	Set firm, realistic limits
Dependency on security object	Place favorite blanket or toy in crib/bed
May ask to sleep with bottle	**Avoid** "bottle mouth syndrome" (caries)
May rebel against going to sleep	Establish bedtime "ritual"
Preschool: 10–12 h/night	May regress in behavior when tired
Gives up afternoon nap	Provide "quiet time" in place of nap
Difficulty falling asleep/nighttime waking	Avoid overstimulation in evening
Fear of dark	Leave night-light on, door open
Enuresis	Occasional accidents are normal
May begin to have nightmares	Comfort child but leave in own bed
School-age: 8–12 h/night	
Nightmares common	Comfort child but leave in own bed
Awakens early in morning	Important that child play/relax before school
May not be aware he/she is tired	Remind about bedtime
Likes to stay up late	"Privilege" of later bedtime can be "awarded" as child gets older
Slumber parties	Permit, as good opportunity to socialize
Adolescent: 10–14 h/night	Needs vary greatly among individuals
Need for sleep increases greatly	Rapid growth rate
May complain of excessive fatigue	Related to rapid growth and overall increased activity

(2) Keep bathroom locked to prevent drowning in toilet.

d. *Burns*
   (1) Turn pot handles *in* when cooking.
   (2) Do *not* allow child to play with electrical appliances.
   (3) Decrease water temperature in house to avoid scald burns.

e. *Poisonings:* most common in 2-yr-olds.
   (1) Consider every nonfood substance a hazard and place out of child's sight/reach.
   (2) Keep all medications, cleaning materials, etc. in clearly marked containers in locked cabinets.
   (3) Instruct in use of syrup of ipecac (see p. 534).

f. *Falls*
   (1) Provide barriers on open windows.
   (2) Avoid gates on stairs—child can strangle on gate.
   (3) Move from crib to bed.

g. *Choking:* avoid food on which child might choke:
   (1) Fish with bones.
   (2) Fruit with seeds or pits.
   (3) Nuts, raisins.
   (4) Hot dogs.
   (5) Chewing gum.
   (6) Hard candy.

III. Preschooler (3–5 yr)
A. **Erikson's theory of personality development**
   1. *Central task:* initiative vs. guilt; central person(s): basic family unit.
   2. *Behavioral indicators*
      a. Attempts to perform activities of daily living (ADL) independently.
      b. Attempts to make things for self/others.
      c. Tries to "help."
      d. Talks constantly: verbal exploration of the world ("Why?").
      e. Extremely active, highly creative imagination: fantasy and magical thinking.
      f. May demonstrate fears: "monsters," dark rooms, etc.
      g. Able to tolerate short periods of separation.
   3. **Parental guidance/teaching**
      a. Encourage child to dress self by providing simple clothing.

b. Remind to go to bathroom (tends to "forget").

c. Assign small, simple tasks or errands.

d. Answer questions patiently, simply; do *not* offer child more information than he or she is asking for.

e. Normal to have "imaginary playmates."

f. Offer realistic support and reassurance with regard to fears.

g. Expose to a variety of experiences: zoo, train ride, shopping, sleigh riding, etc.

h. Enroll in preschool/nursery school program; kindergarten at 5 yr.

4. Additional information about behavioral concerns for each age group may be found in Tables 8.3 and 8.4.

B. Physical growth

1. *Height and weight*

   a. Continued slow, steady growth.

   b. Generally grows more in *height* than weight.

   c. Posture: appears taller and thinner; "lordosis" of toddler gradually *disappears.*

2. *Vital signs:* see Table 8.1.

3. *Teeth*

   a. *All* 20 "baby teeth" present.

   b. Annual dental check-ups, daily brushing.

4. *Vision*

   a. Visual acuity: 20/30 between 3 and 5 yr.

   b. Do vision/hearing screening before kindergarten.

C. DDST/developmental norms

1. *3 yr*

   a. Personal-social

      (1) Dresses without help.

      (2) Plays board/card games.

   b. Fine motor-adaptive

      (1) Picks longer of two lines.

      (2) Copies circle, intersecting lines.

      (3) Draws person, three parts.

   c. Language

      (1) Comprehends "cold," "tired," "hungry."

      (2) Comprehends prepositions: "over," "under."

      (3) Names four colors.

   d. Gross motor

      (1) Broad jumps, jumps in place.

      (2) Balances on one foot.

2. *4 years*

   a. Personal-social

      (1) Brushes own teeth, combs own hair.

      (2) Dresses without supervision.

      (3) Knows own age and birthday.

      (4) Ties own shoes.

   b. Fine motor-adaptive

      (1) Draws person with six body parts.

      (2) Copies square.

   c. Language

      (1) Knows opposite analogies (two of three).

      (2) Defines seven words.

   d. Gross motor

      (1) Balances on each foot for 5 sec.

      (2) Can walk heel-to-toe.

3. *5 years*

   a. Personal-social

      (1) Interested in money.

      (2) Knows days of week, seasons.

   b. Fine motor-adaptive

      (1) Prints name.

   c. Language

      (1) Counts to 10.

      (2) Verbalizes number sequences (e.g., telephone number).

   d. Gross motor

      (1) Attempts to ride bike.

      (2) Rollerskates, jumps rope, bounces ball.

      (3) Backward heel-toe walk.

◆ **D. Nursing interventions/parental guidance:**

1. *Play:* preschool years—associative and cooperative.

   a. Likes to play house, "work," school, firehouse.

   b. "Arts and crafts": color, draw, paint, dot-to-dot, color by number, cut and paste, simple sewing kits.

   c. Ball, rollerskate, jump rope, jacks.

   d. Swimming.

   e. Puzzles, blocks (e.g., Legos).

   f. Tricycle, then bicycle (with/without training wheels).

   g. Simple card games and board games.

   h. Costumes and dress-up: "make-believe."

2. *Safety:* Emphasis now shifts from protective supervision to teaching simple safety rules. Preschoolers are "the great imitators" of parents, who serve as role models now.

   a. Teach child car/*street* safety rules.

   b. Change to "child booster seat" in car at *4 yr or 40 lb or 40 in.*

   c. Teach child not to go with strangers or accept gifts or candy from strangers.

   d. Teach child danger of *fire,* matches, flame: "drop and roll."

   e. Teach child rules of *water* safety; provide swimming lessons.

   f. Provide adult supervision, frequent checks on activity/location. Despite safety teaching, preschooler is still a child and may be unreliable.

IV. School age (6–12 yr)

A. Erikson's theory of personality development

1. *Central task:* industry vs. inferiority; central person(s): school, neighborhood friend(s).

2. *Behavioral indicators*

a. Moving toward complete independence in ADL.

b. May be very competitive—wants to achieve in school, at play.

c. Likes to be alone occasionally, may seem shy.

d. Prefers friends and peers to siblings.

3. *Parental guidance/teaching*

a. Be accepting of the child as he or she *is*.

b. Offer consistent support and guidance.

c. Avoid authoritative or excessive demands on child.

d. Respect need for privacy.

e. Assign household tasks, errands, chores.

4. Additional information about behavioral concerns for each age group may be found in Tables 8.3 and 8.4.

B. Physical growth

1. *Height and weight*

a. Almost *doubles* in weight from 6–12 yr.

b. Period of slow, steady growth.

c. 1–2 in./yr.

d. 3–6 lb/yr.

e. Girls and boys differ very little in size.

2. *Vital signs:* refer to Table 8.1.

3. *Teeth*

a. Begins to lose primary teeth around sixth birthday.

b. Eruption of permanent teeth, including molars; 28 permanent teeth by age 12 yr.

c. Dental screening annually, daily brushing.

4. *Vision and hearing*

a. Should be screened annually—usually in school.

b. 20/20 vision well established between 9–11 yr.

5. *Pubescence* (preliminary physical changes of adolescence)

a. Average age of onset: girls at 10, boys at 12.

b. Beginning of growth spurt.

c. Some sexual changes may start to occur.

C. DDST/developmental norms

1. *6–8 yr*

a. Dramatic, exuberant, boundless energy.

b. Alternating periods: quiet, private behavior.

c. Conscientious, punctual.

d. Wants to care for own needs but needs reminders, supervision.

e. Oriented to time and space.

f. Learns to read, tell time, follow map.

g. Interested in money—asks for "allowance."

h. Eagerly anticipates upcoming events, trips.

i. Can bicycle, swim, play ball.

2. *9–11 years*

a. Worries over tasks; takes things seriously, yet also developing sense of humor—likes to tell jokes.

b. Keeps room, clothes, toys relatively tidy.

c. Enjoys physical activity, has great stamina.

d. Very enthusiastic at work and play; has lots of energy—may fidget, drum fingers, tap foot.

e. Wants to work to earn money: mow lawn, babysit, deliver papers.

f. Loves secrets (secret clubs).

g. Very well behaved outside own home (or with company).

h. Uses tools, equipment; follows directions, recipes.

i. By twelfth birthday: paradoxical stormy behavior, onset of adolescent conflicts.

◆ **D. Nursing interventions/parental guidance:**

1. *Play*

a. Wants to win, likes competitive games.

b. Prefers to play with same-sex children.

c. Enjoys group, team play.

d. Loves to do magic tricks and other "show-off" activities (e.g., puppet shows, plays, singing).

e. Likes to collect things: cards, records.

f. Simple scientific experiments, computer games.

g. Hobbies: needlework, woodwork, models.

h. Enjoys pop music, musical instruments, radio, audio tapes, videos, posters.

2. *Safety*—motor vehicles

a. As passenger: teach to wear safety belt, not distract driver.

b. As pedestrian: teach bike, street safety.

c. Teach how to swim, rules of water safety.

d. Sports: teach safety rules.

e. Adult supervision still necessary; serve as role model for safe activities.

f. Suggest Red Cross courses on first aid, water safety, babysitting, etc.

V. Adolescent (12–18 yr)

A. Erikson's theory of personality development

1. *Central task:* identity vs. role confusion; central person(s): peer group.

2. *Behavioral indicators*

a. Changes in body image related to sexual development.

b. Awkward and uncoordinated.

c. Much interest in opposite sex: females become romantic.

d. Wants to be exactly like peers.

e. Becomes hostile toward parents, adults, family.

f. Concerned with vocation, life after high school.

3. *Parental guidance, teaching*

a. Offer firm but realistic limits on behavior.

b. Continue to offer guidance, support.

c. Allow child to earn own money, control own finances.

d. Assist adolescent to develop positive self-image.

4. Additional information about behavioral concerns for each age group may be found in Tables 8.3 and 8.4.

B. Physical growth

1. *Height and weight*

a. Adolescent growth spurt lasts 24–36 mo.

b. Growth in height commonly *ceases* at 16–17 yr in girls, 18–20 yr in boys.

c. Boys gain more weight than girls, are generally taller and heavier.

2. *Vital signs* approximately those of the adult. See Table 8.1.

3. *Teeth:* 32 permanent teeth by 18–21 yr.

4. *Sexual changes*

a. *Females*

(1) Changes in nipple and areola; development of breast buds.

(2) Growth of pubic hair.

(3) Change in vaginal secretions.

(4) Menstruation—12.8 yr (average).

(5) Growth of axillary hair.

(6) Ovulation.

b. *Males*

(1) Enlargement of genitalia.

(2) Growth of pubic, axillary, facial, and body hair.

(3) Lowering of voice.

(4) Production of sperm; nocturnal emission ("wet dreams").

C. Developmental norms

1. *Motor development*

a. *Early (12–15 yr)*—awkward, uncoordinated, poor posture, decrease in energy and stamina.

b. *Later (15–18 yr)*—increased coordination and better posture; more energy and stamina.

2. *Cognitive*

a. Academic ability and interest vary greatly.

b. "Think about thinking"—period of introspection.

3. *Emotional*

a. Same-sex best friend, leading to strong friendship bonds.

b. Highly romantic period for boys and girls.

c. May be moody, unpredictable, inconsistent.

4. *Social*

a. Periods of highs and lows, sociability and loneliness.

b. Turmoil with parents—related to changing roles, desire for increased independence.

c. Peer group is important socializing agent—conformity increases sense of belonging.

d. Friendships: same-sex best friend advancing to heterosexual "relationships."

◆ **D. Nursing interventions/parental guidance:**

1. *Play*

a. School-related group activities and sports.

b. Develops talents, skills, and abilities.

c. Television—watches soap operas, romantic movies, sports.

d. Develops interest in art, writing, poetry, musical instrument.

e. Girls: increased interest in make-up and clothes.

f. Boys: increased interest in mechanical and electrical devices.

2. *Safety*—motor vehicles (cars and motorcycles)—as *passenger* or as *driver*

a. Encourage driver education; serve as positive role model.

b. Teach rules of safety for water sports.

c. Wants to earn money but still needs guidance: advocate safe job, reasonable hours.

Developmental Disabilities

I. Down syndrome

A. *Introduction:* Down syndrome (trisomy 21; mongolism) is a chromosomal abnormality involving an extra chromosome #21 and resulting in 47 chromosomes instead of the normal 46 chromosomes. As a consequence, the child usually presents with varying degrees of mental retardation, characteristic facial and physical features, and other congenital anomalies. Down syndrome is the most common chromosomal disorder, occurring in approximately 1 of 800 to 1000 live births. Perinatal risk factors include advanced maternal age, especially with the first pregnancy; paternal age is thought to be a related factor.

◆ **B. Assessment:**

1. *Physical characteristics*

a. Brachycephalic (small, round *head*) with oblique palpebral fissures (Oriental *eyes*) and Brushfield's spots (speckling of *iris*)—depressed *nasal* bridge ("saddle nose") and small, low-set *ears*.

b. Mouth

(1) Small oral cavity with protruding tongue causes difficulty sucking and swallowing.

(2) Delayed eruption/misalignment of teeth.

c. Hands

(1) Clinodactyly—in-curved little finger.

(2) Simian crease—transverse palmar crease.

d. Muscles: hypotonic ("floppy baby") with hyperextensible joints.

e. Skin: dry, cracked.

2. Genetic studies reveal an extra chromosome #21 ("trisomy 21").

3. *Intellectual characteristics*

a. Mental retardation—varies from severely retarded to low-average intelligence.

b. Most fall within "trainable" range, or IQ = 36–51 ("moderate mental retardation").

4. *Congenital anomalies/diseases*

a. 30–40% have congenital heart defects: mortality highest in patients with Down syndrome and cyanotic heart disease.

b. GI: tracheoesophageal fistula, Hirschsprung's disease.

c. Thyroid dysfunction, especially hypothyroidism.

d. Visual defects: cataracts, strabismus.

e. Hearing loss.

f. Increased incidence of leukemia.

5. *Growth and development*

a. Slow growth, especially in height.

b. Delay in developmental milestones.

6. *Sexual development*

a. Delayed or incomplete.

b. Females—small number have had offspring (majority have had abnormality).

c. Males—infertile.

7. *Aging*

a. Premature aging, with shortened life expectancy.

b. Death usually before age 40—generally related to respiratory complications: repeated infections, pneumonia, lung disease.

◆ **C. Analysis/nursing diagnosis:**

1. *Risk for aspiration* related to hypotonia.

2. *Altered nutrition, less than body requirements,* related to hypotonia or congenital anomalies.

3. *Altered growth and development* related to Down syndrome.

4. *Self-care deficit* related to Down syndrome.

5. *Altered family processes* related to birth of an infant with a congenital defect.

6. *Knowledge deficit* related to Down syndrome.

◆ **D. Nursing care plan/implementation:**

1. Goal: *prevent physical complications.*

a. Respiratory

(1) Use bulb syringe to clear nose, mouth.

(2) Vaporizer.

(3) Frequent position changes.

(4) Avoid contact with people with upper-respiratory infections.

b. Aspiration

(1) Small, more frequent feedings.

(2) Burp well during/after infant feedings.

(3) Allow sufficient time to eat.

(4) *Position after meals:* head of bed elevated, right side—or on stomach, with head to side.

c. Observe for signs and symptoms of heart disease, constipation/GI obstruction, leukemia, thyroid dysfunction.

2. Goal: *meet nutritional needs.*

▶ a. Suction (before meals) to clear airway.

b. Adapt feeding techniques to meet special needs of infant/child; e.g., use long, straight-handled spoon.

c. Monitor height and weight.

d. As child grows, monitor caloric intake (tends toward obesity).

e. Offer foods *high in bulk* to prevent constipation related to hypotonia.

3. Goal: *promote optimal growth and development.*

a. Encourage parents to enroll infant/toddler in early stimulation program and to follow through with suggested exercises at home.

b. Preschool/school-age: special education classes.

c. Screen frequently, using DDST to monitor development.

d. Help parents focus on "normal" or positive aspects of infant/child.

e. Help parents work toward realistic goals with their child.

4. Goal: *health teaching.*

a. Explain that tongue-thrust behavior is normal and that food should be refed.

b. Before adolescence—counsel parents and child about delay in sexual development, decreased libido, marriage and family relations.

c. In severe cases assist parents to deal with issue of placement/institutionalization.

◆ **E. Evaluation/outcome criteria:**

1. Physical complications are prevented.

2. Adequate nutrition is maintained.

3. Child attains optimal level of growth and development.

II. Attention deficit-hyperactivity disorder (ADHD); behavioral disorder (DSM-IV)

A. *Introduction:* As defined by the American Psychiatric Association (APA), this diagnostic term includes a persistent pattern of inattention or hyperactivity-impulsivity. The exact cause and pathophysiology remain unknown. The major symptoms include a greatly shortened attention span and difficulty in integrating and synthesizing information. This disorder is 10 times more common in boys than girls, with onset before age 7; the diagnosis is based on the child's history rather than on any specific diagnostic test.

◆ **B. Assessment:**

1. The behaviors exhibited by children with ADHD are not unusual behaviors seen in children. The behavior of children with ADHD *differs* from the behavior of non-ADHD children in both quality and appropriateness:
   a. Motor activity is excessive.
   b. Developmentally "younger" than chronological age.
2. Inattention
   a. Does not pay attention to detail.
   b. Does not listen when spoken to.
   c. Does not do what he or she is told to do.
3. Hyperactivity
   a. Fidgets and squirms excessively.
   b. Cannot sit quietly.
   c. Has difficulty playing quietly.
   d. Seems to be constantly in motion, moving or talking.
4. Impulsiveness
   a. Blurts out answers before question is completed.
   b. Has difficulty awaiting turn. Interrupts others.

◆ **C. Analysis/nursing diagnosis:**

1. *Altered thought processes* related to inattention and impulsiveness.
2. *Impaired physical mobility* related to hyperactivity.
3. *Risk for injury* related to impulsivity.
4. *Self-esteem disturbance* related to hyperactivity and impulsivity.
5. *Knowledge deficit* related to behavioral modification program, medications, and follow-up care.

◆ **D. Nursing care plan/implementation:**

1. Goal: *teach family and child about ADHD.*
   a. Provide complete explanation about disorder, probable course, treatment, and prognosis.
   b. Answer questions directly, simply.
   c. Encourage family to verbalize; offer support.
2. Goal: *provide therapeutic environment* using principles of behavior modification.
   a. Reduce extraneous or distracting stimuli.
   b. Reduce stress by decreasing environmental expectations (home, school).
   c. Provide firm, consistent limits.
   d. Special education programs.
   e. Special attention to safety needs.
3. Goal: *reduce symptoms by means of prescribed medication.*
   a. Medications: Ritalin and Cylert—both are CNS stimulants but have a paradoxical calming effect on the child's behavior.
   b. Health teaching (child *and* parents).
      (1) Need to take medication regularly, as ordered. Avoid taking medication

late in the day because it may cause insomnia.
      (2) Need for long-term administration, with decreased need as child nears adolescence.
4. Goal: *provide safe outlet for excess energy.*
   a. Alternate planned periods of outdoor play with schoolwork or quiet indoor play.
   b. Channel energies toward safe, large-muscle activities: running track, swimming, bicycling, hiking.

◆ **E. Evaluation/outcome criteria:**

1. Family and child verbalize understanding of "attention deficit disorders."
2. Therapeutic environment enhances socially acceptable behavior.
3. Medication taken regularly, with behavioral improvements noted.
4. Excess energy directed appropriately.
5. Dietary modification implemented.

❏ Psychosocial-Cultural Functions

Refer to Table 8.5 for information on the nursing care of hospitalized infants and children as it relates to key developmental differences.

❏ Disorders Affecting Fluid-Gas Transport

Cardiovascular Disorders

Congenital Heart Disease (CHD)

I. *Introduction:* There are more than 35 documented types of congenital heart defects, which occur in 4 to 10 per 1000 live births. For the purpose of this review, only six *major* defects are given. These are presented in Figures 8.1 through 8.6. *Note:* The content has been synthesized for ease in review and recall; for additional study aids, the student may wish to refer to Tables 8.6 and 8.7. Unit 2 also contains information on congestive heart failure, and Unit 4 covers the most commonly used drugs, including digoxin and furosemide (Lasix).

◆ **II. Assessment:**

A. Exact cause unknown, but related factors include:

1. Familial history of CHD, especially in siblings, parents.
2. Presence of other genetic defects in infant, e.g., Down syndrome, trisomy 13 or 18.
3. History of maternal prenatal infection with rubella, cytomegalovirus, etc.
4. High-risk maternal factors:
   a. Age: under 18, over 40 yr.
   b. Weight: under 100, over 200 lb.
   c. Maternal insulin-dependent diabetes.

■ **TABLE 8.5   Nursing Care of Hospitalized Infants and Children: Key Developmental Differences**

Age	Assessment: Reaction to Hospitalization	Nursing Care Plan/Implementation: Key Nursing Behaviors
Infant	Difficult to assess needs, pain	Close observation, must look at behavioral cues
	Wants primary caretaker	Rooming-in
Toddler	Separation anxiety	Rooming-in
	Frustration, loss of autonomy	Punching bag, pounding board, clay
	Regression	Behavior modification
	Fears intrusive procedures	Axillary temperatures
Preschooler	Fearful	Therapeutic play with puppets, dolls
	Fantasy about illness/hospitalization (may feel punished, abandoned)	Therapeutic play with puppets, dolls
	Peak of body mutilation fear	Care with dressings, casts, IMs
	Behavior problems: aggressive, manipulative	Clear, consistent limits
	Regression	Behavior modification
School age	Cooperative	Use diagrams, models to teach
	Quiet, may withdraw	Indirect interview: tell story, draw picture
	May complain of being bored	Involve in competitive game with peer. Encourage peers to call, send get well cards, and visit
	Fears loss of control	Provide privacy; allow to make some decisions
	Competitive—afraid of "failing"	Provide tutor prn; get books and homework
Adolescent	Difficulty with body image	Provide own clothes; give realistic feedback
	Does not want to be separated from peers	Telephone in room; liberal visiting; teen lounge
	Rebellious behavior	Set clear rules; form teen "rap groups"

5. Maternal history of drinking during pregnancy, with resultant "fetal alcohol syndrome."
6. Extracardiac defects including tracheo-esophageal fistula, renal agenesis, and diaphragmatic hernia.

B. Most frequent parental complaint: *difficulty feeding.*
 1. Infant must be awakened to feed.
 2. Has weak suck.
 3. May turn blue when eating, especially with cyanotic defects.
 4. Infant takes overly long time to feed.
 5. Falls asleep during feeding, without finishing.

C. Nursing observations
 1. *Most frequent symptom*—tachycardia, as body attempts to compensate for lack of oxygen (hypoxia), i.e., heart rate over 160 beats/min.
 2. Tachypnea, corresponding to heart rate, i.e., respirations over 60 breaths/min.
 3. Cyanosis due to hypoxia:
  a. Not with acyanotic defects (unless CHF is present).
  b. Always with cyanotic defects ("blue babies").
 4. Failure to grow at a normal rate, i.e.,

slow weight gain, height and weight below the norm due to difficulty feeding and hypoxia.
 5. Developmental delays related to weakened physical condition.
 6. Frequent respiratory infections associated with increased pulmonary blood flow or aspiration.
 7. Dyspnea on exertion due to hypoxia, shunting of blood.
 8. Murmurs may or may not be present, e.g., patent ductus arteriosus (PDA) machinery murmur.
 9. Changes in blood pressure, e.g., coarctation-increased blood pressure in arms; decreased blood pressure in legs.
 10. Possible congestive heart failure—refer to Unit 2. *Note:* Infants may *not* demonstrate distended neck veins.
 11. Cyanotic heart defects:
  a. *"Tet. spells"*—choking spells with paroxysmal dyspnea: severe hypoxia, deepening cyanosis; relieved by squatting, or placing infant in knee-chest position, which alters cardiopulmonary dynamics, thus increasing the flow of blood to the lungs.
  b. Clubbing of fingers and toes—due to chronic hypoxia.

■ **FIGURE 8.1** *Atrial septal defect (ASD).* A "hole in the heart," or an abnormal opening between the right and left atria. *White arrows,* unoxygenated blood; *solid arrows,* oxygenated blood; *speckled arrows,* mixed blood. (From Mott SR, Fazekas NF, James SR. *Nursing Care of Children and Families: A Holistic Approach.* Menlo Park, CA: Addison-Wesley, 1985, with permission.)

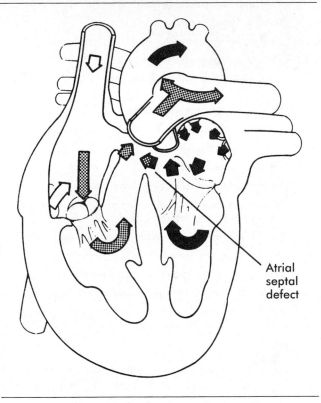

Atrial septal defect

■ **FIGURE 8.2** *Ventricular septal defect (VSD).* A "hole in the heart," or an abnormal opening between the right and left ventricles. *White arrows,* unoxygenated blood; *solid arrows,* oxygenated blood; *speckled arrows,* mixed blood. (From Mott SR, Fazekas NF, James SR. *Nursing Care of Children and Families: A Holistic Approach.* Menlo Park, CA: Addison-Wesley, 1985, with permission.)

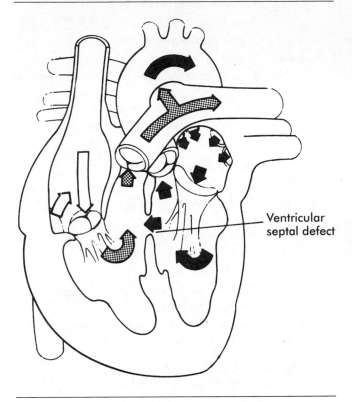

Ventricular septal defect

c. Polycythemia (↑ red blood cells [RBC]) with possible thrombi/emboli formation.

◆ **III. Analysis/nursing diagnosis:**

 A. *Ineffective breathing pattern* related to tachypnea and respiratory infection.

 B. *Activity intolerance* related to tachycardia and hypoxia.

 C. *Altered nutrition, less than body requirements,* related to difficulty in feeding.

 D. *Risk for infection* related to poor nutritional status.

 E. *Knowledge deficit* related to diagnostic procedures, condition, surgical/medical treatments, prognosis.

◆ **IV. Nursing care plan/implementation:**

 A. Goal: *promote adequate oxygenation.*

 1. Administer oxygen per physician's order/prn.

 2. Use loose-fitting clothing; pin diapers loosely to avoid pressure on abdominal organs, which could impinge on diaphragm and impede respiration.

 3. *Position:* neck slightly hyperextended to keep airway patent; place in knee-chest

(squatting) position to relieve "Tet. spell" (choking spell).

 4. Suction prn to clear the airway.

 5. Administer digoxin, per physician's order, to slow and strengthen heart's pumping action (refer to Unit 4 and to Table 8.1 for pediatric pulse rate norms).

 B. Goal: *reduce workload of heart to conserve energy.*

 1. *Position:* infant seat, semi-Fowler's to provide maximum expansion of the lungs.

 2. Provide pacifier to promote psychological rest.

 3. Organize nursing care to provide periods of uninterrupted rest.

 4. Adjust physical activity according to child's condition, capabilities to conserve energy.

 5. Provide diversion, as tolerated, to meet developmental needs yet conserve energy.

 6. Avoid extremes of temperature to avoid the stress of hypothermia/hyperthermia, which will increase the body's demand for oxygen.

 7. Administer diuretics (Lasix), per physician's order, to eliminate excess fluids,

■ **FIGURE 8.3** *Patent ductus arteriosus (PDA).* The ductus between the aorta and the pulmonary artery remains open (or patent). *White arrows,* unoxygenated blood; *solid arrows,* oxygenated blood; *speckled arrow,* mixed blood. (From Mott SR, Fazekas NF, James SR. *Nursing Care of Children and Families: A Holistic Approach.* Menlo Park, CA: Addison-Wesley, 1985, with permission.)

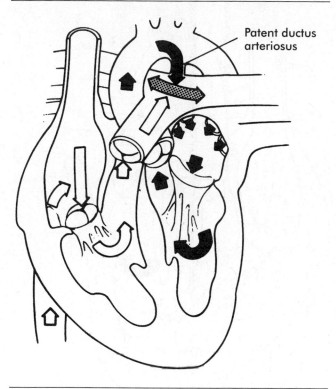

■ **FIGURE 8.4** *Coarctation of the aorta.* A narrowing of the lumen of the vessel (the aorta). *White arrows,* unoxygenated blood; *solid arrows,* oxygenated blood. (From Mott SR, Fazekas NF, James SR. *Nursing Care of Children and Families: A Holistic Approach.* Menlo Park, CA: Addison-Wesley, 1985, with permission.)

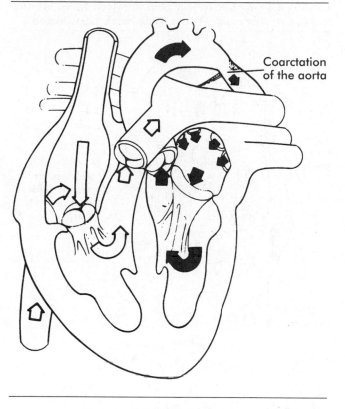

which increase the heart's workload. *Note:* Refer to Unit 4.

C. Goal: *provide for adequate nutrition.*
1. Offer *low-sodium* formula (Lonalac) to minimize fluid retention.
2. Discourage foods with high or added sodium to minimize fluid retention.
3. I&O, daily/weekly weights, and monitor for rate of growth.
▶ 4. Supplement PO feeding with gavage feeding (prn with physician's order) to meet fluid and caloric needs.
5. Encourage foods *high in potassium* (prevent hypokalemia) and *high in iron* (prevent anemia). *Note:* Refer to Unit 3.

D. Goal: *prevent infection.*
1. Universal precautions to prevent infection.
2. Use good handwashing technique.
3. Limit contact with staff/visitors with infections.
4. Monitor for early symptoms and signs of infection; report stat.

E. Goal: *meet teaching needs of patient, family.*
▶ 1. Explain diagnostic procedures: blood tests,

X rays, urine, ECG, echocardiogram, cardiac catheterization.
2. Explain condition/treatment/prognosis. Refer to Table 8.7.
3. Review dietary restrictions, medications.
4. Discuss how to adjust realistically to life with congenital heart disease, activity restrictions, etc.

◆ **V. Evaluation/outcome criteria:**
A. Child's level of oxygenation is maintained, as evidenced by pink color in nailbeds and mucous membranes (for both light- and dark-skinned children) and ease in respiratory effort.
B. Energy is conserved, thus reducing the heart's workload as evidenced by vital signs within normal limits.
C. The child's fluid and caloric requirements are met, allowing for physical growth to occur at normal or near-normal rate.
D. The family (and child, when old enough) verbalize their understanding of the type of CHD, its treatment and prognosis.
E. The family and child demonstrate adequate coping mechanisms to deal with CHD.

■ **FIGURE 8.5** *Tetralogy of Fallot.* **Four defects that occur together: ventricular septal defect, overriding aorta, pulmonic stenosis, right ventricular hypertrophy.** *White arrows,* **unoxygenated blood;** *solid arrows,* **oxygenated blood;** *speckled arrows,* **mixed blood. (From Mott SR, Fazekas NF, James SR.** *Nursing Care of Children and Families: A Holistic Approach.* **Menlo Park, CA: Addison-Wesley, 1985, with permission.)**

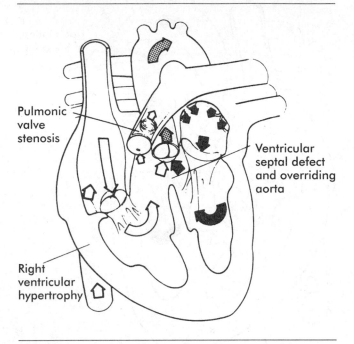

■ **FIGURE 8.6** *Transposition of the great arteries.* **The pulmonary artery arises from the left ventricle, and the aorta arises from the right ventricle.** *White arrows,* **unoxygenated blood;** *solid arrows,* **oxygenated blood. (From Mott SR, Fazekas NF, James SR.** *Nursing Care of Children and Families: A Holistic Approach.* **Menlo Park, CA: Addison-Wesley, 1985, with permission.)**

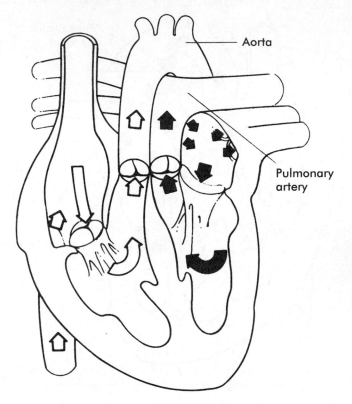

Disorders of the Blood

I. Leukemia

   A. *Introduction:* Known as "cancer of the blood," leukemia is the most common form of childhood cancer, with an incidence of 4/100,000. Acute leukemia is basically a malignant proliferation of white-blood-cell (WBC) precursors triggered by an unknown cause and affecting all blood-forming organs and systems throughout the body. The onset is typically insidious, and the disease is most common in preschoolers (age 2–6 yr), occurring more frequently in boys.

   ◆ **B. Assessment**

      1. Major problem—leukopenia: ↓ WBC/↑ blasts (overproduction of immature, poorly functioning white blood cells).

      2. Bone marrow dysfunction results in:

        a. *Neutropenia:* multiple prolonged infections.

        b. *Anemia:* pallor, weakness, irritability, shortness of breath.

        c. *Thrombocytopenia:* bleeding tendencies (petechiae, epistaxis, bruising).

      3. Infiltration of reticuloendothelial system (RES): hepatosplenomegaly → abdominal pain, lymphadenopathy.

      4. Leukemic invasion of CNS: ↑ ICP/leukemic meningitis.

      5. Leukemic invasion of bone: pain, pathologic fractures, hemarthrosis.

   ◆ **C. Analysis/nursing diagnosis:**

      1. *Risk for infection* related to neutropenia.

      2. *Risk for injury* related to thrombocytopenia.

      3. *Altered nutrition, less than body requirements,* related to loss of appetite, vomiting, mouth ulcers.

      4. *Pain* related to disease process and treatments (e.g., hemarthrosis, bone pain, bone marrow aspiration).

      5. *Activity intolerance* related to infection and anemia.

      6. *Self-esteem disturbance* related to disease process and treatments (e.g., loss of hair with chemotherapy, moon face with prednisone).

      7. *Anticipatory grieving* related to life-threatening illness.

      8. *Knowledge deficit* related to diagnosis, treatment, prognosis.

■ **TABLE 8.6   Comparison of Acyanotic and Cyanotic Heart Disease**

Feature	Acyanotic	Cyanotic
Shunting of blood	L → R	R → L
Cyanosis	Not usual (unless congestive heart failure)	Always; "blue babies"
Surgery	Usually done in one stage—technically simple	Usually done in several stages—technically complex
Prognosis	Very good/excellent	Guarded
Major types	1. ASD (atrial septal defect)	1. Tetralogy of Fallot
	2. VSD (ventricular septal defect)	2. Transposition of the great vessels
	3. PDA (patent ductus arteriosus)	
	4. Coarctation of the aorta	

◆ **D. Nursing care plan/implementation:**
1. Goal: *maintain infection-free state.*
   a. Universal precautions to prevent infection.
   b. Use good handwashing technique.
   c. Ongoing evaluation of sites for potential infection, e.g., gums.
   d. Provide meticulous oral hygiene.
   e. Keep record of vital signs, especially temperature.
   f. Provide good skin care.
   g. Screen staff and visitors—restrict anyone with infection.
   ▶ h. *Protective isolation / reverse isolation* to minimize exposure to potentially life-threatening infection.
   i. Discharge planning: return to school, but isolate from chickenpox or known communicable diseases.
2. Goal: *prevent injury.*
   a. Avoid IMs/IVs if possible, due to bruising and bleeding tendencies.
   b. Do *not* give aspirin or medications containing aspirin, which will interfere with platelet formation, thus increasing the risk of bleeding.
   c. Use soft toothbrush to avoid trauma to gums, which may cause bleeding and infection.
   d. *Avoid* "per rectum" suppositories, due to probable rectal ulcers.
   e. Supervise play/activity carefully to promote safety and prevent excessive bruising or bleeding.
3. Goal: *promote adequate nutrition.*
   a. *Diet:* high calorie, high protein, high iron.
   b. Encourage *extra fluids* to prevent constipation or dehydration.
   c. I&O, daily weights, to monitor fluid and nutritional status.
   d. Allow child to be involved with food selection/preparation; allow child almost any food he or she tolerates, to encourage better dietary intake.
   e. Serve frequent, small snacks to increase fluid and caloric consumption.
   f. Offer dietary supplements to increase caloric intake.
   g. Encourage local anesthetics such as throat lozenges (Chloraseptic) before meals to allow child to eat without pain from oral mucous membrane ulcers.
4. Goal: *relieve pain.*
   a. Offer supportive alternatives: extra company, back rub, etc.
   b. Administer medications, regularly, before pain becomes excessive.
   c. Use bean bag chair for positional changes.
   d. *Avoid* excessive stimulation (noise, light), which may heighten perception of pain.
5. Goal: *promote self-esteem.*
   a. Stress what child can still do to keep the child as independent as possible.
   b. Encourage performance of ADL as much as possible to foster a sense of independence.
   c. Provide diversion/activity as tolerated.
   d. Give lots of positive reinforcement to enhance a sense of accomplishment.
   e. Provide realistic feedback on child's appearance; offer suggestions, such as a wig or cap to cover alopecia secondary to chemotherapy.
   f. Encourage early return to peers/school to avoid social isolation.
6. Goal: *prevent complications related to leukemia / prolonged immobility / treatments.*
   a. Inspect skin for breakdown, especially over bony prominences, due to poor nutritional intake and limited mobility due to bone pain.
   b. Anticipate need for and provide (per physician's order) multiple transfusions of platelets, packed RBCs, etc.
   c. Check for hemorrhagic cystitis; push fluids (especially with cytoxan).

■ **TABLE 8.7 Overview of the Most Common Types of Congenital Heart Disease**

Type of Defect	Medical Treatment	Surgical Treatment	Prognosis
Acyanotic			
ASD (atrial septal defect)	May be closed using devices during cardiac catheterization	Open chest/open heart surgery with closure through patch (recommended age: preschooler).	Excellent, with survival greater than 99%
VSD (ventricular septal defect)	Clinical trials using device closure during cardiac catheterization	*Palliative treatment:* pulmonary banding; *definitive repair:* same as for ASD	Excellent, with 96–99% survival rate
PDA (patent ductus arteriosus)	In newborns—attempt pharmacologic closure with indomethacin (prostaglandin inhibitor)	Open chest: surgical ligation or division (recommended age: 1–2 yr)	Excellent with survival greater than 99%
Coarctation of the aorta	Infants or children with CHF: digitalis and diuretics	Open chest: resection of coarcted portion of aorta with end-to-end anastomosis within first 2 yr of life	Fair—less than 5% mortality
Cyanotic			
Tetralogy of Fallot	None—supportive prn	Often done in *stages* with definitive repair accomplished within first yr of life	Fair—less than 5% mortality
Transposition of the great vessels	None—supportive prn	Often done in *stages* with *definitive repair* within first yr of life.	Guarded—less than 5% mortality

d. Check for constipation or peripheral neuropathy (especially with vincristine). Refer to Unit 6 for specific information on chemotherapy.

7. Goal: *assist child and parents to cope with life-threatening illness.*
   a. Teach rationale for repeated hospitalizations, multiple invasive tests/treatments, long-term follow-up care.
   b. Encourage compliance with all aspects of therapy, to increase chances of survival.
   c. Support family and their coping mechanisms.
   d. Offer factual information regarding ultimate prognosis ("70% cure" for acute lymphocytic leukemia [ALL]).
   e. If death appears imminent, assist family to cope with dying and death.

◆ **E. Evaluation/outcome criteria:**
1. Child is maintained in infection-free state.
2. Injuries are prevented or kept to a minimum.
3. Adequate nutrition is maintained.
4. Child is free from pain or can live with minimum level of pain.
5. Child's self-esteem is maintained; child is treated as living (not dying).
6. Complications are prevented or kept to a minimum.
7. Child and family use positive coping mechanisms to deal with illness.

II. Sickle cell anemia
  A. *Introduction:* Sickle cell anemia is a congenital hemolytic anemia resulting from a defective hemoglobin (Hgb) molecule (hemoglobin S). It is most common in African Americans (8% have sickle cell trait) and in people of Mediterranean descent. The diagnosis is usually made during the toddler or preschool years, during the first crisis episode following an infection. There is also the need to differentiate between *sickle cell trait* (Sickledex test) and *sickle cell anemia* (hemoglobin electrophoresis). Sickle cell anemia has no known cure.

◆ **B. Assessment:**
1. Increased susceptibility to infection (cause: unknown; most common cause of death in children under 5).
2. Inherited as autosomal recessive disorder (see Figure 8.7).
3. Precipitated by conditions of low oxygen tension or dehydration.
4. Signs of anemia:
   a. Pallor (in dark-skinned children, do not rely on pallor alone—check hemoglobin [Hgb] and hematocrit [Hct]).
   b. Jaundice, due to excessive hemolysis.
   c. Irritability, lethargy, anorexia, malaise.
5. Vaso-occlusive crisis: severe pain (variable sites), fever, swelling of hands and feet, joint pain and swelling, all related to hypoxia, ischemia, and necrosis at the cellular level. Most common; non-life-threatening.

6. Splenic sequestration crisis: blood is sequestered (pooled) in spleen; precipitous drop in B/P, ↑ pulse, shock, and ultimately death from profound anemia and cardiovascular collapse.

◆ **C. Analysis/nursing diagnosis:**
1. *Altered tissue perfusion* related to anemia and occlusion of vessels.
2. *Pain* related to vaso-occlusion.
3. *Impaired physical mobility* related to pain, immobility.
4. *Knowledge deficit* related to disease process and treatment (e.g., prevention of sickling or infection; genetic counseling).

◆ **D. Nursing care plan/implementation:**
1. Goal: *prevent sickling.*
   a. *Avoid* conditions of low oxygen tension, which causes RBCs to assume a sickled shape.
   b. Provide continuous extra fluids to prevent dehydration, which causes sluggish circulation.
   c. *Avoid* activities that may result in overheating, to prevent dehydration; suggest appropriate clothes; limit time in sun.
   d. If dehydrated due to acute illness, supplement with IV fluids and additional oral fluids to reestablish fluid balance.
2. Goal: *maintain infection-free state.*
   a. Universal precautions to prevent infection.
   b. Use good handwashing technique.
   c. Evaluate carefully, check continually for potential infection sites, which may either lead to death due to sepsis or precipitate sickle cell crisis.
   d. Teach importance of prevention: adequate nutrition; frequent medical checkups; keep away from known sources of infection.
   e. Stress need to report early signs of infection promptly to physician.
   f. Need to balance prevention of infection with child's need for a "normal" life.
3. Goal: *provide supportive therapy during crisis.*
   a. Provide bedrest/hospitalization during crisis to decrease the body's demand for oxygen.
   b. Relieve pain by administering pain medications as ordered; handle gently and use proper positioning techniques.
   c. Apply heat (*never cold*) to affected painful areas to increase blood flow (vasodilation) and oxygen supply.
   ▶ d. Administer oxygen, as ordered, to relieve hypoxia and prevent further sickling.
   ▶ e. Administer blood transfusions, as ordered, to correct severe anemia.
   f. Monitor fluid and electrolyte balance: I&O, weight, electrolytes.

g. Perform ADL for child if unable to care for own needs; encourage self-care as soon as possible to promote independence.
4. Goal: *teach child and family about sickle cell anemia.*
   a. Provide factual information based on child's developmental level.
   b. When asked, offer information regarding prognosis (no known cure).
   c. Encourage child to live as normally as possible.
   d. Genetic screening and counseling (Figure 8.7).

◆ **E. Evaluation/outcome criteria:**
1. Sickling is prevented or kept to a minimum.
2. Child is maintained in infection-free state.
3. Child/family verbalize that they can cope adequately with crisis.
4. Child/family verbalize their understanding about disease, its management, and its prognosis.

III. Hemophilia

A. *Introduction:* Hemophilia is a bleeding disorder inherited as a sex-linked (X-linked) recessive trait; i.e., it occurs only in males but is transmitted by symptom-free female carriers (Figure 8.8). Hemophilia results in a deficiency of one or more clotting factors, and it is necessary to determine which clotting factor is deficient and to what extent. Classic hemophilia (hemophilia A), a lack of clotting factor VIII, accounts for 75% of all cases of hemophilia.

◆ **B. Assessment:**
1. Major problem is bleeding.
   a. In *newborn* male: abnormal bleeding from umbilical cord, prolonged bleeding from circumcision site.
   b. In *toddler* male: excessive bruising, possible intracranial bleeding, prolonged bleeding from cuts or lacerations.
   c. *General:* hemarthrosis, petechiae, epistaxis, frank hemorrhage anywhere in body, anemia.
2. Need to determine which clotting factor is deficient/missing and extent of deficiency:
   a. *Mild:* child has 5–50% of normal amount of clotting factor.
   b. *Moderate:* child has 1–5% of normal amount of clotting factor.
   c. *Severe:* child has less than 1% of normal amount of clotting factor.

◆ **C. Analysis/nursing diagnosis:**
1. *Risk for injury* related to bleeding tendencies.
2. *Pain* related to hemarthrosis.
3. *Impaired physical mobility* related to bleeding and pain.
4. *Knowledge deficit* related to home care and follow-up.

◆ **D. Nursing care plan/implementation:**

■ **FIGURE 8.7 Genetic transmission of sickle cell anemia.**

(A) Normal parent and parent who carries trait

	A	A
A	AA	AA
S	AS	AS

1:2 (or 2:4) chance offspring will carry trait.

(B) Two parents who carry trait

	A	S
A	AA	AS
S	AS	SS

1:4 chance offspring will be normal.
1:4 chance offspring will have sickle cell anemia.
1:2 (or 2:4) chance offspring will carry trait.

(C) Normal parent and parent with sickle cell anemia

	A	A
S	AS	AS
S	AS	AS

4:4 (100%) chance offspring will carry trait.

(D) Parent with sickle cell anemia and parent who carries trait

	A	S
S	AS	SS
S	AS	SS

1:2 chance offspring will carry trait.
1:2 chance offspring will have sickle cell anemia.

(E) Two parents with sickle cell anemia

	S	S
S	SS	SS
S	SS	SS

4:4 (100%) chance offspring will have sickle cell anemia.

Key AA = normal hemoglobin
     AS = sickle cell trait
     SS = sickle cell disease (anemia)

Note: The odds cited here are for *each* pregnancy.

■ **FIGURE 8.8 Genetic tranmission of hemophilia.**

(A) "Normal" male and female with trait

	X	Y
X*	X*X	X*Y
X	XX	XY

1:4 chance will be female with trait.
1:4 chance will be male with hemophilia.
1:2 (or 2:4) chance will be "normal" female/male.

(B) Male with hemophilia and "normal" female

	X*	Y
X	XX*	XY
X	XX*	XY

1:2 (or 2:4) chance will be female with trait.
1:2 (or 2:4) chance will be "normal" male.

(C) Male with hemophilia and female with trait

	X*	Y
X*	X*X*	X*Y
X	X*X	XY

1:2 (or 2:4) chance will be female with trait.
1:4 chance will be "normal" male.
1:4 chance will be male with hemophilia.

Key XY   = normal male
     X*Y = male with hemophilia
     XX   = normal female
     X*X = female carrying hemophilia trait
     X*X* = female with possible relative lack of
            clotting factor—*not* a true hemophiliac
            (von Willebrand's disease).

Note: The odds cited here are for *each* pregnancy.

1. Goal: *prevent injury and possible bleeding.*
   a. Provide an environment that is as safe as possible, e.g., toys with no sharp edges, child's safety scissors.
   b. Use soft toothbrush to prevent trauma to gums.
   c. When old enough to shave, use only electric razor (no straight-edge razors).
   d. *Avoid* IMs/IVs—but when absolutely necessary, treat as arterial puncture; that is, apply direct pressure to the site for at least 5 min after withdrawing needle.
   e. Do **not** use aspirin or medication containing aspirin (prolongs bleeding/clotting time).
2. Goal: *control bleeding episodes when they occur.*
   a. Local measures: apply direct pressure, elevate, apply ice (vasoconstriction), keep immobilized during acute bleeding episodes only. For epistaxis: child should sit up and lean slightly forward.
   b. Systemic measures: administer clotting factor (Factor VIII, cryoprecipitate) via IV infusion. *Note:* This is a blood product, so a transfusion reaction is possible.
3. Goal: *prevent long-term disability related to joint degeneration.*
   a. Keep immobilized during period of acute bleeding and for 24–48 h afterward to allow blood to clot and to prevent dislodging the clot.
   b. Begin passive range of motion as soon as possible after acute phase.
   c. Administer prescribed pain medications *before* physical therapy sessions.
   d. Begin prescribed exercise program, starting with passive range of motion (ROM) and gradually advancing to active ROM, then full exercise program, as tolerated, to maintain maximum joint function.
   e. **Avoid:** prolonged immobility, braces, splints—which can lead to permanent deformities and loss of mobility.
4. Goal: *promote independence in management of own care.*
   a. Encourage child to assume responsibility for choosing safe activities.
   b. Encourage child to attend regular school as much as possible; provide support through school nurse.
   c. Advise child to wear MedicAlert bracelet.
   d. Caution parents to avoid overprotecting child.
   e. Offer child chance to self-limit activities within appropriate limits (parents can offer guidance).
   f. Assist child to cope with life-threatening disorder with no known cure.

5. Goal: *health teaching.*
   a. Between 9–12 yr of age: child can be taught to self-administer clotting factor IV (before this, family can perform).
   b. As child enters adolescence: begin to discuss issues such as realistic vocations, insurance coverage, genetic transmission (see Figure 8.8).
- **E. Evaluation/outcome criteria:**
  1. Serious injuries are prevented; bleeding is kept to a minimum.
  2. Episodes of bleeding controlled by prompt, effective intervention.
  3. There are no long-term disabilities.
  4. Child is able to manage own care independently, with minimum supervision.

Pulmonary Disorders

I. Cystic fibrosis
A. *Introduction:* Cystic fibrosis is a generalized dysfunction of the exocrine glands that produces multisystem involvement. Although the disorder is inherited as an autosomal recessive defect, the basic biochemical defect is unknown. However, its probable cause is an alteration in a protein or an enzyme, e.g., pancreatic enzyme deficiency. The basic problem is one of *thick, sticky, tenacious mucous secretions that obstruct* the ducts of the exocrine glands, thus affecting their ability to function. Cystic fibrosis is found in all races and socioeconomic groups, although there is a significantly lower incidence in black Americans. It is a chronic disease with no known cure and guarded prognosis; median age at death is 27.6 yr.

- **B. Assessment:**
  1. Newborn: *meconium ileus.*
  2. Frequent, recurrent *pulmonary infections:* bronchitis, bronchopneumonia, pneumonia, and ultimately chronic obstructive pulmonary disease (COPD) due to mechanical obstruction of respiratory tract caused by thick, tenacious mucous gland secretions.
  3. *Malabsorption syndrome:* failure to gain weight, distended abdomen, thin arms and legs, lack of subcutaneous fat due to disturbed absorption of nutrients that results from the inability of pancreatic enzymes to reach intestinal tract.
  4. *Steatorrhea:* bulky, foul-smelling, frothy, fatty stools in increased amounts and frequency (predisposed to rectal prolapse).
  5. Parents may note that child *"tastes salty"* when kissed, due to excessive loss of sodium and chloride in sweat.
  6. *Sweat test* reveals high sodium and chloride levels in child's sweat, unique to children with cystic fibrosis.
  7. Sexual development
     a. *Male:* sterile (due to aspermia).

b. *Female:* difficulty conceiving and bearing children (due to increased viscosity of cervical mucus, which acts as a plug and mechanically blocks the entry of sperm).

◆ **C. Analysis/nursing diagnosis:**

1. *Ineffective breathing patterns* related to thick, viscid secretions.
2. *Altered nutrition, less than body requirements,* related to diarrhea and poor intestinal absorption of nutrients.
3. *Decreased cardiac output* related to COPD and decreased compliance of lungs.
4. *Activity intolerance* related to respiratory compromise.
5. *Self-esteem disturbance* related to body image changes.
6. *Knowledge deficit* related to disease process, treatments, medications, genetics.
7. *Noncompliance* (potential) related to complicated and prolonged treatment regimen.

◆ **D. Nursing care plan/implementation:**

1. Goal: *assist child to expectorate sputum.*
   - ▶ a. Perform postural drainage as prescribed: first thing in morning, between meals, before bedtime.
   - b. Administer nebulizer treatments, expectorants, mucolytics, bronchodilators.
   - c. Provide for exercises that promote position changes and keep sputum moving up and out.
   - d. Encourage high fluid intake to keep secretions liquefied.
   - e. Suction, administer oxygen prn.
2. Goal: *prevent infection.*
   - a. Universal precautions to prevent infection.
   - b. Evaluate carefully, check continually for potential infection (especially respiratory); report to physician promptly.
   - c. Limit contact with staff or visitors with infection.
   - d. Administer antibiotics as ordered, to treat respiratory infections and prevent overwhelming sepsis.
   - e. May be placed on prophylactic antibiotic therapy between episodes of infection.
   - f. Teach importance of prevention of infection at home: adequate nutrition, frequent medical check-ups, stay away from known sources of infection.
3. Goal: *maintain adequate nutrition.*
   - a. *Diet:* well balanced, high calorie and protein to prevent malnutrition.
   - b. Administer *pancreatic enzyme* (viokase, pancreatin) immediately before *every* meal and *every* snack to enhance the absorption of vital nutrients, especially fats.
   - c. If child is unable to swallow tablets, mix pancreatic enzyme powder with cold applesauce.
   - d. Administer water-miscible preparations of fat-soluble vitamins (A, D, E, K), multivitamins, and iron.
   - e. Encourage *extra salt* intake to compensate for excessive sodium losses in sweat.
   - f. Encourage *extra fluid* intake (e.g., Gatorade) to prevent dehydration/electrolyte imbalance.
   - g. Daily I&O and weights to monitor nutritional and hydration status.
   - h. Encourage child to assume gradually increasing responsibility for choosing own foods within dietary restrictions.
4. Goal: *teach child and family about cystic fibrosis.*
   - a. Discuss diagnostic procedures: sweat test, stool specimens.
   - b. Review multiple medications: use, effects, side/toxic effects.
   - c. Stress need to care for pulmonary systems (major cause of mortality/morbidity).
   - ▶ d. Teach various treatments: postural drainage, nebulizers, oxygen therapy, breathing exercise.
   - e. Encourage child to assume as much responsibility for own care as possible: medications, treatments, diet.
   - f. Promote development of healthy attitude toward disease/prognosis (no known cure).
   - g. Refer to appropriate community agencies for assistance with home care.
   - h. Assist with genetic counseling.
   - i. Discuss sexual concerns with adolescent.
5. Goal: *promote compliance with treatment regimen.*
   - a. Encourage child to verbalize anger or frustration at being "different"/body image alterations.
   - b. Suggest alternatives to postural drainage, e.g., yoga/standing on head.
   - c. Offer "rewards" for compliance: going swimming with friends or other types of peer activities.

◆ **E. Evaluation/outcome criteria:**

1. Child can clear own airway, expectorate sputum.
2. Child is maintained in infection-free state.
3. Adequate nutrition is maintained.
4. Child and family verbalize understanding of the disease.
5. Child complies with rigors of treatment.

II. Pediatric respiratory infections

◆ **A. Assessment:** general assessment of infant/child with respiratory distress. *Note:* Additional information about specific respiratory infections may be found in Table 8.8.

1. Restlessness—*earliest* sign of hypoxia.

■ **TABLE 8.8   Pediatric Respiratory Infections**

Name	Definition	Age Group	Etiology	Definitive Clinical Signs and Symptoms	Specifics of Treatment	Prognosis
Bronchiolitis	Acute viral infection of lower respiratory tract (small, low bronchioles), with resultant trapping of air	Infants 2–12 mo (peak at 2–5 mo)	Respiratory syncytial virus	Hyperinflation of alveoli Scattered areas of atelectasis Acute, severe respiratory distress for first 48–72 h, followed by rapid recovery	Supportive care during acute phase: ■ Hospitalization ■ Croup tent ■ Clear liquids	Exellent (less than 1% mortality)
Croup (acute spasmodic laryngitis)	Paroxysmal attacks (spasms of larynx)	6 mo–3 yr	Viral (possible allergy or psychogenic)	Most common onset at night Inspiratory stridor "Croupy" barking cough Dyspnea Anxiety	Teach parents—turn on hot water in bathroom and close door (steam) Common to treat at home	Excellent (but likely to recur)
LTB (laryngotracheo-bronchitis)	Acute infection of lower respiratory tract: larynx, trachea, and bronchi	Children less than 5 yr of age.	Viral (possible secondary bacterial infection)	Inspiratory stridor High fever Signs and symptoms of severe respiratory distress Hoarseness, progressing to aphonia and respiratory arrest without treatment	Hospitalization: ■ Tracheostomy set at bedside ■ Epinephrine/steroids ■ Antibiotics if cultures are positive	Good
Epiglottitis	Extremely acute, severe, and rapid, progressive swelling (due to infection) of epiglottis and surrounding tissue	2–5 yr	Bacterial (*H. influenzae* type b)	Abrupt onset—rapid progression Dyspnea, dysphagia Sit up/chin thrust/mouth open Thick muffled voice Cherry red, swollen epiglottis	*Do not* visualize epiglottis unless airway support is immediately available Will need endotracheal tube or tracheostomy for 24–48 h to maintain patent airway IV ampicillin for 10–14 d to treat bacterial infection IV corticosteroids (e.g., Solucortef) to reduce inflammation	Very good if detected and treated early

2. Difficulty sucking/eating—parents may state the infant or child has "poor appetite."

3. Expiratory grunt, flaring of nasal alae, retractions.

4. Changes in vital signs: fever, tachycardia, tachypnea.

5. Cough: productive/nonproductive.

6. Wheeze; expiratory/inspiratory.

7. Hoarseness or aphonic crying.

8. Dyspnea or prostration.

9. Dehydration—related to increase in sensible fluid loss and poor PO intake.

10. Color change (pallor, cyanosis)—*later* sign of respiratory distress.

◆ **B. Analysis/nursing diagnosis:**

1. *Ineffective airway clearance* related to infection and/or obstruction.

2. *Fluid volume deficit* related to excessive losses through normal routes, discomfort and inability to swallow.

3. *Anxiety* related to hypoxia.

4. *Risk for injury* related to spread of infection.

5. *Knowledge deficit* related to disease process, infection control, home care, and follow-up.

◆ **C. Nursing care plan/implementation:**

1. Goal: *relieve respiratory distress by reducing swelling and edema and liquefying secretions.*

▶ a. Environment: cool, high-humidity croup tent (Table 8.9).

b. Administer oxygen as ordered.

c. *Position:* semi-Fowler's or in infant seat to provide maximum expansion of the lungs; small blanket or diaper roll under neck to keep airway patent; change position at least q2h to prevent pooling of secretions.

▶ d. Suction/postural drainage prn.

e. Pin diapers loosely and use only loose-fitting clothing to avoid pressure on abdominal organs, which could impinge on diaphragm and impede respirations.

f. Administer medications: antibiotics, bronchodilators, steroids.

g. Monitor temperature q4h/prn; reduce fever with acetaminophen, cool sponges, hypothermia blanket.

2. Goal: *observe for potential respiratory failure related to exhaustion or complete airway obstruction.*

a. Place in room near nurses' station for maximum observation.

b. Monitor vital signs: q1h during acute phase, then q4h.

▶ c. Place emergency equipment near bedside prn: endotracheal tube, tracheostomy set.

d. Monitor closely for signs of impending respiratory failure: ↑ rapid, shallow respirations, progressive hoarseness/aphonia, deepening cyanosis.

e. Report adverse changes in condition stat to physician.

3. Goal: *maintain normal fluid balance.*

a. May be NPO initially to prevent aspiration.

b. IVs until severe distress subsides and child is able to suck and swallow.

c. Monitor hydration status: I&O, urine specific gravity, weight.

d. When resuming PO fluids—start with sips of clear liquids, advance slowly as tolerated: "Pedialyte," clear broth, Jell-O, popsicles, fruit juices, ginger ale, cola.

e. **Avoid** milk/milk products, which may cause increased mucous production.

4. Goal: *provide calm, secure environment.*

a. During acute distress: remain with child/family (do not leave unattended).

b. Keep crying to a minimum to prevent severe hypoxia and to reduce the body's demand for oxygen.

c. Avoid painful/intrusive procedures if possible.

d. Organize nursing care to provide planned periods of uninterrupted rest.

e. Allow parents to room-in, and encourage their participation in care of their child to keep the child relatively calm and reduce anxiety.

f. Allow child to keep favorite toy or security object.

5. Goal: *provide parents with teaching, as necessary.*

a. Short term: discuss equipment, treatments, procedures; offer frequent progress reports, answer parents' questions.

b. Long term: how to handle recurrences, how to check temperature at home, medications for fever, when to call physician about respiratory problem.

◆ **D. Evaluation/outcome criteria:**

1. No further evidence of respiratory distress.

2. Resumption of normal respiratory pattern.

3. Normal fluid balance maintained/restored.

4. Parents verbalize their concerns and express confidence in their ability to care for their child after discharge.

III. Apnea-related disorders

A. Apnea of infancy

1. *Introduction:* Apnea of infancy is the unexplained cessation of breathing for 20 sec or longer in an apparently healthy, full-term infant of more than 37 weeks' gestation. It is usually diagnosed by the second month of life and is generally thought to resolve during the first 12–15 mo of life. The exact cause is unknown. The association between apnea of infancy and sudden infant death syndrome (SIDS) is still controversial. However, infants experiencing signifi-

■ **TABLE 8.9   Nursing Care of the Child in a Croup Tent**

Nursing Actions	Rationale
1. Explain purpose of tent to parents and child; stress it is temporary, to make breathing easier	1. Relieves anxiety
2. Inspect tent for cracks, tears. Repair or replace prn	2. Leaks will allow oxygen to escape
3. Place unit at head of bed	3. Child's upper torso and head must be inside tent
4. Cover bed with rubber/plastic sheet	4. Keeps mattress dry
5. Apply extra linen to bed under tent	5. Absorbs extra dampness, wetness
6. Secure metal frame to bedspring, and fasten tent to frame	6. Prevents collapse of tent and keeps it open
7. Fill jar three-fourths with distilled *water*—check q4h	7. Provides *high humidity* to keep secretions moist and liquefied
8. Select "cool mode" by using the control switch	8. Provides *cool air* to reduce swelling and edema
9. Close zippers and tuck in edges tightly	9. Prevents loss of oxygen
10. "Flood" tent with oxygen for 5 min (flow rate = 15 L/min)	10. Raises oxygen concentration
11. Adjust flow rate per physician's order	11. Usual flow rate is 8–10 L/min to maintain 35–40% oxygen concentration
12. Use oxygen analyzer to check concentration at least q2h	12. Oxygen is a drug and must be given per physician's order
13. Place child in tent—stay with child	13. Relieves anxiety
14. Place folded towel/blanket around child's head; stockinette cap for infant's head	14. Keeps child dry and prevents heat loss
15. Cover child with blanket	15. Avoids chilling
16. Selection of toys: (a) Nonflammable (b) Items that can be wiped dry	16. (a) Oxygen is highly combustible (b) Avoids bacterial growth
17. Change child's clothes and bed linens frequently (q4h or prn)	17. High humidity in tent will cause moisture to collect on these items

cant apnea without a known cause are thought to be at high risk for SIDS and must be treated accordingly.

◆ 2. **Assessment:**
   a. Unexplained cessation of breathing (apnea) for 20 sec or longer.
   b. Bradycardia.
   c. Color change: cyanosis or pallor.
   d. Limp, hypotonic.
   ▲ e. Diagnostic tests including cardiopneumogram, pneumocardiogram, and polysomnography.

◆ 3. **Analysis/nursing diagnosis:**
   a. *Ineffective breathing patterns* related to apnea.
   b. *Anxiety, fear* related to apnea and threat of infant's death.
   c. *Knowledge deficit* regarding home care of infant on an apnea monitor and infant cardiopulmonary resuscitation (CPR).

◆ 4. **Nursing care plan/intervention:**
   a. Goal: *maintain effective breathing pattern.*
      (1) Apnea monitor on infant at all times, including at home.
      (2) Place in room near nurses' station for maximum observation with a nurse or parent present at all times.

   ▶ (3) Suction, oxygen, and resuscitation equipment readily available if needed.
      (4) Observe for apnea or bradycardia; note duration and associated symptoms—color change, change in muscle tone.
      (5) If apnea occurs, use gentle stimulation to start infant breathing again. If ineffective, begin CPR (Figures 8.9 to 8.11).
      (6) If suctioning is needed, do it gently for the shortest time and least number of times possible to maintain patent airway. *Note:* Repeated, vigorous suctioning is associated with periods of apnea.
      (7) *Position:* prone, to avoid regurgitation and apnea.
      (8) Feedings: smaller and more frequent; avoid overfeeding, which can lead to reflux and apnea.
   b. Goal: *teach parents how to care for their infant at home* (Table 8.10).
      (1) Thoroughly explain discharge plans to parents; encourage questions and discussion.
      (2) Begin teaching use of apnea monitor and infant CPR techniques sev-

■ **FIGURE 8.9** **Cardiopulmonary resuscitation (CPR) in infants, children, and adults: one-rescuer CPR.** (Modified from Chandra NC, Hazinski MF [eds]. *Textbook of Basic Life Support for Healthcare Providers.* Dallas: American Heart Association, 1994.) *If victim is breathing or resumes effective breathing, place in recovery position: (1) move head, shoulders, and torso simultaneously; (2) turn onto side; (3) leg not in contact with ground may be bent and knee moved forward to stabilize victim; (4) victim should not be moved in any way if trauma is suspected and should not be placed in recovery position if rescue breathing or CPR is required.

	Objectives	ACTIONS		
		Adult (> 8 yr)	**Child (1–8 yr)**	**Infant (< 1 yr)**
A. AIRWAY	1. Assessment: determine unresponsiveness.	Tap or gently shake shoulder.		
		Say, "Are you okay?"		Speak loudly.
	2. Get help.	Activate EMS.	Shout for help. If second rescuer available, have person activate EMS.	
	3. Position the victim.	Turn on back as a unit, supporting head and neck if necessary (4–10 sec).		
	4. Open the airway.	Head tilt/chin lift.		
B. BREATHING	5. Assessment: determine breathlessness.	Maintain open airway. Place ear over mouth, observing chest. Look, listen, feel for breathing (3–5 sec).*		
	6. Give 2 rescue breaths.	Maintain open airway.		
		Seal mouth to mouth.		Mouth to nose/mouth.
		Give 2 slow breaths. Observe chest rise. Allow lung deflation between breaths.		
		1½–2 sec each	1–1½ sec each	
	7. Option for obstructed airway.	a. Reposition victim's head. Try again to give rescue breaths.		
			b. Activate EMS.	
		c. Give 5 subdiaphragmatic abdominal thrusts (the Heimlich maneuver).		c. Give 5 back blows.
				c. Give 5 chest thrusts.
		d. Tongue-jaw lift and finger sweep.	d. Tongue-jaw lift, but finger sweep only if you see a foreign object.	
		If unsuccessful, repeat a, c, and d until successful.		
C. CIRCULATION	8. Assessment: determine pulselessness	Feel for carotid pulse with one hand; maintain head tilt with the other (5–10 sec).		Feel for brachial pulse: keep head-tilt.
CPR	Pulse absent: begin chest compressions: 9. Landmark check.	Run middle finger along bottom edge of rib cage to notch at center (top of sternum).		Imagine a line drawn between the nipples.
	10. Hand position.	Place index finger next to finger on notch.		Place 2–3 fingers on sternum. 1 finger's width below line. Depress ½–1 in.
		Two hands next to index finger. Depress 1½–2 in.	Heel of one hand next to index finger. Depress 1–1½ in.	
	11. Compression rate.	80–100/min	100/min	At least 100/min
	12. Compressions to breaths.	2 breaths to every 15 compressions	1 breath to every 5 compressions	
	13. Number of cycles.	4	20 (approximately 1 min)	
	14. Reassessment.	Feel for carotid pulse.		Feel for brachial pulse.
		If no pulse, resume CPR, starting with compressions.	If alone, activate EMS. If no pulse, resume CPR, starting with compressions.	
	Pulse present; not breathing: begin rescue breathing.	1 breath every 5 sec (12/min)	1 breath every 3 sec (20/min)	

■ **FIGURE 8.10   CPR in infants and children: two-rescuer CPR.** *Note:* Two-rescuer CPR for children ages 1 to 8 years can be performed similarly to that for adults with appropriate changes in chest compressions and ventilations. (Modified from Chandra NC, Hazinski MF [eds]. *Textbook of Basic Life Support for Healthcare Providers.* Dallas: American Heart Association, 1994.)

Step	Objective	Actions
1. AIRWAY	**One rescuer (ventilator):** assessment: determine unresponsiveness.	Tap or gently shake shoulder.
		Shout, "Are you okay?"
	Call for help.	Activate EMS.
	Position the victim.	Turn on back if necessary (4–10 sec).
	Open the airway.	Use a proper technique to open airway.
2. BREATHING	Assessment: determine breathlessness.	Look, listen, and feel (3–5 sec).
	Ventilate twice.	Observe chest rise: 1–1.5 sec/inspiration.
3. CIRCULATION	Assessment: determine pulselessness.	Feel for carotid pulse (5–10 sec).
	State assessment results.	Say, "No pulse."
	Other rescuer (compressor): get into position for compressions.	Hand, shoulders in correct position.
	Locate landmark notch.	Landmark check.
4. COMPRESSION/ VENTILATION CYCLES	**Compressor:** begin chest compressions.	Correct ratio compressions/ventilations: 5:1
		Compression rate: 80–100/min (5 compressions/3–4 sec).
		Say any helpful mnemonic.
		Stop compressing for each ventilation.
	Ventilator: ventilate after every 5th compression and check compression effectiveness. (Minimum of 10 cycles.)	Ventilate 1 time (1.5–2 sec/inspiration).
		Check pulse occasionally to assess compressions.
5. CALL FOR SWITCH	**Compressor:** call for switch when fatigued.	Give clear signal to change.
		Compressor completes 5th compression.
		Ventilator completes ventilation after 5th compression.
6. SWITCH	Simultaneously switch:	
	Ventilator: move to chest.	Move to chest.
		Become compressor.
		Get into position for compressions.
		Locate landmark notch.
	Compressor: move to head.	Move to head.
		Become ventilator.
		Check carotid pulse (5 sec).
		Say, "No pulse."
		Ventilate once (1.5–2 sec/inspiration).
7. CONTINUE CPR	Resume compression/ventilation cycles.	Resume Step 4.

■ **FIGURE 8.11** Procedures for cardiopulmonary resuscitation (A–H) and airway obstruction (I–K). (From Chandra NC, Hazinski MF [eds]. *Textbook of Basic Life Support for Healthcare Providers.* Dallas: American Heart Association, 1994.)

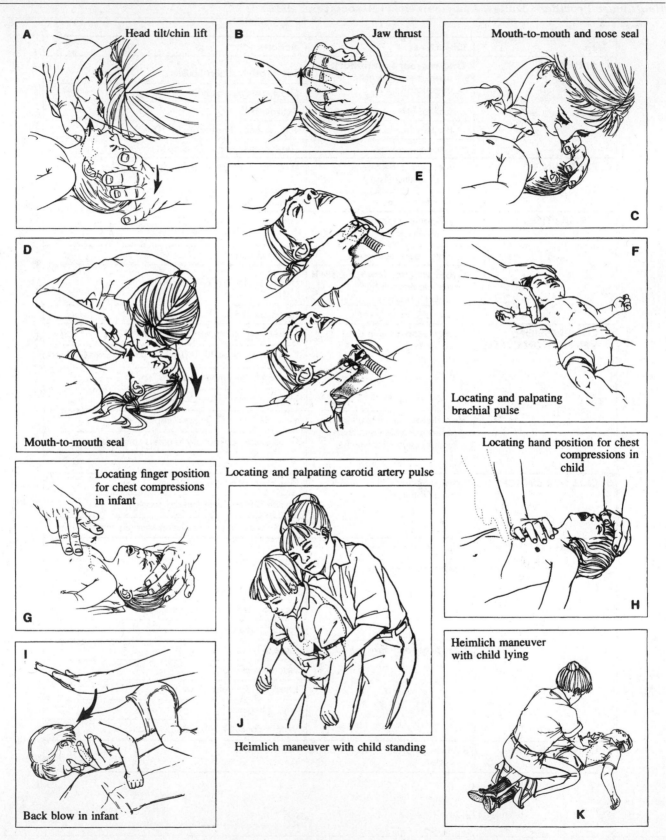

A Head tilt/chin lift

B Jaw thrust

Mouth-to-mouth and nose seal C

D Mouth-to-mouth seal

E

Locating and palpating brachial pulse F

Locating finger position for chest compressions in infant G

Locating and palpating carotid artery pulse

Locating hand position for chest compressions in child H

I Back blow in infant

Heimlich maneuver with child standing J

Heimlich maneuver with child lying K

eral days before discharge; allow parents to handle the monitor and become thoroughly familiar with its use.

(3) Provide parents with emergency response numbers and PHN referral.

(4) Stress need for at least *1 yr of ongoing care* with constant use of monitor.

(5) Discuss need for support and refer to local self-help/support group.

(6) Encourage parents to take time for themselves if a reliable caregiver is available who is trained in use of monitor and infant CPR.

◆ 5. **Evaluation/outcome criteria:**
   a. Effective breathing pattern is established.
   b. Parents verbalize their concerns and express confidence in their ability to care for their infant at home.

B. **Sudden infant death syndrome**
   1. *Introduction:* SIDS is the *sudden, unexpected* death of an apparently healthy infant under 1 yr of age, which remains *unexplained* after a complete postmortem examination. Various theories have been suggested, none proved; research is ongoing. It is the leading cause of death be-

tween 1 mo and 1 yr, affecting 7000 infants annually.

◆ 2. **Assessment:**
   a. Sudden, unexplained death in otherwise "normal" infant; occurs exclusively during sleep.
   b. Note overall appearance of infant (differentiate from child abuse).
   c. Obtain history from parents—note affect or how parents are dealing with grief.

◆ 3. **Analysis/nursing diagnosis:**
   a. *Dysfunctional grieving* related to loss of infant.
   b. *Knowledge deficit* related to SIDS.

◆ 4. **Nursing care plan/implementation:**
   a. *Immediate goal:* support grieving parents.
      (1) Stress that nothing could have been done to prevent the death.
      (2) Allow parents to express grief emotions; provide privacy.
      (3) Offer parents opportunity to see, hold infant.
      (4) Explain purpose of autopsy (physician to obtain consent).
      (5) Contact spiritual advisor: priest, rabbi, minister.
      (6) Assist parents to plan what to tell siblings.
   b. *Ongoing goal:* provide factual information regarding SIDS.
      (1) Offer information that is known about SIDS in simple, direct terms (Table 8.11).
      (2) Answer questions honestly.
      (3) Give parents printed literature on SIDS.

■ **TABLE 8.10   Guidelines for Home Care of Infant on Apnea Monitor**

1. Show the parents how to connect the monitor leads

2. Remind parents to remove the leads unless they are connected to the infant

3. Stress that the infant must be on the monitor whenever respirations are not being directly observed and that a trained person must be present in the home at all times in case the alarm sounds

4. Teach parents **not** to adjust the monitor to eliminate false alarms

5. Explain that the infant will need direct observation whenever loud noises could obscure the monitor alarm, e.g., dishwasher, vacuum

6. Teach parents what to look for when the alarm sounds, i.e., loose monitor leads vs. apnea

7. Teach parents how to assess the infant for an episode of apnea, i.e., lack of respirations, duration, color, muscle tone

8. Teach the parents to first use gentle physical stimulation if the infant experiences an apnea spell, e.g., touching the face or stroking the soles of the feet

9. Demonstrate infant CPR to be used if tactile stimulation is not effective in reestablishing respirations

10. Encourage parents to keep emergency numbers posted near the telephone

11. Explain that monitor will not interfere with normal growth and development. Encourage the parents to promote normal growth and development as much as possible

■ **TABLE 8.11   SIDS: What To Tell Families**

Concern	Facts
Etiology	Unknown (possibly related to delayed maturation of cardiorespiratory system)
Incidence	7000 cases annually; leading cause of death between ages of 1 mo and 1 yr
When	Occurs during *sleep* (nap, night)
Age	Peak at 2–4 mo; 95% of cases occur by age *6 mo*
Sex	More common in boys
Race	More common in blacks & Native Americans
Season	More common in *winter,* peaks in January
Siblings	May have greater incidence
Perinatal	More common in preterm infants, in *multiple* births, and in infants with *low Apgar scores*
Socioeconomic	More common in lower classes
Feeding habits	Lower incidence in breastfed infants

(4) Refer to local/national SIDS foundation group.

  c. *Long-term goal:* assist family to resolve grief.

    (1) Track progress of other siblings.

    (2) Refer to local perinatal bereavement group.

    (3) Consider subsequent pregnancy to be at risk for:

      (a) Attachment/bonding.

      (b) SIDS recurrence.

◆ **5. Evaluation/outcome criteria:**

  a. Parents are able to express their grief and receive adequate support.

  b. Parents raise questions about SIDS and can understand answers.

  c. Family's grief is resolved; in time, normal family dynamics resume.

❏ Disorders Affecting Protective Functions

Immunity and Communicable Diseases

I. Recommended schedule for active immunization of healthy infants and children (Table 8.12).

II. Side effects of immunizations and nursing care (Table 8.13).

III. Contraindications/precautions to immunizations

  A. Child who has a severe febrile illness (e.g., upper respiratory infection (URI), gastroenteritis, or any fever).

  B. Child with alteration in skin integrity: rash, eczema.

  C. Child with alteration in immune system; steroids; chemotherapy, radiation therapy; human immunodeficiency virus (HIV)/acquired immunodeficiency syndrome (AIDS) (no live virus vaccine).

  D. Child with a known allergic reaction to previous immunization or substance in the immunization.

IV. Childhood communicable diseases (Table 8.14). Basic principles of care:

  A. Universal precautions to prevent communicability/infection.

  B. Fever control.

  C. Extra fluids for hydration.

  D. General home care procedures.

Reye's Syndrome

I. *Introduction:* Reye's syndrome, first described as a disease entity in the mid 1960s, is a multisystem disorder primarily affecting children between 6 and 12 years of age. Although **not** truly a "communicable disease," studies have confirmed a relationship between aspirin administration during a viral illness (e.g., chickenpox, flu) and the onset of Reye's syndrome. The exact cause remains unknown. Reye's syndrome is characterized by acute metabolic encephalopathy and fatty degeneration of the visceral organs, particularly the liver. Earlier diagnosis, more sophisticated monitoring equipment, and more aggressive treatment have greatly improved the survival rate of children with Reye's syndrome; recovery is generally rapid in those children who do survive.

◆**II. Assessment:**

  A. Onset typically follows a viral illness, just as child appears to be recovering.

  B. *Early signs and symptoms:*

    1. Rapidly progressing behavioral changes: irritability, agitation, combativeness, hostility, confusion, apathy, lethargy.

    2. Vomiting, which becomes progressively worse.

  C. Rapidly progressive neurologic deterioration:

    1. Cerebral edema and increased intracranial pressure.

■ **TABLE 8.12**   **Recommended Childhood Immunization Schedule**

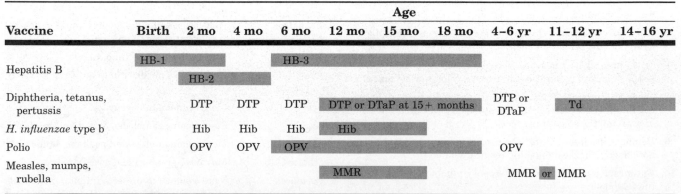

Vaccine	Birth	2 mo	4 mo	6 mo	12 mo	15 mo	18 mo	4–6 yr	11–12 yr	14–16 yr
Hepatitis B	HB-1	HB-2		HB-3						
Diphtheria, tetanus, pertussis		DTP	DTP	DTP	DTP or DTaP at 15+ months			DTP or DTaP	Td	
H. influenzae type b		Hib	Hib	Hib	Hib					
Polio		OPV	OPV	OPV				OPV		
Measles, mumps, rubella					MMR				MMR or MMR	

Note: Vaccines are listed under the routinely recommended ages. Shaded bars indicate range of acceptable ages for vaccination.
The Advisory Committee on Immunization Practices, the American Academy of Pediatrics, and the American Academy of Family Physicians have unified their schedules and simplified what parents and health care professionals should know to ensure children are appropriately vaccinated. A summary can be found in the Centers for Disease Control and Prevention's Jan. 6, 1995, issue of the *Morbidity and Mortality Weekly Report.*

■ **TABLE 8.13 Possible Side Effects of Recommended Childhood Immunizations and Nursing Responsibilities**

Immunization	Assessment: Side Effects	Nursing Responsibilities
Hepatitis B virus	Well tolerated, few side effects	Explain to parents reason for this immunization Consider that cost for three injections may be a factor
Diphtheria	Fever usually within *24–48 h* *Soreness, redness, and swelling* at injection site *Behavioral changes:* drowsiness, fretfulness, anorexia, prolonged or unusual crying	Nursing responsibilities for DTP apply to immunizations for diphtheria, tetanus, and pertussis Instruction for DTP: advise parents of possible side effects
Tetanus	Same as for diphtheria but may include urticaria and malaise All may have delayed onset and last several days *Lump at injection site* may last for weeks, even months, but gradually disappears	Recommend prophylactic use of *acetaminophen* at time of DTP immunization and every 4–6 h for a total of three doses Advise parents to notify practitioner *immediately* of any unusual side effects Before administering next dose of DTP, inquire about reactions
Pertussis	Same as for tetanus but may include loss of consciousness, *convulsions, persistent inconsolable* crying episodes, generalized or focal *neurologic signs,* fever (temperature at or above *40.5°C [105°F]*), systemic allergic reaction	
H. influenzae type b	Mild local reactions (erythema, pain) at injection site Low-grade fever	Advise parents of possible mild side effects
Poliovirus (OPV)	Essentially no immediate side effects Vaccine-associated paralysis rarely occurs within 2 mo of immunization (estimated risk 1:7.8 million doses); more likely to occur in close contact than in OPV recipient	Assess presence of family members *at risk* from trivalent OPV because of immune deficiency states
Measles	Anorexia, malaise, rash, and fever may occur *7–10 d after* immunization Rarely (estimated risk 1:1 million doses), encephalitis may occur	Advise parents of more common side effects and use of *antipyretics* for fever If a persistent fever with other obvious signs of illness occur, have them notify physician immediately
Mumps	Essentially no side effects other than a brief, mild fever	See general comment to parents
Rubella	Fever, lymphadenopathy, or mild *rash* that lasts 1–2 d within a few d after immunization Arthralgia, arthritis, or paresthesia of the hands and fingers may occur about 2 wk *after* vaccination and is more common in *older* children and adults	Advise parents of side effects, especially of time delay before *joint swelling and pain;* assure them that these symptoms will disappear May recommend use of acetaminophen for pain

Source: Wong D. *Whaley and Wong's Nursing Care of Infants and Children* (5th ed). St. Louis: Mosby, 1995. P 557.

2. Alteration in level of consciousness from lethargy through coma, decerebrate posturing, and respiratory arrest.
D. Liver dysfunction, necrosis, and failure:
⚑ 1. Elevated serum alanine aminotransferase (ALT) (serum glutamic-oxaloacetic transaminase [SGOT]), aspartate aminotransferase (AST) (serum glutamate pyruvate transaminase [SGPT]), lactate dehydrogenase (LDH), serum-ammonia levels.
2. Severe hypoglycemia.
3. Increased prothrombin time, coagulation defects, and bleeding.

◆ **III. Analysis/nursing diagnosis:**
A. *Altered cerebral tissue perfusion* related to cerebral edema and increased intracranial pressure.
B. *Altered hepatic tissue perfusion* related to fatty degeneration of the liver.
C. *Risk for injury* related to coagulation defects and bleeding.
D. *Knowledge deficit* related to diagnosis, course of disease, treatment, and prognosis.
◆ **IV. Nursing care plan/implementation:**
A. Goal: *reduce intracranial pressure.*

■ **TABLE 8.14   Communicable Diseases of Childhood**

Disease	Clinical Manifestations	Therapeutic Management/ Complications	Nursing Considerations
Chickenpox (Varicella) Agent: Varicella zoster virus (VZV) Source: Primary secretions of respiratory tract of infected persons; to a lesser degree skin lesions (scabs not infectious) Transmission: Direct contact, droplet (airborne) spread, and contaminated objects Incubation period: 2–3 wk, usually 13–17 d Period of communicability: Probably 1 d before eruption of lesions (prodromal period) to 6 d after first crop of vesicles when crusts have formed	Prodromal stage: Slight fever, malaise, and anorexia for first 24 h; rash highly pruritic; begins as macule, rapidly progresses to papule and then vesicle (surrounded by erythematous base, becomes umbilicated and cloudy, breaks easily and forms crusts); all three stages (papule, vesicle, crust) present in varying degrees at one time Distribution: Centripetal, spreading to face and proximal extremities but sparse on distal limbs and less on areas not exposed to heat (i.e., from clothing or sun) Constitutional signs and symptoms: Elevated temperature from lymphadenopathy, irritability from pruritus	Specific: Antiviral agent acyclovir (Zovirax); varicella-zoster immune globulin (VZIG) after exposure in high-risk children Supportive: Diphenhydramine hydrochloride or antihistamines to relieve itching; skin care to prevent secondary bacterial infection Complications: Secondary bacterial infections (abscesses, cellulitis, pneumonia, sepsis) Encephalitis Varicella pneumonia Hemorrhagic varicella (tiny hemorrhages in vesicles and numerous petechiae in skin) Chronic or transient thrombocytopenia	Maintain strict isolation in hospital Isolate child in home until vesicles have dried (usually 1 wk after onset of disease), and isolate high-risk children from infected children Administer skin care: give bath and change clothes and linens daily; administer topical application of calamine lotion; keep child's fingernails short and clean; apply mittens if child scratches Keep child cool (may decrease number of lesions) Lessen pruritus; keep child occupied Remove loose crusts that rub and irritate skin Teach child to apply pressure to pruritic area rather than scratching it If older child, reason with child regarding danger of scar formation from scratching Avoid use of aspirin; use of acetaminophen controversial
Diphtheria Agent: Corynebacterium diphtheriae Source: Discharges from mucous membranes of nose and nasopharynx, skin, and other lesions of infected person Transmission: Direct contact with infected person, a carrier, or contaminated articles Incubation period: Usually 2–5 d, possibly longer Period of communicability: Variable; until virulent bacilli are no longer present (identified by three negative cultures); usually 2 wk but as long as 4 wk	Vary according to anatomic location of pseudomembrane Nasal: Resembles common cold, serosanguineous mucopurulent nasal discharge without constitutional symptoms; may be frank epistaxis Tonsillar/pharyngeal: Malaise; anorexia; sore throat; low-grade fever; pulse increased above expected for temperature within 24 h; smooth, adherent, white or gray membrane; lymphadenitis possibly pronounced (bull's neck); in severe cases, toxemia, septic shock, and death within 6–10 d Laryngeal: Fever, hoarseness, cough, with or without previous signs listed; potential airway obstruction, apprehensive, dyspneic retractions, cyanosis	Antitoxin (usually IV); preceded by skin or conjunctival test to rule out sensitivity to horse serum Antibiotics (penicillin or erythromycin) Complete bedrest (prevention of myocarditis) Tracheostomy for airway obstruction Treatment of infected contacts and carriers Complications: Myocarditis (second wk) Neuritis	Maintain strict isolation in hospital Participate in sensitivity testing; have epinephrine available Administer antibiotics; observe for signs of sensitivity to penicillin Administer complete care to maintain bedrest Use suctioning as needed Observe respirations for signs of obstruction Administer humidified oxygen if prescribed

Erythema Infectiosum (Fifth Disease)

Agent: Human parvovirus B19 (HPV)

Source: Infected persons

Transmission: Unknown; possibly respiratory secretions and blood

Incubation period: 4–14 d, may be as long as 20 d

Period of communicability: Uncertain but before onset of symptoms in most children; also for about 1 wk after onset of symptoms in children with aplastic crisis

Rash appears in three stages:

I—Erythema on face, chiefly on cheeks, "slapped face" appearance; disappears by 1–4 d

II—About 1 d after rash appears on face, maculopapular red spots appear, symmetrically distributed on upper and lower extremities; rash progresses from proximal to distal surfaces and may last a week or more

III—Rash subsides but reappears if skin is irritated or traumatized (sun, heat, cold, friction)

In children with aplastic crisis, rash is usually absent and prodromal illness includes fever, myalgia, lethargy, nausea, vomiting, and abdominal pain

Symptomatic and supportive: Antipyretics, analgesics, anti-inflammatory drugs; possible blood transfusion for transient aplastic anemia

Complications:

Self-limited arthritis and arthralgia (arthritis may become chronic)

May result in fetal death if mother infected during pregnancy, but no evidence of congenital anomalies

Aplastic crisis in children with hemolytic disease or immune deficiency

Myocarditis (rare)

Isolation of child not necessary, except hospitalized child (immunosuppressed or with aplastic crises) suspected of HPV infection is placed on respiratory isolation and universal precautions

Pregnant women: need not be excluded from workplace where HPV infection is present; should not care for patients with aplastic crises; explain low risk of fetal death to those in contact with affected children

Exanthema Subitum (Roseola)

Agent: Human herpesvirus type 6 (HHV-6)

Source: Unknown

Transmission: Unknown (virtually limited to children between 6 mo–2 yr of age)

Incubation period: Unknown

Period of communicability: Unknown

Persistent high fever for 3–4 d in child who appears well

Precipitous drop in fever to normal with appearance of rash

Rash: Discrete rose-pink macules or maculopapules appearing first on trunk, then spreading to neck, face, and extremities; nonpruritic, fades on pressure, lasts 1–2 d

Associated signs and symptoms: Cervical/postauricular lymphadenopathy, injected pharynx, cough, coryza

Nonspecific

Antipyretics to control fever

Complications:

Recurrent febrile seizures (possibly from latent infection of CNS that is reactivated by fever)

Encephalitis (rare)

Teach parents measures for lowering temperature (antipyretic drugs)

If child is prone to seizures, discuss appropriate precautions, possibility of recurrent febrile seizures

Measles (Rubeola)

Agent: Virus

Source: Respiratory tract secretions, blood, and urine of infected person

Transmission: Usually by direct contact with droplets of infected person

Incubation period: 10–20 d

Period of communicability: From 4 d before to 5 d after rash appears but mainly during prodromal (catarrhal) stage

Prodromal (catarrhal) stage: Fever and malaise, followed in 24 h by coryza, cough, conjunctivitis, Koplik spots (small, irregular red spots with a minute, bluish white center first seen on buccal mucosa opposite molars 2 d before rash); symptoms gradually increase in severity until second d after rash appears, when they begin to subside

Rash: Appears 3–4 d after onset of prodromal stage; begins as erythematous maculopapular eruption on face and gradually spreads downward; more severe in earlier sites (appears confluent) and less intense in later sites (appears discrete); after 3–4 d assumes brownish appearance, and fine desquamation occurs over areas of extensive involvement

Constitutional signs and symptoms: Anorexia, malaise, generalized lymphadenopathy

Vitamin A supplementation

Supportive: Bedrest during febrile period; antipyretics

Antibiotics to prevent secondary bacterial infection in high-risk children

Complications:

Otitis media

Pneumonia

Bronchiolitis

Obstructive laryngitis and laryngotracheitis

Encephalitis

Isolation until fifth d of rash; if hospitalized, institute respiratory precautions

Maintain bedrest during prodromal stage; provide quiet activity

Fever: Instruct parents to administer antipyretics; avoid chilling; if child is prone to seizures, institute appropriate precautions (fever spikes to 40°C [104°F] between fourth and fifth d)

Eye care: Dim lights if photophobia present; clean eyelids with warm saline solution to remove secretions or crusts; keep child from rubbing eyes; examine cornea for signs of ulceration

Coryza/cough: Use cool mist vaporizer; protect skin around nares with layer of petrolatum; encourage fluids and soft, bland foods

Skin care: Keep skin clean; use tepid baths as necessary

continued

■ **TABLE 8.14**   *(Continued)*

Disease	Clinical Manifestations	Therapeutic Management/Complications	Nursing Considerations
Mumps Agent: Paramyxovirus Source: Saliva of infected persons Transmission: Direct contact with or droplet spread from an infected person Incubation period: 14–21 d Period of communicability: Most communicable immediately before and after swelling begins	Prodromal stage: Fever, headache, malaise, and anorexia for 24 h, followed by "earache" that is aggravated by chewing Parotitis: By third d, parotid gland(s) (either unilateral or bilateral) enlarges and reaches maximum size in 1–3 d; accompanied by pain and tenderness Other manifestations: Submaxillary and sublingual infection, orchitis, and meningoencephalitis	Symptomatic and supportive: Analgesics for pain and antipyretics for fever Intravenous fluid may be necessary for child who refuses to drink or vomits because of meningoencephalitis Complications: Sensorineural deafness Postinfectious encephalitis Myocarditis Arthritis Hepatitis Epididymo-orchitis Sterility (extremely rare in adult males)	Isolation during period of communicability; institute respiratory precautions during hospitalization Maintain bedrest during prodromal phase until swelling subsides Give analgesics for pain; if child is unwilling to chew medication, use elixir form Encourage fluids and soft, bland foods; avoid foods requiring chewing Apply hot or cold compresses to neck, whichever is more comforting To relieve orchitis, provide warmth and local support with tight-fitting underpants (stretch bathing suit works well)
Pertussis (Whooping Cough) Agent: *Bordetella pertussis* Source: Discharge from respiratory tract of infected persons Transmission: Direct contact or droplet spread from infected person; indirect contact with freshly contaminated articles Incubation period: 5–21 d, usually 10 d Period of communicability: Greatest during catarrhal stage before onset of paroxysms and may extend to fourth week after onset of paroxysms	Catarrhal stage: Begins with symptoms of upper-respiratory tract infection, such as coryza, sneezing, lacrimation, cough, and low-grade fever; symptoms continue for 1–2 wk, when dry, hacking cough becomes more severe Paroxysmal stage: Cough most often occurs at night and consists of short, rapid coughs followed by sudden inspiration associated with a high-pitched crowing sound or "whoop", during paroxysms cheeks become flushed or cyanotic, eyes bulge, and tongue protrudes; paroxysm may continue until thick mucous plug is dislodged; vomiting frequently follows attack; stage generally lasts 4–6 wk, followed by convalescent stage	Antimicrobial therapy (e.g., erythromycin) Administration of pertussis-immune globulin Supportive treatment: Hospitalization required for infants, children who are dehydrated, or those who have complications Bedrest Increased oxygen intake and humidity Adequate fluids Intubation possibly necessary Complications: Pneumonia (usual cause of death) Atelectasis Otitis media Convulsions Hemorrhage (subarachnoid, subconjunctival, epistaxis) Weight loss and dehydration Hernia Prolapsed rectum	Isolation during catarrhal stage; if hospitalized, institute respiratory precautions Maintain bedrest as long as fever present Keep child occupied during d (interest in play associated with fewer paroxysms) Reassure parents during frightening episodes of whooping cough Provide restful environment and reduce factors that promote paroxysms (dust, smoke, sudden change in temperature, chilling, activity, excitement); keep room well ventilated Encourage fluids; offer small amount of fluids frequently; refeed child after vomiting Provide high humidity (humidifier or tent); suction gently but often to prevent choking on secretions Observe for signs of airway obstruction (increased restlessness, apprehension, retractions, cyanosis) Involve public health nurse if child cared for at home

Poliomyelitis

Agent: Enteroviruses, three types: type 1—most frequent cause of paralysis, both epidemic and endemic; type 2—least frequently associated with paralysis; type 3—second most frequently associated with paralysis

Source: Feces and oropharyngeal secretions of infected persons, especially young children

Transmission: Direct contact with persons with apparent or inapparent active infection; spread is by *fecal-oral* and *pharyngeal-oropharyngeal* routes

Incubation period: Usually 7–14 d, with range of 5–35 d

Period of communicability: Not exactly known; virus is present in throat and feces shortly after infection and persists for about 1 wk in throat and 4–6 wk in feces

May be manifested in three different forms:

Abortive or inapparent—Fever, uneasiness, sore throat, headache, anorexia, vomiting, abdominal pain; lasts a few h to a few d

Nonparalytic—Same manifestations as abortive but more severe, with pain and stiffness in neck, back, and legs

Paralytic—Initial course similar to nonparalytic type, followed by recovery and then signs of central nervous system paralysis

No specific treatment, including antimicrobials or gamma globulin

Complete bedrest during acute phase

Assisted respiratory ventilation in case of respiratory paralysis

Physical therapy for muscles following acute stage

Complications:

Permanent paralysis

Respiratory arrest

Hypertension

Kidney stones from demineralization of bone during prolonged immobility

Maintain *complete bedrest*

Administer mild sedatives as necessary to relieve anxiety and promote rest

Participate in *physiotherapy* procedures (use of moist hot packs and range-of-motion exercises)

Position child to maintain body alignment and prevent contractures or decubiti; use footboard

Encourage child to move; administer analgesics for maximum comfort during physical activity

Observe for *respiratory paralysis* (difficulty in talking, ineffective cough, inability to hold breath, shallow and rapid respirations); report such signs and symptoms to physician; have tracheostomy tray at bedside

Rubella (German Measles)

Agent: Rubella virus

Source: Primarily nasopharyngeal secretions of person with apparent or inapparent infection; virus also present in blood, stool, and urine

Transmission: Direct contact and spread from infected person; indirectly through articles freshly contaminated with *nasopharyngeal secretions, feces, or urine*

Incubation period: 14–21 d

Period of communicability: 7 d before to about *5 d* after appearance of *rash*

Prodromal stage: Absent in children, present in adults and adolescents; consists of low-grade fever, headache, malaise, anorexia, mild conjunctivitis, coryza, sore throat, cough, and lymphadenopathy; lasts for 1–5 d, subsides 1 d after appearance of rash

Rash: First appears on face and rapidly spreads downward to neck, arms, trunk, and legs; by end of first d body is covered with a discrete, pinkish red maculopapular exanthema; disappears in same order as it began and is usually gone by third day

Constitutional signs and symptoms: Occasionally low-grade fever, headache, malaise, and lymphadenopathy

No treatment necessary other than antipyretics for low-grade fever and analgesics for discomfort

Complications:

Rare (arthritis, encephalitis, or purpura; most benign of all childhood communicable diseases; greatest danger is teratogenic effect on fetus

Reassure parents of benign nature of illness in affected child

Employ comfort measures as necessary

Isolate child from *pregnant* women

continued

■ **TABLE 8.14** (*Continued*)

Disease	Clinical Manifestations	Therapeutic Management/ Complications	Nursing Considerations
Scarlet Fever Agent: Group A beta-hemolytic streptococci Source: Usually from nasopharyngeal secretions of infected persons and carriers Transmission: *Direct* contact with infected person or *droplet* spread; *indirectly* by contact with contaminated articles, ingestion of *contaminated milk* or *other food* Incubation period: 2–4 d, with range of 1–7 d Period of communicability: During incubation period and clinical illness approximately 10 d; during first 2 wk of carrier phase, although may persist for months	Prodromal stage: Abrupt high fever, pulse increased out of proportion to fever, vomiting, headache, chills, malaise, abdominal pain Enanthema: Tonsils enlarged, edematous, reddened, and covered with patches of exudate; in severe cases appearance resembles membrane seen in diphtheria; pharynx is edematous and beefy red; during first 1–2 d tongue is coated and papillae become red and swollen (*white strawberry tongue*); by fourth or fifth d white coat sloughs off, leaving prominent papillae (*red strawberry tongue*); palate is covered with erythematous punctate lesions Exanthema: Rash appears within 12 h after prodromal signs; red pinhead-sized punctate lesions rapidly become generalized but are absent on face, which becomes flushed with striking circumoral pallor; rash is more intense in folds of joints; by end of first week desquamation begins (fine, sandpaperlike on torso; sheetlike sloughing on palms and soles), which may be complete by 3 wk or longer	Treatment of choice is a full course of penicillin (or erythromycin in penicillin-sensitive children); fever should subside 24 h after beginning therapy Antibiotic therapy for newly diagnosed carriers (nose or throat cultures positive for streptococci) Supportive measures: Bedrest during febrile phase, analgesics for sore throat Complications: Otitis media Peritonsillar abscess Sinusitis Glomerulonephritis Carditis, polyarthritis (uncommon)	Institute *respiratory precautions until 24 h after* initiation of treatment Ensure compliance with oral antibiotic therapy (intramuscular benzathine penicillin G [Bicillin] may be given if parents' reliability in giving oral drugs is questionable) Maintain *bedrest during febrile phase*; provide quiet activity during convalescent period Relieve discomfort of sore throat with analgesics, gargles, lozenges, antiseptic throat sprays (Chloraseptic), and inhalation of cool mist Encourage fluids during febrile phase; *avoid* irritating liquids (citrus juices) or rough foods; when child is able to eat, begin with *soft diet* Advise parents to consult practitioner if fever persists after beginning therapy Discuss procedures for preventing spread of infection

Source: Adapted from Wong D. *Whaley and Wong's Nursing Care of Infants and Children* (5th ed). St. Louis: Mosby, 1995. Pp 668–677.

1. Child is admitted to pediatric intensive care unit (PICU) for intensive nursing care, continuous observation and monitoring.
2. Monitor neurologic status and vital signs continuously.
3. Assist with/prepare for numerous invasive procedures, including ET tube/mechanical ventilation and intracranial pressure monitor.
4. Monitor closely for the development of seizures; institute seizure precautions.
5. *Position:* elevate head of bed (HOB) 30–45 degrees.
6. Administer medications as ordered:
   a. Osmotic diuretics (e.g., mannitol) to ↓ ICP.
   b. Diuretics (e.g., Lasix) to ↓ CSF production.
   c. Anticonvulsants (e.g., Dilantin, phenobarbital).

B. Goal: *restore and maintain fluid and electrolyte balance, including perfusion of liver.*
1. Administer IV fluids per physician's order—usually 10% glucose (or higher).
2. Strict I&O.
3. Prepare for/assist with Foley catheter placement, CVP, ICP monitor, NG tube, etc.
4. Monitor serum electrolyte lab values.

C. Goal: *prevent injury and possible bleeding.*
1. Observe child for petechiae, unusual bruising, oozing from body orifices or tubes, frank hemorrhage.
2. Check all urine and stool for occult blood.
3. Monitor lab values, including prothrombin time (PT), partial thromboplastin time (PTT), platelets.
4. Administer blood products per physician's order.

D. Goal: *provide parents with thorough understanding of Reye's syndrome.*
1. Primary nurse assigned to provide care and follow through with teaching.
2. Encourage parents' presence, even in PICU—explain all equipment and procedures in simple, direct terms.
3. Provide factual, honest, and complete information re: disease, diagnosis, prognosis.

◆ **V. Evaluation/outcome criteria:**
A. Intracranial pressure is reduced and normal neurologic functioning is restored.
B. Fluid and electrolyte balance is restored.
C. No clinical evidence of bleeding is found.
D. Parents express understanding of Reye's syndrome.

Autoimmune Disorders

Streptococcus Infections/Sequelae

Introduction: Group A beta-hemolytic streptococcus is a common infectious organism that causes illness in children and is highly contagious. In themselves, the diseases caused by streptococcus do not seem very serious: e.g., strep throat, otitis media, impetigo, or scarlet fever. The most common treatment for strep is a full course of antibiotic therapy: 10 d of penicillin (or, if allergic, erythromycin). With adequate therapy, generally no sequelae are seen. If the strep is *not* treated, or is only partially treated, the sequelae include serious systemic diseases, with potentially long-term effects. If the effect is manifested primarily in the heart (carditis), it is acute rheumatic fever. If the effect is manifested primarily in the kidneys, it is acute glomerulonephritis (Figure 8.12).

I. Rheumatic fever
A. *Introduction:* Rheumatic fever is an acute, systemic, inflammatory disease affecting multiple organs and systems: heart, joints, CNS, collagenous tissue, etc. Thought to be autoimmune in nature, it most commonly follows a streptococcus infection (see Figure 8.12) and occurs primarily in school-age children. In addition, it does tend to recur, and the risk of permanent heart damage increases with each subsequent attack of rheumatic fever.
◆ **B. Assessment:**
1. *Major manifestations* (modified Jones criteria)
   a. Carditis: tachycardia, cardiomegaly, murmur, congestive heart failure (CHF).
   b. Migratory polyarthritis: swollen, hot, red, and excruciatingly painful large joints; migratory and reversible.
   c. Sydenham chorea (St. Vitus Dance): sudden, aimless, irregular movements of the extremities; involuntary facial grimaces, speech disturbances, emotional ability, muscle weakness; completely reversible.
   d. Erythema marginatum: reddish pink rash most commonly found on the trunk; nonpruritic, macular, clear center, wavy but clearly marked border; transient.
   e. Subcutaneous nodules: small, round, freely movable, and painless swellings usually found over the extensor surfaces of the hands/feet or bony prominences; resolve without any permanent damage.
2. *Minor manifestations*
   a. Clinical
      (1) Previous history of rheumatic fever.
      (2) Arthralgia.
      (3) Fever—normal in morning, rises in mid-afternoon, normal at night.
   b. Laboratory
      (1) Increased erythrocyte sedimentation rate (ESR).
      (2) Positive C-reactive protein.
      (3) Leukocytosis.
      (4) Anemia.
      (5) Prolonged P-R/Q-T intervals on ECG.
3. Supportive evidence
   a. Recent history of streptococcus infection:

■ **FIGURE 8.12   Sequelae of strep infections.**

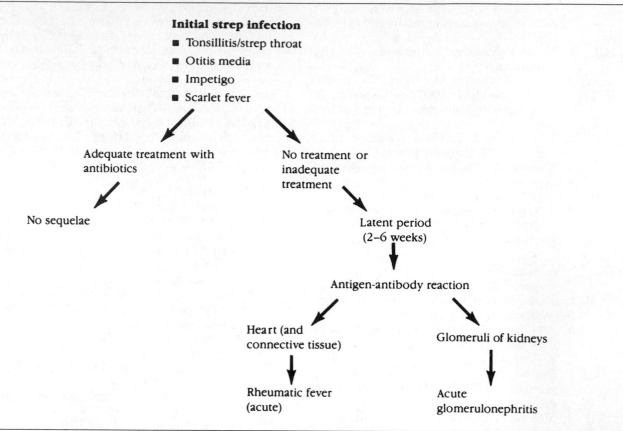

(1) Strep throat/tonsillitis.
(2) Otitis media.
(3) Impetigo.
(4) Scarlet fever.
b. Positive throat culture for streptococcus.
c. Increased ASO titer: indicates presence of streptococcus antibodies; begins to rise in 7 d, reaches maximum level in 4–6 wk.

◆ **C. Analysis/nursing diagnosis:**
  1. *Decreased cardiac output* related to carditis.
  2. *Pain* related to migratory polyarthritis.
  3. *Risk for injury* related to chorea.
  4. *Diversional activity deficit* related to lengthy hospitalization and recuperation.
  5. *Knowledge deficit* related to preventing cardiac damage, relieving discomfort, and preventing injury.
  6. *Ineffective management of therapeutic regimen* with long-term antibiotic therapy and follow-up care.

◆ **D. Nursing care plan/implementation:**
  1. Goal: *prevent cardiac damage.*
    a. Hospitalization, with strict bedrest.
    b. Monitor apical pulse for changes in rate, rhythm, murmurs.
    c. Evaluate tolerance of increased activity by apical rate: if heart rate increases by more than 20 beats/min over resting rate, child should return to bed.
    d. Offer *low-sodium diet* to prevent fluid retention.
    e. Administer oxygen, digoxin/Lasix as ordered (if CHF develops). *Note:* Refer to Unit 2 for additional information on CHF.
  2. Goal: *relieve discomfort.*
    a. Use bed cradle to keep linens from resting on painful joints.
    b. Administer aspirin as ordered to relieve pain.
    c. Move child carefully, minimally—support joints.
    d. *Do not* massage; *do not* perform ROM exercises; *do not* apply splints; *do not* apply heat/cold. All these treatments will cause increased pain and are *not needed*, since *no* permanent deformities will result from this type of arthritis.
  3. Goal: *promote safety and prevent injury related to chorea.*
    a. Use side rails: elevated, padded.
    b. Restrain in bed if necessary.
    c. *No* oral temperatures—child may bite thermometer.

d. Spoon-feed—no forks or knives, to prevent injury to oral cavity.

e. Assist with all aspects of ADL until child can care for own needs.

4. Goal: *provide diversion as tolerated.*

a. Encourage quiet diversional activities: hobbies, reading, puzzles.

b. Get homework, books; provide tutor as condition permits.

c. Encourage contact with peers: telephone calls, letters, cards.

5. Goal: *encourage child and family to comply with long-term antibiotic therapy.*

a. Begin antibiotics immediately, to eradicate any lingering streptococcus infection.

b. Prepare child/family for minimum of 5 yr of IM injections of penicillin.

c. Stress need for exact schedule: every 4 wk.

d. Enlist child's cooperation with therapy, e.g., "hero" badge.

6. Goal: *health teaching.*

a. To encourage compliance with prolonged bedrest—stress that ultimate prognosis depends on amount of cardiac damage.

b. Teach necessity for long-term prophylactic therapy for 5 yr initially (with lifetime follow-up), e.g., during dental work, childbirth, surgery (to prevent subacute bacterial endocarditis [SBE]).

c. Teach rationale: permanent cardiac damage is more likely to occur with subsequent attacks of rheumatic fever.

◆ **E. Evaluation/outcome criteria:**

1. No permanent cardiac damage occurs.

2. Child is free from discomfort or is able to tolerate discomfort.

3. Injuries are avoided.

4. Child's need for diversional activity is met.

5. Child/family comply with long-term antibiotic therapy/prophylactic therapy.

II. Acute glomerulonephritis

A. *Introduction:* Acute glomerulonephritis (AGN) is a bilateral inflammation of the glomeruli of the kidneys and is the most common noninfectious renal disease of childhood. It occurs most frequently in young school-age children, with a peak age of onset of 6–7 yr; it is twice as common in boys as in girls. Like rheumatic fever, acute glomerulonephritis is thought to be the result of an antigen-antibody reaction to a streptococcus infection (see Figure 8.12); however, unlike rheumatic fever, it does *not* tend to recur, since specific immunity is conferred following the first episode of AGN. (Further information about AGN is found in Table 8.19, p. 548.)

◆ **B. Assessment:**

1. Typical concerns from family about urine: change in color/appearance of urine (thick, reddish brown; decreased amounts).

2. Acute edematous phase—usually lasts 4–10 d.

a. Lab examination of urine:
   (1) severe **hematuria.**
   (2) Mild proteinuria.
   (3) Increased specific gravity.

b. **Hypertension**
   (1) Headache.
   (2) Potential hypertensive encephalopathy → seizures, increased intracranial pressure.

c. Mild–moderate edema: chiefly periorbital; increased weight due to fluid retention.

d. General:
   (1) Abdominal pain.
   (2) Malaise.
   (3) Anorexia.
   (4) Vomiting.
   (5) Pallor.
   (6) Irritability.
   (7) Lethargy.
   (8) Fever.

3. Diuresis phase:
   a. Copious diuresis.
   b. Decreased body weight.
   c. Marked clinical improvement.
   d. Decrease in gross hematuria, but miscoscopic hematuria may persist for weeks/months.

◆ **C. Analysis/nursing diagnosis:**

1. *Fluid volume excess* related to decreased urine output.

2. *Pain* related to fluid retention.

3. *Altered nutrition, less than body requirements,* related to anorexia and vomiting.

4. *Impaired skin integrity* related to immobility.

5. *Activity intolerance* related to fatigue.

6. *Knowledge deficit* related to disease process, treatment, and follow-up care.

◆ **D. Nursing care plan/implementation:**

1. Goal: *monitor fluid balance, observing carefully for complications.*

a. Check and record blood pressure at least every 4 h to monitor hypertension.

b. Monitor daily weights.

c. Urine: strict I&O; specific gravity and dipstick for blood every void.

d. Note edema: extent, location, progression.

e. Adhere to fluid restrictions if ordered.

f. Bedrest, chiefly due to hypertension: monitor for possible development of hypertensive encephalopathy (seizures, increased intracranial pressure); report any changes stat to physician.

g. Administer medications as ordered:
   (1) Antibiotics—eradicate any lingering streptococcus infection.
   (2) Antihypertensives, e.g., Apresoline.
   (3) Rarely use diuretics—limited value.

(4) If CHF develops—may use digoxin.

(5) Refer to Unit 4 for additional information on medications.

2. Goal: *provide adequate nutrition.*

a. *Diet: low sodium, low potassium*—to prevent fluid retention and hyperkalemia; *high protein* to replace protein being lost in the urine. Refer to Unit 3 for additional information on diets.

b. Stimulate appetite: offer small portions, attractively prepared; meals with family or other children; offer preferred foods, if possible; encourage parents to bring in special foods, e.g., culturally related preferences.

3. Goal: *provide reasonable measure of comfort.*

a. Encourage parental visiting.

b. Provide for positional changes, give good skin care.

c. Provide appropriate diversion, as tolerated.

4. Goal: *prevent further infection.*

a. Use good handwashing technique.

b. Screen staff, other patients, visitors to limit contact with infectious persons.

c. Administer antibiotics if ordered (usually only for children with positive cultures).

d. Keep warm and dry, stress good hygiene.

e. Note possible sites of infection: ↑ skin breakdown secondary to edema.

5. Goal: *teach child and family about AGN / discharge planning.*

a. Teach how to check urine at home: dipstick for protein and blood. (*Note:* Occult hematuria may persist for months.)

b. Teach activity restriction: no strenuous activity until hematuria is completely resolved.

c. Teach family how to prepare low-sodium, low-potassium diet.

d. Arrange for follow-up care: physician, public health nurse.

e. *Stress:* subsequent recurrences are *rare* because specific immunity is conferred.

◆ **E. Evaluation/outcome criteria:**

1. No permanent renal damage occurs.

2. Normal fluid balance is maintained/restored.

3. Adequate nutrition is maintained.

4. No secondary infections occur.

5. Child/family verbalize their understanding of the disease, its treatment, and its prognosis.

Kawasaki Disease (Mucocutaneous Lymph Node Syndrome)

I. *Introduction:* Kawasaki disease (mucocutaneous lymph node syndrome) is an acute, febrile, multisystem disorder believed to be autoimmune in

nature. Affecting primarily the skin and mucous membranes of the respiratory tract, lymph nodes, and heart, Kawasaki disease has a low fatality rate (<2%), although vasculitis and cardiac involvement (coronary artery changes) may result in major complications in as many as 20–25% of children with this disease. The disease is not believed to be communicable, and the exact cause remains unknown; geographic (living near fresh water) and seasonal (late winter, early spring) outbreaks do occur. Kawasaki disease occurs in both boys and girls between 1 and 14 yr of age; 80% of cases occur in children under the age of 5 yr. It may be preceded by URI or exposure to a freshly cleaned carpet. A complete and apparently spontaneous recovery occurs within 3 to 4 wk in the majority of cases. Treatment, which is primarily symptomatic, does not appear to either enhance recovery or prevent complications, although recent research indicates that life-threatening complications and long-term disability may be avoided or minimized with early treatment (i.e., gamma globulin) to reduce cardiovascular damage.

◆ **II. Assessment:**

A. Abrupt onset with high fever (102°–106°F) lasting more than 5 d that does not remit with the administration of antibiotics.

B. Conjunctivitis—bilateral, nonpurulent.

C. Oropharyngeal manifestations:

1. Dry, red, cracked lips.

2. Oropharyngeal reddening and a "strawberry" tongue.

D. Peeling (desquamation) of the palms of the hands and the soles of the feet; begins at the fingertips and the tips of the toes; as peeling progresses, hands and feet become very red, sore, and swollen.

E. Cervical lymphadenopathy.

F. Generalized erythematous rash on trunk and extremities, without vesicles or crusts.

G. Irritability, anorexia.

H. Arthralgia and arthritis.

I. Panvasculitis of coronary arteries: formation of aneurysms and thrombi; CHF, myocarditis, pericardial effusion, arrhythmias, mitral insufficiency, myocardial infarction (MI).

J. Laboratory tests:

1. Elevated: ESR.

2. Elevated: WBC count.

3. Elevated: platelet count.

◆ **III. Analysis/nursing diagnosis:**

A. *Hyperthermia* related to high, unremitting fever.

B. *Altered oral mucous membrane and impaired swallowing* related to oropharyngeal manifestations.

C. *Impaired skin integrity* related to desquamation.

D. *Fluid volume deficit* related to high fever and poor oral intake.

E. *Altered tissue perfusion* (cardiovascular, potential/actual) related to vasculitis or thrombi.

F. *Knowledge deficit* related to disease course, treatment, prognosis.

◆ **IV. Nursing care plan/implementation:**

A. Goal: *reduce fever.*

1. Monitor rectal temperature every 2 h or prn.

2. Administer **aspirin** (not acetaminophen, Tylenol) per physician's order. (*Note:* Aspirin is the drug of choice to reduce fever; also has anti-inflammatory effect and anti-platelet effect. Dose is 100 mg/kg/d in divided doses q6h. Monitor for signs of salicylate toxicity.)

▶ 3. Tepid sponge baths or hypothermia blanket per physician's order.

4. Offer frequent cool fluids.

5. Apply cool, loose-fitting clothes; use cotton bed linens only (no heavy blankets).

6. Seizure precautions.

B. Goal: *provide comfort measures to oral cavity to ease the discomfort of swallowing.*

1. Good oral hygiene with soft sponge and diluted hydrogen peroxide.

2. Apply petroleum jelly to lips.

3. *Bland* foods in small amounts at frequent intervals.

4. *Avoid* hot, spicy foods.

5. Offer favorite foods from home or preferred foods from hospital selection.

C. Goal: *prevent infections and promote healing of skin.*

1. Monitor skin for desquamation, edema, rash.

2. Keep skin clean, dry, well lubricated.

3. Avoid soap to prevent drying.

4. Gentle handling of skin to minimize discomfort.

5. Provide sheepskin to lie on.

6. Prevent scratching and itching—apply cotton mittens if necessary.

7. Bedrest; elevate edematous extremities.

D. Goal: *prevent dehydration and restore normal fluid balance.*

1. Strict I&O.

2. Monitor urine specific gravity q 8 h for increase (dehydration) or decrease (hydration).

3. Monitor vital signs for fevers, tachycardia, arrhythmia.

4. Monitor skin turgor, mucous membranes, anterior fontanel for dehydration.

5. "Force" fluids.

6. IV fluids per physician's order.

E. Goal: *prevent cardiovascular complications.*

▲ 1. ECG monitor—report arrhythmias or tachycardia.

2. Administer aspirin (see goal A, above) and high-dose IV gamma globulin.

3. Monitor for signs and symptoms of CHF: tachycardia, tachypnea, dyspnea, crackles, orthopnea, distended neck veins, dependent edema.

4. Monitor circulatory status of extremities—check for possible development of thrombi.

▲ 5. Stress need for long-term follow-up, including ECGs and echocardiograms.

◆ **V. Evaluation/outcome criteria:**

A. Fever returns to normal.

B. Oral cavity heals, and child is able to swallow.

C. Skin heals, and no infection occurs.

D. Normal fluid balance is restored.

E. Normal cardiovascular functioning is reestablished, and no complications occur.

F. Parents/child verbalize their understanding of Kawasaki disease.

Bacterial Infections

Introduction: Acute bacterial ear infection (*acute otitis media*) is common in young children, primarily because their eustachian tube is shorter and straighter than the adult's; this allows for ready drainage of infected mucus from URIs directly into the middle ear. In *some* cases, acute otitis media precedes the onset of *bacterial meningitis,* an extremely serious and potentially fatal disease. Bacterial meningitis is a medical emergency, requiring early detection and prompt, aggressive therapy to prevent permanent neurologic damage or death. (Refer to section on Hydrocephalus, p. 552). Serous otitis (chronic) may result in hearing impairment or loss but is not likely to result in meningitis. Refer to Myringotomy, Table 8.15, p. 532.

I. Acute otitis media

◆ **A. Assessment:**

1. Fever.

2. Pain in affected ear. Infant may not complain of pain but may tug at ear, cry, shake head, refuse to lie down.

3. Malaise, irritability, anorexia (possibly vomiting).

4. May have symptoms and signs of URI: rhinorrhea, coryza, cough.

◆ **B. Analysis/nursing diagnosis:**

1. *Pain* related to pressure of pus/purulent material on eardrum.

2. *Risk for injury/infection* related to complication of meningitis.

◆ **C. Nursing care plan/implementation:**

1. Goal: *eradicate infection and prevent further complications (meningitis).* Administer antibiotics as ordered.

2. Goal: *relieve pain and promote comfort.*

a. Administer decongestants as ordered.

b. Offer analgesics/antipyretics to provide symptomatic relief and to decrease fever.

3. Goal: *health teaching.*

a. Teach parents that the child needs to finish all medication, even though child will seem clinically better within 24–48 h.

■ **TABLE 8.15 Pediatric Surgery: Nursing Considerations**

Surgical Procedure	Specific Nursing Care
Tonsillectomy (the most frequently performed pediatric surgical procedure)	*Preoperative:* check bleeding and clotting times *Postoperative:* ■ *Position*—place on abdomen or semiprone with head turned to side to prevent aspiration ■ *Observe for most frequent complication—hemorrhage* (frequent swallowing, emesis of bright red blood, shock) *Prevent bleeding:* ■ Do *not* suction—may cause bleeding ■ Do *not* encourage coughing, clearing throat, or blowing nose—may aggravate operative site and cause bleeding ■ Minimize crying *Decrease pain:* ■ Offer ice collar to decrease pain and for vasoconstriction, but do *not* force ■ Acetaminophen for pain (*no* aspirin) *Nutrition:* ■ NPO initially, then cool, clear fluids such as cool water, crushed ice, flavored icepops, dilute (noncitrus) fruit juice ■ **No** red fluids (punch, Jell-O, icepops), citrus juices, warm fluids (tea, broth), toast, milk/ice cream/pudding, carbonated sodas. Progress to soft, bland *Teach parents/discharge planning:* ■ Signs and symptoms of infection, call physician promptly. ■ 5–10 d postoperatively, expect slight bleeding ■ Continue soft, bland diet as tolerated
Myringotomy ("tubes")	*Postoperative:* ■ *Position*—place with operated ear down, to allow for drainage. Expect moderate amount of purulent drainage initially ■ Keep external ear canal clean and dry *Teach parents/discharge planning:* ■ Need to keep water out of ear—use special earplugs when bathing or swimming ■ "Tubes" will remain in place 3–7 mo and then fall out spontaneously (with healing of eardrum)
Appendectomy	(Observe same principles of preoperative and postoperative care as for adult GI surgery) NPO until bowel sounds return (24–48 h) If appendix ruptured preoperatively or intraoperatively, then *position* in semi-Fowler's and implement wound precautions; administer antibiotics as ordered Monitor for signs and symptoms of peritonitis Typical course: speedy recovery, with discharge in about 2–3 d and excellent prognosis
Herniorrhaphy (umbilical/inguinal)	*Umbilical:* ↑ incidence in black infants *Inguinal:* ↑ incidence in boys *Preoperative:* monitor for possible complications of strangulation Routine postoperative GI surgery care Prognosis—excellent, with discharge 24–48 h postoperatively

b. Review appropriate measures to control fever: antipyretics, cool sponges.

◆ **D. Evaluation/outcome criteria:**
1. Infection is eradicated, no complications.
2. Child appears to be comfortable.

II. Bacterial meningitis

◆ **A. Assessment:**
1. Abrupt onset: initial sign may be a seizure, following an episode of URI/acute otitis media.
2. Chills and fever.
3. Vomiting; may complain of headache, neck pain.
4. Photophobia.
5. Alterations in level of consciousness: delirium, stupor, increased intracranial pressure.
6. Nuchal rigidity.
7. Opisthotonus position: head is drawn backward into overextension.
8. Hyperactive reflexes related to CNS irritability.

◆ **B. Analysis/nursing diagnosis:**
1. *Risk for infection* related to communicability of meningitis.
2. *Risk for injury* related to CNS irritability and seizures.
3. *Pain* related to nuchal rigidity, opisthotonus position, increased muscle tension.
4. *Sensory/perceptual alterations* related to seizures and changes in level of consciousness.
5. *Altered nutrition, less than body requirements,* related to fever and poor oral intake.
6. *Knowledge deficit* regarding diagnostic procedures, condition, treatment, prognosis.

◆ **C. Nursing care plan/implementation:**
1. Goal: *prevent spread of infection.*
   ▶ a. Institute universal precautions.
   b. Enforce strict handwashing.
   ▶ c. Institute and maintain respiratory isolation for minimum of 24 h after starting IV antibiotics, at which time child is no longer considered to be communicable and can come off isolation.
   d. Supervise parents in isolation techniques.
   e. Identify family members and others at high risk: do cultures (*Hemophilus influenzae, Escherichia coli,* etc.); possibly begin prophylactic antibiotics, e.g., rifampin.
   f. Treat with IV antibiotics (as ordered) as soon as possible after admission (after cultures are obtained); continue 10–14 d (until cerebrospinal-fluid [CSF] culture is negative and child appears clinically improved).
   g. Anticipate large-dose IV medications only—administer slowly in dilute form to prevent phlebitis.
   h. Restrain as needed to maintain IV.
2. Goal: *promote safety and prevent injury/seizures.*
   a. Maintain seizure precautions.
   b. Place child near nurses' station for maximum observation; provide private room for isolation.
   c. Minimize stimuli: quiet, calm environment.
   d. Restrict visitors to immediate family.
   e. *Position:* HOB slightly elevated to decrease intracranial pressure. (If opisthotonus: side-lying, for comfort and safety.)
3. Goal: *maintain adequate nutrition.*
   a. NPO or clear liquids initially; supplement with IVs, since child may be unable to coordinate sucking and swallowing.
   b. Offer diet for age, as tolerated—child may experience anorexia (due to disease) or vomiting (due to increased intracranial pressure).
   c. Monitor I&O, daily weights.

◆ **D. Evaluation/outcome criteria:**
1. No spread of infection noted.
2. Safety maintained.
3. Adequate nutrition and fluid intake maintained.
4. Child recovers without permanent neurologic damage, e.g., seizure disorders, hydrocephalus.

III. Infestations
   A. Lice (pediculosis)
   1. *Introduction:* In children, the most common form of lice is pediculosis capitis, or head lice. This parasite feeds on the scalp, and its saliva causes severe itching. Head lice are frequently associated with the sharing of combs and brushes, hats, and clothing; thus, they are more common in girls, especially those with long hair. Lice are also associated with overcrowded conditions and poor hair hygiene.

   ◆ 2. **Assessment:**
   a. Severe itching of scalp.
   b. Visible eggs/nits on shafts of hair.

   ◆ 3. **Analysis/nursing diagnosis:**
   a. *Impaired skin integrity* related to infestation of scalp with lice.
   b. *Risk for impaired skin integrity* related to severe pruritus of scalp.
   c. *Knowledge deficit* related to transmission and prevention of disease and treatment regimen.

   ◆ 4. **Nursing care plan/implementation:**
   a. Goal: *eradicate lice infestation.* Apply Kwell shampoo—rub in for 4–5 min, then comb with fine-tooth comb to remove dead lice and nits (eggs).
   b. Goal: *prevent spread of lice.*
      (1) Wear gloves and cap to protect self.
      (2) Inspect other family members; treat prn with Kwell.
      (3) Wash all clothes and linens to kill any lice that may have fallen off the child's hair.
      (4) Encourage short hair, if acceptable.
      (5) Teach preventive measures: don't share comb, brushes, hats.

   ◆ 5. **Evaluation/outcome criteria:** lice eradicated and do not spread.

   B. Pinworms (enterobiasis)
   1. *Introduction:* In children, the most common parasitic infestation is pinworms. Infestation usually occurs when the child places fingers (and the pinworm eggs) into the mouth. Breaking the anus-to-mouth contamination cycle can best be accomplished by good hygiene, especially handwashing before eating and after toileting. If one family member has pinworms, it is highly likely that other family members are also infested; therefore, treat the entire family to eradicate the parasite. Pin-

worms are easily eradicated with antiparasitic medications.

◆ 2. **Assessment:**
   a. Intense perianal itching.
   b. Visible pinworms in the stool.
   c. Vague abdominal discomfort.
   d. Anorexia and weight loss.

◆ 3. **Analysis/nursing diagnosis:**
   a. *Risk for infection/injury* related to the anus-to-mouth contamination cycle of pinworm infestation, severe rectal itching.
   b. *Knowledge deficit* related to transmission and prevention of disease and treatment regimen.

◆ 4. **Nursing care plan/implementation:**
   a. Goal: *eradicate pinworm infestation.* Treat all family members simultaneously with an antiparasitic agent, e.g., vermox, povan.
   b. Goal: *prevent spread of pinworms.*
      (1) Launder all underwear, bed linens, and towels in hot soapy water to kill eggs.
      (2) Teach family members the importance of good hygiene, especially handwashing before eating (or preparing food) and after toileting. Stress to children to keep their fingers out of their mouths.

◆ 5. **Evaluation/outcome criteria:** Pinworms are eradicated and do not spread; reinfestation does not occur.

Accidents: Ingestions and Poisonings

I. **General principles** of treatment for ingestions and poisonings:
   A. *Prevention:* refer to section on toddler safety, pp. 496–497.
   B. How to induce vomiting:
   1. Drug of choice—syrup of ipecac (available over the counter; does not require a physician's order). Families with young children should keep this medication on hand in case of accidental poisoning.
   2. Dose:
      a. 30 mL for adolescents (over 12 yr of age); repeat dosage once if vomiting has not occurred within 20 min.
      b. 15 mL for children (1–12 yr of age); repeat dosage once if vomiting has not occured within 20 min. *Note:* Do not administer to infants less than 1 yr of age without physician's order.
   3. Follow dose of ipecac with 4–8 oz of tap water or as much water as child will drink. In young children, give water first because child may refuse to drink anything else after tasting the ipecac.

   4. The child *must* vomit the syrup of ipecac to avoid its being absorbed and causing potentially fatal cardiotoxicity, i.e., cardiac arrhythmias, atrial fibrillation, severe heart block. If child does not vomit within 20 min of second dose, manually stimulate gag reflex (use spoon to touch back of throat) or assist with gastric lavage.

   C. When **not** to induce vomiting:
   1. Child is stuporous or comatose.
   2. Poison ingested is a corrosive substance or petroleum distillate.
   3. Child is having seizures.
   4. Child is in severe shock.
   5. Child has lost the gag reflex.

II. **Salicylate poisoning**
◆ A. **Assessment:**
   1. Determine how much aspirin was ingested, when, which type.
   2. Evaluate salicylate levels: normal, 0; therapeutic range = 15–30 mg/dL; *toxic,* >30 mg/dL.
   3. *Early* identification of *mild toxicity:*
      a. Tinnitus (ringing in the ears).
      b. Changes in vision, dizziness.
      c. Sweating.
      d. Nausea, vomiting, abdominal pain.
   4. *Immediate* recognition of salicylate *poisoning:*
      a. Hyperventilation (earliest sign).
      b. Fever—may be quite high (105°–106°F).
      c. Respiratory alkalosis or metabolic acidosis.
      d. *Late* signs: bleeding tendencies, severe electrolyte disturbances, liver or kidney failure.

◆ B. **Analysis/nursing diagnosis:**
   1. *Ineffective breathing patterns* related to hyperventilation/respiratory alkalosis.
   2. *Fluid volume deficit* (dehydration) related to increased insensible loss of fluids through hyperventilation, increased loss of fluids through vomiting, and increased need for fluids due to hyperpyrexia (fever).
   3. *Risk for injury* related to bleeding.
   4. *Anxiety* related to parental/child feelings of guilt, uncertainty as to outcome, invasive nature of treatments.
   5. *Knowledge deficit* regarding accident prevention.

◆ C. **Nursing care plan/implementation:**
   1. Goal: *promote excretion of salicylates.*
      a. If possible, induce vomiting using syrup of ipecac (save, bring to emergency room).
      b. Assist with gastric lavage, if appropriate.
      c. Administer activated charcoal as early as possible.
      d. Assist with hemodialysis, as ordered, to promote excretion of salicylates and fluids.

e. Administer IV fluids, as ordered.
2. Goal: *restore fluid and electrolyte balance.*
   a. Monitor I&O, urinalysis, specific gravity.
   b. Prepare sodium bicarbonate, administer as ordered to correct metabolic acidosis.
   c. Monitor IV fluids and electrolytes.
   d. NPO initially (nasogastric [NG] tube).
3. Goal: *reduce temperature.*
   a. **No** aspirin or acetaminophen, which might further complicate bleeding tendencies or lead to liver or kidney damage.
   ▶ b. Supportive measures: cool soaks, ice packs to armpits/groin, hypothermia blanket.
4. Goal: *prevent bleeding and possible hemorrhage.*
   a. Monitor urine and stools for occult blood.
   ▶ b. Insert NG tube to detect gastric bleeding.
   c. Observe for petechiae, bruising; monitor laboratory values for Hct and Hgb.
   d. Administer vitamin K as ordered to correct bleeding tendencies.
5. Goal: *health education to prevent another accidental poisoning:*
   a. Teach principles of poison prevention.
   b. Stress need to avoid accidental overdose with over-the-counter medications or dosage mix-ups.
   c. Allow child/parents to verbalize guilt, but avoid blaming or scapegoating.

◆ **D. Evaluation/outcome criteria:**
1. Aspirin is successfully removed from child's body without permanent damage.
2. Fluid and electrolyte balance is restored and maintained.
3. Child is afebrile.
4. Bleeding is controlled, no hemorrhage occurs.
5. No further episodes of poisoning occur.

III. Acetaminophen poisoning

◆ **A. Assessment:**
1. Determine how much acetaminophen was ingested, when, and which type.
2. Evaluate acetaminophen levels: normal = 0; therapeutic range = 15–30 µg/mL; toxic = 150 µg/mL 4 h after ingestion.
3. *Initial period* (2–4 h after ingestion): malaise, nausea, vomiting, anorexia, diaphoresis, pallor.
4. *Latent period* (1–3 d after ingestion): clinical improvement with asymptomatic rise in liver enzymes.
5. Hepatic involvement (may last 7 d or may be permanent): pain in right upper quadrant (RUQ), jaundice, confusion, hepatic encephalopathy, clotting abnormalities.
6. Gradual recuperation.

◆ **B. Analysis/nursing diagnosis:**
1. *Altered tissue perfusion* (liver) related to hepatic necrosis.
2. *Fluid volume deficit* related to increased loss of fluids secondary to vomiting and diaphoresis.
3. *Risk for injury* related to bleeding and clotting disorders.
4. *Anxiety* related to parental/child feelings of guilt, uncertainty as to outcome, and invasive nature of treatments.
5. *Knowledge deficit* regarding accident prevention.

◆ **C. Nursing care plan/implementation:**
1. Goal: *promote excretion of acetaminophen.*
   a. If possible, induce vomiting; save, bring to emergency room.
   ▶ b. Assist with gastric lavage, if appropriate.
   c. Administer activated charcoal.
   d. Assist with obtaining acetaminophen level 4 h after ingestion.
2. Goal: *prevent permanent liver damage.*
   a. Treatment must begin as soon as possible; therapy begun later than 10 h after ingestion has no value.
   b. Administer the antidote (acetylcysteine [Mucomyst]) per physician's order. Usually administered through NG tube because of offensive odor. Given as one loading dose and 17 maintenance doses.
   c. Monitor hepatic functioning—assist with obtaining specimens and check results frequently; be aware that liver enzymes will rise and peak within 3 d and then should rapidly return to normal.
3. Goal: *restore fluid and electrolyte balance.*
   a. Monitor vital signs and perform neurologic checks every 2–4 h and prn.
   b. Monitor I&O, urine analysis, including specific gravity, and weight.
   c. Monitor IV fluids as ordered.
4. Goal: *prevent bleeding.*
   a. Assist in monitoring child's PT; notify physician of significant changes.
   b. Monitor urine and stool for occult blood.
   c. Observe for and report any petechiae or unusual bruising.
5. Goal: *health education to prevent another accidental poisoning.* (See goal 5 Nursing care plan/implementation for Salicylate poisoning, at left.)

◆ **D. Evaluation/outcome criteria:**
1. Acetaminophen is successfully removed from child's body.
2. Normal liver functioning is reestablished.
3. Fluid and electrolyte balance is restored and maintained.
4. No further episodes of poisoning occur.

IV. Lead poisoning (plumbism)
   A. *Introduction:* Lead poisoning is a heavy-metal poisoning that occurs from ingestion or inhalation of lead. In children, this is most common in the toddler age group (1–3 yr) and is usually a chronic type of poisoning that occurs as the result of repeated ingestions of

lead. Children who engage in the practice of *pica,* the ingestion of nonnutritive substances, often ingest lead in flecks of lead-based paint from walls, furniture, or toys. In addition, research demonstrates that the parent-child relationship is a significant variable in lead poisoning; typically, there is a lack of adequate parental supervision that enables the child to engage in pica repeatedly over a fairly long time, until symptoms of lead poisoning become evident. (Figure 8.13 shows the pathophysiologic effects of lead poisoning.)

◆ **B. Assessment:**
1. Investigate history of pica (ingestion of nonnutritive substance).
2. Evaluate parent-child relationship.
3. *Chronic lead poisoning:* vague, crampy abdominal pain; constipation; anorexia and vomiting; listlessness.
4. Neurologic, renal, hematologic effects: see Figure 8.13.

5. "Blood-lead line"—bluish black line seen in gums.
6. X rays: lead lines in long bones and flecks of lead in GI tract.
7. Elevated serum-blood-lead levels: toxic ≥20 µg/dL.

◆ **C. Analysis/nursing diagnosis:**
1. *Altered thought processes* related to neurotoxicity.
2. *Activity intolerance* (and *risk for infection*) related to anemia.
3. *Altered urinary elimination* related to excretion of lead by kidneys.
4. *Pain* related to lead poisoning and its treatment.
5. *Knowledge deficit* related to etiology of lead poisoning.

◆ **D. Nursing care plan/implementation:**
1. Goal: *promote excretion of lead.*
   a. Administer chelating agents (EDTA, BAL) as ordered: given as a series of

■ **FIGURE 8.13** *Main effects of lead* on body systems. (From Wong D. *Whaley & Wong's Nursing Care of Infants and Children* [5th ed]. St. Louis: Mosby, 1995. P 696.)

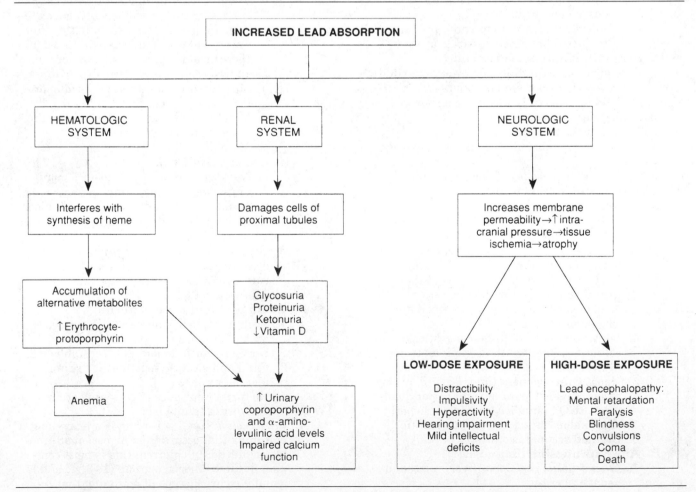

painful, deep IM injections (common dose: 6/d for 5 d).

    b. Monitor kidney function carefully: the treatment itself is potentially nephrotoxic. Maintain adequate oral intake of fluids.

    c. Institute seizure precautions.

2. Goal: *prevent reingestion of lead.*

    a. Determine primary source of poisoning.

    b. Eliminate source from child's environment before discharge.

    c. Follow up with PHN referral.

        (1) Screen other siblings prn.

        (2) Monitor "blood-lead level" of all children in the home.

3. Goal: *assist child to cope with multiple painful injections.*

    a. Prepare child for treatment regimen.

    b. Stress that this is **not** a punishment.

    c. Rotate sites as much as possible.

    d. May use a local anesthetic, e.g., procaine, injected simultaneously with chelating agent to decrease pain of injections.

    e. Apply warm soaks to injection sites: may help lessen pain.

    f. Encourage child to self-limit gross muscle activity (which increases pain).

    g. Offer child safe outlets for anger, fear, frustration—punching bag, pounding board, clay.

    h. Offer opportunity for medical play with empty syringes, etc.

4. Goal: *health teaching.*

    a. Stress (to child and parents) that getting the lead out is the only way to prevent permanent, irreversible neurologic damage (irreversible damage may have *already* occurred).

    b. Teach that the chelating agent binds with the lead and promotes its excretion through the kidneys.

◆ **E. Evaluation/outcome criteria:**

1. Lead is successfully removed from child's body without permanent damage.

2. No further episodes of lead poisoning.

3. Child copes successfully with the disease and its treatment.

Allergic Response: Threats to Health Status

I. Infantile eczema (atopic dermatitis)

    A. *Introduction:* Eczema is an allergic skin reaction, most commonly to foods, e.g., cow's milk or eggs. It is most common in infants and young children (under age 2 yr). Infantile eczema generally undergoes permanent, spontaneous remission by age 3 yr; however, approxi-

mately 50% of children who have had infantile eczema develop asthma during the preschool or school-age years.

◆ **B. Assessment:**

1. Erythematous lesions, beginning on cheeks and spreading to rest of face and scalp.

2. May spread to rest of body, especially in flexor surfaces, e.g., antecubital space.

3. Lesions may ooze or crust over.

4. Severe pruritus, which may lead to secondary infection.

5. Lymphadenopathy near site of rash.

6. Unaffected skin tends to be dry and rough.

7. Systemic manifestations are rare—but child may be irritable, cranky.

◆ **C. Analysis/nursing diagnosis:**

1. *Impaired tissue integrity* related to lesions.

2. *Pain* related to pruritus.

3. *Risk for (secondary) infection* related to breaks in the skin (first line of defense) and itching.

4. *Knowledge deficit* related to care of child with eczema, prognosis, how to prevent exacerbations.

◆ **D. Nursing care plan/implementation:**

1. Goal: *promote healing of lesions.*

    a. Give frequent baths in tepid water with cornstarch, to relieve pruritus, but with **no soap**—apply light coat of baby oil or mineral oil after bath.

    b. Apply wet soaks with Burow's solution (aluminum acetate solution; topical astringent/antiseptic).

    c. Protect child from possible sources of infection; universal precautions to prevent infection.

    d. Absolutely **no immunizations** during acute exacerbations of eczema because of the possibility of an overwhelming dermatitis, allergic reaction, shock, or even death.

    e. Apply topical creams/ointments as prescribed: A&D ointment, hydrocortisone cream to promote healing.

2. Goal: *provide relief from itching/keep child from itching.*

    a. Administer systemic medications as ordered, e.g., Benadryl or Atarax.

    b. Keep nails trimmed short—may need mittens (**preferable** not to use elbow restraints, since the antecubital space is a common site for eczema).

    c. Use clothes and bedlinens that are nonirritating, i.e., pure cotton (**no** wool or blends).

    d. Institute *elimination/hypoallergenic diet:*

        (1) No milk or milk products.

        (2) Change to lactose-free formula, e.g., Isomil.

(3) Avoid eggs, wheat, nuts, beans, chocolate.

e. No stuffed animals or hairy dolls.

3. Goal: *provide discharge planning/teaching for parents and child.*
   a. Include all above information.
   b. Include information on course of disease: characterized by exacerbations and remissions throughout early years.
   c. Include information on prognosis: 50–60% will go into spontaneous (and permanent) remission during preschool years; 40–50% will develop asthma/hayfever during school-age years.

◆ **E. Evaluation/outcome criteria:**
1. Lesions heal well, without secondary infection.
2. Adequate relief from itching is achieved.
3. Parents verbalize understanding of eczema, prognosis, and how to prevent exacerbations.

II. Asthma
A. *Introduction:* Asthma is generally considered a chronic, lower airway disorder characterized by heightened airway reactivity with bronchospasm and obstruction. The exact cause of asthma is unknown; however, it is believed to include an allergic reaction to one or more allergens, psychogenic factors, and perhaps other factors as well. The child usually exhibits other symptoms of allergy, such as infantile eczema or hayfever; in addition, 75% of children with asthma have a positive family history for asthma. The onset is usually before age 5 and remains with the child throughout life, although some children do experience dramatic improvement in their asthma with the onset of puberty.

◆ **B. Assessment:**
1. Expiratory wheeze.
2. General signs and symptoms of respiratory distress, including anxiety, cough, shortness of breath, crackles, cyanosis due to obstruction within the respiratory tract, use of accessory muscles of respirations.
3. Cough: hacking, paroxysmal, nonproductive; especially at night.
4. *Position* of comfort for breathing: sitting straight up, leaning forward, which is the position for optimal lung expansion.

◆ **C. Analysis/nursing diagnosis:**
1. *Ineffective airway clearance* related to bronchospasm.
2. *Anxiety* related to breathlessness.
3. *Knowledge deficit,* actual or potential, related to disease process, treatment, and prevention of future asthmatic attacks.
4. *Activity intolerance* related to dyspnea and bronchospasm.

◆ **D. Nursing care plan/implementation:**
1. Goal: *provide patent airway and effective breathing patterns.*

a. Initiate oxygen therapy, as ordered, to relieve hypoxia, with high humidity (to liquefy secretions).
b. Administer steroids as ordered to reduce inflammation.
c. Administer bronchodilators, as ordered, to relieve the obstruction: epinephrine, aminophylline, theophylline.
d. Carefully regulate flow of aminophylline IV to avoid giving too much medication in too little time.
e. Monitor vital signs closely while giving IV aminophylline, especially pulse and BP, since IV aminophylline can precipitate tachycardia or hypotension as side effects.
f. Observe for signs of aminophylline *toxicity:* prolonged increase in pulse, cardiac arrhythmias, or increasing restlessness.
g. Administer anti-inflammatory medications as ordered to relieve edema: prednisone, decadron.

2. Goal: *relieve anxiety.*
   a. Provide relief from hypoxia (refer to goal 1), which is the chief source of anxiety.
   b. Remain with child, offer support.
   c. Administer sedation as ordered.
   d. Encourage parents to remain with child.

3. Goal: *teach principles of prophylaxis.*
   a. Review home medications, including cromolyn sodium. See Unit 4.
   b. Review breathing exercises.
   c. Discuss precipitating factors and offer suggestions how to avoid.
   d. Introduce need for child to assume control over own care.

◆ **E. Evaluation/outcome criteria:**
1. Adequate oxygenation provided, as evidenced by pink color of nailbeds and mucous membranes and ease in respiratory effort.
2. Anxiety is relieved.
3. Child verbalizes confidence in, and demonstrates mastery of, skills needed to care for own asthma.

Pediatric Surgery: Nursing Considerations

I. In general, basic care principles for children are the same as for adults having surgery.
II. Exceptions:
A. Children should be prepared according to their developmental level and learning ability.
B. Children cannot sign own surgical consent form; to be done by parent or legal guardian.
C. Parents should be actively involved in the child's care.
III. See Table 8.15, which reviews specific nursing care for the most common pediatric surgical procedures.

❏ Disorders Affecting Nutritional Functioning

Insulin-Dependent Diabetes Mellitus (IDDM)

IDDM was formerly called juvenile-onset diabetes. Because diabetes mellitus is fully covered in Unit 2 the information is not repeated here; please refer to Unit 2. Only the differences between the adult and the child are covered in Table 8.16.

Upper Gastrointestinal Anomalies

I. Cleft lip and cleft palate

A. *Introduction:* Cleft lip and cleft palate are congenital facial malformations resulting from faulty embryonic development; there appear to be multiple factors involved in the exact etiology: mutant genes, chromosomal abnormalities, teratogenic agents, etc. The infant may be born with cleft lip alone, cleft palate alone, or with both cleft lip and cleft palate. (Table 8.17 compares these conditions.)

◆ **B. Assessment:**
1. *Cleft lip*—obvious facial defect, readily detectable at time of birth.
2. *Cleft palate*—must feel inside infant's mouth to check for presence of palatal defect and to note extent of defect: soft palate only or soft palate *and* hard palate.
3. *Both*—major problems with feeding: difficult to feed, noisy sucking, swallows excessive amounts of air, prone to aspiration.
4. Parent-infant attachment (bonding) may be adversely affected due to "loss of perfect infant," multiple hospitalizations: note amount and quality of parent-infant interaction.

◆ **C. Analysis/nursing diagnosis:**
1. *Altered nutrition, less than body requirements,* related to physical defect.
2. *Impaired physical mobility* (postoperative) related to postoperative care requirements.
3. *Altered parenting* related to birth of child with obvious facial defect.
4. *Knowledge deficit,* actual or potential, related to treatment and follow-up.

■ **TABLE 8.16   Comparison of Characteristics of Type I and II Diabetes Mellitus**

Characteristic	Type I (IDDM)	Type II (NIDDM)
Age at onset	< 20 yr	> 30 years
Type of onset	Abrupt	Gradual
Sex ratio	Males slightly more than females	Females outnumber males
Percentage of diabetic population	5–8%	85–90%
Heredity:		
Family history	Sometimes	Frequently
HLA	Associations	No associations
Twin concordance	25–50%	90–100%
Ethnic distribution	Primarily whites	Increased incidence in Native Americans and Hispanics
Presenting symptoms	Three Ps* common	May be related to long-term complications
Nutritional status	Underweight	Overweight
Insulin (natural):		
Pancreatic content	Usually 0	> 50% normal
Serum insulin	Low to absent	High or low
Primary resistance	Minimum	Marked
Islet cell antibodies	80–85%	< 5%
Metabolic control	Difficult	Usually easy
Stability	Unstable	Stable
Therapy:		
Insulin	Always	20–30% of patients
Oral agents	Ineffective	Often effective
Diet only	Ineffective	Often effective
Chronic complications	> 80%	Variable
Ketoacidosis	Common	Infrequent

*Polyuria, polydipsia, and polyphagia.
Source: Wong D. *Whaley and Wong's Nursing Care of Infants and Children* (5th ed). St. Louis: Mosby, 1995. P 1765.

■ **TABLE 8.17** Comparison of Cleft Lip and Cleft Palate

	Cleft Lip	Cleft Palate	Both Cleft Lip and Cleft Palate
Incidence	1:800	1:2000	Most common facial malformation
Inheritance	Multifactorial inheritance Male predominance	Associated with syndromes (chromosomal), environmental factors, or teratogens Female predominance	More common among males More common among whites than blacks
Anatomy	Unilateral/bilateral May involve external nose, nasal cartilages, nasal septum, maxillary alveolar ridges, and dental anomalies	Soft palate or hard palate Midline of posterior palate May involve nostril and absence of nasal septal development (communication with oral and nasal cavity)	
Management	Surgical: Z-plasty First few wk of life if no respiratory, oral, or systemic infections occur	Delayed repair: 12–18 mo before development of speech	Lip always repaired before palate to enhance parent-infant attachment, bonding
Short-term problems (before repair)	Feeding, possibly	Feeding: aspiration	
Special postoperative nursing care	Suture line protection and care *Position:* right side or upright in infant seat; *avoid* prone positioning to protect suture line *Special feeding:* Breck feeder or Asepto syringe—sometimes breast—until suture line heals	*Position*—prone, supine, or side-lying *Feeding* cup, Breckfeeder or Asepto syringe; *avoid* spoon, fork (also tongue blade, toothbrush, and other objects that could damage suture line)	O.K. to show parents pictures of "before" and "after" repair
Long-term problems	Social acceptance (depends on success of repair), orthodontic if associated with CP	*Speech*, otitis media, *possible hearing loss*, upper–respiratory tract infections *Orthodontic* Feeding Social acceptance (voice changes, facial appearance if with CL)	

Source: Adapted from Wong D. *Whaley and Wong's Nursing Care of Infants and Children* (5th ed). St. Louis: Mosby, 1995. P 471.

◆ **D. Nursing care plan/implementation:**
1. Goal: *maintain adequate nutrition.*
   a. *Preoperative:* first encourage parents to watch nurse feed infant, then teach parents proper feeding techniques:
   ▶ (1) Use *Breck* feeder or Asepto syringe.
   (2) Deposit formula on back of tongue to facilitate swallowing and to prevent aspiration.
   (3) Rinse mouth with sterile water after feedings, to prevent infection.
   (4) Feed slowly, with child in sitting position, to prevent aspiration.
   (5) Burp frequently, since infant will swallow air along with formula due to the defect.
   (6) Monitor weight.
   b. *Postoperative*
   (1) Begin with clear liquids when child has fully recovered from anesthesia (see Table 8.17).
   (2) Monitor weight gain carefully, to ensure adequate rate of growth.
2. Goal: *promote parent-infant attachment.*
   a. Show no discomfort handling infant; convey acceptance.
   b. Stay with parents the first time they see/hold infant.
   c. Offer positive comments about infant.
   d. Give positive reinforcement to parents' initial attempts at parenting.
   e. Encourage parents to assume increasing independence in care of their infant.
   f. Allow rooming-in on subsequent hospitalizations.
3. Goal: *teach parents regarding feeding and need for long-term follow-up care.*
   a. Teach parents regarding long-term concerns (see Table 8.17).
   b. Make necessary referrals before discharge:
   (1) Specialists: speech, dentition, hearing.
   (2) Public health nurse.
   (3) Social service.
   (4) Disabled children's services for financial assistance.
   (5) Local facial-malformations support group.
   c. Refer parents to genetic counseling services because of mixed genetic/environmental etiology.
   d. Encourage parents to promote self-esteem in infant/child as child grows and develops.

◆ **E. Evaluation/outcome criteria:**
1. Adequate nutrition is provided, and infant grows at "normal" rate for age.
2. Parent-infant attachment is formed.
3. Parents verbalize confidence in their ability to care for infant.

II. Tracheoesophageal fistula
A. *Introduction:* Tracheoesophageal fistula (TEF) is a congenital anomaly resulting from faulty embryonic development; although there are numerous "types" of TEF, the major problem is an anatomic defect that results in an abnormal connection between the trachea (respiratory tract) and the esophagus (GI system) (Figure 8.14). No exact cause has been identified; however, infants born with TEF are often preterm, with a maternal history of polyhydramnios. Diagnosis should be made in the immediate neonatal period, within hours after birth, and preferably before feeding (to avoid aspiration pneumonia). Associated anomalies include CHD, anorectal malformations, and genitourinary anomalies.

◆ **B. Assessment:**
1. Perinatal history: maternal polyhydramnios, preterm infant.
2. *Most important system* affected is *respiratory:*
   a. Shortly after birth, infant has excessive amounts of mucus.
   b. Mucus bubbles or froths out of nose and mouth as infant literally "exhales" mucus.
   c. *"3 Cs": coughing, choking, cyanosis*—because mucus accumulates in respiratory tract.
   d. "Pinks up" with suctioning, only to experience repeated respiratory distress within a short time as mucus builds up again.
   e. Aspiration pneumonia occurs early.
   f. Respiratory arrest may occur.
3. *Second* system affected is GI:
   a. Abdominal distention because excessive air enters stomach with each breath infant takes.
   b. Inability to aspirate stomach contents when attempting to pass NG tube.
   c. If all these signs are not correctly interpreted and feeding is attempted, infant takes 2–3 mouthfuls, coughs and gags, and forcefully "exhales" formula through nostrils.

◆ **C. Analysis/nursing diagnosis:**
1. *Ineffective breathing pattern/ineffective airway clearance* related to excess mucus.
2. *Altered nutrition, less than body requirements,* related to inability to take fluids by mouth.
3. *Anxiety,* related to surgery, condition, preterm delivery, and uncertain prognosis.
4. *Knowledge deficit* regarding discharge care of infant related to gastrostomy tube, feeding.

◆ **D. Nursing care plan/implementation:**
1. Goal: *prepare neonate for surgery.*
   a. Stress to parents that surgery is *only* possible treatment.

■ **FIGURE 8.14** *Five* most common types of *esophageal atresia* and tracheoesophageal fistula. A. Blind pouch at end of esophagus does not communicate with trachea. B. Fistula between esophagus and trachea. C. Distal segment connected to trachea. D and E. Fistula between trachea and esophagus. (From Wong D. *Whaley & Wong's Nursing Care of Infants and Children* [5th ed]. St. Louis: Mosby, 1995. P 480.)

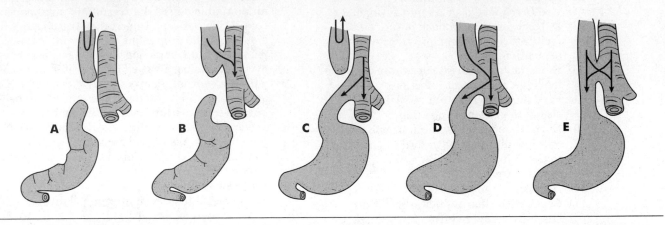

b. Allow parents to see neonate before surgery to promote bonding and attachment.

c. Maintain NPO—provide IV fluids, monitor I&O, NG tube.

d. *Position:* elevate HOB 20–30 degrees to prevent aspiration.

e. Administer warmed, humidified oxygen, as ordered, to relieve hypoxia and to prevent cold stress.

2. Goal: *postoperative—maintain patent airway.*

a. *Position:* elevate HOB 20–30 degrees.

b. Care of chest tubes (open-chest procedure).

c. Care of endotracheal tube/ventilator (neonate frequently requires ventilatory assistance for 24–48 h postoperatively).

d. Monitor for symptoms and signs of pneumonia (most common postoperative complication):
   (1) Aspiration.
   (2) Hypostatic, secondary to anesthesia.

e. Monitor for symptoms and signs of RDS (preterm infant).

f. Use special precautions when suctioning: "suction with marked catheter" to avoid exerting undue pressure on newly sutured trachea.

g. Administer prophylactic/therapeutic antibiotics, as ordered.

h. Administer warmed, humidified oxygen, as ordered; monitor arterial blood gases (ABGs).

3. Goal: *maintain adequate nutrition.*

a. Maintain NPO for 10–14 d, until esophagus is fully healed (offer pacifier).

b. 48–72 h postoperatively: IV fluids only.

c. When condition is stable: begin gastrotomy (G-) tube feedings, as ordered.

(1) Start with small amounts of clear liquids.

(2) Gradually increase to full-strength formula.

(3) *Postoperative:* leave G-tube open and elevated slightly above level of stomach to prevent aspiration if infant vomits.

(4) Offer pacifier ad lib.

d. Monitor weight, I&O.

e. Between *10th and 14th postoperative d:* begin oral feedings.

(1) Start with clear liquids again.

(2) Note ability to suck and swallow.

(3) Offer small amounts at frequent intervals.

(4) May need to supplement postop feeding with G-tube feeding prn.

4. Goal: *prepare parents to successfully care for the infant after discharge.*

a. Teach parents that infant will probably be discharged with G-tube in place; teach care of G-tube at home.

b. Teach parents symptoms and signs of most common long-term problem, i.e., stricture formation.

(1) Refusal to eat solids or swallow liquids.

(2) Dysphagia.

(3) Increased coughing or choking.

c. Stress need for long-term follow-up care.

d. Offer realistic encouragement, because prognosis is generally good.

◆ **E. Evaluation/outcome criteria:**

1. Neonate survives immediate surgical repair without untoward difficulties.

2. Patent airway is maintained; adequate oxygenation is provided.

3. Adequate nutrition is maintained; infant begins to gain weight and grow.

4. Parents verbalize confidence in ability to care for infant on discharge.

III. Pyloric stenosis

A. *Introduction:* Pyloric stenosis is a congenital anomaly of the upper GI tract, but the infant frequently does not present with symptoms until 2–4 wk of age. Basically the condition involves thickening, or hypertrophy, of the pyloric sphincter located at the distal end of the stomach; this causes a mechanical intestinal obstruction that becomes increasingly evident as the infant begins to consume larger amounts of formula during the early weeks of life. Pyloric stenosis is five times more common in boys than girls and is most often found in full-term white infants; the exact etiology remains unknown.

◆ B. **Assessment:**
1. Classic symptom is *vomiting:*
   a. Begins as nonprojectile at 2–4 wk of age.
   b. Advances to projectile at 4–6 wk of age.
   c. Vomitus is nonbile stained (stomach contents only).
   d. Most often occurs shortly after a feeding.
   e. Major problem is the mechanical obstruction of the flow of stomach contents to the small intestine due to the anatomic defect of stenosis of the pyloric sphincter.
   f. *No* apparent nausea or pain, as evidenced by the fact that infant eagerly accepts a second feeding after episode of vomiting.
   g. Metabolic alkalosis develops due to loss of hydrochloric acid.
2. Inspection of abdomen reveals:
   a. Palpable olive-shaped mass in right upper quadrant.
   b. Visible peristaltic waves, moving from left to right across upper abdomen.
3. Weight: fails to gain or loses.
4. Stools: constipated, diminished in number and size—due to loss of fluids with vomiting.
5. Signs of dehydration may become evident (Table 8.18).
6. Upper GI series reveals:
   a. Delayed gastric emptying.
   b. Elongated and narrowed pyloric canal.

◆ C. **Analysis/nursing diagnosis:**
1. *Fluid volume deficit* related to vomiting.
2. *Altered nutrition, less than body requirements,* related to vomiting.
3. *Risk for injury/infection* related to altered nutritional state.
4. *Impaired skin integrity* related to dehydration and altered nutritional state.
5. *Knowledge deficit* related to cause of disease, treatment and surgery, prognosis and follow-up care.

■ **TABLE 8.18 Signs and Symptoms of Dehydration in Infants and Young Children**

Weight loss (most important variable to assess): *mild dehydration* (less than 5% weight loss); *moderate dehydration* (5–9% weight loss); *severe dehydration* (10–15% weight loss)

Skin: gray, cold to touch, poor skin turgor (check skin across abdomen)

Mucous membranes: dry oral buccal mucosa; salivation absent

Eyes: sunken eyeballs; absence of tears when crying

Anterior fontanel (in infant): sunken

Shock: ↑ pulse, ↑ respirations, ↓ BP

Urine: oliguria, ↑ specific gravity, ammonia odor

Alterations in level of consciousness: irritability, lethargy, stupor, coma, possible seizures

Metabolic acidosis (with diarrhea)

Metabolic alkalosis (with vomiting)

Source: Copyright © 1995, GCC. All rights reserved.

◆ D. **Nursing care plan/implementation:**
1. Goal (**preoperative**): *restore fluid and electrolyte balance.*
   a. Generally NPO, with IVs preoperatively: IVs to provide fluids and electrolytes.
   b. Observe and record I&O, including vomiting and stool.
   c. Weight: check every 8 h or daily.
   d. Monitor laboratory data.
2. Goal: *provide adequate nutrition.*
   a. Maintain NPO with IVs for 4–6 h postoperatively, as ordered (*can* offer pacifier).
   b. Follow specific feeding regimen ordered by doctor—generally start with clear fluids in small amounts hourly, increasingly slowly as tolerated. Full feeding schedule reinstated within 48 h. Offer pacifier between feedings.
   c. Fed only by RN for 24–48 h, since vomiting tends to continue in immediate postoperative period.
   d. Burp well—before, during, and after feeding.
   e. *Position* after feeding: high Fowler, turned to right side; minimal handling after feeding to prevent vomiting.
3. Goal (**preoperative and postoperative**): *institute preventive measures to avoid infection or skin breakdown.*
   a. Use good handwashing technique.
   b. Administer good skin care, especially in diaper area (urine is highly concentrated); give special care to any reddened areas.
   c. Give mouth care when NPO or after vomiting.

d. Tuck diaper down below suture line to prevent contamination with urine (post-operatively).

e. Note condition of suture line—report any redness or discharge immediately.

f. Screen staff and visitors for any sign of infection.

4. Goal: *do discharge teaching to prepare parents to care for infant at home.*

a. Teach parents that defect is anatomic and unrelated to their parenting behavior/skill.

b. Demonstrate feeding techniques, and remind parents that vomiting may still occur.

c. Stress that repair is complete; this condition will *never* recur.

d. Instruct parents in care of the suture line: no baths for 10 d, tuck diaper down, report any signs of infection promptly.

e. Offer follow-up referrals as indicated.

◆ **E. Evaluation/outcome criteria:**

1. Infant survives surgical repair without untoward difficulties (including infection/skin breakdown).

2. Adequate nutrition is maintained, and infant begins to grow and gain weight.

3. Parents verbalize confidence in their ability to care for their infant on discharge.

❑ Disorders Affecting Elimination

Gastrointestinal Disorders

I. Lower gastrointestinal anomalies/obstruction

A. Hirschsprung's disease (congenital aganglionic megacolon)

1. *Introduction:* Hirschsprung's disease is a congenital anomaly of the lower GI tract, but the diagnosis is often not established until the infant is 6–12 mo old. The major problem is a functional obstruction of the colon caused by the congenital anatomic defect of lack of nerve cells in the walls of the colon, resulting in the absence of peristalsis. Hirschsprung's disease is four times more common in boys than girls and is frequently noted in children with Down syndrome.

◆ 2. **Assessment:**

a. In the newborn, failure to pass meconium (in addition to other signs and symptoms of intestinal obstruction).

b. *Obstinate constipation*—history of inability to pass stool without stool softeners, laxatives, or enemas; persists despite all attempts to treat medically.

c. Stools, while infrequent, tend to be thin and ribbonlike.

d. Vomiting: bile stained, flecked with bits of stool (breath has fecal odor), due to GI obstruction and eventual backing-up of stools.

e. Abdominal distention can be severe enough to impinge on respirations, due to GI obstruction and retention of stools.

f. Anorexia, nausea, irritability due to severe constipation.

g. Malabsorption results in anemia, hypoproteinemia, and loss of subcutaneous fat.

h. Visible peristalsis and palpable fecal masses may also be detected.

◆ 3. **Analysis/nursing diagnosis:**

a. *Constipation* related to impaired bowel functioning.

b. *Altered nutrition, less than body requirements,* related to poor absorption of nutrients.

c. *Risk for injury/infection* related to malnutrition.

d. *Pain* related to surgery and treatments.

e. *Knowledge deficit* regarding care of the child with a colostomy and follow-up care.

◆ 4. **Nursing care plan/implementation:**

a. Goal (**preoperative**): *promote optimum nutritional status, fluid and electrolyte balance.*

(1) Monitor for signs and symptoms of progressive intestinal obstruction: measure abdominal girth daily.

(2) Administer IV fluids, as ordered—may include hyperalimentation or intralipids.

(3) Daily weights, I&O, urine specific gravity.

(4) Monitor for possible dehydration.

(5) *Diet: low* residue.

b. Goal (**preoperative**): *assist in preparing bowel for surgery.*

(1) Teach parents what will be done and why—enlist their cooperation as much as possible.

▶ (2) Insert NG tube, connect to low suction to achieve and maintain gastric decompression.

(3) *Position:* semi-Fowler's.

▶ (4) Bowel is cleansed with a series of isotonic saline (0.9%) enemas.

(5) Administer oral antibiotics and colonic irrigations to decrease bacteria.

(6) Take axillary temperatures *only.*

(7) If child can understand, prepare for probable colostomy using pictures, dolls (usual age at surgery is 10–16 mo).

c. Postoperative goals: Same as for adult having major abdominal surgery or a colostomy (see Unit 4).

d. Goal (**postoperative**): *discharge teaching to prepare parents to care at home for infant with a colostomy.*
   (1) Home care of colostomy of infant is essentially same as for adult (see Unit 2).
   (2) Teach parents to keep written records of stools: number, frequency, consistency.
   (3) Teach parents to pin/tape diaper below colostomy to prevent irritation.
   (4) Since colostomy is usually temporary, discuss:
      (a) Second-stage repair (closure and pull-through) done when the child weighs about 20 lb.
      (b) Possible difficulties in toilet training.
   (5) Stress need for long-term follow-up care.
   (6) Make referral to PHN if indicated.

◆ 5. **Evaluation/outcome criteria:**
   a. Infant is prepared for surgery and tolerates procedure well.
   b. Postoperative recovery is uneventful.
   c. Parents verbalize confidence in ability to care at home for infant with a colostomy and verbalize their understanding that second surgery will be needed to close the colostomy.

B. Intussusception
   1. *Introduction:* Intussusception is the apparently spontaneous telescoping of one portion of the intestine into another, resulting in a mechanical obstruction of the lower GI tract. There is no known cause, and intussusception is three times more common in boys than girls; the child with intussusception is usually between 3–24 mo of age.

◆ 2. **Assessment:**
   a. Typically presents with sudden onset in healthy, thriving child.
   b. Pain: paroxysmal, colicky, abdominal, with intervals when the child appears normal and comfortable.
   c. Stools: "currant-jelly," bloody, mixed with mucus.
   d. Vomiting due to intestinal obstruction.
   e. Abdomen: distended, tender, with palpable, sausage-shaped mass in RUQ.
   f. *Late signs:* fever, shock, signs of peritonitis as the compressed bowel wall becomes necrotic and perforates.

◆ 3. **Analysis/nursing diagnosis:**
   a. *Fluid volume deficit* related to diarrhea and vomiting.
   b. *Pain* related to bowel-wall ischemia, necrosis, and death.

c. *Risk for injury/infection* related to bowel-wall perforation and peritonitis.
d. *Knowledge deficit* regarding the disease, medical or surgical treatment, and prognosis.

◆ 4. **Nursing care plan/implementation:**
   a. Goal: *assist with attempts at medical treatment.*
   🜊 (1) Explain to parents that a barium enema will be given to the child in an attempt to reduce the telescoping through hydrostatic pressure (succeeds in 75% of cases).
   (2) Stress that, if this treatment is not successful, or if perforation of the bowel wall has already occurred, surgery will be necessary.
   (3) If medical treatment is apparently successful, monitor child for 24–36 h for recurrence before discharge.
   b. *Preoperative and postoperative goals:* same as for adult with major abdominal surgery (see Unit 2).
   c. Goal: *discharge teaching to prepare parents for care of the child at home.*
      (1) Stress that recurrence is rare (10%) and most often occurs within the first 24–36 h after reduction.
      (2) Other teaching: same as for adult going home after bowel surgery (see Unit 2).

◆ 5. **Evaluation/outcome criteria:**
   a. Infant tolerates medical-surgical treatment and completely recovers.
   b. Parents verbalize confidence in ability to care for infant after discharge.

II. Acute gastroenteritis (AGE)
   A. *Introduction:* In infants and young children, gastroenteritis is a very common acute illness that can rapidly progress to dehydration, hypovolemic shock, and severe electrolyte disturbances.

◆ **B. Assessment:**
   1. Diarrhea: often watery, green, explosive, contains mucus and blood.
   2. Abdominal cramping and pain, often accompanied by bouts of diarrhea.
   3. Dehydration: see Table 8.18.
   4. Irritability, restlessness, alterations in level of consciousness.
   5. Electrolyte disturbances: see Unit 2.

◆ **C. Analysis/nursing diagnosis:**
   1. *Fluid volume deficit* related to vomiting and diarrhea.
   2. *Altered nutrition, less than body requirements,* related to AGE and its treatment, i.e., dietary restrictions.
   3. *Pain* related to abdominal cramping, diarrhea.
   4. *Impaired skin integrity* related to diarrhea.
   5. *Altered tissue perfusion* related to dehydration and hypovolemia.

6. *Knowledge deficit* regarding diagnosis, dietary restrictions, treatment.
◆ **D. Nursing care plan/implementation:**
   1. Goal: *prevent spread of infection.*
      a. Universal precautions to prevent infection.
      b. Enforce strict handwashing.
   ▶ c. Institute and maintain *enteric precautions*—follow policies regarding linens, excretions, specimens ("double bag, special tag").
      d. Pin diapers snugly; keep hands out of mouth.
   ⚗ e. Obtain stool culture to identify causative organism; then administer antibiotics as ordered.
      f. Identify family members and others at high risk, obtain cultures.
   2. Goal: *restore fluid and electrolyte balance.*
   💊 a. Administer IV fluids and electrolytes as ordered.
      b. Monitor for appropriate response to therapy: decreased specific gravity, good skin turgor, normal vital signs.
      c. Monitor weight, I&O, specific gravity.
      d. Oral feedings—oral rehydration therapy (ORT) with Pedialyte or comparable solution; resume normal diet as quickly as possible.
      e. Ongoing assessment of stools: note *a*mount, *c*olor, *c*onsistency, *t*iming ("*ACCT*").
   3. Goal: *maintain or restore skin integrity.*
      a. Frequent diaper changes (use cloth diapers).
      b. Keep perineal area clean and dry.
   💊 c. Apply protective ointments, e.g., petroleum jelly, A&D ointment.
      d. If feasible, expose reddened buttocks to air (but *not* with explosive diarrhea).
   4. Goal: *provide discharge teaching to parents.*
      a. Careful review of diet to be followed at home.
      b. Review principles of food preparation and storage to prevent infection.
      c. Instruct in disposal of stools at home.
      d. Emphasize importance of good hygiene.
◆ **E. Evaluation/outcome criteria:**
   1. No spread of infection noted.
   2. Fluid and electrolyte balance normal.
   3. No skin breakdown noted.
   4. Parents verbalize understanding of home care.

Genitourinary Disorders

I. Hypospadias
   A. *Introduction:* Hypospadias is a congenital anatomic defect of the male genitourinary tract, readily detected at birth through simple visual

examination. In hypospadias, the urethral opening is located on the ventral surface of the penile shaft; this makes voiding in the standing position virtually impossible, and serious psychological problems could therefore occur. Ideally, staged surgical repair should be completed by 6–18 mo of age, before body image is developed or castration fears are evident.
◆ **B. Assessment:**
   1. Urethral opening is located on ventral surface of penis.
   2. May be accompanied by "chordee"—ventral curvature of the penis due to a fibrous band of tissue.
   3. (Rare) ambiguous genitalia, resulting in need for chromosomal studies to determine sex of neonate.
◆ **C. Analysis/nursing diagnosis:**
   1. *Altered urinary elimination* related to congenital anatomic defect of penis.
   2. *Pain* related to surgery and treatments.
   3. *Self-esteem disturbance* related to anatomic defect in penis and resulting disturbance in ability to void standing up.
   4. *Knowledge deficit* related to condition, surgeries, outcome.
◆ **D. Nursing care plan/implementation:**
   1. Goal: *promote normal urinary function.*
      a. Teach family that surgery is done in several stages, beginning in the early months of life and finishing by age 18 mo.
      b. Provide age-appropriate information to child regarding condition, surgery.
      c. *Preoperative* teaching with child should include: simulate anticipated postoperative urinary drainage apparatus and dressings on dolls; allow child to handle and play with them *now*, but stress need *not* to touch postoperatively.
   ▶ d. *Postoperatively:* Monitor urinary drainage apparatus; note hourly urine output, color, appearance (should be clear yellow, no blood).
   2. Goal: *promote self-esteem.*
      a. Do not scold child if he exposes penis, dressings, catheters, etc.
      b. Reassure parents that preoccupation with penis is normal and will pass.
      c. Encourage calm, matter-of-fact acceptance of, and *avoid* strict discipline for, this behavior, which could negatively affect the child.
◆ **E. Evaluation/outcome criteria:**
   1. Child is able to void in normal male pattern.
   2. Child does not experience disturbances in self-concept and has normal self-esteem.

II. Wilms' tumor (nephroblastoma)
   A. *Introduction:* Wilms' tumor, a malignant tumor of the kidney, is the most common form of renal cancer in children. Peak incidence occurs

at 3 yr of age, with a slightly higher incidence in boys than girls. Ninety percent of the cases occur unilaterally; the treatment of choice is nephrectomy (and adrenalectomy) followed by chemotherapy and radiation.

◆ **B. Assessment:**

1. Most common sign: abdominal mass (firm, nontender).
2. Most often first found by parent changing diaper; felt as a mass over the kidney area.
🜎 3. Intravenous pyelogram (IVP) confirms the diagnosis.
4. Metastasis occurs most frequently to the lungs: pain in chest, cough, dyspnea.

◆ **C. Analysis/nursing diagnosis:** *altered urinary elimination* (other diagnoses depend on stage of tumor and presence of metastasis—similar to adult with cancer).

◆ **D. Nursing care plan/implementation:**

1. Goal: *promote normal urinary function.*
   a. Inform family that surgery is scheduled as soon as possible after confirmed diagnosis (within 24–48 h).
   b. Explain to family that the preferred surgical approach is nephrectomy (and adrenalectomy).
   c. *Preoperative: Do not palpate abdomen* because the tumor is highly friable, and palpation increases the risk of metastasis.
   d. *Postoperative nursing care:* similar to care of adult with nephrectomy (see Unit 2).
   e. *Postop care also includes long-term radiation* therapy and chemotherapy (actinomycin D, vincristine, adriamycin; see Unit 2).
2. Goal: *discharge teaching to prepare parents to care for child at home.*
   a. Teach parents need for long-term followup care with specialists: oncologist, urologist.
   b. Answer questions regarding prognosis, offering realistic hope.
      (1) Child with localized tumor: 90% survival rate.
      (2) Child with metastasis: 50% survival rate.

◆ **E. Evaluation/outcome criteria:**

1. Child is able to maintain normal urinary elimination.
2. Parents verbalize their understanding of home care for the child.

III. Nephrosis. Nephrosis (idiopathic nephrotic syndrome) is a chronic renal disease having no known cause, variable pathology, and no known cure. It is thought that several different pathophysiologic processes adversely affect the glomerular membranes of the kidneys, resulting in increased permeability to protein. This "leakage" of protein into the urine results in massive *proteinuria,* severe *hypoproteinemia,* and total body

edema. A chronic disease, nephrosis often has its onset during the preschool years but is characterized by periods of exacerbation and remission throughout the childhood years.

The nursing care plan for the child with nephrosis is very similar to that for the adult with compromised renal functioning. The reader should refer to Units 3 and 4 for additional information about dietary restrictions and medications; also, refer to Table 8.19 for a chart comparing nephrosis and nephritis.

❏ Disorders Affecting Comfort, Rest, Activity, and Mobility

Musculoskeletal Disorders

Orthopedic conditions in infants and children are many and varied, but treatment is based on basic principles of nursing care. Table 8.20 and Figures 8.15 and 8.16 offer a quick review of the major pediatric orthopedic conditions.

Neuromuscular Disorders

I. Cerebral palsy

A. *Introduction:* Cerebral palsy (CP) is the most common permanent physical disability of childhood. It is a neuromuscular disorder of the pyramidal motor system resulting in the major problem of impaired voluntary muscle control. The damage appears to be fixed and nonprogressive, and the cause is unknown. However, although a variety of factors have been implicated in the etiology of CP, it is now known that CP results more commonly from prenatal brain abnormalities.

◆ **B. Assessment:**

1. Most common type of cerebral palsy— spastic.
   a. Delayed developmental milestones.
   b. Tongue thrust with difficulty swallowing and sucking. Poor weight gain. Aspiration may occur.
   c. Increased muscle tone: "scissoring" (legs crossed, toes pointed).
   d. Persistent neonatal reflexes.
   e. Associated problems:
      (1) Mental retardation in 30% of children with cerebral palsy (70% are normal).
      (2) Sensory impairment: vision, hearing.
      (3) Orthopedic conditions: congenital dysplasia of hip, club foot.
      (4) Dental problems: malocclusion.
      (5) Seizures.

◆ **C. Analysis/nursing diagnosis:**

1. *Ineffective airway clearance* related to hyperactive gag reflex and possible aspiration.

■ **TABLE 8.19   Comparison of Nephrosis and Acute Poststreptococcal Glomerulonephritis**

Factor	Nephrosis (Nephrotic Syndrome)	Acute Poststreptococcal Glomerulonephritis (APSGN)
Illness type	Chronic	Acute
Illness course	Characterized by periods of exacerbations and remissions over many yr	Predictable, self-limiting, typically lasting 4–10 d (acute edematous phase)
Cause	Unknown	Group A beta-hemolytic streptococcus
Age at onset	2–4 yr	Early school age, peak at 6–7 yr
Sex	More common in boys	More common in boys
Major signs and symptoms	Syndrome with variable pathology: massive proteinuria, hypoalbuminemia, severe edema, hyperlipidemia	Hematuria, hypertension
Treatment	Symptomatic—no known cure	Penicillin (EES), antihypertensives
Diet	↓ *sodium,* ↑ *protein*	↓ *sodium,* ↓ *potassium,* ↑ *protein*
Fluid restrictions	Seldom necessary	Necessary if output is significantly reduced
Specific nursing care	Treat at home if possible; good skin care; prevent infection	Treat in hospital during acute phase; monitor vital signs, especially BP; on discharge, stress need to restrict activity until microscopic hematuria is gone
Prognosis	Fair; subject to long-term steroid treatment and social isolation related to frequent hospitalizations/confinement during relapses; 20% suffer chronic renal failure	Good; stress that recurrence is *rare,* since specific immunity *is* conferred

2. *Altered nutrition, less than body require-ments,* related to difficulty sucking and swallowing.
3. *Fluid volume deficit* related to difficulty sucking and swallowing.
4. *Impaired verbal communication* related to difficulty with speech.
5. *Sensory/perceptual alterations* related to potential vision and hearing defects.
6. *Risk for injury* related to difficulty controlling voluntary muscles.
7. *Self-esteem disturbance* related to disability.
8. *Note:* Because the level of disabilities with CP can vary, the nurse must select those diagnoses that apply, and clearly specify the individual child's limitations in any diagnostic statements.

◆ **D. Nursing care plan/implementation:**
1. Goal: *maintain patent airway.*
   a. Have suction and oxygen readily available.
   b. Use feeding and positioning techniques to maintain patent airway.
   c. Institute prompt, aggressive therapy for URIs, to prevent the possible development of pneumonia.
2. Goal: *promote adequate nutrition.*
   a. *Diet:* high in calories (to meet extra energy demands).
   b. Ensure balanced diet of basic foods that can be easily chewed.

c. Provide feeding utensils that promote independence.
   d. Relaxed mealtimes, decreased emphasis on manners, cleanliness.
   e. Monitor I&O, weight gain.
3. Goal: *facilitate verbal communication.*
   a. Refer to speech therapist.
   b. Speak slowly, clearly to child.
   c. Use pictures or actual objects to reinforce speech.
4. Goal: *prevent injury.* Refer to safety throughout growth and development section, pp. 494–495, 496–497, 498, 499, 500.
   a. Use individually designed chairs with restraints for positioning and safety.
   b. Provide protective helmet to prevent head trauma.
   c. Implement seizure precautions.
5. Goal: *provide early detection of and correction for vision and hearing defects.*
   a. Arrange for screening tests.
   b. Assist family with obtaining corrective devices: eyeglasses, hearing aids.
6. Goal: *promote locomotion.*
   a. Encourage "infant stimulation" program to assist infant in reaching developmental milestones.
   b. Refer to physical therapy for exercise program.
   c. Incorporate play into exercise routine.

■ **TABLE 8.20   Common Pediatric Orthopedic Conditions**

Condition	Definition	Age at Onset/ Sex Difference	Treatment	Nursing Considerations
Club foot	Downward, inward rotation of one or both feet: talipes equinovarus (95%)	Newborn (congenital); twice as common in boys	Series of casts changed weekly followed by Denis Browne splint and then corrective shoes (severe cases—surgery)	Care of child in cast/brace Stress need for follow-up Encourage compliance
Congenital hip dysplasia	Abnormal development of hip joint (most frequently unilateral)	Newborn (congenital); more common in girls	*Newborn*—double or triple diapers, Frejka pillow splint; *older infant or toddler*—possible surgery, spica cast	Early identification Care of child in traction/ cast Encourage compliance Check for other anomalies, e.g., spina bifida
Osteomyelitis	Most frequently occurring bone infection among children	5–14 yr; twice as common in boys	Blood cultures to diagnose causative organisms— select appropriate antibiotic; bedrest, immobilization with splint or cast	Care of child in splint/cast Provide diversion Pain medications/ antibiotics as ordered
Legg-Calvé-Perthes	Aseptic necrosis of the head of the femur (cause unknown)	*Peak:* 4–8 yr; *range:* 3– 12 yr; five times more common in boys; ten times more common in whites than nonwhites	Conservative therapy lasts 2–4 yr, usually begins with bedrest and traction, followed by non-weight-bearing devices such as brace, cast	Early identification Care of child in traction/ cast Provide diversion Assist child and family to cope with child's prolonged immobility
Juvenile rheumatoid arthritis	Chronic systemic inflammatory disease (cause unknown)	*Peak:* 2–5 yr and 9–12 yr; more common in girls	Prevent joint deformity by exercise, splints, medications (steroids, ASA, IM gold); relieve symptoms (as per adult with arthritis)	Care of child in brace/ splint Provide diversion Encourage compliance
Scoliosis	Lateral curvature of the spine (cause unknown)	Adolescence; more common in girls	Milwaukee brace; halo-pelvic traction; Harrington rod	Care of child in traction/ cast/brace Teach that brace is worn 23 h/d, 7 d/wk for 1–2 yr (no exceptions) Encourage compliance Promote positive self-image
Osteosarcoma	Most frequently occurring bone cancer among children	Adolescence (10–25 yr); more common in boys and men	Amputation → prosthesis; intensive chemotherapy with high-dose methotrexate	Prepare child for loss of limb Help cope with prosthesis, life-threatening illness Assist with grieving process

d. Use devices that promote locomotion: parallel bars, crutches, and braces.
e. Surgical approach may be needed to relieve contractures.
7. Goal: *encourage independence in ADL.*
  a. Adapt clothing, feeding utensils, etc. to facilitate self-help.

b. Encourage child to perform ADL as much as possible; offer positive reinforcement.
c. Assist parents to have realistic expectations for their child; avoid excessively high expectations that might increase frustration.

■ **FIGURE 8.15** Signs of developmental *dysplasia of the hip*. **A.** Asymmetry of gluteal and thigh folds. **B.** Limited hip abduction as seen in flexion. **C.** Apparent shortening of the femur, as indicated by the level of the knees in flexion. **D.** Ortolani click (if infant is under 4 wk of age). **E.** Positive Trendelenburg sign or gait (if child is weight bearing). (From Wong D. *Whaley & Wong's Nursing Care of Infants and Children* [5th ed]. St. Louis: Mosby, 1995. P 466.)

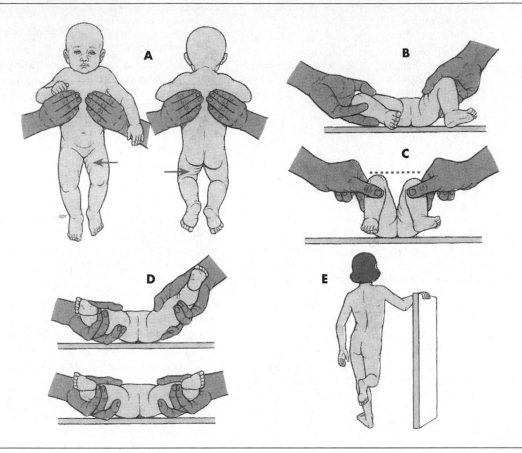

8. Goal: *promote self-esteem*.
   a. Praise child for each accomplishment or for sincere effort.
   b. Help child dress and groom self daily in an attractive "normal" manner for developmental level and age.
   c. Encourage child to form friendships with children with similar problems.
   d. Enroll child in "special ed" classes to meet his or her needs.
   e. Encourage parents to expose child to wide variety of experiences.

◆ **E. Evaluation/outcome criteria:**
   1. Patent airway and adequate oxygenation maintained.
   2. Adequate nutrition maintained, and child begins to grow and gain weight.
   3. Child has an acceptable means of verbal communication.
   4. Safety is maintained.
   5. Vision and hearing within normal limits using corrective devices prn.
   6. Child is as mobile as possible, given disabilities.
   7. Child is performing ADL, within capabilities.

8. Child has positive self-image/self-esteem.

II. Spina bifida (myelodysplasia)
   A. *Introduction:* Three different types of spina bifida:
   1. Spina bifida occulta—a "hidden" bony defect without herniation of the meninges or cord; not visible externally, no symptoms are present, no treatment is needed.
   2. Meningocele—Table 8.21.
   3. Myelomeningocele—see Table 8.21. Most serious type of spina bifida and also most common.

The remainder of this section deals with *myelomeningocele* exclusively.

◆ **B. Assessment:**
   1. Congenital defect.
   2. Readily detected by visual inspection in delivery room: round, bulging sac filled with fluid, usually in lumbosacral area.
   3. Sensation and movement: complete lack below the level of the lesion.
   4. Urinary: retention, with overflow incontinence.
   5. Fecal: constipation, fecal impaction, oozing of liquid stool around impaction.

■ **FIGURE 8.16** *Defects of the spinal column.* A. Normal spine. B. Kyphosis. C. Lordosis. D. Normal spine in balance. E. Mild scoliosis in balance. F. Severe scoliosis not in balance. G. Rib, hump, and flank asymmetry in flexion caused by rotary component. (From Wong D. *Whaley & Wong's Nursing Care of Infants and Children* [5th ed]. St. Louis: Mosby, 1995. P 1846.)

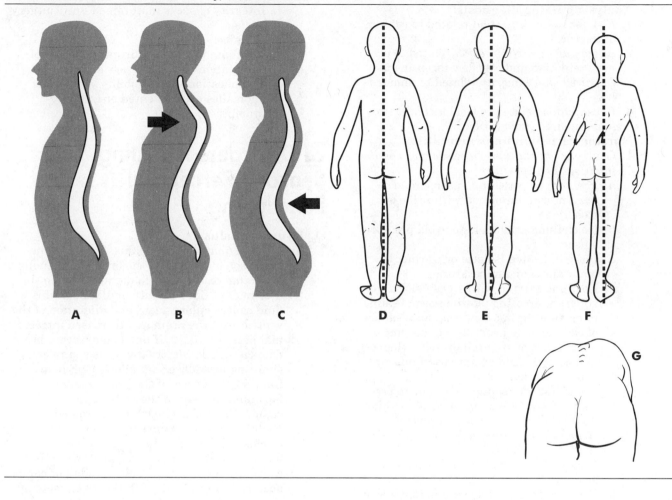

■ **TABLE 8.21   Comparison of Two Major Types of Spina Bifida**

Dimension	Meningocele	Myelomeningocele
Contents of sac	Meninges and CSF	Meninges, cerebrospinal fluid, spinal cord
Transillumination	Present	Absent
Percentage of total cases	25%	75%
Motor function	Present	Absent
Sensory function	Present	Absent
Urinary/fecal incontinence	Absent	Present
Associated orthopedic anomalies	Rare	*Congenital hip dysplasia, club foot*
Other anomalies	Rare	*Hydrocephalus (90–95%)*
Treatment	Surgery	Surgery
Major *short-term* complication	Infection (meningitis)	Infection (meningitis)
Major *long-term* complication	None	Chronic urinary tract infection → renal disease/failure
Prognosis	Excellent	Guarded

6. 90–95% develop signs and symptoms of hydrocephalus (see p. 552).
7. May have associated orthopedic anomalies: club foot, congenital hip dysplasia.

◆ **C. Analysis/nursing diagnosis:**
1. *Risk for injury/infection* related to rupture of the sac.
2. *Altered urinary elimination* related to urinary retention and overflow incontinence.
3. *Impaired skin integrity* related to immobility.
4. *Constipation* related to fecal incontinence and impaired innervation.

◆ **D. Nursing care plan/implementation:**
1. Goal: *prevent rupture of the sac and possible infection (preoperative).*
   a. *Position:* no pressure on sac; prone to prevent contamination with urine or stool.
   b. No clothing or diapers to avoid pressure on sac.
   c. Place in heated isolette or warmer to maintain body temperature.
   d. Keep sac covered with sterile moist non-adherent dressing (sterile normal saline) to prevent drying, cracking, and leakage of CSF; change every 2–4 h; document appearance of sac each dressing change to note signs and symptoms of infection, leaks, abrasions, or irritation.
   ▶ e. Enforce strict aseptic technique to prevent infection (leading cause of morbidity/mortality in neonatal period).
2. Goal: *prevent infection in postoperative period.*
   a. *Position:* prone, side-lying, or partial side-lying.
   b. Use myelomeningocele apron (specific type of dressing) to prevent urine or stool from contaminating suture line.
   c. Administer antibiotics as ordered.
   d. Use strict aseptic techniques in dressing changes; universal precautions to prevent infection.
3. Goal: *prevent urinary retention and UTI.*
   a. Monitor I&O, offer extra fluids to flush kidneys.
   b. Keep urethral meatus clean of stool to prevent ascending bacterial infection.
   c. Monitor urinary output for retention.
   d. Administer antibiotics/urinary tract antiseptics as ordered.
4. Goal: *prevent complications of prolonged immobility or associated orthopedic anomalies.*
   a. *Position:* hips abducted.
   b. Use positional devices, rotating pressure mattress/flotation mattress.
   c. Refer to physical therapy for ROM exercises.
   d. Make necessary referrals for care of possible club foot/congenital hip dysplasia.

5. Goal: *monitor for possible development of hydrocephalus.* Occurs in 90–95% of infants born with myelomeningocele.

◆ **E. Evaluation/outcome criteria:**
1. Integrity of sac is maintained until surgery is done.
2. No infection occurs.
3. Adequate patterns of urinary and bowel elimination with necessary support.
4. Complications of immobility, orthopedic anomalies are prevented or treated promptly.

❏ Disorders Affecting Sensory-Perceptual Functioning

I. Hydrocephalus
   A. *Introduction:* Hydrocephalus, known to the layperson as "water on the brain," is actually a syndrome resulting from disturbances in the dynamics of CSF. The accumulation of this fluid causes enlargement and dilatation of the ventricles of the brain and increased intracranial pressure (ICP). If untreated, severe brain damage will result; treatment is a surgical shunting procedure that allows CSF to drain from the ventricles of the brain to another, less harmful area within the body: jugular vein, right atrium of the heart, or peritoneal cavity. Hydrocephalus can develop as the result of a congenital malformation (e.g., Arnold-Chiari malformation), can be associated with other congenital defects (e.g., spina bifida), or can be acquired secondary to infection (e.g., meningitis), trauma, or neoplasm.

◆ **B. Assessment:**
1. Head: increased circumference—earliest sign of hydrocephalus in the infant (more than 1 in./mo).
2. Fontanels: tense and bulging without head enlargement.
3. Veins: dilated scalp veins.
4. "Setting-sun" sign: sclera visible above pupil; pupils are sluggish with unequal response to light.
5. Cry: shrill, high pitched.
6. Developmental milestones: delayed.
7. Reflexes: persistence of neonatal reflexes; hyperactive reflexes.
8. Feeds poorly.
9. *Signs of ↑ ICP:*
   a. Vomiting.
   b. Irritability.
   c. Seizures.
   d. ↓ pulse.
   e. ↓ respirations.
   f. ↑ blood pressure.
   g. Widened pulse pressure.

10. History may reveal other CNS defects (e.g., spina bifida), infection (e.g., meningitis), trauma, or neoplasm.

◆ **C. Analysis/nursing diagnosis:**
1. *Altered cerebral tissue perfusion* related to increased intracranial pressure.
2. *Impaired skin integrity* related to enlarged head size and lack of motor coordination.
3. *Altered nutrition, less than body requirements,* related to anorexia and vomiting.
4. *Anxiety* related to diagnosis and uncertain outcome.
5. *Knowledge deficit* regarding care of the child with a shunt and follow-up care.

◆ **D. Nursing care plan/implementation:**
1. Goal: *monitor neurologic status.*
   a. Measure head circumference daily, and note any abnormal increase.
   b. Perform neurologic checks at least every 4 h to monitor for signs of ↑ ICP.
   c. Report signs of ↑ ICP **stat** to physician.
   d. Assist with diagnostic procedures/treatments: ventricular tap, computed tomography (CT) scan, etc.
2. Goal: *health teaching to reduce parental anxiety.*
   a. Do preoperative teaching regarding the shunt procedure: stress need to remove excessive CSF to relieve pressure on brain; done as soon as possible after diagnosis is established.
   b. Stress early diagnosis and prompt shunting procedure to minimize the risk of long-term neurologic complications.
   c. Offer realistic information regarding prognosis:
      (1) Surgically treated, with continued follow-up care = 80% survival rate.
      (2) Of these survivors, 50% are completely normal and 50% have some degree of neurologic disability (such as inattentiveness or hyperactivity).
3. Goal: *provide postoperative shunt care.*
   a. *Position:*
      (1) Flat in bed for 24 h, to prevent subdural hematoma.
      (2) Gradually increase the angle of elevation of HOB, as ordered by surgeon.
      (3) On the unoperative side, to prevent mechanical pressure and obstruction to shunt.
   b. Monitor head circumference daily to note any abnormal increase that might indicate malfunctioning shunt.
   c. Monitor vital signs; monitor for signs of ↑ ICP.
   d. Monitor for possible complications:
      (1) Infection.
      (2) Malfunction of shunt: ↑ ICP.

4. Goal: *provide discharge teaching to parents regarding home care of the child with a shunt.*
   a. Stress need for long-term follow-up care.
   b. Discuss feeding techniques, care of skin (especially scalp), need for stimulation.
   c. Prepare parents for shunt revisions to be done periodically as child grows.
   d. Teach parents signs and symptoms of shunt malfunctioning (i.e., of ↑ ICP or infection) and to report these promptly to physician.
   e. Encourage parents to enroll infant in "early infant stimulation" program to maximize developmental potential.
   f. Stress need to monitor development at frequent intervals, make referrals prn.

◆ **E. Evaluation/outcome criteria:**
1. Neurologic functioning is maintained or improved.
2. Adequate nutrition is maintained.
3. No impairment of skin integrity occurs.
4. Parents' anxiety is relieved; they verbalize understanding of how to care for child after discharge.

II. Febrile seizures
A. *Introduction:* Febrile seizures are transient neurologic disorders of childhood, affecting perhaps as many as 3% of all children. Although the exact cause of febrile seizures remains uncertain, they seem to be a relatively transient problem that occurs exclusively in the presence of high, spiked fevers. Children in the infant and toddler stages (6 mo–3 yr) appear to be most susceptible to febrile seizures, and they are twice as common in boys as in girls. There also appears to be an increased susceptibility within families, suggesting a possible genetic predisposition. *Note:* Epilepsy is discussed in Unit 2.

◆ **B. Assessment:**
1. History usually reveals presence of URI or gastroenteritis.
2. Occurs with a sudden rise in fever: often spiked and quite high (102°F or higher) vs. prolonged temperature elevation.

◆ **C. Analysis/nursing diagnosis:**
1. *Risk for injury* related to seizures.
2. *Knowledge deficit* related to prevention of future seizures, care of child having a seizure and possible long-term effects.

◆ **D. Nursing care plan/implementation:**
1. Goal: *reduce fever/prevent further increase in fever.*
   a. Administer antipyretics, as ordered: acetaminophen only (*not* aspirin).
   b. Use cool, loose, cotton clothes to decrease heat retention.
   c. Sponge with tepid water 20–30 min.
   d. Encourage child to drink cool fluids.
   e. Monitor temperature hourly.

f. Minimize stimulation, frustration for child.

2. Goal: *teach parents regarding care of child who experiences febrile seizure.*

   a. Discuss how to prevent seizures from recurring: best method is to prevent temperature from rising over 102°F (see goal 1).

   b. Discuss how to handle seizures if they do recur: prevent injury, maintain airway, etc.

   c. Answer questions simply and honestly:
      (1) 25% of children with one febrile seizure will experience a recurrence.
      (2) 75% of recurrences occur within 1 yr.
      (3) Reassure parents of the benign nature of febrile seizures; 95–98% of children with febrile seizures do not develop epilepsy or neurologic damage.

◆ **E. Evaluation/outcome criteria:**

1. Fever is kept below 102°F; additional seizures are prevented.

2. Parents verbalize their understanding of how to care for child at home.

❑ Questions

Select the one best answer for each question.

1. The best position for the delivery room nurse to place a newborn with myelomeningocele at the lumbosacral area in is:
   1. Prone.
   2. Supine.
   3. Side-lying.
   4. Trendelenburg.

2. A school-age child with rheumatic fever complains of severe joint pains in the knees and ankles. The best method to provide relief would be for the nurse to:
   1. Give a warm bath or shower.
   2. Apply splints to the affected joints.
   3. Refer the child to physical therapy.
   4. Place a bed cradle over the child's legs.

3. A hospitalized school-age child is very quiet and seldom talks to the staff. The nurse can best communicate with this child by saying:
   1. "I've noticed you seem very quiet. Is anything troubling you?"
   2. "Let's tell each other a secret; you start by telling me what you are thinking."
   3. "It must be awfully hard to be away from home. Let's call your mom!"
   4. "Draw me some pictures of the things you've seen and done while you've been in the hospital."

4. Three of the following signs or symptoms indicate an improvement in the condition of a toddler with laryngotracheobronchitis. Which one indicates a *worsening* and should be promptly reported to the physician?
   1. Apical pulse = 118.
   2. Increase in appetite.
   3. Progressive hoarseness.
   4. Pink nailbeds.

5. The nurse reviews a toddler's immunizations with the parents and finds that the child has had all immunizations recommended during the toddler years. The nurse should advise the parents that, at 4–6 years of age, the child should next receive:
   1. MMR (measles, mumps, rubella).
   2. Hepatitis B.
   3. Hemophilus influenza type b.
   4. MMR (measles, mumps, rubella) and polio.

6. Which is the *most common* complaint by parents about infants with heart disease?
   1. Frequent, severe respiratory infections.
   2. "Slower" development.
   3. "Stunted" growth.
   4. Difficult to feed.

7. The nurse in the newborn nursery should plan any interventions with a newborn with myelomeningocele based on the knowledge that the major *short-term* complication the child is most likely to suffer is:
   1. Hydrocephalus.
   2. Meningitis.
   3. Mental retardation.
   4. Paraplegia.

8. The physician orders Tylenol elixir for a 14-month-old with a fever of 102°F. Considering this child's developmental level and her diagnosis, which would be the best approach by the nurse?
   1. Give her the medicine cup and tell her the "pretty red syrup" will taste sweet like candy.
   2. Mix the medication with 4 oz of apple juice and allow her to drink it through a "crazy straw."
   3. Put the medication into a brightly colored plastic cup and give her a chance to drink it herself.
   4. Raise her to a sitting position, bring the medicine cup to her lips, and tell her kindly but firmly to drink it.

9. A toddler is to be placed in a croupette. The nurse should plan to perform which nursing action?
   1. Remove all toys from the crib.
   2. Withhold all liquids and solids temporarily.
   3. Monitor oxygen concentration daily and record in notes.
   4. Evaluate the toddler's reaction to oxygen therapy in terms of vital signs and color.

10. The nurse should review principles of care with a 12-year-old child with asthma. Which comment by the child would require additional teaching by the nurse?
    1. "I keep all my stuffed animals on my bookcase now."
    2. "I have aluminum miniblinds on the windows in my room."
    3. "I gave my cat to my best friend."
    4. "I joined the swim team at school."

11. A mother asks the nurse about the normal time for the onset of menstruation. The nurse would be most correct in advising her that menses usually begin at age:
    1. 11½ years.
    2. 12 years.
    3. 12½ years.
    4. 13 years.

12. In doing an infant's admission examination, the nurse notes all the following abnormal findings. Which one is the *most common sign* of heart disease the *nurse* should assess?
    1. Circumoral cyanosis.
    2. Hypertension.
    3. Diastolic murmur.
    4. Tachycardia.

13. To "flood" the croupette with oxygen before placing a toddler in the tent, the nurse should initially adjust the oxygen flow rate to:

1. 2–3 L/min.
2. 4–5 L/min.
3. 8–10 L/min.
4. 15 L/min.

14. A 2-year-old is admitted to the hospital with acute bilateral otitis media. Her temperature is 103°F, and she has tremors in her arms and legs. In addition to a spinal tap to rule out bacterial meningitis, the doctor orders all the following. Which order should the nurse perform *first?*
   1. Respiratory isolation.
   2. IV 5% dextrose in 0.45 normal saline solution at 35 mL/h.
   3. Tylenol 120 mg PO q4h.
   4. Seizure precautions.

15. The doctor orders an IV to infuse at 35 mL/h; a pediatric microdrip chamber is hanging. How many drops per minute should the nurse regulate the IV to infuse?
   1. 5–6.
   2. 7–8.
   3. 9–10.
   4. 35.

16. A 7-year-old who has had leukemia for 2 years was in primary remission for 18 months but recently experienced infections, epistaxis, and abdominal petechiae. The doctor suspects she is no longer in remission and admits her to the hospital. In reviewing her admitting blood work, the nurse notes all the following. Which finding should the nurse interpret as the probable cause of her infections?
   1. Anemia.
   2. Leukopenia.
   3. Neutropenia.
   4. Thrombocytopenia.

17. A school-age child with rheumatic fever develops heart failure and is placed on digoxin, Lasix, and potassium. The chief purpose for giving potassium is to:
   1. Enhance the cardiogenic effect of digoxin.
   2. Potentiate the diuretic action of Lasix.
   3. Prevent hypokalemia.
   4. Pharmacologically induce hyperkalemia.

18. Two hospitalized school-age children complain that they are "bored." The nurse should offer them:
   1. A game of "Monopoly" or "Life."
   2. Workbooks, paper, and pencils.
   3. Some books from the hospital library.
   4. A chance to stay up late and watch TV.

19. A 12-year-old is admitted to the hospital in status asthmaticus, for the second time. In planning care for this child, the nurse must first assess:
   1. What she knows about asthma.
   2. How she usually cares for herself.
   3. What she knows about hospitalization.
   4. How she feels about becoming a teenager.

20. When the nurse begins teaching a teenager with diabetes about insulin, which one fact should be stressed to this teen and the family?
   1. Properly controlled dietary management, along with hypoglycemic agents, may eventually be used.
   2. Exogenous insulin will be necessary for the rest of the child's life.
   3. Activity level, nutritional intake, and state of health will necessitate daily modifications in the insulin dose.
   4. Due to the need for insulin, the child should no longer participate in active sports.

21. In doing a 3-year-old's admission history, the nurse notes all the following signs of hemophilia. The hallmark, or classic sign, of hemophilia is:
   1. Excessive hematoma formation.
   2. Hemarthrosis.
   3. Prolonged bleeding from lacerations.
   4. Intracranial bleeding.

22. The nurse performs a Denver Developmental Screening Test (DDST) on a 3-year-old. Which behavior should the nurse expect this child to be capable of doing?
   1. Going up stairs on alternate feet.
   2. Pedalling a bicycle.
   3. Dressing without supervision.
   4. Tying shoelaces.

23. While admitting an infant, the nurse notes all the following abnormal findings. Which one is considered the classic sign of Hirschsprung's disease?
   1. Abdominal distention.
   2. Anorexia.
   3. Constipation.
   4. Vomitus flecked with feces.

24. The best way for a nurse to perform a DDST on a 9-month-old is to:
   1. Take the infant from the mother and ask her to wait in the child's room.
   2. Take the infant from the mother and ask her to come with them to the testing area.
   3. Briefly talk first with the mother, then take the infant to the testing area alone.
   4. Ask the infant's mother to carry the child to the testing area.

25. For an infant with severe chronic CHF, the formula the nurse should plan to offer would be:
   1. Isomil.
   2. Lofenalac.
   3. Lonalac.
   4. Similac 27 with iron.

26. The parents of a school-age child with leukemia tell the nurse that their daughter frequently has nightmares, and they wonder how to handle this. The nurse would be most correct in advising them to:
   1. Comfort her, but leave her in her own bed.
   2. Comfort her by bringing her into their bed.
   3. Consult a child psychologist to determine why she has recurring sleep disturbances.
   4. Encourage the child to keep a written record of her dreams and discuss them with her primary nurse during hospitalization.

27. Before giving a child digoxin, which pulse would the nurse be most correct in assessing?
   1. Apical.
   2. Brachial.
   3. Pedal.
   4. Radial.

28. A 4½-year-old is admitted to the pediatrics unit for the third, and final, surgical procedure to correct his congenital hypospadias. When admitting this child to the hospital, the nurse should assess all of the following. Which information will be the most important to the nursing plan of care for this child?
   1. His developmental level.
   2. His knowledge level regarding hypospadias.
   3. His previous experience with illness and hospitalization.
   4. His parents' plans for rooming-in.

29. A hospitalized 4-year-old wakes up crying at 2 A.M. and says, "I want my mommy now." The nurse should:

1. Pick him up and rock him for a little while.
2. Talk softly to him while rubbing his back, but leave him in his crib.
3. Gently but firmly tell him to go back to sleep.
4. Call his mother and ask her to come to the hospital.

30. The nurse does discharge teaching with the mother of a preschooler with epiglottitis before his discharge. Which statement by the mother indicates that she has *correctly* understood the nurse's teaching?
    1. "I'm so glad that he is all better now."
    2. "I will keep him home from preschool for the rest of this month."
    3. "I'm still worried that he will get sick again when we get home."
    4. "I will get a portable tank of oxygen for him before he comes home."

31. After flooding a croupette for 5 minutes, the nurse should readjust the flow rate of oxygen. To maintain an oxygen concentration of 35–40%, the nurse should now adjust the oxygen flow rate to:
    1. 2–3 L/min.
    2. 4–5 L/min.
    3. 8–10 L/min.
    4. 15 L/min.

32. A toddler tries to pull her IV out, and the nurse determines she must be restrained to maintain the IV site. Which restraint would the nurse be most correct in applying?
    1. Posey jacket.
    2. Elbow.
    3. Mummy.
    4. Clove-hitch.

33. A lumbar puncture is performed on a child by the doctor. After the procedure, the nurse should position the child:
    1. Flat in bed, with no pillow.
    2. Flat in bed, with a small pillow.
    3. In semi-Fowler's position.
    4. Semiprone, with head to the side.

34. When the parents of a newborn with myelomeningocele visit the nursery for the first time, they make no comments about the baby's spinal sac. Instead, they offer many positive observations about size, color, hair, and appearance. The nurse would be most correct in interpreting the parents' behavior as:
    1. Attachment.
    2. Denial.
    3. Immaturity.
    4. Love.

35. The pediatrician orders syrup of ipecac for a toddler who has ingested a harmful substance. Generally, the nurse *should* administer this medication only if the child is:
    1. Alert and reactive.
    2. Convulsing.
    3. Comatose.
    4. Known to have swallowed a corrosive substance.

36. The mother of a preschooler who will have his third, and final, surgical procedure to correct congenital hypospadias questions the need for another surgical procedure while he is still so young. The nurse should stress that:
    1. It is the mother's right to refuse surgery at any time.
    2. It's in her son's best interest to follow the doctor's recommendations.
    3. He can have this third, and final, surgery any time before the onset of puberty.

4. This type of surgery is usually timed to precede kindergarten.

37. After the nurse completes preoperative teaching with a preschooler, which would be the *best* method for evaluating the effectiveness of the teaching?
    1. Ask him to draw a picture of what he will look like after surgery.
    2. Using puppets, ask him to show the nurse what he has learned about his surgery.
    3. Tell him that this is a test and he must repeat what he has learned about his operation.
    4. Suggest his parents check on their child's level of understanding and report back to the nurse.

38. The nurse should withhold a 6-year-old's digoxin and notify the physician if the child's pulse was *below*:
    1. 80 beats/min.
    2. 90 beats/min.
    3. 100 beats/min.
    4. 110 beats/min.

39. A 13-year-old is admitted to the hospital in sickle cell crisis with severe pain in her legs and abdomen. She asks the nurse why the doctor ordered oxygen for her when she has no trouble breathing. The nurse would be *most* correct in telling her that the main therapeutic effect of oxygen for her is to:
    1. Reverse sickling of RBCs.
    2. Prevent further sickling.
    3. Prevent respiratory complications.
    4. Increase the oxygen-carrying capacity of RBCs.

40. A 9-year-old is admitted to the hospital with a second attack of rheumatic fever. In doing an admission assessment on this child, which group of symptoms would the nurse most likely find?
    1. Petechiae, malaise, and joint pain.
    2. Chorea, anemia, and hypertension.
    3. Tachycardia, erythema marginatum, and fever in late afternoon.
    4. Subcutaneous nodules, dependent edema, and conjunctivitis.

41. A school-age child has leukemia. Considering her diagnosis and her health-teaching needs, the nurse would be most correct in advising this child to:
    1. Skip brushing her teeth at this time.
    2. Brush her teeth with a soft toothbrush only.
    3. Brush her teeth with a firm toothbrush only.
    4. Rinse her mouth with an antiseptic solution instead of brushing her teeth.

42. The mother of a hospitalized 3-year-old tells the nurse that he is a very poor eater at home. The best recommendation the nurse can make to increase his nutritional intake would be to:
    1. Provide him with a child-size table.
    2. Use plastic cups and plates with cartoon characters he likes.
    3. Offer him small portions of his favorite foods.
    4. Allow him to feed himself.

43. A 3-year-old with hemophilia is to be discharged, and the nurse has completed teaching with the child's parents. Which statement by the parents indicates they may have misunderstood the nurse's teaching regarding his care?
    1. "If he gets a fever, we will only give him acetaminophen, not aspirin."
    2. "We will be sure to supervise him carefully so that he doesn't experience another bleeding episode."
    3. "I'll order a MedicAlert bracelet for him as soon as we get home."

4. "It's a relief to know that his little sister will not get this disease too."

44. An infant with CHF takes 1¼ oz of formula in 20 minutes. The doctor ordered 2 oz of formula q 3 h. The *best* action for the nurse to take at this time would be to:
1. Ask his mother to feed him when she arrives.
2. Burp him and try to stimulate him to suck.
3. Continue feeding him slowly, allowing him as much time as he needs to finish.
4. Stop the feeding, and request an order for gavage feedings prn.

45. The mother of a 4-year-old with epiglottitis tells the nurse that she does not even know what epiglottitis is. The nurse would be most correct in telling her that it is:
1. An infection of the upper respiratory tract related to allergy and excessive mucous production.
2. A potentially life-threatening infection that requires prolonged intensive care.
3. A mild form of croup that is usually treated at home.
4. A swelling in the throat that can lead to total airway obstruction if not treated promptly.

46. On admission, a preschooler is carrying a soiled and worn-looking "Cookie Monster" stuffed animal. His mother states that this is his favorite toy. The most appropriate action for the nurse to take at this time is to:
1. Offer him a choice of another stuffed animal from the hospital playroom.
2. Place Cookie Monster somewhere in his room where he can see it but not touch it.
3. Suggest his mother bring him a new Cookie Monster stuffed animal.
4. Tell him that he can keep Cookie Monster in the bed with him.

47. In reviewing a preschooler's admission history and laboratory results, the nurse should know that the two most common findings in children with nephrosis are:
1. Generalized edema and proteinuria.
2. Hyperlipidemia and periorbital edema.
3. Hypertension and hematuria.
4. Oliguria and anorexia.

48. The number one priority during the nurse's admission assessment of a school-age child with rheumatic fever is the child's:
1. Weight.
2. Apical pulse rate.
3. Developmental level.
4. ESR.

49. In planning care for a teenager in sickle cell crisis, the nurse should base any actions on the knowledge that pain in vaso-occlusive crisis is *primarily* due to:
1. Increased RBC destruction.
2. Hepatosplenomegaly.
3. Occlusion of small blood vessels.
4. Sequestration of blood.

50. A teenager is preparing his first dose of insulin. The physician orders 14 U of NPH insulin; the teen draws up 13 U and shows it to the nurse. The nurse should base any response on the knowledge that:
1. This is his first attempt and he did come close to the exact dose.
2. At his age, he cannot be expected to make such fine discriminations in dosage.
3. He must draw up the exact amount before administration.
4. Teenagers like him often antagonize adults subconsciously.

51. Between meals, the nurse should place an infant with CHF in which position?
1. In an infant seat with head elevated.
2. Prone with head turned to side.
3. Supine with head slightly hyperextended.
4. Side-lying with the head of the bed elevated 30°.

52. The doctor attempts to shine a light through a myelomeningocele sac and notes "no transillumination." The nurse should interpret this finding to mean that the sac:
1. Can be easily repaired.
2. Cannot be evaluated by this technique.
3. Contains meninges and CSF.
4. Contains meninges, CSF, and the spinal cord.

53. After administering syrup of ipecac to a toddler, the nurse should also give:
1. Four ounces of warm milk.
2. Activated charcoal powder.
3. As much water as the child will drink.
4. A slice of dry toast.

54. After placing a toddler in a croup tent, the nurse should adjust the plastic canopy so that:
1. The edges are tucked tightly under the linen.
2. The edges are lying loosely on top of the linen.
3. The crib rails are raised and the canopy edges are over them.
4. The crib rails are lowered and the canopy edges are inside them.

55. In what position should the nurse place a child in status asthmaticus?
1. Knee-chest.
2. High Fowler's.
3. Lateral Sims'.
4. Supine, with neck hyperextended.

56. A teenager hospitalized with diabetes goes to the teen lounge and becomes very boisterous and aggressive, starting a fight with another teen. The *first* question the nurse should consider is:
1. "Should he be sent to his room?"
2. "Did he eat breakfast today?"
3. "What did the other teen do to him?"
4. "Does he miss his own friends?"

57. The nurse has completed discharge teaching with the parents of an infant with ventricular septal defect (VSD) and CHF. Which one statement by the mother would indicate the need for additional teaching by the nurse?
1. "I'll be sure to dress him in loose-fitting clothes."
2. "I'll try to keep my house as warm as I can for him."
3. "I'll be at the clinic in 3 days for his appointment."
4. "I'll put him in his playpen at least once a day."

58. A 7-month-old infant is admitted to the pediatrics unit with moderate dehydration secondary to AGE. The physician writes all the following orders for this infant. Which one should the nurse implement *first*?
1. Universal precautions.
2. IV of 5% dextrose in ⅓ normal saline solution at 25 mL/h.
3. Urine specific gravity stat and q4h.
4. Stool culture every shift × 3.

59. The *best* advice the nurse can give to parents to handle a toddler's temper tantrums would be to:
1. Allow the toddler to make her own choices.
2. Ignore this behavior.
3. Change the setting in which they occur.
4. Give in to the toddler's demands, to nurture autonomy.

60. A 3-year-old is admitted to the hospital with classic hemophilia (factor VIII deficiency). Which admission procedure by the nurse will probably be the most frightening for this child?
    1. Blood pressure.
    2. Rectal temperature.
    3. Urine specimen.
    4. Weight.

61. In writing a nursing care plan for a 7-year-old child with leukemia, the nurse should include all of the following goals. Which goal is *most* important and should receive *top* priority?
    1. Maintain infection-free state.
    2. Prevent injury.
    3. Promote adequate nutrition.
    4. Meet developmental needs.

62. The physician orders sterile moist soaks to a myelomeningocele sac. The major reason for this treatment is to:
    1. Promote comfort.
    2. Prevent infection.
    3. Relieve pressure.
    4. Stimulate neural development.

63. The night before surgery, as he is getting ready for bed, a preschooler asks his father to "check under the bed for monsters." The nurse would be most correct in advising his father to:
    1. Ask the child to talk more about these monsters.
    2. Leave a light on and let the child check for himself.
    3. Make a game of checking under his bed.
    4. Tell him that monsters are only make-believe.

64. Following surgery to correct hypospadias, a toddler returns to the unit with a Foley catheter in place. The nurse should expect the drainage to have:
    1. A clear yellow appearance.
    2. Small clots of blood or mucus.
    3. Gross hematuria in moderate amounts.
    4. A brownish tinge.

65. A 6-year-old with cystic fibrosis is to receive replacement pancreatic enzymes several times daily. The best time for the nurse to plan to administer this medication is:
    1. After every meal or snack.
    2. Between meals and after every snack.
    3. Immediately before meals or snacks.
    4. With meals and before snacks.

66. In addition to administering oxygen, the nurse can also relieve the pain experienced by a teenager in sickle cell crisis by:
    1. Applying warm compresses.
    2. Applying cold compresses.
    3. Performing passive ROM exercises.
    4. Performing ADL as needed.

67. The nurse observes a nursing student fastening an infant's diaper snugly around his abdomen; the infant has CHF. The nurse should:
    1. Ask the student to loosen his diaper.
    2. Do or say nothing, as this is expected behavior for a student.
    3. Loosen the diaper after the student leaves the room.
    4. Praise the student for outstanding attention to detail.

68. Which statement by the parents of a preschooler with nephrosis indicates that they have fully understood the nurse's teaching?
    1. "We will keep him away from other children so he doesn't get a relapse."

    2. "We're so glad this is all over and we don't have to worry any more."
    3. "When we get home, we're going to find it hard to keep him in bed."
    4. "We will watch him for any signs of this starting up again."

69. A child with leukemia is receiving vincristine. The nurse should observe this child closely for the side effect of:
    1. Diarrhea.
    2. Diplopia.
    3. Hemorrhagic cystitis.
    4. Peripheral neuropathy.

70. A 6-year-old with cystic fibrosis refuses to swallow the replacement pancreatic enzymes tablets (e.g., Viokase). The best course of action for the nurse would be to:
    1. Check with the doctor about discontinuing this medication.
    2. Crush the tablets and mix with 1 teaspoon of cold applesauce.
    3. Dissolve the tablets in 4 oz of warm milk.
    4. Offer the child a "special treat" for swallowing the tablets "like a big kid."

71. A school-age child experiences the following signs or symptoms of rheumatic fever. The nurse should plan any interventions based on the knowledge that the only one that may result in *permanent* damage is:
    1. Sydenham's chorea.
    2. Migratory polyarthritis.
    3. Carditis.
    4. Erythema marginatum.

72. The best roommate for a 9-year-old girl with rheumatic fever would be:
    1. An 8-year-old girl with impetigo.
    2. A 9-year-old girl with a tonsillectomy.
    3. A 10-year-old girl with a concussion.
    4. An 11-year-old girl with a fractured elbow.

73. The nurse should be aware that the most important nursing diagnosis in caring for a child with diabetes is:
    1. High risk for injury related to insulin deficiency.
    2. Altered family processes related to situational crisis (child with chronic disease).
    3. Knowledge deficit related to care of a child with diabetes.
    4. Altered body image related to treatment of diabetes.

74. An infant with myelomeningocele is scheduled to have surgery to close the sac. The mother asks the nurse if the baby will be able to move her legs following this operation. The best response for the nurse to make would be:
    1. "Not usually, although we can always hope for a miracle."
    2. "There is no way to predict. All we can do is watch her closely."
    3. "No, the surgery is done mainly to prevent infection."
    4. "Yes, the surgery will restore her ability to move her legs."

75. The best method to prevent the spread of infection from an infant with AGE to other staff members or visitors would be:
    1. Double bagging all linens.
    2. Obtaining stool cultures.
    3. Strict handwashing.
    4. Wearing disposable gloves.

76. At 7 months of age, an infant exhibits the following skills. The nurse should know that the most recently acquired skill is probably the ability to:

1. Roll over.
2. Sit up.
3. Bear some weight on legs.
4. Pick up objects with palmar grasp.

77. The most appropriate person to administer a preoperative series of cleansing enemas to a 9-month-old with Hirschprung's disease would be his:
    1. Primary nurse.
    2. Mother.
    3. Student nurse.
    4. Nursing assistant.

78. On admission, the nurse would expect a 14-month-old to demonstrate which two *early* signs of laryngotracheobronchitis (LTB)?
    1. Dyspnea and cyanosis.
    2. Hoarseness and tachycardia.
    3. Expiratory wheeze and low-grade fever.
    4. Metallic cough and inspiratory stridor.

79. A diagnosis of bacterial meningitis is confirmed, and the child assumes an opisthotonus position. In which position should the nurse now place this child?
    1. Prone.
    2. Supine.
    3. Side-lying.
    4. Trendelenburg.

80. In planning a roommate for a hospitalized 12-year-old girl, the nurse should realize that a child of this developmental level will:
    1. Probably prefer another girl her own age.
    2. Most likely seek out opportunities to socialize with teenagers.
    3. Enjoy being with either a girl or boy, as long as they're the same age.
    4. Feel helpful if given the opportunity to look after a slightly younger child.

81. In teaching a teenager how to prevent further episodes of sickle cell crisis, the nurse should stress the need to *avoid:*
    1. Moderate emotional stress.
    2. Cool weather.
    3. Swimming in public pools.
    4. Extra fluid consumption.

82. If a child who was given syrup of ipecac has not vomited within 30 minutes, the nurse should:
    1. Stimulate the gag reflex using his or her fingers.
    2. Wait another 30 minutes before doing anything else.
    3. Assume the danger is past and no further treatment is needed at this time.
    4. Repeat the dose a second time.

83. The physician orders "increasing activity as tolerated" for a school-age child with rheumatic fever. After getting her up into an armchair, the nurse should monitor how well she tolerates this increase in activity by checking her:
    1. Apical pulse rate.
    2. Breath sounds.
    3. Degree of restlessness.
    4. Lips and nailbeds.

84. About a week after discharge, a newly-diagnosed teen-aged diabetic and his mother return to the clinic for a check-up. His mother states, "I'm worried he will make a mistake, so I've been giving him his insulin." The nurse should:
    1. Allow the teenager and his mother to work this out on their own.
    2. Assist his mother to understand that he must assume this responsibility.

3. Encourage his mother to continue working closely with him.
4. Realize that this is an appropriate response by the mother.

85. The mother of a hospitalized infant with CHF asks the nurse why he is sucking on a pacifier. The nurse would be most correct in telling her:
    1. "He seems to like it."
    2. "Most infants prefer a pacifier to their thumb."
    3. "This is to keep him from crying."
    4. "We give all hospitalized infants a pacifier."

86. The first night in the hospital, a 3-year-old hemophiliac suffers an episode of epistaxis. In which position should the nurse place this child?
    1. Prone, with head turned to side.
    2. Semi-Fowler's with two pillows.
    3. Sitting up with head tilted backward.
    4. Sitting up and leaning forward slightly.

87. Nursing care for a toddler while she is in the croupette includes which of the following?
    1. Giving her a bald plastic doll.
    2. Removing her blanket and pajamas.
    3. Restraining her arms and legs.
    4. Restricting visitors to her immediate family.

88. The mother of a child with cystic fibrosis tells the nurse that she is thinking of getting pregnant again but is worried that her next child might also have cystic fibrosis. Because her child does have this disease, the nurse should advise this mother that a second child:
    1. Could be even more severely affected than her first child.
    2. Might also have the disease.
    3. Should be "normal," or disease-free.
    4. Would only carry the trait.

89. A child has had asthma since age 6. In reviewing this child's history, which one factor should the nurse realize may be related to the development of the asthma?
    1. Strep throat/tonsillitis at age 2.
    2. Eczema at age 3½.
    3. Paternal death at age 5.
    4. Pneumonia at age 7.

90. Which one behavior should the nurse expect a 5-month-old with CHF to be capable of demonstrating?
    1. Rolling over from stomach to back.
    2. Sitting with support.
    3. Pincer grasp.
    4. Bearing some weight on legs.

91. Following surgery to close the myelomeningocele sac, the nurse should place the infant on her:
    1. Abdomen, with head 10 degrees lower than hips.
    2. Abdomen, with head of bed elevated 30 degrees.
    3. Abdomen, with hips 10 degrees lower than head.
    4. Abdomen, flat in bed.

92. Parents of an infant with Hirschsprung's disease ask the nurse how their baby got the disease. The nurse would be most correct in advising them that:
    1. Their baby was born with this condition.
    2. It is the result of the meconium ileus the baby experienced as a newborn.
    3. Their baby spontaneously developed this condition.
    4. It often occurs following the introduction of solid foods due to a genetically inherited metabolic defect.

93. As a toddler recovers from meningitis, the nurse should watch carefully for which *long-term* complication?
    1. Encephalitis.
    2. Hydrocephalus.

3. Learning disabilities.
4. Mental retardation.

94. In reviewing what he would do if he experienced a hypoglycemic episode, a teenager correctly states that he would eat a piece of candy or drink a glass of orange juice. The nurse should then instruct him to follow this concentrated sweet with:
   1. A Dextrostix test.
   2. A urine dipstick for glucose.
   3. A glass of milk.
   4. 5 U of regular insulin.

95. The mother of a child hospitalized with asthma asks the nurse what causes asthma. The nurse would be most correct in telling her the cause is:
   1. Unknown.
   2. Allergies.
   3. Stress.
   4. Multiple factors.

96. Long-term follow-up care is being planned for a school-age child with rheumatic fever before discharge from the hospital. This *must* include:
   1. Indefinite antibiotic therapy.
   2. Immunization against future attacks.
   3. Cardiac rehabilitation program.
   4. Home-bound tutoring.

97. A preschooler has been admitted with a tentative diagnosis of epiglottitis. A medical student tells the nurse that she wants to look down this child's throat to visualize the epiglottis. The nurse would be most correct in:
   1. Asking the child's mother if she objects to the medical student checking her child.
   2. Telling the medical student that she absolutely cannot do this.
   3. Promising the child a special treat for "opening real wide for the doctor."
   4. Helping restrain the child so the medical student can get a better look.

98. A preschooler with nephrosis is started on prednisone. If the prednisone is having the expected therapeutic effect, the nurse should expect that this child will:
   1. Experience mood swings.
   2. Have sugar in the urine.
   3. Gain weight.
   4. Feel better.

99. A toddler who is being placed in a croupette cries and tries to cling to her mother. Her mother asks the nurse if she can climb into the crib and lie in the tent with the toddler. The nurse's best response would be:
   1. "Do you always let her have her way like this?"
   2. "I'll have to check with her doctor first."
   3. "No, that would not be safe for you or her."
   4. "It may help her calm down; let's give it a try."

100. In a 2-week-old infant, the earliest sign of hydrocephalus the nurse would observe is:
   1. Bulging anterior fontanel.
   2. Increasing head circumference.
   3. Shrill, high-pitched cry.
   4. Sunset eyes.

101. A child with leukemia who is receiving chemotherapy develops oral ulcers. The most appropriate nursing intervention would be to:
   1. Encourage her to use viscous lidocaine (Xylocaine) before meals.
   2. Offer her lukewarm liquids, such as tea or broth.
   3. Crush two tablets of aspirin in warm water and instruct her to gargle with this solution.
   4. Allow her to eat or drink foods of her own choosing.

102. A preschooler with nephrosis has a swollen scrotal sac. Which nursing action would be most effective in relieving discomfort?
   1. Apply zinc oxide to scrotum qid.
   2. Cleanse scrotum with warm water only.
   3. Sprinkle medicated powder on scrotum.
   4. Support scrotum on folded diapers.

103. The surgeon orders a preoperative series of cleansing enemas for an infant with Hirschsprung's disease. The nurse should expect the solution ordered for these enemas to be:
   1. Soapsuds enema (SSE).
   2. Normal saline.
   3. Pediatric Fleets.
   4. Tap water.

104. In doing the admission assessment, the nurse should expect to find which signs of dehydration in an infant?
   1. Fever and bradycardia.
   2. Irritability and sunken eyeballs.
   3. Hypotension and anuria.
   4. Dry mucous membranes and bulging anterior fontanel.

105. If a toddler were to develop hydrocephalus, which would be the *earliest* sign(s) the nurse would most likely note?
   1. Irritability and poor feeding.
   2. Increasing head circumference.
   3. Headache and diplopia.
   4. Ruptured retinal vessels.

106. The mother of a child with cystic fibrosis asks the nurse if the child will be allowed to participate in any team sports now that he is starting school. The nurse would be most correct in advising her that he can participate in:
   1. Softball.
   2. Tennis.
   3. Soccer.
   4. Swimming.

107. Parents of a child with sickle cell anemia both have the sickle cell trait. In counseling these parents about having another child, the nurse would be most correct in telling them that future pregnancies will have a:
   1. 1:4 chance of producing a child with sickle cell anemia.
   2. 1:2 chance of producing a child with sickle cell anemia.
   3. 1:4 chance of producing a child with sickle cell trait.
   4. 4:4 chance of producing a child with sickle cell anemia.

108. A hemophiliac is to receive cryoprecipitate (Factor VIII). During the infusion of this medication, the nurse should plan to observe this patient for which one of the following potential complications?
   1. Emboli formation.
   2. Fluid volume overload.
   3. Onset of AIDS.
   4. Transfusion reaction.

109. A preschooler with epiglottitis is admitted to the hospital and is to receive Solucortef 100 mg IV q6h. The main purpose for this medication is to:
   1. Provide mild sedation.
   2. Reduce swelling.
   3. Relieve pain.
   4. Treat infection.

110. A child with leukemia is being discharged, and the doctor suggests an immediate return to school. The nurse should be sure to teach the parents to keep this child home if any classmates develop:

1. Impetigo.
2. Strep throat.
3. Pneumonia.
4. Chickenpox.

111. In discharge teaching with the parents of an infant with VSD and CHF, which one visitor should the nurse discourage from touching or holding this infant?
1. His aunt, who has lupus.
2. His grandmother, who has a slight cold.
3. His father, who is a drug addict.
4. His 3-year-old sister, who is in nursery school.

112. In monitoring a toddler for response to syrup of ipecac, the nurse should base any actions on the knowledge that ipecac is potentially:
1. Cardiotoxic.
2. Hepatotoxic.
3. Nephrotoxic.
4. Neurotoxic.

113. A mother who lost her first-born to SIDS tells the nurse that she plans to breastfeed her second baby to prevent this from happening again. The nurse should base any response on the knowledge that:
1. Breastfeeding does *not* prevent SIDS.
2. Breastfeeding *does* seem to prevent SIDS.
3. SIDS occurs *more* frequently in infants who are bottlefed.
4. Breastfeeding is contraindicated for *siblings* of infants who died from SIDS.

114. Normally, an infant's birthweight doubles by the age of 6 months and triples by the age of 1 year. By what age should the nurse expect the birthweight to *quadruple?*
1. 18 months.
2. 2 years.
3. 2½ years.
4. 3 years.

115. A mother asks the nurse how tall her child will be when grown up. What answer should the nurse offer?
1. "This is virtually impossible to predict."
2. "It will be double the child's height at 2 years of age."
3. "It will be triple the child's height at 18 months of age."
4. "Add 2 feet to the child's height at 4 years of age."

116. The only childhood communicable disease for which there is *not* currently a recommended routine immunization is:
1. Chickenpox.
2. Smallpox.
3. Parotitis.
4. Rubeola.

117. In teaching principles of poison control to a group of mothers, the nurse would be most correct in stressing that the age group most likely to suffer from accidental ingestions is:
1. 6–18 months.
2. 12 months–2½ years.
3. 2–4 years.
4. 3–5 years.

118. In deciding which *one* type of accident prevention to discuss *first* with the parents of a toddler, the nurse should base the choice on the knowledge that most deaths in children under age 3 are caused by:
1. Aspiration/suffocation.
2. Falls.
3. Motor vehicles.
4. Poisonings.

119. The following four children are patients in the pediatrics unit. Which one should the nurse anticipate will be *most* affected by separation from parents?
1. A 6-week-old with pyloric stenosis.
2. A 19-month-old with salicylate poisoning.
3. A 3½-year-old with hypospadias.
4. A 5-year-old with hemophilia.

120. In assessing the development of a 5-year-old, the nurse would not expect the child to be able to:
1. Name primary colors.
2. Count to 100.
3. Know the days of the week.
4. Give telephone number and address.

❑ Answers/Rationale

1. **(1)** Place the infant with a myelomeningocele on her stomach in a prone position to avoid pressure on the sac, which could cause tears, leaks, and infection. The side-lying position **(3)** might be an acceptable second choice, depending on the exact size and location of the sac. Placing the infant on her back **(2)** is absolutely contraindicated, since this would lead to immediate rupture of the sac. Trendelenburg position **(4)** is unnecessary for this infant. **IMP,3,SECE**

2. **(4)** For a child experiencing migratory polyarthritis, even the weight of a single sheet can cause excruciating pain; therefore, a bed cradle will help keep the linens off the child's joints and provide symptomatic relief. This child is most likely on absolute bedrest, thus making a bath or shower **(1)** out of the question. Splints or a referral to physical therapy **(2, 3)** is unnecessary, because this type of arthritis causes no permanent deformities. **IMP,1,PhI**

3. **(4)** Projective techniques seem to work best with school-age children in getting them to share their thoughts, feelings, and experiences. Direct questioning **(1)** often proves too threatening, causing the child to become even quieter. Challenging the child directly to "tell secrets" **(2)** is also too threatening and will likely cause the child to refuse to speak about anything. Finally, calling the child's mother **(3)** will not necessarily assist the child to communicate with the nurse. **IMP,7,PsI**

4. **(3)** Progressive hoarseness, followed by aphonia, is an ominous sign of impending airway obstruction and respiratory arrest secondary to edema and inflammation. This must be promptly reported to the physician, who will probably do an emergency tracheostomy. An apical pulse of 118 **(1)** is normal for a toddler; pink nailbeds **(4)** indicate a satisfactory level of oxygenation. Finally, as the toddler begins to improve, appetite should also pick up **(2)**. **EV,6,PhI**

5. **(4)** At preschool age (4–6 years), the child should receive immunizations for DTP, OPV, and MMR. MMR **(1)** is not wrong, but it is less complete. Hepatitis **(2)** is completed by 18 months, and *Hemophilus influenzae* **(3)** is completed by 15 months. **IMP,1,HPM**

Key to codes following rationales Nursing process: **AS,** Assessment; **AN,** Analysis; **PL,** Plan; **IMP,** Implementation; **EV,** Evaluation. Category of human function: **1,** Protective; **2,** Sensory-perceptual; **3,** Comfort, Rest, Activity, and Mobility; **4,** Nutrition; **5,** Growth and Development; **6,** Fluid-Gas Transport, **7,** Psychosocial-Cultural; **8,** Elimination. Client need: **SECE,** Safe, Effective Care Environment; **PhI,** Physiological Integrity; **PsI,** Psychosocial Integrity; **HPM,** Health Promotion/Maintenance. See appendices for full explanation.

6. **(4)** Typically, the majority of parents of infants with CHD will complain about the infant's being very difficult to feed: must be woken up to feed, has weak suck, may turn blue with feeding, takes an overly long time to feed but falls asleep before finishing. Because of the weak suck, and altered cardiopulmonary dynamics, the infant is also prone to aspiration, pneumonia, and various respiratory infections **(1)** as well, although parents often do not make the connection between these factors. In addition, because of the difficulty in feeding the infant, the infant typically presents with developmental delays **(2)** and a slow rate of growth **(3)**, although again this is not what the majority of parents of infants with CHD complain about. **AN,6,PhI**

7. **(2)** The major short-term complication that infants with myelomeningocele face is infection following a tear or rupture of the sac. Hydrocephalus **(1)** does occur in 90% of these cases, usually following closure of the sac, but it is thought to be part of the CNS defect rather than a "complication." Likewise, paraplegia **(4)** is part of the symptom complex these patients present with, rather than a "complication." Finally, mental retardation **(3)** may or may not occur, but if it does occur it is a long-term complication. **AN,3,PhI**

8. **(4)** As a toddler, this child will probably assert her autonomy by refusing to take this medication. The best approach is to be firm yet kind, and always calm. No child should be told medicine is (like) candy **(1)**. Medication should be mixed with no more than one teaspoon of any nonessential food or beverage **(2)**. This toddler will probably not drink this medication by herself **(3)**, and the nurse should not offer her this choice because, if she refuses, then a "power" struggle will follow. **IMP,5,HPM**

9. **(4)** If the toddler responds well to oxygen therapy, she should show clinical improvement in terms of pink lips and nailbeds and normal vital signs, especially pulse. "All" toys do not have to be removed from her crib **(1)**, nor will she have to be NPO **(2)**, although she will probably be somewhat anorexic and prefer clear, cool liquids initially. Oxygen concentrations should be monitored and recorded at least every 2 hours **(3)**. **PL,6,SECE**

10. **(1)** Children with asthma should have no stuffed animals in their rooms, because they tend to collect dust, so more teaching would be needed. Additional measures to "allergy proof" the room and home should include using only aluminum miniblinds rather than curtains **(2)** and having no pets in the home **(3)**. Moderate exercise such as swimming **(4)** is recommended. **EV,1,HPM**

11. **(3)** The average age for the onset of menstruation for American females is 12½ years of age; girls between 10 and 16 years can begin to menstruate within the normal range **(1, 2, 4)**. **IMP,5,PsI**

12. **(4)** The majority of infants with CHD present with tachycardia, or a heart rate above 160 beats/min; this is often the first sign of CHD that the nurse can assess. Circumoral cyanosis **(1)**, hypertension **(2)**, and diastolic murmur **(3)** all may or may not be present, depending on the type and severity of the defect. **AS,6,PhI**

13. **(4)** To "flood" the croupette with oxygen means to raise the oxygen concentration to that level ordered by the physician; in general, the flow rate should be adjusted to 15 L/min, the tent should be closed and tucked in, and the nurse should wait about 15 minutes before checking the concentration and readjusting the flow.

Lower flow rates **(1, 2, 3)** would result in lower-than-required oxygen concentrations. **IMP,6,SECE**

14. **(1)** In caring for a patient with a potentially contagious condition such as meningitis, the first priority is protecting the nurse and other patients by observing appropriate infection control measures, in this case, respiratory isolation. All other nursing care measures would then follow in the appropriate order **(2, 3, 4)**. **AN,1,SECE**

15. **(4)** With a pediatric microdrip chamber, the number of mL/hour = number of drops/minute. Therefore, if the physician orders 35 mL/hour, the IV should infuse at 35 drops/minute. Any other flow rate would be incorrect **(1, 2, 3)**. **IMP,1,SECE**

16. **(3)** Neutropenia is an abnormal decrease in the number of neutrophils, the specific type of WBC responsible for phagocytosis and bacterial destruction; as such, the infection in a leukemic patient is most commonly related to neutropenia. Leukemic patients may also suffer from anemia **(1)**, leukopenia **(2)**, or thrombocytopenia **(4)**, although these blood dyscrasias will result in other signs or symptoms of leukemia. **AN,1,PhI**

17. **(3)** Clients receiving digoxin in addition to Lasix are particularly prone to developing hypokalemia, which can result in digoxin toxicity and potentially fatal cardiac dysrhythmias. Potassium supplements are frequently administered to avoid this problem rather than for any of the other reasons cited here **(1, 2, 4)**. **AN,1/5,PhI**

18. **(1)** School-age children are notoriously competitive, and they particularly enjoy the challenge of board games such as "Monopoly" or "Life." Although schoolwork is important and should receive due consideration **(2)**, it will not relieve their boredom. Likewise, books or TV **(3, 4)** are less effective diversions for the school-age child. **IMP,7,PsI**

19. **(3)** In working with children in hospitals, the most important factor for the nurse to assess first is the child's experience with illness and hospitalization. This is of special importance with this child, who has been hospitalized previously. After this most important factor, the nurse would continue the admitting assessment by determining what she knows about asthma **(1)**, how she usually cares for herself **(2)**, and how she feels about becoming a teenager **(4)**. **AN,7,PsI**

20. **(2)** Because the beta cells of the islets of Langerhans of the pancreas will never again produce a sufficient quantity of insulin, this teenager will remain dependent on insulin injections (exogenous insulin) for the rest of his life. Juvenile diabetics can never rely on hypoglycemic agents to control diabetes **(1)**, since these drugs work by stimulating the pancreas, and in this case the stimulation would have absolutely no effect. *Daily* modifications would generally not be necessary **(3)**, although periodic adjustments in insulin dosage would be needed as this teenager grows. He can continue to participate in sports **(4)**, but he should be taught to take some extra foods on those days he is active in sports. **IMP,4,PhI**

21. **(2)** Hemarthrosis, or bleeding into a joint either spontaneously or following an injury, is considered the hallmark, or most typical sign, of hemophilia. If hemarthrosis is not treated properly or adequately, permanent joint deformities may result. Other signs of hemophilia include prolonged bleeding from a relatively minor injury **(3)**, excessive or unusual hematoma formation **(1)**, and intracranial bleeding following a closed head injury **(4)**. **AN,6,PhI**

22. **(1)** Three-year-olds should be able to coordinate the brain and gross motor activity necessary to go up stairs using alternate feet. They should also be able to pedal "Big Wheels" or a tricycle but *not* a bicycle **(2)**. Three-year-olds should also be able to get dressed *with* supervision but not without it **(3)**. They should not be ready to master tying shoelaces **(4)** for another year or two. **AN,6,HPM**

23. **(3)** The classic sign of Hirschsprung's disease is obstinate constipation that persists despite all efforts at treatment. Other symptoms may also occur but are not generally considered specific to Hirschsprung's disease as much as they indicate intestinal obstruction: abdominal distention **(1)**, anorexia **(2)**, and vomiting **(4)**. **AN,8,PhI**

24. **(4)** The instruction manual of the DDST clearly states that the parent should accompany the child who is to have the DDST and that the examiner should do everything possible to establish rapport with the parent and the child. With a 9-month-old, this should include allowing the parent to hold the child rather than separating them for the purpose of testing **(1, 2, 3)**. **IMP,5,HPM**

25. **(3)** An infant with severe chronic CHF should be on a low-sodium formula, Lonalac. Isomil **(1)** is a lactose-free formula that contains a normal amount of sodium. Lofenalac **(2)** is the formula used to treat infants with PKU and also contains a normal amount of sodium. Similac 27 with iron **(4)** is most frequently used for preterm infants and also contains a normal amount of sodium. **PL,6,SECE**

26. **(1)** Most psychologists would recommend that a child be offered comfort in the form of a hug, kiss, or cuddle; however, the child should be left in his or her own bed to avoid overdependence on the parents or possible psychosexual conflicts caused by entering the parents' bed **(2)**. For the school-age child, nightmares are a common occurrence and can be accepted as a normal part of growth and development; therefore, no professional intervention is necessary at this time **(3)**. It could be very difficult for this child to keep written records of her dreams **(4)**; in fact, such an expectation might lead to even more severe sleep disturbances for her. **IMP,5,HPM**

27. **(1)** Before administering digoxin to a child, the nurse should auscultate the apical pulse for a full minute to most accurately evaluate cardiac rate and rhythm. Other pulse sites **(2, 3, 4)** are less accurate in children. **AS,6,SECE**

28. **(3)** In working with children in hospitals, the most important factor for the nurse to assess first is what that child's experience with illness and hospitalization has been thus far. This is of special importance with this child, who has previously had two hospitalizations and surgeries; the nurse needs to know if these were positive experiences for this child and how he was able to cope with them. After this, the nurse would continue the admitting assessment by determining the child's developmental level **(1)**, what the child already knows about hypospadias **(2)**, and whether the child's parents plan to room-in with him **(4)**. **PL,8,PsI**

29. **(2)** Hospitalized preschoolers often regress in their behavior and want "mommy," but this is obviously not practical all the time. The nurse should try to soothe the child back to sleep during the middle of the night. Calling the mother to come right in **(4)** would be inappropriate, since the family should not be called in the absence of a genuine emergency. The nurse should also not pick the child up **(1)**, because hospitalized preschoolers frequently reject everyone except their "mommy." Simply insisting the child go back to sleep **(3)** is not enough, since he needs some degree of comfort at this time. **IMP,7,PsI**

30. **(1)** Although the abrupt onset and critical nature of this illness is very frightening for parents, the child is expected to make a total recovery before discharge. The parents should be aware of this very positive diagnosis. Although discharge instructions from the physician may include some rest at home, there is no need for the child to miss almost a month of school **(2)**. The parents should not worry about the child's getting sick again **(3)** or having oxygen in the home **(4)**; again, the excellent prognosis should be stressed. **EV,6,HPM**

31. **(3)** To maintain an oxygen concentration of 35–40%, the flow rate should now be adjusted to 8–10 L/min; this is the usual concentration ordered for a croup tent. Other flow rates would result in higher or lower concentrations **(1, 2, 4)**. **IMP,6,SECE**

32. **(4)** To restrain a toddler receiving IV therapy, clove-hitch restraint to two or more limbs is most effective in maintaining the IV site. A posey jacket **(1)** would allow the toddler use of her hands with which to pull at her IV. Elbow restraints **(2)** would still allow the toddler to stand and twist at the IV tubing. A mummy restraint **(3)** would be unnecessarily restrictive for a toddler. **IMP,1,SECE**

33. **(1)** The best position for patients who have had a spinal tap is perfectly flat in bed, with no pillow at all. Such patients are prone to headaches due to the loss of CSF during the spinal tap; until the fluid is naturally replaced by the body, a flat position will minimize cerebral irritation and minimize headache; thus, **(2)** is incorrect. Elevating the HOB **(3)** will increase headache and is not recommended. There is no need to place the child semiprone **(4)** at this time. **IMP,1,SECE**

34. **(2)** The usual response to the birth of a defective infant is denial, often manifest in the parents' "refusing" to acknowledge the problem; this is a normal response, at least initially. The parents' comments about their infant, in view of this serious defect, should not be interpreted as attachment **(1)**, immaturity **(3)**, or love **(4)**. **EV,7,PsI**

35. **(1)** With a child who has suffered an ingestion, vomiting should be induced only if the child is fully alert and reactive. If the child has any alterations in level of consciousness, such as seizures **(2)** or coma **(3)**, vomiting may cause an aspiration pneumonia. Further, if the child has swallowed a corrosive substance **(4)**, the substance that burned once going down will burn a second time coming up if vomiting is induced. **AN,1,SECE**

36. **(4)** Because hypospadias interferes with the child's ability to void in the normal male standing position, the corrective surgery is usually timed to be completed before the child starts kindergarten. The main reason is to avoid other children making fun of the little boy's having to sit to void. Developmental and psychological factors thus play a crucial role in the timing of this surgery, and other explanations **(1, 2, 3)** are either incorrect or inappropriate for this child. **IMP,8,PhI**

37. **(2)** When doing preoperative teaching with preschoolers, the best method is to use puppets (doctor, nurse, hospital set-up) to "act out" what the child can expect to happen. For evaluating the teaching, the nurse can then ask the child to use puppets to give a return demonstration of what was learned; this enables the nurse to clarify any misconceptions or answer any lingering

questions the child might still have. Most preschoolers will not be able to *accurately* draw pictures regarding the factual information of preop teaching **(1)**, although this might be a good way to get at feelings about the surgery or hospital. A preschooler probably has had limited experience with "tests" **(3)**. The nurse should not rely on the parents to evaluate the preop teaching **(4)**, since they are not professionals and are most likely too involved emotionally. **EV,1,PsI**

38. **(1)** The lower limit of a normal pulse rate for a 6-year-old is 75–80 beats/min; the nurse would be most correct in withholding the child's digoxin and notifying the physician if the pulse were below 80. A pulse rate of from 90 to 110 **(2, 3, 4)** would be considered within normal limits for a 6-year-old, and the nurse would be correct in administering the medication as ordered. **EV,6,SECE**

39. **(2)** Sickling of RBCs occurs under conditions of low oxygen tension; giving this child oxygen will prevent further sickling of RBCs, but it will not reverse the sickling of cells that has already occurred **(1)**. The oxygen is not given to prevent any respiratory complication **(3)**, nor will the oxygen have an effect on the oxygen-carrying capacity of the RBCs **(4)**. **IMP,6,PhI**

40. **(3)** The most common symptom in children with rheumatic fever is tachycardia due to cardiac involvement; in addition, these children may develop a rash, "erythema marginatum," and a characteristic fever, which spikes in the late afternoon. They do not usually present with petechiae **(1)**, hypertension **(2)**, or conjunctivitis **(4)**. **AS,1,PhI**

41. **(2)** Children with leukemia often experience bleeding gums due to thrombocytopenia; in addition, chemotherapy may cause oral mucous membrane ulceration. Therefore, the nurse would be most correct in advising this child to brush her teeth with a soft toothbrush only. Using a firm toothbrush **(3)** might cause a break in the gums, leading to infection. Rinsing her mouth only **(4)** might also lead to infection, since this would not necessarily clean the gums and teeth adequately; likewise, infection might be caused by not brushing her teeth **(1)**. **IMP,1/6,PhI**

42. **(4)** For a child just leaving the toddler period of autonomy and just entering the preschool period of initiative, the best suggestion to improve his nutritional intake would be to allow the child to feed himself. Other suggestions would supplement and enhance this one primary consideration **(1, 2, 3)**. **IMP,5,HPM**

43. **(2)** It would be impossible to supervise a hemophiliac child so carefully that any other bleeding episodes would be prevented; further, to attempt to do so would cause the parents to restrict the child totally, resulting in extreme overprotection. An acceptable alternative response would be to prevent "major" episodes of bleeding or to promptly recognize signs of a bleeding episode that would require medical intervention. The other statements **(1, 3, 4)** are all correct responses by the parents, indicating they have probably understood the nurse's teaching regarding the child's care. **EV,6,HPM**

44. **(4)** Infants with CHF should be given about 15–20 minutes per feeding; if the infant is unable to finish the feeding, or if the infant becomes cyanotic or experiences respiratory distress during the feeding, gavage feeding should be used to avoid exhausting the infant and possibly precipitating an episode of apnea. No attempts should be made to continue the feeding **(1, 2, or 3)**. **IMP,6,PhI**

45. **(4)** Epiglottitis is a bacterial infection of the epiglottis resulting in swelling and obstruction; without prompt, aggressive treatment, it can progress rapidly, resulting in respiratory arrest within 6–8 hours of onset. Although this condition does require hospitalization and is potentially life-threatening, the ICU stay is usually less than 5 days **(2, 3)**. There is no allergic cause of epiglottitis **(1)**. **IMP,6,PhI**

46. **(4)** When a preschooler has a favorite "security object," be it a blanket or a doll or a stuffed animal, that child should be allowed to keep the security object, even during hospitalization. This will promote the child's sense of trust and security, thus helping to make the hospitalization a more positive experience. Offering the child another toy **(1)**, putting the toy where he can see it but not touch it **(2)**, or giving him a new Cookie Monster **(3)** will not take the place of the child's old but well-loved original Cookie Monster. **IMP,7,PsI**

47. **(1)** Nephrosis (nephrotic syndrome) is a chronic syndrome characterized by variable pathology and questionable prognosis. In general, most children with nephrosis do present with severe, total body edema and 4+ proteinuria, along with hypoproteinemia. Hypertension and hematuria **(3)**, and hyperlipidemia and periorbital edema **(2)**, are more common in acute glomerulonephritis. The child with nephrosis seldom presents with severe oliguria **(4)**, although occasionally this may occur; anorexia **(4)** may or may not occur, depending on the severity of the exacerbation. **AN,8,PhI**

48. **(2)** Carditis is the only manifestation of rheumatic fever that can lead to permanent damage; the best way to evaluate a child for the presence of carditis is to monitor her apical pulse at least q4h. Her growth and development **(1, 3)** and her ESR **(4)** deserve secondary consideration after checking her apical pulse. **AN,1,PhI**

49. **(3)** The pain in vaso-occlusive crisis is due primarily to the clumping together of RBCs, which blocks small blood vessels, thus causing tissue ischemia, necrosis, and death. Although there may be increased RBC destruction **(1)** and hepatosplenomegaly **(2)**, this is not the primary cause of this child's pain. Sequestration of blood does not normally occur with sickle cell anemia **(4)**. **PL,6,PhI**

50. **(3)** From the very first attempt by a child to administer his or her own insulin, the nurse should stress the need to administer exact amounts as ordered by the physician. The child should learn from the start that "close" is not "correct" **(1)**. A teenager can and should be capable of drawing up the exact amount **(2)**. Drawing up an incorrect dose does not mean this teen is trying to antagonize the nurse, consciously or subconsciously **(4)**. **EV,4/5,PsI**

51. **(1)** As with an adult with CHF, the infant should be positioned in a chair/infant seat, in semi-Fowler's position, to provide for maximum expansion of the lungs and to assist the heart. Placing him on his stomach **(2)** might be an acceptable second choice, providing he can tolerate this position. He should never be placed on his back **(3)**, even with his head slightly hyperextended, because of the possibility of aspiration and other respiratory complications. A side-lying position **(4)** would not allow for maximum expansion of the lungs; an infant seat is more appropriate. **IMP,6,SECE**

52. **(4)** Transillumination, or the procedure of shining a light through the sac, is the usual means for evaluating the contents of the sac. When there is "no transillumination" (the light cannot shine through the sac), this

indicates the presence of solid material, or the spinal cord, within the sac. Thus (2) and (3) are incorrect. Transillumination has no bearing on determining whether the sac can be easily repaired (1). **AN,3,PhI**

53. (3) Syrup of ipecac is an emetic used to induce vomiting following ingestion of a harmful substance; the usual dose in children is 10–15 mL PO followed by at least 200 mL of water. The water is thought to enhance the emetic effect of ipecac and stimulate emptying of the stomach, thus ridding the body of the harmful substance. Activated charcoal (2) will neutralize the emetic effect and should not be given with ipecac, although in some cases it may be given after vomiting has occurred. Milk or toast (1, 4) has little or no effect and will neither help nor harm, although, if the child does vomit, they may increase the risk of aspiration. **IMP,1,SECE**

54. (1) Because oxygen is heavier than room air, it will settle to the bottom of the croupette and leak out unless the edges are tucked in tightly. If the edges are lying loosely on top of the linens (2), the oxygen will escape, resulting in lower concentrations than ordered. The crib rails should be raised for safety, not lowered (4); and again the edges should be tucked in tightly, not draped over the rails (3). **IMP,6,SECE**

55. (2) The preferred position for asthmatics is high Fowler's, or sitting up straight, which allows for maximum expansion of the lungs. Other positions would not allow for the maximum expansion of the lungs (1, 3, 4) and would only contribute to this child's hypoxia. **IMP,6,SECE**

56. (2) Juvenile diabetics are extremely brittle, or difficult to control, and prone to episodes of hypoglycemia or ketoacidosis. If this teenager were to experience a hypoglycemic episode, the earliest symptoms would often be behavioral: irritability, personality changes, etc. If this teen becomes disruptive, the nurse should first ask if he has eaten his breakfast, how much he ate, and when; other areas (1, 3, 4) would be appropriate to explore *after* this primary consideration. **AN,4,PhI**

57. (2) Extremes of temperatures, either too warm or too cold, should be avoided for infants with CHD, since this increases the body's demand for oxygen, thus increasing the workload of the heart. The mother would need no further teaching if she correctly stated that this infant should be dressed in loose-fitting clothing (1), should be brought back to the clinic for regularly scheduled appointments (3), and should be placed in a safe play area to stimulate development (4). **EV,6,HPM**

58. (1) With a patient with a potentially contagious infection such as AGE, the first priority is protection of the nurse and other patients by observing appropriate infection control measures. Other interventions can then be safely implemented without risk of cross-contamination (2, 3, 4). **AN,3,SECE**

59. (2) The general recommendation to make to parents on how to handle temper tantrums is to ignore this behavior because attention to a tantrum can reinforce undesirable behavior. If a parent allows a child to make a choice (1) and then does not follow through with this choice either because of personal preference or because the choice is unsafe, then tantrums will increase. Changing settings (3) is often a catalyst for a tantrum as the child is moved from one area to another, e.g., from the park to home. Finally, giving in to a toddler's demands (4) is unrealistic; parents should offer only allowable choices to their toddler and then allow the toddler to follow through with these choices. **IMP,5,HPM**

60. (2) Toddlers typically fear those procedures that are "intrusive," that is, where something goes into their bodies. Therefore, a rectal temperature would most likely evoke the most anxiety in a 3-year-old. Generally, a 3-year-old would be relatively cooperative with getting weighed (4) and giving a urine specimen (3), although having BP taken might also be somewhat threatening (1). **AN,7,HPM**

61. (1) The leading cause of morbidity and mortality in children with leukemia is infection; therefore, preventing infection is the most important nursing care plan goal. Preventing injury (2), promoting adequate nutrition (3), and meeting developmental needs (4) are other, less important goals for the leukemic child. **PL,1/6,SECE**

62. (2) The chief purpose of the moist soaks is to prevent tears or leaks in the sac, which could lead to infection, the number one cause of death during the neonatal period. Promoting comfort (1) and relieving pressure (3) are not reasons for ordering moist soaks for this infant. It is *not* possible to stimulate neural development (4), which is permanently and irreversibly arrested before birth. **AN,3,SECE**

63. (3) Preschoolers are in the age of fantasy or magical thinking. By making a game of "checking for monsters," a potentially frightening situation is relieved, and the child may even begin to realize that there "really" are no monsters. Asking the child to talk about his monsters (1) may make him believe they are real and that his father also believes in them. It would be too frightening to the child to have to look for these monsters by himself (2). Telling a preschooler that his fantasies are not real (4) would not be enough to convince him and might make him become even more convinced they are indeed real! **IMP,5,HPM**

64. (1) The surgical repair for hypospadias is done on the urethra primarily and also on the urethral meatus. Postoperatively, a urinary drainage apparatus (Foley or suprapubic) will be in place, and the urine is expected to have a clear yellow appearance. There should normally be no blood or mucus (2, 3, 4), which would indicate hemorrhage or infection if present. **EV,8,PhI**

65. (3) To be most effective, pancreatin (Viokase) should be administered immediately before every meal and every snack; this will facilitate the absorption of fats and proteins contained within the meal. The enzyme will have little or no therapeutic value if given at other times (1, 2, 4). **PL,6,SECE**

66. (1) Warmth causes vasodilatation, thus relieving the occlusion of small vessels and preventing tissue damage. Cold (2) would never be used, since it causes vasoconstriction. Performing ROM exercises (3) or ADL (4) would not relieve pain. **IMP,6,SECE**

67. (1) An infant with CHF should be wearing loose-fitting clothes, including diapers, to avoid pressure on the abdominal organs, which could impinge on his diaphragm and impede his respiratory effort. The student nurse should loosen his diaper, and she should know the rationale for this action as well. The nurse should not take care of this after the student leaves (3), since the student will repeat the mistake without the nurse's intervention; in addition, pinning the diaper snugly is inappropriate for an infant with CHF (2, 4), and the nurse has the final responsibility for the care this infant receives. **EV,6,PhI**

68. **(4)** Nephrosis is characterized by periods of exacerbations and remissions that occur throughout the childhood years. The child's parents should watch him closely for exacerbations, which should be reported promptly to the physician. The child should be encouraged to play with other children, not to stay away from them **(1)** to avoid feelings of social isolation. It is not "over" **(2)**, and the child will need to be watched carefully for periods of exacerbation. Once the child is discharged, he will generally not need to remain in bed **(3)** but rather can convalesce at home with alternating periods of activity and rest. **EV,8,HPM**

69. **(4)** Vincristine is an antineoplastic *Vinca* alkaloid, which has the major side effect of peripheral neuropathy; this may be manifested in numbness, tingling, footdrop, paresthesia, etc. In addition, vincristine may also cause constipation, not diarrhea **(1)**. Hemorrhagic cystitis **(3)** may be caused by cyclophosphamide (Cytoxan), not vincristine. Vincristine does not cause visual changes **(2)**. **IMP,6,PhI**

70. **(2)** Viokase is an enzyme; as such, it will begin to break down whatever food or liquid it is mixed with. However, for maximum therapeutic effect, the enzymatic action should be delayed until the medication reaches the stomach. The best food to mix with Viokase is the cold applesauce. The applesauce should be cold because cold delays the enzymatic action, which is most effective at 98.6°F. Applesauce is used because of its high fiber content, which also delays the enzymatic action of the Viokase. Any other foods or liquids the Viokase might be mixed with **(3)** would be less than ideal. Viokase cannot simply be discontinued **(1)** because a child has difficulty swallowing it; this medication must continue to be taken for the rest of the child's life. It is not appropriate to bribe a child **(4)** with a reward for desired behavior; children should never be bribed or threatened into taking medication. **IMP,6/7,SECE**

71. **(3)** Carditis can lead to permanent, irreversible cardiac damage, specifically, mitral valvular stenosis. The other manifestations of rheumatic fever **(1, 2, 4)** are transient and do not leave any permanent effects. **PL,1,PhI**

72. **(4)** A child with rheumatic fever will be in the hospital for a relatively longer time and will be confined to bed most of the time. The ideal roommate would be another child of the same sex and same developmental level who will also be in the hospital for some time and confined to bed. The best choice is the young girl with the fractured elbow, who will probably be in traction and also on bedrest. The child with a tonsillectomy **(2)** or the child with a concussion **(3)** will most likely be in the hospital for a very short time and will be out of bed. The child with impetigo, caused by streptococcus **(1)**, would be a most unsatisfactory roommate for this child, since she might reinfect her with strep. **IMP,1/5,HPM**

73. **(1)** The most important nursing diagnosis relates to physiologic integrity (i.e., maintaining a normal blood-sugar level). Other diagnoses **(2, 3, 4)** would be correct but not necessarily of primary concern. **EV,4,PhI**

74. **(3)** Parents often hope that the surgery done to close the sac will also help the infant move her legs; it is very important to stress the permanent, irreversible nature of the nerve damage. Surgery will *not* enable the infant to regain motor or sensory functioning; surgery is done primarily to prevent infection. Parents should not be told the infant will move her legs after surgery **(4)** or offered false hope **(1 or 2)**. **IMP,3,HPM**

75. **(3)** The best means to prevent any type of infection in any type of setting is good handwashing. Other techniques are secondary **(1, 2, 4)**. **AN,8,SECE**

76. **(2)** At 7 months of age, an infant may either sit with some support or sit alone; either behavior is commonly acquired at this age. Rolling over **(1)** is usually found in infants around 3–4 months of age, whereas weight bearing **(3)** and the palmar grasp **(4)** are commonly found in infants between the ages of 4 and 6 months. **AN,5,HPM**

77. **(2)** As a 9-month-old with a chronic bowel problem, this infant has probably become accustomed to his mother's administering suppositories or enemas. In addition, fear of strangers is common in this age group. Considering these factors, this infant's mother should at least be offered the opportunity to administer or assist with the enemas. If this is not feasible, another qualified person could take her place **(1, 3, 4)**. **AN,5/6,HPM**

78. **(4)** Early in the course of LTB, children most commonly exhibit inspiratory stridor, a harsh-pitched crowing sound made on inspiration, and a croupy, barking, metallic cough. As the condition worsens and respiratory efforts increase, there may be dyspnea and cyanosis **(1)**, tachycardia and hoarseness **(2)** progressing to aphonia. Fever up to 104°F is also common, but an expiratory wheeze is not **(3)**. **AN,6,PhI**

79. **(3)** The opisthotonus position occurs in children with severe meningitis due to the pressure on the spinal cord; the child's head is drawn back and the spine is arched backward in an attempt to minimize pressure on the cord. When the child assumes this position, the nurse should place the child in a side-lying position for safety and comfort. Any other position would not work as well **(1, 2, 4)**. **IMP,1,SECE**

80. **(1)** Younger teenage girls in particular prefer the company of other young girls; this is the age of the "best friend," and a definite preference for same-sex, same-age companions. As such, this child would not necessarily seek out older or younger children **(2, 4)** nor would she have "no preference" regarding the sex of her companion **(3)**. **AN,7,PsI**

81. **(3)** Crises are precipitated by conditions of low oxygen tension; this may include infection, which could easily be picked up by swimming in public pools. Other sources of low oxygen tension might include *severe* emotional stress **(1)**, *extremely* cold or windy weather **(2)**, or dehydration **(4)**, as well as high altitudes. **IMP,6,PsI/PhI**

82. **(4)** With children who have received a 10-mL dose of syrup of ipecac, if vomiting has not occurred within 30 minutes, the dose can and should be repeated once more. Although the first dose is generally effective in the majority of cases, a second dose is almost always 100% effective. If the child does not vomit after a second dose, manual stimulation of the gag reflex or gastric lavage must be promptly initiated to avoid toxic effects of ipecac. The nurse should never use fingers to stimulate the gag reflex **(1)**, especially in a toddler, because of the danger of receiving a human bite. Ipecac works within 15–30 minutes, and waiting another 30 minutes will not be helpful **(2)**. If the child does not vomit at all, thus not removing either the ipecac or the ingested substance(s), there is the danger of ipecac toxicity as well as poisoning from the ingested substance **(3)**. **IMP,1,SECE**

83. **(1)** Due to this child's carditis, the best means for the nurse to evaluate how well she tolerates any increase in activity would be by monitoring her apical pulse

rate. Any increase in her pulse rate over 15–20 beats/min would indicate that she is not tolerating the increase in activity and would be an indication for returning her to bed immediately. Any other method of evaluating her tolerance of increasing activity would be less effective **(2, 3, 4)**. **IMP,1/6,PhI**

84. **(2)** The newly diagnosed teenaged diabetic must assume responsibility for his own care as soon as possible; diabetes is a chronic disease with no known cure that this teen will have to live with for the rest of his life. The nurse should discourage his mother from being overly protective of him or from assuming this responsibility **(1, 3, 4)**. **IMP,5/7,HPM**

85. **(3)** The use of a pacifier for an infant with CHF will promote true psychological rest for him, thus reducing his body's demand for oxygen and reducing the workload of his heart. This is the *most* important reason that this infant should be offered the pacifier; although it may also be true that he seems to like the pacifier **(1)**, this is not the main reason he should be given one. **(2)** and **(4)** are too generalized and not necessarily true. **IMP,5/6,PsI**

86. **(4)** Contrary to popular belief, the best position for the nurse to place a child with a nosebleed in is sitting up and leaning forward slightly, with head remaining above the level of the heart; this position will allow the blood to drain freely from the nose and prevent aspiration. Sitting up with the head tilted backward **(3)** will predispose the child to swallowing or aspirating blood, as will a semi-Fowler's position **(2)**. The prone position **(1)** might be an acceptable second choice if the child were too weak to sit up without assistance. **IMP,6,SECE**

87. **(1)** While in the croupette, toddlers should be allowed only those toys that can be dried off easily; all stuffed animals, dolls with hair, etc. are not allowed, since they will harbor moisture and bacteria. While in the croupette, the child and the linens will also get damp or wet, and the nurse should implement measures to prevent chilling. Pajamas and blankets should be changed q4h or prn **(2)**. There is no need to restrain a child in the croupette **(3)**, since all working parts are safely outside the croupette. Finally, there is also no need to restrict visitors **(4)**. **IMP,6,SECE**

88. **(2)** Cystic fibrosis is inherited as an autosomal recessive disorder. The fact that these parents have a child with CF means that they are carriers of the trait, and each subsequent pregnancy might result in a child who also has CF. It would not be correct to advise the mother that a second child would only carry the trait **(4)** or would be normal **(3)**, although there is a possibility these might occur; the parents should be fully advised of the odds of this happening. In addition, it would needlessly worry the parents to tell them a second child might be more severely affected **(1)**, although this is also a possibility. **IMP,6,HPM**

89. **(2)** About half the children with eczema during the toddler or preschool years develop asthma during the schoolage or teenage years. Asthma seems to have little or no relation to strep throat or tonsillitis **(1)**. The father's death undoubtedly would have affected this child, but it occurred 1 year before the onset of the asthma **(3)**. The pneumonia experienced at age 4 might have been related to the asthma, but was not the cause of it **(4)**. **AN,1/5,SECE**

90. **(1)** Considering this infant's diagnosis, the nurse should anticipate that he will most likely have at least some developmental delays; most infants would begin

to roll over by 3 months of age, but at 5 months he should be doing this now. Sitting **(2)** is normally found around 6 months of age; he will most likely *not* be capable of this behavior at 5 months. A pincer grasp **(3)** is normally found at 9–12 months of age, and again he will most likely *not* be capable of this behavior either. Finally, weight bearing **(4)** is typically noted in healthy infants 4–6 months of age; but considering this infant's diagnosis, he may or may not be capable of this more strenuous behavior. **AS,5/6,HPM**

91. **(1)** The infant is placed on her abdomen, postoperatively, to prevent trauma or pressure to the sutured area on her back. In addition, the infant's head should be positioned 10 degrees lower than her hips to prevent the pressure of circulating CSF from affecting the suture line on the lower back. An obvious contraindication to this position is if increased intracranial pressure is present, in which case the infant would be positioned flat in bed **(4)**. In general, the head is never higher than the hips **(2 or 3)** during the immediate postoperative period for this type of surgery. **IMP,3,SECE**

92. **(1)** Hirschsprung's disease is a congenital condition. It does not "develop spontaneously," although the diagnosis may not be made until symptoms have been present for several months and some attempts at conservative medical treatment (enemas, stool softeners, etc.) have been made **(3)**. In the newborn with Hirschsprung's disease, there may be an episode of meconium ileus **(2)**, but this occurs as a result of the Hirschsprung's disease rather than as the cause of it. Finally, there is no known metabolic defect **(4)**. **IMP,8,PhI**

93. **(2)** As healing of the pathways of the CSF occurs following an episode of meningitis, scar tissue naturally forms; this may lead to noncommunicating hydrocephalus. The hydrocephalus might then lead to learning disabilities **(3)** or mental retardation **(4)**. Encephalitis **(1)** may occur in conjunction with the meningitis, but it is not a complication. **AS,1,PhI**

94. **(3)** Because concentrated sweets will cause a rise in blood sugar, followed by a precipitous drop, the nurse should teach this patient that he should follow up this concentrated sweet with a complex carbohydrate such as a glass of milk. The complex carbohydrate will help maintain a consistent level of blood sugar, thus avoiding the precipitous drop. Any other action would be inappropriate at this time **(1, 2, 4)**. **IMP,4,PhI**

95. **(4)** There are multiple factors involved in the etiology of asthma, including an allergic predisposition **(2)**, precipitation by severe emotional or physical stress **(3)**, and other factors yet to be determined **(1)**. **IMP,1,PhI**

96. **(1)** Long-term follow-up care for children with rheumatic fever most frequently includes antibiotic therapy with penicillin or erythromycin on an exact schedule for an indefinite time, or a minimum of 5 years. There is no way to immunize against future attacks **(2)**. This child will be sent home on severely restricted activity, and cardiac rehabilitation programs are out of the question at this time **(3)**. Home-bound tutoring would be fine, after a while, but it is not a priority at this time **(4)**. **IMP,1,PhI**

97. **(2)** In suspected cases of epiglottitis, the visualization of the epiglottis is strictly contraindicated, since it may precipitate laryngospasm and immediate respiratory arrest. It is a nursing responsibility to inform any less knowledgeable health care providers of this danger; any other action **(1, 3, 4)** would be inappropriate at this time. **IMP,6,PhI**

98. (4) There is no known cure for nephrosis; rather, treatment is aimed at providing symptomatic relief. To that effect, prednisone—an anti-inflammatory corticosteroid—is given to relieve symptoms rather than effect a cure. If prednisone has the expected therapeutic effect, the patient should report "feeling better" as symptoms are relieved. *Side* effects of prednisone therapy may also include mood swings (1), glucosuria (2), and fluid retention with weight gain (3). **EV,8,SECE**

99. (4) Toddlers will suffer the most if separated from their mothers; a croupette is a particularly frightening experience, as explanations are difficult. If the toddler will calm down with her mother in the croupette with her, this will decrease her body's need for oxygen. There is no need to check with the physician (2), nor would it be "unsafe" (3). Considering the child is hospitalized and most likely frightened by the strange equipment, there is no reason to question the parent's handling of the situation (1). **IMP,5/6,PsI**

100. (2) In infants, the earliest sign of hydrocephalus is increasing head circumference, which occurs as the suture lines separate and the fontanels widen to accommodate the extra fluid within the skull. Later signs would indicate that no further accommodation can occur and brain tissue is being destroyed; these signs might include bulging anterior fontanel (1), shrill, high-pitched cry (3), and sunset eyes (4). **AN,3,PhI**

101. (1) Viscous lidocaine (Xylocaine) is a topical anesthetic that is often used with leukemic patients; by numbing the mouth, pain due to oral ulcers is relieved, and the child may eat better. The leukemic child with oral ulcers should not be offered lukewarm liquids, which may serve as media for bacterial growth (2). The leukemic child with bleeding tendencies should never be offered aspirin for pain (3). Allowing this child to choose her own menu (4) would not necessarily relieve the pain due to her oral ulcers. **IMP,6,PhI**

102. (4) As generalized edema progresses, in males the scrotal sac can become extremely swollen, tender, and painful. The best nursing intervention is to place soft, folded diapers under the scrotum while the child is lying in bed. Zinc oxide (1) or medicated powder (3) will have little beneficial effect because the problem is mechanical rather than on the skin itself. Cleansing the scrotum (2) is important to prevent infection, since all edematous tissue needs special care to prevent skin breakdown; however, this will not relieve the child's discomfort. **IMP,8,PhI**

103. (2) The only solution that should be used in doing cleansing enemas for a child with Hirschsprung's disease is normal saline, because the child will retain some of this fluid, which will be absorbed through the bowel wall. As an isotonic solution, normal saline will not alter the fluid balance like a nonisotonic solution almost certainly would (1, 3, 4). **AN,8,SECE**

104. (2) Signs of dehydration in infants would include irritability and sunken, dry eyeballs due to fluid loss. Fever may be present, and tachycardia, not bradycardia (1) is also common. Low blood pressure often results, followed by oliguria; anuria (3) is rare and would be an ominous sign of renal failure. Finally, the oral buccal mucosa may be quite dry, and the anterior fontanel may be sunken, not bulging (4). **AS,8,PhI**

105. (1) If a toddler were to develop hydrocephalus, the first sign would most likely be irritability and poor feeding due to increased intracranial pressure. The head circumference would not increase (2), since the fontanels have closed. Headaches or double vision might occur

(3), but a toddler is not likely to complain of them. Ruptured retinal vessels (4) is a later sign of increased intracranial pressure. **AN,1,PhI**

106. (4) The best exercise for a child with cystic fibrosis is swimming, which provides needed exercise at an activity level that is not overly taxing for the child. Softball, tennis, and soccer (1, 2, 3) are all generally thought to be too strenuous for a child with CF. **IMP,5/6,HPM**

107. (1) Because sickle cell anemia is inherited as an autosomal recessive disorder, if both parents have the trait, any future pregnancies would have a 1:4 chance of producing a child with sickle cell anemia (2, 4). In addition, each pregnancy would have a 1:2 chance of producing a child with the trait (3), or a 1:4 chance of producing a normal child. **IMP,6,PhI**

108. (4) Cryoprecipitate, or Factorate, is a blood product; a type and crossmatch may be ordered for the child before the IV administration of this medication. As with any blood product, the child should be closely observed for possible transfusion reaction. Given the relatively small volume of fluid to be administered, it would not usually cause fluid volume overload (2). Although there has been some discussion about administering multiple IV medications in the hemophiliac and the linkage to AIDS (3), this is not a concern during the actual administration of the medication but rather a long-term concern. Finally, emboli formation (1) can occur with any IV administration and is not specific to cryoprecipitate, although the nurse would need to take the necessary precautions to prevent this possibility. **PL,6,SECE**

109. (2) Solucortef is a corticosteroid/anti-inflammatory, used in epiglottitis to relieve swelling and edema. Solucortef does not provide sedation (1) or relieve pain (3), and the bacterial infection is treated with antibiotics (4). **AN,6,SECE**

110. (4) Although any infection can be life-threatening to a child with leukemia, chickenpox presents a particular danger, since the child may develop encephalitis or sepsis. Infections such as impetigo (1), streptococcus (2), or pneumonia (3) are less specific dangers. **IMP,1/6,PhI**

111. (2) Because infants with VSD and CHF do have a tendency toward respiratory infections, he should have limited contact with visitors with URIs, such as the grandmother with her slight cold. In fact, her slight cold might mean an episode of pneumonia for this infant. Lupus (1) in the aunt is not contagious, nor is the father's drug addiction (3). His sister (4) should be allowed to see and touch him, unless she herself is sick. **IMP,6,SECE**

112. (1) The chief danger of ipecac's being absorbed into the body is potentially fatal cardiotoxicity, which can cause cardiac arrhythmias, atrial fibrillation, or severe heart block. There is minimal effect on the liver (2), kidneys (3), or CNS (4). **AN,1,PhI**

113. (1) The most recent research indicates that there is no relationship, either positive or negative, between breastfeeding and the occurrence of SIDS; there is roughly the same incidence of SIDS in infants who are breastfed or bottlefed (2, 3, 4). **IMP,5,PhI**

114. (3) Generally, infants who weigh 7 lb at birth will weigh 28 lb, or quadruple their birthweight, by 2½ years of age. Consequently the other listed ages are incorrect (1, 2, 4). **EV,5,PhI**

115. (2) The general rule of thumb to predict a child's height as an adult is to double the child's height at 2

years of age. The other answers **(1, 3, 4)** are incorrect. **IMP,5,HPM**

116. **(1)** The only communicable childhood disease for which there is not currently a recommended routine immunization is chickenpox, although there is ongoing testing of a newly developed vaccine. Recently, the U.N. World Health Organization officially listed smallpox as "eradicated," making immunization no longer necessary, although a vaccine had been available **(2)**. The immunization for measles (rubeola) **(4)**, mumps (parotitis) **(3)**, and rubella (german measles) is currently available and is recommended to be given first at 12–15 months of age, followed by a booster at either 4–6 years of age or 11–12 years of age. **AN,1,HPM**

117. **(2)** Poisoning is most common in toddlers, who have the motor skills necessary to reach the poisons yet lack the intelligence to know not to ingest the poison. The other answers **(1, 3, 4)** are, therefore, incorrect. **AN,1,SECE**

118. **(3)** In children under 3 years, most accidental deaths are related to motor vehicles in which the child is a passenger; other types of accidents are not as common or not as likely to result in death **(1, 2, 4)**. **AN,1,SECE**

119. **(2)** Toddlers always suffer when separated from their parents, more so than any other age group **(1, 3, 4)**. In fact, the years between ages 1 and 3 are when children are most likely to suffer separation anxiety. **AN,7,PsI**

120. **(2)** Five-year-olds may count up to 20 or 25, but seldom beyond this. They should be able to name colors such as red, green, and blue **(1)**. In addition, they should be able to give their phone number and address **(4)** and have a better sense of temporal relationships, as evidenced by their ability to name days of the week, months of the year, and seasons **(3)**. **AS,5,PsI**

Unit 9

Ethical and Legal Aspects in Nursing

❏ Nursing Ethics

Nursing ethics involves rules and principles to guide right conduct in terms of moral duties and obligations to protect the rights of human beings. In nursing, ethical codes provide professional standards and formal guidelines for nursing activities to protect both the nurse and the patient.

I. Code of ethics—serves as a frame of reference when judging priorities or possible courses of action. *Purposes:*
  A. To provide a basis for regulating relationships between nurse, patient, coworkers, society, and profession.
  B. To provide a standard for excluding unscrupulous nursing practitioners and for defending nurses unjustly accused.
  C. To serve as a basis for nursing curricula.
  D. To orient new nurses and the public to ethical professional conduct.

ANA Code for Nurses

1. The nurse provides services with respect for human dignity and the uniqueness of the client unrestricted by considerations of social or economic status, personal attributes, or the nature of health problems.
2. The nurse safeguards the client's right to privacy by judiciously protecting information of a confidential nature.
3. The nurse acts to safeguard the client and the public when health care and safety are affected by the incompetent, unethical, or illegal practice of any person.
4. The nurse assumes responsibility and accountability for individual nursing judgments and actions.
5. The nurse maintains competence in nursing.
6. The nurse exercises informed judgment and uses individual competence and qualifications as criteria in seeking consultation, accepting responsibilities, and delegating nursing activities to others.
7. The nurse participates in activities that contribute to the ongoing development of the profession's body of knowledge.
8. The nurse participates in the profession's efforts to implement and improve standards of nursing.
9. The nurse participates in the profession's efforts to establish and maintain conditions of employment conducive to high-quality nursing care.
10. The nurse participates in the profession's effort to protect the public from misinformation and misrepresentation and to maintain the integrity of nursing.
11. The nurse collaborates with members of the health professions and other citizens in promoting community and national efforts to meet the health needs of the public.

Source: American Nurses Association. *1985 Code for Nurses, with Interpretive Statements.* Kansas City, MO: American Nurses Association. Reprinted with permission. (Interpretive statements for each portion of the above Code for Nurses are available from ANA.)

II. Bioethics—a philosophical field that applies ethical reasoning process for achieving clear and convincing reasons to issues and dilemmas (conflicts between two obligations) in health care.*
  A. Purpose of applying ethical reflection to nursing concerns:
    1. Improve quality of professional nursing decisions.

*From Davis AJ. Ethical Dilemmas in Nursing. Recorded at JONA and Nurse Educator's 1981 Joint Leadership Conference.

2. Increase sensitivity to others.
3. Offer a sense of moral clarity and enlightenment.

B. Framework for analyzing an ethical issue:
1. Who are the relevant participants in the situation?
2. What is the required action?
3. What are the probable and possible consequences of the action?
4. What is the range of alternative actions or choices?
5. What is the intent or purpose of the action?
6. What is the context of the action?

C. Principles of bioethics:
1. *Autonomy*—the right to make one's own decisions.
2. *Nonmalfeasance*—the intention to do no wrong.
3. *Beneficence*—the principle of attempting to do things that benefit others.
4. *Justice*—the distribution, as fairly as possible, of benefits and burdens.
5. *Veracity*—the intention to tell the truth.
6. *Confidentiality*—the social contract guaranteeing another's privacy.

III. Patient rights*

A. Right to appropriate treatment.
B. Right to individualized treatment plan, subject to review and reassessment.
C. Right to active participation in treatment, with the risk, side effects, and benefits of all medication and treatment (and alternatives) to be discussed.
D. Right to give and withhold consent (exceptions: emergencies and when under conservatorship).
E. Right to be free of experimentation unless following recommendations of the National Commission on Protection of Human Subjects.
F. Right to be free of restraints except in an emergency.
G. Right to human environment.
H. Right to confidentiality.
I. Right of access to personal treatment record.
J. Right to as much freedom as possible to exercise constitutional rights of association (e.g., having visitors) and expression.
K. Right to information about these rights in both written and oral form, presented in an understandable manner at outset and periodically thereafter.
L. Right to assert grievances through a grievance mechanism that includes the power to go to court.
M. Right to obtain advocacy assistance.
N. Right to criticize or complain about conditions or services without fear of retaliatory punishment or other reprisals.
O. Right to referral to complement the discharge plan.

IV. Conflicts and problems
A. *Personal values versus professional duty*—nurses have the right to refuse to participate in those areas of nursing practice that are against their personal values, as long as a patient's welfare is not jeopardized. Example: therapeutic abortions.
B. *Nurse versus agency*—conflict may arise regarding whether or not to give out needed information to a patient or to follow agency policy, which does not allow it. Example: an emotionally upset teenager asks a nurse about how to get an abortion, a discussion which is against agency policy.
C. *Nurse versus colleagues*—conflict may arise when determining whether to ignore or report others' behavior. Examples: you see another nurse steal medications; you know that a peer is giving a false reason when requesting time off; or you observe an intoxicated colleague.
D. *Nurse versus patient/family*—conflict may stem from knowledge of confidential information. Should you tell? Example: patient or family member relates a vital secret to the nurse.
E. *Conflicting responsibilities*—to whom is the nurse primarily responsible when needs of the agency and the patient differ? Example: an MD asks a nurse not to list all supplies used for patient care, as the patient cannot afford to pay the bill.
F. *Ethical dilemmas*—stigma of diagnostic label (e.g., AIDS, schizophrenic, addict); involuntary psychiatric confinement; right to control individual freedom; right to suicide; right to privacy and confidentiality.

V. Trends in nursing practice
A. Overall characteristics:
1. Some trends are subtle and slow to emerge; others are obvious and quickly emerge.
2. Trends may conflict; some will prevail, others get modified by social forces.
B. General trends:
1. *Broadened focus of care*—from care of ill to care of sick and healthy, from care of individual to care of family. Focus on prevention of illness, promotion of optimum level of health, holism.
2. *Increasing scientific base*—in bio-social-physical sciences, not mere reliance on intuition, experience, and observation.
3. *Increasingly complex technical skills* and use of *technologically advanced equipment,* such as monitors and computers.
4. *Increased independence* in use of judg-

---

*From Davis AJ. Ethical Dilemmas in Nursing. Recorded at JONA and Nurse Educator's 1981 Joint Leadership Conference.

ment, such as teaching nutrition in pregnancy and providing primary prenatal care.

5. *New roles,* such as *nurse-clinician,* require advanced skills in a particular area of practice. Examples: psychiatric nurse consults with staff about problems; *primary care* nurse takes medical histories and does physical assessment; one nurse coordinates 24-h care during hospital stay; *independent nurse practitioner* has her or his own office in community where patients come for care; case management.

6. *Community nursing services* rather than hospital based; needs of the healthy are served as well as those of the ill.

7. *Development of nursing standards* to reflect specific nursing functions and activities.

   a. Ensure *safe* standard of care to patients and families.

   b. Provide criteria to measure *excellence* and *effectiveness* of care.

C. Trends in care of childbearing family

1. *Consumerism*

   a. Consumer push for humanization and individualization of health care during the childbearing cycle to reflect patient's role in decision making, preferences, and cultural diversity.

   b. Emphasis on family-centered care (including father, siblings, grandparents).

   c. Increase in options available for conduct of birth experience and setting for birth: birthing homes, alternative birth center (ABC) in hospitals; birthing chairs; side-lying position for birth; family-centered cesarean birth; health care provider (MD, RN, lay midwife); length of postpartum stay.

   d. Increased consumer awareness of legal issues, patient's rights.

   e. Major nursing role: patient advocate.

2. *Social trends*

   a. Alternative life-styles of families—single parenthood, communal living, surrogate motherhood, marriages without children.

   b. Earlier sexual experimentation—availability of assistance to emancipated minors.

   c. Increase in number of older (>38 yr) primiparas.

   d. Legalization of abortion; availability to emancipated minors.

   e. Smaller families.

   f. Rising divorce rates.

3. *Technologies*

   a. Development of genetic and bioengineering techniques.

   b. Development of prenatal diagnostic

techniques, with options for management of each pregnancy.

   c. In-vitro fertilization and embryo transplantation.

D. Trends in community mental health (1960s–1990s):

1. Shift from institutional to community-based care.

2. Preventive services.

3. Consumer participation in planning and delivery of services.

4. Original 12 essential services (1975) reduced to 5 (indicated by asterisk [*]) (1981).

   *a. 24-h inpatient care.

   *b. Outpatient care.

   *c. Partial hospitalization (day or night).

   d. Emergency care.

   *e. Consultation and education.

   f. Follow-up care.

   g. Transitional services.

   h. Services for children and adolescents.

   i. Services for elderly.

   *j. Screening services (courts).

   k. Alcohol abuse services.

   l. Drug abuse services.

5. Protecting human rights of persons in need of mental health care.

6. Developing an advocacy program for chronically mentally ill.

7. Improving delivery of services to underserved and high-risk populations (e.g., minorities).

E. ANA Standards of Clinical Nursing Practice:

Standards of Clinical Nursing Practice

The ANA Standards of Clinical Nursing Practice address the following standards of care and standards of professional performance:

1. Use of *nursing process:* assessment, nursing diagnosis, outcome identification, planning, implementation, evaluation.

2. Quality of care.

3. Performance appraisal review.

4. Continuing education.

5. Collegiality; peer review.

6. Ethics.

7. Interdisciplinary collaboration.

8. Research.

9. Resource utilization—utilization of community health systems.

Source: Complete description in American Nurses Association. *1991 Standards of Clinical Nursing Practice.* Washington, DC: American Nurses Association. Reprinted with permission. (Rationale and assessment factors for the above Standards of Clinical Nursing Practice are available from the ANA.)

Ethical/Legal

F. *Four levels* of nursing practice:
1. *Promotion of health* to increase level of wellness. Example: provide dietary information to reduce risks of coronary artery diseases.
2. *Prevention of illness or injury.* Example: immunizations.
3. *Restoration of health.* Example: teach how to change dressing, care for wound.
4. *Consolation of dying*—assist person to attain peaceful death.

G. *Five components* of nursing care:
1. *Nursing care activities*—assist with basic needs, give medications and treatments; observe response and adaptation to illness and treatments; teach self-care; guide rehabilitation activities for daily living.
2. *Coordination of total patient care*—all health team members should work together toward common goals.
3. *Continuity of care*—when the location of care is transferred.
4. *Evaluation of care*—flexibility and responsiveness to changing needs: patients' reactions and perceptions of their needs.
5. *Delegate responsibility and direct nursing care provided by others*—based on particular patient/family needs and on skills of other nursing personnel.

H. *Three main nursing roles* in relation to care of patients and their families. The emphasis of each role varies with the situation, with adaptation of skills and modes of care as necessary.
1. *Therapeutic role* (instrumental). Function: work toward "cure" in acute setting.
2. *Caring role* (expressive). Function: provide support through human relations, show concern, demonstrate acceptance of differences.
3. *Socializing role.* Function: offer distractions and respite from focus on illness.

❏ Nursing Organizations

I. International Council of Nurses (ICN)
A. *Purpose:* to provide a medium through which national nursing associations can work together, share common interests. Formed in 1899.
B. *Functions:*
1. Serves as representatives of and spokespersons for nurses at international level.
2. Promotes organization of national nurses' associations.
3. Assists national organizations to develop and improve services for public health practice of nursing and social/economic welfare of nurses.

II. World Health Organization (WHO)—special intergovernmental agency of the UN, formed in 1948.

A. *Purpose:* to bring all people to the highest possible level of health.
B. *Functions:* provides assistance in the form of education, training, improving health standards, fighting disease, and reducing water pollution in member countries.

III. American Nurses Association (ANA)—national professional association in the U.S., composed of the nurses' associations of the 50 states, Guam, Virgin Islands, Puerto Rico, and Washington, D.C.
A. *Purpose:* to foster high standards of nursing practice and promote the education and welfare of nurses.
B. *Functions:* officially represents professional nurses in this country and internationally; defines practice of nursing; lobbies and promotes legislation affecting nurses' welfare and practice.

IV. National League for Nursing (NLN)—composed of both individuals and agencies.
A. *Purpose:* to foster the development and improvement of all nursing services and nursing education.
B. *Functions:*
1. Provides educational workshops.
2. Assists in recruitment for nursing programs.
3. Provides testing services for both RN and LPN (LVN) nursing programs.

❏ Legal Aspects of Nursing

I. Definition of terms
A. *Common law:* accumulation of law as a result of judicial court decisions.
B. *Civil law* (private law): law that derives from legislative codes and deals with relations between private parties.
C. *Public law:* concerns relationships between an individual and the state. The thrust of public law is to attain what are deemed valid public goals, such as reporting child abuse.
D. *Criminal law:* concerns actions against the safety and welfare of the public, such as robbery. It is part of the public law.
E. *Informed consent:* implies that significant benefits and risks of any procedure, as well as alternative methods of treatment, have been explained; person has had time to ask questions and have these answered; person has agreed to the treatment voluntarily and is legally competent to give consent; and communication is in a language known to the patient.
F. *Reasonably prudent nurse:* nurse must react as a reasonably prudent nurse trained in that specialty area would react. For example, if a nurse works with fetal monitors, she must know how to use the monitors,

know how to read the strips, and know what actions to take based on the findings.

II. Nursing licensure—mandatory licensure required in order to practice nursing.

   A. *Nurse Practice Act:* each state has one to protect nurses' professional capacity, to legally control nursing through licensing, and to define standards of professional nursing.

   B. *American Nurses Association (1980):* "The practice of nursing means the performance for compensation of professional services requiring substantial specialized knowledge of the biological, physical, behavioral, psychological, and sociological sciences and of nursing theory as the basis for assessment, diagnosis, planning, intervention, and evaluation in the promotion and maintenance of health; the casefinding and management of illness, injury, or infirmity; the restoration of optimum function; or the achievement of a dignified death. Nursing practice includes but is not limited to administration, teaching, counseling, supervision, delegation, and evaluation of practice and execution of the medical regimen, including the administration of medications and treatments prescribed by any person authorized by state law to prescribe. Each registered nurse is directly accountable and responsible to the consumer for the quality of nursing care rendered" (American Nurses Association. *The Nursing Practice Act; Suggested State Legislation.* Kansas City, MO: American Nurses Association, 1980. P 6. Reprinted with permission).

   C. *Revoking a license:* Board of Examiners in each state in the U.S. and each province in Canada has the power to revoke licenses for just cause, such as incompetence in nursing practice, conviction of crime, drug addiction, obtaining license through fraud, or hiding criminal history.

III. Crimes and torts

   A. *Crime:* an act committed in violation of societal law and punishable by fine or imprisonment. A crime does not have to be intended (as in giving a patient an accidental overdose that proves to be lethal).

      1. *Felonies:* crimes of a serious nature (such as murder) punishable by imprisonment of longer than 6 mo.

      2. *Misdemeanors:* crimes of a less serious nature (such as shoplifting), usually punishable by fines or short prison term or both.

   B. *Tort:* a wrong committed by one individual against another or another's property. Fraud, negligence, and malpractice are torts (such as losing a patient's hearing aid or bathing the patient in water that burns her or him).

      1. *Fraud:* misrepresentation of fact with intentions for it to be acted upon by another person (such as falsifying college transcripts when applying for a graduate nursing program).

      2. *Negligence:* "Omission to do something that a reasonable person, guided by those *ordinary* considerations which ordinarily regulate human affairs would *do,* or doing something which a reasonable and prudent person would *not* do" (Creighton H. *Law Every Nurse Should Know.* Philadelphia: Saunders, 1986). Types of negligent acts related to:

         a. Sponge counts: incorrect counts or failure to count.

         b. Burns: heating pads, solutions, steam vaporizers.

         c. Falls: siderails left down, baby left unattended.

         d. Failure to observe and take appropriate action—forgetting to take vital signs and check dressing in a newly postoperative patient.

         e. Wrong medicine, wrong dose and concentration, wrong route, wrong patient.

         f. Mistaken identity—wrong patient for surgery.

         g. Failure to communicate—ignore, forget, fail to report complaints of patient or family.

         h. Loss of or damage to patient's property—dentures, jewelry, money.

      3. *Malpractice:* part of the law of negligence as applied to the *professional* person; any professional misconduct, unreasonable lack of skill, or lack of fidelity in professional duties, such as accidentally giving wrong medication or forgetting to give correct medication or instilling wrong strength of eyedrops into the patient's eyes. Proof of intent to do harm is not required in acts of commission or omission.

IV. Invasion of privacy—compromising a person's right to withhold self and own life from public scrutiny. Implications for nursing—avoid unnecessary discussion of patient's medical condition; patient has a right to refuse to participate in clinical teaching; obtain consent prior to teaching conference.

V. Libel and slander—wrongful action of communication that damages person's reputation by print, writing, or pictures (libel), or by spoken word using false words (slander). Implications for nursing—make comments about patient only to another health team member caring for that patient.

VI. Privileged communications—information relating to condition and treatment of patient requires confidentiality and protection against invasion of privacy. This applies only to court proceedings. Selected person does not have to reveal in court a patient's communication to him or her. The purpose of privileged communication is to encourage the patient to communicate honestly with the treating practitioner. It is the patient's privilege at any time to permit the professional to release information.

Therefore, if the patient asks the nurse to testify, the nurse must truthfully give all information. However, if the nurse is a witness against the patient, without the patient's permission to release information, the nurse must keep the information confidential by invoking the privileged communication rule if the state law recognizes it and if it applies to the nurse.

VII. Assault and battery—violating a person's right to refuse physical contact with another.
   A. Definitions
      1. *Assault*—the attempt to touch another or the threat to do so.
      2. *Battery*—physical harm through willful touching of person or clothing.
   B. Implications for nursing—need to obtain consent to treat, with special provisions when patients are underage, unconscious, or mentally ill.

VIII. Good Samaritan Act—protects health practitioners against malpractice claims resulting from assistance provided at scene of an emergency (unless there was willful wrongdoing) as long as the level of care provided is the same as any other reasonably prudent person would give under similar circumstances.

IX. Nurses' responsibilities to the law
   A. A nurse is liable for nursing acts, even if directed to do something by an MD.
   B. A nurse is not responsible for the negligence of the employer (hospital).
   C. A nurse is responsible for refusing to carry out an order for an activity believed to be injurious to the patient.
   D. A nurse cannot legally diagnose illness or prescribe treatment for a patient. (This is the MD's responsibility.)
   E. A nurse is legally responsible when participating in a criminal act (such as assisting with criminal abortions or taking medications from patient's supply for own use).
   F. A nurse should reveal patient's confidential information only to appropriate health care team members.
   G. A nurse is responsible for explaining nursing activities but not for commenting on medical activities in a way that may distress the patient or the MD.
   H. A nurse is responsible for recognizing and protecting the rights of patients to refuse treatment or medication, and for reporting their concerns and refusals to the MD or appropriate agency people.
   I. A nurse needs to respect the dignity of each patient and family.

Questions Most Frequently Asked by Nurses about Nursing and the Law

I. Taking orders
   A. *Should I accept verbal phone orders from an MD?* Generally, no. Specifically, follow your hospital's by-laws, regulations, and policies regarding this. Failure to follow the hospital's rules could be considered negligence.
   B. *Should I follow an MD's orders if (a) I know it is wrong, or (b) I disagree with his or her judgment?* Regarding (a)—no, if you think a reasonable, prudent nurse would not follow it; but first inform the MD and record your decision. Report it to your supervisor. Regarding (b)—yes, because the law does not allow you to substitute your nursing judgment for a doctor's medical judgment. Do record that you questioned the order and that the doctor confirmed it before you carried it out.
   C. *What can I do if the MD delegates a task to me for which I am not prepared?* Inform the MD of your lack of education and experience in performing the task. Refuse to do it. If you inform him or her and still carry out the task, both you and the MD could be considered negligent if the patient is harmed by it. If you do not tell the MD and carry out the task, you are solely liable.

II. Obtaining patient's consent for medical and surgical procedures: *Is a nurse responsible for getting a consent for medical/surgical treatment?* Obtaining consent requires explaining the procedure and risks involved, which is the MD's responsibility. A nurse may accept responsibility for *witnessing* a consent. This carries with it little legal liability other than obtaining the correct signature and describing the patient's condition at time of signing.

III. Patient's records
   A. *What should be written in the nurse's notes?* All facts and information regarding a person's condition, treatment, care, progress, and response to illness and treatment. Purpose of record: factual documentation of care given to meet legal standards; used to refute unwarranted claims of negligence or malpractice.
   B. *How should data be recorded?* Entries should:
      1. State time given.
      2. Be written and signed by caregiver or supervisor who observed action.
      3. Follow chronologic sequence.
      4. Be accurate, precise, and clear.
      5. Be legible.
      6. Use universal abbreviations.

IV. Confidential information

  A. *If called on the witness stand in court, do I have to reveal confidential information?* It depends on your state, as each state has its own laws pertaining to this. Consult a lawyer. Inform the judge and ask for specific directions before relating in court information that was given to you within a confidential, professional relationship.

  B. *Am I justified in refusing (on the basis of "invasion of privacy") to give information about the patient to another health agency to which a patient is being transferred?* No. You are responsible for providing continuity of care when the patient is moved from one facility to another. Necessary and adequate information should be transferred between professional health care workers. The patient's consent for this exchange of information should be obtained. Circumstances under which confidential information can be released include:

  1. By authorization and consent of the patient.
  2. By order of the court.
  3. By statutory mandate, as in reporting cases of child abuse or communicable diseases.

V. Liability for mistakes—yours and others.

  A. *Is the hospital or the nurse liable for mistakes made by the nurse while following orders?* Both the hospital and the nurse can be sued for damage if a mistake made by the nurse injures the patient. The nurse is responsible for his or her own actions. The hospital would be liable, based on the doctrine of *respondeat superior.*

  B. *Who is responsible if a nursing student or another staff nurse makes a mistake? The supervisor? The instructor?* Ordinarily the instructor and/or supervisor would not be responsible unless the court thought the instructor and/or supervisor was negligent in supervising or in assigning a task beyond the capability of the person in question. No one is responsible for another's negligence unless he or she contributed to or participated in that negligence. Each person is personally liable for his or her own negligent actions and failure to act as a reasonably prudent nurse.

  C. *Am I responsible for injury to a patient by a staff member who was observed (but not reported) by me to be intoxicated while giving care?* Yes, you may be responsible. You have a duty to take reasonable action to prevent a patient's injury.

VI. Good Samaritan Act: *For what would I be liable if I voluntarily stopped to give care at the scene of an accident?* You would be protected under the Good Samaritan Act and required to live up to reasonable and prudent nursing stan-

dards in those specific circumstances. You would not be treated by the law as if you were performing under professional standards of properly sterile conditions, with proper technical equipment.

VII. Leaving against medical advice (AMA): *Would I or the hospital be liable if a client left "AMA," refusing to sign the appropriate hospital forms?* None of the involved parties would ordinarily be liable in this case as long as (a) the medical risks were explained, recorded, and witnessed, and (b) the patient is a competent adult. The law permits patients to make decisions that may not be in their own best health interest. You cannot interfere with the right and exercise of the decision to accept or reject treatment.

VIII. Restraints: *Can I put restraints on a patient who is combative even if there is no order for this?* Only in an emergency, for a limited time, for the limited purpose of protecting the patient from injury, not for convenience of personnel. Notify attending MD immediately. Consult with another staff member, obtain patient's consent if possible, document facts and reasons, get coworker to witness the record. Apply restraints properly; check frequently to ensure they do not impair circulation, cause pressure sores, or other injury. Remove restraints at the first opportunity, and use them only as a last resort after other reasonable means have not been effective. Restraints of any degree may constitute false imprisonment. Freedom from unlawful restraint is a basic human right protected by law.

IX. Wills: *What do I do when a patient asks me to be a witness to her or his will?* There is no legal obligation to participate as a witness, but there is a moral and ethical obligation to do so. You should not, however, help draw up a will as this could be considered practicing law without a license. You would be witnessing that (a) the patient is signing the document as her or his last will and testament; (b) at that time, to the best of your knowledge, the patient (testator) was of sound mind, was lucid, and understood what she or he was doing (i.e., she or he must not be under the influence of drugs or alcohol or otherwise unable to know what she or he is doing); and (c) the testator was under no overt coercion, as far as you could tell, but was acting freely, willingly, and under her or his own impetus.

X. Disciplinary action

  A. *For what reasons may the RN license be suspended or revoked?*

  1. Obtaining license by fraud (omission of information, false information).
  2. Negligence and incompetence.
  3. Substance abuse.
  4. Conviction of crime (state or federal).
  5. Practicing medicine without a license.

6. Practicing nursing without a license (expired, suspended).
7. Allowing unlicensed person to practice nursing or medicine.
8. Giving patient care while under the influence of alcohol or other drugs.
9. Habitually using drugs.
10. Discriminatory and prejudicial practices in giving patient care (pertaining to race, color, sex, age, or ethnic origin).

B. *What could happen to me if I am proven guilty of professional misconduct?*
1. License may be revoked.
2. License may be suspended.
3. Behavior may be censured and reprimanded.
4. You may be placed on probation.

C. *Who has the authority to carry out any of the above penalties?* The State Board of Registered Nursing that granted your license.

D. *I am the head nurse. One of my nursing aides has a history of failing to appear to work and not giving notice of or reason for absence. How should I handle this?* An employee has the right to know hospital policies, what is expected of an employee, and what will happen if an employee does not meet the expectations stated in his or her job description or in hospital policies and procedures. As a head nurse, you need to document behavior factually, clearly, and concisely, as well as any discussion and decision about future course of action. The employee needs the chance to read and sign it. The head nurse then sends a copy to her or his supervisor.

XI. **Floating:** *Is a nurse hired to work in psychiatry obligated to cover in ICU when the latter is understaffed?* The issue is the hiring contract (implied or expressed). The contract is a composite of the mutual understanding by involved parties of rights and responsibilities, any written documents, and hospital policies. If the nurse was hired as a psychiatric nurse, he or she could legally refuse to go to the ICU. If the hospital intends to float personnel, such a policy should be clearly stated during the hiring process. Also at this time the employer should determine the employee's education, skills, and experience. On the other hand, if emergency staffing problems exist, a nurse should go to the ICU regardless of personal preference.

XII. **Dispensing medication:** *Can a nurse legally remove a drug from a pharmacy when the pharmacy is closed (during the night) if the MD insists that the nurse go to the pharmacy to get the specifically prescribed medication immediately?* Within the legal boundaries of the Pharmacy Act, a nurse may remove one dose of a particular drug from the pharmacy for a particular patient during an unanticipated emergency within a limited time and availability of resources.

However, the hospital should have a written policy for the nurse to follow and should authorize a specific person to use the services of the pharmacy under certain circumstances.

XIII. **Illegible orders:** *What should I do if I cannot decipher the MD's handwriting when she or he persists in leaving illegible orders?* Talk to the MD regarding the dangers of your giving the wrong amount of the wrong medication via the wrong route at the wrong time. If that does not help, follow appropriate channels. Do not follow an order you cannot read. You will be liable for following orders you thought were written.

XIV. **Heroic measures:** *The wife of a terminally ill patient approaches me with the request that heroic measures not be used on her husband. She has not discussed this with him but knows that he feels the same way. Can I act on this request?* No. The patient is the only one who can legally make the decision as long as he or she is mentally competent.

XV. **Medication:** *An MD orders pain medication prn for a patient. The patient asks for the medication, but when I question her she says the pain "isn't so bad." If in my judgment the patient's pain is not severe, am I legally covered if I give half of the pain medication dosage ordered by the MD?* A nurse cannot substitute his or her judgment for the MD's. If you alter the amount of medication prescribed by the MD without a specific order to do so, you may be liable for practicing medicine without a license.

XVI. **Malfunctioning equipment:** *At the end-of-shift report the nurse going off duty tells me that the tracheal suctioning machine is malfunctioning and describes how she got it to work. Should I plan to use the machine in the evening shift and follow her suggestions about how to make it work?* Do not plan to use equipment that you know is not functioning properly. You could be held liable since you could reasonably foresee that proper functioning of equipment would be needed for your patient. You have been put on notice that there are defects. Report this to the supervisor or person responsible for maintaining equipment in proper working order.

Ethical and Legal Considerations in Intensive Care of the Acutely Ill Neonate

I. **Responsibilities of the health agency**
A. Provide an NICU or transfer to another hospital.
B. *Personnel—adequate number trained in neonate diseases, special treatment, and equipment.*
C. Equipment—adequate supply on hand, functioning properly (especially temperature regulator in incubator, oxygen analyzer, blood–gas machine).

II. Dying infants

  A. Decision regarding resuscitation in cardiac arrest, with brain damage from cerebral anoxia. It is difficult to predict the effect of anoxia in infancy on the child's later life.

  B. Decision to continue supportive measures.

  C. Issue of euthanasia, such as in severe myelomeningocele at birth.

  1. Active euthanasia (giving overdose).

  2. Passive euthanasia (not placing on respirator).

III. Extended role of nurse in NICU—may raise issues of nursing practice versus medical practice, as when a nurse draws blood samples for blood gas determinations without prior order. To be legally covered:

  A. The nurse must be trained to perform specialized functions.

  B. The functions must be written into the nurse's job description.

IV. Issue of negligence—such as cross-contamination in nursery.

V. Issue of malpractice—such as assigning care of critically ill infant on respirator to untrained student or aide.

  A. May be liable for inaccurate bilirubin studies for neonatal jaundice; may be legally responsible if brain damage occurs in absence of accurate laboratory tests.

  B. May be liable for brain damage in infant due to respiratory or cardiac distress. Nurse needs to make sure that there are frequent blood gas determinations to ensure adequate oxygen to prevent brain damage. Nurse also needs to make sure that the infant is not receiving too high a concentration of oxygen, which may lead to retrolental fibroplasia.

Legal Aspects of Psychiatric Care

I. Four sets of criteria to determine criminal responsibility at time of alleged offense

  A. *M'Naghten Rule* (1832)—a person is not guilty if:

  1. Person did not know the *nature and quality* of the act.

  2. Person could not distinguish right from wrong—if person did not know what he or she was doing, person did not know it was wrong.

  B. *The Irresistible Impulse Test* (used together with M'Naghten Rule)—person knows right from wrong, but:

  1. Driven by *impulse* to commit criminal acts regardless of consequences.

  2. Lacked premeditation in sudden violent behavior.

  C. *American Law Institute's Model Penal Code (1955) Test*

  1. Not responsible for criminal act if person lacks capacity to "appreciate" the wrongfulness of it or to "conform" conduct to requirements of law.

  2. Excludes "an abnormality manifested only by repeated criminal or antisocial conduct"—namely, psychopathology.

  3. Includes "knowledge" and "control" criteria.

  D. *Durham Test* (Product Rule—1954): accused not criminally responsible if act was a "product of mental disease." Discarded in 1972.

II. Types of admissions

  A. *Voluntary:* person, parent, or legal guardian applies for admission; person agrees to receive treatment and to follow hospital rules; civil rights are retained.

  B. *Involuntary:* process and criteria vary among states (Figure 9.1).

III. Legal and civil rights of hospitalized patients—the right to:

  A. Wear own clothes, keep and use personal possessions and reasonable sum of money for small purchases.

  B. Have individual storage space for private use.

  C. See visitors daily.

  D. Have reasonable access to confidential phone conversations.

  E. Receive unopened correspondence and have access to stationery, stamps, and a mailbox.

  F. Refuse: shock treatments, lobotomy.

IV. Concepts central to community mental health (Community Mental Health Act, 1980)

  A. *Systems* perspective: scope of care moves beyond the individual to the community, with

■ **FIGURE 9.1 Typical procedure for involuntary commitment.**

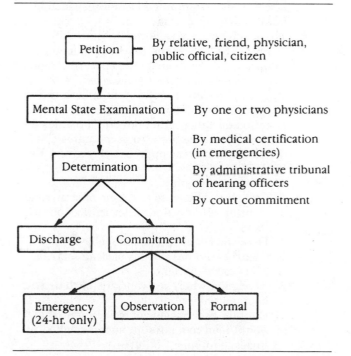

influences from biologic, psychological, and sociocultural forces.

B. Emphasis on *prevention: primary* (reduce incidents by preventing harmful social conditions); *secondary* (early identification and treatment of disorders to reduce duration); *tertiary* (early rehabilitation to reduce impairment from disorders).

C. *Interdisciplinary collaboration:* flexible roles based on unique areas of expertise.

D. *Consumer participation and control.*

E. *Comprehensive services:* outpatient care, partial hospitalization, 24-h hospitalization and emergency care; consultation and education; screening services.

F. *Continuity of care.*

Legal Aspects of Preparing a Patient for Surgery

I. No surgical procedure, however minor, can proceed without the voluntary, informed, and written consent of the patient.

A. Surgical permits are witnessed by the physician, nurse, or other authorized person.

B. Surgical permits protect the patient against unsanctioned surgery and also protect the surgeon and hospital staff against claims of unauthorized operations.

C. Informed consent means that the operation has been fully explained to the patient, including possible complications and disfigurements, as well as whether any organ or parts of the body are to be removed.

D. Adults and emancipated minors may sign their own operative permits if they are mentally competent; permission for surgery of minor children and incompetent or unconscious adults must be obtained from a responsible family member or guardian.

E. The signed operative permit is placed in a prominent place on the patient's chart and accompanies the patient to the operating room.

F. *Legal issues in the emergency room: record keeping* plays an essential role in both the prevention and defense of malpractice suits. Detailed documentation not only provides for continuity of care but also perpetuates evidence that care was appropriately given. Records should:
1. Be written legibly.
2. Clearly note events and time of occurrence.
3. Contain all lab slips and results of other tests.
4. Describe events and clients objectively.
5. Clearly note physician's parting instructions to the patient.
6. Be signed where appropriate, such as with doctor's orders.
7. Contain descriptions of every event that might lead to a lawsuit, such as fights, injuries, equipment failures.

G. *Consent*—although there is no law requiring written consent before performing medical treatment, all elective procedures can only be performed if the patient has been fully informed and voluntarily consents to the procedure.
1. If informed consent cannot be obtained because of the patient's condition and immediate treatment is necessary to save life or safeguard health, the emergency rule can be applied. This rule implies consent. However, if time allows, it is advisable to obtain either oral or written informed consent from someone who has authority to act for the patient.
2. Verbal consents should be recorded in detail, witnessed and signed by *two* individuals.
3. Written or verbal consent can be given by alert, coherent, or otherwise competent adults, by parents, legal guardian, or person in loco parentis (one standing in for the parent with the parent's rights, duties, and responsibilities) of minors or incompetent adults.
4. If the minor is 14 yr old or older, consent must be acquired from the minor as well as from the parent or legal guardian. Emancipated minors can consent for themselves.

❑ Questions

Select the one best answer for each question.

1. A physician orders the elixir form of a medication. The nurse, familiar only with the injectable form of the medication, believes the order is incorrect. The nurse should:
   1. Ask the two physicians who are currently on the unit whether the medication should be given as the nurse understood the order.
   2. Ask the head nurse if the order is correct.
   3. Call the physician who ordered the medication.
   4. Contact the nursing supervisor about the problem.

2. A patient had been receiving a drug by injection over a number of weeks. As the clinical symptoms changed, the physician wrote an order on the patient's order sheet changing the mode of administration from injection to oral. When the nurse on the unit, who had been off duty for several days, was preparing to give the medication by injection, the patient objected and referred the nurse to the physician's new orders. The nurse should:
   1. Go back to the order sheet and check for the order.
   2. Talk with the nurse who had taken care of this particular patient while he or she had been off duty.
   3. Talk with the head nurse about the advisability of using oral rather than injectable medications.
   4. Check the order sheet for the changed order and then speak with the attending physician concerning the changed order.

3. A nurse had been caring for a patient whose vital signs had previously been unstable. The nurse had not had a coffee break or a lunch break all day. By 2 P.M. the patient had been stable for a number of hours. The physician in charge had seen the patient and had told the

nurse that the patient appeared "much improved." The nurse should:

1. Leave for lunch break.
2. Forego lunch break because of the patient's previous unstable condition.
3. Arrange to eat lunch in the patient's room.
4. Discuss the situation with the nurse in charge of the unit and determine who should cover the patient while the staff nurse is at lunch.

4. In a certain hospital, whenever there are patients in the recovery room, two nurses are usually present. The hospital policy expects the nurses to take their breaks before patients arrive from surgery. On this particular day, there are two nurses on duty and two patients in the recovery room who have had minor surgeries performed that morning. One nurse had not had a coffee break that morning. That nurse should:

1. Stay because hospital policy expects there to be two nurses in attendance while there are patients in the recovery room.
2. Leave for coffee break because there are only two patients in the recovery room and one nurse can handle two patients quite easily.
3. Talk with the nursing supervisor and secure permission from him or her.
4. Leave to get coffee and come right back.

5. While driving down a freeway, a nurse spots an overturned car with the driver lying next to the car. The nurse:

1. May drive on without stopping, or stop and render emergency first aid, without liability.
2. May stop, start to render aid, and then leave, without liability.
3. Must stop at the scene of an accident and render first aid.
4. May stop and render aid, but if he or she performs a medical act, he or she may be charged with illegal practice of medicine.

6. A patient is terminally ill and has asked the nurse to witness a will. Which statement is true?

1. The nurse has a legal obligation to act as a witness to a will.
2. The nurse should help the patient draw up a will.
3. The nurse should make sure that the patient is of sound mind, is lucid (not under the influence of drugs or alcohol), and understands what he or she is doing.
4. Only lawyers or family members can act as a witness to a will. If the nurse acts as a witness, the will may automatically be declared invalid.

7. A patient, just returned from the recovery room, complains of pain that is "not too severe" and requests pain medication. The nurse notes that the patient has been given pain medication in the recovery room. Which statement indicates the best action to take?

1. Administer the dosage the physician had ordered on a prn basis.
2. Consult the physician and let him or her know that the patient is requesting medication for pain that is "not too severe."
3. Give half of the pain medication dosage ordered as prn by the physician.
4. Chart that the patient was complaining of pain but that it was "not too severe."

8. When a nurse is being sued for malpractice, what will occur?

1. The nurse's license will be revoked or suspended *automatically.*

2. The nurse will automatically be put on probation until the matter is cleared up.
3. The nurse will automatically be charged with a crime.
4. The State Board of Registered Nurses will be notified of the suit, and, depending on the offense and outcome of the suit, it might hold a hearing to determine the status of the license.

9. A nurse's license will be revoked or she or he will be put on probation for which reason?

1. The nurse lost a malpractice suit.
2. The nurse was found guilty of practicing while under the influence of drugs or alcohol.
3. The nurse was accused of negligence.
4. The nurse gave a wrong medication.

10. A nurse who applies restraints on a patient *may* be held liable by the patient for restraint of freedom of movement (false imprisonment) if the nurse:

1. Does not immediately obtain an order from the physician.
2. Does so after other means to subdue the patient have failed.
3. Tries but fails to obtain the patient's consent.
4. Applies restraints for the convenience of the personnel.

11. The nurse has been working with a terminally ill male patient for weeks. The patient is lucid. His wife pleads with the nurse not to use heroic measures on her husband but to let him die "with dignity." The nurse should:

1. Tell the wife that she needs to talk with the attending physician, patient (if possible), and other significant people about her concerns.
2. Act on the wife's request.
3. Ignore the wife's request and proceed with the patient's care.
4. Tell the wife that to do as she requested would be equivalent to murdering the patient.

12. A physician calls the unit, wishing to leave an important order. A new nurse answers the phone so that the senior nurses may continue their conversation. The new nurse does not know the physician nor the patient to whom the order pertains. The nurse should:

1. Take the telephone order.
2. Refuse to take the telephone order.
3. Ask the charge nurse or one of the other senior staff nurses to take the telephone order.
4. Ask the physician to call back after the nurse has read the hospital policy manual.

13. Which statement concerning consent is *false*?

1. If an informed consent is not obtained from the patient, then the nurse, doctor, and/or hospital may be liable for assault.
2. One need only obtain a general consent to treatment.
3. In an emergency a nurse may do what she or he can do to save life and limb, even in cases in which she or he has no consent.
4. Consent may be given by conduct as well as expressed words.

14. A nurse gave a patient the wrong medication. The patient was seriously injured. The patient sued. Who will most likely be held liable?

1. The nurse.
2. No one, because it was just an accident.
3. The hospital.
4. The nurse and the hospital.

15. The supervisor of a cardiovascular unit, responsible for checking staffing patterns, assigned a particular staff nurse to work on the unit because that nurse had many

years of experience on that unit. That evening, this staff nurse made a treatment error and a patient was injured. Who is liable?

1. The staff nurse.
2. The staff nurse and the supervisor.
3. The staff nurse and the hospital.
4. The staff nurse, the supervisor, and the hospital.

16. Nurse A noticed that Nurse B was intoxicated while giving care. However, Nurse A did not report this fact to the supervisor. That same day, Nurse B made a medication error and a patient was injured. Who *may* be held responsible?

1. Nurse B (the one intoxicated).
2. Nurse A, Nurse B, and the hospital.
3. Nurse A (the one who did not report Nurse B).
4. Nurse B (the one intoxicated) and the hospital.

17. A graduate nurse who was new to a unit was caring for an elderly patient. The physician on call ordered a treatment that the nurse had not heard of. The nurse should:

1. Inform the physician of the nurse's lack of education and experience and refuse to do the treatment without supervision.
2. Inform the physician of the nurse's lack of education and experience and then proceed to perform the treatment.
3. Refuse to perform the treatment.
4. Carry out the treatment to the best of the nurse's ability.

18. Which is *not* true about informed consent?

1. Obtaining consent is the responsibility of the physician.
2. A nurse may accept responsibility for witnessing a consent form.
3. A physician subjects himself or herself to liability if he or she withholds any facts that are necessary to form the basis of an intelligent consent.
4. If a nurse witnesses a consent for surgery, the nurse is, in effect, indicating that the patient is "informed."

19. The day nurse tells the night nurse that the suction equipment in a patient's room is not working properly. The night nurse, who will be working with this patient, should:

1. Follow the day nurse's suggestions on how to get the malfunctioning equipment to work.
2. Continue to use the malfunctioning machine, hoping that it will function for the night shift.
3. Ask the supervisor how to work with the malfunctioning equipment.
4. Replace the equipment or report it to whomever is responsible for maintaining equipment in proper working condition.

20. A competent adult patient has refused treatment and wishes to leave AMA (against medical advice). The patient has also refused to sign any of the appropriate AMA forms. Which statement is inaccurate?

1. The physician and/or hospital is always liable for any injury that might occur as a result of the patient's decision to leave AMA.
2. The law usually permits competent adult patients to make decisions that may not be in their own best health interest.
3. Even if the patient is a competent adult, the law may interfere with the patient's decision to refuse medical treatment if the patient has small children that need care.
4. The physician might be held liable if it can be proved that the patient did not receive sufficient information about risks involved with leaving AMA.

21. The only Spanish-speaking nurse in the emergency room admitted a 6-year-old child. The child's mother explained in Spanish that she had removed two ticks from the child the previous day. The child was now running a very high temperature and had a rash on the abdomen. The nurse reported the information to the emergency room physician, who did not speak Spanish. The nurse failed to tell the doctor about the ticks. The physician diagnosed the child as having measles. Over the course of the day, the child's health deteriorated until the child died. Who is liable?

1. The nurse.
2. The nurse and the physician.
3. The nurse and the hospital.
4. The physician.

22. A nurse was on weekend call for the operating room. Late Saturday night, the nursing supervisor called the nurse to say that they were expecting an emergency appendectomy within the hour. While gowning the surgeon, the nurse smelled alcohol on the doctor's breath. The nurse mentioned this to the anesthesiologist, who also admitted smelling alcohol on the surgeon. Both the nurse and the anesthesiologist felt the surgeon was somewhat unstable on his feet. However, neither the nurse nor the other doctor said anything. If the patient had been injured during the surgery, who would have been liable?

1. Nurse, anesthesiologist, surgeon, and hospital.
2. Nurse and surgeon.
3. Surgeon and hospital.
4. Hospital, surgeon, and anesthesiologist.

23. A child about 11 months old was brought by her mother to a hospital for examination, diagnosis, and treatment. The child was seen by a nurse and physician. At the time, the child was suffering from a comminuted spiral fracture of the right tibia and fibula that gave the appearance of having been caused by twisting. The child also had numerous bruises and burns on her body. In addition, she had a nondepressed linear fracture of the skull in the process of healing. When approached, the child demonstrated fear and apprehension. The mother had no explanation for the child's wounds. No further X rays were taken, and the child was released to the mother without report to concerned agencies. One month later the child was brought in again by the mother and was seen by a different physician. The second physician correctly diagnosed the battered-child syndrome and filed the proper reports. The child was placed in a foster home, and the foster home filed suit. Who may be liable?

1. First nurse, first doctor, and hospital.
2. First doctor.
3. No one.
4. First nurse.

24. While getting a patient ready for surgery, the nurse removed the patient's dentures. The nurse wrapped the dentures in a towel so as not to break them and left them on the bedside stand. While the nurse was out of the room, two nursing aides stripped the bed and threw all the linen, including the towel, in the laundry hamper. Upon returning from surgery, the patient requested the dentures. However, the nurse and nursing aides were unable to find them. Who is liable?

1. The nurse.
2. The nurse and the hospital.
3. The nurse and nursing aides.
4. The nurse, nursing aides, and hospital.

25. A teenage girl who had complained of dizziness the previous day wanted to take a shower. The physician gave permission for the patient to shower with assistance. The nurse started to get the girl out of bed and over to the shower. The nurse questioned the patient about her dizziness. The girl replied that she was not dizzy. The mother then said that she would watch her daughter in the shower and help her back to bed. The nurse then left the room. While the nurse was out, the patient fainted getting back into bed. The patient injured her head. Who is liable?
    1. The nurse.
    2. The doctor, nurse, and hospital.
    3. The nurse and the hospital.
    4. No one.

26. What does the Durham Test state about the accused?
    1. The same thing as the M'Naghten Rule.
    2. Accused is not criminally responsible if the act was the product of mental disease.
    3. Accused is not criminally responsible if the act was a result of impulsiveness.
    4. Accused is not criminally responsible if he or she does not appreciate the wrongfulness of the act.

27. What does voluntary admission require of the individual?
    1. The individual must ask to be admitted to a psychiatric hospital and must agree to abide by its rules.
    2. The request for hospitalization needs to originate with the individual to be admitted.
    3. The individual needs to make written application to a hospital, agree to treatment, and agree to abide by the rules.
    4. The individual needs to be responsible for the hospital bill.

28. Standards of practice for psychiatric mental health nursing have been developed by:
    1. A joint commission of psychiatric nurses and psychiatrists.
    2. Psychiatric nurses who are members of the American Nurses Association.
    3. A panel of representative psychiatric nurses in the U.S.
    4. The Division on Psychiatric and Mental Health Nursing Practice of the American Nurses Association.

29. The standards of practice for psychiatric mental health nursing are organized around:
    1. Different models of treatment.
    2. Rights of the clients.
    3. The nursing process.
    4. Legal aspects of treatment.

30. The Community Mental Health Centers Amendments of 1975, Title III of Public Law 94–63:
    1. Cut the flow of funds to community mental health centers and set forth general guidelines for service.
    2. Extended the flow of funds to community mental health centers and set forth specific guidelines for service.
    3. Cut the flow of funds to community mental health centers and set forth specific guidelines for service.
    4. Extended the flow of funds to community mental health centers and set forth general guidelines for service.

31. Congress, in the Mental Health Centers Act of 1974, also stated that it wanted to:
    1. Increase federal operation funds to centers and have centers under federal support.

    2. Provide funding on a declining basis at the federal level and encourage the goal of independence from federal support.
    3. Provide funding on a declining basis at the federal level but maintain federal control.
    4. Get out of the community mental health business.

32. The principal recommendation of the Report of the President's Commission on Mental Health, 1978, was:
    1. The federal government should get out of mental health.
    2. The government should upgrade the old federal grant program for community mental health to encourage the creation of necessary services where they are inadequate and to increase the flexibility of communities planning a comprehensive network of services.
    3. Community mental health programs should strictly adhere to the provision of specific services to all communities.
    4. A new federal grant program should be established for community mental health to encourage the creation of necessary services where they are inadequate and to increase the flexibility of communities planning a comprehensive network of services.

33. For nurses to control their own profession, they need to demonstrate:
    1. Expertise in implementing patient care levels already determined by law.
    2. The ability to participate in the drafting of health care laws that directly reflect patient care levels.
    3. The ability to participate in the drafting of laws at all levels and in all areas of health care.
    4. Neutrality by ignoring political power, thus being free from political influence in giving health care.

34. The ICN's Code for Nurses, "Ethical Concepts Applied to Nursing," approved by the Council of Nurse Representatives in 1973, states that:
    1. The professional body of nurses of a particular country carries the responsibility for nursing practice and for maintaining competence.
    2. The hospital employing the nurse carries the responsibility for nursing practice and for maintaining competence.
    3. The laws of the country in which the nurse works carry the responsibility for nursing practice and for maintaining competence.
    4. The individual nurse carries personal responsibility for nursing practice and for maintaining competence by continual learning.

35. The National Health Planning and Resource Development Act of 1974 allows:
    1. Physicians the largest representation on local and state health care boards that make decisions about health care.
    2. Hospital administrators the largest representation on local and state health care boards that make decisions about health care.
    3. The consumer the largest representation on local and state health care boards that make health care decisions.
    4. Health professionals as a group the largest representation on local and state health care boards that make health care decisions.

❑ Answers/Rationale

1. (3) The nurse would be negligent for any untoward effects of the drug if she or he failed to contact the physi-

cian who ordered the drug before the nurse administered it. In *Norton* v. *Argonaut Insurance Co.* [144 So. 2nd 249 (La. Ct. App. 1962)], the court stated that it was the responsibility of the nurse to clarify the order with the physician *involved,* not with other nurses (**Nos. 2 and 4**). **No. 1** is incorrect because the doctors on the unit are not the ones who wrote the order. **IMP,7,SECE**

2. **(4)** Although **No. 1** is a correct answer, No. 4 is the *best* answer because the nurse would validate the changed order and learn the physician's rationale for the change. In *Larrimore* v. *Homeopathic Hospital Association* [54 Del. 449, 181 A. 2d 573 (1962)], the court found that the nurse who went ahead and gave the medication was negligent. The courts went on to say that the jury could find the nurse negligent by applying ordinary common sense to establish the applicable standard of care. **Nos. 2 and 3** are incorrect because talking with nurses is not the direct way to clarify and validate an order. **IMP,7,SECE**

3. **(4)** The nurse would come back to the patient revitalized after having a lunch break, and the patient would be covered the whole time the nurse is away. In deciding that the nurse would not be negligent to leave such a patient, the court would emphasize that the question of liability should be determined in light of the circumstances as they existed at the time. When the nurse left the patient, it was not foreseeable that an increased risk to the patient would result. On the contrary, the patient would be looked after, and the nurse's needs would also be met. *Child* v. *Vancouver General Hospital* [71 W.W.R. 656 (1979)]. **No. 1** does not provide for patient's care. **Nos. 2 and 3** are not necessary actions, for the patient's condition at the time did not warrant the nurse's foregoing lunch or eating in the patient's room. **IMP,7,SECE**

4. **(1)** In a court of law, hospital policy may be used to set the standard of care by which the nurses' actions are judged. Since the hospital policy states that two nurses must be in attendance while patients are in the recovery room, both the nurse who left (**Nos. 2 and 4**) and the supervisor who authorized the nurse's absence (**No. 3**) would be held liable for any untoward effect on the patient. *Laidlaw* v. *Lions Gate Hospital* [70 W.W.R. 727 (1969)]. **IMP,7,SECE**

5. **(1)** The court has stated that no one is obliged by law to assist a stranger, even if he or she can do so by a word and without the slightest danger to himself or herself. Hence, **No. 3** is incorrect. But once one has undertaken to give assistance, the law imposes on him or her a duty of care toward the person assisted. Hence **No. 2** is incorrect. The court also states that under emergency circumstances, a nurse, like any other person, may perform a medical act to preserve life and limb. Either law or custom exempts such actions from coming within the medical practice acts. This, then, would rule out **No. 4**. **PL,7,SECE**

6. **(3)** Anyone can act as a witness. **No. 1** is incorrect because a nurse has no legal obligation to participate as a witness, only a moral and ethical obligation. **No. 2** would also be incorrect because only a lawyer or the patient can draw up a will. If the nurse draws up the will, she or he could be charged with practicing law without a license. If a nurse does act as a witness, he or she should determine that the patient is of sound mind or the will could be declared invalid—not because the nurse acted as a witness (**No. 4**) but because the patient was not of sound mind. **EV,7,SECE**

7. **(2)** The physician should be notified of the patient's complaints, and the new orders should be established. This is what the courts would consider prudent under the circumstances and what a reasonable nurse should do. **No. 1** would not be the best choice because the patient had already been given pain medication in the recovery room, and another full dose might be too much. Without further information, this is a very dangerous choice, and the nurse would be held liable for any untoward effects. **No. 3** would also be incorrect because a nurse cannot substitute his or her judgment for the physician's without consulting the physician first. If a nurse alters the amount prescribed without an order from the physician, the nurse could be charged with practicing medicine without a license. **No. 4** is incomplete. A nurse must chart the patient's complaints but must also indicate what was done about them. **IMP,7,SECE**

8. **(4)** Only the State Board of Registered Nurses has the authority to revoke or suspend a license. This can occur only after the nurse has been given a fair hearing before an impartial hearing body. Hence, **Nos. 1, 2, and 3** are incorrect because they assume a penalty should be applied before the State Board is notified. **EV,7,SECE**

9. **(2)** All State Practice Acts list "guilty of practicing while under the influence of drugs or alcohol" as a reason for revocation of a license or for putting a nurse on probation. **Nos. 1, 3, and 4** may cause revocation of a license; however, other circumstances would have to be considered first, such as the frequency with which these had occurred. **EV,7,SECE**

10. **(4)** Freedom from unlawful restraint is a basic human right. Restraints of any type may constitute false imprisonment. False imprisonment is an actionable tort for which a nurse may be held liable by a patient. The patient may have an actionable case of false imprisonment if the restraints were applied for staff convenience only. Most likely the nurse would not be held liable for false imprisonment even if the nurse does not immediately obtain an order from the physician for the restraints. However, **No. 1** is not the *best* choice. Restraints should be used only in emergency situations, for a limited time, for the limited purpose of protecting the patient, and not for the convenience of the staff. Even though the patient's consent (**No. 3**) is not usually obtainable under the circumstances, the nurse should try in order to avoid being held liable for false imprisonment. However, these restraints should only be applied as a last resort (**No. 2**). **EV,7,SECE**

11. **(1)** This type of case is an example of the most difficult medical ethical and legal questions today. The answers are ambiguous at best. However, in this case No. 1 would be best since neither the nurse (**No. 3**), the wife (**No. 2**), nor the doctor can make that decision as long as the patient is a competent adult. **No. 4** is incorrect because the nurse's values should not supersede the wife's concerns for her husband's welfare. **IMP,7,HPM**

12. **(3)** Get a senior nurse who knows the policies, the patient, and the doctor. Generally speaking, a nurse should not accept telephone orders. However, if it is nec-

---

Key to codes following rationales Nursing process: **AS,** Assessment; **AN,** Analysis; **PL,** Plan; **IMP,** Implementation; **EV,** Evaluation. Category of human function: **1,** Protective; **2,** Sensory-perceptual; **3,** Comfort, Rest, Activity, and Mobility; **4,** Nutrition; **5,** Growth and Development; **6,** Fluid-Gas Transport; **7,** Psychosocial-Cultural; **8,** Elimination. Client needs: **SECE,** Safe, Effective Care Environment; **PhI,** Physiologic Integrity; **PsI,** Psychosocial Integrity; **HPM,** Health Promotion/Maintenance; *,* Nursing process step or client need *not applicable.* See appendices for full explanation.

essary to take one, follow the hospital's policy regarding telephone orders. Failure to follow hospital policy could be considered negligence. In this case, the nurse was new and did not know the hospital's policy concerning telephone orders. The nurse was also unfamiliar with the doctor and the patient. Therefore the nurse should not take the order unless (a) no one else is available and (b) it is an emergency situation. **Nos. 1 and 2** are both incomplete, as they do not take into account the mitigating circumstances described above. Since the doctor has said that the order is important, the nurse should not delay the doctor while she or he reads the manual; hence, **No. 4** is incorrect. **IMP,7,SECE**

13. **(2)** *Assault* is the unjustifiable attempt to touch another person or the threat to do so in such circumstances as to cause the other reasonably to believe that it will be carried out. The lack of informed consent is an important part of the meaning of assault. Consent is a defense to an action for assault. However, if the treatment or procedure goes beyond the patient's consent (as it probably would if consent was only to "general" treatment, as in No. 2), the nurse, the doctor, and/or the hospital may be liable. Hence, **No. 1** is a true statement. In an emergency situation in which the nurse is trying to save the patient's life, if the patient does not or cannot consent to treatment, the nurse usually will not be held to have assaulted the patient. Hence, **No. 3** is also a true statement. Consent may be given by conduct as well as by expressed words, as in **No. 4**. For example, in a case in which a person held up his arm to be vaccinated, the court said he had consented. However, it is best to get the consent in writing, specifically outlining the treatment or procedure to be performed. The consent will most likely be deemed invalid, however, if the patient is a child, is mentally incompetent, or is intoxicated. **EV,7,SECE**

14. **(4)** *Both* the nurse and the hospital can be sued for damages if a mistake the nurse makes injures the patient. The nurse is always responsible for his or her own actions. The hospital, as the employer, will be vicariously liable under the *respondeat superior doctrine*—the employer is liable for the negligent conduct of its nurses when the act was committed within the scope of employment. **Nos. 1 and 3** are incomplete; **No. 2** is incorrect. **EV,7,SECE**

15. **(3)** The hospital is *always* initially held liable under the theory of *respondeat superior*—vicarious liability of the employer. **Nos. 2 and 4** are incorrect because the supervisor would *not* be responsible unless the court thought that the supervisor was negligent in supervising or assigning a task beyond the capabilities of another. In this case, the staff nurse had had numerous years of experience on the cardiovascular unit. Without further data, the supervisor would not be considered negligent for assigning this nurse to the cardiovascular unit. **No. 1** is incomplete. **AN,7,SECE**

16. **(2)** This answer includes all parties: the hospital, Nurse A, and Nurse B. The hospital, as the employer, might be held liable under the theory of *respondeat superior*—vicarious liability. Nurse B would be held responsible since each nurse is personally liable for his or her own negligent actions. Nurse A might also be held responsible since every nurse is obligated to act so that patients are safe from injury. In this case, Nurse A knew of B's intoxicated state. Nurse A did not act as a *reasonably prudent nurse* in failing to inform a supervisor. **Nos. 1, 3, and 4** are incomplete. **AN,7,SECE**

17. **(1)** If the nurse informs the physician and still carries out the treatment **(No. 2)**, both the nurse and the physician could be held liable if the patient is negligently harmed. The nurse would be liable for not acting as a reasonably prudent nurse, and the physician would be liable because he or she knew of the nurse's lack of knowledge and did not step in to protect the patient. If the nurse does not tell the physician and still carries out the treatment **(No. 4)**, the nurse would be solely liable. The nurse should not refuse to perform the treatment **(No. 3)** unless she or he has no supervision. **IMP,7,SECE**

18. **(4)** The nurse who witnesses a consent for surgery or other procedure is witnessing only that the signature is that of the purported person and that the person's condition is as indicated at the time of signing. The nurse is not witnessing that the patient is "informed." **Nos. 1, 2, and 3** are all true statements. **AN,7,SECE**

19. **(4)** As a nurse, you should *not* plan to use equipment that you know is malfunctioning. You could be held liable since you were on notice and could reasonably foresee that properly functioning equipment would be needed by your patient. Hence, **Nos. 1, 2, and 3** are incorrect. **IMP,7,SECE**

20. **(1)** This is the *only clearly false* option. Neither the physician nor the hospital would ordinarily be liable if (a) the medical risk is explained and a full report concerning the incident is documented and (b) the patient is a competent adult. The court does not usually interfere with one's right to refuse treatment, as in **No. 2**. However, the court will closely scrutinize a situation in which the patient's refusal to accept treatment results in death or in the patient's inability to care for children. If the children might be left as wards of the court, the court may force the patient to accept treatment, as in **No. 3**. Hence, **Nos. 2, 3, and 4** do not apply, as they are true. **EV,7,SECE**

21. **(3)** The court in *John Ramsey, Jr. et al.* v. *Physicians Memorial Hospital, Inc. et al.* stated: ". . . evidence supported finding that the failure of nurse to notify physician of client history involving removal of ticks from one of the children constituted a violation of her duties as a nurse, and failure to relate the information to the physician was the contributing proximate cause of death of the child." The hospital is *also* held liable under the doctrine of *respondeat superior* for the negligent conduct of its nurses when committed within the scope of their employment. Hence, **No. 1** is incomplete because it doesn't include the hospital. The physician would most likely *not* be held liable because of the language barrier and the nurse's clear failure to communicate. Hence, **Nos. 2 and 4** are incorrect. **EV,7,SECE**

22. **(1)** Both nurses and doctors are under a duty to protect the safety of their patients. In this case, the patient's safety was potentially jeopardized, yet neither the anesthesiologist nor the nurse reported the situation. Therefore, if something had happened to the patient during surgery, the court could have made a good argument that all were negligent. Hence, **Nos. 2, 3, and 4** are incomplete. What can a nurse do in a situation as described here? First, for the nurse's own safety, he or she should prepare a summary of the incidents. The nurse might also consult with nurse colleagues who have worked with the physician, as they could confirm or deny the problem and possibly offer support. Second, the nurse should report the incident to the supervisor and director of nursing, who have a liaison with the surgical/medical staff. If the action is not pursued successfully,

the nurse can bring the problem to the attention of the hospital administrator. Again, if no action is forthcoming, the nurse may seek out a board member who might be sensitive to the situation. In any case, these are difficult situations that may arise. There is no easy solution. **AN,7,SECE**

23. **(1)** Most state statutes provide that every hospital to which any person is brought who is suffering from any injuries inflicted by another must report the fact immediately to the local law enforcement authorities. Most state statutes also impose the same duty on other health care professionals, school officials and teachers, child care supervisors, and social workers. Hence **Nos. 2 and 4** are incomplete; **No. 3** is incorrect. From *Landeros* v. *Flood* as well as other cases, it seems clear that the responsibility of professional people—doctors, nurses, and others who must deal with injured children—includes the duty to report suspicious evidence to the proper authorities. **AN,7,SECE**

24. **(2)** However, it could be argued that **No. 1** is correct. The nurse's liability for the negligent loss of or damage to a patient's property is based on the nurse's duty as a person, trained or untrained, to act as a reasonable and ordinary, prudent person. In this case, the nurse put the dentures in a towel without a label. The nurse might reasonably expect that aides would be stripping the linen after the patient left for surgery. Therefore, this act was not that of an ordinary prudent person. The nurse would be liable. Since the nurse is liable, the hospital, as employer, *might* also be held liable. This would be for court determination. Since the aides had no knowledge of the dentures, and they were acting reasonably, they would not be liable for the lost dentures. Hence, **Nos. 3 and 4** are incorrect. **AN,7,SECE**

25. **(4)** Although No. 4 is best, this is a very close case. When family members help with a hospitalized patient, liability becomes complicated. Where members of the nursing team offer to assist patients in bathing, feeding, etc., and an apparently capable family member prefers to assist the patient, this is usually acceptable and neither the hospital nor the health care team is liable. Thus, **Nos. 1, 2, and 3** can be eliminated as correct choices. However, the nurse should never assume that the presence of a family member obviates the nurse helping the patient. **EV,7,SECE**

26. **(2)** The Durham Test says that a person is not criminally responsible if the act was a product of mental disease. **No. 1** is incorrect because the M'Naghten Rule states that a person is insane if he or she cannot determine right from wrong. **No. 3** is wrong because it is *not* what the Durham Test states. **No. 4** is wrong because it is an interpretation of the M'Naghten Rule. *,7,SECE

27. **(3)** The request must be in writing. **Nos. 1 and 2** are true but incomplete. **No. 4** has nothing to do with voluntary admission. **EV,7,SECE**

28. **(4)** This division of the ANA sets the standards; therefore, **No. 1** cannot be correct. **Nos. 2 and 3** are also incorrect, although they may be part of No. 4. *,7,SECE

29. **(3)** **Nos. 1, 2, and 4** may be referred to in the standards, but the standards were organized around the nursing process. *,7,SECE

30. **(2)** The Amendments extended the flow of funds and set forth specific guidelines for service. **No. 1** is incorrect because it did not cut funds or set general guidelines. **No. 3** is incorrect because it did not cut funds. **No. 4** is incorrect because it did not set general guidelines. *,7,SECE

31. **(2)** Congress intended to provide funding on a declining basis and to encourage independence from federal support. **No. 1** is incorrect because Congress does not want centers under continual federal support. **No. 3** is incorrect because it did not want to maintain federal control. **No. 4** is incorrect because although Congress wanted declining funding and control, it remains interested in community mental health centers. *,7,*

32. **(4)** This was the principal recommendation. **No. 1** is incorrect. **No. 3** is incorrect because the commission wanted flexibility in services. **No. 2** is incorrect because the commission did not want to upgrade the old grant; it wanted to provide a new one. *,7,*

33. **(3)** Nurses, for control and better health care, should be active at all levels and in all areas of health care. **No. 1** passively carries out others' ideas. **No. 2** is too limited in scope. **No. 4** is also passive, with an additional loss of control. **EV,7,SECE**

34. **(4)** This is what the document states. *Other* choices do not give the individual nurse primary responsibility. *,7,SECE

35. **(3)** The Act states that the boards must be composed of 60% *consumers* who are not affiliated with any health professional group; hence, **Nos. 1, 2, and 4** are incorrect. *,7,*

Unit 10

Practice Test

❏ Introduction

The **Practice Test** is a *follow-up assessment* tool designed to assess areas of improvement from your initial self-assessment using the **Pre Test.** Take the **Practice Test** immediately after reading the specific *content* areas related to your individual problem areas as identified by the **Pre Test.** Determine that you are now able to meet the goal of 75% correct answers in this integrated exam.

After taking this **Practice Test,** use the units in this book again to fill in any "gaps" this test reveals in your preparation. Then take the **Final Test** to assess your readiness for NCLEX-RN.

❏ Questions

Select the one best answer for each question.

1. For an adolescent boy, the main life-stage task is:
   1. Developing a sense of trust in others and in his environment.
   2. Finalizing his goals and plans for the future.
   3. Striving to attain independence and identity.
   4. Resolving inner conflicts and turmoil.
2. A child lying on the stretcher during admission suddenly complains of nausea and begins to vomit. The nurse should immediately:
   1. Turn the child's head to the side.
   2. Suction the child's oropharynx.
   3. Raise the head of the stretcher.
   4. Insert an NG tube.
3. A woman is in active labor; her membranes ruptured spontaneously 2 hours ago. While auscultating for the point of maximum intensity (PMI) of fetal heart tones before applying an external fetal monitor, the nurse counts 100 beats per minute. Which action should the nurse take *immediately?*
   1. Examine the woman for signs of a prolapsed cord.
   2. Turn the woman on her left side to increase placental perfusion.
   3. Take the woman's radial pulse while still auscultating the FHR.
   4. Start oxygen by mask to reduce fetal distress.
4. The nurse explains that a sigmoidoscopy involves:
   1. Instillation of a radiopaque dye into the lower gastrointestinal tract.
   2. Insertion of a rigid instrument that allows for direct visual examination of the anal canal, rectum, and sigmoid colon.
   3. Insertion of a fiber-optic scope that allows for direct visualization of the sigmoid colon, transverse colon, and ileocecal valve.
   4. Surgical removal of polyps and biopsy of suspicious gastrointestinal mucosa.
5. A viable 7-pound, 12-ounce boy is born. Apgar scores are 7 and 9. In assessing the baby, the nurse notes he appears slightly cyanotic. What should the nurse perform *first?*
   1. Wrap him in another blanket, to reduce heat loss.
   2. Stimulate him to cry, to increase oxygenation.
   3. Aspirate his mouth and nose with bulb syringe.
   4. Elevate his head to promote gravity drainage of secretions.
6. A 32-year-old mother of three adolescents has increased her consumption of alcoholic beverages to 24 oz of 80-proof drinks per day. She gets angry with the children very quickly, cries spontaneously several times every day, and complains of headaches constantly. In planning her care, what would be considered the *least* appropriate nursing intervention?
   1. Stimulating her to work at a concrete task.
   2. Encouraging her to cry.
   3. Providing her with someone to talk to.
   4. Isolating her from stimuli.
7. The nurse explains to a patient that bronchitis is characterized by:
   1. Hypertrophy of the bronchial mucous glands and the production of mucoid sputum sometimes difficult to expectorate.
   2. Bronchoconstriction and edema of the wall of the bronchioles.
   3. Exudate in the alveoli.
   4. Increasing lung stiffness.

8. Which assessment finding indicates a need for further assessment of a pregnant woman's general health status at 18 weeks' gestation?
   1. Rheumatic fever at age 12.
   2. Rubella titer negative.
   3. Family history of multifetal births.
   4. Treatment for chlamydial infection prior to pregnancy validation.

9. If a child's nasogastric tube is functioning properly after an emergency appendectomy, the nurse should expect to make which observation?
   1. There is no drainage on the surgical dressing.
   2. The child's abdomen is soft.
   3. The child is able to swallow saliva.
   4. There are bowel sounds in all four quadrants.

10. At 38 weeks' gestation, a woman's cervix is dilated 4 cm and effaced 60%. She speaks no English and has no prenatal record. Which nursing diagnosis is least likely to prove a problem during this woman's labor and birth?
    1. *Pain* related to uterine contractions and fear.
    2. *Impaired verbal communication* related to language barrier.
    3. *Anxiety/fear* related to poor communication and labor.
    4. *Altered nutrition, less than body requirements*.

11. The nurse plans care for an adolescent based on the knowledge that this patient least needs:
    1. External control on his or her behavior by adults.
    2. Limit setting based on fear and reprimands.
    3. Adult role models for identification.
    4. Stable relationships and interactions.

12. A patient has been admitted to the hospital with acute rheumatoid arthritis. The hands are painful and edematous, and there is severe pain in the left hip. The temperature is 101°F orally; pulse, 96; respirations, 22. ASA gr̄x qid has been ordered. The nurse can expect this patient's temperature and pulse to be elevated because of:
    1. Increased fluid losses.
    2. Inflammation of the hand and hip joints.
    3. Stress response.
    4. Side effect of salicylate therapy.

13. Which factor should the nurse identify as the most probable cause of a child's lice?
    1. The child washes her hair only once a week.
    2. The child shares her comb and brush with her friend.
    3. The child wears a hat to school every day.
    4. The child's hair is long, thick, and curly.

14. A 45-year-old man is assessed as having an obsessive-compulsive disorder. Which behavior would the nurse *least* expect him to exhibit?
    1. Working 50- to 60-hour weeks.
    2. Smoking two packs of cigarettes a day.
    3. Showing flexibility in decision making.
    4. Exhibiting a low level of concentration.

15. The nurse knows that a colostomy begins functioning:
    1. Immediately.
    2. Two to 3 days postoperatively.
    3. One week postoperatively.
    4. Two weeks postoperatively.

16. A woman is seen in clinic complaining of amenorrhea, fatigue, urinary frequency, and morning nausea. She states that her LMP was 7 weeks ago and that her menses have been normal except for one episode following a spontaneous abortion at 8 weeks' gestation. She states she has a 5-year-old boy and 3-year-old twin girls at home. Which would accurately describe this woman if she is pregnant now?
    1. Gravida 4 para 2.
    2. Gravida 5 para 3.
    3. Gravida 4 para 3.
    4. Gravida 3 para 2.

17. The *least* appropriate nursing intervention for a client experiencing alcohol withdrawal delirium would be:
    1. Reinforcing time, place, and person.
    2. Providing consistent and concrete answers to questions.
    3. Administering ordered vitamins and glucose.
    4. Applying and maintaining physical restraints.

18. The nurse is discussing nutrition in pregnancy with a group of women in the prenatal clinic. Which comment indicates a lack of understanding that requires the nurse's intervention?
    1. "I'll be drinking six to eight glasses (1500–2000 mL) of water, milk, and juices every day."
    2. "Since I am overweight, I am maintaining a weight gain of two-thirds of a pound a week during the last 5 months of pregnancy."
    3. "Since our nutrient needs can't be met through dietary sources, I am taking plenty of vitamin and mineral supplements."
    4. "Since I am a vegetarian, I am working with a registered dietitian to plan meals with complementary protein combinations."

19. Following above-the-knee amputation, a patient verbalizes feelings of decreased self-worth and of being less of a person. Acceptance of the surgery is largely dependent on:
    1. What the doctor says.
    2. How the patient's family is reacting.
    3. How the nursing staff reacts and responds to the patient's behavior.
    4. The patient's ability to grieve.

20. After being in a community mental health day treatment center for 3 weeks, an adolescent client has become apathetic and withdrawn. He generally sits alone and stares into space. The most appropriate nursing intervention would include:
    1. Selecting a group activity for him to participate in.
    2. Stimulating self-growth by providing challenging activities for him.
    3. Allowing him to spend at least 3 hours a day in his room, for inner reflection.
    4. Encouraging staff members to sit with him during group activities until he socializes voluntarily.

21. The nurse recognizes that the pattern of pulmonary dysfunction reflected by increased total lung capacity (TLC), functional residual capacity (FRC), and residual volume (RV) is characteristic of:
    1. Restrictive lung disease.
    2. Obstructive lung disease.
    3. Vascular lung disease.
    4. A combination of restrictive and obstructive lung disease.

22. A 15-year-old girl is seen in clinic with complaints of severe vulvovaginal itching, burning on urination, and thin, watery vaginal discharge for the past 4 days. During the history and physical examination, she appears very embarrassed and upset. Looking at the floor, she admits to being sexually active. She says, "Do you think I'm pregnant, or have something awful? How can I tell my mother?" Which nursing diagnosis is *least likely* to apply in this situation?

1. *Anxiety/fear* related to the perceived possibility of diagnosis of pregnancy or sexually transmitted disease.
2. *Ineffective individual coping* related to situational crisis.
3. *Self-esteem disturbance* related to inability to reconcile expectations of peers and family; situational crisis.
4. *Powerlessness* related to life-style of helplessness.

23. A patient, age 25, has been scheduled for surgery to remove the lesions at the footplate of the stapes, associated with *otosclerosis*. A patient who is scheduled for a *stapedectomy* should be told to expect:
    1. Tinnitus for several weeks after surgery.
    2. Rhinitis as the edema from surgery resolves.
    3. The hearing loss to continue for a while.
    4. Showering and swimming not to be permitted.

24. A 16-year-old boy hospitalized in a psychiatric unit for 10 days disappears from the hospital after an argument with a staff member. He is found walking about a mile from the hospital grounds. In planning care for him after this incident, the nurse would consider which factor most significant?
    1. His need to be reprimanded for his deviant behavior.
    2. His need to be medicated to calm him down.
    3. His need to be listened to in order to identify his feelings.
    4. His need to understand the consequences of his actions.

25. The physician orders prednisone, 10 mg every morning, for a patient with rheumatoid arthritis. Which precaution should the nurse advise the patient of during predischarge teaching?
    1. Take oral preparations of prednisone before meals.
    2. Never stop or change the amount of the medication without medical advice.
    3. Have periodic complete blood counts while on the medication.
    4. Wear sunglasses if exposed to bright light for an extended period of time.

26. External fetal monitor tracings show consistent fetal decelerations of uniform shape, which begin with the contraction and return to baseline as the contraction subsides. What is the correct interpretation of these data?
    1. Acute fetal distress.
    2. Uteroplacental insufficiency.
    3. Umbilical cord compression.
    4. Physiologic fetal bradycardia.

27. A woman with active tuberculosis (TB) wants to become pregnant. The nurse knows that further teaching is necessary when the woman states:
    1. "Pulmonary TB may jeopardize my pregnancy."
    2. "Spontaneous abortion may occur in one out of five women who are infected."
    3. "I can get pregnant after I have been free of TB for 6 months."
    4. "I know that I may not be able to have close contact with my baby until contagion is no longer a problem."

28. The nurse can increase the ventilatory efficiency of a patient with COPD by positioning the patient as follows:
    1. High Fowler's.
    2. Prone.
    3. Sitting up and leaning slightly forward.
    4. Trendelenburg.

29. During the adolescent period, the *least* important task to complete is:
    1. Developing an individualized personality.
    2. Attaining adequate defense mechanisms.
    3. Establishing an ego identity.
    4. Refining and stabilizing the superego.

30. The nurse would position a patient with *ruptured appendix* in:
    1. Semi-Fowler's.
    2. Trendelenburg.
    3. Left Sims'.
    4. Dorsal recumbent.

31. A woman wants to breastfeed her baby. Which hormone, normally secreted during the postpartum period, influences both the milk ejection reflex and uterine involution?
    1. Estrogen.
    2. Progesterone.
    3. Relaxin.
    4. Oxytocin.

32. A 7-year-old is admitted to the burn unit in serious condition with deep partial-thickness burns over her head, face, neck, and anterior chest. On her first night in the hospital, the nurse enters her room and finds her crying softly and moaning in pain. Recognizing the extent of her injuries, the nurse should:
    1. Do nothing at this time.
    2. Offer her two acetaminophen (Tylenol) pills as ordered and a glass of warm milk.
    3. Give her an IM injection of 40 mg of meperidine HCl (Demerol) as ordered.
    4. Inject 25 mg of meperidine HCl (Demerol) as ordered via her central IV line.

33. Suddenly, during a labor contraction, a woman's water breaks. Which assessment finding indicates a deviation from normal labor patterns?
    1. Issue of colored amniotic fluid.
    2. The woman complains of nausea and vomits.
    3. Fetal bradycardia with contractions.
    4. The woman becomes diaphoretic and irritable.

34. The most important nursing intervention in planning care for a woman with increasing symptoms of depression and alcoholism would include:
    1. Referring her to an alcohol rehabilitation program.
    2. Identifying how she has coped with anxiety in the past.
    3. Arranging for inpatient hospitalization.
    4. Requesting a prescription for an antidepressant.

35. What should the nurse recognize as an *inappropriate* method of treating *hyperthyroidism?*
    1. Subtotal thyroidectomy.
    2. Administration of propylthiouracil.
    3. Radioiodine therapy.
    4. Administration of thyroglobulin.

36. A pregnant woman returns for a routine visit at 12 weeks' gestation. Which nursing assessment could the nurse use to verify the EDB and estimate uterine/fetal growth?
    1. Leopold's maneuvers.
    2. Weight-gain pattern.
    3. Vital signs and fetal heart tones.
    4. Height of the fundus.

37. A teenage boy has a history of setting fires. His arson attempts may exhibit which behavior?
    1. Acting out.
    2. Depression.
    3. Paranoia.
    4. Mania.

38. Which statement by the nurse correctly describes a wheeze?
    1. A high-pitched musical sound produced by airflow in narrowed bronchioles.
    2. Rarely considered pathologic.
    3. A medium-pitched sonorous sound produced by airflow in obstructed bronchi.
    4. A high-pitched crowing sound produced by edema in the trachea.

39. A 32-year-old woman is diagnosed as having a mood disorder. What drug is usually administered in treating such disorders?
    1. Lithium (lithium carbonate).
    2. Librium (chlordiazepoxide HCl).
    3. Prolixin (fluphenazine hydrochloride).
    4. Mellaril (thioridazine).

40. The primary purpose of the nurse performing passive range-of-motion exercises to an acute rheumatoid arthritis patient's affected limbs is to:
    1. Prevent contractures and limited range of motion.
    2. Continually evaluate the patient's functional abilities.
    3. Assess the patient's pain tolerance.
    4. Evaluate the effectiveness of drug therapy.

41. A pregnant woman's last menstrual period began on April 3. Which is an accurate estimate of her EDB?
    1. January 3.
    2. January 10.
    3. January 27.
    4. December 10.

42. After 24 hours of hospitalization for a suicide attempt, the client begins to verbalize more and has interacted with other clients on the inpatient psychiatric unit. The nurse should realize that this increase in energy level may indicate that the client:
    1. Needs less individual attention.
    2. Needs more individual attention.
    3. Needs a decrease in antidepressant medications.
    4. Is presently motivated to get well.

43. The appropriate nursing action with a patient experiencing expressive aphasia following a CVA would be:
    1. Help the patient and family accept this permanent disability.
    2. Associate words with physical objects.
    3. Wait indefinitely for the patient to verbalize.
    4. Tell the family that the patient cannot communicate.

44. Which action by the nurse would be most helpful in preparing a 5-year-old for cardiac catheterization?
    1. Describe the procedure in very simple terms.
    2. Take the child to the lab to observe such a procedure.
    3. Answer only those questions the child asks.
    4. Use puppets to dramatize the procedure for the child.

45. The number of first-time pregnancies in women between the ages of 35 and 40 years has increased by 40%. The nurse conducting a parent education class for these women, in the last trimester of pregnancy, needs to include discussion of:
    1. Energy and stamina to meet demands of parenting.
    2. Feeling troubled by pregnancy and being less adjusted during the last trimester of pregnancy.
    3. The longer labor experienced by older mothers.
    4. The greater number of labor/birth complications experienced by older mothers.

46. The nurse explains to a patient that the colostomy appliance for a double-barrel colostomy should be changed:
    1. Every day.
    2. When drainage leaks through the seal.
    3. Once a week.
    4. At a time selected by the visiting nurse.

47. A woman in labor expresses concern about her baby's status. If the nurse identifies the presence of early decelerations, which intervention should be instituted?
    1. Elevate the woman's hips, and start oxygen by mask.
    2. Lower the head of the bed, and place the woman in supine position.
    3. Mark the tracing in red, and check for dislodged electrode.
    4. Reassure the woman that this represents a normal tracing.

48. A patient is scheduled for a temporary colostomy due to severe diverticulitis. Preoperative preparation of this patient includes administration of neomycin SO_4. The nurse expects that this antibiotic will:
    1. Combat postoperative wound infection.
    2. Decrease bacterial count of the colon.
    3. Reduce the size of the suspected tumor before surgery.
    4. Stimulate peristalsis and facilitate action of cleansing enemas.

49. A 35-year-old woman takes an overdose of sleeping pills and alcohol. She is brought to the emergency room in an ambulance called by a neighbor, who discovered her unconscious on the living room sofa. Upon admission, she is unconscious. Her vital signs are TPR 98–60–10 and BP 90/50. Her reflexes are dull. The emergency room nurse's initial response should include:
    1. Administering a central nervous system stimulant.
    2. Paging the resident on call.
    3. Maintaining a patent airway.
    4. Assessing her neurologic signs.

50. After nebulizer treatment with isoproterenol (Isuprel), the following pulmonary function data were obtained:

	TLC	FRC	RV	VC	FEV_1
Before treatment	7000	5000	4200	2800	2000
After treatment	7000	4000	3000	3800	2500

The nurse would conclude that the change in lung volumes indicates:
    1. Improvement.
    2. Deterioration.
    3. No change.
    4. Data inadequate to decide.

51. A vaginal examination disclosed several painful red papules on the inner surfaces of the labia minora and in the vagina. Lesions were extremely painful on gentle touch with an applicator. Discharge had a very foul odor. Inflammatory regional lymph nodes were easily palpated. With which infectious organism are these assessment findings associated?
    1. *Trichomonas vaginalis*.
    2. *Candida albicans*.
    3. Herpesvirus type 2.
    4. *Neisseria gonorrhoeae*.

52. A 15-year-old boy in a day treatment center begins to mutilate his forearms with lighted cigarettes and scratch his wrists with thumbtacks and staples he finds on the unit. What is the *least* appropriate nursing goal?

1. Supervising him closely.
2. Avoiding confrontations regarding his behavior.
3. Removing all items that could be used for destructive purposes.
4. Assisting him to increase his self-esteem.

53. A woman asks the nurse what makes a pregnancy test "turn positive." The nurse's best response is based on the knowledge that the biologic marker for pregnancy tests is:
    1. Human placental lactogen.
    2. Human chorionic gonadotropin.
    3. Luteinizing hormone.
    4. Alpha-fetoprotein.

54. A woman who speaks no English is in active labor, with moderate to strong contractions every 2–3 minutes, lasting 45 seconds. She appears very frightened. By which modality can the nurse convey caring and allay anxiety?
    1. Asking her husband to translate all interactions.
    2. Touching, smiling, and speaking in a calm, assured voice.
    3. Speaking slowly, loudly, and clearly, to facilitate her understanding.
    4. Offering to notify the doctor on call.

55. After an adolescent has been in a mental health day treatment center for a year and a half, the professional staff are considering discharging him. The client asks the nurse whether he must tell other people that he has been in a mental health center. The most appropriate response the nurse could make would be:
    1. "Yes, especially to all future school officials."
    2. "Yes, especially to all prospective employers."
    3. "No, this is an individual decision."
    4. "No, there is no specific requirement."

56. A peripheral iridectomy is the surgical procedure of choice following an acute episode of closed-angle glaucoma. Which nursing measure is *inappropriate* for a patient who has had an *iridectomy*?
    1. Instill eyedrops to mobilize the affected pupil by alternate dilatation and constriction.
    2. Ambulate the patient as soon as possible after the surgery.
    3. Reinforce the surgical dressing as needed to prevent infection.
    4. If ordered, instruct the patient to massage the affected eye.

57. A pregnant woman complains of constipation. What should the nurse recommend to relieve her symptoms of constipation?
    1. Regular bedtime use of mild laxatives like mineral oil.
    2. Limit fluid intake to 1000 mL daily.
    3. Increase dietary intake of fresh fruit and salads.
    4. Begin Kegel exercises to increase tone.

58. In monitoring the postop course of an adolescent who has had surgery for a ruptured appendix, the nurse would be most correct in expecting that this patient will:
    1. Have severe pain for 24 hours.
    2. Be discharged within 48 hours.
    3. Make a slow, steady recovery.
    4. Make a fairly rapid and complete recovery.

59. An adolescent may exhibit depression differently from an adult. An adolescent who is depressed is most likely to exhibit which behavior?
    1. Withdrawal.
    2. Apathy.
    3. Violence.

4. Regression.

60. The nurse needs to know that the woman likely to be at highest risk for pelvic inflammatory disease (PID) is one who:
    1. Uses an intrauterine device (IUD) for contraception.
    2. Acquired gonorrhea from a fomite.
    3. Has had multiple sex partners.
    4. Drinks one alcoholic beverage per day (e.g., one glass of wine).

61. Nursing actions that will facilitate a COPD patient's medical therapy include:
    1. Limiting fluid intake to prevent volume overload and right-sided heart failure.
    2. Oral and endotracheal suctioning as necessary.
    3. Instructing the patient in deep breathing and coughing techniques as well as pursed-lip exhalations.
    4. Maintenance of bedrest and activity restrictions to reduce acidosis.

62. When a newborn is nearly 24 hours old, a nursing assessment notes that the infant's skin is dry and flaking and that there are several areas of an apparent macular rash. The nurse charts this as:
    1. Erythema toxicum.
    2. Milia.
    3. Icterus neonatorum.
    4. Multiple hemangiomas.

63. What is a reliable index of the exercise tolerance of a patient who has rheumatoid arthritis?
    1. Pulse and respiratory rate.
    2. Occurrence and duration of pain in the affected joint.
    3. Mobility of joints.
    4. Decreased redness and swelling of joints.

64. In planning nursing care for a hospitalized suicidal client, what is the *least* appropriate nursing action?
    1. Searching personal effects for toxic agents.
    2. Removing straps from clothing.
    3. Placing the client in small groups for observation.
    4. Removing sharp objects from the environment.

65. In positioning a child with burns of the head, face, neck, and anterior chest during her recovery, the nurse should:
    1. Avoid head flexion.
    2. Keep the child as still as possible.
    3. Avoid sitting the child up in a chair.
    4. Place two firm pillows under the child's head.

66. A woman in labor, with an interest in using Lamaze for labor and birth, appears tired, tense, and uncomfortable. She complains that her back aches, the monitor "bothers" her, and she wants people to leave her alone and let her rest. Which nursing intervention, implemented by the nurse, demonstrates *proper* nursing judgment?
    1. Offer to get an order for some pain medication.
    2. Reposition the woman and apply sacral pressure.
    3. Turn monitor off audible reading.
    4. Darken room and leave her alone for 5 minutes.

67. A patient's laboratory work reveals: Hct 50%, Hgb 17, HCO_3 32. Arterial blood gases: pH 7.38, Po_2 65, Pco_2 55. The nurse's interpretation of this patient's blood gases is that he or she has:
    1. Uncompensated respiratory acidosis.
    2. Compensated respiratory acidosis.
    3. Uncompensated metabolic alkalosis.
    4. Compensated metabolic alkalosis.

68. An adolescent boy's parents have decided that they would rather have him placed outside of the home

when he is discharged from the mental health day treatment center. The most appropriate intervention the nurse could make would include:

1. Asking his parents to reassess their feelings about this decision.
2. Suggesting that his parents discuss this decision with the entire family.
3. Referring his parents to a social worker to assist in finding an alternative placement.
4. Assisting his parents in finding an appropriate discharge placement.

69. Which laboratory test result or parameter(s) would be increased on assessment of a patient with acute rheumatoid arthritis?
1. Hemoglobin and hematocrit.
2. Sedimentation rate and C-reactive protein.
3. Wasserman test result.
4. Platelet count.

70. Anticipatory guidance may be indicated to assist expectant parents achieve the normal developmental tasks of the beginning family. What is *least likely* to cause anxiety and stress at 18 weeks' gestation?
1. Economic demands of having a child.
2. Change in intrafamily relationships.
3. Increasing awareness of the need to be responsible for another individual (the baby).
4. Feelings of having to "compete" for attention.

71. The teaching plan for a patient with COPD should emphasize:
1. Smoking and alcohol restrictions.
2. Nutrition, fluid balance, and ways to stop smoking.
3. Vocational rehabilitation programs available in the community.
4. Activity restrictions and pulmonary physiology.

72. To establish a relationship with a 14-year-old boy who is hospitalized in a private, coed, inpatient mental hospital unit, what would be inappropriate for the nurse to consider?
1. Boys in early adolescence feel threatened by female authority figures.
2. Enforced inactivity will deprive the adolescent of a major avenue for relieving frustration.
3. Impulse control is a major problem for males.
4. Fear and ambivalence will usually dissipate with the passage of time.

73. A woman in labor begins to push. Vaginal examination reveals the cervix is dilated 8 cm. For which reason does the nurse tell her to pant with her "pains"?
1. To increase oxygenation of the fetus during transitional phase.
2. Pushing on an incompletely dilated cervix may cause cervical edema and may prolong labor.
3. Hyperventilating will make her dizzy, reduce pain, and encourage complete dilatation.
4. To reduce stress on the fetal head during internal rotation.

74. A pregnant woman states, "I don't feel like myself lately." Further assessment identifies feelings of discomfort due to mood swings, tingling, tender breasts, and fluctuating sexual desire. Which nursing diagnosis is *most* appropriate?
1. *Body-image disturbance* related to second trimester physiologic and psychological adaptations.
2. *Altered nutrition, less than body requirements,* related to increased need for vitamin B_6 during pregnancy.
3. *Ineffective individual coping* related to perceived need to alter life-style, role change.

4. *Personal identity disturbance* related to introspection and self-focusing.

75. An adolescent client in a mental health day treatment center exhibits frequent outbursts of maladaptive behavior. He started hitting other clients and even struck a nurse. In assessing this client's behavior, the nurse should consider which fact to be most relevant?
1. Hitting others makes him feel satisfied because he is in control of the situation.
2. Hitting others provides him with an escape from feelings of hopelessness.
3. Hitting others is his mechanism for alleviating anxiety.
4. Hitting others allows him to instill fear in others.

76. Chronic obstructive pulmonary disease can progress to respiratory failure. A patient with emphysema becomes increasingly drowsy, tachypneic, and tachycardic. The nurse should first:
1. Prepare IV aminophylline.
2. Position the patient in high Fowler's.
3. Give 2 liters of O_2 per nasal cannula.
4. Administer 60% O_2 via mask.

77. A pregnant woman complains her nausea is very "bothersome" in the morning, when she must prepare breakfast for her family. Which action should the nurse recommend?
1. Avoid eating before retiring.
2. Drink a glass of fruit juice immediately on rising.
3. Eat one or two soda crackers before rising.
4. Make and eat her breakfast first.

78. A child is to have daily debridement and whirlpool therapy for burns. In cleansing the burns, the nurse should use sterile:
1. 4×4 gauze pads.
2. Cotton balls.
3. Washcloths.
4. Telfa pads.

79. A patient with a history of alcohol abuse is hospitalized after an overdose of sleeping pills. The nurse should be aware that in the first 72 hours following admission to the hospital she is most likely to exhibit:
1. Withdrawal delirium.
2. Suspiciousness.
3. Mood swings.
4. The use of coping mechanisms such as reaction formation.

80. A patient has a smoking history of 25 years, and a recent episode of 5 days of increased breathlessness. On physical examination, he is found to have a barrel chest, medium-pitched rhonchi, and wheezes in the right upper lobe and both lower lung lobes. The nurse observes that this patient demonstrates the "increased work of breathing" during this acute period by:
1. Increasing the rate and depth of his respirations.
2. Increasing diaphragmatic excursion.
3. Using pursed-lip exhalations.
4. Using accessory muscles for ventilation.

81. A pregnant woman complains of severe "charley horses" during the night. Which action should the nurse recommend to provide symptomatic relief?
1. Drink a glass of milk at bedtime.
2. Extend affected leg, and dorsiflex the foot.
3. Increase dietary intake of vitamin C.
4. Mild exercise every evening, such as walking.

82. Two days before above-the-knee amputation, an adult patient expresses a desire to learn more about the surgery and outcome. Preoperative teaching is directed toward:

   1. Discussing the possibility of another vocation.

   2. Learning crutch walking.

   3. Instruction in postoperative exercises.

   4. Encouraging the patient to verbalize fears and concerns.

83. A 14-year-old boy with a history of setting fires has developed a homosexual relationship with a 16-year-old boy. In planning care, the nurse should *primarily*:

   1. Avoid confronting him about his attention-getting behavior.

   2. Validate his rationale for establishing the relationship.

   3. Explore his thoughts, feelings, and attitudes.

   4. Enforce limits on interactions between the two patients.

84. A male adolescent (age 15) complains of having nothing to do while he is recovering from an appendectomy. The nurse should:

   1. Ask him to place routine lab slips in the charts.

   2. Refer him to the tutor and arrange for him to get his school books and homework.

   3. Bring in several board games, and encourage him and his 14-year-old roommate to start playing with one of them.

   4. Introduce him to the two 15-year-old girls in the room next door.

85. Health teaching for a woman infected with *Trichomonas vaginalis* should include:

   1. "Abstain from intercourse until lesions heal."

   2. "Penicillin is the drug of choice for treatment."

   3. "Therapy is curative."

   4. "The organism is associated with later development of hydatidiform mole."

86. Which statement by the nurse correctly describes a double-barrel colostomy?

   1. It is the least common type of colostomy, and it discharges liquid or unformed stool.

   2. A single loop of the transverse colon is exteriorized and supported by a glass rod. There are two openings, a proximal loop and a distal loop.

   3. It has two stomas. A proximal loop discharges feces, and a distal loop discharges mucus.

   4. It is most often permanent and is done to treat disorders of the sigmoid colon.

87. When administering lithium to a client with a mood disorder, what is the *least* relevant consideration?

   1. If the client's urinary output decreases significantly, diuretics should be ordered.

   2. The client needs to be given a complete physical examination prior to administering the drug.

   3. If the client experiences nausea, vomiting, and muscle weakness, the dosage may need regulating.

   4. If the client exhibits symptoms of mania during the first 10 days of receiving the drug, haloperidol (Haldol) may also be administered.

88. A woman in labor suddenly screams and shouts in Spanish. Her husband translates that she has a "terrible pain in her calf," a charley horse. What should the nurse do *immediately*?

   1. Inform the doctor that the woman has signs of thrombophlebitis.

   2. Administer oxygen by mask to expedite conversion of muscle lactic acid.

   3. Straighten the woman's knee and dorsiflex her foot.

   4. Turn the woman on her left side to increase placental perfusion.

89. A 7-year-old child is fitted for a pressure stockinette to cover her head, face, and neck to minimize scarring as her burns are healing. To help the child cope with her injuries, treatment, and recuperation, the nurse should ask her parents to bring:

   1. Her favorite toys and stuffed animals.

   2. Some of her friends for a short visit.

   3. Her favorite foods, including pizza and ice cream.

   4. Colorful scarves and hats.

90. A 14-year-old boy is likely to experience several biologic and psychosocial changes at this time. Which behavior would the nurse expect to see?

   1. An increase in imaginative thinking.

   2. An increased ability to learn by rote.

   3. An increase in academic achievement.

   4. An increased ability to cope with frustration.

91. The nursing goal for a non-English-speaking woman who has just given birth is demonstration of confidence and competence in caring for her newborn. Which modality will be most effective in facilitating and evaluating her achievement of this goal?

   1. Giving her a booklet in her language, describing basic techniques of baby care.

   2. Discussing the pattern and procedures of basic newborn care with her.

   3. Demonstrating basic baby care procedures and having her perform them with her husband.

   4. Referring her to the Public Health Department nurses in her community.

92. The nurse identifies methods to reduce flatus and odor for a patient with a double-barrel colostomy. What would be the *least* effective method to achieve this?

   1. Avoid eating broccoli and cabbage.

   2. Utilize *Banish* deodorant drops in bottom of appliance.

   3. Put pinhole in appliance to let flatus escape.

   4. Empty feces and gas from appliance as necessary.

93. A woman in labor says, "I can't stand it any longer. I have to push." On vaginal examination, her cervix has dilated to 8 cm and the head is at station 0. For which reason should the nurse encourage this woman to pant, or breathe naturally, with her contractions?

   1. Pushing now could cause the cord to prolapse.

   2. She should increase her oxygen level before completion of the first stage.

   3. Pushing before complete dilatation may cause cervical edema and may prolong labor.

   4. Panting will speed cervical dilatation.

94. Pulmonary function data were collected on a patient. The results were:

	TLC	FRC	RV	VC	FEV$_1$
Predicted	6000	3000	2000	4000	3000
Observed	7000	5000	4200	2800	2000

The nurse's analysis of these data reveals:

   1. Hyperinflation.

   2. Hyperventilation.

   3. Hyperpnea.

   4. Hypercapnia.

95. The nurse should teach the parents of a child with lice that to prevent other members of the family from getting lice:

   1. The child should sleep alone and in her or his own bed.

   2. All family members should get a very short haircut.

   3. The child should wear a hair net for a few days.

   4. All family members should comb their hair with a fine-toothed comb after regular shampooing.

96. An 18-year-old with acting-out behaviors has been living in a group home for the past 2 months. He has

asked permission to visit a friend in the psychiatric hospital. The nurse should:
1. Allow him to visit.
2. Assess his motives.
3. Ask his parents' permission.
4. Consult with the hospital staff.

97. Which nursing intervention should be implemented to reduce a pregnant woman's stress in the first trimester regarding her feelings about mood swings, tingling, tender breasts, and fluctuating sexual desire?
   1. Validate normalcy of emotional lability.
   2. Recommend high-protein, high-vitamin diet.
   3. Refer her to a psychologist for counseling.
   4. Reinforce positive feelings about the pregnancy.

98. A complication of chronic obstructive pulmonary disease is the possible rupture of an emphysematous bleb. The nurse suspects that the patient has a right tension pneumothorax. What signs would the nurse expect to see?
   1. Flushed appearance from elevated blood pressure.
   2. Tracheal deviation to the unaffected side.
   3. Hyporesonance on the affected side.
   4. Medial shift of the heart.

99. A 15-year-old's behavior is becoming increasingly combative. He hits other clients as well as the nursing staff at least once or twice each day. What is an inappropriate nursing goal?
   1. Helping him develop impulse control.
   2. Helping him manage his feelings appropriately.
   3. Helping him learn socially acceptable behavior.
   4. Helping him internalize his feelings.

100. To reduce symptoms of early morning stiffness in a patient who has rheumatoid arthritis, the nurse can encourage the patient to:
   1. Take a hot tub bath or shower in the morning.
   2. Put joints through passive ROM before trying to move them actively.
   3. Sleep with a hot pad.
   4. Take two aspirins before arising, and wait 15 minutes before attempting locomotion.

❑ Answers/Rationale

1. (3) The adolescent is striving to attain a sense of independence and identity. Trust (**No. 1**) is usually developed during infancy and matures as the individual develops. Goals and plans (**No. 2**) are made during the adolescent period, but they are rarely finalized realistically until late adulthood. During this period, inner conflicts (**No. 4**) are rarely resolved and are usually heightened. **EV,5,HPM**

2. (1) To prevent aspiration, the first and immediate action the nurse should take is to turn the child's head to the side. All of the other actions (**Nos. 2, 3, and 4**) may also prevent aspiration but will take considerably longer and are not effective immediately. **IMP,1,SECE**

3. (3) Taking the mother's pulse while listening to the FHR will differentiate between the maternal and fetal

Key to codes following rationales Nursing process: **AS**, Assessment; **AN**, Analysis; **PL**, Plan; **IMP**, Implementation; **EV**, Evaluation. Category of human function: **1**, Protective; **2**, Sensory-perceptual; **3**, Comfort, Rest, Activity, and Mobility; **4**, Nutrition; **5**, Growth and Development; **6**, Fluid-Gas Transport; **7**, Psychosocial-Cultural; **8**, Elimination. Client needs: **SECE**, Safe, Effective Care Environment; **PhI**, Physiologic Integrity; **PsI**, Psychosocial Integrity; **HPM**, Health Promotion/Maintenance. See appendices for full explanation.

heart rates and rule out fetal bradycardia. **No. 1** is wrong because although the cord may prolapse at any time before the oncoming head occludes the cervix, the most common time of occurrence is when the membranes rupture. **No. 2** is wrong because fetal bradycardia has not yet been determined; the nurse needs to differentiate maternal from fetal heart rate. **No. 4** is wrong because if the fetal heart rate is normal, there is no need for supplemental oxygen therapy. **IMP,6,HPM**

4. (2) Sigmoidoscopy involves the insertion of a rigid instrument into the anus that allows direct visualization of the anal canal, rectum, and sigmoid colon. The patient is usually prepared for this procedure with enemas or rectal suppositories. **No. 1** is an example of a lower GI study. **No. 3** describes a colonoscopy, and **No. 4** describes two of the procedures that can be accomplished with a colonoscope. **IMP,8,SECE**

5. (3) Gentle aspiration of mucus helps maintain a patent airway, required for effective gas exchange. **No. 1** is wrong because the first priority is a patent airway. **No. 2** is wrong because the baby may aspirate mucus, which would occlude the airway. **No. 4** is wrong because gravity drainage is accomplished in head-dependent position. **IMP,6,SECE**

6. (4) Isolation may lead to withdrawal and depression. She needs positive reinforcement and reassurance to increase her self-esteem. Isolation may also lead to an increase in her drinking and depression. Based on the symptoms she is exhibiting, involving her in simple, concrete tasks (**No. 1**) may help her feel useful. Crying (**No. 2**) helps her alleviate anxiety through the physical expression of her feelings. Encouraging the verbalization of her feelings (**No. 3**) will demonstrate that someone cares for her enough to listen, and may decrease her anxiety level. **PL,7,PsI**

7. (1) The basic pathophysiologic changes associated with chronic bronchitis are hypertrophy of the mucous glands lining the bronchi and the production of increased amounts of mucus (sometimes thick and difficult to expectorate) that tend to narrow the airway and trap air distal to the mucus. Bronchoconstriction and edema of the bronchial walls (**No. 2**) are characteristic of *asthma*. Exudate in the alveoli (**No. 3**) and increasing lung stiffness (**No. 4**) are consistent with *pneumonia*. **IMP,6,PhI**

8. (1) Definitive (30%) increase in blood volume occurs at this point in pregnancy; rising cardiac load imposes stress on the heart valves (e.g., mitral stenosis) affected during the episode of rheumatic fever. **No. 2** is wrong because *first-trimester* rubella infection presents the greatest hazard to the fetus, and immunization should be planned for the immediate postpartum period. **No. 3** is wrong because diagnosis of multifetal pregnancy would be based *not* on discussions of *general* health status but on physical evidence (fundal height, ultrasound). **No. 4** is wrong because once treatment is ended, infection is gone. **AS,1,PhI**

9. (2) The main purpose of a nasogastric tube is to drain fluid and gas from the stomach; if it is functioning properly, the child's abdomen should be soft, and the tube should drain stomach contents, including bile. The nasogastric tube will not affect the drainage on the dressing (**No. 1**) or the bowel sounds (**No. 4**). The child may complain of a sore throat from this tube, but it should not affect the ability to swallow saliva (**No. 3**). **EV,8,PhI**

10. (4) Although hydration may be affected by the physiologic stress of labor, the duration is insufficient to sig-

nificantly affect nutritional status. **No. 1** is wrong because discomfort generally does accompany labor. **No. 2** is wrong because the inability to communicate clearly affects nurse-patient relationships and may induce or augment anxiety. **No. 3** is wrong because labor *is* commonly accompanied by anxiety. **AN,5,HPM**

11. **(2)** Limits *do* need to be set but they should be based on *mutual respect* rather than fear. Adult (or external) controls on behavior **(No. 1)** are essential and must be consistent. Role models serve to stimulate the identification process **(No. 3)** both consciously and unconsciously. Stable relationships **(No. 4)** are essential if the adolescent is to mature and develop a sense of trust. **PL,5,HPM**

12. **(2)** Fever and increased pulse rates occur in rheumatoid arthritis due to the systemic inflammatory process of this dysfunction. If the fever is high or prolonged, increased fluid losses could occur due to insensible water loss **(No. 1)**; however, the effects on body temperature would be secondary to the primary inflammatory response. Though the stress response **(No. 3)** does increase pulse rate, normally it does not significantly affect body temperature. **No. 4** is incorrect because salicylates have an antipyretic effect. **EV,3,PhI**

13. **(2)** Lice are spread by direct or indirect contact: sharing combs and brushes, sharing hats, sleeping together, etc. It is generally unrelated to frequency of hair washing **(No. 1)**, wearing a hat **(No. 3)**, or having long hair **(No. 4)**. **AS,1,HPM**

14. **(3)** Most obsessive-compulsive individuals are highly inflexible and resist change because change stimulates anxiety and they are unable to cope with stress. **Nos. 1, 2, and 4** are all likely behaviors. **AS,7,PsI**

15. **(2)** The stomas will begin to secrete mucus within 48 hours, and the proximal loop should begin to drain fecal material within 72 hours. Ileostomies **(No. 1)** begin to drain immediately. **Nos. 3 and 4** are incorrect because peristalsis generally returns within 48–72 hours postoperatively. **EV,8,PhI**

16. **(1)** History of three pregnancies plus current pregnancy (gravida 4). Parity refers to the number of pregnancies carried to viability, *not* the number of babies. Two pregnancies were carried past viability (para 2). This formula does not allow for indicating the number of abortions or living children. **Nos. 2, 3, and 4** are wrong based on the definitions of gravida and parity. **AS,5,HPM**

17. **(4)** The psychological effect of being restrained can be severe. Therefore any form of restraint should be applied as a last resort. Isolating the client from other clients during the initial adjustment period would serve to decrease stimuli and possibly prevent the need for restraints. **Nos. 1, 2, and 3** are all more appropriate interventions. **IMP,7,PsI**

18. **(3)** The nurse needs to check out what "plenty of vitamins and mineral supplements" means. Hypervitaminosis has an *adverse* effect on the woman's immune system response and fetal development. **No. 1** is not the answer because 1500–2000 mL of fluids per day *is* recommended. **No. 2** is not the answer because the recommended weight gain, with a good diet, *is* two-thirds of a pound per week for the last 6 months of pregnancy. **No. 4** is not the answer because a registered dietitian *is* recommended to assist vegetarian women with complementary protein combinations. **EV,4,HPM**

19. **(4)** The loss of a limb is significant. The patient facing the amputation must deal with self-perception, incorporate the changes in body image, and be allowed to grieve. The nurse must be sensitive to the patient's stage of grieving and provide information as asked for, at a level consistent with the patient's ability to comprehend. Although the attending physician **(No. 1)**, family **(No. 2)**, and nursing staff **(No. 3)** may affect the patient's perception of a situation, the work of grieving is primarily personal, with movement both forward and backward as the patient progresses through the stages. **AN,7,PsI**

20. **(4)** The adolescent *initially* needs staff's help in one-to-one socialization. He *next* must be stimulated by the staff to participate in minimally demanding group activities **(No. 1)**. Allowing him a minimum of 3 hours of isolated behavior **(No. 3)** will probably increase his withdrawal. Perhaps the nurse could establish a behavior-modification program involving a trade-off of 15 minutes alone for every 45 minutes spent socializing and interacting with others. If activities are too challenging **(No. 2)**, he may become frustrated and feel incompetent, which would lead to a decrease in self-esteem. **PL,7,PsI**

21. **(2)** Increased lung volumes (TLC, FRC, RV) and decreased airflow—vital capacity (VC) and forced expiratory volume in 1 second (FEV_1)—are functional problems consistent with obstructive lung disease. In restrictive lung disease **(No. 1)**, volumes generally are decreased. Vascular lung disease **(No. 3)** has no effect on ventilatory capacity but directly affects diffusion of gases; that is, pulmonary infarction decreases blood flow to the lungs, so some alveoli that are ventilated are no longer perfused. Restrictive lung disease is incorrect in **No. 4**. **AN,6,PhI**

22. **(4)** Adolescents rarely demonstrate a life-style characterized by helplessness; rather, they are striving to gain control over their own lives. **No. 1** is wrong because the teenager *has* verbalized anxiety and fear over possible diagnoses. **No. 2** is wrong because the threat of adolescent pregnancy evidently presents a situational crisis for her. **No. 3** is wrong because either diagnosis *will* provide her with evidence that she failed to meet family expectations, and precipitates situational crisis. **AN,7,PsI**

23. **(3)** Stapedectomy is the surgical procedure for the treatment of otosclerosis. Its success cannot be determined in the immediate postoperative period. The patient must be told that hearing is affected for a while after surgery because of edema. Tinnitus **(No. 1)** is a postoperative complication that must be reported, but is *not* expected. The resolution of postoperative edema **(No. 2)** does *not* result in rhinitis. Once the ear has healed, normal activities *are* permitted, including showering and swimming **(No. 4)**. With an upper respiratory infection, deep-sea diving and flying are usually restricted. **IMP,2,SECE**

24. **(3)** The adolescent client is probably very frightened and angry. He needs to feel that his side will be considered if he is to cope effectively with these feelings and with his behavior. **Nos. 1, 2, and 4** are all staff oriented and provide little psychological support for the client as an individual striving for independence. **AN,7,PsI**

25. **(2)** In preparing the patient for discharge on prednisone therapy, the nurse should caution him or her to (a) take oral preparations after meals; (b) remember that routine checks of vital signs, weight, and lab studies are critical; (c) never stop or change the amount of medication without medical advice; and (d) store the medication in a light-resistant container. **No. 1** is in-

correct because prednisone, as well as other medications given in rheumatoid arthritis therapy, is irritating to the GI tract and should be taken after meals. **No. 3** is incorrect because although fluid, electrolyte, and serum-glucose levels need frequent evaluation during prednisone therapy, CBCs need regular checking if the patient is on phenylbutazone (Butazolidin), oxyphenbutazone (Tandearil), or ibuprofen (Motrin) therapy. **No. 4** is a precaution given to patients on hydroxychloroquine SO_4 (Plaquenil) or chloroquine (Aralen) therapy. **IMP,4,SECE**

26. **(4)** Early decelerations represent the normal fetal response to head compressions during contractions. **No. 1** is wrong because head compression does not cause fetal distress. **Nos. 2 and 3** are wrong because there are no signs of late or variable decelerations. **AN,6,PhI**

27. **(3)** Intervention is needed when the woman thinks that she needs to wait only 6 months after being free of TB before she can get pregnant. She needs to wait 1½–2 years after she is declared to be free of TB before she should attempt pregnancy. **No. 1** is not the answer because pregnancy *may* be jeopardized by TB. **No. 2** is not the answer because spontaneous abortion *does* occur in one of five women who are infected. **No. 4** is not the answer because she will *not* have close contact with her baby until contagion is no longer a problem. **EV,1,SECE**

28. **(3)** The position that allows for the greatest amount of lung expansion is sitting up and leaning slightly forward. This position can be facilitated by allowing the patient to rest his or her arms on a bedside table. The position that also facilitates lung expansion, but not to the same degree, is high Fowler's **(No. 1)**. Both the prone position **(No. 2)** and the Trendelenburg position **(No. 4)** tend to decrease full lung expansion due to increased pressure of abdominal contents on the diaphragm. **IMP,6,SECE**

29. **(4)** The superego may never be completely refined or stabilized. Some individuals may achieve an optimal level of functioning some time in late adulthood; however, rarely will the superego become stabilized during adolescence. As stated in **No. 1**, the individual does strive to develop an independent and unique personality during adolescence. To maintain a steady state of functioning, the adolescent must learn to use defense mechanisms **(No. 2)** in an appropriate manner. Developing a positive ego identity **(No. 3)** is one of the major goals of adolescence. **PL,5,HPM**

30. **(1)** The patient is placed in a semi-Fowler's position to promote the flow of drainage to the pelvic region, where a localized abscess can be drained or be resolved by the body's normal defenses. The elevated position also keeps the infection from spreading upward in the peritoneal cavity. **Nos. 2, 3, and 4** are incorrect because none of them elevates the trunk of the body. **IMP,3,SECE**

31. **(4)** Contraction of the milk ducts and the let-down reflex occur under the stimulation of oxytocin released by the posterior pituitary gland. **Nos. 1, 2, and 3** are wrong because these hormones have no effect on the let-down reflex or uterine involution. **AN,5,PhI**

32. **(4)** The nurse should know that deep partial-thickness (second-degree) burns cause severe pain. The nurse should also know that during the first 48–72 hours following a serious burn, there is a very poor peripheral circulation due to hypovolemia; therefore, medications should be given via the IV route. PO **(No. 2)** and IM **(No. 3)** medications are generally contraindicated dur-

ing this time. To do nothing **(No. 1)** would be inappropriate, given the nature and extent of her injuries. **IMP,3,SECE**

33. **(1)** Normal amniotic fluid is essentially colorless; any color may signify fetal or maternal problems. For example, green amniotic fluid indicates meconium released due to fetal hypoxia; bloody amniotic fluid may indicate abruptio placentae. **No. 2** is wrong because nausea with or without emesis *is common* in labor, due to physiologic stress. **No. 3** is wrong because fetal bradycardia *commonly* manifests at contraction acme, due to head compression. **No. 4** is wrong because diaphoresis and irritability *are* signs of transitional phase of labor. **AS,5,PhI**

34. **(2)** Past coping mechanisms are important in assessing the client's ability to return to a steady state of functioning. Strengths and weaknesses in the client's ability to rationally assess and cope with her feelings need to be explored. Referrals may need to be made **(No. 1)**, but an initial assessment of the client needs to be completed first. Inpatient hospitalization may be needed **(No. 3)**; however, the assessment of her ability to cope with the situation may assist in identifying whether hospitalization is needed. Obtaining a prescription for an antidepressant at this time **(No. 4)** may prove to be detrimental. Even if she does not decide to overdose, medication without psychological support is generally ineffective. **IMP,7,PsI**

35. **(4)** Thyroglobulin (Proloid) is a purified extract of pig thyroid and is utilized in the treatment of *hypothyroidism*. **Nos. 1, 2, and 3** *are* current methods for treating Graves' disease, or hyperthyroidism. **IMP,3,SECE**

36. **(4)** At 12 weeks' gestation, fundus should be palpable at the pubic symphysis. **No. 1** is wrong because of inability to palpate due to current uterine size and position. **No. 2** is wrong because weight-gain patterns provide no information regarding uterine or fetal growth. **No. 3** is wrong because maternal vital signs are not diagnostic of gestational age or uterine growth, and fetal heart tones may be heard with a Doppler as early as 9–10 weeks. **AS,5,SECE**

37. **(1)** Acting out is the expression through behavior (rather than through words) of emotions that occur when the client relives or reproduces the feelings, wishes, or conflicts that are operating unconsciously. He may be feeling frustrated, angry, ambivalent, etc., for numerous reasons, such as conflict between himself and his parents, a reaction to parents' marital conflicts, sibling rivalry, or frustration due to poor self-esteem. By definition, **Nos. 2, 3, and 4** are incorrect. **AS,7,PsI**

38. **(1)** A wheeze is a high-pitched, musical chest sound produced by airflow in narrowed bronchioles. It is primarily an expiratory sound and is always, *not* rarely **(No. 2)**, considered pathologic. *Rhonchi* are medium-pitched sonorous sounds **(No. 3)** produced by airflow obstruction in larger airways. *Stridor* is a high-pitched crowing sound **(No. 4)** on inspiration and is due to an upper-airway obstruction, such as edema, adhesions, or tracheal hypertrophy. **IMP,6,PhI**

39. **(1)** Lithium is used to treat affective disorders. Thioridazine (Mellaril) **(No. 4)** is a major tranquilizer used to treat schizophrenia. Thioridazine has been used to treat the manic phase of bipolar affective disorders, but it is not the primary drug. Chlordiazepoxide HCl (Librium) **(No. 2)** is a minor tranquilizer used to relieve the mild or moderate anxiety usually associated with affective and somatoform disorders. Fluphenazine HCl (Prolixin) **(No. 3)** is a long-acting psychotropic

used primarily to treat schizophrenia. It can be administered biweekly in an injection for a long-term effect. **IMP,7,PsI**

40. **(1)** The *primary* purpose of passive range-of-motion exercises is to prevent contractures and decreased range of motion. *Secondarily,* passive range-of-motion exercises assist the nurse in evaluating functional abilities **(No. 2)**, pain tolerance **(No. 3)**, and the effectiveness of drug therapy **(No. 4)**. **IMP,3,SECE**

41. **(2)** By calculation of EDB using Nägele's rule of counting back 3 months and adding 7 days to the date of LMP: 4th month − 3 months = 1st month (January); third day plus 7 days = tenth day; January 10 is her EDB. **No. 1** is wrong because of failure to add 7 days to LMP. **No. 3** is wrong because 7 days were subtracted from date of LMP. **No. 4** is wrong because of counting back 4 months instead of 3. **AN,5,HPM**

42. **(2)** An increase in the client's energy level may provide enough motivation to make another suicide attempt. Generally, depressed clients do not kill themselves because their energy level is very low. Therefore the one-to-one relationship needs to be maintained and stressed at this time. **Nos. 1, 3, and 4** are dangerous assumptions at this time. **EV,7,PsI**

43. **(2)** The patient needs an opportunity to receive word images. Point to the object and clearly enunciate its name, e.g., "spoon." Also, the expressive aphasia patient needs the chance to practice repeating words. Begin with simple words, such as *yes* and *no,* and then progress to complete phrases. Recovery from aphasia depends on the area of the brain involved and the extent of damage. There may be spontaneous recovery or improvement with speech therapy 2 years after the stroke. To consider the impairment permanent **(No. 1)** would be premature. **No. 3** is incorrect because waiting may increase the patient's frustration. Try to anticipate the patient's needs to reduce feelings of helplessness. The nurse plays an important part in showing the family members how to communicate and in not discouraging communication **(No. 4)**. **IMP,2,HPM**

44. **(4)** A preschooler would probably respond best to the use of puppets to dramatize the procedure. Any description of the procedure alone **(No. 1)**, no matter how simple, would probably not be enough to enable most preschoolers to understand what will happen to them. Taking a patient to the operating room or the catheterization lab **(No. 2)** would probably be unnecessarily frightening for any patient, especially a child. The child may not ask any questions himself or herself **(No. 3)**; and if the child does not, then the nurse would be unable to do any teaching. **IMP,5,PsI**

45. **(1)** The nurse needs to address the amount of energy and stamina needed to meet the demands of parenting. Older women have commented that the lack of energy and stamina came as a surprise. **No. 2** is incorrect because older women tend to be less troubled by pregnancy and remain better adjusted during the last trimester. Older mothers, as a group, do not have longer labor **(No. 3)**, nor with good prenatal care, do they show a greater number of labor/birth complications **(No. 4)**. **PL,5,HPM**

46. **(2)** Appliance should be changed every 2–3 days or as soon as there is leakage. Drainage can excoriate the skin; therefore, a new appliance needs to be applied as soon as leakage appears. **No. 1** is wrong because every day is too often; there will be damage to the skin from pulling the appliance off so often. **No. 3** is wrong because 1 week is too long for the skin to go without be-

ing examined and cleansed. **No. 4** is incorrect; the visiting nurse does not determine when the appliance should be changed. **PL,8,SECE**

47. **(4)** Early decelerations represent the normal fetal response to contractions. **No. 1** is wrong because this action would be taken to relieve possible cord compression. **No. 2** is wrong because use of the Trendelenburg position is not necessary. **No. 3** is an inaccurate interpretation of the assessment data. **IMP,5,SECE**

48. **(2)** Neomycin sulfate is used preoperatively because it is poorly absorbed in the intestinal tract and acts to decrease the bacteria count in the colon. As the result of this action, postoperative infection is reduced **(No. 1)**. Neomycin does not reduce tumor size **(No. 3)** or directly affect peristalsis **(No. 4)**. **EV,8,PhI**

49. **(3)** The first priority with any unconscious client is to maintain a patent airway. The nurse would need a physician's order to administer any medication or stimulant **(No. 1)**, which may not be appropriate in this situation. The emergency room nurse would see that the attending resident was paged **(No. 2)**, but this task could be delegated while the nurse administered primary care. Monitoring neurologic signs **(No. 4)** is also essential but can be done after ensuring that the client can breathe. **IMP,6,PhI**

50. **(1)** Treatment with bronchodilators such as isoproterenol will decrease bronchoconstriction, *improving* the movement of air in and out of the lungs. **Nos. 2, 3, and 4** are incorrect because these pulmonary function studies indicate that the patient has been able to increase inspiratory capacity by 1000 mL (VC 2800–3800) and expiratory capacity (RV decreased, FRC decreased, and FEV_1 increased). **EV,6,PhI**

51. **(3)** Painful, red, papular lesions associated with foul-smelling vaginal discharge are characteristic of herpesvirus type 2 infection. **No. 1** is wrong because discrete lesions do not accompany trichomonal infections; discharge usually is thin, frothy, and gray or yellow-green and usually has a foul odor (like rotting fish). **No. 2** is wrong because monilial vaginal infections produce a characteristic white, cheesy discharge. **No. 4** is wrong because gonorrhea in women is often totally asymptomatic or may produce a purulent vaginal discharge. **AS,1,PhI**

52. **(2)** Confrontation *could* help the 15-year-old client identify the inappropriateness of mutilation and other destructive behaviors as attention-getting devices. **Nos. 1, 3, and 4** *are* all *appropriate* interventions. **PL,7,PsI**

53. **(2)** Human chorionic gonadotropin (HCG) is the biologic marker used in pregnancy tests. This hormone is produced by the fertilized ovum and the chorionic villi, and maintains the corpus luteum's production of estrogen and progesterone for the first 8–10 weeks of pregnancy. The hormone reaches maximum level at 50–70 days. **No. 1** is incorrect because human placental lactogen is produced by the *placenta.* Luteinizing hormone **(No. 3)** is the primary anterior pituitary hormone during the *second "half"* of the *menstrual cycle.* Alpha-fetoprotein **(No. 4)** is a biologic marker for assessing for open neural tube *defects* in the *fetus.* **IMP,5,HPM**

54. **(2)** Touch, facial expression, and tone of voice may be used effectively to reduce anxiety, apprehensions, and fear in situations where verbal communication is inhibited by language barriers. **No. 1** is wrong because the continual use of an intermediary (her husband) may impede establishing the rapport necessary for a successful labor experience. **No. 3** is wrong because incom-

prehensible words become no more understandable if spoken slowly or distinctly; loud voices are disconcerting during labor. **No. 4** is inappropriate because the *nurse,* not the MD, is there to provide ongoing care and allay anxiety. **PL,7,PsI**

55. **(3)** Although there *are* several specific forms that elicit disclosure of this information, there is no law that mandates disclosure **(No. 4)**. The client has to make this decision independently. The nurse should provide therapeutic support for whatever he decides. **Nos. 1 and 2** are untrue statements. **IMP,7,PsI**

56. **(3)** An iridectomy is performed in the upper segment of the iris and is covered by the upper eyelid, as normally. The excision in the iris is occluded, which decreases discomfort. Infection is less likely since bacteria are carried in the tears, by gravity, to the lower cul-de-sac. The need for a dressing is usually indicated, to decrease infection or eye movement. Since infection is *not* likely and mobilization of the eye **(No. 1)** *is* desirable to prevent posterior synechiae (adhesion of iris to cornea or lens), no dressing is needed. **Nos. 2 and 4** *are* appropriate actions. Massage of the eye, if ordered, encourages continuous flow of fluids through the surgical opening. **IMP,2,SECE**

57. **(3)** Increased dietary bulk and adequate fluids relieve symptoms of constipation naturally, by stimulating peristalsis. **No. 1** is wrong because regular use of laxatives reduces normal bowel functions; mineral oil contributes to loss of fat-soluble vitamins A, D, and E. **No. 2** is wrong because *adequate* fluid intake is needed to avoid dry, packed stools associated with constipation. **No. 4** is wrong because Kegel exercises increase sphincter control and do *not* encourage defecation. **PL,8,HPM**

58. **(4)** Adolescents who have had an appendectomy are expected to make a complete, rapid recovery; they should have *minimal* to moderate pain during the first 24 hours **(No. 1)**. Discharge time frame varies, not necessarily within 48 hours, or after a *slow* recovery **(Nos. 2 and 3)**. **EV,8,PhI**

59. **(3)** Hostility and aggression are considered the underlying factors in the psychogenesis and psychodynamics of depression. The adolescent is in a stage of development where he or she experiences extensive anger due to frustration. The adolescent has a greater energy level because of the increased libidinal energy available in his or her system. To expend this energy, many adolescents act out their feelings of depression in violent ways rather than become withdrawn, apathetic, or regressive **(Nos. 1, 2, and 4)**. **AS,7,PsI**

60. **(3)** PID is more common in women who have multiple sex partners. **No. 1** is incorrect because there is an increased incidence of *infection (not* PID) in women during the first month after insertion of an IUD. Gonorrhea **(No. 2)** can cause PID *whether* it is acquired through skin-to-skin contact *or* from a fomite (a fomite is a nonliving material on which disease-producing organisms can be conveyed, e.g., bed linens or washcloths). **No. 4** is incorrect because a pattern of *heavy* alcohol consumption is associated with certain nutritional deficiencies (e.g., vitamin B complex) that decrease a person's immune responsiveness to vaccines and depress the cell-mediated and humoral lymphocytic activity. **AN,1,HPM**

61. **(3)** Deep breathing, coughing, and pursed-lip exhalations are all techniques that the nurse can teach the patient to improve ventilation. *Adequate* fluid intake **(No. 1)** is essential for keeping sputum liquefied; however, very hot and very cold drinks should be avoided since they may cause bronchospasm. Patients with COPD also need to be taught to avoid exposure to infections, early signs of infection, and the need to seek medical intervention promptly should symptoms occur. **Nos. 2 and 4** are not indicated in this patient's therapy. **IMP,6,PhI**

62. **(1)** Erythema toxicum is the normal, nonpathologic macular newborn rash. **No. 2** is wrong because milia are small white nodules due to clogged sebaceous glands. **No. 3** is wrong because *icterus neonatorum* is the term for normal physiologic jaundice of the newborn, which occurs 48–72 hours after birth. **No. 4** is wrong because hemangiomas are small elevated clusters of capillaries ("stork bites"). **IMP,5,HPM**

63. **(2)** Patients should not be encouraged to do exercises to the point of unusual pain, and pain should not last longer than one-half hour after exercise. If pain lasts longer than this, the exercises are too strenuous. **No. 1** is incorrect because pulse and respiratory rates are affected not only by physical stress but by emotional or psychological stress as well. **Nos. 3 and 4** indicate that therapy has been effective. **EV,3,PhI**

64. **(3)** The client should be placed under one-to-one, not group, observation to ensure effective protection against suicidal behaviors. **Nos. 1, 2, and 4** are all appropriate actions. **IMP,7,PsI**

65. **(1)** In positioning the child during recovery, the nurse should avoid those positions where contractures and flexion deformities may occur. With burns on the neck, the nurse should keep the neck extended and help the child avoid flexing the neck **(No. 4)**. Keeping the child still **(No. 2)** will predispose him or her to complications of immobility. There is no reason why the child cannot sit in a chair (with help as needed) during recovery **(No. 3)**. **IMP,3,SECE**

66. **(2)** The woman is demonstrating signs of beginning transition. Sacral pressure and backrubs assist in reducing her discomfort at this time. **No. 1** is wrong because assessment indicates irritability, not pain. Further, she has expressed a desire to use Lamaze for labor and birth. **No. 3** is wrong because it is important to maintain continual assessment of fetal status during the transitional stage. **No. 4** is wrong because the woman should be attended continually during transition. **IMP,3,SECE**

67. **(2)** To read blood gases, first note the pH. In this case, pH is 7.38, which is within the normal range (7.35–7.45) but is on the acidotic side. Next, look at the PCO_2 and HCO_3 to see which one is causing the shift to acidosis. In this case the PCO_2 is 55 (acidosis) and the HCO_3 is 32 (alkalosis). Therefore, the patient has compensated respiratory acidosis because the kidneys have been able to conserve enough bicarbonate to keep pH within normal range. In this case a pH below 7.35 would indicate uncompensated respiratory acidosis **(No. 1)**. If the patient had uncompensated metabolic alkalosis **(No. 3)**, then pH would be above 7.45. If the patient had compensated metabolic alkalosis **(No. 4)**, pH would be between 7.41 and 7.45. **AN,6,PhI**

68. **(2)** Although the adolescent's parents may perceive this as a parental decision, it is important for the entire family to be included in the decision-making process because the entire family system will be affected by this change. Asking the parents to reassess their feelings **(No. 1)** may help them evaluate the situation, but it avoids facing the issue as a family decision. A referral may be appropriate **(Nos. 3 and 4)**; however, all

parties involved in the decision must be listened to before making a referral or searching for an alternative placement. **IMP,7,PsI**

69. **(2)** In rheumatoid arthritis both the erythrocyte sedimentation rate and C-reactive protein levels are increased. Anemia is common, so hemoglobin and hematocrit are usually decreased, not increased (**No. 1**). The Wasserman test result (**No. 3**) is normally negative. The platelet count (**No. 4**) is not affected either. **AN,1,SECE**

70. **(4)** During pregnancy, attention is focused on the expectant parents; feelings of competition for attention with the baby arise during the *postpartum* period. **No. 1** is wrong because pressures of present and anticipated expenses associated with childbearing *do* impose stress on the family. **No. 2** is wrong because both expectant parents *must adjust* to changing relationships between themselves and their extended families. **No. 3** is wrong because both parents may *experience* stress on recognizing the need to be totally responsible for the health and development of a baby and the concomitant need to change their life-styles to meet those obligations. **AN,7,PsI**

71. **(2)** Although it is not possible to make a patient stop smoking, the patient should be presented with information about methods used by other people who were successful in stopping. Although most people are aware of the deleterious effects of smoking, patients need to be reminded of the relationship between smoking and their present condition. Fluid intake and nutrition need to be discussed and adapted to individual needs. Patients should be able to identify drugs, giving the name, correct dosage, timing, and potential side effects. Alcohol in moderation is not restricted (**No. 1**). Vocational rehabilitation should be present as an option but not emphasized (**No. 3**). Activities should be encouraged to tolerance (**No. 4**). **IMP,6,SECE**

72. **(4)** The passage of time will *not* help him cope effectively with his feelings of fear and ambivalence. These feelings are a normal part of the maturation process, and *only* with effective limit setting and psychological support will the adolescent's ability to cope be strengthened. In early adolescence boys generally are intolerant of female authority figures (**No. 1**). They perceive these females as a threat to their emerging masculine identity. Adolescents need physical activity to alleviate tension (**No. 2**). Males in general have problems dealing with impulse control (**No. 3**) and need consistent limits set on their behaviors. **AN,7,PsI**

73. **(2)** Pushing before complete dilatation may result in edema of the cervix and increase the resistance to be overcome by the oncoming head. **No. 1** is wrong because panting is recommended to reduce the urge and ability to push. **No. 3** is wrong because hyperventilating has no effect on cervical dilatation. **No. 4** is wrong because the open fontanels and flexibility of the sutures of the fetal head reduce pressure imposed by the force of uterine contractions. **PL,6,SECE**

74. **(1)** This woman's behavior typifies patterns expressed during the second trimester. **No. 2** is wrong because her symptoms are related both to fluctuating hormone levels and to psychological reevaluation of self and marriage. **Nos. 3 and 4** are wrong because of the *physiologic* component of her symptoms. **AN,7,PsI**

75. **(2)** Hitting others provides the adolescent with an outlet for feelings of hopelessness and despair. Although this behavior may not make a person feel happy or satisfied, it does provide a defense against feeling unhappy. **Nos. 1, 3, and 4** are not primary motivations of this behavior. **AN,7,PsI**

76. **(2)** Position the conscious patient sitting upright in a supported, forward-leaning position (high Fowler's, orthopneic) to improve ventilation and oxygenation. A calm and reassuring approach will decrease hyperactivity of the patient and oxygen need. Acute respiratory failure is a medical emergency. Aminophylline (**No. 1**) is indicated to combat bronchospasm, but it is *not an independent nursing* action. Low-flow oxygen (2 L) is also administered to the patient in respiratory failure; however, nasal cannulas (**No. 3**) do not provide predictable O_2 concentrations. A Venturi mask would be more appropriate. **No. 4** is incorrect because the higher concentration of O_2 (60%) may lead to respiratory depression unless the patient is maintained on controlled mechanical ventilation. **AN,6,PhI**

77. **(3)** Dry soda crackers will absorb gastric juices and increase blood sugar, thereby reducing nausea. **No. 1** is wrong because eating before retiring has no effect on morning nausea. **No. 2** is wrong because drinking fruit juice on an empty stomach may increase nausea. **No. 4** is wrong because demands of physical activity may increase nausea. **IMP,4,HPM**

78. **(1)** The best topical cleansing material to use in debriding burns are sterile 4×4 gauze pads. Cotton balls (**No. 2**) may pull and stick to burned tissue. Washcloths (**No. 3**) are too harsh and may damage new healing tissue. Telfa pads (**No. 4**) are too smooth and will not cleanse the area as well as gauze pads. **IMP,7,SECE**

79. **(1)** Individuals who have used alcohol habitually over an extended time period usually exhibit symptoms of withdrawal delirium when the alcohol intake is severely decreased or curtailed. **Nos. 2, 3, and 4** are less likely reactions. **AS,7,PsI**

80. **(4)** Indications of respiratory distress and the increased work of breathing in this patient are characterized by the use of the accessory muscles of respiration, the sternocleidomastoid and trapezius muscles. Using these muscles enables the patient to *increase the size* of the thorax, thus allowing air to move in. Patients with chronic bronchitis and air trapping generally are not able to increase the depth of breathing (**No. 1**) by increasing diaphragmatic excursion (**No. 2**). Some patients may be using pursed-lip exhalations (**No. 3**), but these help maintain open airways for the expulsion of gases. **AS,6,PhI**

81. **(2)** "Charley horse" pain (cramp in gastrocnemius muscle) is due to sudden spasm and acute flexion of leg muscles; it is relieved by dorsiflexing the foot, which reduces the muscle spasm. **No. 1** is wrong because such action will not eliminate the possibility of muscle spasm during pregnancy. **No. 3** is wrong because the actions of vitamin C do not affect muscle spasms. **No. 4** is wrong because exercise does not prevent muscle spasm. **PL,3,HPM**

82. **(3)** Although the patient expresses a willingness to learn, apprehension will limit the ability to assimilate much. The patient must be taught specific arm and leg exercises, including frequent repositioning onto the abdomen to prevent contracture. Prior to discharge, alternate vocational pursuits (**No. 1**) may be discussed, as indicated. In the *postoperative* period the focus changes to crutch walking (**No. 2**). Encouraging the patient to verbalize fears and concerns (**No. 4**) is not a specific teaching strategy but rather an intervention designed

to give support as well as identify potential problems. **PL,1,HPM**

83. (3) His thoughts, feelings, and attitudes toward sexual relationships need to be explored to assess his level of maturity in deciding his sexual preference. *Confrontation,* rather than avoidance of confrontation (No. 1), could help him identify his use of homosexual behavior as an attention-seeking device. Validation of his rationale for seeking homosexual relationships (No. 2) may be identified more appropriately through exploring his thoughts, feelings, and attitudes regarding his sexual orientation. Enforcing limits on his relationships (No. 4) will only make him angry and is in any case an invasion of his right to privacy and freedom of choice. As long as neither client is forcing himself on the other, their relationship should not be interfered with. However, if it is determined that for some appropriate reason this relationship is detrimental to either individual's optimal level of functioning, then limits should be set. **PL,7,PsI**

84. (3) A male adolescent will most likely prefer the companionship of another boy close to his age. Although he may be interested in girls (No. 4), being introduced to them would not necessarily prove helpful for him. Adolescents cannot be relied on to place materials into hospital charts (No. 1). Because his recovery is expected to be quite rapid and complete, he will miss little school, and there is no need to get him involved with in-hospital tutoring (No. 2); he can easily catch up with his schoolwork when he gets home. **IMP,5,PsI**

85. (1) Abstinence will eliminate any unnecessary pain during intercourse and will reduce the possibility of transmitting infection to one's sexual partner. No. 2 is wrong because the current drug of choice is acyclovir (Zovirax). No. 3 is wrong because currently available therapy is only palliative; the virus remains in the body after symptoms subside. No. 4 is wrong because hydatidiform mole has a genetic basis. **IMP,1,HPM**

86. (3) A double-barrel colostomy has two stomas that may or may not be separated by skin. The proximal loop discharges feces, and the distal loop discharges mucus. The closure of this temporary colostomy usually occurs in approximately 6 months. No. 1 is an example of an ascending colostomy, No. 2 describes a transverse loop colostomy, and No. 4 describes a descending colostomy. **PL,8,PhI**

87. (1) Lithium is excreted through the kidneys. Consequently, the kidneys must function adequately to avoid lithium toxicity. Diuretics should *not* be given concurrently with lithium because they may potentiate sodium and fluid depletion, which may lead to lithium toxicity. Haloperidol (Haldol) (No. 4) is a major tranquilizer that is sometimes administered simultaneously with lithium during the first week to 10 days to control manic symptoms. Nausea, vomiting, and muscle weakness (No. 3) are all possible side effects of lithium. They indicate a need for close observation and regulation of the drug if they disrupt the person's level of functioning. Every client should be screened prior to the administration of any medication (No. 2). However, since lithium is a drug that is taken over a long period of time, blood levels must be consistently regulated and physical examinations routinely scheduled (i.e., every 3 months initially, then every 6 months once the client appears to be regulated). **EV,7,PsI**

88. (3) Sudden spasm and extreme flexion of the calf muscles are relieved by forcibly extending the muscle by hyperextension of the knee and dorsiflexion of the foot.

No. 1 is wrong because her complaint is due to muscle spasm. No. 2 is wrong because relief is accomplished by stretching the muscle; the pain is not due to lowered levels of oxygen in the muscle. No. 4 is wrong because increasing placental perfusion will be ineffective in relieving the muscle spasm. **IMP,3,PhI**

89. (4) To help the child cope with body-image changes associated with her burns, the nurse should work with her parents to help her with her physical appearance. Colorful scarves and hats will cover her hairless scalp and pressure stockinette, making her look more like other school-age children. It may also boost her morale. Stuffed animals (No. 1) may harbor bacteria and be a possible source of infection. Her friends (No. 2) will probably not be allowed to visit in the hospital, especially in the burn unit, which is a frightening place for most children. They can call her or send cards and pictures instead; they can visit her when she returns home. Favorite foods (No. 3) won't specifically help the child cope with her injuries and treatment; thus, this is not a good choice. **IMP,5,PsI**

90. (1) Adolescents are preoccupied with their changing bodies, their relationships, and their fantasies. Although they have difficulty with rote learning (No. 2), they have an increased potential for imaginative thinking. During this period they are less able to concentrate on their academic work (No. 3), which leads to increased feelings of frustration that are usually *not* accompanied by an increased ability to cope (No. 4). **EV,7,HPM**

91. (3) Assisting the mother to develop basic skills in infant care under comfortable professional supervision is the most effective way of increasing a woman's confidence and competence in caring for her infant. No. 1 is wrong because although the booklet is a helpful adjunct to teaching, skills are most effectively gained by actual experience. *Note:* Always sensitively assess her ability to read. No. 2 is wrong because clear, meaningful communication is inhibited by the language barrier, and actual experience in providing care will be of most assistance to her. No. 4 is wrong because basic infant care techniques should be mastered before the mother leaves the hospital with her newborn. **PL,7,HPM**

92. (3) Putting a pinhole in the appliance is the least effective method because it allows flatus to escape immediately and the patient has no control. No. 1 is incorrect because foods that cause increased flatus, such as cabbage and broccoli, *should* be avoided. No. 2 is incorrect because any deodorant that is safe for mucous membranes *can* be utilized, or the patient can purchase appliances that have an odor barrier. No. 4 is incorrect because emptying the appliance *does* protect the seal since extra weight from a full pouch will pull at a seal; once the seal is broken, odor can escape. **PL,8,PhI**

93. (3) Pushing on an incompletely dilated cervix may contribute to development of cervical edema and/or lacerations. No. 1 is wrong because an engaged head occludes the cervix. Neither panting nor normal breathing increases oxygen level (No. 2). No. 4 is wrong because breathing patterns do *not* affect cervical dilatation. **AN,5,HPM**

94. (1) The observed total lung capacity (TLC), functional residual capacity (FRC), and residual volume (RV) are all increased over expected values. These values indicate that the patient is hyperinflated, a common phenomenon with air obstruction and air trapping. Hyperventilation is characterized by an increase in P_{O_2} and

pH (**No. 2**). Hyperpnea is simply an increase in respiratory rate (**No. 3**). Hypercapnia is identified when P_{CO_2} is elevated (**No. 4**). **AN,6,SECE**

95. (**1**) Lice are spread by direct or indirect contact; the child should sleep alone to prevent other family members from also getting lice. In addition, the family should be taught to wash the linens in hot soapy water to kill any lice that are on them. Having the family all get short haircuts (**No. 2**), or use a fine-toothed comb (**No. 4**), or having the child wear a hair net (**No. 3**) would not necessarily prevent the other family members from getting lice. **IMP,1,HPM**

96. (**2**) The 18-year-old may have valid reasons for wanting to visit his friend, but allowing him to visit without assessing his motives (**No. 1**) may prove detrimental to him, to his friend, and to the staff. His parents (**No. 3**) essentially relinquished their decision-making authority by allowing him to live in the group home. The hospital staff would have to be consulted prior to his visit, regardless of his motive. However, **No. 4** is too vague, in that it does not specify what issues would be covered in the consultation. **IMP,7,PsI**

97. (**1**) Understanding the reasons for disconcerting symptoms, and receiving assurance of their normalcy, assist in coping. **No. 2** is wrong because although diet may improve the general sense of well-being, diet will *not affect feelings* generated by the developmental tasks of pregnancy. **No. 3** is wrong because the woman is demonstrating *normal* behavioral changes associated with the first trimester of pregnancy. **No. 4** is wrong because it does not address the problem. **PL,7,PsI**

98. (**2**) Indications of mediastinal shift and tension pneumothorax include cyanosis, severe dyspnea, and deviation of the trachea and larynx from the normal midline position toward the side of the chest *opposite* the pneumothorax (the unaffected side). Because no blood is available for cardiac output, the blood pressure is absent, not elevated (**No. 1**). **No. 3** is incorrect because the lung has collapsed on the affected side, resulting in tympany on percussion, reduced or absent breath sounds, and *hyperresonance*. With a right tension pneumothorax, the heart will shift *laterally* from the normal midclavicular line. If the *left* lung were involved, the heart would shift medially (**No. 4**). **AS,6,PhI**

99. (**4**) It is important for the angry client to express his feelings overtly. Internalizing them would cause increased feelings of frustration and anxiety and would therefore be counterproductive. **Nos. 1, 2, and 3** *are* all appropriate goals. **PL,7,PsI**

100. (**1**) A hot tub bath or shower in the morning helps many patients limber up and reduces the symptoms of early morning stiffness. Cold and ice packs are used to a lesser degree, though some patients state that cold decreases localized pain, particularly during acute attacks. Passive ROM exercises (**No. 2**) may be helpful, but this is not the response of choice. Sleeping with a hot pad (**No. 3**) may cause localized injury. Some patients, however, have found electric blankets helpful in reducing early morning stiffness. Taking salicylates on an empty stomach (**No. 4**) may increase gastric irritation and distress. **IMP,3,SECE**

Practice Test

What Is the Test?

The **Final Test** is a multiple-choice exam designed to assess your baseline nursing knowledge and evaluate your ability to apply that knowledge to various clinical situations and to items presented in a simulated NCLEX-RN exam. Self-analysis of your scores will help you prioritize what to study by identifying your individual problem areas.

Written to reflect the content framework and the purpose of the NCLEX-RN Test Plan, ". . . to measure a candidate's ability to practice safely and effectively as a Registered Nurse in an entry-level position," the **Final Test** can be used as preparation and review for the licensure examination. It can also be used for review by *nurses returning to active practice* as well as by *graduates of foreign nursing schools* who are preparing for qualifying examinations.

Each question on the **Final Test** was field tested in a pilot test given to NCLEX-RN candidates representing a wide geographic distribution as well as various types of nursing programs.

Selection of Content and Distribution of the Questions

The **Final Test** is composed of 200 content-integrated, multiple-choice questions, each with four options. *One* of the answers is most complete and therefore the best choice. The other three answers (distractors) are not always wrong but are usually not as complete or as important as the best answer.

Using a nursing process framework, the questions on the **Final Test** reflect nursing situations that involve different clinical areas and diagnoses. As on the NCLEX-RN, the number of questions for each content area varies. The percentage distribution of items in this test related to client needs follows the NCLEX-RN blueprint (see Unit 1, Orientation, for percentages).

Based on the blueprint for the *Test Plan for The National Council Licensure Examination* (NCLEX-RN)

published by the National Council of State Boards of Nursing, Inc., the **Final Test** assesses your knowledge, skills, and abilities in the five phases of the *nursing process:* Assessment (AS), Analysis (AN), Plan (PL), Implementation (IMP), Evaluation (EV), and four areas of *client needs:* Safe, Effective Care Environment (SECE), Physiologic Integrity (PhI), Psychosocial Integrity (PsI), and Health Promotion and Maintenance (HPM). Each question in the **Final Test** has also been classified according to the categories of human functions listed in Appendix G.

Timing

Allow about 1 minute per question. Time yourself and plan to complete the 200-question test in no more than 3½ hours. Simulate test-taking conditions by having uninterrupted time of 3½ hours, or divide the exam into two sessions of 100 questions for 1 hour and 45 minutes for each session.

Test Results

When you check your answers, keep track not only of how many are incorrect, but also how many are incorrect in *each category* of nursing process, client needs, and human functions.

Suggestions for Further Study

You can use your test results, in combination with the appendices, to assess your NCLEX-RN strengths and weaknesses.

I.	When you have problems with *types* of questions	Refer to Appendix:
	A. Nursing process	
	1. Definitions/Descriptions	B
	2. Index to nursing process *questions*	C

II.	When you have problems with *content*/subject areas	Refer to Appendix:

A. Client needs

1. Definitions/Descriptions .... D
2. Index to *content* .... E
3. Index to *practice questions that cover these content areas* .... F

B. Human functions

1. Definitions/Descriptions .... G
2. Index to *content* .... H
3. Index to *practice questions that cover these content areas* I

You now have an individualized evaluation with which to develop your plan for *what* you need to study and *where* to find the material for further study. Our good wishes for your success!

❑ Questions

Select the one best answer for each question.

1. Which statement by the nurse would correctly characterize essential hypertension?
   1. Forty percent of the American adult population is affected by hypertension.
   2. Essential hypertension is more severe in men than women.
   3. American blacks develop hypertension at an earlier age than whites but have a lower mortality rate.
   4. Given newer screening devices, most hypertensive persons are now being detected.

2. In assessing a woman's reasons for suspecting she may be 3 months' pregnant, the most relevant question for the nurse to ask would be:
   1. "Are you currently taking oral contraceptives?"
   2. "When was your last menstrual period?"
   3. "How much weight have you gained?"
   4. "Have you been pregnant before?"

3. When caring for a child who has experienced severe burn(s) of the oral cavity and possibly of the esophagus, pharynx, and larynx, the primary nursing intervention should be:
   1. Observe for symptoms of shock.
   2. Check airway for signs of obstruction.
   3. Maintain adequate hydration by offering small amounts of clear liquid.
   4. Initiate intravenous therapy immediately.

4. A patient with a history of substance abuse is admitted to the hospital; he was brought there by police when he was found on school property running around in the nude with several other students. He appeared to be hallucinating. The nurse who admits this patient to the unit should be primarily concerned with:
   1. Providing a general orientation to the unit.
   2. Maintaining a quiet environment.
   3. Taking precautions against seizures.
   4. Taking vital signs every 4 hours.

5. A patient with a history of severe abdominal cramping and vomiting a moderate amount of blood arrives at the emergency room. The nurse's *primary* concern should be:
   1. Observing for signs and symptoms of shock.
   2. Immediately paging the physician on call.
   3. Filling out the appropriate assessment tool.
   4. Immediately administering CPR.

6. The nurse considers information regarding smoking cigarettes and marijuana essential for pregnant women because it is well established that these activities may lead to:
   1. Retarded infants.
   2. Low-birthweight infants.
   3. Deformed infants.
   4. Malnourished infants.

7. The nurse finds a post-MI patient slumped on the siderails of his bed. He does not respond when the nurse shakes his shoulders or loudly calls his name. The nurse's next action is to:
   1. Call for help and note the time.
   2. Clear the airway.
   3. Give two sharp thumps to precordium.
   4. Administer two quick breaths.

8. Postop orders include "IV of D5 ¼ NS at 75 mL per hour." At 7:00 P.M., a new 1000-mL bag of fluid is hung. If the IV infuses at the prescribed rate, how much fluid should be left in the bag at 7:00 A.M.?
   1. 100 mL.
   2. 900 mL.
   3. Nothing should be left; bag should be empty.
   4. Not enough information given to determine this.

9. As a cardiac patient gets up to use the commode, he turns ashen and diaphoretic. Vital signs are as follows: BP 128/60, pulse 42, respirations 24. ECG shows patterns of complete heart block. The nurse knows that the patient's signs and symptoms are related to:
   1. Inability of heart to increase its rate during exertion.
   2. Insufficient blood flow to the coronary arteries.
   3. Increased stroke volume.
   4. Inability of the circulatory reflexes to increase venous return.

10. A woman is in labor; she and the father learn that the fetus is in the transverse position. The father tells the nurse that they had counted on his being with her throughout their baby's birth. The nurse's most therapeutic response would be to:
    1. Refer him to the attending physician for permission to attend the birth.
    2. Assess whether he has attended childbirth education classes.
    3. Check with the attending physician and relay the response to the couple.
    4. Tell the father to dress and meet the nurse in the cesarean room.

11. Parents of an infant on an apnea monitor ask the nurse what the monitor will do. The nurse's most appropriate response would be:
    1. "It will stimulate your baby's breathing."
    2. "It will monitor your baby's vital signs."
    3. "It will sound an alarm if your baby's breathing stops."
    4. "It will maintain your baby's respirations."

12. Preoperative teaching includes deep breathing and coughing. What is the *least* desired outcome of the teaching plan? The patient:
    1. States the rationale for repeating these exercises every 1–2 hours postoperatively.
    2. Demonstrates coughing technique.
    3. Inhales through both nose and mouth and raises abdomen with each respiration.
    4. States she recognizes the need to repeat exercises until she is feeling light-headed.

13. A patient's blood gases are as follows: P_{O_2} 85, P_{CO_2} 37, pH 7.35, HCO_3 19. The nurse's analysis of this patient's blood gases indicate:

1. Compensated metabolic acidosis.
2. Hyperventilation.
3. Uncompensated metabolic acidosis.
4. Alveolar hypoventilation.

14. In doing a child's admission assessment, the nurse should be alert to note which signs/symptoms of chronic lead poisoning?
    1. Irritability and seizures.
    2. Dehydration and diarrhea.
    3. Bradycardia and hypotension.
    4. Petechiae and hematuria.

15. A woman is hospitalized with mild preeclampsia. In planning the woman's care during this hospitalization, which nursing order is *least* likely to be implemented?
    1. Vital signs and FHR and rhythm q4h while awake.
    2. Daily weight.
    3. Deep-tendon reflexes once per shift.
    4. Absolute bedrest.

16. The nurse prepares a patient for tracheostomy based on the knowledge that the purpose of a tracheostomy is to:
    1. Decrease patient anxiety by increasing the size of the airway.
    2. Provide more controlled ventilation and ease removal of secretions the patient is unable to handle.
    3. Provide increased cerebral oxygenation, thereby preventing further respiratory depression.
    4. Facilitate nursing care, since tracheal tubes have fewer side effects than nasotracheal tubes.

17. A teenage boy with a history of substance abuse is hospitalized for hallucinatory behavior. His mother is very upset. She is in the waiting room crying uncontrollably. The most appropriate nursing action would be to:
    1. Provide privacy for her.
    2. Ask the physician to order diazepam (Valium) for her.
    3. Contact her husband.
    4. Offer to sit with her.

18. The pressure dressing placed after modified mastectomy encircles the patient's chest and fits very snugly. The nurse should anticipate difficulty in which postoperative nursing function?
    1. Maintaining good body alignment.
    2. Initiating arm exercises.
    3. Promoting deep breathing and coughing.
    4. Taking vital signs.

19. The nurse must be on the alert constantly for anaphylaxis, an immediate hypersensitivity reaction, characterized by local reactions such as:
    1. Angioedema.
    2. Cardiovascular collapse.
    3. Nausea, vomiting, diarrhea.
    4. Asthmalike symptoms.

20. If the first day of a pregnant woman's last menstrual period (LMP) was July 10, what is her baby's expected date of birth (EDB)?
    1. April 17.
    2. May 30.
    3. March 14.
    4. June 1.

21. At 7:00 A.M., the night nurse hangs a new 500-mL bag of D5 ½ NS and adjusts the flow rate to 35 mL/h per MD order. If the IV infuses at the proper rate, how much fluid should be left in the bag when the day nurse makes rounds at 11:30 A.M., halfway through the shift?
    1. 160 mL.
    2. 250 mL.

3. 340 mL.
4. Unable to determine.

22. An adolescent patient with a history of substance abuse asks the nurse, "Have you ever used drugs?" The most appropriate nursing response would be:
    1. "Yes, once I tried grass."
    2. "Why do you want to know?"
    3. "How will my answer help you?"
    4. "No, I don't think so."

23. A woman is in labor; her membranes are ruptured by the attending physician. The nurse should expect the amniotic fluid to:
    1. Be clear in color.
    2. Have a slightly pungent odor.
    3. Have a thick consistency.
    4. Turn litmus paper blue.

24. The nurse should know that the majority of amputations are attributed to:
    1. Chemical burns.
    2. Diabetic ulcers.
    3. Arteriosclerosis obliterans.
    4. Bone tumors.

25. A 15-year-old is admitted to the hospital with a compound fracture of the left tibia and patella following a minibike accident. The fractures are repaired surgically, and a long leg cast is applied. During the first night in the hospital, the patient complains of severe pain in the left leg. At this time, it would be most appropriate for the nurse to:
    1. Obtain more information about the characteristics of the pain.
    2. Give the patient a dose of "Demerol 50 mg IM prn q4–6h" as ordered.
    3. Reassure the patient that the pain will diminish in a few days.
    4. Distract the patient by turning on the television.

26. When caring for a child who has received a diazepam (Valium) "IV push" × 2 during a procedure, which vital sign should the nurse evaluate *first*?
    1. Temperature.
    2. Pulse.
    3. Respirations.
    4. Blood pressure.

27. Several weeks after the funeral of one of her twin infants, a mother tells the public health nurse that she is experiencing difficulty producing enough breast milk to satisfy the other infant. The most appropriate response for the nurse to make would be:
    1. "You probably have a virus and should see a doctor right away."
    2. "Your baby is probably reacting to the loss of a sibling and not sucking long enough to stimulate an adequate supply."
    3. "Milk production may decrease with an increase in stress."
    4. "The lactation ducts may be occluded."

28. When parents ask how their baby might have gotten pyloric stenosis, the nurse should tell them that:
    1. Their baby was born with this condition.
    2. Their baby acquired it due to a formula allergy.
    3. Their baby was normal at birth and it developed spontaneously.
    4. There is no way to determine this preoperatively.

29. Morphine sulfate, 0.6 mg, has been ordered to relieve the chest pain of a patient who has had an anterior MI. The nurse would give this narcotic to:
    1. Increase the threshold for pain tolerance and decrease arterial resistance.

2. Increase arterial resistance and reduce apprehension and anxiety as well as pain.
3. Relieve apprehension, anxiety, and pain and stimulate medullary respiratory centers.
4. Reduce venous capacitance and reduce pain threshold.

30. A pregnant woman with severe preeclampsia is at 38 weeks' gestation; she is in active labor, with contractions every 10 minutes, and her membranes ruptured 45 minutes ago. Her husband is with her. The nurse's primary intervention would be to:
1. Teach the couple about the stages of labor.
2. Prepare the woman for birth.
3. Assess the couple's degree of preparation.
4. Answer any questions the couple may have.

31. In preparing preop injections for a 3-year-old, which size needle would the nurse be most correct in selecting to administer the IM injection?
1. 25 G, ⅝ in.
2. 21 G, 1 in.
3. 18 G, 1 in.
4. 18 G, 1½ in.

32. The physician orders the insertion of a permanent pacemaker for a patient with complete heart block. In preparing a preoperative teaching plan for this patient, the nurse would initially:
1. Assess the patient's interest in learning about the procedure and current understanding.
2. Invite the patient's family to join the preoperative teaching session.
3. Ascertain from the physician the amount of information she or he has given the patient.
4. Have the operative permit signed, then institute the teaching plan.

33. Following administration of preoperative medication, it is important for the nurse to:
1. Position the patient in high Fowler's position to improve ventilation.
2. Let the patient know she will be asleep when she leaves the unit.
3. Tell the patient that a nurse will be there when she returns.
4. Get the patient up to the bathroom when she complains of bladder fullness.

34. In the first few hours after cardiac catheterization, which nursing measure would be most essential?
1. Checking pedal pulse in the extremity used for the cut-down.
2. Encouraging the patient to cough and deep breathe hourly.
3. Keeping the patient sedated to maintain the pressure dressing.
4. Monitoring the patient's urine output.

35. The nurse has established the unresponsiveness of a patient. After the airway is opened, the next nursing action would be to:
1. Look, listen, and feel for breathing.
2. Pinch the patient's nostrils and give two full breaths.
3. Check the patient's carotid pulse for 5–10 seconds.
4. Finger sweep the patient's mouth for any foreign object.

36. While the nurse is changing a CVP dressing, the patient becomes tachypneic and complains of chest pain. The nurse suspects the symptoms are related to an air embolism. The first nursing priority would be to position the patient:
1. In Trendelenburg.

2. On the left side, head down.
3. On the right side, head up.
4. Supine, in high Fowler's.

37. A pregnant woman with severe preeclampsia is at 38 weeks' gestation. She is in the transitional phase of the first stage of labor. During this time the nurse would expect her to be:
1. Irritable.
2. Excited.
3. Euphoric.
4. Serious.

38. An adolescent patient's girlfriend comes to visit him in the hospital. The nurse suspects that they may become intimate. What is the most appropriate nursing intervention?
1. Don't allow his girlfriend to visit.
2. Inform the couple that "necking" is prohibited.
3. Provide privacy from staff and other clients.
4. Allow visitation with supervision.

39. A patient is to be discharged on a 2-g sodium diet. The nurse would know that the patient understands the dietary limitations if he or she selected:
1. Filet of sole, tossed salad with lemon juice, coffee.
2. Chow mein, fried rice, tea.
3. Canned tomato soup, unsalted crackers, skim milk.
4. Two hot dogs with mustard, macaroni salad, ginger ale.

40. A patient complains of increasing shortness of breath with exercise. On physical examination, he is found to be moderately overweight, and has BP 152/105, pulse 81, respirations 16, and fine basilar crackles in both lung fields, and the PMI (point of maximal impulse) is shifted to the left and down by 1.5 cm. The best explanation the nurse could offer this patient is that his shortness of breath is most likely related to:
1. Inadequate functioning of the left ventricle.
2. Insufficient blood return to the right side of the heart.
3. Asynergistic pumping of the left ventricle.
4. Obesity and sedentary life-style.

41. The best approach for the nurse to take in administering a preop injection to a preschooler would be to:
1. Ask her mother to explain the injection to her.
2. Simply give the injection as quickly as possible without telling her anything, as it may scare her.
3. Give her a short and simple explanation immediately before giving the injection.
4. Tell her she must have the injection and then her mother can read her a story.

42. The nurse explains that the *primary* objective of a preoperative skin prep is:
1. To clean the skin of excess oils and hair.
2. To prevent postoperative infection by sterilizing the skin.
3. To prevent postoperative infection by reducing the number of microorganisms on the skin.
4. To provide a clear field for the incision.

43. Since a patient who hallucinates is not in touch with reality, the most appropriate nursing intervention would be to:
1. Maintain a safe environment.
2. Establish a trusting relationship.
3. Orient the patient to time, place, and person.
4. Isolate the patient from other patients.

44. Which hobby will most likely be restricted for an adult following recovery from pacemaker insertion?
1. Swimming.
2. Fashioning lamps from driftwood and metal.

3. Operating ham radio.

4. Playing golf.

45. During the first 24–48 hours after admission, the most appropriate diet for a patient who has GI bleeding is likely to be:

1. NPO.

2. Clear liquids.

3. A soft, bland diet.

4. Skim or regular milk.

46. If a woman is pregnant for the second time, but her first pregnancy did not reach viability, what would be her parity?

1. 1-0-0-1.

2. 0-0-1-0.

3. 0-1-0-0.

4. 0-1-0-1.

47. After determining that a patient is pulseless, the nurse would begin adult one-person CPR at a minimum compression rate of:

1. 60 compressions per minute.

2. 80 compressions per minute.

3. 90 compressions per minute.

4. 100 compressions per minute.

48. A patient has had an appendectomy, following a ruptured appendix. During postop care, the nurses' notes in this patient's chart should include documentation of:

1. Teaching to prevent dumping syndrome and to promote early ambulation.

2. Frequent mouth care and dressing changes, including drainage.

3. Bowel sounds, intake and output, and the need for a low-residue diet.

4. Dressing changes, intake and output, and bowel sounds.

49. Three hours after admission to the CCU for anterior myocardial infarction (MI), a patient develops increasing ventricular ectopy, followed by a short burst of ventricular tachycardia. The first nursing action is to:

1. Notify the attending physician.

2. Increase the flow of O_2 from 4 to 8 liters.

3. Administer a bolus of lidocaine, per order.

4. Repeat the morphine sulfate, per order.

50. Sudden infant death syndrome (SIDS) occurs most frequently when which factor is involved?

1. White.

2. Low birthweight.

3. Midrange socioeconomic status.

4. Breastfeeding.

51. After a patient returns from surgery following craniotomy, the nurse knows that the optimum positioning of a neurosurgery patient, unless otherwise indicated, would be:

1. Flat on back.

2. Head elevated 30 degrees.

3. Head elevated 45 degrees.

4. Head elevated 90 degrees.

52. Immediately before a woman is to give birth, her husband expresses anxiety about staying with her. The *most* appropriate response the nurse could make would be:

1. "Many people feel frightened at this time."

2. "You'll do fine, don't worry."

3. "Think of your wife. How will she feel if you don't stay?"

4. "Once things get going, you'll forget about being afraid."

53. Which type of anesthesia should the nurse anticipate will be used for an amputation?

1. IV regional.

2. Spinal.

3. General intravenous and inhalation anesthesia.

4. Muscle relaxant.

54. To facilitate the proper drying of a long leg cast, the nurse should include which measure in the plan of care?

1. Leave the cast exposed to the air.

2. Encourage the patient to remain in one position.

3. Place the patient on a bedboard.

4. Use only tips of the fingers to handle the cast.

55. Which nursing care procedure is *least* important during the period prior to insertion of the pacemaker?

1. Providing sedation to relieve anxiety and promote relaxation as needed.

2. Instituting arm and leg range-of-motion exercises to prevent postinsertion complications.

3. Establishing an intravenous line and having emergency equipment and medications available.

4. Weighing the patient and instituting intake and output records.

56. On turning a patient who has had a right modified mastectomy to her left side, the nurse notes a moderately large amount of serosanguineous drainage on the bedsheets. The nurse should:

1. Remove the dressing to ascertain the origin of the bleeding.

2. Milk the Hemovac tubing, using a downward motion.

3. Note vital signs, reinforce the dressing, and notify the surgeon immediately.

4. Recognize that this is a frequent occurrence with this type of surgery.

57. Immediately following birth, an infant's condition is assessed. His respirations do not establish readily, he is slightly cyanotic, and there is some muscle flaccidity. The most appropriate nursing action would be to:

1. Initiate CPR immediately.

2. Clear airway and administer oxygen.

3. Reassure the parents.

4. Check the mother's chart for her last medication (drug, time, and amount).

58. Which nursing action is essential to prevent hypoxemia during tracheal suctioning?

1. Removal of oral and nasal secretions.

2. Encouraging the patient to deep breathe and cough to facilitate removal of upper-airway secretions.

3. Administer 100% oxygen to reduce the effects of airway obstruction during suctioning.

4. Auscultate the lungs to determine the baseline data to assess the effectiveness of suctioning.

59. An expectant couple is informed that a cesarean will be performed immediately. The couple inquire whether the mother must be put to sleep. The most appropriate nursing response would be to:

1. Refer the couple to the anesthesiologist.

2. Ask the attending physician to explain the procedure to the couple.

3. Tell the couple that she probably will receive general anesthesia.

4. Inform the couple that most women who have a cesarean birth receive spinal anesthesia.

60. A client is hospitalized for substance abuse and hallucinatory behavior. In assessing this client's mother, the nurse would expect her initial reaction to be:

1. Anger.

2. Denial.

3. Acceptance.

4. Shock.

61. What should the nurse see in the vomitus that is characteristic of infants with pyloric stenosis?
    1. Stomach contents only.
    2. Stomach contents plus bile.
    3. Stomach contents streaked with blood.
    4. Stomach contents with flecks of feces.

62. At 36 weeks, a pregnant woman's preeclamptic condition changes: she has hyperreflexia, generalized edema, and ataxia. If she begins to have a convulsion, the nurse's *primary* action should be:
    1. Maintain patent airway.
    2. Observe for bowel or bladder evacuation.
    3. Administer cardiac pulmonary resuscitation.
    4. Maintain a safe environment.

63. An assessment finding in a patient with an MI that would be an early indicator of the extent of tissue necrosis in the heart is:
    1. The duration of sinus tachycardia.
    2. CPK and ALT[SGOT] enzyme measures.
    3. The duration of chest pain.
    4. The occurrence of primary ventricular fibrillation.

64. Which system should the nurse monitor carefully for possible toxic effects of EDTA?
    1. Neurologic.
    2. Renal.
    3. Cardiovascular.
    4. Hematologic.

65. The nurse knows that a modified radical mastectomy involves removal of:
    1. The breast only.
    2. The breast and axillary nodes.
    3. The breast, pectoralis major muscle, and axillary lymph nodes.
    4. The breast, underlying chest muscle, axillary lymph nodes, and internal mammary lymph nodes.

66. An adolescent patient's friend brings him a marijuana cigarette. The nurse finds the cigarette under the patient's pillow. The most appropriate nursing action would be to:
    1. Ignore the situation.
    2. Inform the police.
    3. Discuss the incident with the patient's parents.
    4. Confront the patient.

67. On the first postoperative day following an above-the-knee amputation, a patient's surgeon ordered rehabilitation exercises to begin. Which is most important for the nurse to initiate *first?*
    1. External rotation of the stump.
    2. Hyperextension of the thigh and stump.
    3. Lifting the buttock and stump off the bed while the patient is lying flat on the back.
    4. Arm exercises to prepare for crutch walking.

68. A toddler is admitted to the hospital with severe eczema lesions on his face, scalp, neck, and arms. The best nursing intervention to prevent him from scratching the affected areas would be to apply:
    1. Clove-hitch restraints to his hands.
    2. Elbow restraints to his arms.
    3. Mittens to his hands.
    4. A posey jacket to his torso.

69. During the first stage of labor, maternal and fetal vital signs need to be closely monitored. The best time to observe maternal vital signs is:
    1. Immediately before a contraction.
    2. Between contractions.
    3. Immediately after a contraction.
    4. Any time the mother feels totally comfortable.

70. A child admitted to rule out intussusception is scheduled for a barium enema. The nurse should teach the child's parents that the major purpose of this procedure is to:
    1. Confirm the diagnosis.
    2. Reduce the telescoping.
    3. Ease the passage of stool.
    4. Provide symptomatic relief.

71. If a woman is 3 months' pregnant, what symptom or symptoms would the nurse's assessment most likely discover?
    1. Quickening.
    2. Lightening.
    3. Breast tingling and tenderness.
    4. Nausea and vomiting.

72. A patient is to have a breast biopsy and possible mastectomy. Before going to see this patient the morning of surgery, the nurse assigned to assist her in the final preparations for surgery should first:
    1. Prepare the preoperative medication.
    2. Check to be sure the operative permit has been signed.
    3. Check to see if the preoperative laboratory reports have been placed in the chart.
    4. Check the diet orders to be sure the patient has been placed on the NPO list.

73. The attending physician and anesthesiologist decide to administer spinal anesthesia for a cesarean birth. The nurse knows the amount of anesthesia used will be as minimal as possible because spinal anesthesia:
    1. Produces severe fetal depression.
    2. Causes maternal hypotension.
    3. Rapidly crosses the placenta.
    4. Depresses maternal respirations.

74. A client's mother asks the nurse what caused her son to take drugs. The most therapeutic response would be:
    1. "He probably wanted to be like his peers."
    2. "Inappropriate limits were probably set on his behavior."
    3. "It involves many factors."
    4. "He felt isolated and unloved."

75. At 2:30 A.M., the nurse hangs a 1000-mL bottle of IV fluid. If the IV infuses at 110 mL per hour as ordered, how much fluid should infuse by 6:00 A.M.?
    1. 385 mL.
    2. 500 mL.
    3. 615 mL.
    4. 740 mL.

76. When teaching the parents about an apnea monitor, the nurse should stress:
    1. "Always respond to the monitor alarm immediately."
    2. "Initiate CPR whenever the alarm sounds."
    3. "A responsible adult must remain in the room with the infant at all times."
    4. "Call the emergency room during any episodes of apnea."

77. On admission to the recovery room, a patient is very restless. Her respirations are deep and somewhat irregular; she startles easily and moans when the nurse touches her. The best nursing action is:
    1. Continue to stimulate her by telling her the operation is over.
    2. Raise the siderails and remain quietly in attendance.
    3. Administer meperidine (Demerol) HCl, 100 mg IM.
    4. Check her nailbeds for cyanosis.

78. On the third day of hospitalization following an anterior MI, a patient becomes increasingly restless. Pulse

rate has increased to 126 beats per minute. The first nursing action is to:
1. Do a partial physical assessment, which includes vital signs, pulmonary auscultation, and cognitive functions.
2. Ask if the patient is upset, since depression is common on the third day of hospitalization.
3. Readminister oxygen per nasal catheter (prongs or tongs) at 6 liters, as restlessness is an early sign of cerebral hypoxia.
4. Decrease the rate of intravenous infusion to prevent fluid volume overload.

79. While observing a patient throughout a blood transfusion, the nurse should be alert to which possible sign of a hemolytic reaction?
1. Urticaria.
2. Polyuria.
3. Flank pain.
4. Hypothermia.

80. A patient is awaiting the insertion of a pacemaker. His blood pressure is 128/60. Which medication should the nurse have available during this patient's preoperative period?
1. Lidocaine (Xylocaine).
2. Atropine sulfate.
3. Digoxin.
4. Propranolol hydrochloride (Inderal).

81. In considering the equipment for Bryant's traction, the nurse should expect to see:
1. A Kirschner wire in the fractured femur.
2. A Steinmann pin in the fractured femur.
3. Adhesive material taped to the skin of both legs.
4. Adhesive material taped to the skin of the fractured leg only.

82. In providing health teaching for an expectant couple, what should the nurse tell them is a *probable* sign of pregnancy?
1. Fetal heart sounds.
2. Positive pregnancy test.
3. Fetal movements felt by examiner.
4. Outline of fetus on sonogram.

83. The physician suspects that a patient has a peptic ulcer. The nurse should expect the physician to order which diet after the first 48–72 hours?
1. Small feedings of bland food.
2. Frequent feedings of clear liquids.
3. A regular diet given frequently in small amounts.
4. NPO.

84. A patient tells the nurse that he sees big white ants crawling all over the wall. The most appropriate nursing response would be:
1. "Where are they? I'll kill them for you."
2. "You must be seeing things."
3. Silence.
4. "I don't see any ants; but you seem afraid."

85. In assisting a patient to prepare for immediate surgery, what would the nurse do?
1. Remove the patient's wedding band.
2. Begin exploring the patient's fears and anxieties about surgery.
3. Assist in removing dentures and nail polish.
4. Remind the patient to void following preoperative medication.

86. A patient is to be discharged on the antihypertensive drug reserpine. The nurse's instructions to avoid intermittent hypotension would include:
1. "Rise slowly from sitting or lying."
2. "Ingest alcohol to prevent hypotension."

3. "Avoid cold weather, which precipitates attacks."
4. "Exercise to decrease sudden vasodilation."

87. The nurse administers preop medication, atropine (0.15 mg) IM. Fifteen minutes later, the patient is breathing rapidly and has a flushed, red face. The nurse should:
1. Administer the atropine antidote stat.
2. Give the patient a cool sponge bath.
3. Tell the patient these are normal side effects of atropine.
4. Page and advise the surgeon of the patient's condition prior to transporting the patient to the operating room.

88. The nurse has discussed important aspects of breastfeeding with a new mother. To evaluate the effects of the teaching, the nurse asks her to put it in her own words. Which response indicates a need for further teaching?
1. "Rest and relaxation are essential."
2. "An adequate diet is important."
3. "Large breasts produce more milk."
4. "Birth control is necessary throughout breastfeeding if I don't want to become pregnant."

89. A patient who has had a modified mastectomy begins to demonstrate some early signs of shock, such as increased pulse, cool, clammy skin, and restlessness. The nurse could enhance venous return by:
1. Administering oxygen via mask to reduce restlessness.
2. Keeping trunk flat and raising foot of bed.
3. Placing her in Trendelenburg position.
4. Wrapping her entire body in warmed blankets.

90. In discussing what clothes a toddler with eczema should wear, both in the hospital and at home, the nurse would be most correct in teaching the mother that this child should wear only:
1. Cotton.
2. Linen.
3. Natural wool.
4. Polyester blend.

91. The physician orders a soapsuds enema for a woman in preterm labor, whose membranes have ruptured. The most appropriate nursing action would be to:
1. Administer the enema as soon as possible.
2. Recheck the order for the type of enema.
3. Refuse to administer the enema because this is a preterm labor and membranes have ruptured.
4. Ask the physician to check the fetal position prior to giving the enema.

92. While doing chest compressions during CPR on an adult, the nurse hears a "cracking" sound. The appropriate response would be to:
1. Stop chest compressions immediately and ventilate only.
2. Compress no more than 1½ in.
3. Check for proper hand placement and continue.
4. Have someone else who is not as strong do compressions.

93. A pregnant woman verbalizes concern about the possibility of having to remain hospitalized for the next 8 weeks because of her preeclampsia. The *most* therapeutic response the nurse could make would be:
1. "It may not be that bad if you keep busy."
2. "Tell me how you are feeling."
3. "I'll sit with you a while."
4. "Maybe you should tell your doctor how you are feeling."

94. A patient should be able to describe signs of pacemaker malfunction. Which behavior would indicate that this goal has been met?
    1. Counts pulse correctly and identifies need to monitor rate daily.
    2. Counts pulse correctly and identifies the significance of drainage or discoloration around the battery insertion site.
    3. Counts pulse correctly, states the estimated life of the battery, and understands need of prophylactic replacement.
    4. Counts pulse correctly and identifies need to report rate changes and symptoms such as dizziness, palpitations, and hiccoughs.

95. A pregnant woman is in early labor; she has a history of smoking cigarettes and marijuana, although she stopped when she learned she was pregnant. Her husband expresses some concern over his wife's previous smoking habits. The nurse should inform him that:
    1. Although she no longer smokes, she was exposed to cigarette and marijuana smoke, which could affect her pregnancy.
    2. She is assured of a healthy infant because she stopped smoking as soon as she knew she was pregnant.
    3. The early labor is probably due to her smoking marijuana.
    4. Alcohol is considered much safer than marijuana.

96. A patient with a left leg fracture is to be taught the three-point gait prior to discharge. This patient should be given which instruction by the nurse?
    1. "Advance your right crutch, swing the left foot forward, advance the left crutch, and then bring the right foot forward."
    2. "Move your right crutch and left foot forward together, and then swing the right foot and left crutch in one movement."
    3. "While partially bearing weight on your left leg, advance both crutches and then bring your right leg forward."
    4. "Using one movement, advance your left foot and both crutches and then bring your right leg forward."

97. Immediately postoperative, after general anesthesia, a patient has an airway in place and is in a supine position. To prevent airway obstruction, the nurse should:
    1. Leave the airway tube in and turn the patient's head to the side.
    2. Maintain the patient's present position.
    3. Remove the airway tube and turn the patient's head to the side.
    4. Remove the airway tube and maintain the patient's prone position.

98. A patient with a history of substance abuse asks the nurse not to tell anyone that he was smoking a marijuana joint in his hospital room, and he promises that he'll never do it again. The nurse should realize that this patient is *mostly:*
    1. Being sincere and wanting to change.
    2. Seeking attention.
    3. Being manipulative.
    4. Trying to avoid punishment.

99. The nurse can expect increased restlessness in a patient with tachycardia following an anterior myocardial infarction because:
    1. Decreased ventricular filling time results in decreased venous return and cerebral edema.
    2. Palpitations result in anxiety.

3. Decreased ventricular filling time always results in decreased cardiac output and tissue perfusion.
4. A significant decrease in stroke volume may occur, causing a decrease in cardiac output.

100. To evaluate a woman's understanding of the discussion about Down syndrome, the nurse would ask her to explain the syndrome in her own words. Which response indicates a need for further health teaching?
    1. "Down syndrome is an abnormality that can result from an extra chromosome."
    2. "Only children born to older women have Down syndrome."
    3. "A test can be done to diagnose Down syndrome while the fetus is still in utero."
    4. "Down syndrome includes a form of mental retardation."

101. A patient is to have an above-the-knee (AK) amputation for severe vascular insufficiency and gangrene of the foot. The best explanation by the nurse for why the patient is to have this amputation would be:
    1. The degree of vascular insufficiency is extensive.
    2. AK amputees are better suited for a prosthesis.
    3. The higher the amputation, the less energy required for rehabilitation of balance and walking.
    4. Below-the-knee amputation heals less successfully.

102. The proper method of suctioning a tracheostomy tube includes:
    1. Suctioning only while inserting the catheter.
    2. Suctioning only while withdrawing the catheter.
    3. Suctioning during both insertion and withdrawal of the catheter.
    4. Suctioning on insertion only if secretions are copious.

103. In assessing a woman in labor following the administration of spinal anesthesia, the nurse should realize that if she can wiggle her toes:
    1. The effect of the spinal anesthesia has dissipated.
    2. She may still become hypotensive.
    3. This behavior is essentially meaningless.
    4. She is prone to hypertension.

104. To help a preschooler cope most effectively with repeated painful injections of EDTA, the nurse should:
    1. Teach his mother the importance of bringing him his favorite toys.
    2. Encourage him to spend most of the day in the playroom, engaged in free play.
    3. Offer him the opportunity for therapeutic play.
    4. Allow him to play with other preschool children as much as he wants.

105. Which arm position will best facilitate venous return on the operative side of a patient who has had a modified mastectomy, and reduce the occurrence of lymphedema?
    1. Semi-Fowler's position with the elbow flexed and the arm across the chest.
    2. Low Fowler's position with the arm elevated so that the hand and elbow are slightly higher than the shoulder.
    3. High Fowler's position with the elbow flexed and the right hand positioned next to the head.
    4. Adduction of the shoulder, extension of the elbow, and flexion of the wrist.

106. The most important aspect of treatment for a client who is a substance abuser is:
    1. Teaching the client about the hazards of taking drugs.
    2. Informing the client that using drugs is illegal.
    3. Encouraging the client to want to change behavior.

4. Assisting the client to develop alternative coping mechanisms.

107. Two hours after a child returns to the unit following cardiac catheterization, the dressing is soaked with bright red blood. The nurse first reinforces the dressing. What should the nurse do next?
    1. Check vital signs.
    2. Increase the flow rate of the IV.
    3. Place the child in reverse Trendelenburg position.
    4. Notify the cardiologist.

108. New parents express concern about when they can resume intercourse. After validating the information with the physician, the nurse would inform the couple that:
    1. Generally it is a good idea to wait until after the sixth-week postpartum check-up.
    2. If there are no unforeseen problems, 3 weeks is usually the recommended waiting time.
    3. The couple may have sex as soon as they arrive home from the hospital, as long as the mother feels up to it.
    4. The couple should wait until the mother ceases to breastfeed.

109. A patient is awaiting the insertion of a permanent pacemaker because of complete heart block. The nurse knows that isoproterenol hydrochloride (Isuprel) is used for this patient because of which effect?
    1. Beta-mimetic.
    2. Cardiac glycoside.
    3. Anticholinergic.
    4. Beta-blocker.

110. A pregnant woman is hospitalized for preeclampsia. She and her husband express anxiety about having limited insurance, which may not cover this hospitalization. The *most* appropriate nursing intervention would be to:
    1. Refer the couple to social services for possible assistance.
    2. Initiate a family-counseling referral.
    3. Provide supportive counseling.
    4. Assess the couple's needs through discussion.

111. A patient has had an above-the-knee amputation on his left side. While being repositioned onto his abdomen, the patient states that he can't turn because his "left foot is causing him too much pain." The first response by the nurse should be:
    1. To insist he lie on his abdomen.
    2. To ignore his comment and state that he or she will return later.
    3. To discuss the principle of phantom pain postamputation.
    4. To offer some form of pain control.

112. During a predischarge teaching session for a patient who has had a permanent pacemaker inserted, the patient's wife states, "Don't worry, I'll be sure that he obeys the doctor's orders to the letter." The nurse's best response would be:
    1. "I can see that with your help, he should do just fine."
    2. "Are you worried?"
    3. "I'm not worried. You both have a lot of common sense."
    4. "This has been a difficult period for both of you. Can you foresee any problems with these instructions?"

113. In planning initial care for an adolescent client who is a substance abuser, the nurse should:
    1. Be very direct with the client.

2. Allow the client to make all the decisions about his or her care.
    3. Help the client to feel very secure to prevent anxiety.
    4. Encourage the client to begin to depend on others.

114. Upon his return from the OR at 11:30 A.M., a patient has 425 mL left in an IV bag of 5% dextrose and ½ NS. The postop MD orders include "IV to infuse at 320 mL every 8 hours." When should the nurse anticipate having to change the IV bag?
    1. 3:00 P.M.
    2. 6:00 P.M.
    3. 9:00 P.M.
    4. 12:00 midnight.

115. The nurse's assessment of a patient in pulmonary edema would reveal:
    1. Rapid respiration, frequent cough, flushed face.
    2. Persistent cough, rapid respiration, hemoptysis.
    3. Dyspnea, hacking cough, purulent sputum.
    4. Air hunger, orthopnea, elevated temperature.

116. Prior to entering a patient's room, the nurse should wash her or his hands for a minimum of:
    1. 10 seconds.
    2. 30 seconds.
    3. 45 seconds.
    4. 60 seconds.

117. The nurse in the recovery room is monitoring the patient's vital signs every 15 minutes. Which change should be reported immediately to the surgeon?
    1. Dry, cool skin.
    2. A systolic blood pressure that drops 20 mm Hg or more.
    3. A diastolic pressure below 70.
    4. A pulse rate that increases and decreases with respirations.

118. The preoperative medications ordered by the anesthesiologist are morphine sulfate, 15 mg, and atropine SO_4, 0.4 mg, subcutaneously. The nurse can expect to give these drugs:
    1. Right before the patient leaves for surgery.
    2. 45–60 minutes before anesthetic induction.
    3. 20–30 minutes before anesthetic induction.
    4. 10–15 minutes before anesthetic induction.

119. The nurse knows that a person with a peptic ulcer who is on a bland diet may *lack* which essential nutrient?
    1. Vitamin C.
    2. Carbohydrates.
    3. Protein.
    4. Vitamin A.

120. When assessing a client who has been abusing amphetamines, the nurse would expect to see which symptom?
    1. Bradycardia.
    2. Increased irritability.
    3. Hypotension.
    4. Constipation.

121. Which action is *least* likely to be within the role and legal responsibilities of the nurse who is assisting with an amniocentesis?
    1. Informing the woman about the risks involved in amniocentesis.
    2. Explaining/reinforcing how the procedure will be done.
    3. Monitoring the fetal heart rate.
    4. Observing the woman for signs of bleeding or contractions after the procedure is completed.

122. When noticing that a patient's IV site appears red and swollen, the nurse should:
    1. Apply warm soaks.

2. Decrease the flow rate.
3. Elevate the IV site.
4. Remove the IV.

123. Two weeks after a cast is applied, a foul odor is detected at the lower end of the cast. A window is made in the cast over the infected area and an antibiotic is prescribed. After 3 days on antibiotic therapy, which effect would be most indicative of a therapeutic response?
1. White blood cell count is 7900 per mm³.
2. Temperature is 99.4°F.
3. No complaints of pain.
4. Appetite is fairly good.

124. On completion of a nursing assessment, the nurse concludes that the patient is showing signs of increased intracranial pressure. Data to support this conclusion would include:
1. Decreased blood pressure, tachycardia, tachypnea.
2. Increase in level of consciousness.
3. Dilation of the pupil on the side opposite the hematoma.
4. Bradycardia, increased pulse pressure, and Biot's breathing.

125. Ten days after the birth of their infant, a new father is concerned about the mother's mood. He states that she is tearful and apathetic and does not eat much. What would be the nurse's most appropriate response?
1. "Many women experience some degree of depression after the birth of a baby."
2. "I will suggest a psychiatric referral to assist her in coping with this crisis."
3. "I will notify the physician of your concern and ask the physician to prescribe an antidepressant for her."
4. "You need to be patient since these symptoms will dissipate."

126. A diabetic patient is NPO prior to surgery. An appropriate nursing measure on the day of surgery is:
1. To withhold the daily insulin dose.
2. To administer the daily insulin dose.
3. To administer the insulin and request that the patient drink a glass of juice.
4. To request specific orders regarding insulin administration.

127. A patient with hallucinatory behavior constantly asks the nurse to bring him french fries and a piece of apple pie. The nurse should realize that this patient is probably:
1. Starving.
2. Hallucinating.
3. Disoriented.
4. Playing a game.

128. In caring for a patient with a double-lumen tracheostomy tube, the inner cannula should be removed and cleansed with hydrogen peroxide and normal saline:
1. Only as necessary.
2. Every 2–4 hours.
3. Once a day.
4. Never—do not remove the inner cannula for any reason.

129. Assessment of a woman in labor reveals the following: 4-cm dilated cervix, intact membranes, mild to moderate contractions every 4–6 minutes, alert affect. The nurse determines that this woman is in which stage of labor?
1. First.
2. Second.
3. Third.

4. Fourth.

130. The best antimicrobial agent for the nurse to use in handwashing is:
1. Soap and water.
2. Isopropyl alcohol.
3. Hexachlorophene (PhisoHex).
4. Chlorhexidine gluconate (CHG)(Hibiclens).

131. The nurse knows that the proper technique for two-person CPR includes:
1. Two full breaths followed by five compressions.
2. A brief pause between rescue breathing and compressions.
3. Rescuers changing positions every 5 minutes to prevent fatigue.
4. A slower rate than is used in one-person CPR.

132. A patient is taking nitroglycerin to control angina. Patient teaching regarding administration of nitroglycerin includes the importance of notifying the physician if repeated doses do not relieve chest pain. Additional information would include:
1. Notifying the physician if headaches occur.
2. Storing the medication in the refrigerator.
3. Taking nitroglycerin prophylactically before exercise.
4. Ingesting the tablets with liquid.

133. The mother of a recently deceased infant insists on seeing the infant's body before leaving the hospital. The most therapeutic nursing action includes:
1. Arranging for her to see the infant's body.
2. Discussing this with the family's priest.
3. Informing the father that seeing the infant's body would be detrimental to the mother's health.
4. Telling the parents that hospital policy forbids her seeing the infant's body.

134. A woman is to have a cesarean birth. Her partner asks the nurse whether he will see any gore or blood during the operation. The most realistic response would be:
1. "I'm not sure."
2. "It depends on the technique the physician uses."
3. "Probably not, because a drape keeps the operation from view by both of you, if you sit by her head."
4. "Yes, blood and tissue will be all over the table."

135. If a patient's antihypertensive drug therapy is effective, the nurse would expect:
1. A greater decrease in systolic than diastolic pressure.
2. A greater decrease in diastolic than systolic pressure.
3. An approximately equal decrease in both systolic and diastolic pressures.
4. Little change in blood pressure initially, but pulse will slow.

136. When teaching a 3-year-old about a procedure, the nurse should realize that the *most* important factor influencing the child's ability to learn is:
1. Chronologic age.
2. Developmental level.
3. Present state of anxiety.
4. Previous experience with illness and hospitalization.

137. What will the nurse encourage a patient who has had a modified right mastectomy to do as appropriate *initial* therapy 24 hours after surgery?
1. Self-feeding and hair combing.
2. Passive/active flexion and extension of the elbow and pronation and supination of the wrist.
3. Abduction and external rotation of the right shoulder.

4. Early ambulation and active extension and flexion of the elbow.

138. When teaching a young mother about a decrease in her milk production, the nurse should:
    1. Recommend weaning the baby onto formula.
    2. Assess the mother's feelings about breastfeeding.
    3. Refer the mother to La Leche League.
    4. Suggest supplemental feedings of glucose water.

139. Besides enhancing pacemaker automaticity and facilitating AV conduction during heart block, what other effect of isoproterenol (Isuprel) would the nurse look for?
    1. Increased peripheral vascular resistance.
    2. Decreased automaticity of Purkinje fibers.
    3. Decreased bronchoconstriction.
    4. Decreased oral secretion.

140. A pregnant woman at 29 weeks' gestation is concerned about her weight gain of 15 pounds during this pregnancy. The nurse will most likely determine that this woman is primarily concerned about:
    1. The baby's nutrition status.
    2. Her own body image.
    3. Her need to diet.
    4. Her need to gain more weight.

141. A patient who has had a myocardial infarction states that he can hardly get his breath. His vital signs are BP 100/70, apical pulse 126, respirations 26. Pulmonary crackles and rhonchi are heard halfway up his chest. The first nursing action is to:
    1. Administer morphine sulfate to allay the patient's apprehension.
    2. Assist the patient to a sitting position and lower his legs.
    3. Remove excess pulmonary secretions with suction.
    4. Administer oxygen at 10 liters, per mask instead of nasal catheter.

142. When a woman is in labor, which action requested by the nurse could cause a problem to the woman?
    1. Empty her bladder.
    2. Lie on her back to facilitate adequate ventilation.
    3. Not bear down until she enters the second stage.
    4. Breathe slowly and evenly.

143. A husband blames his wife for their son's problems with substance abuse, saying, "I always know you were too easy on him. You see what giving him his way has done!" In understanding the father's response, the nurse should realize that this behavior indicates a nursing diagnosis of defensive coping as evidenced by:
    1. Guilt.
    2. Sublimation.
    3. Projection.
    4. Displacement.

144. The doctor orders Burow's solution soaks for a toddler with eczema. In order to gain his cooperation with this treatment, the nurse should tell him:
    1. "Let's do this real fast and then you can see mommy and daddy."
    2. "You don't want to have to stay here forever, do you? Let's make you all better now!"
    3. "This medicine will help you get better so you can go home. Help me pour some on your arms."
    4. "This is magic medicine that will make all your boo-boos go away. Don't you want to chase away those boo-boos?"

145. When teaching parents how to provide CPR for their infant, it is important to stress:
    1. Applying systematic pressure to the chest with the heel of the hand.

2. Compressing the chest at a rate of 100 compressions per minute.
3. Placing the resuscitator's mouth over the infant's mouth to ensure an adequate seal.
4. Blowing forcefully into the infant's air passages to fully inflate the lungs.

146. When planning to teach a client about the side effects of amphetamines, the nurse should emphasize that:
    1. Withdrawal from these drugs usually causes death.
    2. The body develops a tolerance to these drugs.
    3. An overdose of these drugs induces sleepiness.
    4. Physiologic dependence may develop.

147. While preparing a patient's preoperative medication, the nurse notes that the atropine SO_4 on hand is in a strength of 0.6 mg/mL. The prescribed dosage is 0.4 mg. The correct amount of atropine to administer is:
    1. 1.5 mL.
    2. 1 mL.
    3. 10 minims.
    4. 8 minims.

148. If a pregnant woman remains essentially healthy, the nurse's health teaching about safeguards to maintain throughout pregnancy should be for her to:
    1. Stop working by week 32 of gestation.
    2. Avoid intercourse.
    3. Avoid alcohol and smoking.
    4. Eat a minimum of three full meals each day.

149. Given a diagnosis of pulmonary edema, the nurse knows that a patient's dyspnea is the result of:
    1. Increased lung compliance due to mechanical congestion.
    2. Decreased CO_2 retention.
    3. Decreased venous return.
    4. Fluid shift from systemic circulation to lungs.

150. The nurse realizes that the discharge of green amniotic fluid may indicate:
    1. Rh or ABO incompatibility.
    2. Fetal distress occurred approximately 36 hours ago.
    3. Recent or current hypoxia.
    4. Abruptio placentae has occurred.

151. The rationale for using humidified oxygen with tracheal tubes is that:
    1. It is a traditional procedure.
    2. It is a means of providing fluid intake.
    3. It decreases insensible water loss.
    4. The natural humidifying pathway has been bypassed.

152. Parents of a 6-month-old infant bring him in for a physical examination; all of his immunizations are up-to-date. This infant should receive three of the following immunizations at this time; which immunization should he not receive?
    1. Hepatitis B.
    2. Diphtheria, tetanus, and pertussis (DTP).
    3. *H. influenza* type b.
    4. Measles, mumps, rubella.

153. An IV rate is to be regulated to keep vein open (KVO). The nurse knows that the longest possible time that a single 1000-mL bottle or bag can infuse safely is:
    1. 24 hours.
    2. 5 hours.
    3. 18 hours.
    4. 12 hours.

154. The nurse should know that the best position to check an adolescent for scoliosis is:
    1. Standing up straight.
    2. Lying flat on the stomach.
    3. Standing and bending 90 degrees at the waist.

4. Sitting in a straight-back chair.

155. A unit of blood is ordered for a patient, when the BP drops to 90/60. What is the most important safeguard prior to administering blood?
    1. Refrigerate unit of blood until immediately before giving.
    2. Agitate the blood so it is well mixed.
    3. Carefully check labeled blood against patient's wristband.
    4. Infuse the blood through a blood warmer.

156. Potassium chloride is to be added to an infant's intravenous fluids. Before adding this electrolyte, the nurse should determine that:
    1. The infant has voided recently.
    2. Moro reflex is present.
    3. Respiratory rate is between 25 and 40.
    4. Mucous membranes are moist.

157. A young woman describes experiencing a heavy vaginal discharge and severe itching for the past 3 days. She is diagnosed as having *Trichomonas vaginalis* infection. Health teaching for this woman should include dosage, administration, and signs and symptoms of side effects of which medication as treatment for this condition?
    1. Tetracycline.
    2. Erythromycin.
    3. Nystatin.
    4. Metronidazole.

158. Immediately on returning to the recovery room, a patient's above-the-knee amputation stump should initially be:
    1. Elevated on a pillow to reduce occurrence of edema and hemorrhage.
    2. Placed in Buck's traction to prevent skin and muscle retraction.
    3. Firmly bandaged to a padded board to prevent contractures.
    4. Wrapped in an Ace bandage to reduce edema formation.

159. When a postop patient is admitted following an appendectomy, the *first* action the nurse should take is to:
    1. Attach nasogastric tube to suction.
    2. Calculate the IV flow rate and adjust the drip.
    3. Monitor vital signs.
    4. Check patient's ID band.

160. The nurse planning to administer a unit of blood to a child should know that after it is removed from the refrigerator, the blood should be transfused within:
    1. Six hours.
    2. Two hours.
    3. Four hours.
    4. One hour.

161. In observing women in the latent phase of the first stage of labor, the nurse would expect to see which behavior?
    1. Tendency to hyperventilate.
    2. Euphoria, excitement, and talkativeness.
    3. Fairly quiet and introverted behavior.
    4. Irritability and crying.

162. To which postoperative complication is a patient who has had a modified mastectomy predisposed because of the nature of her surgery?
    1. Peripheral thrombophlebitis.
    2. Wound dehiscence.
    3. Atelectasis.
    4. Paralytic ileus.

163. In teaching a couple about preparation for childbirth, the nurse should *first*:

1. Evaluate the couple's knowledge base of childbirth techniques.
2. Assess the couple's level of readiness to learn.
3. Consult a childbirth nurse practitioner regarding what to tell the couple.
4. Refer the couple to a Lamaze childbirth class.

164. Following surgery for a ruptured appendix, the nurse should place the patient in a semi-Fowler's position primarily to:
    1. Fully aerate the lungs.
    2. Promote drainage and prevent subdiaphragmatic abscesses.
    3. Splint the wound.
    4. Facilitate movement and reduce complications from immobility.

165. The nurse assessing a person who has a history of substance abuse would expect to find which characteristic?
    1. A very assertive individual.
    2. A very dependent individual.
    3. A very mature individual.
    4. A very aggressive individual.

166. The earliest signs of whole blood transfusion reaction a nurse would monitor for are:
    1. Headache and elevated temperature.
    2. Hypertension and flushing.
    3. Urticaria and wheezing.
    4. Oliguria and jaundice.

167. The nurse caring for a patient recovering from GI bleeding should:
    1. Plan care so the patient can receive at least 8 hours of uninterrupted sleep each night.
    2. Monitor vital signs every 2 hours.
    3. Make sure that the patient takes food and medications at prescribed intervals.
    4. Provide milk every 2–3 hours.

168. To monitor a patient's fluid volumes more closely, a CVP line has been inserted via the right subclavian vein. The nurse needs to know that CVP assesses the pressure in:
    1. The left atrium.
    2. The right atrium.
    3. The left ventricle.
    4. The right ventricle.

169. A patient is diagnosed as being mildly hypertensive. In assessing this patient's BP, the nurse most likely finds that the resting diastolic pressure is:
    1. Between 110 and 120 mm Hg.
    2. Between 90 and 100 mm Hg.
    3. Between 120 and 140 mm Hg.
    4. Between 100 and 115 mm Hg.

170. A patient has had a permanent pacemaker inserted, with the pacing catheter introduced into the right external jugular vein and positioned in the right ventricle. Which nursing care activity is the nurse's first priority in the *early* postimplantation period?
    1. Restricting activity to prevent pacing catheter displacement.
    2. Monitoring the ECG continually, noting rhythm, rate, appearance, and amplitude of pacing spike.
    3. Implementing passive range-of-motion exercise to the right arm to prevent "frozen shoulder."
    4. Maintaining sterile dressings over the operative site to prevent infection.

171. A client takes secobarbital (Seconal) whenever he feels "too stressed," such as whenever he has an exam or feels too pressured, which happens at least four or five times a week. The nurse should be aware that large doses of secobarbital can cause:

1. Tachycardia.
2. Hypertension.
3. Assaultive behavior.
4. Increased respirations.

172. The nurse knows that angina pectoris, which occurs after eating, may be due to:
    1. Incomplete digestion of fats due to a decrease in pancreatic enzyme, thereby increasing reflux.
    2. Local blood flow regulators that shunt blood to gut during digestion, thereby decreasing coronary artery perfusion pressures.
    3. Abdominal distention from swallowing air during eating, thereby decreasing diaphragmatic excursion and arterial P_{O_2}.
    4. Decreased heart rate and blood pressure resulting in increased myocardial oxygen consumption.

173. A toddler is diagnosed as having iron deficiency anemia. In addition to teaching the parents to give this toddler Fer-In-Sol (ferrous sulfate) between meals, the nurse should also instruct them to give this medication with:
    1. Orange juice.
    2. Milk.
    3. Apple juice.
    4. Prune juice.

174. The nurse knows that the desired effects of morphine SO_4 and atropine SO_4 have been achieved when:
    1. Pain is relieved and anxiety is reduced.
    2. Secretions are decreased and sensitivity to stimuli is reduced.
    3. Sleep occurs and oral secretions are reduced.
    4. Sensitivity to pain is reduced and muscular relaxation occurs.

175. A woman in labor has a history of undiagnosed vaginal bleeding. Which procedure may be *contraindicated* on her arrival in the labor room?
    1. Initiating intravenous therapy.
    2. Taking her blood pressure.
    3. Examining her vaginal canal.
    4. Monitoring FHR.

176. The mother of a child with eczema asks the nurse if she can bathe the child in the bathtub at home. The best response by the nurse would be:
    1. "It would probably be a good idea to check with your doctor first."
    2. "Perhaps in a week to 10 days you can begin tub baths; until then, a sponge bath will be adequate."
    3. "No, baths are not generally permitted for children with eczema."
    4. "Yes, frequent baths will help dry the lesions."

177. Crepitus in the neck and upper chest of a patient who has a new tracheostomy in place is caused by:
    1. Air from a displaced tracheal tube.
    2. An inadequately inflated tracheostomy cuff.
    3. An overinflated tracheostomy cuff.
    4. Edema from the trauma of surgery.

178. An expectant couple is concerned about what effect preeclampsia may have on the fetus. Which indicator or test of fetal well-being should the nurse teach the couple to expect most commonly during the rest of the prenatal period?
    1. Nonstress test.
    2. Amniocentesis.
    3. L/S ratio.
    4. Fetal blood gases.

179. The nursing aide caring for a child in Bryant's traction reports that the child's buttocks are resting on the mattress. The nurse would be most correct in telling the aide that:
    1. This is where the buttocks should be.
    2. The buttocks should be slightly off the mattress.
    3. This is the responsibility of the nurse.
    4. The child will need special skin care to avoid pressure areas or breakdown.

180. Which nursing intervention for a patient with a Hemovac is *inappropriate*?
    1. Observing and recording the amount and color of the drainage.
    2. Maintaining suction by emptying and recompressing the apparatus regularly.
    3. Increasing suction by attaching the Hemovac to wall suction as the drainage increases.
    4. Preventing traction on the drainage tubes by repositioning the Hemovac each time the patient is repositioned.

181. An adolescent boy was admitted for substance abuse and hallucinations. This client's mother asks the nurse to talk with her son's father when he arrives at the hospital. She says that she is afraid of what the father might say to the boy. The most appropriate nursing intervention would be to:
    1. Inform the mother that she and the father can work through this problem themselves.
    2. Refer the mother to the hospital social worker.
    3. Agree to talk with the mother and the father together.
    4. Suggest that the father and son work things out.

182. Following an amputation, a nursing measure to help reduce the size of the stump once the surgical wound is healed is:
    1. Elevation of the stump on a pillow when reclining.
    2. Pushing the stump against a hard surface.
    3. Wrapping moist, warm soaks on the thigh.
    4. Applying an elastic bandage.

183. The nurse would interpret a patient's central venous pressure (CVP) as normal if the pressure were:
    1. 4–10 cm H_2O.
    2. 20–30 mm Hg.
    3. 10–20 cm H_2O.
    4. 7–14 mm Hg.

184. The nurse working with a family that is using an apnea monitor should know that the monitor's most problematic side effect is:
    1. Sounding the alarm whenever the infant moves around the crib.
    2. Overprotectiveness by the parents.
    3. Developmental lag in the infant.
    4. Unreliability of the monitor.

185. During an adolescent's hospitalization for treatment of substance abuse, the nurse must be able to handle a variety of behavior problems. In implementing care for this client, which action would be the *least* appropriate?
    1. Allowing the client to select some of the food he or she wants to eat.
    2. Restricting activity level.
    3. Encouraging friends to visit.
    4. Closely monitoring behavior.

186. The nurse knows that following administration of nitroglycerin a patient's angina will be relieved because the drug:
    1. Constricts cardiac chambers to reduce workload.
    2. Stimulates the heart rate to increase blood supply to the myocardium.
    3. Increases myocardial contractility.

4. Decreases workload of the heart through lowering the systemic blood pressure.

187. A patient is hospitalized with a BP of 170/100, difficulty breathing, dizziness, and weakness. The nurse establishing this patient's care should consider:
    1. Ensuring that a different nurse takes care of the patient each day to prevent hospital fatigue.
    2. Planning care to allow for periods of activity.
    3. Identifying any misconceptions the patient may have regarding hypertension.
    4. Instructing the patient to report only major symptoms to the physician.

188. In planning for discharge, the nurse should inform a patient who has had a right modified mastectomy of actions that may increase lymphedema. Which activity is *most likely* to increase symptoms?
    1. Wearing gloves for household tasks or gardening.
    2. Carrying heavy groceries in her right arm.
    3. Wearing dresses with elasticized sleeves.
    4. Driving to and from work.

189. A woman is in preterm labor and is bleeding. She requests a sip of water after being in labor for 2 hours in the hospital. The most appropriate nursing action would be:
    1. Checking the physician's orders.
    2. Giving her a small sip of water.
    3. Offering her ice chips.
    4. Telling her she cannot have fluids at this time.

190. A mother states that the pediatrician told her that her son has numerous allergies, including milk allergies. The nurse should offer him which formula?
    1. Lofenalac.
    2. Lonalac.
    3. Similac with iron.
    4. Isomil.

191. What would receive the *least* emphasis in the nurse's predischarge education plan for a patient who has had a permanent pacemaker inserted?
    1. Rationale for pacemaker implantation.
    2. Pacemaker function and signs indicating malfunction.
    3. Therapeutic program, including medication, diet, activity schedule, and safety precautions.
    4. Necessity for periodic follow-up visits to physician.

192. The nurse needs to know that SIDS usually occurs:
    1. Within 2–4 weeks after birth.
    2. Between 2 and 4 months after birth.
    3. More than 6 months after birth.
    4. Between 6 and 9 months after birth.

193. A patient's vital signs are BP 124/84, apical pulse 100 and regular, respirations 24. Given that this patient's normal BP is 144/96 and average pulse is 80, the nurse concludes that the present vital signs are related to:
    1. Increased vagal stimulation of SA node.
    2. Arrhythmias.
    3. Cardiogenic shock.
    4. Sympathetic nervous system response.

194. The nurse must recognize the side effects of morphine and atropine administration, which include:
    1. Bradycardia, anorexia, and decreased urine output.
    2. Hypertension, nausea, vomiting, tachycardia.
    3. Hypotension, cotton mouth, nausea, and vomiting.
    4. Dryness, cotton mouth, constricted pupils, and bradycardia.

195. In planning discharge care for a patient after treatment for hypertension, the nurse should emphasize:
    1. Medication scheduling and side effects.
    2. Need to change jobs.

3. Importance of smoking less.
4. Sexual activity restrictions.

196. The MD orders an IV of D5W at 40 mL/h. A 500-mL bag, with a pediatric microdrip chamber, is hung at 11:00 A.M. At 3:15 P.M., the nurse notes that the bag has 100 mL left. What should be the nurse's initial action?
    1. Readjust the flow rate to 40 microdrops per minute.
    2. Hang a new 500-mL bag of fluid.
    3. Maintain the flow rate at 20 microdrops per minute until the IV is back on schedule.
    4. Notify the physician.

197. The nurse knows that the *primary* advantage of Hemovac wound suction is that it:
    1. Exerts high, even suction.
    2. Allows easy mobility because it is lightweight.
    3. Speeds wound healing by removing excess fluids.
    4. Reduces the occurrence of postoperative infection.

198. The nurse would expect to find drug abuse *least* prevalent in:
    1. An upper socioeconomic family.
    2. An elderly individual.
    3. A lower socioeconomic family.
    4. An adolescent.

199. After a toddler has been in the hospital 1 week, she refuses to talk with anyone, including her family. She sits in the corner of her crib crying and rocking back and forth. The most important nursing intervention at this time should be to:
    1. Establish a one-to-one relationship with her to develop trust.
    2. Assign different staff to work with her each day to promote socialization.
    3. Ignore her behavior because it probably indicates normal regression.
    4. Refer her to the Pediatric Clinical Nurse Specialist for further evaluation.

200. Among the elderly, what is the most common postoperative complication following amputation?
    1. Hemorrhage and shock.
    2. Pulmonary embolus.
    3. Disseminated intravascular clotting.
    4. Thrombophlebitis.

❏ Answers/Rationale

1. **(2)** Hypertension is considerably more severe in men than women and tends to occur more frequently at an earlier age. **No. 1** is incorrect because currently it is estimated that 20–25 million Americans (about 10% of the population) have hypertension. The low percentage is due largely to non-detection related to the slow onset and lack of specific symptoms in its early stages. **No. 3** is incorrect because the prevalence in *every* age group is higher for American blacks than for whites. Likewise, the severity of hypertension in black men is three times that in white men and the severity in black women is almost six times that experienced by white

---

Key to codes following rationales Nursing process: **AS**, Assessment; **AN**, Analysis; **PL**, Plan; **IMP**, Implementation; **EV**, Evaluation. Category of human function: **1**, Protective; **2**, Sensory-perceptual; **3**, Comfort, Rest, Activity, and Mobility; **4**, Nutrition; **5**, Growth and Development; **6**, Fluid-Gas Transport; **7**, Psychosocial-Cultural; **8**, Elimination. Client need: **SECE**, Safe, Effective Care Environment; **PhI**, Physiologic Integrity; **PsI**, Psychosocial Integrity; **HPM**, Health Promotion/Maintenance. See appendices for full explanation.

women. Mortality rates for the American black population with hypertension are twice those of the white hypertensive population. **No. 4** is incorrect because in many individuals hypertension goes undetected and untreated. **AN,6,PhI**

2. **(2)** The date of the woman's last period is the most relevant question to ask in performing the initial assessment, because it will assist the nurse in making a preliminary determination of possible pregnancy. **No. 1** is incorrect: Whether the woman is presently taking oral contraceptives may be relevant, but it would be more pertinent to assess what general type of birth control the couple may be using and if they have been using it effectively. **Nos. 3 and 4** are incorrect: Whether she has been pregnant before and how much weight she has gained are both relevant to performing the assessment, but not essential to determining whether she is pregnant at the present time. **AS,5,HPM**

3. **(2)** Adequate oxygenation is foremost in importance. **No. 1** is incorrect because the primary intervention should be to ensure a patent airway, *followed* by observation for signs and symptoms of shock. **No. 3** is incorrect: liquids would be contraindicated because of the child's burns and possible shock. **No. 4** is incorrect because a medical order would be needed to initiate intravenous therapy. **IMP,1,PhI**

4. **(3)** Patients who abuse drugs react in various ways, depending on the amount and type of drug taken, the combination of drugs, and individual factors such as overall general health and age. However, seizures are common shortly after the ingestion of drugs such as narcotics and stimulants. Seizures may also accompany the withdrawal from drugs. **No. 1** is incorrect because the patient is not even in touch with reality. **No. 2** is incorrect because maintaining a quiet environment is of secondary importance to taking precautions against seizures. **No. 4** is incorrect because taking vital signs is of secondary importance to taking precautions against seizures. However, vital signs should be taken as soon as possible, to establish a baseline, and retaken at least every 1–2 hours thereafter until the patient is stable. **PL,7,PsI**

5. **(1)** Because the patient has experienced some gastric bleeding, he or she should be observed closely for symptoms of shock. **No. 2** is incorrect because paging the physician is secondary to the close monitoring of the patient's vital signs for symptoms of shock. **No. 3** is incorrect because completing the appropriate assessment tool may be done when the patient is under less stress. **No. 4** is incorrect because CPR is not indicated at this time—the patient is not experiencing cardiac or respiratory failure. **AS,6,PhI**

6. **(2)** The one factor that has been highly correlated to smoking cigarettes and marijuana is low birthweight. **Nos. 1, 3, and 4** are incorrect because retardation, deformation, and malnourishment do not have a high correlation to smoking cigarettes and marijuana. **EV,5,HPM**

7. **(1)** Having established, by stimulating the patient, that he or she is unconscious rather than asleep, the nurse should immediately call for help. This may be done by dialing the operator from the patient's phone and giving the hospital code for cardiac arrest and the patient's room number to the operator, or if a phone is not available, by pulling the emergency call button. Noting the time is important baseline information for cardiac arrest procedure. **No. 2** is incorrect because clearing the airway follows an unsuccessful attempt to

ventilate. **No. 3** is incorrect because checking the pulse follows after the airway has been established and ventilation has begun. **No. 4** is incorrect because initial ventilation includes two full breaths. **IMP,6,PhI**

8. **(1)** If the IV infuses at the prescribed rate of 75 mL per hour from 7:00 P.M. to 7:00 A.M., or 12 hours, 75 mL $\times$ 12 hours = 900 mL infused. If a 1000-mL bag were hung and 900 mL infused, 1000 $-$ 900 = 100 mL *left* in the bag. **Nos. 2 and 3** are incorrect calculations. **No. 4** is incorrect because there *is* enough information to determine this (see above calculation). **EV,6,SECE**

9. **(1)** The inherent rate of ventricular excitable tissue is between 20 and 40 and does not increase significantly with exertion in complete heart block. **Nos. 2 and 3** are incorrect because this phenomenon results in decreased cardiac output despite increased diastolic filling time, coronary artery blood flow, and stroke volume with each ventricular contraction. **No. 4** is incorrect because the decreased cardiac output results in stimulation of circulatory reflexes to increase venous return, which produces peripheral vasoconstriction, the cause of the patient's pallor and diaphoresis. **AN,6,PhI**

10. **(3)** Depending on the hospital, this is a physician's decision, especially in cases where the fetus, as well as the mother, may be in danger. **No. 1** is incorrect because time may not permit a physician *referral* to occur. **No. 2** is incorrect because although some hospitals and/or physicians require childbirth classes as a prerequisite to attending the birth, others do not require it. **No. 4** is incorrect because it is an inappropriate nursing action without a physician's approval. **IMP,7,HPM**

11. **(3)** The apnea monitor will sound an alarm during any periods of apnea to warn the parents or caretakers. **No. 1** is incorrect. Although the alarm may startle the infant and stimulate breathing, it should not be relied on for this function. **No. 2** is incorrect because the monitor screen displays the infant's respirations (and pulse, with some monitors) but not temperature. **No. 4** is incorrect because the monitor will not maintain the infant's respirations. **IMP,2,SECE**

12. **(4)** To repeat the breathing exercises until the patient is light-headed is inappropriate. It indicates hyperventilation, which may lead to tetany due to loss of volatile hydrogen ions. Patients *should,* however, be able to supply a rationale for deep breathing and coughing techniques **(No. 1)**, as well as demonstrate them correctly **(No. 2)**. **No. 3** is also a desirable outcome. **EV,6,SECE**

13. **(1)** The patient's pH is within normal range (pH 7.35–7.45). Therefore even though the serum bicarbonate level is reduced, indicating metabolic acidosis, the lungs have been able to excrete enough CO_2 to keep the total pH within normal range. **No. 2** is incorrect because P_{CO_2} in hyperventilation is reduced (<40 mm Hg), but serum bicarbonate levels are usually normal. **No. 3** is incorrect because a pH *below* 7.35 would represent uncompensated metabolic acidosis. **No. 4** is incorrect because in alveolar hypoventilation the P_{CO_2} is elevated and the condition of respiratory acidosis exists. **EV,6,PhI**

14. **(1)** Lead poisoning primarily affects the CNS, causing increased intracranial pressure. This results in irritability and changes in level of consciousness, as well as seizure disorders, hyperactivity, and learning disabilities. **No. 2** is incorrect because lead poisoning may affect the GI tract and cause constipation, *not* diarrhea. **No. 3** is incorrect because lead poisoning may also

cause anemia and tachycardia, *not* bradycardia. **No. 4** is incorrect because lead poisoning does not cause bleeding tendencies. **AS,1,PhI**

15. **(4)** Although reducing environmental stimuli and activity is necessary for a woman with mild preeclampsia, she will most probably have bathroom privileges. **No. 1** is incorrect because her vital signs and fetal heart rate and rhythm should be assessed at least once per shift during the time she is awake. **No. 2** is incorrect because her daily weight is an indicator of her response to treatment and loss of edema. **No. 3** is incorrect because deep-tendon reflexes assist in assessing the degree of CNS hyperirritability. **IMP,6,SECE**

16. **(2)** The purpose of a tracheostomy is to provide more controlled ventilation and to ease removal of respiratory secretions. When long-term therapy is indicated, it reduces or prevents respiratory fatigue. A tracheostomy is done when intubation is necessary for longer than 3–5 days, when the patient is unable to handle respiratory secretions, or if there is upper-airway obstruction. **No. 1** is incorrect because although anxiety will be decreased when ventilation is improved, this is not the primary purpose for a tracheostomy. **No. 3** is incorrect because desired effects of improving ventilation include improved cerebral oxygenation. **No. 4** is incorrect because a side effect of tracheostomy is increased risk of pulmonary infection, which is not true in the case of endotracheal intubation, though both may cause injury to mucous membranes. **PL,6,PhI**

17. **(4)** Acknowledging her presence and discomfort is most important to provide emotional support. **No. 1** is incorrect: Privacy is important if she requests it; however, assuming that she wants to be isolated may cause feelings of rejection and loneliness. **No. 2** is incorrect because an assessment of her overall level of functioning and coping abilities needs to be performed *before* any medication is prescribed. It is also the doctor's decision to give medication. **No. 3** is incorrect: Such a decision needs to be discussed with her. **IMP,7,PsI**

18. **(3)** Tight pressure dressing, discomfort, and fear of tearing the incision tend to limit chest expansion and the patient's willingness to cough. The nurse can assist the patient in this procedure by helping her sit upright and by supporting (with her hand) both the anterior and the posterior chest wall at the incisional site. Frequent turning will also facilitate mobilization of secretion and the prevention of atelectasis. **No. 1** is incorrect because the dressing is on the chest wall and will not interfere with body alignment. **No. 2** is incorrect because arm exercises initially will be isometric and can be done with the dressing in place. **No. 4** is incorrect because vital signs should be checked on the *inoperative* arm. **EV,6,PhI**

19. **(1)** A local hypersensitivity reaction is angioedema, a redness and swelling. **No. 2** is incorrect because cardiovascular collapse is a systemic reaction. **No. 3** is incorrect because nausea with vomiting and diarrhea represents a systemic reaction. **No. 4** is incorrect because asthmalike symptoms also represent a systemic reaction. **AS,1,SECE**

20. **(1)** According to Nägele's rule (LMP − 3 months + 7 days), the calculations would be: 7/10 − 3 months = 4/10 + 7 days = 4/17. Nägele's rule assumes that the woman has a 28-day cycle and that pregnancy occurred on the fourteenth day. If the woman's cycle is longer or shorter than 28 days, appropriate adjustments must be made. Only about 4–5% of women give birth on the EDB plus or minus 7 days. (*Hint:* A simpler method is,

from the LMP, to count forward 9 months and add 7 days.) **Nos. 2, 3, and 4** are incorrect calculations. **AN,5,HPM**

21. **(3)** If the IV infusion was at the prescribed rate of 35 mL/hour for 4½ hours, from 7:00 A.M. to 11:30 A.M., 35 mL × 4.5 hours = 157.5 mL absorbed. If 500 mL was hung at 7:00 A.M., and approximately 160 mL was infused, 500 − 160 = 340 mL left in the bag at 11:30 A.M. **Nos. 1 and 2** are incorrect calculations. **No. 4** is incorrect; see above calculation. **EV,6,SECE**

22. **(3)** The patient may perceive this as avoidance, but it is more important to redirect back to the patient, especially in light of the manipulative behaviors of drug abusers and adolescents. **Nos. 1 and 4** are incorrect because they provide information about the nurse's personal life that is irrelevant to the maintenance of a therapeutic relationship. **No. 2** is incorrect because it plays into the patient's manipulation. **IMP,7,PsI**

23. **(4)** Amniotic fluid is alkaline, which makes litmus paper turn blue. **No. 1** is incorrect because the fluid is usually milky or opaque with small white flecks (vernix caseosa), not clear. **No. 2** is incorrect because no offensive odor is usually apparent. **No. 3** is incorrect because most fluid has a thin consistency, not thick. **EV,6,HPM**

24. **(3)** Although some complete or partial amputations may result from trauma **(No. 1)**, the majority are necessitated by arteriosclerosis obliterans. **No. 2** is incorrect because long-standing complications of diabetes mellitus are peripheral vascular insufficiency and infections, which in turn may increase the likelihood of amputation. **No. 4** is incorrect because bone tumors, particularly of the knee, necessitate amputation less often than arteriosclerosis obliterans. **AN,3,PhI**

25. **(1)** Initially, the nurse must obtain more information about the patient's pain prior to giving medication. **No. 2** is incorrect because if the pain were due to compression of the leg by a cast that is too tight, medicating the patient could result in serious neurovascular complications. **Nos. 3 and 4** are incorrect because offering reassurance or distraction is not appropriate at this time, or a sufficient nursing intervention. **IMP,3,PhI**

26. **(3)** Diazepam is a CNS depressant, and in children and elderly adults, it may depress the respiratory center. Thus, when the patient returns to the unit, the nurse should first evaluate respirations. **Nos. 1, 2, and 4** are incorrect. After determining that the patient is breathing adequately, the nurse can then evaluate the temperature, pulse, and blood pressure. **EV,1,SECE**

27. **(3)** Many times the physiologic response to stress may be a decrease in milk production. This may rectify itself over time, provided the anxiety is controlled. However, as long as the system is under prolonged, intense stress, the milk supply will probably remain diminished. **Nos. 1 and 4** are incorrect because the nurse does not have physiologic evidence to substantiate the probability of a virus or of occluded lactation ducts. **No. 2** is incorrect because the surviving infant is probably too young to react physiologically to the twin's death. However, it is possible that the infant is experiencing some emotional trauma in response both to the increase in familial tension and to not hearing or seeing the other twin. **IMP,5,HPM**

28. **(1)** Pyloric stenosis is a congenital anatomic defect that the infant is born with, although symptoms may take several weeks to develop. **No. 2** is incorrect because pyloric stenosis is not acquired due to a formula allergy. **No. 3** is incorrect because pyloric stenosis does not de-

velop after birth. **No. 4** is incorrect because the presence of pyloric stenosis is well known before surgery. **IMP,4,PhI**

29. **(1)** Morphine sulfate acts on subcortical brain levels not only to inhibit perception of pain and to decrease apprehension and anxiety by inducing euphoria, but also to decrease sympathetic nervous system stimulation, thereby reducing peripheral arterial resistance and increasing venous capacitance. A side effect of this last action is hypotension. **No. 2** is incorrect because morphine reduces arterial resistance. **No. 3** is incorrect because a second side effect of morphine is respiratory *depression*. **No. 4** is incorrect because it describes actions directly opposite to the effects of morphine. **PL,6,PhI**

30. **(4)** In this case the nurse's calm, assured manner would be most therapeutic. It would serve to decrease the couple's anxiety and to facilitate an effective admission, labor, and birth. **No. 1** is incorrect because the couple's anxiety level would probably interfere with effective learning at this time. However, reinforcing any previously learned material and answering questions may be used. **No. 2** is incorrect because although the woman is in active labor, she is not ready to give birth at this time. **No. 3** is incorrect because assessing the couple's level of preparation would be done in conjunction with answering questions. It would be more important to assess their level of readiness rather than preparation at this time. **IMP,5,HPM**

31. **(2)** In selecting the correct needle to administer an IM injection to a preschool child, the nurse should always look at the child and use judgment in evaluating muscle mass and amount of subcutaneous fat. In this case, in the absence of further data, the nurse would be most correct in selecting a needle gauge and length appropriate for the "average" preschool child. A medium-gauge needle (21 G) that is 1 in. long would be most appropriate. **No. 1** is incorrect because a ⅝ in. needle would be too short. A 25 G needle would be too thin to use on most preschool children. **No. 3** is incorrect because an 18 G needle would be too large (wide) to use on most preschool children and would be better suited for a school-age child or an adolescent. **No. 4** is incorrect because a 1½-in. needle would be too long. An 18 G needle would also be too large (wide) to use on most preschool children and would be better suited for a school-age child or an adolescent. **IMP,1,SECE**

32. **(1)** Before beginning any teaching plan, the nurse must assess the patient's current understanding of the procedure, as well as his or her interest and ability to comprehend different facets of it. The physician has generally given the patient an outline of the facts as to why the procedure is necessary. **No. 2** is incorrect because the patient's husband, wife, or significant others may be invited to join the teaching session *if* the clinical situation allows; otherwise they should be informed separately. **No. 3** is incorrect because several intervening variables, such as anxiety and decreased cerebral perfusion, may be affecting the patient's ability to absorb information. Therefore, it is frequently necessary not only to reinforce information given by the physician but also to reexplain the procedure. **No. 4** is incorrect because *following* explanations of the procedure, the operative permit is signed, thereby assuring *informed* consent. **IMP,7,SECE**

33. **(3)** When the patient knows what to expect or who will care for her on return from the operating room, anxiety decreases. **No. 1** is incorrect because it would be diffi-

cult for the patient to relax in high Fowler's position, and at this time there is no documented evidence of respiratory distress. **No. 2** is incorrect because the patient may be drowsy but may not be asleep. Assuring her that she will be asleep gives her false information. **No. 4** is incorrect because the patient should void *before* medication is given, not after. **IMP,1,PhI**

34. **(1)** When cardiac catheterization is performed, a cutdown must be performed on a major artery in either an arm or a leg; thus, essential nursing care following this procedure involves checking the pulse in the affected extremity to be sure there is adequate circulation. **No. 2** is incorrect because following cardiac catheterization, during which the patient does not receive anesthesia, deep breathing is unnecessary and coughing is contraindicated, as it may cause hemorrhage at the cut-down site. **No. 3** is incorrect because there is no need to sedate the patient following this procedure, although bedrest for several hours is usually recommended. **No. 4** is incorrect because in general, cardiac catheterization should have little or no effect on urine output; therefore, there would be no specific need to monitor urine output. **IMP,1,SECE**

35. **(1)** After opening the airway by head tilt and chin lift, the nurse must look, listen, and feel for any movement of air. Often opening the airway may be all that is needed. Giving two breaths **(No. 2)** is done after establishing breathlessness, followed by checking the pulse **(No. 3)**. Finger sweeps **(No. 4)** are only done if ventilation is unsuccessful and back blows have been done. **IMP,1,SECE**

36. **(2)** The nurse should quickly turn the patient onto the left side, lowering the head of the bed to minimize the chance of air bubbles entering the cerebral circulation, and notify the physician. **No. 1** is incorrect because, alone, Trendelenburg is insufficient; the air must be trapped in the right ventricle (left-side position). **No. 3** is incorrect because turning the patient to the right side, head up, would facilitate movement of the air embolism through the circulation and potentially to the brain. **No. 4** is incorrect because supine, in high Fowler's position would facilitate movement of the air embolism through the circulation and potentially to the brain. **IMP,6,SECE**

37. **(1)** The woman is more apt to become irritable, uncooperative, and discouraged during the transitional phase. **Nos. 2 and 3** are incorrect because excitement and euphoria are associated with the latent phase, *not* the transitional phase. **No. 4** is incorrect because seriousness is associated with the active phase, *not* the transitional phase. **EV,5,HPM**

38. **(4)** Although the nurse suspects that this behavior may occur, there is no valid concern unless the couple's behavior becomes inappropriate. The nurse needs to realize that kissing is a normal part of adolescence. **No. 1** is incorrect because some privacy may be provided; however, periodic supervision is warranted because the patient is an adolescent. However, the patient still needs companionship. **No. 2** is incorrect because he needs to feel trusted in order to develop into an independent and mature person. **No. 2** serves only to highlight mistrust, and the couple may already feel that intimacy is inappropriate in this setting. **No. 3** is incorrect because privacy is needed, but with some supervision to promote responsible behavior. **IMP,7,PsI**

39. **(1)** Fresh fish with scales would be permitted on a mildly restricted (2 g) to an extremely restricted (200 mg) sodium diet. Only shellfish are restricted. **Nos. 2,**

3, and 4 are incorrect because foods to be avoided on a sodium-restricted diet include ethnic foods, particularly Chinese, which is usually prepared with soy sauce; commercially prepared soups, such as canned tomato soup; and hot dogs, which are a commercially prepared meat. **EV,4,PhI**

40. **(1)** During exercise there is a general increase in vaso-motor tone, which increases venous return. To meet the increased metabolic needs of the body, the heart normally increases its rate and stroke volume. In this patient's case, left ventricular hypertrophy has compromised his heart's ability to increase its efficiency during exercise. Therefore, even though his heart rate is increased, the stroke volume does not increase sufficiently, so the increased venous return tends to back up into the pulmonary vasculature. This results in the perception of increased work of breathing, or shortness of breath. **No. 2** is incorrect because venous return is increased with exercise. **No. 3** is incorrect because asynergistic cardiac contractions occur when a portion of the heart is noncontractile, as with myocardial infarction with ventricular aneurysm. **No. 4** is not correct because obesity and sedentary life-style are contributing factors to physiologic phenomena underlying his symptoms. **AN,6,PhI**

41. **(3)** The best approach in administering an injection to a preschooler is to give a short, simple explanation immediately before giving the injection, being truthful that it will hurt. This helps maintain the child's sense of trust in the nurse. **No. 1** is incorrect because the nurse should not rely on the mother to give an appropriate explanation. **No. 2** is incorrect because the nurse should not give the injection without telling the child anything. **No. 4** is incorrect because the nurse should not attempt to bribe the child. **IMP,5,PsI**

42. **(3)** Skin preps are designed primarily to reduce the occurrence of postoperative infections by reducing the number of microorganisms on the skin and by removing any hair that may tend to harbor these organisms. **No. 1** is incorrect because cleaning excess oils and hairs is a *secondary* objective of a skin prep. **No. 2** is incorrect because skin preps do *not* sterilize the skin or kill all the microorganisms. **No. 4** is incorrect because providing a clear field is a *secondary* objective of a skin prep. **PL,1,SECE**

43. **(1)** It is of paramount importance to prevent the patient from hurting himself or herself or others. **No. 2** is incorrect because the nurse cannot establish a trusting relationship at this time since the patient is unable to communicate effectively. **No. 3** is incorrect because the patient cannot be oriented to time, place, and person until he or she is able to communicate. **No. 4** is incorrect because to isolate the patient is only one aspect of maintaining a safe environment, which will prevent the patient from harming others, as well as protect the patient from overstimulation. **PL,2,PsI**

44. **(3)** Patients with permanent pacemakers are cautioned to avoid all sources of high electronic output because they may cause pacemaker malfunction. Other sources of high electronic output include older, noninsulated microwave ovens, running car engines, and dental drills. **Nos. 1 and 4** are incorrect because activities such as swimming and golf can be resumed usually after 5 weeks. **No. 2** is incorrect because creative hobbies such as fashioning lamps are indicated as long as precautions are taken to avoid electrical shocks. **IMP,6,SECE**

45. **(1)** The patient is kept NPO until shock and bleeding are controlled. Often a nasogastric tube is inserted to drain off blood and to provide a route for antacid therapy. **No. 2** is incorrect because a liquid diet is started after shock and bleeding have been controlled. **No. 3** is incorrect because a soft, bland diet is started after a liquid diet has begun. **No. 4** is incorrect because milk is not given; it increases gastric acid production. **IMP,4,PhI**

46. **(2)** The "formula" for determining parity is *TPAL: T* is the number of *t*erm pregnancies (38+ weeks); *P* is the number of *p*reterm pregnancies (20–37 weeks); *A* is the number of *a*bortions (pregnancies that do not reach viability, 20–22 weeks' gestation); *L* is the number of *l*iving children. This woman's first pregnancy ended in abortion and she has no living children. Her parity is T = 0, P = 0, A = 1, L = 0; or 0-0-1-0. **Nos. 1, 3, and 4** are not correct according to this formula. **AN,5,HPM**

47. **(2)** One-person or two-person CPR for adults is done at a minimum rate of 80 compressions per minute (up to a rate of 100). Sixty compressions per minute (**No. 1**) is no longer considered adequate in CPR. **Nos. 3 and 4** are both within the range of acceptable rates; however, the question asks for the *minimum* rate. **IMP,6,SECE**

48. **(4)** Following an appendectomy, the nurses' notes in the patient's chart should include the dressing changes, input and output, and return of bowel sounds. **No. 1** is incorrect because dumping syndrome is not a common complication following an appendectomy. **No. 2** is incorrect: Mouth care and dressing changes should be noted but are not as critical as charting input and output and bowel sounds. **No. 3** is incorrect: Following a ruptured appendectomy, a patient will be NPO initially and then gradually advanced; a low-residue diet is not routine. **IMP,8,SECE**

49. **(3)** Lidocaine is the treatment of choice in this situation. Ventricular tachycardia is a serious arrhythmia. It must be treated at once because (a) it may compromise cardiac output and (b) it is considered a precursor of ventricular fibrillation. **No. 1** is incorrect because standing coronary care unit orders generally cover the administration of lidocaine in this situation, so it is not necessary to notify the physician to obtain a verbal order. **No. 2** is incorrect because O_2 flow rate is increased only if clinical signs indicate the patient is in distress, which is unlikely with a short burst of ventricular tachycardia. **No. 4** is incorrect because recent research data indicate that morphine sulfate may stabilize the threshold for ventricular fibrillation, but it is not the drug of choice in this situation. **IMP,6,PhI**

50. **(2)** SIDS occurs most frequently in low-birthweight, preterm infants, and in the lower, not middle (**No. 3**), socioeconomic groups. **No. 1** is incorrect because SIDS occurs most frequently in blacks and Native Americans, not whites. **No. 4** is incorrect because SIDS has a lower incidence in breastfed infants. **AS,5,HPM**

51. **(2)** Elevation of 20–30 degrees is the optimum position to reduce intracranial pressure, aid venous drainage from the brain, and facilitate respiration. **No. 1** is incorrect because flat on the back may increase the chance of aspiration. A lateral or semiprone position may be indicated in the early postoperative period if there are no signs of cerebral edema. **Nos. 3 and 4** are incorrect because they may increase the amount of hip flexion and can contribute to an increase in intracranial pressure. **PL,2,SECE**

52. **(1)** Providing reassurance that it is normal for most people to fear the unknown may bolster the husband's

confidence. If more time were available, the nurse would try to explore his fears and provide emotional support. **No. 2** is inappropriate because it provides false reassurance, which may merely increase his anxiety. **No. 3** is incorrect because it may stimulate feelings of guilt. **No. 4** is incorrect because it may not necessarily be true and may provide false reassurance. **IMP,7,PsI**

53. **(3)** The choice of anesthesia depends on the surgeon's choice and the patient's condition. **No. 1** is incorrect because IV regional blocks may not provide adequate blockage of impulses for this procedure, and the patient would be awake. **No. 2** is incorrect: Though a spinal anesthetic may be used, the sawing of the bone can be very distressing to the patient, so usually a general anesthetic is preferred. **No. 4** is incorrect because muscle relaxants are administered in conjunction with general anesthesia. **PL,1,SECE**

54. **(1)** The cast should be fully exposed to the air to help it dry properly. **No. 2** is incorrect because the patient should be turned every 2 hours to help the cast to dry, not remain in one position. **No. 3** is incorrect because the cast should be elevated and placed on pillows rather than a bedboard. **No. 4** is incorrect because the cast should be handled with the palms of the hands to avoid pressure and making indentations with the fingers. **PL,3,PhI**

55. **(4)** Weighing the patient and instituting intake and output records are admission procedures; therefore, they are the least important. **No. 1** is incorrect: Providing sedation to relieve anxiety and promote relaxation *is* a greater priority than weighing the patient and instituting records. **No. 2** is incorrect: Instituting arm and leg range-of-motion exercises *is* a greater priority than weighing and instituting records. **No. 3** is incorrect: Establishing an intravenous line *is* a greater priority than weighing the patient and instituting records. **PL,6,SECE**

56. **(3)** Pressure dressings are never removed **(No. 1)**, but if saturated, they should be reinforced with sterile dressings. The possibility of hemorrhage is ever-present, and signs of increased bleeding should be immediately reported to the surgeon. This is not a normal occurrence. Vital signs and Hemovac drainage and function should also be assessed. **No. 2** is incorrect: Hemovacs may be irrigated, but generally they are not milked. **No. 4** is incorrect because this is not a normal occurrence. **IMP,6,PhI**

57. **(2)** Providing and maintaining a patent airway and administering oxygen immediately are essential to establish regular respirations. **No. 1** is incorrect because CPR may not be necessary if respirations are adequately established. **No. 3** is incorrect because reassuring the parents is not appropriate now. No one can accurately predict the outcome at this point. **No. 4** is incorrect because checking the mother's chart for type of drug, amount, and time given is more appropriately the job of a second staff member in attendance. The neonate may be a candidate for naloxone HCl (Narcan). **IMP,6,SECE**

58. **(3)** Pre- and postsuctioning ventilation with 100% oxygen is important in reducing hypoxemia, which occurs when the flow of gases in the airway is obstructed by the suctioning catheter. **No. 1** is incorrect because it describes the nursing action while suctioning the patient with an *endotracheal* tube rather than a tracheal tube. **No. 2** is incorrect because it is a proper nursing action prior to suctioning the patient with an endotra-

cheal tube, *rather than* a tracheal tube. **No. 4** is incorrect; although it is a correct nursing procedure prior to suctioning any patient, it does not *prevent* hypoxemia. **IMP,6,SECE**

59. **(2)** This response allows the couple to become informed without infringing on the physician's role. The physician can then decide either to inform the couple of the procedure to be used or to have the anesthesiologist inform them. **No. 1** is incorrect because time is limited and the physician may decide to inform the couple himself or herself. **Nos. 3 and 4** are incorrect because it is not the nurse's role to discuss anesthesia of choice. **IMP,3,HPM**

60. **(4)** In addition to the shock of the immediate crisis, the mother probably has never accepted the fact that her son was extensively involved with drugs. **No. 1** is incorrect because it will take time to develop as she takes in the implications of the situation. **No. 2** is incorrect because this is part of the shock process. **No. 3** is incorrect because acceptance is unrealistic at this time. **AS,7,PsI**

61. **(1)** In pyloric stenosis, the pyloric sphincter at the distal end of the stomach is thickened, or stenotic. This sphincter blocks the flow of formula into the small intestine, causing vomiting; it also blocks the flow of bile back into the stomach. Thus, the infant with pyloric stenosis characteristically vomits only stomach contents, not bile **(No. 2)**, blood **(No. 3)**, or feces **(No. 4)**. **AS,4,PhI**

62. **(1)** The primary nursing action would be to maintain a patent airway to ensure oxygen for the woman and fetus. **No. 2** is incorrect because although observing bowel and bladder functioning may also be important for a thorough assessment of the convulsion, it is of lower priority than providing a patent airway or ensuring safety. **No. 3** is incorrect: CPR may be needed if the woman progresses into cardiac arrest; however, in implementing CPR, maintaining a patent airway is again the foremost priority. **No. 4** is incorrect: Providing a safe environment is an important *second* priority. **PL,2,SECE**

63. **(2)** Although ECG changes can be utilized to identify the site, extent of changes, and acuteness of an infarct, the extent of the injury is usually approximated by the peak levels of serial enzymes (CPK, ALT [SGOT], LDH). Of these enzymes, CPK-MB or CPK2 gives the most specific information about the amount of myocardial necrosis. **No. 1** is incorrect because sinus tachycardia may result from a number of factors, including emotional responses and heart failure. **No. 3** is incorrect because the duration of chest pain is dependent not only on the extent of tissue ischemia but also on other factors, such as affective responses and muscle spasm. **No. 4** is incorrect because primary ventricular fibrillation does not indicate the extent of infarct; fibrillation occurs due to metabolic changes in the ischemic area. **AS,6,PhI**

64. **(2)** EDTA and BAL work by binding to the heavy metal lead and promoting its excretion via the kidneys. Renal toxicity may occur as a result. The nurse should force fluids and monitor kidney function carefully. The other choices are incorrect because calcium disodium edetate (EDTA) and dimercaprol (BAL) do not adversely affect the neurologic system **(No. 1)**, the cardiovascular system **(No. 3)**, or the hematologic system **(No. 4)**. **EV,8,PhI**

65. **(2)** Modified radical mastectomy consists of removal of the breast and all or selected lymph nodes with preser-

vation of the pectoralis major muscle. The other choices are incorrect because they are examples of a simple mastectomy (**No. 1**), classic radical mastectomy (**No. 3**), and supraradical mastectomy (**No. 4**). **AS,3,SECE**

66. (4) Being direct with the adolescent about this issue is extremely important because the incident violates hospital policy, the law, treatment, and parents' rules. The patient should be directly confronted and the incident discussed with the patient and the medical staff. The health team will decide whether it is in the patient's best interest to inform the parents and/or the police. **No. 1** is incorrect because avoidance will merely perpetuate the situation. **Nos. 2 and 3** are incorrect because whether to inform the police or the parents is a health team decision. **IMP,7,PsI**

67. (4) The day following surgery, the patient who has had an above-the-knee (AK) amputation is turned on his or her abdomen for a short period. Thereafter, he or she is turned to the prone position at least three times daily. While in this position, the patient should practice push-up exercises that strengthen arm and shoulder muscles, thereby facilitating both transfer procedures and preparation for crutch walking. **No. 1** is incorrect; sandbags or blanket rolls are used after this surgery to *prevent* outward rotation of the stump. **No. 2** is incorrect because hyperextension of the thigh and stump is encouraged for patients with *below-the-knee* amputations only. Patients with AK amputations may perform this exercise only on medical orders, as it tends to put undue stress on the suture line. **No. 3** is incorrect because the patient is taught at a later time to lift the buttocks and stump off the bed while in a supine position, an exercise that develops abdominal muscles necessary for stabilizing the pelvis when the patient stoops or bends. **IMP,3,SECE**

68. (3) The purpose of restraints for this child is to keep him from scratching the affected areas. Mitten restraints would prevent him from scratching, while allowing him the most movement permissible. **No. 1** is incorrect because clove-hitch restraints would needlessly restrict the toddler's movements. **No. 2** is incorrect because elbow restraints are generally inappropriate for children with eczema, as the inner aspect of the arm is usually affected. **No. 4** is incorrect because a posey jacket would not prevent the child from scratching the affected areas. **IMP,1,PhI**

69. (2) Contractions may affect the pulse, BP, and respiratory rate. If possible, take vital signs between contractions. **No. 1** is incorrect because immediately prior to a contraction the mother is usually very excited and apprehensive. **No. 3** is incorrect because after a contraction she may feel more comfortable, but her vital signs may be altered due to the contraction itself. **No. 4** is incorrect because if the nurse waits for the mother to feel totally comfortable, she or he may never be able to assess the maternal vital signs. **PL,5,HPM**

70. (1) The definitive diagnosis of intussusception is based on a barium enema, which clearly demonstrates the telescoping of the bowel wall, which blocks the flow of the barium. **No. 2** is incorrect because although a secondary effect may be a nonsurgical reduction of the telescoping (which may occur due to hydrostatic pressure), this is uncertain and is not the main reason the procedure is performed. **Nos. 3 and 4** are incorrect because a barium enema is not administered to ease the passage of stool or provide symptomatic relief. **IMP,8,SECE**

71. (3) These are common symptoms of pregnancy. Eighty percent of pregnant women experience breast tingling sensation during the first few weeks of gestation. **No. 1** is incorrect because quickening usually is not perceived until the sixteenth to eighteenth week of gestation. **No. 2** is incorrect because lightening usually occurs about 2 weeks before labor in the nullipara, and with the onset of labor in subsequent pregnancies. **No. 4** is incorrect because nausea and vomiting are not necessarily experienced by all women. **AS,5,HPM**

72. (2) Before any operative procedure can proceed, however minor, a voluntary, informed consent must be given. **No. 1** is incorrect: The nurse's *third* step is to check the time and the type of preoperative medication. **No. 3** is incorrect because before the nurse initiates preoperative care, charts should be checked *first* for operative consent and *second* for laboratory results, noting any abnormalities. **No. 4** is incorrect: The nurse must verify an informed consent in the chart *prior to* checking to be sure the patient has been placed on the NPO list. Once done, it is followed up by checking for the sign on the patient's bed when the nurse goes to help the patient prepare. **IMP,7,SECE**

73. (2) Hypotension is even more severe when there has been bleeding. **No. 1** is incorrect because one of the advantages of spinal anesthesia is that it causes very little fetal depression. **No. 3** is incorrect because if administered properly, *very little* anesthesia should cross the placenta. **No. 4** is incorrect because it is *irrelevant* unless the mother has an adverse reaction to the anesthesia. **AN,6,SECE**

74. (3) There are no definite answers, as there are many possible causes of drug abuse. Many times not even the abuser can say why he or she began using drugs. **No. 1** is incorrect because although peer pressure may be a contributing factor, the nurse lacks validation. **No. 2** is incorrect because inappropriate limits is an invalidated assumption that would need to be explored further. **No. 4** is incorrect because although feelings of isolation and of being unloved may be contributing factors, the nurse again lacks validation. **IMP,7,PsI**

75. (1) If the IV infuses at the proper rate, 110 mL per hour, from 2:30 A.M. to 6:00 A.M., 110 mL × 3.5 hours = 385 mL infused. **Nos. 2, 3, and 4** are incorrect calculations. **EV,6,SECE**

76. (1) If the alarm sounds, the parents should always respond immediately. **No. 2** is incorrect because they should first check the infant's breathing and, if the infant is not breathing, they must start CPR immediately to prevent brain damage. However, if the infant is breathing normally when the alarm sounds, then something technical is responsible for the alarm, and it would be inappropriate to begin CPR. **No. 3** is incorrect because having to remain with the infant at all times would defeat the alarm's purpose. The adult can leave the room if the infant is being monitored correctly. **No. 4** is incorrect because in terms of follow-up care, the physician and/or emergency room should be contacted, but only after the apnea has been successfully resolved; it is *not* appropriate to call the emergency room *while* the infant is apneic. **IMP,2,SECE**

77. (2) Anesthesia is divided into four stages. Most surgical procedures are carried out in Stage III, during which time the patient is unconscious and reflexes are depressed. As the patient eliminates the anesthetic agent, she or he goes into Stage II, which is the stage of delirium or excitement. Respirations are exaggerated and irregular, and muscle tone is increased. To

prevent injury during this stage, nursing measures are designed to reduce stimulation by maintaining a quiet, well-regulated environment. **No. 1** is incorrect because continued stimulation will only increase restlessness. **No. 3** is incorrect because pain medication may delay elimination of the anesthetic secondary to decreased respiratory excursion. **No. 4** is incorrect because while nailbeds should always be checked for signs of hypoxia, cyanosis only occurs with severe respiratory *depression*. **IMP,3,SECE**

78. **(1)** An early indication of cardiac decompensation is tachycardia. Therefore, the patient's vital signs, mentation, and pulmonary status should be assessed to rule out this complication of myocardial infarction. Other causes of tachycardia are hypovolemia, anxiety, and pain. Assessment of pain and emotional status can be determined during cognitive assessment. **Nos. 2, 3, and 4** are incorrect because actions such as encouraging verbalization of feelings, administering oxygen, and decreasing the rate of intravenous infusion will be determined by the nurse's assessment of vital signs. **IMP,6,PhI**

79. **(3)** Signs and symptoms of a hemolytic reaction usually include chills, shaking, fever, red (or black) urine, headache, and flank pain. **No. 1** is incorrect because urticaria is not a common sign in a hemolytic reaction, although it is common with an allergic reaction. **Nos. 2 and 4** are incorrect because neither polyuria nor hypothermia is a common sign in a hemolytic reaction. **AS,6,PhI**

80. **(2)** Both atropine and isoproterenol (Isuprel) are kept available in the preoperative period as drugs of choice should the ventricular rate decrease further. Isoproterenol enhances pacemaker automaticity and facilitates AV conduction in heart block. Atropine acts to enhance AV conduction by inhibiting parasympathetic nervous system innervation of the AV node. **No. 1** is incorrect because lidocaine is an antiarrhythmic utilized to depress myocardial automaticity. Therefore, this drug would not be indicated should the patient's ventricular rate decrease in the preinsertion period. **No. 3** is incorrect because digoxin enhances vagal stimulation of the AV node, decreasing conduction through the node, and therefore would not be indicated should the patient's ventricular rate decrease in the preinsertion period. **No. 4** is incorrect because propranolol is a beta-blocker that depresses cardiac contractility and heart rate. This drug would not be indicated should the patient's ventricular rate decrease in the preinsertion period. **PL,6,PhI**

81. **(3)** Bryant's traction is a form of skin traction used in infants and toddlers with fractured femurs; when applied correctly, adhesive material should be taped to the skin of both legs. **Nos. 1 and 2** are incorrect because skeletal traction in the form of a Kirschner wire or Steinmann pin is not used in Bryant's traction. **No. 4** is incorrect because adhesive material should be taped to the skin of both legs, not one leg. **AS,3,SECE**

82. **(2)** Positive pregnancy test results are considered among the *probable* signs of pregnancy (with the exception of the bioassay test for the beta subunit of HCG, which is accurate). **Nos. 1, 3, and 4** are incorrect because hearing fetal heart sounds, feeling fetal movements, and seeing the fetus are all *positive* signs of pregnancy, not probable signs. **IMP,5,HPM**

83. **(1)** Bland feedings should be given in small amounts on a frequent basis to neutralize the hydrochloric acid and to prevent overload. **No. 2** is incorrect because

clear liquids may not control the amount of acid in the stomach, would be monotonous, and may lack all the necessary nutrients. **No. 3** is incorrect because a regular diet may overload the system. **No. 4** is incorrect: NPO would promote the production of free acid in the stomach and increase the symptoms. **PL,4,PhI**

84. **(4)** This response does not contradict the patient's perceptions, is honest, and shows empathy. **No. 1** is incorrect because it "humors" the patient and is dishonest and nontherapeutic. **No. 2** is incorrect because it makes fun of the patient. **No. 3** is incorrect because it avoids the situation and makes the patient feel that the nurse does not care. **IMP,2,PsI**

85. **(3)** Dentures, hairpins, and combs need to be removed. Nail polish needs to be removed so cyanosis can be easily monitored by observing nailbeds. **No. 1** is incorrect because the wedding band is taped securely to the finger, not removed. **No. 2** is incorrect because in the short time available before surgery, although the patient should be allowed to voice concerns and should be given any needed support, time will not permit an extensive exploration of the basis of the patient's concerns. **No. 4** is incorrect because the patient should void prior to receiving medication, not afterward. **IMP,1,SECE**

86. **(1)** Hypertensive patients should be cautioned to make position changes slowly to prevent intermittent postural hypotension. **No. 2** is incorrect because alcohol may contribute to hypotension, not prevent it. **No. 3** is incorrect because cold causes vasoconstriction, not vasodilation associated with hypotension. **No. 4** is incorrect because exercise will increase, not decrease vasodilation. **IMP,6,PhI**

87. **(3)** Atropine is a cholinergic blocker (parasympatholytic) used preoperatively to diminish secretions and to block cardiac vagal reflexes. Normal side effects include dry mouth; hot, dry, flushed skin; and tachycardia or palpitations. Thus, the patient can be safely told that these are normal, expected effects of atropine; in fact, this probably should have been included in the preop instructions, before the patient even received the medication. **No. 1** is incorrect because it would be unnecessary to administer the atropine antidote, which is physostigmine salicylate. **No. 2** is incorrect because it would be inappropriate to bathe the patient at this time. **No. 4** is incorrect because it would be unnecessary to page the surgeon. **EV,1,SECE**

88. **(3)** The actual size of the breasts is not as important as the amount of glandular tissue, because it is not the adipose tissue but the secreting tissues of the mammary glands that produce the milk. **Nos. 1 and 2** are incorrect responses because adequate diet and rest *are* essential to promoting lactation. **No. 4** is incorrect because she may ovulate and could become pregnant while lactating. **EV,4,HPM**

89. **(2)** Having the legs elevated (20 degrees) in a straight line, and the trunk horizontal, improves venous return to the heart and prevents abdominal viscera from impinging on the diaphragm. **No. 1** is incorrect because oxygen administration may have a palliative effect but does not affect venous return. **No. 3** is incorrect because the Trendelenburg position, after initially increasing blood flow to the brain, initiates a reflex mechanism that causes cerebral vasoconstriction. **No. 4** is incorrect: Wrapping the patient in blankets will cause dilatation of the peripheral vasculature, which will further decrease venous return. **IMP,6,PhI**

90. **(1)** To prevent exacerbating the eczema, it is generally recommended that the child wear pure, natural cotton clothing only. **Nos. 2, 3, and 4** are incorrect because linen, wool, and polyester blends are more likely to cause worsening of the eczema. **IMP,1,PhI**

91. **(3)** Enemas are not administered when there is vaginal bleeding or preterm labor or when the fetus is in an abnormal presentation or position. **No. 1** is incorrect for the same reason. **No. 2** is incorrect: Soapsuds enemas are contraindicated because they are potentially dangerous due to their physiologic incompatibility with the lower gastrointestinal tract. **No. 4** is incorrect: Though the fetal position needs to be assessed prior to administering an enema, enemas are not administered in these circumstances. **IMP,1,SECE**

92. **(3)** Broken ribs may occur *even with proper CPR technique,* particularly when performed on the elderly. The nurse should check that the hands are positioned properly, then continue CPR even if the cracking continues. Broken ribs will heal, whereas stopping compressions **(No. 1)** will likely result in the patient's death. Compressing less than the standard of 1½ to 2 in. **(No. 2)** will be ineffective on an adult. Individual strength **(No. 4)** is irrelevant; proper hand position and depth are essential for anyone doing CPR. **EV,1,SECE**

93. **(2)** This response is open-ended and will elicit the most information. **No. 1** is incorrect because it merely provides false reassurance and trivializes her feelings. **No. 3** is incorrect: Although it may be a therapeutic response, it is a short-term intervention unless the nurse consistently sits with the woman for a while every day. If possible, the same nurse should be assigned to her each day. **No. 4** is an inappropriate nursing intervention because the nurse *can* work in conjunction with the physician to provide psychological support. **IMP,7,PsI**

94. **(4)** Periodic checks on pacemaker function are essential and may be accomplished by pulse taking, frequent ECGs, or telephone transmission of ECG. Generally rate changes greater than $+/-15$ beats should be reported to the physician; so should symptoms such as syncope, dizziness, hiccoughs (diaphragmatic stimulation), dyspnea, chest pain, and fluid retention. **No. 1** is incorrect because it is incomplete. The patient must also report rate changes and symptoms. **No. 2** is incorrect because drainage and discoloration refer to indicators of infection. **No. 3** is incorrect: Although estimating battery life indicates that the patient understands the battery pack has a limited life expectancy, the answer is incomplete. **EV,6,PhI**

95. **(1)** This is the most appropriate and honest response. However, it is essential to answer the question clearly, without stimulating unnecessary fear. **No. 2** is incorrect because there is no way to guarantee the birth of a healthy infant. Furthermore, the woman smoked early in her pregnancy, the period of organogenesis when the conceptus is most susceptible to teratogenic effects. **No. 3** is incorrect: There is no way to absolutely validate this. **No. 4** is incorrect because there are no definitive data to support such a claim. **IMP,1,SECE**

96. **(4)** In the three-point gait, both crutches and the affected "bad" leg and foot are moved together, with the unaffected "good" leg and foot following. **Nos. 1 and 2** are incorrect because the crutches are both moved simultaneously, not independently. **No. 3** is incorrect because the patient should not bear any weight on the fractured leg when using the three-point gait. **IMP,3,HPM**

97. **(1)** The airway tube should remain in place and the patient's head should be turned to the side to prevent obstruction of the airway by the tongue and to allow secretions to drain from the mouth. **No. 2** is incorrect because the head is not turned to the side. **Nos. 3 and 4** are incorrect because the airway tube should never be removed until the patient is alert enough to begin attempting to eject it. Leaving the airway tube in after this point may cause vomiting due to stimulation of the gag reflex. **IMP,6,SECE**

98. **(3)** Attempting to control the situation and do as he pleases is most likely his primary goal, in light of his history of drug abuse. Bending the rules for a severe violation of hospital policy, his treatment, and the law is not justified. For **No. 1** to be correct, the nurse would need further evidence of the patient's desire to change, such as overt, consistent changes in his pattern of behavior and open verbalization of his feelings. **Nos. 2 and 4** are incorrect because they are aspects of manipulation. **AN,7,PsI**

99. **(4)** Tachycardia decreases diastole, which decreases ventricular filling time and stroke volume. A significant decrease in stroke volume will result in a concomitant fall in cardiac output and tissue perfusion. Decreased cerebral perfusion and cellular hypoxia will result in signs of increased restlessness, anxiety, apprehension, and irritability. **No. 1** is incorrect because to prime the pump, venous return is enhanced by the activation of circulatory reflexes, not depressed. **No. 2** is incorrect because tachycardia is the result of increased sympathetic nervous system stimulation of the heart and may result in the patient's awareness of his or her heartbeat, thus increasing anxiety. **No. 3** is incorrect because decreased cardiac output and tissue perfusion only occur at very high rates or when myocardial contractility is compromised, as with myocardial infarction. **EV,6,PhI**

100. **(2)** Down syndrome is due to chromosomal aberration and, although trisomy 21 is more common in infants of older women, another form, mosaicism, occurs in pregnancies of women of all ages. **No. 1** is incorrect because an extra chromosome *is* implicated in the development of Down syndrome. **No. 3** is incorrect because amniocentesis at or after 16 weeks' gestation *can* successfully identify the presence of this abnormality. **No. 4** is incorrect because varying degrees of mental retardation *do* accompany Down syndrome. **EV,5,HPM**

101. **(1)** Above-the-knee amputations are often necessary because of the extent of the disease. The most critical factor in determining the level of the amputation is the adequacy of the arterial blood supply. **No. 2** is incorrect because it describes the advantages associated with a below-the-knee amputation. **No. 3** is incorrect because an above-the-knee amputation requires *more* energy for rehabilitation and walking. **No. 4** is incorrect because a below-the-knee amputation not only heals faster than does an above-the-knee amputation, but it is less painful postsurgically, less psychologically disturbing, and less prone to contractures. **IMP,6,PhI**

102. **(2)** Suction is applied only after the catheter is in place and ready for withdrawal. Applying suction intermittently, as well as rotating the suction catheter, assist in reducing the negative pressure effects of suctioning. Suctioning should be limited to periods of 10–15 seconds. **Nos. 1, 3, and 4** are incorrect because of the negative effects these actions would have on patient aeration. **IMP,6,SECE**

103. **(2)** Wiggling the toes indicates that the motor block caused by the spinal is wearing off. However, the autonomic block is still present, and the woman may experience hypotension (not hypertension, **No. 4**). **No. 1** is incorrect because the autonomic block is still present even though the effects of the anesthesia are wearing off. **No. 3** is incorrect because wiggling the toes indicates that the motor block caused by the spinal is wearing off, and is therefore not meaningless. **No. 4** is incorrect because the woman may experience hypotension. **EV,2,PhI**

104. **(3)** The most effective intervention to help preschoolers cope with painful experiences during hospitalization is to offer the opportunity for therapeutic play with puppets or dolls and medical equipment. This type of play experience allows the child to "act out" his frustrations and anger in a safe, controlled manner, enabling him to work through his feelings about a difficult experience. **Nos. 1, 2, and 4** are incorrect because playing with his own toys, engaging in free play, and playing with other children are not as effective as offering an opportunity for therapeutic play. **IMP,5,PsI**

105. **(2)** Low Fowler's to semi-Fowler's position with the arm elevated on pillows so that the wrist and elbow are slightly higher than the shoulder best facilitates venous return, reducing the occurrence of edema. Some physicians may order that the patient be positioned so that the hand is raised above the head. **Nos. 1, 3, and 4** are incorrect because venous return is not enhanced, or muscle contractures may possibly develop. **IMP,6,SECE**

106. **(3)** The treatment of drug abuse is only effective if the client is motivated to make changes in style and pattern of living. Although the hazards of drugs (**No. 1**), the fact that using drugs is illegal (**No. 2**), and developing alternative coping mechanisms (**No. 4**) are all significant components to be incorporated in health teaching, the client must first be motivated to learn. **PL,7,PsI**

107. **(1)** After marking the original dressing (to indicate the extent of the bleeding) and reinforcing the dressing (to prevent infection), the nurse should check the vital signs to determine if the bleeding episode has had any effect on the child's physiologic status. **No. 2** is incorrect because in general the nurse should never change the flow rate of the IV without a physician's order. **Nos. 3 and 4** are incorrect because *after* checking vital signs, depending on the status of the bleeding and the vital signs, the nurse might change the patient's position and notify the cardiologist. **IMP,6,PhI**

108. **(2)** All physicians and institutions have their own guidelines. However, 3 weeks is generally appropriate if the lochia has decreased and becomes fairly clear in color, and if there are no other problems. **No. 1** is incorrect because 6 weeks is longer than is usually necessary. **No. 3** is incorrect because "when they arrive home" is too soon. **No. 4** is incorrect because waiting until breastfeeding ceases is longer than is usually necessary. **IMP,5,HPM**

109. **(1)** Isoproterenol is categorized as a beta-mimetic, in that its action simulates beta-adrenergic discharge. Actions include increased strength of cardiac contraction, increased heart rate, and decreased venous pooling, which increases venous return. An additional effect of isoproterenol is increased myocardial consumption resulting from increased rate and contractility. Isoproterenol is not a cardiac glycoside (**No. 2**) like *digoxin,* an

anticholinergic (**No. 3**) like *atropine,* or a beta-blocker (**No. 4**) like *propanolol.* **AS,6,PhI**

110. **(4)** An effective assessment of the couple's needs is obtained through discussing the couple's own perceptions of those needs. **Nos. 1 and 2** are incorrect: Although referral to social services or family counseling may be an appropriate action once a thorough assessment is complete, it should never precede discussion with the couple. **No. 3** is incorrect: Although supportive counseling may be an appropriate action once a thorough assessment is complete, it also should never precede discussion with the couple. **IMP,7,PsI**

111. **(3)** Phantom limb pain or sensation is an unpleasant complication that sometimes follows amputation. This phenomenon is not completely understood but is believed to result from afferent nerve fibers (sensory) severed during surgery. The pain in the limb may be identical to that perceived by the patient before surgery. The patient needs to be aware of the nature of this discomfort. Sometimes the sensation will disappear if the patient looks at the stump and recalls that the limb has been amputated. In cases where discomfort persists, alcohol may be injected into the nerve endings for temporary relief, the nerve endings may be removed, or on rare occasions reamputation may be required. **Nos. 1 and 2** are incorrect because they negate the patient's perceptions of discomfort and avoid the issue. **No. 4** is incorrect: An explanation of the phenomenon and other palliative measures should *precede* the administration of a narcotic. **IMP,2,PhI**

112. **(4)** Conflicts concerning discharge instructions following myocardial infarction and pacemaker insertion are common. When the nurse prepares a patient for discharge, it is important to recognize that both patient and spouse may have several fears they have not verbalized. Allow time for and encourage verbalization of feelings. Likewise, be sure that discharge instructions are feasible for the individual's life-style; if they are not, work out a plan of modification with the patient, family, and physician. Referral to a community health nurse or local cardiac rehabilitation support group may also facilitate the rehabilitation. **Nos. 1, 2, and 3** are incorrect because they cut off the patient's and spouse's range of response and may therefore preclude obtaining pertinent data. **IMP,7,PsI**

113. **(1)** Straightforward, direct communication is needed to keep the client from manipulating his or her care. The nurse needs to be honest and to set very firm limits. **No. 2** is incorrect because an adolescent drug abuser tends to be very manipulative; however, allowing the client to *assist* in the decision-making process is essential. **No. 3** is incorrect because too much security will foster dependence. The client needs to identify and begin to cope with the anxiety, although anxiety generally cannot be eliminated entirely. **No. 4** is incorrect because drug abusers are already characteristically very dependent individuals. **PL,7,PsI**

114. **(3)** Per MD order, the IV should infuse at 320 mL every 8 hours or 40 mL per hour. Thus, if there is 425 mL left in the IV and it runs at 40 mL per hour, the present bag should last 10 hours, or from 11:30 A.M. to 9:30 P.M. The nurse should plan to change the bag at 9:00 P.M., before it runs out completely. **Nos. 1 and 2** are incorrect because changing it earlier would waste IV fluid, which is costly. **No. 4** is incorrect because changing it later would mean the IV would run out completely, and may result in an embolism or a clogged IV line. **IMP,6,SECE**

115. (2) As the capillary pressure in the lungs increases from cardiac decompensation, fluid pours from the circulatory system, across the capillary membrane into the alveoli, bronchi, and bronchioles. Typical manifestations include a respiratory rate as high as 60–70 breaths per minute and a persistent cough with expectoration of large amounts of frothy, blood-tinged sputum (hemoptysis). **No. 1** is incorrect because the patient's face will be pale, not flushed. **No. 3** is incorrect because the cough is productive, not hacking, and purulent sputum would be seen with an infection such as pneumonia. **No. 4** is partially correct, except the patient in pulmonary edema will show signs of shock and be cold, most likely with a subnormal temperature. **AS,6,PhI**

116. (1) To be sure a typical antimicrobial will have the desired effect, it must be in contact with the skin for a minimum of 10 seconds. **Nos. 2, 3, and 4** are incorrect because durations longer than 10 seconds are not necessary. **IMP,1,SECE**

117. (2) A drop in the systolic blood pressure of 20 mm Hg or more below the preoperative blood pressure is indicative of impending shock. Shock may be due to hemorrhage, vasodilation caused by anesthesia, insufficient fluid replacement, or abnormal clotting. **No. 1** is incorrect because skin may be dry and cool in the immediate postoperative period because of normal temperature-regulating mechanisms, that is, vasoconstriction due to skin exposure in the operating room. **No. 3** is incorrect because a diastolic reading below 70 mm Hg is significant only if it is abnormal for the patient and is accompanied by a drop in systolic or a narrowing pulse pressure. **No. 4** is incorrect because pulse rates normally increase and decrease with respirations to some extent because changes in intrathoracic pressures affect venous return. This phenomenon, however, is more evident in children. **EV,6,PhI**

118. (2) To reduce anxiety and ensure ease of induction, a preoperative medication should be administered 45–60 minutes prior to anesthesia. Siderails should be raised after administration of medication, as the patient will begin to feel drowsy and light-headed. **Nos. 1, 3, and 4** are incorrect because giving medication less than 45–60 minutes prior to induction of anesthesia would not allow sufficient time for the medication to reach its peak effect. **PL,1,SECE**

119. (1) The patient should be given diluted orange juice to ensure an adequate supply of ascorbic acid (vitamin C). **Nos. 2, 3, and 4** are incorrect because carbohydrates, protein, and vitamin A can be easily obtained by ensuring a variety of foods in the bland diet. **EV,4,PhI**

120. (2) Although in moderation these drugs produce feelings of well-being and alertness, an overdose of amphetamines causes an increase in tension and irritability. **Nos. 1 and 3** are incorrect because an increase in the heart rate and blood flow is exhibited, as these drugs stimulate the release of norepinephrine. **No. 4** is incorrect because diarrhea, not constipation, is a common side effect. **EV,7,PhI**

121. (1) Obtaining consent and informing the woman about the risks involved are legally the physician's role. The nurse's role is to reinforce the physician's teaching and to confirm that the information has been given to the woman. **No. 2** is an incorrect response because it is an appropriate nursing action to reinforce the physician's teaching and to confirm that the information has been given to the woman. **Nos. 3 and 4** are incorrect because monitoring the fetal heart rate and observing for bleeding are both appropriate nursing actions. **PL,7,SECE**

122. (4) If it appears that the patient's IV has infiltrated (site is red and swollen), the only acceptable action by the nurse would be to remove the IV line. **No. 1** is incorrect: *After* removing the IV line, the nurse might apply warm soaks if the area appeared reddened. **No. 2** is incorrect because the nurse should not increase or decrease the flow rate without a physician's order. **No. 3** is incorrect because elevating the site would further slow the flow rate, although IV fluids would continue to drip into tissue and might cause damage to the surrounding area. **IMP,1,SECE**

123. (1) The most objective measure of the effectiveness of an antibiotic is a return of the white blood cell count to normal. **No. 2** is incorrect because a low-grade temperature may indicate a lingering infection. **Nos. 3 and 4** are incorrect because no pain and a good appetite are both good clinical indicators, but not as objective or as clearly measurable as the white blood cell count. **EV,1,PhI**

124. (4) The classic vital sign changes in increased intracranial pressure are known as the Cushing's reflex. The pressure on the vasomotor center in the brain produces a slowing of the heart rate (bradycardia), an increase in the pulse pressure in an attempt to increase cerebral perfusion pressure, and an irregular breathing pattern (e.g., Biot's or ataxic, Cheyne-Stokes, apneustic). **No. 1** is incorrect because the vital sign changes indicate shock and are just the opposite of increased intracranial pressure. **No. 2** is incorrect because the level of consciousness, rather than increasing, will decrease, which may be indicated by an unconscious patient becoming nonresponsive to painful stimuli. **No. 3** is incorrect because pupil dilation will occur when there is compression of cranial nerve III (oculomotor) on the same side as the injury or hematoma, not the opposite side. **EV,2,PhI**

125. (1) Many women experience some slight to moderate depression. Sleep deprivation and an inadequate support system may contribute to the "blues." **No. 2** is incorrect: If the behaviors become severe (i.e., persistent over a long period of time and increasingly exaggerated), *then* professional help should be initiated. **No. 3** is incorrect because a physician's referral may not be necessary and it is not the nurse's job to ask the physician to prescribe antidepressants; medication may not even be needed. **No. 4** is incorrect because the new father should be informed that patience, understanding, *and help* with housework *and care* of the infant are needed, and may help decrease some of the mother's anxiety. **IMP,7,PsI**

126. (4) All insulin-dependent diabetics are to receive daily insulin. However, the physician should write specific orders for insulin coverage on the day of surgery. The reason for this is that both the physical and the psychological stresses of surgery tend to increase serum-glucose levels via glycogenolysis, and the patient's usual insulin may be insufficient. **No. 1** is incorrect because all insulin-dependent diabetics are to receive daily insulin. **No. 2** is incorrect because the physical and psychological stresses of surgery tend to increase serum-glucose levels via glycogenolysis, and the patient's usual insulin may be insufficient. Frequently, a rainbow coverage of regular insulin is ordered to supplement or temporarily replace daily doses of NPH or other longer-acting insulins. **No. 3** is incorrect because the patient is not given fluids before surgery, particu-

larly if a general anesthetic is to be administered. **IMP,4,SECE**

127. **(3)** The patient is disoriented to time, place, and person. He needs constant monitoring and comprehensive support. **No. 1** is incorrect: Although he may be physiologically hungry, this is difficult to validate since he is confused. **No. 2** is incorrect because although he may be hallucinating, the information given here merely indicates that he is disoriented. **No. 4** is incorrect because he does not appear to be in touch with reality. **AN,2,PsI**

128. **(2)** During the early postinsertion period, the inner cannula is removed using aseptic technique every 2–4 hours for cleansing. If secretions are copious or very viscous, more frequent cleansing may be necessary. If the patient is receiving oxygen therapy or is on mechanical ventilation, these treatments are continued through the outer cannula. **No. 1** is incorrect because routine cleansing is done, even when it appears unnecessary. **No. 3** is incorrect because once a day is not frequent enough. **No. 4** is incorrect because the cannula *must* be removed for cleansing. **PL,1,SECE**

129. **(1)** The first stage is the stage of the cervix. The woman's cervix is dilated only 4 cm, with contractions occurring every 4–6 minutes, and she is alert. **No. 2** is incorrect because the second stage is the stage from a 10-cm dilated cervix to full birth of the baby. **No. 3** is incorrect because the third stage is the stage of the placenta. **No. 4** is incorrect because the fourth stage is the period of recovery, usually the first 2 hours after birth. **AN,5,HPM**

130. **(4)** CHG is a highly effective antimicrobial ingredient, especially when it is used consistently over time. **No. 1** is incorrect because soap and water, while recommended for most general patient care, is not an antimicrobial. **No. 2** is incorrect because alcohol will degerm skin rapidly but because of its drying effect on the skin, it is not recommended for repeated washing. **No. 3** is incorrect because hexachlorophene acts primarily on gram-positive bacteria and has also been associated with neurotoxicity; it is no longer recommended. **IMP,1,SECE**

131. **(2)** The person doing compressions should allow for a full breath to be given before starting the compressions. Without the pause, the patient will not receive sufficient ventilation. The ratio is *one* full breath to five compressions, not two breaths (**No. 1**). The persons doing CPR may change positions *as needed;* the protocol does *not* specify the time (**No. 3**). The compression rate for two-person CPR is the *same* as the rate for one-person CPR: 80–100 compressions per minute (not slower, **No. 4**). **IMP,1,SECE**

132. **(3)** Patients must be taught to place a nitroglycerin tablet under the tongue prior to exercising, eating a large meal, emotionally stressful events, or sexual activity. **No. 1** is incorrect because headaches following drug use are to be expected, but lessen over time. The physician does not need to be notified unless repeated dosages (3–5 tablets) do not relieve the pain. **No. 2** is incorrect because the medication should be stored in a dark bottle in a dry location. Refrigeration is not appropriate. **No. 4** is incorrect because the tablet is placed under the tongue and allowed to dissolve completely, and the saliva is retained briefly before swallowing. Swallowing whole with liquid will negate the drug's effectiveness. **PL,1,SECE**

133. **(1)** This is a health team decision that needs to be supported by the hospital administration in order to assist the family in working through the grieving process. **No. 2** is incorrect because it may be a violation of the family's privacy. The priest's input may be considered, if the family requests it. **No. 3** is incorrect because it is an inappropriate assumption that would need further validation. **No. 4** is incorrect because it should not be standard policy in any hospital today. It is essential for many families to see the deceased in order to work through their grief. **IMP,7,PsI**

134. **(3)** In most cesareans a drape is used and one can see very little "gore" or blood. **No. 1** is incorrect because the nurse needs to find out what the procedure usually involves. **No. 2** is incorrect because in almost all hospitals a drape of some type is used. **No. 4** is incorrect because it is not true. **IMP,7,HPM**

135. **(3)** Both systolic and diastolic pressures should decrease as the result of the pharmacologic interventions. **No. 1** is incorrect because vasodilation and decreases in fluid volume decrease peripheral resistance, thereby lowering the diastolic pressure. **No. 2** is incorrect for the same reason, but a concomitant drop in systolic pressure also occurs because the left ventricle is delivering its stroke volume at considerably less resistance. **No. 4** is incorrect because the goal of antihypertensive drug therapy is to lower pressure, not slow pulse. **EV,6,HPM**

136. **(3)** Anxiety is a significant factor; if it is too high, anxiety would negatively affect the child's ability to learn. Although the child's chronologic age (**No. 1**), developmental level (**No. 2**), and previous experiences (**No. 4**) are important for the nurse to assess in relation to the teaching style or techniques to be used, they are all *less* important in terms of the child's ability to learn. **AN,5,PsI**

137. **(2)** The earliest exercises initiated are passive range of motion of the elbow, wrist, and hand; these exercises are begun on the first postoperative day. As the patient is able, she is encouraged to put those joints through active range of motion. These exercises assist in maintaining function and in reducing lymphedema. Progression to other exercises, such as hair combing and wall reaching, is dependent on wound healing, grafts, presence of drainage tubes, and the patient's tolerance. **Nos. 1, 3, and 4** are incorrect responses; they are implemented after a modified mastectomy, but are not appropriate *initial* therapy. **PL,3,PhI**

138. **(2)** Any recommendation must be based on an assessment of the mother. This will ensure that her needs are met at an appropriate level and may prevent unnecessary stress and feelings of guilt at a later time. **No. 1** is incorrect. It may be appropriate if she thinks she would rather wean or if the combination of breastfeeding and supplemental feeding proves inadequate for the infant or mother. **No. 3** is incorrect. It may be appropriate if the mother has experienced a similar situation; however, this referral should be initiated only after assessing and validating the need and appropriateness with the patient and with the La Leche League. **No. 4** is incorrect. It may be appropriate after assessing the mother's feelings about breastfeeding; however, the supplemental feedings will need to be validated with a physician, and they will probably consist of some type of formula rather than glucose water. **PL,4,HPM**

139. **(3)** Actions of isoproterenol include relaxation (dilatation) of smooth muscles in the bronchi, skeletal muscle vasculature, and alimentary tract, and thus decreased bronchoconstriction. **No. 1** is incorrect: Increased pe-

ripheral vascular resistance is the action of norepinephrine (Levophed) or metariminol (Aramine). **No. 2** is incorrect: Decreased automaticity of Purkinje fibers is the action of digoxin. **No. 4** is incorrect: Decreased oral secretion is the anticholinergic effect of a drug like atropine. **EV,6,PhI**

140. **(2)** Throughout pregnancy, especially after the second trimester, most women express anxiety over their change in body image. The nurse must be aware of the need to provide positive reinforcement and encouragement in order to facilitate and maintain the woman's self-esteem. **No. 1** is incorrect because during this stage of pregnancy the mother is very self-focused. **No. 3** is incorrect because most women realize that dieting during pregnancy is contraindicated unless prescribed by a physician. **No. 4** is of no concern to the pregnant woman because she is gaining plenty of weight. **AN,7,HPM**

141. **(2)** While summoning the physician, the nurse should ensure that the patient's head is elevated. A sitting position bent slightly forward is best (a bedside table with pillows can be used for the patient to rest on), as it allows for the greatest lung expansion and gravity aids in shifting fluids toward the bases of the lungs. Lowering the legs tends to decrease venous return by pooling blood in the periphery. **No. 1** is incorrect because morphine SO_4 may be given only per physician order. **No. 3** is incorrect because suctioning at this time is not indicated. **No. 4** is incorrect: Supplemental oxygen *may* be given while awaiting medical orders, but *initial* nursing actions should be directed toward decreasing venous return and improving ventilation. **IMP,6,PhI**

142. **(2)** The woman in labor is instructed to lie on her *side* to promote relaxation, to prevent supine hypotension, and to facilitate anterior rotation of the fetal head. Therefore, to tell the woman to lie on her back would cause a problem to the woman. **No. 1** *is* an appropriate action. A full bladder may impede progress or result in trauma to the bladder. **No. 3** *is* an appropriate action. Bearing down prior to the second stage is fruitless and serves only to expend energy and possibly damage the cervical opening. **No. 4** *is* an appropriate action. Slow, even breathing promotes adequate ventilation for the maternal and fetal systems and controls some anxiety. **EV,1,SECE**

143. **(4)** He is essentially blaming the situation on his son's mother because he is unable to cope effectively with his own feelings at this time. **No. 1** is incorrect because it is usually not a coping mechanism because it does not help a person cope with anxiety or other feelings. **No. 2** is incorrect because sublimation involves rechanneling a destructive or instinctual impulse that is socially unacceptable into an acceptable outlet, such as channeling anger into sports. **No. 3** is incorrect because it involves denying one's own thought or emotion and seeing that thought or emotion in others. **AN,7,PsI**

144. **(3)** To best gain the cooperation of a toddler, the nurse should help her or him focus on how the treatment will help the toddler go home and the nurse should also use distraction. **Nos. 1, 2, and 4** are incorrect because the nurse should never bribe, threaten, or lie to the child. **IMP,5,PsI**

145. **(2)** The rate for cardiac compressions for infants is 100 per minute. **No. 1** is incorrect because pressure should be evenly applied with the fingers over the middle third of the sternum, not with the heel of the hand.

No. 3 is incorrect because to form a seal, the resuscitator should place his or her mouth over the mouth and nose of the infant. **No. 4** is incorrect because once the seal over the airway is made, the rescuer need only use gentle, not forceful puffs of air to inflate lungs. **IMP,6,SECE**

146. **(2)** There is no physiologic dependence, but the person has to increase the dose to receive the same effect because the body develops a tolerance. **No. 1** is incorrect because withdrawal usually leads to severe exhaustion. **No. 3** is incorrect because overdoses induce hyperactivity within the system. **No. 4** is incorrect because psychological, not physiologic, dependence develops from increased tolerance. **IMP,7,SECE**

147. **(3)** Correct medication administration is very important. When the medication order is of a different strength from the supplies at hand, using the following formula will be helpful in determining the correct dose:

$$\frac{\text{desired}}{\text{available}} \times \frac{\text{quantity}}{\text{on hand}} = \frac{0.4}{0.6} \times \frac{15 \text{ minims}}{1}$$

$$= \frac{2}{3} \times \frac{15}{1}$$

$$= \frac{30}{3}$$

$$= 10 \text{ minims}$$

Nos. 1, 2, and 4 are inaccurate calculations. **IMP,1,PhI**

148. **(3)** Alcohol and smoking are thought to present dangers to the fetus. **No. 1** is incorrect: Many women *do* work until they are about to give birth. **No. 2** is incorrect because intercourse *is* permissible in the absence of vaginal bleeding. **No. 4** is incorrect because *caloric requirements* for growth need to be maintained. **IMP,5,HPM**

149. **(4)** The patient's dyspnea is due to a shift of fluid from systemic circulation to lungs. With left ventricular failure, blood backs up in the pulmonary vasculature, causing increased pulmonary pressure and exudation of fluids into the interstitial space, alveoli, and bronchioles—that is, pulmonary edema. **No. 1** is incorrect because the mechanical congestion of the lungs decreases expandability (compliance) and increases the work of breathing; that is, the patient becomes aware of his or her efforts at breathing (dyspnea). **No. 2** is incorrect because pulmonary edema also decreases the amount of pulmonary membrane available for the diffusion of gases, thereby decreasing arterial oxygen and increasing the likelihood of CO_2 retention. **No. 3** is incorrect because venous return is increased, not decreased. **AN,6,PhI**

150. **(3)** Green fluid is usually seen when the fetus is or has recently been in distress and hypoxic. **No. 1** is incorrect because Rh or ABO incompatibility may result in a *yellow* fluid. **No. 2** is incorrect because fetal distress that occurred 36 hours ago also may result in a yellow fluid. **No. 4** is incorrect because abruptio placentae usually results in a port wine–colored fluid. **AN,6,PhI**

151. **(4)** The natural pathway of humidification, the upper respiratory tract, has been bypassed. Therefore, to prevent drying out of the mucous membranes of the bronchi, as well as crusting of secretions, humidification by nebulization is provided. **No. 1** is incorrect: Although supplying humidification during oxygen therapy has become standard, it is not a rationale for its use. **Nos. 2 and 3** are incorrect because they are not specific to

this question, though probably true to some extent. **AN,6,SECE**

152. **(4)** Measles, mumps, and rubella are first given at 12–18 months, and repeated at either 4–6 years or 11–12 years. Hepatitis B **(No. 1)**, DTP **(No. 2)**, and *H. influenzae* type b **(No. 3)** *should* all be given at 6 months. **IMP,1,HPM**

153. **(1)** The likelihood of product contamination after opening the bottle or bag increases over time, but the bottle or bag can hang safely for a maximum of 24 hours. Bottles or bags used for intermittent IV medications should be timed and dated, and not left hanging at the bedside for over 24 hours. The use of the heparin lock has decreased the need for KVO IVs, and medications are administered with 50-mL or 100-mL single-use solution bags. **Nos. 2, 3, and 4** are incorrect because the times are all too soon and would unnecessarily increase the cost of hospitalization. **EV,6,SECE**

154. **(3)** To effectively screen for the S-shaped lateral curvature of scoliosis, the nurse should ask the adolescent to stand and bend over at the waist 90 degrees. The nurse should look for unevenness of the shoulders or hips, or any curves or humps, which require further follow-up and evaluation. **Nos. 1, 2, and 4** are incorrect because no other position is recommended. **AS,3,HPM**

155. **(3)** Some of the most serious reactions occurring with blood transfusions are the result of human error. To reduce human error, it is essential for two nurses to verify that the patient's name and hospital number on the blood bag correspond exactly to that on the wristband. **Nos. 1, 2, and 4** are incorrect because while they are proper safeguards, they are not the *first* priority. **IMP,6,SECE**

156. **(1)** Prior to adding potassium chloride to any IV line, the nurse must check that the patient's kidneys are functioning to avoid potassium overload and hyperkalemia. **Nos. 2, 3, and 4** are incorrect because it is not necessary to check reflexes, respiratory rate, or mucous membranes prior to adding potassium to the IV line. **AN,8,SECE**

157. **(4)** Metronidazole (Flagyl) is the drug of choice in treating trichomonal vaginitis. **Nos. 1 and 2** are incorrect because tetracycline and erythromycin are ineffective against *Trichomonas* infection and are more commonly used in treating bacterial disease. **No. 3** is incorrect because nystatin has little effect on *Trichomonas vaginalis,* but is the drug of choice for *Candida* infection. **IMP,1,PhI**

158. **(1)** To reduce bleeding and edema, the stump is elevated for the first 24 hours; after 24 hours, however, hip flexion contracture may occur with prolonged elevation. **No. 2** is incorrect because this procedure is not used for amputations. **No. 3** is incorrect because this procedure is used with a below-the-knee amputation, to prevent contractures in the knee joint. **No. 4** is incorrect: This is a standard postoperative procedure *initiated by the surgeon in the operating room* to facilitate shrinkage of the stump and to prevent edema. **IMP,3,SECE**

159. **(4)** When a nurse is admitting a new patient to the unit, the first action the nurse should take is to correctly identify the patient. If the patient is fully awake and alert, the nurse can ask the patient for his or her name; if the patient is a newly postop patient, still under the influence of anesthesia and medication, the nurse should first check the ID band. After identifying the patient, the nurse could *then* proceed to monitor vital signs **(No. 3)**, check the IV **(No. 2)**, and attach the Salem sump tube to suction **(No. 1)**. **IMP,1,SECE**

160. **(3)** Refrigerating blood assists in delaying the growth of bacteria. The blood must be administered within 4 hours (not 6 hours, **No. 1**), but not so rapidly that the patient experiences overload **(Nos. 2 and 4)**. **IMP,6,SECE**

161. **(2)** Euphoria, excitement, and talkativeness are all seen initially when the woman is fairly energetic and anxious to have labor begin. **No. 1** is incorrect because a tendency to hyperventilate usually occurs during the midactive phase. Introverted behavior **(No. 3)** and irritability or crying **(No. 4)** usually occur in the transitional or deceleration period of the active phase of the first stage. **EV,5,HPM**

162. **(3)** Splinting of the incision, as well as tight pressure dressings, tend to reduce lung expansion and ventilation. As a result, mucus can block off small bronchioles, causing atelectasis or collapse of distal alveoli. **No. 1** is incorrect because peripheral thrombophlebitis is always a threat if the patient's legs are not exercised. In most patients, early ambulation prevents its occurrence. **No. 2** is incorrect because wound dehiscence is more likely to occur with abdominal surgeries. **No. 4** is incorrect because paralytic ileus is more likely to occur with abdominal surgeries, though it may occur as the result of the effects of anesthesia on autonomic nervous system function, or hypokalemia. **AN,6,PhI**

163. **(1)** In evaluating the couple's present knowledge base of childbirth and childbirth techniques, the nurse will be able to set up a more efficient and effective program of learning for the couple. The couple may have already investigated resources and may need more validation than primary health teaching. **No. 2** is incorrect; a *secondary* goal would be to meet the couple at their level of readiness to ensure optimal learning. **No. 3** is incorrect: If unsure of the information, the nurse may consult or refer to a specialist in the area. **No. 4** may be inappropriate if the couple desires an alternative method. **AS,5,HPM**

164. **(2)** Following surgery for a ruptured appendix, the patient should be placed in a semi-Fowler's position to promote drainage and to prevent possible complications, such as diaphragmatic abscess. **No. 1** is incorrect: This position will help to aerate the patient's lungs by allowing for maximum expansion, but it is not the *primary* reason for this position. **No. 3** is incorrect because this position will *not* help splint the incision. **No. 4** is incorrect because this position will *not* help facilitate movement or necessarily reduce complications. **PL,1,PhI**

165. **(2)** Drug abusers tend to be excessively dependent and passive, become easily frustrated, and cannot cope with anxiety. **Nos. 1, 3, and 4** are incorrect because assertive, mature, or aggressive individuals are generally able to externalize their feelings and fears or to cope effectively with stress. **AS,7,PsI**

166. **(1)** The earliest indications of blood transfusion reactions are headache, chills, and elevation of temperature. The skin may also become pale and cool, and hypotension may develop quickly. Respirations generally increase in rate and depth. Should symptoms occur, stop transfusion, notify physician, and send a stat urine specimen to the lab for analysis. **No. 2** is incorrect: Hypertension and flushing are not indicators of a transfusion reaction. **No. 3** is incorrect: Wheezing and urticaria may occur, but are *not the earliest* indications of blood transfusion reaction. **No. 4** is incorrect because

oliguria and jaundice are *late* signs of transfusion reaction, *secondary* to *hemolysis* of red blood cells. **EV,6,PhI**

167. (3) Food and drug therapy will prevent the accumulation of hydrochloric acid or will neutralize and buffer the acid that does accumulate. **No. 1** is incorrect because 8 hours would be too long without food/medication. **No. 2** is incorrect because monitoring vital signs every 2 hours is not indicated unless bleeding or shock continues and if those symptoms are present, vital signs should be taken more frequently. **No. 4** is incorrect: Milk is not a food of choice because it increases gastric acid production. **PL,4,SECE**

168. (2) Central venous pressure (CVP) is a reflection of pressures in the right atrium and systemic veins. While CVP is the least sensitive indicator of left ventricular end-diastolic pressures (increased with decreased ventricular compliance due to myocardial infarction and left ventricular failure), the CVP line is a safer one than a pulmonary artery (PA) line. In addition, it can be used to estimate blood volumes, obtain venous blood samples, and administer fluids. **No. 1** is incorrect: A PA line reflects left atrial pressure. **No. 3** is incorrect: A PA line indirectly reflects left ventricular pressure. **No. 4** is incorrect because right ventricular pressure is not measured by a CVP line. **AS,6,SECE**

169. (2) The patient with mild hypertension usually has a diastolic pressure of between 90 and 100 mm Hg. **No. 1** is incorrect because diastolic pressures of 110–120 mm Hg are considered moderately hypertensive. **No. 3** is incorrect because diastolic pressures of 120–140 mm Hg are considered severely hypertensive. **No. 4** is incorrect because diastolic pressures of 100–115 cross over two levels of hypertension; persons with these diastolic pressures would probably be considered to have mild to moderate hypertension. **AS,6,PhI**

170. (1) Each of these activities (restricting activity, monitoring ECG, implementing passive range-of-motion, maintaining sterile dressings) is a priority in the early postinsertion period. However, since a transvenous approach was used with this patient, it is essential that activities be restricted for the first few days to reduce the risk of catheter dislodgement. To monitor for this complication, periodic comparisons of his or her current rhythm strip should be made, with the tracing taken at the time of insertion. Changes in either the pacemaker artifact or pacemaker-initiated QRS indicate a change in position. While this may not always be significant, it becomes so if the pacemaker fails to capture, causing a decrease in heart rate and cardiac output. **Nos. 2, 3, and 4** are incorrect because *restricting activity* is the nurse's first priority. **PL,6,PhI**

171. (3) With large dosages of secobarbital there may be an increase in anger or a deep sleep, depending on the individual's reaction. Secobarbital, a barbiturate, causes a depression of the CNS, so its effects usually include bradycardia (not tachycardia, **No. 1**), hypotension (not hypertension, **No. 2**), and depressed respiration (not increased respirations, **No. 4**). **EV,7,SECE**

172. (2) Blood flow to the intestines is increased following ingestion of meals, to facilitate digestion and absorption. As a result of this circulatory shift, other organs receive less volume. This blood shift is partially responsible for feelings of sleepiness and lethargy following large meals. If a patient has a large atheromatous plaque in one of the coronary arteries, the decreased pressure and flow of blood may result in transient is-

chemia. **No. 1** is incorrect because decreased pancreatic enzyme secretion results in diarrhea and steatorrhea (large amounts of fats in the stools). **No. 3** is incorrect: Swallowing air during eating can produce an uncomfortable feeling of fullness that can be relieved by eructation (belching), but should not decrease arterial oxygenation. **No. 4** is incorrect because a decrease in heart rate and blood pressure will decrease rather than increase myocardial oxygen consumption. **AN,6,PhI**

173. (1) Liquid iron preparations such as Fer-In-Sol should be given with a citrus juice to enhance the absorption of the iron. **No. 2** is incorrect because milk may actually block the absorption of iron. **No. 3** is incorrect because apple juice will not enhance the absorption of iron. **No. 4** is incorrect because prune juice will not enhance the absorption of iron (however, since iron does cause constipation, prune juice may be given to treat or prevent this side effect). **IMP,4,SECE**

174. (2) The desired effect of morphine in this situation is to reduce sensitivity to stimuli in order to allay apprehension and in some cases, to induce drowsiness. Atropine acts to dry oral and bronchial secretions, reducing the hazards of aspirations during anesthetic induction. **No. 1** is incorrect because while morphine effectively relieves pain, pain relief is usually not an objective in administering a preoperative medication. **No. 3** is incorrect because drowsiness, not sleep, may result. **No. 4** is incorrect because morphine is not a muscle relaxant. **EV,3,PhI**

175. (3) Examining her vaginal canal is contraindicated initially because of her preadmission history of bleeding. **No. 1** is incorrect: Initiating IV therapy *is* imperative, to have a line available for any ordered medications or fluids. **Nos. 2 and 4** are incorrect because taking her blood pressure and monitoring FHR *are* essential to establish baseline data and to monitor the mother's and infant's status. **IMP,1,SECE**

176. (4) Frequent baths will help lesions crust over, dry, and heal; thus bathing more frequently than usual is recommended. However, no soap should be used, as it will cause excessive drying and cracking of both the affected areas and the healthy skin. **No. 1** is incorrect because it is inappropriate for the nurse to tell the mother to check with the doctor first. The nurse can and should handle this question, since teaching is part of the nurse's responsibility. **No. 2** is incorrect because it would be incorrect for the nurse to advise the mother that sponge baths are recommended for 10 days. **No. 3** is incorrect because it would also be incorrect for the nurse to advise the mother that baths are not permitted. **IMP,1,HPM**

177. (1) Crepitus in the neck or upper chest is a sign that the tracheal tube is no longer in place and is delivering oxygen into the interstitial or mediastinal space. This condition may severely impair ventilation of the lungs. **No. 2** is incorrect because an inadequately inflated cuff creates an air leak around the tracheal tube. **No. 3** is incorrect because an overinflated cuff can cause necrosis of the trachea. **No. 4** is incorrect because edema is characterized by fluid, not air, in the tissues. **AN,6,PhI**

178. (1) The procedure most commonly used in assessing fetal well-being is the nonstress test, which provides valuable data without inducing hazard to mother or fetus. **No. 2** is incorrect because amniocentesis is used selectively, that is, in cases where the information gained is vital to fetal survival. **No. 3** is incorrect because the lecithin-sphingomyelin (L/S) ratio is an indi-

cator of fetal lung maturity; it would require amniocentesis. **No. 4** is incorrect because determination of fetal blood gases is not a common procedure and is most often done on scalp blood when the mother is in labor. **AS,5,SECE**

179. **(2)** In Bryant's traction, the hips and buttocks should be raised slightly (1 in.) above the mattress, not resting on the mattress **(No. 1)**, for the traction to be effective. **No. 3** is incorrect because although the nurse is ultimately "responsible," the aide should be commended for having brought this concern to the nurse's attention. **No. 4** is incorrect: Though it is true that this child will need special skin care due to prolonged immobility, the nurse should first take measures to correct the problem with the traction. **IMP,3,SECE**

180. **(3)** The Hemovac is a portable suction system that provides low negative pressure (30–45 mm Hg) to gently remove excess fluid and debris from the wound. It does not require attachment to any other suction system. **Nos. 1, 2, and 4** are incorrect because they *are* standard and appropriate nursing measures. **IMP,6,SECE**

181. **(3)** By agreeing to talk with both parents, the nurse can provide emotional support and further assess and validate the family's needs. **No. 1** is incorrect because it lacks empathy and makes the mother feel rejected. **No. 2** is incorrect: It may be an appropriate action *after* doing further assessment. **No. 4** is incorrect because this suggestion should be made only, if after further assessment and discussion with the physician and social worker, the health team thinks it is appropriate. However, at this time it is inappropriate. **IMP,7,PsI**

182. **(4)** After the stump has healed, an elastic bandage is applied to it to produce shrinkage and a conical shape. It is a compression dressing, with maximal compression at the distal end of the stump and minimal compression at the proximal end. The stump is wrapped with a clean bandage each day and rewrapped four times each day to maintain compression. **No. 1** is incorrect: Elevation of the stump *after* the first 24 hours is always contraindicated because of the risk of flexion contracture in the hip. **No. 2** is incorrect: Pushing the stump against a hard surface will facilitate toughening the skin for weight bearing once the prosthesis is applied, but it does not facilitate either reduction in size or shaping of the stump. **No. 3** is incorrect: Warm, moist soaks may be applied to reduce phantom pain discomfort, but they are *not applicable* to this situation. **IMP,3,SECE**

183. **(1)** Central venous pressures of 4–10 cm H_2O are normal. Some clinicians consider up to 15 cm H_2O to be normal, but pressures over 15 cm H_2O **(No. 3)** clearly indicate hypervolemia or heart failure. **Nos. 2 and 4** are incorrect because CVP is measured by water, not mercury. **EV,6,SECE**

184. **(2)** Many parents become "slaves" to the monitor and become overprotective to the infant. **No. 1** is incorrect because faulty alarms should only occur if the electrodes are not properly placed. **No. 3** is incorrect: The monitor should have very little effect on the infant's developmental level, provided it is used appropriately and the infant is environmentally stimulated. **No. 4** is incorrect because most apnea monitors are reliable if properly used. **EV,2,SECE**

185. **(3)** Encouraging friends to visit is inappropriate because they may bring drugs or encourage the client to act out by leaving the hospital or taking drugs. Visitation should not be completely curtailed, but should be very closely monitored. **No. 1** allows the client to feel he or she has some control over care, which is especially important during adolescence. **No. 2** helps the client regain strength and decreases stimuli in the immediate environment. **No. 4** allows the nurse to monitor care more closely. **IMP,7,PsI**

186. **(4)** Nitroglycerin causes vasodilation and a decrease in systemic blood pressure, which subsequently decreases the amount of work the heart must perform. **No. 1** is incorrect because constriction of the cardiac chambers would increase cardiac resistance and workload. **No. 2** is incorrect because nitroglycerin does not increase heart rate. That effect would be seen with isoproterenol (Isuprel) or atropine. **No. 3** is incorrect because to increase myocardial contractility, digoxin would be given. **AN,6,PhI**

187. **(3)** Understanding the condition will increase the patient's compliance with the treatment regimen. **No. 1** is incorrect because it is important to provide consistency in assigning nurses to care for the person with hypertension, to minimize stress and provide constant and consistent reinforcement of care and health teaching. **No. 2** is incorrect: The nurse should plan care to reduce the number of situations that create or increase physical stress. **No. 4** is incorrect because the patient must report minor symptoms as well as major ones. **PL,7,PsI**

188. **(2)** Carrying anything heavy, such as groceries or even a purse, on the affected side may increase the occurrence of lymphedema. **No. 1** is incorrect because wearing gloves for household tasks or gardening is encouraged to prevent lymphedema or possible infection *if* the skin is broken. **No. 3** is incorrect because elasticized sleeves *may* be worn if they are *not tight*. However, any constricting garment or jewelry should be avoided. **No. 4** is incorrect because driving, particularly if the affected arm is kept high on the steering wheel, should *not* increase lymphedema. **IMP,3,SECE**

189. **(1)** Fluid orders vary among hospitals, physicians, and childbirth methods. Since the woman is in preterm labor and is bleeding, the orders will probably maintain her NPO with an IV. **Nos. 2 and 3** are incorrect because giving her a small sip of water or ice chips may be contraindicated at this time. **No. 4** is incorrect because the physician may allow sips of water or ice chips. **IMP,6,HPM**

190. **(4)** Infants or children with milk allergies should be offered a lactose-free formula such as Isomil. **Nos. 1, 2, and 3** are incorrect because these formulas are lactose based and are contraindicated for infants or children with milk allergies. **IMP,4,SECE**

191. **(1)** The rationale for pacemaker implantation is presented in the preinsertion period and is reinforced in the postinsertion period and therefore, receives the least emphasis in the predischarge plan. **Nos. 2, 3, and 4** are incorrect because they *are* essential components of a predischarge teaching plan, as the patient must focus on management of the pacemaker, and they all receive great emphasis. **PL,6,SECE**

192. **(2)** SIDS usually occurs within the first year of life. The peak time appears to be between 2 and 4 months after birth. **No. 1** is incorrect because SIDS rarely occurs before 4 weeks after birth. **Nos. 3 and 4** are incorrect because SIDS is comparatively unusual after 6 months of age; 90% of all cases occur by 6 months of age. **AS,5,HPM**

193. **(4)** Baroreceptors in the carotid sinus and aortic arch constantly monitor and respond to variations in blood

pressure. Decreased cardiac output results in a drop of blood pressure. These receptors transmit afferent signals to the cardiovascular center in the medulla. Activation of these centers results in increased vasoconstriction, heart rate, and force of cardiac contraction via adrenergic efferents in the sympathetic nervous system. **No. 1** is incorrect because vagal stimulation of the SA node decreases heart rate. **No. 2** is incorrect because arrhythmias generally produce an irregularity in heart rhythm. **No. 3** is incorrect because these vital signs do not indicate shock at this time. **AN,6,PhI**

194. **(3)** Morphine sulfate acts not only to reduce pain and anxiety by blocking the activity of the reticular substance in the brain stem, but also to relax vascular smooth muscle, thereby decreasing blood pressure. Nausea and vomiting are common adverse side effects of this medication. Atropine is an anticholinergic whose drying effects tend to cause the patient to complain that the mouth feels like cotton. **Nos. 1 and 4** are incorrect because atropine also blocks vagal effects on the heart, increasing pulse rate, not decreasing it. **No. 2** is incorrect because blood pressure is decreased, not increased. **EV,1,SECE**

195. **(1)** Teaching regarding medications is essential if the patient is going to recognize side effects. The patient must be told that medications must continue even though he or she "feels" fine. **No. 2** is incorrect because changing jobs is unrealistic in most cases. The patient should be taught stress-reduction or relaxation techniques to better handle work-related stress. **No. 3** is incorrect because the patient should quit smoking, not just lessen the amount. **No. 4** is incorrect because there are generally no limitations on sexual activities merely due to hypertension; unless restrictions are warranted because of an individual's specific condition, this is considered irrelevant when teaching the average hypertensive patient. **PL,6,PsI**

196. **(1)** If the IV infused at the correct rate of 40 mL/hr from 11:00 A.M. to 3:15 P.M., the patient should have received 170 mL of IV fluid; because the patient has received twice the prescribed amount, the nurse should *first* correct the rate, *then* notify the physician **(No. 4)**. (The nurse should also check at this time to see if the IV line is being affected by the position of the limb.) If after contacting the physician, a new rate is ordered, only then would the nurse adjust the rate to a level lower than originally prescribed **(No. 3)**. **No. 2** is incorrect because there is no reason to hang a new bag at this time. **IMP,6,SECE**

197. **(3)** The primary advantage of Hemovac suction is that it removes excess fluid and debris from the wound site

that could retard tissue granulation and healing. If serum is allowed to accumulate under the skin, the pressure can cause sloughing of tissue flaps. **No. 1** is incorrect because the Hemovac exerts low even pressure. **No. 2** is incorrect because the Hemovac is also lightweight (which is an advantage in postoperative ambulation), but this is *not* its *primary* advantage. **No. 4** is incorrect because the removal of excess sera reduces the likelihood of postoperative infection but is a *secondary* advantage. **PL,1,PhI**

198. **(2)** Although drug abuse may be found at every age level, the elderly seem least likely to abuse substances. This is probably due to generational differences in cultural norms and morals. (It was thought that one was "weak" or "sick" to rely on drugs to escape problems.) However, many times the elderly use alcohol as an escape mechanism. **Nos. 1 and 3** are incorrect because drug abuse is found among all socioeconomic classes. **No. 4** is incorrect because many adolescents use drugs to escape reality, cope with stress, identify with their peers, etc. The reasons for abuse vary from individual to individual, depending on their particular needs. **AN,7,PsI**

199. **(1)** The toddler is probably experiencing severe separation anxiety and is exhibiting symptoms of despair. A consistent one-to-one relationship will develop trust in the nurse; in addition, rooming-in by her mother should be encouraged. **No. 2** is incorrect because assigning different staff would increase anxiety stemming from feelings of uncertainty and lack of trust. **No. 3** is incorrect because ignoring the behavior may worsen her age-related separation anxiety. **No. 4** is incorrect: Referral to the Pediatric Clinical Nurse Specialist may not be necessary at this time, as long as appropriate interventions are implemented. **IMP,5,PsI**

200. **(2)** The most common complication occurring in the postoperative period is pulmonary embolus. This is a particularly significant problem in elderly patients with a history of vascular insufficiency. Therefore, an antiembolism stocking is applied to the unaffected limb, and early physiotherapy and ambulation with a walker are encouraged. **No. 1** is incorrect because hemorrhage and shock are always potential problems after *any* surgery. To assess for this problem in *this* case, any bright red drainage on the stump dressing should be outlined so that the rate of bleeding can be determined. **No. 3** is incorrect because disseminated intravascular clotting is a problem associated with *prolonged shock*. **No. 4** is incorrect because thrombophlebitis tends to occur with *long bedrest* and can be prevented. **EV,6,PhI**

Appendix A
Laboratory Values

Test	Normal Values	Possible Significance	
		Increases	**Decreases**
Hematology			
Aspartate amino-transferase (AST)—formerly called serum glutamic oxaloacetic transaminase (SGOT)	8–20 U/L	Myocardial infarction, cardiac surgery, hepatitis, cirrhosis, trauma, severe burns, progressive muscular dystrophy, infectious mononucleosis, acute renal failure	
Bleeding time—indication of hemostatic efficiency	1–9 min	Hemorrhagic purpura, acute leukemia, aplastic anemia, DIC, oral anticoagulant therapy	
Hematocrit—volume of packed red blood cells/100 mL of blood	*Men:* 45% (38–54%) *Women:* 40% (36–47%)	Dehydration, polycythemia, congenital heart disease	Anemia, hemorrhage, leukemia, dietary deficiencies
Hemoglobin—oxygen-combining protein	*Men:* 14–18 g/dL *Women:* 12–16 g/dL	Same as for Hematocrit	Same as for Hematocrit
Partial thromboplastin time (PTT)—tests coagulation mechanism; Stage I deficiencies	*APTT:* 30–40 sec *PTT:* 60–70 sec	Deficiency of factors VIII, IX, X, XI, XII; anticoagulant therapy	Extensive cancer, DIC
Platelets—thrombocytes	150,000–400,000/mm^3	Polycythemia, postsplenectomy, anemia	Leukemia, aplastic anemia, cirrhosis, multiple myeloma, chemotherapy
Prothrombin time—tests extrinsic clotting; Stages II and III	11–15 sec	Anticoagulant therapy, DIC, hepatic disease, malabsorption	Digitalis therapy, diuretic reaction, vitamin K therapy
Red blood cell count—number of circulating erythrocytes in 1 μL of whole blood	*Men:* 4.5–6.2 million/μL *Women:* 4.0–5.5 million/μL	Polycythemia vera, anoxia, dehydration	Leukemia, hemorrhage, anemias, Hodgkin's
Sedimentation rate—speed at which red blood cells settle in uncoagulated blood	*Men:* 0–15 mm/h *Women:* 0–20 mm/h	Acute bacterial infection, cancer, infectious disease, numerous inflammatory states	Polycythemia vera, sickle cell anemia

Appendices

continued

		Possible Significance	
Test	**Normal Values**	**Increases**	**Decreases**
White blood cell count—number of leukocytes in 1 µL	5000–10,000 µL	Leukemia, bacterial infection, severe sepsis	Viral infection, overwhelming bacterial infection, lupus erythematosus, antineoplastic chemotherapy
White blood cell differential—enumeration of individual leukocyte distribution			
Neutrophils	55–70%	Bacterial infection, tumor, inflammation, stress, drug reaction, trauma, metabolic disorders	Acute viral infection, anorexia nervosa, radiation therapy, drug induced, alcoholic ingestion
Eosinophils	1–4%	Allergic disorder, parasitic infestation, eosinophilic leukemia	Acute or chronic stress; excess ACTH, cortisone, or epinephrine; endocrine disorder
Basophils	25–100/µL, or 0–1%	Myeloproliferative disease, leukemia	Anaphylactic reaction, hyperthyroidism, radiation therapy, infections, ovulation, pregnancy, aging
Lymphocytes	20–40%	Chronic lymphocytic leukemia, infectious mononucleosis, chronic bacterial infection, viral infection	Leukemia, systemic lupus erythematosus, immune deficiency disorders
Blood Chemistry Alkaline phosphatase (ALP)	30–85 U/L	Hyperparathyroidism, Paget's disease, cancer with bone metastasis, obstructive jaundice, cirrhosis, infectious hepatitis, rickets	Malnutrition, scurvy, celiac disease, chronic nephritis, hypothyroidism
Amylase	56–190 IU/L	Acute pancreatitis, mumps, duodenal ulcer, pancreatic cancer, perforated bowel	Advanced chronic pancreatitis, chronic alcoholism
Bilirubin, serum	*Direct:* 0.1–0.3 mg/dL *Indirect:* 0.2–0.8 mg/dL *Total:* 0.1–1.0 mg/dL	Massive hemolysis, low-grade hemolytic disease, cirrhosis, obstructive liver disease, hepatitis, biliary obstruction, erythroblastosis fetalis.	
Calcium, serum	9.0–10.5 mg/dL, or 4.5–5.6 mg/dL, ionized	Hyperparathyroidism, multiple myeloma, bone metastasis, bone fracture, thiazide-diuretic reaction, milk-alkali syndrome	Hypoparathyroidism, renal failure, pregnancy, massive transfusion
Carbon dioxide	24–30 mEq/L	Emphysema, salicylate toxicity, vomiting	Starvation, diarrhea
Chloride, serum	90–110 mEq/L	Hyperventilation, diabetes insipidus, uremia	Heart failure, pyloric obstruction, hypoventilation, vomiting, chronic respiratory acidosis
Cholesterol (total serum)	< 200 mg/dL	Hypercholesterolemia, hyperlipidemia, myocardial infarction, uncontrolled diabetes mellitus, high-cholesterol diet, atherosclerosis, stress, glomerulonephritis (nephrotic stage), familial	Malnutrition, cholesterol-lowering medication, anemia, liver disease, hyperthyroidism
Creatinine, serum	*Men:* 0.6–1.2 mg/dL *Women:* 0.5–1.1 mg/dL	Chronic glomerulonephritis, nephritis, congestive heart failure, muscle disease	Debilitation

continued

Test	Normal Values	Possible Significance	
		Increases	**Decreases**
Creatine kinase (CK) (creatine phospho-kinase [CPK])	*Men:* 12–70 U/mL (55–170 U/L) *Women:* 10–55 U/mL (30–135 U/L)	Acute myocardial infarction, acute CVA, convulsions, surgery, muscular dystrophy, hypokalemia	
Isoenzymes			
CPK-MM/CK-MM	100%	Muscular dystrophy, delirium tremens, surgery, hypokalemia, crush injuries, hypothyroidism	
CPK-MB/CK-MB	0%	Acute myocardial infarction, cardiac defibrillation, myocarditis, cardiac ischemia	
CPK-BB/CK-BB	0%	Pulmonary infarction, brain surgery, CVA, pulmonary embolism, seizures, intestinal ischemia	
Fibrinogen, serum	0.2–0.4 g/100 mL or 200–400 mg/dL	Pneumonia, acute infection, nephrosis, rheumatoid arthritis	Cirrhosis, toxic liver necrosis, anemia, obstetric complications, DIC, advanced carcinoma
Glucose (fasting)	80–120 mg/100 mL	Acute stress, Cushing's syndrome, hyperthyroidism, acute or chronic pancreatitis, diabetes mellitus, hyperglycemia	Addison's disease, liver disease, reactive hypoglycemia, pituitary hypofunction
Glycosylated hemo-globin (HbA$_{1c}$)	4.0–7.0%	Newly diagnosed or poorly controlled diabetes mellitus	
Iron-binding capacity (total)	25–420 µg/L	Lead poisoning, hepatic necrosis	Iron deficiency anemia, chronic blood loss
Lactic dehydrogenase (LDH)	40–90 U/L 115–225 IU/L	Myocardial infarction, pernicious anemia, chronic viral hepatitis, pneumonia, pulmonary emboli, CVA, renal tissue destruction	
LDH-1	17–27%		
LDH-2	27–37%		
LDH-3	18–25%		
LDH-4	3–8%		
LDH-5	0–5%		
Phosphorus, inorganic, serum	3.0–4.5 mg/dL	Chronic glomerular disease, hypoparathyroidism, milk-alkali syndrome, sarcoidosis	Hyperparathyroidism, rickets, osteomalacia, renal tubular necrosis, malabsorption syndrome, vitamin D deficiency
Potassium, serum	3.5–5.0 mEq/L	Diabetic ketosis, renal failure, Addison's disease, excessive intake	Thiazide diuretics, Cushing's syndrome, cirrhosis with ascites, hyperaldosteronism, steroid therapy, malignant hypertension, poor dietary habits, chronic diarrhea, diaphoresis, renal tubular necrosis, malabsorption syndrome, vomiting
Protein, serum (albumin/globulin)	*Total:* 6.4–8.3 g/dL *Albumin:* 3.5–5.0 g/dL *Globulin:* 2.3–3.5 g/dL	Dehydration, multiple myeloma	Chronic liver disease, myeloproliferative disease, burns
Sodium, serum	138–144 mEq/L	Increased intake, either orally or IV; Cushing's syndrome, excessive sweating, diabetes insipidus	Addison's disease, sodium-losing nephropathy, vomiting, diarrhea, fistulas, tube drainage, burns, renal insufficiency with acidosis, starvation with acidosis, paracentesis, thoracentesis, ascites, heart failure, SIADH

continued

Appendices

Test	Normal Values	Possible Significance	
		Increases	**Decreases**
T₃ uptake	24–34%	Hyperthyroidism, thyroxine-binding globulin (TBG) deficiency	Hypothyroidism, pregnancy, TBG excess
Thyroxine	5–12 µg/dL	Hyperthyroidism, pregnancy	Hypothyroidism, renal failure
Serum glutamic oxal-oacetic transami-nase (SGOT)—see AST			
Urea nitrogen, serum (BUN)	10–20 mg/dL	Acute or chronic renal failure, heart failure, obstructive uropa-thy, dehydration	Cirrhosis, malnutrition
Uric acid, serum	*Men:* 2.1–8.5 mg/dL *Women:* 2.0–6.6 mg/dL	Gout, chronic renal failure, starva-tion, diuretic therapy	
Blood Gases Bicarbonate (HCO₃)	21–28 mEq/L	Metabolic alkalosis	Metabolic acidosis
pH, serum	7.35–7.45	Metabolic alkalosis–alkali inges-tion, respiratory alkalosis–hyper-ventilation	Metabolic acidosis–ketoacidosis, shock, respiratory acidosis–alve-olar hypoventilation
Oxygen pressure (PO₂), whole blood, arterial	80–100 mm Hg	Oxygen administration in the ab-sence of severe lung disease	Chronic obstructive lung disease, severe pneumonia, pulmonary embolism, pulmonary edema, respiratory muscle disease
Carbon dioxide pres-sure (PCO₂), whole blood, arterial	35–45 mm Hg	Primary respiratory acidosis, loss of H⁺ through nasogastric suc-tioning or vomiting	Primary respiratory alkalosis
Immunodiagnostic Studies Carcinoembryonic an-tigen	< 5 ng/mL	Cancer of colon, lung, metastatic breast, pancreas, stomach, pros-tate, ovary, bladder, limbs; also neuroblastoma, leukemias, osteo-genic carcinoma; noncancer con-ditions such as hepatic cirrhosis, uremia, pancreatitis, colorectal, polyposis, peptic ulcer disease, ulcerative colitis, regional enteri-tis	
Urinalysis pH	4.8–8.0	Metabolic alkalosis	Metabolic acidosis
Specific gravity	1.010–1.030	Dehydration, pituitary tumor, hy-potension	Distal renal tubular disease, poly-cystic kidney disease, diabetes insipidus, overhydration
Glucose	Negative	Diabetes mellitus	
Protein	Negative	Nephrosis, glomerulonephritis, lu-pus erythematosus	
Casts	Negative	Nephrosis, glomerulonephritis, lu-pus erythematosus, infection	
Red blood cells	Negative	Renal calculi, hemorrhagic cystitis, tumors of the kidney	
White blood cells	Negative	Inflammation of the kidneys, ure-ters, or bladder	
Color	Normal yellow	*Abnormal:* red to reddish brown—hematuria; brown to brownish gray—bilirubinuria or urobilinu-ria; tea colored—possible ob-structive jaundice	*Almost colorless:* chronic kidney disease, diabetes insipidus, dia-betes mellitus
Sodium	40–220 mEq/L/24 h	Salt-wasting renal disease, SIADH, dehydration	Heart failure, primary aldosteron-ism

continued

Test	Normal Values	Possible Significance	
		Increases	Decreases
Chloride	110–250 mEq/24 h	Chronic obstructive lung disease, dehydration, salicylate toxicity	Gastric suction, HF, emphysema
Potassium	25–120 mEq/L/24 h	Diuretic therapy	Renal failure
Creatinine clearance	90–139 mL/min		Renal disease
Hydroxycorticosteroids	2–10 mg/24 h	Cushing's disease	Addison's disease
Ketosteroids	*Men:* 7–25 mg/24 h	Hirsutism, adrenal hyperplasia	Thyrotoxicosis, Addison's disease
	Women: 4–15 mg/24 h		
Catecholamines (VMA)	*Epinephrine:* 0.5–20.0 µg/24 h	Pheochromocytoma, severe anxiety, numerous medications	
	Norepinephrine: 15–80 µg/24 h		
Urine Tests **Shilling test**	Excretion of 8–40% or more of test dose should appear in urine		Gastrointestinal malabsorption, pernicious anemia

Appendix B

NCLEX-RN Test Plan: Nursing Process Definitions/Descriptions

The phases of the nursing process include:

I. Assessment: establishing a database.
   A. *Gather objective and subjective information relative to the client:*
   - Collect information from the client, significant others, and/or health care team members; current and prior health records; and other pertinent resources.
   - Utilize assessment skills appropriate to client's condition.
   - Recognize *symptoms* and significant findings.
   - Determine client's ability to assume care of daily health needs.
   - Determine health team member's ability to provide care.
   - Assess environment of client.
   - Identify own or staff reactions to client, significant others, and/or health care team members.
   B. *Confirm data:*
   - Verify observation or perception by obtaining additional information.
   - Question prescriptions and decisions by other health care team members when indicated.
   - Observe condition of client directly when indicated.
   - Validate that an appropriate client assessment has been made.

   C. *Communicate information gained in assessment:*
   - Document assessment findings thoroughly and accurately.
   - Report assessment findings to relevant members of the health care team.

II. Analysis: identifying actual or potential health care needs and/or problems based on assessment.
   A. *Interpret data:*
   - Validate data.
   - Organize related data.
   - Determine *need for additional* data.
   - Determine client's unique needs and/or problems.
   B. *Formulate client's nursing* diagnoses:
   - Determine significant relationship between data and client needs and/or problems.
   - Utilize *standard taxonomy* for formulating nursing diagnoses.
   C. *Communicate results of analysis:*
   - *Document client's nursing diagnoses.*
   - Report results of analysis to relevant members of the health care team.

III. Planning: setting goals for meeting client's needs and designing strategies to achieve these goals.
   A. *Prioritize nursing diagnoses:*
   - Involve client, significant others, and/or health care team members when establishing nursing diagnoses.
   - Establish priorities among nursing diagnoses.
   - Anticipate needs and/or problems on the basis of established priorities.

Source: National Council of State Boards of Nursing. *NCLEX-RN Test Plan.* Chicago, IL: The National Council of State Boards, 1994.

Appendices

B. *Determine goals of care:*
- Involve client, significant others, and/or health care team members in setting goals.
- Establish *priorities among goals.*
- Anticipate needs and/or problems on the basis of established priorities.

C. *Formulate outcome criteria for goals of care:*
- Involve client, significant others, and/or health care team members in formulating outcome criteria for goals of care.
- Establish *priorities* among *outcome criteria* for goals of care.
- Anticipate needs and/or problems on the basis of established priorities.

D. *Develop plan of care and modify as necessary:*
- Involve the client, significant others, and/or health care team members in designing strategies.
- Individualize the plan of care based on such information as *age, gender, culture, ethnicity and religion.*
- Plan for client's safety, comfort, and maintenance of optimal functioning.
- Select nursing interventions for delivery of client's care.
- Select *appropriate teaching* approaches.

E. *Collaborate with other health care team members when planning delivery of client's care:*
- Identify health or social resources available to the client and/or significant others.
- Select appropriate health care team members when planning assignments.
- Coordinate care provided by health care team members.

F. *Communicate plan of care:*
- Document plan of care thoroughly and accurately.
- Report plan of care to relevant members of the health care team.
- Review plan of care with client.

IV. **Implementation: initiating and completing actions necessary to accomplish the defined goals.**
A. *Organize and manage client's care:*
- Implement a plan of care.
- Arrange for a client care conference.

B. *Counsel and teach client, significant others, and/or health care team members:*
- Assist client, significant others, and/or health care team members to recognize and manage stress.
- Facilitate client relationships with significant others and health care team members.
- *Teach* correct principles, procedures, and techniques for maintenance and promotion of health.
- Provide client with health status information.
- Refer client, significant others, and/or health care team members to appropriate *resources.*

C. *Provide care to achieve established goals of care:*
- Use safe and appropriate techniques when administering client care.
- Use precautionary and *preventive* interventions in providing care to client.
- *Prepare client for surgery,* delivery, or other procedures.
- Institute *interventions* to compensate for *adverse* responses.
- Initiate *lifesaving interventions* for emergency situations.
- Provide an environment conducive to attainment of goals of care.
- Adjust care in accord with client's expressed or implied needs, problems, and/or preferences.
- Stimulate and motivate client to achieve self-care and independence.
- Encourage client to follow a treatment regime.
- Assist client to maintain optimal functioning.

D. *Supervise and coordinate the delivery of client's care provided by nursing personnel:*
- Delegate nursing interventions to appropriate nursing personnel.
- Monitor and follow up on delegated interventions.
- Manage health care team members' reactions to factors influencing therapeutic relationships with clients.

E. *Communicate nursing interventions:*
- Record actual client responses, nursing interventions, and other information relevant to implementation of care.
- Provide complete, accurate reports on assigned client(s) to relevant members of the health care team.

V. **Evaluation: determining the extent to which goals have been achieved and interventions have been successful.**
A. *Compare actual outcomes with expected outcomes of care:*
- Evaluate responses (expected and unexpected) in order to determine the degree of success of nursing interventions.
- Determine impact of therapeutic interventions on the client and significant others.
- Determine need for modifying the plan of care.
- Identify factors that may interfere with the client's ability to implement the plan of care.

B. *Evaluate the client's ability to implement self-care:*
- Verify that tests *or measurements are performed correctly* by the client and/or other care givers.
- Ascertain client's and/or others' understanding of information given.

C. *Evaluate health care team members' ability to implement client care:*
- Determine impact of teaching on health care team members.
- Identify factors that might alter health care team members' response to teaching.

D. *Communicate evaluation findings:*
- Document client's response to therapy, care, and/or teaching.
- Report client's response to therapy, care, and/or teaching to relevant members of the health care team.
- Report and document others' responses to teaching.
- Document other caregivers' responses to teaching.

The practice questions in this book (end-of-unit questions, **Pre Test, Practice Test,** and **Final Test**) are coded as to the phase of the nursing process being tested; the codes are found following the answer/rationale for each question. *Key to nursing process codes:*

AS	Assessment
AN	Analysis
PL	Planning
IMP	Implementation
EV	Evaluation

For an index to questions relating to each phase of the nursing process, see Appendix C.

Appendices

Appendix C

Index: Questions Related to Nursing Process

Use this index to locate practice questions throughout the book, on each of the five phases of the nursing process.

Unit	Assessment (AS) Question #	Analysis (AN) Question #	Plan (PL) Question #	Implementation (IMP) Question #	Evaluation (EV) Question #
Unit 1 Orientation and Pre Test	1, 10, 27, 32, 43, 53, 57, 73, 92, 99, 111, 112, 113, 114, 161, 162, 167, 176, 177, 183, 185, 190, 195, 198	2, 3, 5, 6, 9, 13, 15, 16, 18, 20, 26, 28, 30, 36, 38, 46, 48, 50, 59, 62, 65, 71, 72, 74, 80, 82, 84, 102, 104, 105, 107, 109, 115, 117, 118, 121, 125, 126, 129, 130, 138, 141, 144, 150, 151, 155, 159, 160, 164, 166, 169, 178, 182, 184, 186, 196, 200	8, 11, 12, 17, 21, 22, 41, 51, 61, 67, 79, 81, 85, 87, 89, 95, 103, 106, 110, 116, 127, 134, 135, 143, 148, 152, 156, 157, 165, 173, 187	4, 7, 19, 23, 24, 25, 29, 31, 33, 34, 35, 37, 40, 42, 44, 45, 52, 54, 56, 58, 60, 64, 66, 68, 70, 75, 76, 77, 78, 83, 86, 88, 96, 98, 100, 101, 108, 119, 120, 122, 123, 124, 128, 131, 132, 133, 136, 137, 139, 145, 146, 147, 153, 154, 158, 163, 168, 170, 172, 174, 175, 179, 180, 181, 189, 191, 193, 197, 199	14, 39, 47, 49, 55, 63, 69, 90, 91, 93, 94, 97, 140, 142, 149, 171, 192, 194
Unit 2 Nursing Care of the Acutely Ill and the Chronically Ill Adult	4, 13, 35, 41, 53, 72, 77, 78, 79, 84, 90, 98	5, 8, 9, 10, 11, 15, 17, 19, 22, 23, 29, 30, 32, 37, 39, 45, 56, 58, 65, 71, 74, 80, 82, 85, 86, 93, 95	2, 3, 6, 12, 20, 21, 27, 38, 40, 44, 62, 75, 81	1, 7, 14, 18, 24, 25, 26, 28, 36, 42, 43, 46, 48, 49, 52, 54, 55, 57, 59, 60, 63, 69, 70, 73, 89, 92, 97	16, 31, 33, 34, 47, 50, 51, 61, 64, 66, 67, 68, 76, 83, 87, 88, 91, 94, 96
Unit 3 Review of Nutrition	8		2, 4, 5, 7, 9	1, 3, 6	
Unit 4 Review of Pharmacology	1, 11, 20, 29	14, 19, 23, 35, 36, 37, 41, 44, 47, 50	2, 4, 9, 13, 27, 31, 33, 39, 40, 45, 49	3, 6, 8, 12, 16, 21, 22, 24, 25, 26, 30, 32, 38, 46, 48, 51, 52, 53, 54, 55	5, 7, 10, 15, 17, 18, 28, 34, 42, 43
Unit 5 Common Diagnostic Procedures, Treatments, and Nursing Care	9	1, 2, 3, 6	8, 12	4, 5, 10, 11	7, 13
Unit 6 Nursing Care of Behavioral and Emotional Problems Throughout the Life Span	4, 15, 39, 45, 52, 71, 102, 108, 128, 136, 143	8, 9, 12, 20, 25, 27, 36, 37, 38, 40, 41, 43, 44, 46, 47, 53, 55, 56, 57, 60, 62, 63, 65, 69, 70, 72, 76, 78, 80, 83, 99, 103, 104, 106, 107, 110, 111, 112, 113, 114, 123, 125, 127, 129, 130, 132, 137, 147	1, 10, 17, 21, 26, 29, 32, 33, 34, 49, 59, 64, 67, 73, 74, 75, 81, 89, 91, 92, 98, 105, 115, 117, 118, 124, 138, 140, 141	2, 3, 5, 6, 7, 11, 13, 14, 16, 19, 22, 23, 24, 28, 30, 31, 35, 42, 50, 51, 54, 58, 61, 66, 68, 77, 79, 84, 85, 86, 87, 88, 90, 94, 96, 97, 100, 101, 119, 120, 121, 122, 126, 133, 134, 135, 142, 145, 146	18, 48, 82, 93, 95, 109, 116, 131, 139, 144

Appendices

Appendix D

NCLEX-RN Test Plan: Client Needs Definitions/Descriptions

The latest NCLEX-RN test plan follows the categories of client needs described below.

❏ Safe, Effective Care Environment

See also Appendix G, Categories of Human Functions Definitions/Descriptions—*Protective Functions*.

The nurse meets client needs for a safe and effective care environment by providing and directing nursing care that promotes achievement of the following client needs:

- **Coordinated care**—coordinating, supervising, and/or collaborating with all other health care team members to facilitate integrated client care, including activities related to ethical and legal issues.
- **Environmental safety**—manipulating the care delivery setting to protect clients, family, and/or significant others, and health care personnel.
- **Safe and effective treatment and procedures**—preparing and/or caring for clients undergoing diagnostic procedures and invasive therapies.

Knowledge, Skills, and Abilities

To meet client needs for a safe, effective care environment, the nurse should possess knowledge, skills, and abilities that include but are not limited to the following areas:

Source: National Council of State Boards of Nursing. *NCLEX-RN Test Plan.* Chicago, IL: The National Council of State Boards, 1994.

- Advance directives
- Basic principles of management
- Client rights
- Confidentiality
- Continuity of care
- Environmental and personal safety
- Expected outcomes of various treatment modalities
- General and specific protective measures
- Informed consent
- Interpersonal communications
- Knowledge and use of special equipment
- Principles of teaching and learning
- Principles of quality improvement
- Principles of group dynamics
- Spread and control of infectious agents
- Staff education

❏ Physiologic Integrity

See also Appendix G, Categories of Human Functions Definitions/Descriptions—*Sensory-Perceptual; Comfort, Rest, Activity, and Mobility; Nutrition; Fluid-Gas Transport; Elimination.*

The nurse meets the physiologic integrity needs of clients with potentially life-threatening and/or chronically recurring physiologic conditions, and of clients at risk for the development of complications or untoward effects of treatments or management modalities by providing and directing nursing care that promotes achievement of the following client needs:

- **Physiologic adaptation**—managing and providing care during the acute and chronic phases of existing conditions, including emergency situations.
- **Reduction of risk potential**—reducing the potential of clients to develop complications and/or health

Appendices

647

problems. Also included are those activities that involve monitoring changes in status and the administration of medications and parenteral fluids.
- **Provision of basic care**—assisting in the performance of activities of daily living including those which have been modified because of health deviations.

Knowledge, Skills, and Abilities

To meet client needs for physiologic integrity, the nurse should possess knowledge, skills, and abilities that include but are not limited to the following areas:

- Activities of daily living
- Body mechanics
- Comfort interventions
- Drug administration
- Effects of immobility
- Expected and unexpected response to therapies
- Intrusive procedures
- Managing emergencies
- Normal body structure and function
- Nutritional therapies
- Pathophysiology
- Pharmacologic actions
- Skin and wound care
- Use of special equipment

❏ Psychosocial Integrity

See also Appendix G, Categories of Human Functions Definitions/Descriptions—*Psychosocial-Cultural Functions.*

The nurse meets client needs for psychosocial integrity in stress and crisis-related situations throughout the life span by providing and directing nursing care that promotes achievement of the following client needs:

- **Psychosocial adaptation**—managing and providing for needs of clients with acute or chronic psychiatric disorders, including chemical dependency.
- **Coping and/or adaptation**—promoting client's ability to cope, adapt, and/or problem solve situations related to illness or stressful events.

Knowledge, Skills, and Abilities

To meet client needs for psychosocial integrity, the nurse should possess knowledge, skills, and abilities that include but are *not limited* to the following areas:

- Accountability
- Behavior norms
- Chemical dependency
- Communication skills
- Community resources
- Cultural, religious, and spiritual influences on health

- Family systems
- Mental health concepts
- Principles of teaching and learning
- Psychodynamics of behavior
- Psychopathology
- Treatment modalities

❏ Health Promotion and Maintenance

See also Appendix G, Categories of Human Functions Definitions/Descriptions—*Growth and Development, Nutrition.*

The nurse meets client needs for health promotion and maintenance throughout the life span by providing and directing nursing care that promotes achievement within clients and their significant others of the following needs:

- **Continued growth and development throughout the life span**—assisting clients through the stages of *normal growth and development,* from birth to death (includes routine newborn care and normal pre-, intra-, and postpartum care).
- **Self-care and support systems**—(1) providing assistance to clients and families and/or significant others to promote client self-care; or (2) supporting families and/or significant others in order to enhance the overall management of client care, including self-care related teaching provided in any care delivery environment.
- **Prevention and early treatment of disease**—managing and providing for needs of clients for prevention and early detection of health problems and disease.

Knowledge, Skills, and Abilities

To meet client needs of health promotion and maintenance, the nurse should possess knowledge, skills, and abilities that include but are not limited to the following areas:

- Adaptation to altered health states
- Birthing and parenting
- Communication skills
- Community resources
- Concepts of wellness
- Death and dying
- Disease prevention
- Family systems
- Family planning
- Growth and development including aging
- Health care screening
- Life-style choices
- Principles of immunity
- Principles of teaching and learning
- Reproduction and human sexuality

The practice questions in this book (end-of-unit questions, **Pre Test, Practice Test,** and **Final Test**) are coded as to the client need being tested; the codes are found following the answer/rationale for each question. *Key to client need codes:*

SECE   Safe, Effective Care Environment
PhI   Physiologic Integrity
PsI   Psychosocial Integrity
HPM   Health Promotion and Maintenance

For an index to *questions* relating to each client need, see Appendix F.

For page references for specific *topics to review* relating to each client need, see Appendix E.

Appendices

Appendix E

Index: Content Related to Client Needs (Detailed Knowledge, Skills, and Abilities)

The following outline of content (nursing knowledge, skills, and abilities) is organized in terms of **four categories of client need:** *Safe, Effective Care Environment* (SECE), *Physiologic Integrity* (PhI), *Psychosocial Integrity* (PsI), and *Health Promotion/Maintenance* (HPM). Included in the outline of topics are 11 numbered **subcategories** and corresponding task statements. These items are derived from study of nursing tasks and are used in the development of the NCLEX-RN test plan.

Students who have taken and evaluated their performance on the **Pre Test, Practice Test,** or **Final Test** in this book will find this outline a useful guide for a concentrated review of specific problem topics. **Repeat NCLEX-RN test takers** will also find this outline to be a useful guide for review of their areas of weakness. Refer to the pages listed in the right column for review of content in a particular topic.

Appendices

For an index to *questions* relating to each client need, see Appendix F.

Appendices

Appendix F

Index: Questions Related to Client Needs

To *practice questions* in each of the four categories of client *needs* that are tested on NCLEX-RN, refer to the questions listed.

Unit	Safe, Effective Care Environment (SECE) Question #	Physiologic Integrity (PhI) Question #	Psychosocial Integrity (PsI) Question #	Health Promotion and Maintenance (HPM) Question #
Unit 1 Orientation and Pre Test	6, 12, 18, 19, 20, 22, 23, 26, 28, 31, 35, 37, 39, 42, 45, 52, 53, 54, 58, 60, 61, 64, 67, 68, 69, 70, 71, 74, 75, 77, 78, 81, 86, 87, 89, 90, 93, 96, 97, 101, 103, 105, 108, 109, 110, 112, 118, 119, 120, 123, 124, 133, 134, 136, 137, 139, 146, 148, 154, 156, 158, 161, 165, 169, 170, 171, 172, 173, 175, 180, 181, 188, 191, 197	1, 2, 3, 4, 5, 7, 9, 10, 13, 16, 21, 27, 29, 30, 32, 34, 36, 38, 40, 41, 43, 44, 55, 56, 59, 72, 73, 79, 80, 82, 84, 88, 92, 94, 100, 107, 111, 113, 114, 121, 130, 131, 138, 141, 143, 144, 147, 150, 153, 155, 159, 160, 162, 166, 167, 168, 176, 177, 178, 182, 183, 185, 186, 190, 192, 195, 200	8, 11, 24, 25, 33, 46, 50, 51, 66, 83, 85, 91, 95, 102, 104, 106, 117, 122, 132, 140, 142, 145, 152, 157, 174, 179, 184, 187, 199	14, 15, 17, 47, 48, 49, 57, 62, 63, 65, 76, 98, 99, 115, 116, 135, 149, 151, 163, 164, 189, 193, 194, 196, 198
Unit 2 Nursing Care of the Acutely Ill and Chronically Ill Adult	1, 2, 7, 14, 15, 19, 20, 21, 24, 25, 26, 28, 34, 37, 38, 40, 43, 46, 54, 57, 60, 62, 63, 69, 75, 81, 88, 94	4, 5, 6, 8, 10, 11, 12, 13, 16, 17, 18, 22, 23, 27, 29, 30, 31, 32, 33, 35, 36, 39, 41, 44, 45, 47, 49, 50, 51, 55, 56, 58, 61, 64, 65, 66, 67, 68, 70, 71, 72, 74, 77, 78, 79, 80, 82, 83, 84, 85, 87, 89, 90, 91, 92, 93, 95, 96, 97, 98	3, 9, 42, 48, 52, 53, 73, 76, 86	59
Unit 3 Review of Nutrition		1, 2, 3, 4, 5, 6, 7, 8, 9		
Unit 4 Review of Pharmacology	21, 23, 24, 25, 27, 28, 44, 48, 49, 50, 51, 52, 53, 55	1, 2, 3, 4, 5, 6, 7, 8, 9, 10, 11, 12, 13, 14, 15, 16, 17, 18, 19, 20, 29, 30, 31, 32, 33, 34, 35, 36, 37, 38, 39, 40, 41, 42, 43, 45, 46, 47	54	22, 26

continued

Appendices

Unit	Safe, Effective Care Environment (SECE) Question #	Physiologic Integrity (PhI) Question #	Psychosocial Integrity (PsI) Question #	Health Promotion and Maintenance (HPM) Question #
Unit 5 Common Diagnostic Procedures, Treatments, and Nursing Care	10, 12	1, 2, 3, 4, 5, 6, 7, 9, 10, 11, 13		
Unit 6 Nursing Care of Behavioral and Emotional Problems Throughout the Life Span	11, 22, 24, 26, 29, 49, 50, 51, 59, 61, 81, 96, 98, 118, 133, 145, 146, 147	1, 10, 57, 99, 102, 108, 143, 144	2, 3, 4, 5, 6, 7, 8, 9, 13, 14, 17, 19, 20, 21, 23, 25, 27, 28, 30, 32, 33, 34, 35, 36, 37, 38, 39, 40, 41, 42, 43, 44, 45, 46, 47, 48, 52, 54, 55, 56, 60, 62, 63, 64, 65, 66, 67, 68, 69, 70, 71, 72, 73, 74, 75, 76, 77, 78, 79, 80, 82, 83, 84, 85, 86, 87, 89, 91, 92, 93, 94, 95, 97, 100, 101, 103, 104, 105, 106, 107, 109, 110, 111, 113, 114, 115, 117, 119, 120, 121, 122, 123, 124, 125, 126, 127, 128, 129, 130, 131, 135, 136, 139, 140, 141, 142	12, 15, 16, 18, 31, 53, 58, 88, 90, 112, 116, 132, 134
Unit 7 Nursing Care of Childbearing Family	3, 12, 67	9, 13, 16, 23, 29, 31, 37, 41, 42, 45, 46, 58, 72, 76, 79, 81	21, 28, 44	1, 2, 4, 5, 6, 7, 8, 10, 11, 14, 15, 17, 18, 19, 20, 22, 24, 25, 26, 27, 30, 32, 33, 34, 35, 36, 38, 39, 40, 43, 47, 48, 49, 50, 51, 52, 53, 54, 55, 56, 57, 59, 60, 61, 62, 63, 64, 65, 66, 68, 69, 70, 71, 73, 74, 75, 77, 78, 80, 82, 83, 84
Unit 8 Nursing Care of Children and Families	1, 9, 13, 14, 15, 25, 27, 31, 32, 33, 35, 38, 51, 53, 54, 55, 58, 61, 62, 65, 66, 70, 75, 79, 82, 86, 87, 89, 91, 98, 103, 108, 109, 111, 117, 118	2, 4, 6, 7, 12, 16, 17, 20, 21, 23, 36, 39, 40, 41, 44, 45, 47, 48, 49, 52, 56, 64, 67, 69, 71, 73, 78, 81, 83, 92, 93, 94, 95, 96, 97, 100, 101, 102, 104, 105, 107, 110, 112, 113, 114	3, 11, 18, 19, 28, 29, 34, 37, 46, 50, 80, 81, 85, 99, 119, 120	5, 8, 10, 22, 24, 26, 30, 42, 43, 57, 59, 60, 63, 68, 72, 74, 76, 77, 84, 88, 90, 106, 115, 116
Unit 9 Ethical and Legal Aspects in Nursing	1, 2, 3, 4, 5, 6, 7, 8, 9, 10, 12, 13, 14, 15, 16, 17, 18, 19, 20, 21, 22, 23, 24, 25, 26, 27, 28, 29, 30, 33, 34			11
Unit 10 Practice Test	2, 4, 5, 23, 25, 27, 28, 30, 32, 35, 36, 40, 46, 47, 56, 65, 66, 69, 71, 73, 78, 94, 100	7, 8, 9, 12, 15, 21, 26, 31, 33, 38, 48, 49, 50, 51, 58, 61, 63, 67, 76, 80, 86, 88, 92, 98	6, 14, 17, 19, 20, 22, 24, 34, 37, 39, 42, 44, 52, 54, 55, 59, 64, 68, 70, 72, 74, 75, 79, 83, 84, 87, 89, 96, 97, 99	1, 3, 10, 11, 13, 16, 18, 29, 41, 43, 45, 53, 57, 60, 62, 77, 81, 82, 85, 90, 91, 93, 95

continued

Unit	Safe, Effective Care Environment (SECE) Question #	Physiologic Integrity (PhI) Question #	Psychosocial Integrity (PsI) Question #	Health Promotion and Maintenance (HPM) Question #
Unit 11 Final Test	8, 11, 12, 15, 19, 21, 26, 31, 32, 34, 35, 36, 42, 44, 47, 48, 51, 53, 55, 57, 58, 62, 65, 67, 70, 72, 73, 75, 76, 77, 81, 85, 87, 91, 92, 95, 97, 102, 105, 114, 116, 118, 121, 122, 126, 128, 130, 131, 132, 142, 145, 146, 151, 153, 155, 156, 158, 159, 160, 167, 168, 171, 173, 175, 178, 179, 180, 182, 183, 184, 188, 190, 191, 194, 196	1, 3, 5, 7, 9, 13, 14, 16, 18, 24, 25, 28, 29, 33, 39, 40, 45, 49, 54, 56, 61, 63, 64, 68, 78, 79, 80, 83, 86, 89, 90, 94, 99, 101, 103, 107, 109, 111, 115, 117, 119, 120, 123, 124, 137, 139, 141, 147, 149, 150, 157, 162, 164, 166, 169, 170, 172, 174, 177, 186, 193, 197, 200	4, 17, 22, 38, 41, 43, 52, 60, 66, 74, 84, 93, 98, 104, 106, 110, 112, 113, 125, 127, 133, 136, 143, 144, 165, 181, 185, 187, 195, 198, 199	2, 6, 10, 20, 23, 27, 30, 37, 46, 50, 59, 69, 71, 82, 88, 96, 100, 108, 129, 134, 135, 138, 140, 148, 152, 154, 161, 163, 176, 189, 192

For an index to *topics* relating to each client need, see Appendix E.

Appendices

Appendix G

Categories of Human Functions Definitions/Descriptions

Protective Functions

Client's ability to maintain defenses and prevent physical and chemical trauma, injury, infection, and threats to health status. Examples: communicable diseases (including sexually transmitted diseases), immunity, physical trauma and abuse, asepsis, safety hazards, poisoning, skin disorders, and preoperative care and postoperative complications.

Sensory-Perceptual Functions

Client's ability to perceive, interpret, and respond to sensory and cognitive stimuli. Examples: auditory, visual, and verbal impairments, sensory deprivation, sensory overload, aphasia, brain tumors, laryngectomy, organic brain syndrome, body image, reality orientation, learning disabilities, and seizure disorders.

Comfort, Rest, Activity, and Mobility Functions

Client's ability to maintain mobility, desirable level of activity, and adequate sleep, rest, and comfort. Examples: joint impairment, body alignment, pain, sleep disturbances, activities of daily living, neuromuscular impairment, musculoskeletal impairment, and endocrine disorders that affect activity.

Nutrition

Client's ability to maintain the intake and processing of essential nutrients. Examples: normal nutrition, diet in pregnancy and lactation, obesity, conditions such as diabetes, gastric disorders, and metabolic disorders that affect primarily the nutritional status.

Growth and Development

Client's ability to maintain maturational processes throughout the life span. Examples: child-bearing, child-rearing, conditions that interfere with the maturation process, maturational crises, changes in aging, psychosocial development, sterility, and conditions of the reproductive system.

Fluid–Gas Transport Functions

Client's ability to maintain fluid–gas transport. Examples: fluid volume deficit and overload, cardiopulmonary diseases, acid-base balance, cardiopulmonary resuscitation, anemias, hemorrhagic disorders, leukemias, and infectious pulmonary diseases.

Psychosocial-Cultural Functions

Client's ability to function in intrapersonal, interpersonal, intergroup, and sociocultural relationships. Examples: grieving, death and dying, psychotic and neurotic behaviors, self-concept, therapeutic communication, group dynamics, ethical-legal aspects, community resources, spiritual needs, situational crises, and substance abuse.

Elimination Functions

Client's ability to maintain functions related to relieving the body of waste products. Examples: conditions of the gastrointestinal system, such as vomiting, diarrhea, constipation, ulcers, neoplasms, colostomy, and hernia; conditions of the urinary system, such as kidney stones, transplants, renal failure, and prostatic hypertrophy.

The practice questions in this book (end-of-unit questions, **Pre Test, Practice Test,** and **Final Test**) are coded as to the category of human function being tested; the codes are found following the answer/rationale for each question. *Key to category of human function codes:*

1   Protective
2   Sensory-Perceptual
3   Comfort, Rest, Activity, and Mobility
4   Nutrition
5   Growth and Development
6   Fluid–Gas Transport
7   Psychosocial-Cultural
8   Elimination

For an index to *questions* relating to each human function, see Appendix I.

For page references of specific *topics to review* relating to each client need, see Appendix H.

Appendix H

Index: Content Related to Categories of Human Functions

These eight categories of human functions/concepts provide detailed examples of *content* areas incorporated under the four areas of client needs.

For an index to *questions* relating to each category of human function, see Appendix I.

Appendices

Appendix I

Index: Questions Related to Categories of Human Functions

This index lists *practice questions* for you to use in reviewing *categories of human functions* (which are detailed examples of what is covered by the four broad client needs categories).

Unit	Protective Functions (1) Question #	Sensory Perceptual Functions (2) Question #	Comfort, Rest, Activity, and Mobility Functions (3) Question #	Nutrition (4) Question #	Growth and Development (5) Question #	Fluid-Gas Transport Functions (6) Question #	Psycho-social-Cultural Functions (7) Question #	Elimination Functions (8) Question #
Unit 1 Orientation and Pre Test	19, 23, 37, 42, 43, 52, 53, 54, 60, 69, 70, 74, 75, 87, 90, 97, 110, 120, 125, 126, 128, 134, 135, 139, 156, 167, 170, 186, 191	21, 38, 77, 111, 124, 147, 148, 163, 180	7, 15, 17, 18, 22, 26, 41, 45, 68, 89, 96, 99, 101, 108, 136, 138, 160, 190, 197	3, 6, 20, 27, 30, 34, 36, 44, 56, 59, 82, 100, 103, 118, 141, 143, 145, 162, 166, 168, 175, 193	14, 47, 48, 49, 57, 58, 62, 63, 76, 98, 107, 115, 116, 141, 151, 189, 194, 196, 198	2, 10, 12, 13, 28, 29, 31, 32, 35, 64, 71, 72, 73, 78, 79, 80, 84, 86, 88, 92, 93, 94, 105, 109, 113, 114, 119, 121, 123, 127, 130, 131, 133, 137, 146, 150, 153, 159, 161, 164, 165, 171, 172, 176, 178, 181, 182, 183, 185, 192, 195, 200	8, 11, 24, 25, 33, 46, 50, 51, 65, 66, 83, 85, 91, 95, 102, 104, 106, 117, 122, 129, 132, 140, 142, 152, 157, 174, 179, 184, 187, 199	1, 4, 5, 9, 16, 39, 40, 55, 61, 67, 81, 112, 144, 154, 155, 158, 169, 173, 177
Unit 2 Nursing Care of the Acutely Ill and Chronically Ill Adult	8, 21, 22, 28, 46, 64, 81, 88	2, 11, 26, 31, 36, 51, 56, 59, 60, 61, 63, 65, 67, 77, 98	6, 16, 18, 24, 27, 30, 45, 49, 50, 55, 62, 69, 70, 74, 75, 78, 79, 80, 82, 83, 84, 90, 93	1, 7, 10, 12, 19, 25, 29, 39, 44, 68, 72, 73, 96, 97		4, 15, 17, 20, 23, 32, 33, 35, 37, 38, 40, 41, 47, 58, 66, 85, 87, 91, 92, 94, 95	3, 9, 42, 48, 52, 53, 76, 86	5, 13, 14, 34, 43, 54, 57, 71, 89
Unit 3 Review of Nutrition				1, 2, 3, 4, 5, 6, 7, 8, 9				
Unit 4 Review of Pharmacology	22, 24, 30, 31, 32, 37, 38, 44, 45, 46, 51, 52, 53, 55	10, 21, 26	1, 3, 14, 17, 39	9, 13, 16, 23, 27	29, 33, 34, 35, 36, 54	4, 5, 6, 11, 12, 25, 47, 48, 49, 50	40, 41, 42, 43	2, 7, 8, 15, 18, 19, 20, 28
Unit 5 Common Diagnostic Procedures, Treatments, and Nursing Care				5, 6, 7, 8, 12		2, 3, 4, 13		1, 9, 10, 11

continued

Appendices

Unit	Protective Functions (1) Question #	Sensory Perceptual Functions (2) Question #	Comfort, Rest, Activity, and Mobility Functions (3) Question #	Nutrition (4) Question #	Growth and Development (5) Question #	Fluid-Gas Transport Functions (6) Question #	Psycho-social Cultural Functions (7) Question #	Elimination Functions (8) Question #
Unit 9 Ethical and Legal Aspects in Nursing							1, 2, 3, 4, 5, 6, 7, 8, 9, 10, 11, 12, 13, 14, 15, 16, 17, 18, 19, 20, 21, 22, 23, 24, 25, 26, 27, 28, 29, 30, 31, 32, 33, 34, 35	
Unit 10 Practice Test	2, 8, 13, 27, 51, 60, 69, 78, 82, 85, 95	23, 43, 56	12, 30, 32, 35, 40, 63, 65, 66, 81, 88, 100	18, 25, 77	1, 10, 11, 16, 29, 31, 33, 36, 41, 44, 45, 47, 53, 62, 84, 89, 93	3, 5, 7, 21, 26, 28, 38, 49, 50, 61, 67, 71, 73, 76, 80, 94, 98	6, 14, 17, 19, 20, 22, 24, 34, 37, 39, 42, 52, 54, 55, 59, 64, 68, 70, 72, 74, 75, 79, 83, 87, 90, 91, 96, 97, 99	4, 9, 15, 46, 48, 57, 58, 86, 92
Unit 11 Final Test	3, 14, 19, 26, 31, 33, 34, 35, 42, 53, 68, 85, 87, 90, 91, 92, 95, 116, 118, 122, 123, 128, 130, 131, 132, 142, 147, 152, 157, 159, 164, 175, 176, 194, 197	11, 43, 51, 62, 76, 84, 103, 111, 124, 127, 184	24, 25, 54, 59, 65, 67, 77, 81, 96, 137, 154, 158, 174, 179, 182, 188	28, 39, 45, 61, 83, 88, 119, 126, 138, 167, 173, 190	2, 6, 20, 27, 30, 37, 41, 46, 50, 69, 71, 82, 100, 104, 108, 129, 136, 144, 148, 161, 163, 178, 192, 199	1, 5, 7, 8, 9, 12, 13, 15, 16, 18, 21, 23, 29, 36, 40, 44, 47, 49, 55, 56, 57, 58, 63, 73, 75, 78, 79, 80, 86, 89, 94, 97, 99, 101, 102, 105, 107, 109, 114, 115, 117, 135, 139, 141, 145, 149, 150, 151, 153, 155, 160, 162, 166, 168, 169, 170, 172, 177, 180, 183, 186, 189, 191, 193, 195, 196, 200	4, 10, 17, 22, 32, 38, 52, 60, 66, 72, 74, 93, 98, 106, 110, 112, 113, 120, 121, 125, 133, 140, 143, 146, 165, 171, 181, 185, 187, 198	48, 64, 70, 156

For an index to *topics* relating to each client need, see Appendix H.

Appendices

Appendix J

Common Acronyms and Abbreviations

a	Before (*ante*)
Ab	Antibody/Abortion
Abd	Abdomen/Abdominal
ABG	Arterial blood gas
ac	Before meals (*ante cibum*)
ADH	Antidiuretic hormone
ad lib	As much as desired (*ad libitum*)
ADLs	Activities of daily living
AFB	Acid-fast bacillus
Afib	Atrial fibrillation
Aflutter	Atrial flutter
AFP	Alpha-fetoprotein
AG	Antigen
AIDS	Acquired immunodeficiency syndrome
AK (or AKA)	Above-the-knee (amputation)
ALL	Acute lymphocytic (lymphoblastic) leukemia
AMA	Against medical advice
A&O × 3	Alert, oriented to person, place, time
AP	Anteroposterior/Alkaline phosphatase
ARC	AIDS-related complex
ARDS	Adult respiratory distress syndrome
ARF	Acute renal failure
ASA	Acetylsalicylic acid (aspirin)
ASAP	As soon as possible
ASD	Atrial septal defect
AV	Atrioventricular/Arteriovenous/Aortic valve
AVB	Atrioventricular block
AVM	Arteriovenous malformation
bid	Twice daily (*bis in die*)
BK (or BKA)	Below-the-knee (amputation)
BM	Bowel movement/Bone marrow
BMR	Basal metabolic rate
BP	Blood pressure
BPH	Benign prostatic hypertrophy

bpm	Beats per minute
BRP	Bathroom privileges
BUN	Blood urea nitrogen
c̄	With (*cum*)
CA	Carcinoma/Cancer
CABG	Coronary artery bypass graft operation (×1,2,3,4 = number of grafts)
CAD	Coronary artery disease
CBC	Complete blood count
CC	Chief complaint
cc	Cubic centimeter
CCU	Cardiac (intensive) care unit
CF	Cystic fibrosis
CHD	Congenital heart disease
CHF	Congestive heart failure
CMV	Cytomegalovirus
CNS	Central nervous system/Coagulase-negative staphylococcus
C/O	Complains of
COPD	Chronic obstructive pulmonary disease
CPK	Creatine phosphokinase
CPR	Cardiopulmonary resuscitation
CRF	Chronic renal failure/Cardiac risk factors
CRP	C-reactive protein
CSF	Cerebral spinal (cerebrospinal) fluid
CVA	Cerebrovascular accident/Costovertebral angle
CVP	Central venous pressure
Δ	Change (Greek letter delta)
D/C	Discharge/Discontinue
D&C	Dilatation and curettage
DI	Diabetes insipidus
DIC	Disseminated intravascular coagulation
Dig	Digitalis
DM	Diabetes mellitus
DNR	Do not resuscitate

Source: Fine P. *The Wards: An Introduction to Clinical Clerkships.* Boston: Little, Brown, 1994.

Appendices

DOA	Dead on arrival		INH	Isoniazid
DOB	Date of birth		I&O	Intake and output
DOE	Dyspnea on exertion		IPPB	Intermittent positive pressure breathing
DPT	Diphtheria, pertussis, and tetanus		IUD	Intrauterine device
DRG	Diagnosis-related group		IV	Intravenous
DTs	Delirium tremens		IVC	Inferior vena cava
DTR	Deep-tendon reflex		IVP	Intravenous pyelogram/Intravenous push
D5W/D$_5$W	5% dextrose in water			
Dx	Diagnosis			
			JRA	Juvenile rheumatoid arthritis
ECG	Electrocardiogram (purist's version)			
Echo	Echocardiogram		KUB	Kidneys, ureters, bladder (flat/upright abdominal X ray)
ECT	Electroconvulsive therapy			
EDB	Estimated date of birth			
EEG	Electroencephalogram		LLL	Left lower (lung) lobe
EKG	Electrocardiogram (common version)		LLQ	Left lower quadrant
EMG	Electromyogram		LMP	Last menstrual period
EMT	Emergency medical technician		LOC	Loss of consciousness
ENT	Ear, nose, and throat		LPN	Licensed practical nurse
ER	Emergency room		LUL	Left upper (lung) lobe
ESR	Erythrocyte sedimentation rate		LUQ	Left upper quadrant
ETOH	Alcohol (ethanol)			
			MAP	Mean arterial pressure
FBS	Fasting blood sugar		MCL	Midclavicular line
FEV$_1$	Forced expiratory volume in 1 second		Med	Medication
FRC	Functional residual capacity		MI	Myocardial infarction
FTT	Failure to thrive		MMR	Measles, mumps, rubella
FUO	Fever of unknown origin		MOM	Milk of magnesia
FVC	Forced vital capacity		Mono	Mononucleosis
Fx	Fracture		MR	Mitral regurgitation/Mental retardation
			MRI	Magnetic resonance imaging
g	Gram		MS	Mental status/Mitral stenosis/Multiple sclerosis/Morphine sulfate
G	Gravida			
GB	Gallbladder			
GC	Gonococcus/Gonorrhea			
GI	Gastrointestinal		NA	Not applicable
gr	Grain		NG	Nasogastric
GTT	Glucose tolerance test		NIDDM	Non-insulin-dependent diabetes mellitus
gtt(s)	Drop(s) (*guttae*)			
GU	Genitourinary		NL	Normal
GYN	Gynecologic		NOC	Night (nocturnal)
			NPH	Neutral-protamine-Hagedorn (intermediate-acting insulin)
HAV	Hepatitis A virus			
HCG	Human chorionic gonadotropin		NPO	Nothing by mouth (*nil per os*)
Hct	Hematocrit		NS	Normal saline
HDL	High-density lipoprotein		NSAID	Nonsteroidal anti-inflammatory drug
HEENT	Head, eyes, ears, nose, throat		NSR	Normal sinus rhythm
Hgb	Hemoglobin		NTG	Nitroglycerin
HIV	Human immunodeficiency virus		N/V	Nausea, vomiting
HMO	Health maintenance organization		NVD	Nausea, vomiting, diarrhea
HOB	Head of bed			
HR	Heart rate		O$_2$	Oxygen
hs	Bedtime (*hora somni*)		OB	Obstetrics
Hx	History		OD	Right eye (*oculus dextro*)/Overdose
			OOB	Out of bed
ICP	Intracranial pressure		O&P	Ova and parasites
ICU	Intensive care unit		OR	Operating room
I&D	Incision and drainage		OS	Left eye (*oculus sinistro*)/Opening snap
IDDM	Insulin-dependent diabetes mellitus		OT	Occupational therapy
Ig	Immunoglobulin		OU	Both eyes (*oculo utro*)
IM	Intramuscular			

P	Para/Pulse
p̄	Post (after)
PA	Posterior-anterior/Physician's assistant/Pulmonary artery
PAC	Premature atrial contraction
PAF	Paroxysmal atrial fibrillation
PAO_2	Alveolar oxygen pressure
PaO_2	Arterial partial pressure of oxygen
PAS	Para-aminosalicylic acid
PAT	Paroxysmal atrial tachycardia
pc	After meals (*post cibum*)
PCA	Patient-controlled analgesia pump
PCP	*Pneumocystis carinii* pneumonia/Phencyclidine
PDA	Patent ductus arteriosus
PEEP	Positive end-expiratory pressure
PERRL(A)	Pupils equally round and reactive to light (and accommodation)
PID	Pelvic inflammatory disease
PKU	Phenylketonuria
PMI	Point of maximum impulse
PMS	Premenstrual syndrome
PND	Paroxysmal nocturnal dyspnea
PO	By mouth (*per os*)
PPD	Purified protein derivative (TB skin test)
PPO	Preferred provider organization
prn	When necessary (*pro re nata*)
PSA	Prostate-specific antigen
Pt	Patient
PT	Prothrombin time/Physical therapy
PTA	Prior to admission
PTCA	Percutaneous transluminal coronary angioplasty
PTT	Partial thromboplastin time
PUD	Peptic ulcer disease
PVC	Premature ventricular contraction
q	Each, every (*quaque*)
qd	Each day
qhs	Every night before sleep
qid	Four times a day (*quarter in die*)
qod	Every other day
R	Respirations
RA	Rheumatoid arthritis/Right atrium
RBC	Red blood cell
RHD	Rheumatic heart disease
RLL	Right lower (lung) lobe
RLQ	Right lower quadrant
RML	Right middle (lung) lobe
R/O	Rule out
ROM	Range of motion
ROS	Review of systems

RUL	Right upper (lung) lobe
RUQ	Right upper quadrant
Rx	Prescription/Therapy/Treatment
s̄	Without (*sine*)
S_1	First heart sound
S_2	Second heart sound
S_3	Third heart sound
S_4	Fourth heart sound
SBE	Subacute bacterial endocarditis
SC	Subcutaneously
SGA	Small for gestational age
SIADH	Syndrome of inappropriate antidiuretic hormone
SICU	Surgical intensive care unit
SIDS	Sudden infant death syndrome
SL	Sublingually
SLE	Systemic lupus erythematosus
SOB	Short(ness) of breath
SQ	Subcutaneously
S/S	Signs, symptoms
Stat	Immediately (*statim*)
STD	Sexually transmitted disease
SVG	Spontaneous vaginal delivery
Sx	Symptoms
T	Temperature
T&A	Tonsillectomy and adenoidectomy
TB	Tuberculosis
TIA	Transient ischemic attack
TID	Three times a day (*ter in die*)
TKO	To keep open
TLC	Total lung capacity/Tender loving care
TPN	Total parenteral nutrition
TPR	Temperature, pulse, respirations
TSH	Thyroid-stimulating hormone
TURP	Transurethral resection of prostate
TV	Total volume/Tidal volume
Tx	Treatment
UA	Urinalysis
UGI	Upper gastrointestinal
UQ	Upper quadrant
URI	Upper respiratory infection
UTI	Urinary tract infection
UV	Ultraviolet
VC	Vital capacity
Vfib (VF)	Ventricular fibrillation
VS	Vital signs
VSD	Ventricular septal defect
WBC	White blood count/White blood cells
WNL	Within normal limits
w/o	Without

Appendices

Appendix K

Quick Guide to Common Clinical Signs

Many clinical signs have been named for the physicians who first described them, or the phenomena they resemble. Following is a list of some of the most common clinical signs, for use as a quick reference as you review.

Babinski reflex Dorsiflexion of the big toe after stimulation of the lateral sole; associated with corticospinal tract lesions.

Blumberg's sign Transient pain in the abdomen after approximated fingers pressed gently into abdominal wall are suddenly withdrawn—rebound tenderness; associated with peritoneal inflammation.

Brudzinski's sign Flexion of the hip and knee induced by flexion of the neck; associated with meningeal irritation.

Chadwick's sign Cyanosis of vaginal and cervical mucosa; associated with pregnancy.

Chvostek's sign Facial muscle spasm induced by tapping on the facial nerve branches; associated with hypocalcemia.

Cheyne-Stokes respiration Rhythmic cycles of deep and shallow respiration, often with apneic periods; associated with central nervous system respiratory center dysfunction.

Coppernail's sign Ecchymoses on the perineum, scrotum, or labia; associated with fracture of the pelvis.

Cullen's sign Bluish discoloration of the umbilicus; associated with acute pancreatitis or hemoperitoneum, especially rupture of fallopian tube in ectopic pregnancy.

Doll's eye sign Dissociation between the movements of the head and eyes: as the head is raised the eyes are lowered, and as the head is lowered the eyes are raised; associated with global-diffuse disorders of the cerebrum.

Fluid wave Transmission across the abdomen of a wave induced by snapping the abdomen; associated with ascites.

Goldstein's sign Wide distance between the great toe and the adjoining toe; associated with cretinism and trisomy 21.

Harlequin sign In the newborn infant, reddening of the lower half of the laterally recumbent body and blanching of the upper half, due to a temporary vasomotor disturbance.

Hegar's sign Softening of the fundus of the uterus; associated with the first trimester of pregnancy.

Homans' sign Pain behind the knee, induced by dorsiflexion of the foot; associated with peripheral vascular disease, especially venous thrombosis in the calf.

Kehr's sign Severe pain in the left upper quadrant, radiating to the top of the shoulder; associated with splenic rupture.

Kernig's sign Inability to extend leg when sitting or lying with the thigh flexed on the abdomen; associated with meningeal irritation.

Knie's sign Unequal dilatation of the pupils; associated with Graves' disease.

Kussmaul's respiration Paroxysmal air hunger; associated with acidosis, especially diabetic ketoacidosis.

McBurney's sign Tenderness at McBurney's point (located two-thirds of the distance from the umbilicus to the anterior-superior iliac spine); associated with appendicitis.

Osler's sign Small painful erythematous swellings in the skin of the hands and feet; associated with bacterial endocarditis.

Source: Macklis RM, et al. *Introduction to Clinical Medicine* (3rd ed). Boston: Little, Brown, 1994.

Psoas sign   Pain induced by hyperextension of the right thigh while lying on the left side; associated with appendicitis.

Setting-sun sign   Downward deviation of the eyes so that each iris appears to "set" beneath the lower lid, with white sclera exposed between it and the upper lid; associated with increased intracranial pressure or irritation of the brain stem.

Tinel's sign   Tingling sensation felt from light percussion on the radial side of the palmaris longus tendon; associated with carpal tunnel syndrome.

Williamson's sign   Markedly diminished blood pressure in the leg as compared with that in the arm on the same side; associated with pneumothorax and pleural effusions.

Appendix L

Memory Aids

Acid-base—*"RAMS"* (*Respiratory Alternate, Metabolic Same*)

	Respiratory (alternate)		Metabolic (same)	
Acidosis	$\downarrow$ pH	$\uparrow$ Pco_2	$\downarrow$ pH	$\downarrow$ HCO_3
Alkalosis	$\uparrow$ pH	$\downarrow$ Pco_2	$\uparrow$ pH	$\uparrow$ HCO_3

Alcohol withdrawal: clinical features—*"HITS"*[a]
Hallucinations (visual, tactile)
Increased vital signs and insomnia
Tremens → delirium tremens (potentially lethal)
Shakes/Sweats/Seizures/Stomach pains (nausea, vomiting)

Angina: precipitating factors—*"3 Es"*
Eating
Emotion
Exertion (Exercise)

Anorexia nervosa: clinical features—*"ANOREXIC"*[a]
Adolescent females/Amenorrhea
NGT alimentation (most severe cases)
Obsession with losing weight/becoming fat though underweight
Refusal to eat ($\geq$ 5% die)
Electrolyte abnormalities (e.g., $\downarrow$ K$^+$, cardiac arrhythmia)
$\uparrow$ e**X**ercise
Intelligence often above average/Induced vomiting
Cathartic use (and diuretic abuse)

Arterial occlusion: symptoms—*"6 Ps"*
Pain
Pale
Pulseless
Paresthesia
Poikilothermic
Paralysis

Blood glucose *(rhyme)*

Symptom	Implication
Cold and **clammy** . . .	give hard **candy.**
Hot and **dry** . . .	glucose is **high.**

Cancer: focus of patient care—*"CANCER"*
Chemotherapy
Assess body image disturbance (related to alopecia)
Nutritional needs when N/V present
Comfort from pain
Effective response to Tx? (Evaluate)
Rest (for patient and family)

Car seats for children—*"Rule of 4s"*
Use if under:
4 years old, or
40 pounds, or
40 in. tall

Cholecystitis: risk factors—*"5 Fs"*
Female
Fat
Forty
Fertile
Fair

---

[a]From Rogers PT. *The Medical Student's Guide to Top Board Scores.* Boston: Little, Brown, 1996.

Cleft lip: nursing care plan (postoperative)— *"CLEFT LIP"*
Crying, minimize
Logan bow
Elbow restraints
Feed with Breck feeder
Tent, croup

Liquid (sterile water), rinse after feeding
Impaired feeding (no sucking)
Position—*never* on abdomen

Cognitive disorders: assessment of difficulties— *"JOCAM"*
Judgment
Orientation
Confabulation
Affect
Memory

Coma: causes—*"A-E-I-O-U TIPS"*[b]
Alcohol, acidosis (hyperglycemic coma)
Epilepsy (also electrolyte abnormality, endocrine problem)
Insulin (hypoglycemic shock)
Overdose (or poisoning)
Uremia and other renal problems

Trauma; temperature abnormalities (hypothermia, heat stroke)
Infection (e.g., meningitis)
Psychogenic ("hysterical coma")
Stroke or space-occupying lesions in the cranium

Cushing's syndrome: symptoms—*"3 Ss"*
Sugar (hyperglycemia)
Salt (hypernatremia)
Sex (excess androgens)

Diabetes—*"3 Ps"* (or *"3 poly's"*): signs and symptoms
Polydipsia (very thirsty)
Polyphagia (very hungry)
Polyuria (urinary frequency)

Diarrhea: diet—*"BRAT"*
Banana
Rice (cereal)
Applesauce
Toast/Tea

Dystocia: etiology—*"3 Ps"* (see p. 448)
Power
Passageway
Passenger

Dystocia: general aspects (maternal)—*"3 Ps"* (see p. 448)
Psych
Placenta
Position

Eardrops: administering—*UP/DOWN*

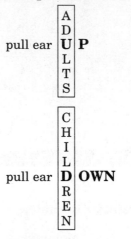

pull ear ADULTS **UP**

pull ear CHILDREN **D**OWN

Episiotomy assessment—*"EDEMA"*
Edema
Drainage
Ecchymosis (and redness)
Mobility, impaired
Approximation of skin

Eye medications
My**d**riatic = **d**ilated pupils
Mio**t**ic = **t**iny (constricted) pupils

Hormonal contraceptives: symptoms to report— *"ACHES"*
Abdominal pain (liver, gallbladder)
Chest pain, short of breath (clot in lungs or heart)
Headaches (CVA, hypertension)
Eye problems
Severe leg pain (thromboembolic)

Hypertension: complications—*"4 Cs"*
CHF (congestive heart failure)
CVA (cardiovascular accident)
CAD (coronary artery disease)
CRF (chronic renal failure)

Hypertension: nursing care plan—*"I TIRED"*
Intake and output (urine)

Take blood pressure
Ischemia attack, transient (watch for TIAs)
Respiration, pulse
Electrolytes
Daily weight

---

[b]From Caroline NL. *Emergency Care in the Streets* (5th ed). Boston: Little, Brown, 1995.

Hypoglycemia: signs and symptoms—*"DIRE"*
Diaphoresis
Increased pulse
Restless
Extra hungry

IUD: potential problems with use—*"PAINS"*[c]
Period (menstrual: late, spotting, bleeding)
Abdominal pain, dyspareunia
Infection (abnormal vaginal discharge)
Not feeling well, fever or chills
String missing

Manipulation: nursing plan—promote *"3 Cs"*
Cooperation
Compromise
Collaboration

Medication administration—*"5 rights"*
RIGHT medication
RIGHT dosage
RIGHT route
RIGHT time
RIGHT patient

Mental retardation: nursing care plan—*"3 Rs"*
Regularity (provide routine and structure)
Reward (positive reinforcement)
Redundancy (repeat)

Regularity (provide routine and structure)
Reward (positive reinforcement)
Redundancy (repeat)

Regularity (provide routine and structure)
Reward (positive reinforcement)
Redundancy (repeat)

Pain: assessment—*"PQRST"*[d] (see Table 2.30, p. 159)

What	**P**rovokes the pain?
What is the	**Q**uality of the pain?
Does the pain	**R**adiate?
What is the	**S**everity?
What is the	**T**iming of the pain?

Pain: management—*"ABCs"*
Ask about the pain
Believe when patients say they have pain
Choices—let patients know their choices
Deliver what you can, when you said you would
Empower/Enable patients' control over pain

Postoperative complications: order—*"4 Ws"*
Wind (pulmonary)
Wound
Water (urinary tract infection)
Walk (thrombophlebitis)

Schizophrenia: primary symptoms—*"4 As"*
Associative looseness
Affect
Ambivalence
Autism

Sprain: nursing care plan—*"ICE"*
Immobilize (and rest)
Cool (with ice)
Elevate

Stool assessment—*"ACCT"*
Amount
Color
Consistency
Timing

Tracheoesophageal fistula: assessment—*"3 Cs"*
Coughing
Choking
Cyanosis

Traction: nursing care plan—*"TRACTION"*
Trapeze bar overhead to raise and lower upper body
Requires free-hanging weights; body alignment
Analgesia for pain, prn
Circulation (check color and pulse)
Temperature (check extremity)
Infection prevention
Output (monitor)
Nutrition (alteration related to immobility)

Transient ischemic attacks: assessment—*"3 Ts"*
Temporary unilateral visual impairment
Transient paralysis (one-sided)
Tinnitus → vertigo

Trauma care: complications—*"TRAUMA"*
Thromboembolism/Tissue perfusion, altered
Respiration, altered
Anxiety related to pain and prognosis
Urinary elimination, altered
Mobility impaired
Alterations in sensory-perceptual functions and skin integrity (infections)

[c]Modified from Hatcher RA, et al. *Contraceptive Technology: 1994–1996* (16th ed). New York: Irving Publishers, 1994.

[d]From Caroline NL. *Emergency Care in the Streets* (5th ed). Boston: Little, Brown, 1995.

Appendices

Wernicke-Korsakoff syndrome (alcohol-associated neurologic disorder)—"COAT RACK"[e]
Wernicke's encephalopathy (acute phase): clinical features

Confusion
Ophthalmoplegia
Ataxia
Thiamine is an important aspect of Tx

Korsakoff's psychosis (chronic phase): characteristic findings

Retrograde amnesia (↓ recall of some old memories)
Anterograde amnesia (↓ ability to form new memories)
Confabulation
Korsakoff's psychosis

[e]From Rogers PT. *The Medical Student's Guide to Top Board Scores.* Boston: Little, Brown, 1996.

Index

Index